Oxford Clinical Practice Series

NEUROINTENSIVE CARE

The Oxford Clinical Practice Series covers an array of resources providing essential evidence-based, up-to-date information and key clinical references that will enhance the clinical knowledge of healthcare practitioners and medical students across the globe.

Oxford Clinical Practice Series
NEUROINTENSIVE CARE

Edited by
Hemanshu Prabhakar

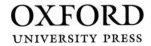

OXFORD
UNIVERSITY PRESS

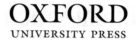

OXFORD
UNIVERSITY PRESS

Oxford University Press is a department of the University of Oxford.
It furthers the University's objective of excellence in research, scholarship,
and education by publishing worldwide. Oxford is a registered trademark of
Oxford University Press in the UK and in certain other countries.

Published in India by
Oxford University Press
2/11 Ground Floor, Ansari Road, Daryaganj, New Delhi 110 002, India

ISBN-13: 978-0-19-948143-9
ISBN-10: 0-19-948143-1

Typeset in Adobe Garamond Pro 10.5/13
by Transistics Data Technologies, Kolkata 700 091
Printed in India by Nutech Print Services India

To my grandparents
Karam Chand and Indrawati Prabhakar
Vidya Sagar and Savitri Agnihotri

Contents

x

PART XX   APPENDIX

Foreword

It is a privilege to have been asked to write the Foreword to this book, *Neurointensive Care*. The field of neurointensive care has changed considerably in recent years, largely as a result of advances in technology enabling improved imaging and monitoring of the brain in health and disease. As a result, we now have not only a better understanding of alterations in brain function during acute neurological disease processes, but also of how systemically critical illnesses, such as sepsis, affect brain function. The neurointensive care patient management has also improved and books such as this are important to enable physicians to become up-to-date with the latest changes and recommendations for best practice.

The book is divided into two parts, the first covering the theoretical and management aspects of a wide range of neurological conditions, and the second including an interesting selection of individual case studies. Within the first part, there is a section on clinical procedures,

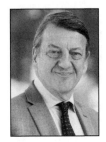

supported by videos, which provides useful practical information for the intensivist. At the end of the book, there is a helpful Appendix of various scales and scores used in the care of neurointensive care patients.

The chapters are clearly presented, well-illustrated, and written by an international group of experts in the field. The book will certainly be useful to everyone interested in the neurological aspects of intensive care.

Jean-Louis Vincent
Professor, Intensive Care Medicine,
Dept of Intensive Care, Erasme Univ Hospital,
Université Libre de Bruxelles, Belgium
Former President, World Federation of Societies of
Intensive and Critical Care Medicine (WFSICCM)

Preface

Neurocritical care is the intensive care management of patients with life-threatening neurological and neurosurgical illnesses such as massive stroke, bleeding in or around the brain (subarachnoid haemorrhage, intracerebral haemorrhage, subdural haemorrhage, and intraventricular haemorrhage), brain tumours, brain trauma, status epilepticus, nerve and muscle diseases (such as myasthenia gravis and Guillain-Barre syndrome), spinal cord disorders, and cardiopulmonary complications of brain injury. Neurocritical care units specialize in managing the unique needs of such critically ill patients.

This volume comprises a comprehensive review of all possible neurological conditions which one may encounter while practicing neurointensive care. The topics covered range from understanding the history and origin of neuro-intensive care to topics such as psychological and nursing care. Issues related to palliative care have also been discussed. Some of the commonly performed procedures in the neuro-intensive care unit have also been discussed. Clinical scales and scores that are commonly used in the neurologic ICU have also been compiled. This book will serve as a quick reference guide to all intensivists managing neurosurgical patients. It would be useful for general intensivists who occasionally have to manage neurologic patients, trainees, and fellows.

The book has a straightforward and systematic approach to various clinical problems encountered during intensive care management of neurologic patients. The book is unique as it has a problem-based approach to all neurological diseases and not a disease- or condition-based approach.

The authors have done an exceptional work of writing the chapters in the simplest manner for the targeted audience. I am grateful to all the contributors who have made this work possible in such a magnificent way.

Acknowledgements

I wish to acknowledge the support of the administration of the All India Institute of Medical Sciences (AIIMS), New Delhi, in allowing me to conduct this academic task.

I thank the faculty and staff of my Department of Neuroanaesthesiology and Critical Care for their support.

I also acknowledge the efforts of Dr Jayeeta Bannerjee and Oxford University Press.

Editor and Contributors

Hemanshu Prabhakar

Professor, Department of Neuroanesthesiology and Critical Care, All India Institute of Medical Sciences, New Delhi, India

Sanchit Ahuja

Fellow, Cleveland Clinic, Cleveland, OH, USA

Başak Akça

Assistant Professor, Hacettepe University Faculty of Medicine, Department of Anesthesiology and Reanimation, Ankara, Turkey

Oguzhan Arun

Associate Professor, Selcuk University Faculty of Medicine, Department of Anesthesiology and Reanimation, Konya, Turkey

Swati Bajpai

PhD Scholar, Clinical Neuropsychology, Neuroscience Center, All India Institute of Medical Sciences, New Delhi, India

Hossam El Beheiry

Associate Professor, Trillium Health Partners, Mississauga, ON, Canada

Amanda Moraska Benson

Associate Staff – Anesthesiology & Critical Care; Assistant Professor of Anesthesiology, CCLCM, Cleveland Clinic, Cleveland, OH, USA

Karen Berger

Clinical Pharmacy Manager, New York-Presbyterian Hospital, Weill Cornell Medical Center, New York, NY, USA

Rita Bertuetti

Consultant, Department of Anesthesia, Critical Care Medicine and Emergency, PiazzaleOspedaliCivili, Brescia, Italy

Richard D. Betzold

Division of Trauma, Emergency General Surgery, and Surgical Critical Care, Department of Surgery, Section of Surgical Sciences, Nashville, TN, USA

Dharmendra Singh Bhadauria

Associate Professor, Department of Nephrology, Sanjay Gandhi Postgraduate Institute of Medical Sciences (SGPGIMS), Lucknow, India

P. S. Bhat

Professor and Head of Department, Department of Psychiatry, Armed Forces Medical College, Pune, India

Brittany D. Bissell

Critical Care Pharmacist, Medical Intensive Care Unit/Pulmonary, University of Kentucky HealthCare, Lexington, KY, USA

Parmod K. Bithal

Consultant, Neuroanesthesia, King Fahad Medical City, Riyadh, Saudi Arabia

Hanson Bow
Resident at the Department of Neurologic Surgery, Vanderbilt Medical Center, Nashville, TN, USA

Gretchen M. Brophy
Professor of Pharmacotherapy & Outcomes Science and Neurosurgery, Virginia Commonwealth University, Richmond, VA, USA

Bilal Butt
Assistant Professor of Neurology, Southern Illinois University, Springfield, Illinois, USA

Amber Castle
Manager, Education & Residencies, PGY-1 Residency Program Director, Yale New Haven Hospital, Pharmacy Department, New Haven, CT, USA

Onuma Chaiwat
Associate Professor, Department of Anesthesiology, Faculty of Medicine, Siriraj Hospital, Mahidol University, Bangkok, Thailand

Diana Greene Chandos
Assistant Professor, Department of Neurology, The Ohio State University College of Medicine, OH, USA

Katleen Chester
Clinical Pharmacist Specialist, Marcus Stroke and Neuroscience Center, Department of Pharmacy and Drug Information, Grady Health System; Atlanta, Georgia, USA

Aaron Cook
Associate Adjunct Professor, University of Kentucky, USA

Vicky Davies
Principal Dietitian for Neurosciences, Development Officer: Critical Care Group of the BDA, The Walton Centre, Liverpool, UK

Caroline Der-Nigoghossian
Clinical Pharmacy Manager, New York-Presbyterian Hospital/The Allen Hospital, New York, NY, USA

Kinjal Desai
Medical Stroke Director, Vascular Neurologist & Neurointensivist, Neurohospitalist, Clearlake Regional Medical Center, Webster, Texas, USA

Judith Dinsmore
Consultant Neuroanaesthetist, St George's University Hospitals NHS Foundation Trust, London, UK

NG Shu Hui Elizabeth
Senior Resident, Department of Anaesthesia, National University Hospital, Singapore

Nazzareno Fagoni
Professor, Department of Anesthesia, Critical Care Medicine and Emergency, Spedali Civili University Hospital, Brescia, Italy

Ehab Farag
Professor of Anesthesiology, Cleveland Clinic Lerner College of Medicine; Staff Anesthesiologist, Department of General Anesthesiology & Section of Neuroanesthesiology, Cleveland Clinic, Cleveland, OH, USA

David F. Gaieski
Associate Professor, Department of Emergency Medicine, Sidney Kimmel School of Medicine, Thomas Jefferson University, Philadelphia, PA, USA

Kevin T. Gobeske

Neurocritical Care Fellow,
Department of Neurology,
Mayo Clinic, School of Medicine,
Rochester, MN, USA

Nicolai Goettel

Staff Anesthesiologist and Intensivist,
Department of Anesthesia, Surgical
Intensive Care, Prehospital Emergency
Medicine and Pain Therapy, University
Hospital, Basel, Switzerland

Svetlana A. Gracheva

Assistant Professor, Burnazian Scientific
State Centre of Federal Medical and
Biological Agency of Russian Federation,
Russia

Chantel Gray

Fellow, Anesthesia Critical Care, Surgical
ICU, Anesthesiology Institute, Cleveland
Clinic, Cleveland, OH,USA

Kristy Greene

Clinical Pharmacist Specialist, Emory
University Hospital Midtown, Atlanta,
Georgia, USA

Sandeep Grover

Additional Professor, Department
of Psychiatry, PGIMER, Chandigarh,
India

Mohan Gurjar

Additional Professor, Department
of Critical Care Medicine,
Sanjay Gandhi Postgraduate Institute
of Medical Sciences (SGPGIMS),
Lucknow, India

Shahreyar Hafeez

Assistant Professor, Neurocritical Care,
Department of Neurosurgery,
UT Health Science Center, San Antonio,
TX, USA

Matthew Hallman

Assistant Professor, University
of Washington, Department of
Anesthesiology and Pain Medicine,
Seattle, WA, USA

Lucy He

Resident Physician, Department of
Neurological Surgery, Vanderbilt
University Medical Center, Nashville,
TN, USA

Christopher Patrick Henson

Assistant Professor, Department of
Anesthesiology, Division of Critical Care
Anesthesiology; Medical Director, OR
Holding Room and PACU, Vanderbilt
University Medical Center, Nashville,
TN, USA

Archana Hinduja

Assistant Professor, Department of
Neurology, Ohio State University Wexner
Medical Center, Columbus, OH, USA

Theresa Human

Neuroscience Clinical Specialist,
Washington University, Barnes Jewish
Hospital, Department of Clinical
Pharmacy, Washington, USA

Aaron M. Joffe

Professor, Department of Anesthesiology
and Pain Medicine, University of
Washington, Seattle, WA, USA

Nicholas J. Johnson

Acting Assistant Professor of Medicine,
Division of Emergency Medicine;
Attending Physician, Neurocritical Care
Service & Medical Intensive Care Unit,
University of Washington/Harborview
Medical Center, Seattle, WA, USA

Garima Joshi

PhD Scholar, Clinical Neuropsychology,
Neuroscience Center, All India Institute of
Medical Sciences, New Delhi, India

Gaurav Kakkar

Fellow, The Walton Centre for Neurosciences , Liverpool, UK; Associate Director, Neuroanaesthesia & Neurocritical Care, Medanta-The Medicity, Gurgaon, India

Peter Kaplan

Professor, Johns Hopkins Bayview Medical Center, Baltimore, MD, USA

Indu Kapoor

Assistant Professor, Department of Neuroanesthesiology and Critical Care, All India Institute of Medical Sciences, New Delhi, India

S. Omar Kazmi

Neurocritical Care Fellow, Division of Vascular Neurology & Neurocritical Care, Department of Neurology, Baylor College of Medicine, Texas, USA

Ankur Khandelwal

Senior Resident, Department of Neuroanesthesiology and Critical Care, All India Institute of Medical Sciences, New Delhi, India

Ashish Khanna

Staff Intensivist, SICU & Center for Critical Care; Assistant Professor of Anesthesiology; Staff Anesthesiologist, Department of General Anesthesiology, Staff Department of Outcomes Research, Cleveland Clinic, Cleveland, OH, USA

Sarah M. Khorsand

Clinical Fellow, Division of Critical Care Medicine, Department of Anesthesiology & Pain Medicine, University of Washington School of Medicine, Seattle, WA, USA

Matthew A. Kirkman

Assistant Professor Neurocritical Care Unit, The National Hospital for Neurology and Neurosurgery, University College London Hospitals, London, UK

Lauren Koffman

Assistant Professor, Department of Neurology and Department of Anesthesiology and Critical Care Medicine, Johns Hopkins University School of Medicine, Baltimore, MD, USA

Sundar Krishnan

Associate Professor, Department of Anesthesia, Division of Critical Care, University of Iowa Hospitals and Clinics, Iowa City, IA, USA

Avinash B. Kumar

Medical Director Neuroscience ICU; Professor Anesthesiology & Critical Care; Professor Neurology, Vanderbilt University Medical Center, Nashville, TN, USA

Nicola Latronico

Professor of Anesthesia and Critical Care Medicine, Department of Anesthesia, Critical Care Medicine and Emergency, PiazzaleOspedaliCivili, Brescia, Italy

Abhijit Lele

Associate Professor, Department of Anesthesiology and Pain Medicine; Adjunct Associate Professor, Department of Neurosurgery; Associate Faculty, Harborview Injury Prevention and Research Center; Director, Neurocritical Care Service, Neuroscience ICU; Director, Quality Improvement, Neurocritical Care Service, Harborview Medical Center, Seattle, WA, USA

Mhoira Leng

Palliative care physician and medical director, Makerere University Palliative Care Unit, Kampala, Uganda, Africa; Cairdeas International Palliative Care Trust, Scotland, UK

Ne-Hooi Will Loh

Consultant, Department of Anaesthesia, National University Hospital, Singapore

Andrey Yu Lubnin

Professor, Burdenko Neurosurgical Research Institute of Ministry of Health of Russian Federation, Russia

Kevin Luk

Assistant Professor, Divisions of Critical Care Medicine and Neuroanesthesiology & Perioperative Neurosciences, Department of Anesthesiology & Pain Medicine, Harborview Medical Center/ University of Washington School of Medicine, Seattle, WA, USA

Charu Mahajan

Assistant Professor, Department of Neuroanesthesiology and Critical Care, All India Institute of Medical Sciences, New Delhi, India

Jason Makii

Clinical Assistant Professor; Manager, Clinical Services; Residency Program Director, PGY-2 Critical Care, Department of Pharmacy Services, University Hospitals Cleveland Medical Center, Cleveland, OH, USA

Edward M. Manno

Vice Chair of Clinical Affairs Department of Neurology; Professor of Neurology and Neurosurgery, Northwestern University, Feinberg School of Medicine, IL, USA

Casey C. May

Clinical Pharmacist, Department of Pharmacy, University of Alabama at Birmingham Hospital, AL, USA

Merrick Miles

Assistant Professor Anesthesiology and Critical Care, Anesthesiology Department, Vanderbilt Medical Center, Nashville, TN, USA

Christopher Morrison

Critical Care Clinical Specialist, Memorial Hospital West, Pembroke Pines, Florida, USA

Jeffrey J. Mucksavage

Clinical Assistant Professor; Clinical Pharmacist – Neurocritical Care, University of Illinois Hospital and Health Sciences System, College of Pharmacy, Chicago, USA

Priya Nair

Consultant Neuroanaesthetist and Intensivist, The Walton Centre NHS Foundation Trust, Lower Lane, Liverpool, UK

Roy Neeley

Assistant Professor, Department of Anesthesia, Division of Critical Care, Vanderbilt University, Nashville, TN, US

Ashima Nehra

Additional Professor, Clinical Neuropsychology, Neurosciences Centre; Head, Division of Clinical Psychology, Department of Psychiatry, All India Institute of Medical Sciences, New Delhi, India

Lena Nyholm

CCRN, PhD, Neurocritical Care Unit, Uppsala University Hospital, Department of Neurosurgery, Uppsala University, Sweden

Kent Owusu

Specialty Practice Pharmacist, Neurocritical Care, Yale New Haven Hospital, Pharmacy Department, New Haven, CT, USA

Mayur B. Patel

Division of Trauma, Emergency General Surgery, and Surgical Critical Care, Department of Surgery, Section of Surgical Sciences, Nashville, TN, USA

Konstantin Popugaev

Deputy Director, Head of Regional Vascular Centre, Sklifosovsky Research Institute of Emergency Medicine, Moscow, Russia

Shobana Rajan

Vice Chair of Education; Associate Director of Neuroanesthesiology, Allegheny Health Network, Cleveland Clinic, Cleveland, OH, USA

Manee Raksakietisak

Associate Professor; Chair of Neuroanesthesia Unit, Faculty of Medicine Siriraj Hospital, Mahidol University, Thailand

G. S. Umamaheswara Rao

Senior Professor, Department of Neuroanaesthesia, National Institute of Mental Health and Neurosciences (NIMHANS), Bangalore, INDIA

Frank A. Rasulo

Professor, Department of Anesthesia, Critical Care Medicine and Emergency, Piazzale Ospedali Civili, Brescia, Italy

Emanuele Rossetti

Professor, Pediatric Intensive Care unit, DEA-ARCO Department, Bambino Gesu Children's hospital, IRCCS, Rome, Italy

Dominic Rosso

Lecturer, University of Toronto, Toronto, ON, Canada

Toni Sabbouh

Research Assistant, Ohio State University, Wexner Medical Center, Columbus, Ohio, USA

Altan Sahin

Hacettepe Üniversitesi Tıp Fakültesi, Anesteziyoloji ve Reanimasyon A.D, Algoloji B.D., Ankara, Turkey

Nahel N. Saied

Professor of Anesthesia and Critical Care; Director Critical Care Anesthesiology, UAMS, Nashville, TN, USA

Alexander S. Samoilov

Professor, Burnazian Scientific State Centre of Federal Medical and Biological Agency of Russian Federation, Russia

Ahmad Sawalha

Research Scholar, Department of Neurology, The Ohio State University College of Medicine, OH, USA

Megha Uppal Sharma

Consultant, Artemis Hospitals, Gurugram, Haryana, India

Ashleigh Sherrington

Consultant, St George's University Hospitals, NHS Foundation Trust, UK

Charu Singh

Professor, Department of Pain and Palliative Medicine, Amrita Institute of Medical sciences, Kochi, Kerala, India

Vasudha Singhal

Senior Consultant, Medanta—The Medicity, Gurgaon, Haryana, India

Sanjeev Sivakumar

Neurocritical Care Fellow, Division of Vascular Neurology and Neurocritical Care, Department of Neurology, Baylor College of Medicine, Houston, TX, USA

Keaton Smetana

Specialty Practice Pharmacist, The Ohio State University Wexner Medical Center, Columbus, OH, USA

Mike Souter

Professor of Anesthesiology & Pain Medicine, Neurological Surgery, University of Washington, USA

Kalpana Srivastava

Scientist 'G', Dept of Psychiatry, Armed Forces Medical College, Pune, India

Jose I. Suarez

Professor and Director Neurosciences Critical Care, Departments of Anesthesiology and Critical Care Medicine, Neurology, and Neurosurgery, Johns Hopkins University School of Medicine Baltimore, USA

Priyadarshini Sundararajan

Consultant Anesthetist, Dr.Sundararajan Super Specialty Hospital, Salem, India

Monica S. Tandon

Director-Professor, Govind Ballabh Pant Institute of Postgraduate Medical Education and Research, New Delhi, India

Eljim P. Tesoro

Clinical Pharmacist, Neurosciences; Clinical Associate Professor, College of Pharmacy; Director, PGY2 Residency in Critical Care Pharmacy, University of Illinois Hospital & Health Sciences System, IL, USA

Anneli Thelandersson

Department of Physiotherapy and Occupational Therapy, Sahlgrenska University Hospital, Gothenburg, Sweden

Srinivas Thota

Assistant Professor of Anesthesiology and Pain management, Upstate Medical University/State University of New York, Syracuse, New York, USA

Sudha Thota

Consultant Radiologist, Buffalo MRI, Amherst, New York, USA

Concezione Tommasino

Associate Professor of Anesthesiology and Intensive Care, Department of Biomedical, Surgical and Odontoiatric Sciences, University of Milano, Italy

Michel Torbey

Chair, Department of Neurology, University of New Mexico, Albuquerque, New Mexico, USA

Swagata Tripathy

Associate Professor (Critical Care), Department of Anesthesia, All India Institute of Medical Sciences, Bhubaneswar, India

Filiz Uzumcugil

Assistant Professor, Hacettepe University School of Medicine, Department of Anesthesiology and Reanimation, Ankara, Turkey

Yvonne Valzani

Consultant, Area ad Alta Intensità di cura, Policlinico Sant'Orsola-Malpighi, Bologna, Italy

Chitra Venkateswaran

Professor, Consultant in Psycho Oncology, Department of Pain and Palliative Medicine, Amrita Institute of Medical sciences, Kochi, Kerala, India

Sarah Wahlster

Assistant Professor, Department of Neurology, Harborview Medical Center, University of Washington School of Medicine, Seattle, WA, USA

James Wang

Resident, Department of Neurology, University of Washington School of Medicine, Seattle, WA, USA

Kyle D. Weaver

Assistant Professor, Department of Neurological Surgery, Vanderbilt University Medical Center, Nashville, TN, USA

Sheena M. Weaver

Assistant Professor, Department of Anesthesiology, Division of Critical Care Medicine, Vanderbilt University Medical Center, Nashville, TN, USA

Aaron Yengo-Kahn

Resident Physician, Department of Neurological Surgery, Vanderbilt Medical Center, Nashville, TN, USA

Aysun Ankay Yilbas

Assistant Professor, Hacettepe University Faculty of Medicine, Department of Anesthesiology and Reanimation, Ankara, Turkey

Thassayu Yuyen

Attending physician, Department of Anesthesiology, Faculty of Medicine, Siriraj Hospital, Mahidol University, Bangkok, Thailand

Maxim V. Zabelin

Professor, Burnazian Scientific State Centre of Federal Medical and Biological Agency of Russian Federation, Moscow, Russia

Wendy Ziai

Department of Neurology; Department of Anesthesiology and Critical Care Medicine, Johns Hopkins University School of Medicine, Baltimore, MD, USA

Megan Zielke

Clinical Pharmacy Specialist, Penn Presbyterian Medical Center, Philadelphia, PA, USA

Argyro Zoumprouli

Consultant, St George's University Hospitals NHS Foundation Trust, London, UK

Abbreviations*

5-HT	5-hydroxytryptamine	AMP	adenosine monophosphate
ABC	airway, breathing, and circulation	AMS	altered mental state
ABG	arterial blood gases	AMSAN	acute motor-sensory axonal neuropathy
ABI	acute brain injury		
ABP	arterial blood pressure	APACHE 2	Acute Physiology and Chronic Health Evaluation 2
ACA	anterior cerebral artery		
ACCESS	Acute Candesartan Celexetil Therapy in Stroke Survivors	aPTT	activated partial thromboplastin time
		ARDS	acute respiratory distress syndrome
ACE	angiotensin converting enzyme	ARF	acute renal failure
AChR	acetylcholine receptor	ASA	American Society of Anesthesiologist
ACL	acetylcholine	aSAH	aneurysmal subarachnoid haemorrhage
ACoA	anterior communicating artery	aSCI	acute spinal cord injury
ACPO	acute colonic pseudo-obstruction	ASIA	American Spinal Injury Association
ACS	acute coronary syndrome	ASPEN	American Society for Parenteral and Enteral Nutrition
ACTH	adrenocorticotropin hormone		
ADC	apparent diffusion coefficient	ATP	adenosine-5-triphosphate/adenosine triphosphate
ADQI	acute dialysis quality initiative		
ADP	adenosine diphosphate	AVDO$_2$	anteriovenous oxygen difference
ADR	alpha–delta ratio	AVM	arteriovenous malformation
AED	anti-epileptic drug	AVP	arginine vasopressin
AF	atrial fibrillation/flutter	BA	basilar artery
AFC	aggressive fever control	BAEP	brainstem auditory evoked potentials
AGI	acute gastric injury	BAO	basilar artery occlusion
AHTR	acute hypotensive transfusion reaction	BASICS	Basilar Artery International Cooperation Study
AI	adrenal insufficiency		
AICA	anterior inferior cerebellar artery	BBB	blood–brain barrier
AIDP	acute inflammatory demyelinating polyradiculoneuropathy	BCAA	branched chain amino acids
		BIPAP	bi-level positive airway pressure
AIDS	acquired immunodeficiency syndrome	BIPLED	bilateral independent periodic lateralized epileptiform discharge
AIS	Abbreviated Injury Scale		
AIS	acute ischaemic stroke	BIS	bispectral index
AKI	acute kidney injury	BMI	body mass index
ALE	autoimmune limbic encephalitis	BMR	basal metabolic rate
ALI	acute lung injury	BP	blood pressure
ALF	acute liver failure	BPS	Behavioural Pain Scale
AMAN	acute motor axonal neuropathy	BTF	Brain Trauma Foundation
AMP	amplitude	BS	Beçhet's Syndrome
AMP	amino-3-hydroxy-5-methyl-4-isoxazolepropionate	BV	Bacterial Ventriculitis
		CA	cardiac arrest

*This list consolidates abbreviations used in the book. There may be instances of duplication of an abbreviation by virtue of a difference in its full form. Readers are advised to refer to the list contextually.

CA	cerebral autoregulation		CSD	cortical spreading depression
CAE	carotid endarterectomy		CSF	cerebrospinal fluid
CaO$_2$	arterial oxygen content		CSV	continuous spontaneous ventilation
CALCULATE	Critical care Pressure Ulcer Assessment made Easy		CSW	cerebral salt wasting
			CSWS	cerebral salt wasting syndrome
CAM-ICU	Confusion Assessment Method for the ICU		CT	computed tomography
			CTA	computed tomography angiography
CBC	complete blood chemistry		CTO	cervicothoracic orthosis
CBF	cerebral blood flow		CTV	computed tomography venogram
CBV	cerebral blood volume		CVC	central venous catheter
CCB	calcium channel blockers		CVR	cerebrovascular resistance
CCP	critical closing pressure		CVT	cerebral venous thrombosis
CCT	computerized cognitive training		CVVH	continuous venovenous haemofiltration
CEA	carotid endarterectomy			
cEEG	continuous electroencephalography		CVVHD	continuous venovenous haemodialysis
CFC	conventional fever control		CVVHDF	continuous venovenous haemodiafiltration
CHS	cerebral hyperperfusion syndrome			
CI	confidence interval		CYP	cytochrome
CIM	critical illness myopathy		DAI	diffuse axonal injury
CINCH	cooling in intracerebral haemorrhage		DART	Dementia Assessment by Rapid Test
CIP	critical illness polyneuropathy		DAT	direct antiglobulin test
CIV	continuous intravenous infusion		DAVF	dural arteriovenous fistula
CjO$_2$	jugular venous oxygen content		DBP	diastolic blood pressure
CKD	chronic kidney disease		DCI	delayed cerebral ischaemia
CLABSI	central line associated blood stream infections		DHA	docosahexaenoic acid
			DHC	decompressive hemicraniectomy
CMD	cerebral microdialysis		DI	diabetes insipidus
CMRglu	cerebral metabolic rate for glucose		DIT	diet-induced thermogenesis
CMRO$_2$	cerebral metabolic rate of oxygen		DNA	deoxyribonucleic acid
CMV	continuous mandatory ventilation		DOAC	direct oral anticoagulant
CMS	colistimethate sodium		dROR	dynamic rate of regulation
CNS	central nervous system		DRS	Disability Rating Scale
CO	carbon monoxide		DSA	digital subtraction angiography
CO	cardiac output		DSMB	data safety monitoring board
CO$_2$	carbon dioxide		DTR	deep tendon reflex
COMBI	Centre for Outcome Measurement in Brain Injury		dTT	dilute thrombin time
			DVT	deep vein thrombosis
COPD	chronic obstructive pulmonary disease		DWI	diffusion-weighted imaging
CPAP	continuous positive airway pressure		EAC	external auditory canal
CPC	Cerebral Performance Category scale		EASI	Everyday Abilities Scale for India
CPM	continuous passive motion		ECASS	European Cooperative Acute Stroke Study
CPOT	Critical-Care Pain Observation Tool			
CPP	cerebral perfusion pressure		ECG	electrocardiography
CPR	cardiopulmonary resuscitation		ECMO	extracorporeal membrane oxygenation
CRASH	Corticosteroid Randomization after Significant Head Injury		ECOG	electrocorticography
			ECPR	extracorporeal cardiopulmonary resuscitation
CRRT	continuous renal replacement therapy			
CRS	Coma Remission Scale		ECT	ecarin clotting time
CS	carotid siphon		ECT	electroconvulsive therapy
CS	compression stockings		EDH	extradural haematoma
CSA	compressed spectral arrays		EDP	effective downstream pressure

EDV	end diastolic volume
EEG	electroencephalography
EF	executive function
ELISA	enzyme-linked immunoabsorbent assay
EMG	electromyography
EMT	endovascular mechanical thrombectomy
ENG	electroneurography
ENLS	Emergency Neurological Life Support
EP	evoked potentials
EPA	eicosapentaenoic acid
EPF	electrophysiological study
EPO	erythropoietin
EPUAP	European National Pressure Ulcer Advisory Panel
ERI	Early Rehabilitation Index
ESBL	extended-spectrum beta-lactamase
ESV	end systolic volume
ETCO$_2$	end tidal CO$_2$
ETT	endotracheal tube
eVA	extracranial vertebral artery
EVD	external ventricular drain
FADH$_2$	flavin adenine dinucleotide
FAITH	fluid balance, aperients, investigations and results, therapies, and hydration status
FAST HUG	feeding, analgesia, sedation, thromboembolic prophylaxis, head of bed elevation, ulcer prophylaxis, and glycaemic control
FDA	Food and Drug Administration
FDG	fluorodioxyglucose
FFP	fresh frozen plasma
FiO$_2$	fraction of inspired oxygen
FIM	functional independence measure
FIRDA	frontal intermittent rhythmic delta activity
FLAIR	fluid-allenuated inversion recovery
FNHTR	febrilenon-haemolytic transfusion reaction
FOUR	Full Outline of Unresponsiveness
FVC	forced vital capacity
GABA	gamma-aminobutyric acid
GAD	generalized anxiety disorder
GAMES	Glyburide Advantage in Malignant Edema and Stroke
GBM	glioblastoma multiforme
GBS	Gullain-Barré syndrome
GCE	global cerebral oedema
GCS	Glasgow Coma Scale

GCS	graded compression stockings
GCSE	Generalized convulsive Status epilepticus
GFR	glomerular filtration rate
GI	gastrointestinal
GLUTI	glucose transporter
GOS	Glasgow Outcome Scale
GOS-E	Glasgow Outcome Scale-Extended
GP	glycoprotein
GPED	generalized periodic epileptiform discharge
GRV	gastric residual volume
HART	highly active retroviral therapy
Hct	haematocrit
HD	haemodialysis
HHS	Hunt and Hess Scale
HHTR	hyperhaemolytic transfusion reaction
HIE	hypoxic-ischaemic encephalopathy
HIF	hypoxia inducible factor
HINTS	Head Impulse, Nystagmus and Test for Skew deviation
HIPA	heparin-induced platelet aggregation
HIT	heparin-induced thrombocytopenia
HLA	human leucocyte antigen
HMSE	Hindi Mental Status Examination
HOPE Act	HIV Organ Policy Equity Act
HPAA	hypothalamo-pituitary-adrenal axis
HR	hazard ratio
HSV	herpes simplex virus
HTR	haemolytic transfusion reaction
HTS	hypertonic saline
IAH	intra-abdominal hypertension
IAP	intra-abdominal pressure
IAT	intra-arterial thrombolysis
IBW	ideal body weight
IC	indirect calorimetry
ICA	internal carotid artery
ICD	implantable cardioverter defibrillator
ICD	International Classification of Diseases
ICDSC	Intensive Care Delirium Screening Checklist
ICH	intracerebral haemorrhage
ICP	intracranial pressure
ICTuS	Intravascular Cooling in the Treatment of Stroke
ICU	intensive care unit
ICUAW	ICU-acquired weakness
IDSA	Infectious Diseases Society of America
IH	intracranial hypertension
IHD	intermittent haemodialysis

ILMA	intubating laryngeal mask airway		NAD⁺	nicotinamide adenine dinucleotide (oxidized)
IMV	intermittent mandatory ventilation		NADH	nicotinamide adenine dinucleotide (reduced)
INR	international normalized ratio			
IPC	intermittent pneumatic compression		NADPH	nicotinamide adenine dinucleotide phosphate
IRIS	immune reconstitution inflammatory syndrome		NAT	non-accidental trauma
IR-PEP	inspiratory resistance positive expiratory pressure		NCCU	neurocritical care unit
			NCS	Nociception Scale
ISUIA	International Study of Unruptured Intracranial Aneurysm		NCSE	Neurobehavioural Cognitive Status Examination
IVC	inferior vena cava		NCSE	nonconvulsive status epilepticus
IVIG	intravenous immunoglobulin		NEMC-PCR	New England Medical Center Posterior Circulation Registry
JVP	jugular venous pressure			
LD	loading dose		NEST	Neuropsychological Evaluation Screening Tool
LD	lumbar drain			
LMA	lyrangeal mask airway		NFNSS	World Federation of Neurological Surgeons Scale
LMWH	low molecular weight heparin			
LOS	length of stay		NIC	neurointensive care
LPR	lactate–pyruvate ratio		NICE	National Institute for Health and Care Excellence
LSW	last seen well			
LV	left ventricle		NICU	neurointensive care unit
LVEDV	LVend-diastolic volume		NIF	negative inspiratory force
LVOT	left ventricular outflow tract		NIHSS	National Institutes of Health Stroke Scale
MAC	manually assisted cough			
MAC	multi-access catheter		NINDS	National Institute of Neurological Disorders and Stroke
MAP	mean arterial pressure			
MCA	middle cerebral artery		NIPPV	non-invasive positive pressure ventilation
MDD	major depressive disorder			
MEG	magnetoencephalography		NIRS	near-infrared spectroscopy
MEP	maximal expiratory pressures		NMDA	N-methyl-D-aspartate
MFV	mean flow velocity		NMES	neuromuscular electrical stimulation
MG	myasthenia gravis		NMS	neuroleptic malignant syndrome
MGFA	Myasthenia Gravis Foundation of America		NNT	number needed to treat
			NO	nitric oxide
MI-E	mechanical in-exsufflation		NOS	nitric oxide synthase enzymes
MIP	maximal inspiratory pressure		NPE	neurogenic pulmonary oedema
MLS	midline shift		NPPB	normal perfusion pressure breakthrough
MMSE	Mini Mental State Examination			
MoCA	Montreal Cognitive Assessment		NRBM	non-rebreather mask
MOF	multiple organ failure		NS	normal saline
MRA	magnetic resonance angiography		NSAID	non-steroidal anti-inflammatory drug
MRC	Medical Research Council		NSE	neuron-specific enolase
MRI	magnetic resonance imaging		NSM	neurogenic stunned myocardium
mRMR	measured resting metabolic rate		NVPS	Nonverbal Pain Scale
mRS	modified Rankin scale		O₂ER	oxygen extraction ratio
MS	multiple sclerosis		OA	ophthalmic artery
MTT	mean transit time		OCF	occipital condyle fracture
MuSK-MG	muscle-specific tyrosine kinase type myasthenia gravis		ODS	osmotic demyelination syndrome
			OEF	oxygen extraction fraction
NaCl	sodium chloride		OHCA	out-of-hospital cardiac arrest
NAD	nicotinamide adenine dinucleotide			

ONS	optic nerve sheath
ONSD	optic nerve sheath diameter
OPO	organ procurement organization
OR	operating room
OSUMC	Ohio State University Medical Center
OTPD	organs transplanted per donor
OTT	onset to treatment time
PaO$_2$	pressure of arterial oxygen
PaCO$_2$	arterial carbon dioxide partial pressure
PAD Guidelines	Pain, Agitation, and Delirium Guidelines
PAID	paroxysmal autonomic instability with dystonia
PAST	Preliminary Aphasia Screening Test
PbrO$_2$	partial brain tissue oxygen tension
PbtO$_2$	brain tissue oxygen tension
PCA	patient-controlled analgesic
PCA	posterior cerebral artery
PCoA	posterior communicating artery
PCR	polymerase chain reaction
PDT	percutaneous dilatational tracheostomy
PE	plasma exchange
PE	phenytoin equivalents
PE	pulmonary embolism
PEEP	positive end expiratory pressure
PEG	percutaneous endoscopic gastrostomy
PEP	positive expiratory pressure
PET	positron emission tomography
PFO	patent foramen ovale
PGE$_2$	prostaglandin E$_2$
pH	acidity level
PI	pulsatility index
PICA	posterior inferior cerebella artery
PICC	peripherally inserted central catheter
PID	peri-injury depolarization
PIV	peripheral IV
PLED	periodic lateralized epileptiform discharges
PLR	passive leg raising
PML	progressive multifocal leukoencephalopathy
PN	parenteral nutrition
PNS	peripheral nerve stimulation
POCUS	point-of-care ultrasound
POLST	Physicians Orders for Life Sustaining Treatment
PONV	postoperative nausea and vomiting
PPV	pulse pressure variation
PPV	positive predictive values
PRBC	packed red blood cells

PRES	posterior reversible encephalopathy syndrome
PRIS	propofol-related infusion syndrome
pRMR	predicted resting metabolic rate
PRx	pressure reactivity index
PSH	paroxysmal sympathetic hyperactivity
PSU	Penn State University
PTT	partial thromboplastin time
PVC	premature ventricular contraction
PVC	pulmonary vascular resistance
PVS	persistent vegetative state
pVT	pulseless ventricular tachycardia
qEEG	quantitative electroencephalography
RA	radial artery
RAP	right atrial pressure
RASS	Richmond Agitation-Sedation Scale
RCT	randomized controlled trial
RESCUEicp	Randomised Evaluation of Surgery with Craniectomy for Uncontrollable Elevation of Intracranial Pressure
RI	resistance index
RMR	resting metabolic rate
RNA	ribonucleic acid
RNS	reactive nitrogen species
RNS	repetitive nerve stimulation
ROM	range of motion
ROS	reactive oxygen species
ROSC	return of spontaneous circulation
RQ	respiratory quotient
RR	relative risk
RRT	renal replacement therapy
rScO$_2$	regional cerebral oxygen saturation
RSBI	rapid shallow breathing index
RSE	refractory status epilepticus
RSI	rapid sequence intubation
rtPA	recombinant tissue plasminogen activator
RV	right ventricle
RVR	rapid ventricular response
RyR	ryanodin receptor
SAFE	Saline versus Albumin Fluid Evaluation
SAH	subarachnoid haemorrhage
SAS	Sedation-Agitation Scale
SBP	systolic blood pressure
SCA	superior cerebellar artery
SCCM	Society of Critical Care Medicine
SCI	spinal cord injury
SCr	serum creatinine
SDH	subdural haematoma
SE	status epilepticus

SEPS	subdural evacuating port system	TLC	triple lumen catheter
SFEMG	single-fibre electromyography	TMD	tympanic membrane displacement
SHINE	Stroke Hyperglycaemia Insulin Network Effort	TMP-SMX	trimethoprim-sulfamethoxazole
		TMS	transcranial magnetic stimulation
SIADH	syndrome of inappropriate secretion of antidiuretic hormone	TNF	tumour necrosis factor
		TOF	time-of-flight (MRA)
sICH	spontaneous intracerebral haemorrhage	TOF	train of four
SIMV	synchronized intermittent mandatory ventilation	TOI	tissue oxygenation index
		tPA	tissue plasminogen activator
SIP	Sickness Impact Profile	TPN	total parenteral nutrition
SIRS	systemic inflammatory response syndrome	TRALI	transfusion-related acute lung injury
		TRH	thyrotropin-releasing hormone
SIRPID	stimulus-induced periodic, rhythmic, or ictal discharge	TRIM	transfusion-related immunomodulation
$SjvO_2$	jugular venous oxygen saturation	tSCI	traumatic spinal cord injury
SNP	single nucleotide polymorphism	TTE	Transthoracic echocardiogram
SOFA	Sequential Organ Failure Assessment	TTM	Targeted Temperature Management
SPECT	single photon emission computed tomography	TV	tidal volume
		UCNS	United Sates Council of Neurological Subspecialty
SpO_2	arterial oxyhaemoglobin saturation		
SRMD	stress-related mucosal disorder	UFH	unfractionated heparin
SSEP	somatosensory evoked potential	US	United States
SSI	surgical site infection	UTI	urinary tract infection
SSS	superior sagittal sinus	UUN	urinary urea nitrogen
STEMI	ST elevation myocardial infarction	VA	vertebral artery
STOP	Stroke Prevention Trial in Sickle Cell Anaemia	VAP	ventilator-associated pneumonia
		VBG	venous blood gases
SUDEP	sudden unexpected death in epilepsy	VC	vital capacity
SVT	sinus venous thrombosis	V-CMV	volume-controlled mandatory ventilation
SVV	stroke volume variation		
TACO	transfusion-associated circulatory overload	VEGF	vascular endothelial growth factor
		VF	ventricular fibrillation
TA-GVHD	transfusion-associated graft versus host disease	VP	ventriculoperitoneal
		VRG	ventral respiratory group
TAMG	thymoma-associated myasthenia gravis	VT	ventricular tachycardia
TBI	traumatic brain injury	VTE	venous thromboembolism
TCCD	transcranial colour-coded duplex	vWf	von Willebrand factor
TCD	transcranial Doppler	VZV	varicella-zoster virus
TEE	total energy expenditure	WD	dicrotic wave
TH	therapeutic hypothermia	WGAP	Working Group on Abdominal Problems
THRR	transient hyperemic response ratio		
THRT	transient hyperemic response test	WHO	World Health Organization
TIA	transient ischaemic attack	WHOQOL	World Health Organization Quality of Life
TICA	terminal internal carotid artery		
TIPS	transjugular intrahepatic portosystemic shunting	WP	percussion wave
		WT	tidal wave

1

Introduction to and History of Neurointensive Care

P. K. Bithal and H. Prabhakar

ABSTRACT

Neurointensive care (NIC) is an emerging sub-specialty that attained importance after it was proved beyond doubt that care of traumatic brain injury (TBI) patients in a specialized NIC unit improves outcomes. This improvement may be the outcome of combination of multiple attributes, one of them being management of critically sick neurological patients by a dedicated neurointensive care team, including full time neurointensivist. Care by neurointensivist significantly reduces the in-hospital mortality and shortens the length of hospital stay, though it may not influence the long term outcome favourably.

KEYWORDS

Neurointensive care (NIC); history; evolution; critical care; neurosurgery; neuroanesthesia.

Neurointensive care (NIC) is a fledgling subspeciality that integrates neurology, neurosurgery, intensive care medicine, and neuroanaesthesia. It attained importance after it was proven beyond doubt that care of traumatic brain injury (TBI) patients in a specialized NIC unit improves health outcomes. This improvement may be the outcome of a combination of multiple attributes, one of them being the management of critically ill neurological patients by a dedicated neurointensive care team, including full-time neurointensivists. Dedicated care by neurointensivists significantly reduces in-hospital mortality and shortens the length of hospital stay, though it may not necessarily influence the long-term outcomes favourably. NIC is a specialized unit which specifically focuses on critical care management of patients with acute neurological diseases such as TBI, subarachnoid haemorrhage, postoperative care of neurosurgical patients, hypoxic brain injury, and central causes of brain damage following neurosurgery, etc. In the current scenario, this specialty is making rapid strides aided by the introduction of advanced therapies based on various techniques and technologies exclusively directed to monitor brain physiology and

biochemistry. One of the most significant benefits of treatment of neurologically critical patients in the NIC unit is the availability of complex management strategies for these patients in this area which is beyond the realm of care in the general intensive care unit. With further advancements, NIC has also assumed the management of neurological conditions such as acute ischaemic stroke, which were not traditionally thought to be its part. With a rapid progress in this field, the main challenge now faced by NIC is resuscitation and management of traumatic and vascular brain injuries, previously given up as fatal.

The precise time when a neurocritical care unit became a reality is a matter of debate and conjecture.[1] However, in the modern era, this discipline came into being in the second half of the twentieth century.

The history of NIC has remained unravelled. The genesis of this specialty began probably in the prehistoric period and dates back to antiquity, which is documented in the Edwin Smith surgical Papyrus (Figure 1.1).

This text named after a nineteenth century Egyptologist who purchased the document in Luxor or Thebes in 1862, is an unfinished textbook on physical injuries written in circa 1600 BC.[2] The Edwin Smith Papyrus is a unique treatise containing the oldest known description of signs and symptoms of spinal column and spinal cord injuries.[3] This ancient record not only forms the fountainhead of many anatomical and physiological concepts of the nervous system, but also forms the basis for development of modern objective clinical thinking, firmly laying the foundation of modern medicine more than a thousand years before Hippocrates. The Papyrus text instructs physicians to examine the patient and look for revealing physical signs that may indicate the outcome of injury.[4] It has elucidated 48 case reports, including 27 head trauma and 6 spinal cord injuries, many with documented interventions.[2]

The oldest recorded neurosurgical operation was reported in ancient Egypt circa 3000 BC and consisted of traction reduction which was used successfully to reverse a paralysing cervical spine injury of an early Egyptian leader (Osiris).[5] Other authors believe that the earliest known neurosurgical procedures most probably originated in the Neolithic Era, which has been proven by the discovery of a trephined (or trepanned) skull dating back to 10,000 BC.[2] Figure 1.2 presents three trepanned skulls from the Copacabana Peninsula.

Hippocrates in his work has stated and advised prophylactic trepanation for managing certain head traumas, including skull fractures and brain contusions, but the rationale for this was not clearly explained. Hippocrates was the first to systematically document skull fractures and emphasised on the significance of history taking and careful physical examination.[6] Subsequently, Aulus Aurelius Cornelius Celsus of Alexandria promoted the work of Hippocrates, approximately 300 years later.[2]

Aulus made contributions to the work of Hippocrates by describing epidural and subdural removal of haematoma using trepanation. In the second century another great physician, Galen of Pergamon, further expanded on the technique of trepanation and described novel innovative tools.[7] This era also marked the beginning of initial management of spinal cord injuries. Hippocrates too, is credited for applying traction in the early treatment of such injuries. Thereafter, Celsus and Galen further advanced the understanding of the pathophysiology of spinal cord injuries by recognising that damage to the spinal marrow or cord, and not the vertebrae leads to neurological deficits.[8] There was no noteworthy progress in medicine during the medieval period. However, during this era, Canon of Medicine by the famous Persian intellectual Avicenna was widely used for text literature throughout Europe until the eighteenth century.[9] He may have been the first person to realize that stroke was due to the blockage of cerebral vessels, offering remedies for the management of acute stroke including venesection.[10]

In the beginning of the twentieth century all patients regardless of criticality of disease were treated in common general wards. The necessity of creating separate space for critically ill patients was deeply felt by the physicians during the Scandinavian poliomyelitis epidemics of 1940s and 1950s. These epidemics also proved that intermittent positive pressure breathing was more effective in saving a life rather than cuirass or tank ventilators which formed the mainstay of managing patients with respiratory failure until then. These poliomyelitis epidemics acted as the catalyst for the development of dedicated respiratory units—the first true intensive care units (ICU) to treat patients with respiratory failure.[2,11–13] Another reason to reserve separate space from the general care wards in hospital was the rapidly increasing number of complex surgical procedures and ensuing high complication rates. This led to the establishment of many specialized care ICUs simply as centres demanding more care.[14] Later, with the development of respiratory and cardiac ICUs, a decrease in mortality rate among mechanically ventilated patients treated in the traditional general hospitals compared to those in new ICUs became an eye opener and provided convincing evidence for the establishment of these units despite higher costs.[15]

Management of neurosurgical patients in the ICU in the modern era takes us back to the work of Walter and Dandy at the John Hopkins Hospital in the 1930s.[16] They are credited for their concept of establishment of special units for the postoperative care of neurosurgical patients. However, initially, patients with neurological diseases or following craniospinal surgeries were managed in a general ICU, even though it was felt that treatment of these patients in a general ICU was not comprehensive. Owing to special requirements for the satisfactory treatment of the neurosurgical patients and also better outcomes, other patients hospitalized with diagnoses of TBI, spinal cord trauma, cerebrovascular accident, poorly controlled epilepsy, encephalitis, and neuromuscular conditions endangering life were also thought to be deserving candidates for management in the NIC unit.

During the 1970s and the 1980s, progress in neuroanaesthesiology facilitated highly complex operative neurosurgical interventions requiring higher level of care in the immediate and early postoperative period. Patients were taken care of in dedicated areas of neurological wards managed by skilled nursing staff, trained in close monitoring to detect neurological deterioration. These wards had round the clock access to neurosurgical support services in the event of neurologic deterioration of a patient. In the United States (US), Allan Ropper (neurologist), Sean Kennedy (neuroanaesthetist), and Nicholas Zervas (neurosurgeon) set up the first combined neurological and neurosurgical ICU at the Massachusetts General Hospital in Boston, and their collaboration led to the publication of the first text book on Neurocritical Care.[1] In 1971, the Society of Critical Care Medicine (SCCM) was founded to promote the speciality and define core competencies. The three founding physicians of SCCM came from different medical specialities: cardiology, anaesthesiology, and trauma surgery.[16]

Subsequent to the establishment of the SCCM, in 2002 the international and multidisciplinary Neurocritical Care Society was created and in 2004, the first journal dedicated to neurointensive care (called *Neurocritical Care*) was published. Over a period of time, NIC has broadened its horizon to provide comprehensive care for all potentially life-threatening conditions of the central nervous system (CNS) and neuromuscular diseases. Managing the complex interaction between the brain and other body systems is the cornerstone of NIC, which has evolved from its original focus on the CNS into a subspecialty encompassing all aspects of care of a neurologically ill patient. This realization of necessity has resulted in the establishment of NIC units worldwide.[17] Neurocritical care was formally recognized by the United States Council of Neurological Subspecialty (UCNS) in 2005 and this led to the accreditation of neurointensivists in the US.[18]

Assessment and management of intracranial pressure (ICP) remains to be one of the main responsibilities of neurointensivists practising today. Cushing published a landmark study demonstrating the 'Cushing response', which is a response to raised ICP, a triad of hypertension, bradycardia, and irregular respiration. The recognition of this triad of symptoms remains crucial to clinical intensive care.[19]

In 1965, Lundberg and colleagues published the first report of continuous ICP monitoring using a ventricular cannula.[20] These authors demonstrated variations in ICP in patients with TBI and provided a targeted approach for the management of raised ICP. Fibre-optic transducer-tipped monitors were introduced in the 1980s. Current studies examine the use of silver or antibiotic-coated catheters to reduce the risks of ventriculitis, a serious complication of intraventricular ICP monitoring.[21]

The importance of various agents that would lower cerebrospinal fluid (CSF) pressure temporarily and also decrease brain volume was known to neurosurgeons. Since Wilikins, Weed and McKibben[22] demonstrated that various hypertonic solutions could achieve this goal, many

agents have been examined.[23] The use of hypertonic urea for this purpose was proposed by Fremont Smith and Forbes.[24] However, sterile hypertonic urea intravenous preparation was difficult, but when lyophilized urea and invert sugar became available, it found wide acceptance.[25] In view of its propensity to cause rebound increases in CSF pressure and brain volume, neurosurgeons were not satisfied with its use. Besides, these agents had many other adverse effects because of which they failed to maintain their popularity among the neurosurgeons.

In 1930, the correlation between barbiturates and lowered ICP was identified by Horsley.[26] Mannitol was first used in dogs in 1961; subsequently, Wise and Chater published their report of lowering CSF pressure in a clinical setting in 1962.[27] Extensive experience of using mannitol in animals and clinical settings thus established its inertness and lack of toxicity.[2,28]

The management of critical neurologic patients on ICP monitoring was observed to have many drawbacks. Therefore, in order to overcome these shortcomings, multimodal monitoring was introduced a few decades ago. The term 'multimodal monitoring' refers to keeping a check on multiple parameters of brain physiology and chemistry that can be influenced by medical/surgical intervention. Multimodal monitoring can provide crucial information of brain physiology and metabolism at the bedside. Advancements in technology has seen the introduction of new techniques to monitor brain oxygen. These monitoring techniques have helped in the efficient management of patients in NIC units by predicting brain ischaemia/secondary injury to the brain. Near infrared spectroscopy (NIRS) was described in the 1970s. It has been found to be useful in monitoring cerebral ischaemia during carotid endarterectomy as well as in the management of TBI patients in NIC units. Jugular venous oxygen saturation helps the intensivists in identifying global cerebral ischaemia. Brain tissue oxygen tension monitoring was introduced in the 1990s. All these techniques of brain oxygen determination are most useful in TBI patients (to predict prognosis), though they are also being studied in other neurological conditions in the NIC setup. In 1982, Aaslid and colleagues introduced clinical transcranial Doppler (TCD) examination of the intracranial arteries.[29] TCD has made it possible to monitor cerebral vasospasm and confirm brain death at the bedside in an NIC unit.

The cerebral microdialysis principle was first employed in the early 1960s, when push-pull cannulas[30] and dialysis sacs[31] were implanted into rodent brains to directly study the tissue biochemistry. It was introduced into clinical practice in the 1990s during thalmotomy intended to relieve tremors in Parkinson's disease.[32] This technique continuously measures cerebral chemistry and metabolism. Various quantifiable markers of brain metabolism give information before the patient develops signs and symptoms of brain ischaemia/secondary injury. Additionally, changes in various measured markers have been shown to be early predictors of cerebral vasospasm in subarachnoid haemorrhage.[33]

In 1995, the National Institute of Neurological Disorders and Stroke supported the use of intravenous tissue plasminogen activator for ischaemic stroke and it showed improved outcomes in treated patients at 3 months.[34] A major role of the neurointensive care team now is to admit patients following neuroradiological interventional procedures like embolization, carotid stenting, clot retrieval, post recombinant tissue plasminogen activator (rt-PA) therapy, etc.

In the year 1934, therapeutic breakthrough for myasthenia gravis came when Mary Walker, an assistant house officer at a hospital for poor in London suburban area, administered an injection of physostigmine to patients with myasthenia gravis and observed dramatic improvement. She postulated in her letter to the *Lancet* describing her findings that physostigmine inhibits the action of esterase that destroys acetylcholine.[35]

One of the criteria that reduction of antibodies ameliorates the disease was provided by a technique called plasma exchange (PE) or plasmapheresis. This technique was tested on patients in the early 1950s to separate blood components. With further improvements in cell separator equipment in the late 1960s, PE therapy became popular in the 1970s for many antibody mediated autoimmune diseases like myasthenia gravis, Guillain-Barré syndrome, etc.

Thus NIC speciality is a relatively young and evolving field which has generated tremendous interest among neurologists and neuroanaesthesiologists. As diagnostic and therapeutic modalities continue to be developed and refined, it is evident that highly trained individuals with in-depth knowledge of the nervous system physiology are crucial for the favourable outcome in patients. As the field moves forward at a rapid pace, advances will hopefully continue to keep abreast of the development of new technologies and improved clinical trial designs.

REFERENCES

1. Bleck TP. Historical aspects of critical care and nervous system. *Crit Care Clin* 2009;25:153–64.
2. Korbakis G, Bleck T. The evolution of neurocritical care. *Crit Care Clin* 2014;30:657–61.
3. van Middendorp JJ, Sanchez GM, Burredge AL. The Edwin Smith papyrus: a clinical reappraisal of the oldest known document on spinal injuries. *Eur Spine J* 2010;19:1815–23.
4. Stiefel M, Shaner A, Shaefer SD. The Edwin Smith papyrus: the birth of analytical thinking in medicine and otolaryngology. *Laryngoscope* 2006;116:182–8.
5. Filler AG. A historical hypothesis of the first recorded neurosurgical operation: Isis, Osiris, Thoth and the origin of the djed cross. *Neurosurg Focus* 2007;23:1E6.
6. Rose FC. The history of head injuries: an overview. *J Hist Neurosci* 1997;6:154–80.
7. Kshettry VR, Midea SA, Batjer HH. The management of cranial injuries in antiquity and beyond. *Neurosurg Focus* 2007;23:E8.
8. Lifshutz J, Colohan A. A brief history of therapy for spinal cord injury. *Neurosurg Focus* 2004;16:E5.
9. Rahimi SY, McDonnel DE, Ahmadian A, Vender JR. Medieval neurosurgery: contributions from the Middle East, Spain and Persia. *Neurosurg Focus* 2007;23:E14.
10. Zargaran A, Zarshenas MM, Karimi A, Yarmohammadi H, Borhani-Haghighi A. Management of stroke as described by Ibn Sina (Avicenna) in the Canon of Medicine. *Int J Cardiol* 2013:169:233–7.
11. Anderson EW, Ibsen B. The anesthetic management of patients with poliomyelitis and respiratory paralysis. *BMJ* 1954;2:786–8.
12. Berthelsen PG, Cronqvist M. The first intensive care unit in the world: Copenhagen 1953. *Acta Anaesthesiol Scand* 2003;47:1190–5.
13. Lassen HC. A preliminary report on the 1952 epidemic of poliomyelitis in Copenhagen with special reference to the treatment of acute respiratory insufficiency. *Lancet.* 1953;1:37–41.
14. Hilberman M. The evolution of the intensive care unit. *Crit Care Med* 1975;3:159–65.
15. Rogers RM, Weiler C, Ruppenthal B. Impact of the respiratory intensive care unit on survival of patients with acute respiratory failure. *Chest* 1972;62:94–7.
16. Grenvik A, Pinsky MR. Evolution of intensive care unit as a clinical center and critical care medicine as a discipline. *Crit Care Clin* 2009;25:239–50.
17. Howard RS, Kullmann DM, Hirsch NP. Admission to neurological intensive care: who, when and why? *J Neurol Neurosurg Psychiatry* 2003;74(Suppl):iii2–iii9.
18. Mayer SA, Coplin WM, Chang C, et al. Core curriculum and competencies for advanced training in neurological intensive care. United Council of Neurologic Subspecialties guidelines. *Neurocrit Care* 2006;5:159–65.
19. Cushing H. Concerning a definite regulatory mechanism of the vasomotor centre which controls blood pressure during cerebral compression. *Johns Hopkins Hospital Bulletin* 1901;12:290–2.
20. Lundberg N, Troupp H, Lorin H. Continuous recording of the ventricular fluid pressure in patients with severe

acute brain injury: a preliminary report. *J Neurosurg* 1965;22:581–90.

21. Keong NC, Bulters DO, Richards HK, et al. The SILVER (silver impregnated line versus EVD. Randomized trial): a double blind, prospective, randomized controlled trial of an intervention to reduce the rate of external ventricular drain infection. *Neurosurgery* 2012;71:394–403.

22. Wilkins RH, Weed LH, McKibben PS. Neurosurgical classic-XXXII. *J Neurosurg* 1965;22:404–19.

23. Hays AN, Lazaridis C, Neyens R, Nicholas J, Gay S, Chalela JA. Osmotherapy: Use among neurointensivists. *Neurocrit Care* 2011;14:222–8.

24. Fremont-Smith F, Forbes HS. Intraocular and intracranial pressure: an experimental study. *Arch Neurol Psychiatry* 1927;18:550–64.

25. Andrews RJ, Bringas JR. A review of brain retraction and recommendations for minimizing intraoperative brain injury. *Neurosurgery* 1994;35:172–3.

26. Horsley JS. The intracranial pressure during barbital narcosis. *Lancet* 1937;229:141–3.

27. Wise BL, Chater N. The value of hypertonic mannitol solution to decrease brain mass and lowering cerebrospinal fluid pressure. *J Neurosurg* 1962;19:1038–43.

28. Tan G, Zhou J, Yuan D, Sun S. Formula for use of mannitol in patients with intracranial haemorrhage and high intracranial pressure. *Clin Drug Invest* 2008;28:81–7.

29. Aaslid R, Markwalder TM, Nornes H. Noninvasive transcranial Doppler ultrasound recording of flow velocity in basal cerebral arteries. *J Neurosurg* 1982;57:769–74.

30. Gaddun JU. Push pull cannulae. *J Physiol* 1961;155:1–2.

31. Bito L, Davson H, Levin E, Murray M, Snider N. The concentration of free amino acids and other electrolytes in cerebrospinal fluid, in vivo dialysis of brain and blood plasma of the dogs. *J Neurochem* 1966;13:1057–67.

32. Meyerson BA, Linderoth B, Karlsson H, Ungerstedt U. Microdialysis in human brain: extracellular measurements in the thalamus of Parkinsonian patients. *Life Sci* 1990;46:301–8.

33. Bellander BM, Cantais E, Enblad P, et al. Consensus meeting on microdialysis in neurointensive care. *Intens Care Med* 2004;30:2166–9.

34. The National Institute of Neurologic Disorders and stroke rt-PA Stroke study Group. Tissue plasminogen activator for acute ischaemic stroke. *N Eng J Med* 1995;333:1581–7.

35. Walker MB. The treatment of myasthenia gravis with physostigmine. *Lancet* 1934;1:1200–1.

Part I

Basic Principles of Neurointensive Care

Editor: Judith Dinsmore

2

Cerebral Blood Flow and Dynamics

A. Zoumprouli

ABSTRACT

The brain requires a lot of energy to support its functions. Although it represents only 2 of the body mass of an average adult, it consumes almost 25% of the body's glucose and around 20% of oxygen. Glucose is the main source of energy for the brain and thus a tight regulation of glucose metabolism is critical for maintenance of its physiology.

The brain utilizes almost all its energy for active transport of ions to sustain and restore the membrane potentials discharged during the process of excitation and conduction.

Under normal conditions, the demand for energy by the brain is parallel to the supply to the substrate. Investigations support that there is a tight coupling between the processes that consume energy and those that supply the substrate. Therefore, anatomical and physiological mechanisms are in place to ensure that the blood flow to the normal brain is adequate.

KEYWORDS

Cerebral blood flow; cerebrovascular circulation; cerebral autoregulation; Circle of Willis; astrocytes; brain ischaemia; neurovascular coupling; blood pressure; glucose; hypercapnia; hypocapnia.

INTRODUCTION

The brain requires significant amounts of energy to support its functions. Although it represents only 2% of the body mass of an average adult, it consumes almost 25% of the body's glucose and accounts for around 20% oxygen utilization. Glucose is its main source of energy and thus tight regulation of glucose metabolism [through generation of adenosine triphosphate (ATP)] is critical for the maintenance of normal physiology. The brain has a negligible reserve of oxygen, which is utilized, almost entirely for the oxidation of carbohydrates.[1]

In addition, its ability to generate energy is low and as a result the small reserves of energy are depleted rapidly following sudden interruption to the blood and substrate delivered. The brain uses almost all its energy for active transport of ions to sustain and restore the membrane potentials discharged during the process of excitation and conduction. A small amount of energy is consumed for the formation of neurotransmitters.

Under normal conditions, the demand for energy by the brain is parallel to the supply to the substrate. There is investigative evidence to support the presence of a tight coupling between the processes that consume energy and those that supply the substrate. Therefore, anatomical and physiological mechanisms are in place to ensure that the blood flow to the normal brain is maintained.[2] Table 2.1 shows the numerical data of cerebral blood supply.

CEREBRAL CIRCULATION

The blood supply to the brain originates from the aorta and is provided solely by the two common carotids and the two vertebral arteries.

The common carotid arteries are derived from the aortic arch and as they enter the skull they form the internal carotid arteries (anterior circulation). The vertebral arteries are branches of the subclavian arteries. The basilar artery (posterior circulation) originates from the confluence of the vertebral arteries at the lower

Table 2.1 Cerebral blood supply in numbers

Parameter	Value
Percentage of brain utilization of total body oxygen at rest	20%
Percentage of cardiac output used by the brain	15%–20%
Total blood flow through the brain (adult)	750–1000 ml/min
Total blood flow through the brain (adult)	54 ml/100 g brain tissue/min
Total blood flow through the brain (child)	105 ml/100 g brain tissue/min
Cerebral blood flow (whole brain)	55–60 ml/100 g brain tissue/min
Cerebral blood flow (grey matter)	75 ml/100 g brain tissue/min
Cerebral blood flow (white matter)	45 ml/100 g brain tissue/min

pontine border. The two circulations (anterior and posterior) give rise to branches that create a polygonal anastomotic circle that connects the anterior and posterior circulation; the circle of Willis.[3]

The arrangement of arteries into the circle of Willis supplies the brain and surrounding structures with blood through a system that creates collaterals to allow equalization of pressure. If one vessel is blocked or narrowed, blood flow from the other arteries is preserved in order to avoid cerebral ischaemia.

The classic 'normal' circle is present only in 30%–50% of brains and is often incomplete (especially in young adults and females). Although there is some anastomoses between the terminal branches of these arteries, the 'watershed' areas (where the blood supply from two vessels meet) are vulnerable to decreases in perfusion. Global cerebral ischaemia produces maximal ischaemic lesions in these zones.[4]

It is noteworthy that there is an extensive autonomic nerve supply to the cerebral arteries, however, its precise purpose is not well known and it is still controversial. The innervation system can be divided into two components: that which innervates the extraparenchymal vessels and that influencing the intraparenchymal arteries.

The extraparenchymal vessels (before the vessels enter the pia) are innervated by the superior cervical, sphenopalatine, otic, and trigeminal ganglions. Vasoactive substances that they release on the arterial walls include: norepinephrine, neuropeptide Y, acetylcholine (ACh), nitric oxide, substance P nitric oxide synthase,

peptide histidine isoleucine, and neurokinin A. The intraparenchymal vessels receive their innervation from the nucleus basalis, locus coeruleus or raphe nucleus. These neurons send projection fibres to cortical vessels and the astrocytes that surround them. The arterioles and capillary endothelial cells, neurons, pericytes, astrocytes and microglia together constitute a functional unit that is often referred to as a neurovascular unit. Upon electrical or chemical stimulation these subcortical areas control cerebral blood flow (CBF) via secretion of noradrenaline, 5-hydroxytryptamine (5-HT), ACh or gamma-aminobutyric acid (GABA). Receptors for these vasoactive mediators are found on the capillary endothelium, smooth muscle cells, and astrocytes. The latter allows modulation of microvascular tone according to changes in neuronal activity.[3]

CEREBRAL PERFUSION PRESSURE

In order to describe CBF, the flow-in-a-tube model can be used if it is assumed that the flow is laminar, constant and uniform, and the tube has a thin wall that cannot distend. Under these conditions, Ohm's law describes that flow is proportional to the difference in pressure between the two ends of the tube (ΔP) divided by the resistance to flow (R): Flow = $\Delta P/R$. In every organ, the pressure responsible for flow through the organ is the difference between the arterial and venous pressure. Since the brain is within a closed cavity, the downstream pressure is not necessarily the pressure in the jugular veins. Furthermore, as the intracranial pressure can affect the pial veins and venous sinuses, it becomes a significant component of the equation. Therefore, the cerebral perfusion pressure (CPP) becomes the difference between mean arterial pressure (MAP) and mean intracranial pressure (ICP) or mean jugular venous pressure (JVP), whichever is higher[5]:

$$CPP = MAP - ICP$$
$$CPP = MAP - JVP$$

PHYSIOLOGICAL CONSIDERATIONS OF CEREBRAL BLOOD FLOW

The only significant arteriovenous differences that have been found in the brain are for the substrates glucose (glu) and oxygen (O_2), and the metabolic product, carbon dioxide (CO_2). Water is also produced but has never been measured. Lactate and pyruvate are produced occasionally—mainly under conditions of cerebral vascular insufficiency and rarely under normal conditions. In a normal adult brain the O_2 consumption and CO_2 production are equal giving a respiratory quotient (RQ) of 1.0. The normal adult brain consumes 156 micromoles (µmol)/100 g brain tissue/min of O_2 at rest.

If it is accepted that for every µmol of glucose, 6 µmol of O_2 is consumed in order to achieve complete oxidation, then the calculated glucose used should be 26 µmol/100 g brain tissue/min. In contrast, the measured glucose utilization in the brain is 31 µmol/100 g brain tissue/min. For complete oxidation, the actual ratio O_2:glu is 5.5. What happens to this excess glucose is not clear. It is assumed that some of this may be used for the synthesis of chemical substances in the brain.

At rest, the brain is not homogenous with regard to perfusion and metabolic rates. In general, grey matter values are 4–5 times higher than white matter. Positron emission tomography (PET) in human beings has proven that energy metabolism is linked to local functional activity and metabolic demand, which adjusts to the local/regional CBF.[6] Activation of the brain results in increased CBF. This happens through 'capillary recruitment', but as brain capillaries are open at all times this 'recruitment' actually represents changes in flow rates and a more homogenous distribution of flow. During functional activation, the relationship between regional CBF and cerebral metabolic rate for glucose (CMRglu) is linear. Glucose consumption rate is greater than the rate of increase in oxygen consumption. This close correlation of CBF and CMRglu (and, to a lesser extent, the cerebral metabolic rate of oxygen [$CMRO_2$]) demands highly dynamic and finely tuned mechanisms. The local glucose and O_2 delivery and CO_2 removal adapt to the actual demand of active brain regions. This adaptation appears to happen via regulation of cerebrovascular resistance: the contractile mechanism of precapillary arterioles. The key event of this contraction-relaxation cycle is the increase in intracellular free calcium (Ca^{2+}) ions. It is still unclear which products of metabolism mediate changes in calcium concentration and/or opening of the calcium channels. The classical theory that calcium mobilization is mediated by vasoactive metabolic products such as lactate and hydrogen ions (H^+), or adenosine has recently been replaced by the 'neuronal' hypothesis that suggests neuronal energy demand is communicated to the vasculature within the neurovascular unit. This can happen either directly or through astrocytes (can release vasoactive factors) in an anticipatory manner by vasoactive neurotransmitters or products of synaptic signalling. Vasodilation occurs independently of glucose metabolism-induced signalling. It is possible that both mechanisms coexist; neurovascular coupling regulated by feed-forward signalling may be supplemented or modulated by metabolism-dependent mechanisms (Table 2.2).[7–10]

Table 2.2 Cerebral oxygen consumption and glucose utilization in a normal young adult

Function	Value
O_2 consumption	156 (µmol/100 g brain tissue/min)
Glucose utilization	31 (µmol/100 g brain tissue/min)
O_2: glucose ratio	5 (mol/mol)
Glucose equivalent of O_2 consumption	26b (µmol glucose/100 g brain tissue/min)
CO_2 production	156 (µmol/100 g brain tissue/min)
Cerebral respiratory quotient	0.97

AUTOREGULATION

There is an impressive stability in blood flow to the normal human brain despite the wide fluctuations in CPP. Thus, the normal brain is considered to have the ability to autoregulate. Autoregulation is present in most of the vascular beds but is particularly well developed in the brain because of the need for constant blood supply and water homeostasis. Cerebral autoregulation can be visualized as a curve with three key elements: the lower limit, the upper limit, and the plateau.[1,11] The lower and upper limits are sharp inflection points. They represent the boundaries of pressure independent flow. In normal adults, CBF is maintained at 50 ml/100 g/min of brain tissue (provided CPP remains within the range of 60–150 mmHg) by altering cerebrovascular resistance (CVR). Outside these CPP limits CBF becomes linearly dependent on MAP. These numbers represent means that have been calculated from various groups of subjects without any range of distribution.

Cerebral ischaemia can occur below the lower inflection point of the autoregulation curve. The position of the lower inflection point is also affected by the mechanism of hypotension (haemorrhagic vs drug-induced). Initially, the reduction of CBF is counterbalanced by an increase in oxygen extraction from the blood. When the capacity for increased oxygen extraction is less than the reduction in perfusion, we start seeing clinical signs/symptoms of ischaemia. This occurs when MAP falls below 60% of the lower autoregulatory threshold.[12] At the upper inflection point of the curve, outside autoregulation limits, acute changes in blood pressure create excessive intravascular pressure, which overcomes myogenic vasoconstriction (smooth muscles in arterioles) and causes forced dilatation of the cerebral vessels. This decreases CVR and as a result CBF increases by up to 400% (autoregulatory breakthrough). The decreased CVR increases hydrostatic pressure on the endothelium, which leads to vasogenic oedema formation. This is the underlying mechanism in conditions such as hypertensive encephalopathy, posterior reversible encephalopathy, and eclampsia.

Arterial Carbon Dioxide

Alterations in arterial carbon dioxide partial pressure ($PaCO_2$) have been recognized as having a potent influence on CVR. An increase in the $PaCO_2$ to 80 mmHg (10.6 kPa) will approximately double CBF. Further increase in $PaCO_2$ does not have an effect, possibly because of maximum vessel dilatation.

Decreasing the $PaCO_2$ to 20 mmHg (2.7 kPa) reduces the flow by almost half. Further reductions of $PaCO_2$ do not seem to produce any subsequent change in CBF. Several mechanisms have been suggested to be involved in hypercapnic vasodilation: extracellular pH, prostanoids, and nitric oxide (NO). However, the major mechanism in human beings appears to be related to a direct effect of extracellular hydrogen ions on the smooth muscles of cerebral arteries and arterioles.[13]

Arterial carbon dioxide partial pressure also has an effect on the autoregulation curve. The autoregulation should be regarded as dynamic (mobile) when nonperfusion pressure mechanisms are involved. This effect is clinically significant. The combined vasodilatory effect of hypotension and hypercapnia could cause a rightward shift of the lower point. Hypercapnia may also shift the upper point of the curve leftwards. In addition, the plateau also shifts upwards due to overall vasodilation and it is shortened. It is noteworthy that these changes depend on the degree of hypercapnia. In severe hypercapnia the pressure-flow relationship is linear.

In animal models of haemorrhagic hypotension, when MAP is reduced to 50 mmHg, the CBF response to hypocapnia is lost. In drug-induced hypotension models, CBF response is attenuated but not lost completely.[13-16]

Hypocapnia also has an effect on cerebrovascular pressure reactivity but there are not many studies that address this aspect. Whilst the plateau descends because of vasoconstriction, the lower point appears to be unchanged. There are no data to define the effect of hypocapnia on the upper point of the autoregulation curve (Figure 2.1).

Effect of Oxygen

The brain has a very high metabolic demand for oxygen compared to other organs, and thus, it is not surprising that acute hypoxia is a potent dilator of cerebral circulation. A hypoxia-induced drop in ATP levels opens up ATP-sensitive potassium channels on smooth muscle causing hyperpolarization and vasodilation. Animal studies have shown that CBF remains unchanged until the partial pressure of arterial oxygen falls below 50 mmHg (6.6 kPa). However, human studies using transcranial Doppler (TCD) suggest that the threshold for cerebral vasodilation is as high as 58 mmHg $PaCO_2$ (around 89–90% SpO_2). The relationship is non-linear because the sigmoidal shape of the haemoglobin-O_2 dissociation curve determines tissue oxygen delivery.

Chronic hypoxia increases capillary density through activation of angiogenic pathways. This adaptation increases cerebral blood volume and flow.

Increases in arterial oxygen tension causes only slight changes in CBF; the administration of 100% O_2 (at 1 Atm) will decrease flow by approximately 10%.[17,18]

MEASUREMENT OF CEREBRAL FLOW

Numerous techniques have been used to measure blood flow to the brain. Some of them will be discussed below.

Classic Kety–Schmidt Technique

The classic Kety–Schmidt technique was the first method used for estimation of CBF in human beings in 1945. It is considered the gold standard. Low concentration (15%) of the inert inhaled nitrous oxide (N_2O) was used as a tracer. The calculations are based on the Fick principle, which states that 'the quantity of a substance uptake by an organ per unit time is equal to the product of the blood flow through that organ' and the arteriovenous concentration is the difference of this substance ($Qt = Ft \times (Ca - Cv)$), where Qt is the quantity of substance taken up per unit time; Ft is the blood flow per unit time; and Ca and Cv are the arterial and venous concentrations of the substance. For the measurement of CBF, the subject inhales 15% N_2O present in the air for 10 minutes. Meanwhile the arterial and jugular bulb blood samples are taken and analysed for N_2O content. The initial difference between the arterial and venous concentrations of N_2O decreases as the brain takes up the tracer. After 10–15 minutes the brain and cerebral blood reach equilibrium. The amount of N_2O delivered to or removed by the brain thus equals the CBF multiplied by the arterial or venous concentrations, respectively. The value of global CBF calculated has been reproduced with newer techniques. The technique is simple, repeatable, and can be used in conscious human beings. Limitations include the inability to discriminate variations between different areas of the brain (grey vs white matter) and the assumption that the sampled jugular venous blood reflects pure cerebral venous drainage.[19]

Radioactive Inert Gases

The introduction of radioactive inert gases (krypton-85 and xenon-133) eliminates the need for arterial and venous cannulation since the rate at which the isotope leaves the brain could be calculated by monitoring the decay in radioactivity. The radioactive gas is injected into the internal carotid artery and attains equilibrium rapidly. On stopping the injection, the rate of clearance will depend on the blood flow. The inert gas clearance has two advantages compared with the Kety–Schmidt technique; first, the flow can be calculated from a graphical analysis of the clearance curves and the result can be obtained rapidly. The second advantage of the method is the ability to calculate regional blood flow. It is possible to focus on small cones of tissue and demonstrate variations of flow due to discrete lesions (tumours, infarcts) by using small detectors appropriately. The technique is adequately sensitive to detect changes in regional CBF due to functional activity. Apart from the need for carotid puncture, the other disadvantages include anaesthetic properties of xenon and the radioactive nature of the tracer.[20,21]

Xenon Computed Tomography

Xenon has a remarkable property of freely crossing the blood-brain barrier. Stable xenon also absorbs X-rays and is used to enhance images that are obtained with standard computed tomography (CT). In this technique, a short period of 33% xenon gas inhalation is used. Computed tomography of the brain is performed before and during the inhalation. The resultant changes in the absorption coefficients of the X-rays depend on the solubility of xenon and perfusion of the tissue. These differences in addition to measurements of the end-tidal concentration of xenon can be used to calculate absolute values of local CBF. The technique produces functional mapping of blood flow with excellent anatomical specificity. Patients should be given supplemental oxygen and subjected to continuous monitoring of oxygen saturation.[22]

Table 2.3 Clinical and research applications of transcranial doppler

Clinical	Research
Subarachnoid haemorrhage and cerebral vasospasm	Cerebral autoregulation
Intracranial steno-occlusive disease	Cerebral vasoreactivity
Acute ischaemic stroke	Neurovascular coupling
Collateral flow	Traumatic brain injury
Sickle cell disease	Intraoperative TCD monitoring
Brain death	
Detection of microemboli	

Transcranial Doppler Sonography

Transcranial Doppler sonography is a non-invasive technique, which measures the velocity of blood flow in major intracranial arteries in real time. The test is performed by placing the probes extracranially. Ultrasound can be generated by a piezoelectric crystal and focused into a beam using a lens. Transcranial Doppler sonography produces a 2 megahertz (MHz) signal that allows better penetration of the bone. The velocity of the flowing blood is determined by calculating the shift in frequency between the transmitted ultrasound and the reflected one. Transcranial Doppler sonography currently has clinical and research applications (Table 2.3).[23]

Near Infrared Spectroscopy (NIRS)

Measurements of local CBF can be obtained using the near infrared spectroscopy (NIRS) technique with oxyhaemoglobin as a tracer. If there is a sudden increase in the arterial saturation of haemoglobin, the resultant increase in cerebral oxyhaemoglobin concentration can be detected and measured. The rate of cerebral haemoglobin delivery can be calculated (mmol/min) and this can be converted to CBF (ml/100 g/min). The technique offers real-time measurements that are non-invasive, non-operator dependent, and easily reproducible.[24]

CONCLUSIONS

Under normal conditions, the demand for energy by the brain is parallel to the supply to the substrate. Investigations support that there is a tight coupling between the processes that consume energy and those that supply the substrate. Therefore, anatomical and physiological mechanisms are in place to ensure that the blood flow to the normal brain is adequate.

REFERENCES

1. Lassen NA. Cerebral blood flow and oxygen consumption in man. *American Physiological Society* 1959;39(2):183–238.

2. Sokoloff L. The metabolism of the central nervous system in vivo. In: Field J, Magoun HW, Hall VE Eds. *Handbook of Physiology*, Section I, Neurophysiology. vol. 3. American Physiological Society, Washington D.C., 1960; pp. 1843–64.

3. Cipolla MJ. *The Cerebral Circulation* (2nd ed). Morgan & Claypool Life Sciences: United States 2016.

4. Liebeskind DS. Collateral circulation. *Stroke* 2003;34:2279–84.

5. The Brain Trauma Foundation. Guidelines for cerebral perfusion pressure. *J Neurotrauma* 2000;17:507–11.

6. Paulson OB, Hasselbalch SG, Rostrup E, Knudsen GM, Pelligrino D. Cerebral blood flow response to functional activation. *J Cereb Blood Flow Metab* 2009;30(1):2–14.

7. Koehler RC, Roman RJ, Harder DR. Astrocytes and the regulation of cerebral blood flow. *Trends in Neurosciences* 2009;32(3):160–9.

8. Hamel E. Perivascular nerves and the regulation of cerebrovascular tone. *J Appl Physiol* 2005;100(3):1059–64.

9. Filosa JA, Bonev AD, Nelson MT. Calcium dynamics in cortical astrocytes and arterioles during neurovascular coupling. *Circ Res* 2004;95(10):e73–81.

10. Attwell D, Buchan AM, Charpak S, Lauritzen M, MacVicar BA, Newman EA. Glial and neuronal control of brain blood flow. *Nature* 2010;468(7321):232–43.

11. Paulson OB, Strandgaard S, Edvinsson L. Cerebral autoregulation. *Cerebrovascular and Brain Metabolism Reviews* 1990;2(2):161–92.

12. Drummond JC. The lower limit of autoregulation. *Anesthesiology* 1997;86(6):1431–3.

13. Coles JP, Minhas PS, Fryer TD, et al. Effect of hyperventilation on cerebral blood flow in traumatic head injury: Clinical relevance and monitoring correlates. *Crit Care Med* 2002;30(9):1950–9.

14. Rozet I, Vavilala MS, Lindley AM, Visco E, Treggiari M, Lam AM. Cerebral autoregulation and CO$_2$ reactivity in anterior and posterior cerebral circulation during sevoflurane anesthesia. *Anesth Analg* 2006;102(2):560–4.

15. Marion DW, Bouma GJ. The use of stable xenon-enhanced computed tomographic studies of cerebral blood flow to define changes in cerebral carbon dioxide vasoresponsivity caused by a severe head injury. *Neurosurgery* 1991;29(6):869–73.

16. Meng L, Gelb AW. Regulation of cerebral autoregulation by carbon dioxide. *Anesthesiology* 2015;122(1):196–205.

17. Gupta AK, Menon DK, Czosnyka M, Smielewski P, Jones JG. Thresholds for hypoxic cerebral vasodilation in volunteers. *Anesth Analg* 1997;85(4):817–20.

18. Masamoto K, Tanishita K. Oxygen transport in brain tissue. *J Bimech Eng* 2009;131(7):074002.

19. Kety SS, Schmidt CF. The nitrous oxide method for the quantitative determination of cerebral blood flow in man: theory, procedure and normal values. *J Clin Invest* 1948;27(4):476–83.

20. Waltz A, Wanek A, Anderson R. Comparison of analytic methods for calculation of cerebral blood flow after intracarotid injection of 133 Xe. *J Nucl Med* 1972;13(1):66–72.

21. Munck O, Lassen NA. Bilateral cerebral blood flow and oxygen consumption in man by use of Krypton 85. *Cir Res* 1957;5(2):163–8.

22. Gur D, Yonas H, Good WF. Local cerebral blood flow by xenon-enhanced CT: current status, potential improvements, and future directions. *Cerebrovascular and Brain Metabolism Reviews* 1989;1(1):68–86.

23. Reinstrup P, Ryding E, Asgeirsson B, Hesselgard K, Unden J, Romner B. Cerebral blood flow and Transcranial Doppler Sonography measurements of CO$_2$-Reactivity in acute traumatic brain injured patients. *Neurocrit Care* 2012;20(1):54–9.

24. Kim MN, Durduran T, Frangos S, et al. Noninvasive measurement of cerebral blood flow and blood oxygenation using near-infrared and diffuse correlation spectroscopies in critically brain-injured adults. *Neurocrit Care* 2009;12(2):173–80.

3

Cerebrospinal Fluid Dynamics

J. Dinsmore

ABSTRACT

The cerebrospinal fluid (CSF) provides buoyancy, mechanical protection to the brain and a stable ionic environment. The choroid plexus produces approximately 80% of the CSF. The CSF is produced at a rate of 0.3–0.5 ml/min or 500–600 ml/day and is renewed about four times a day. In adults the total volume is about 150 ml. CSF formation involves a complex array of transporters and channels in the choroidal epithelium. It is an active, energy-dependent process. The main determinants of secretion are Na^+/K^+-ATPase and carbonic anhydrase activity. Traditional teaching describes the CSF circulating through the ventricular system into the spinal canal and subarachnoid spaces across the arachnoid granulations and back into the blood stream. The CSF space is a dynamic pressure system. The CSF pressure is the result of a dynamic equilibrium between CSF formation, CSF absorption, and resistance to flow.

KEYWORDS

Cerebrospinal fluid (CSF); choroid plexus; secretion; circulation; dynamics; intracranial pressure.

INTRODUCTION

The cerebrospinal fluid (CSF) is a clear, colourless fluid, which bathes the central nervous system. It has several physiological functions such as providing buoyancy to gravity and mechanical protection to the brain against sudden movements and external trauma. The CSF provides a stable ionic environment for the brain, supplying nutrients such as neuropeptides and removing waste products of metabolism and drugs. It may also aid neuronal communication by transporting hormones and neurotransmitters to different areas of the brain. Finally, it acts as a compensatory mechanism to increasing intracerebral volume through displacement of CSF into the spinal spaces and increasing absorption.

CEREBROSPINAL FLUID PRODUCTION

Choroid Plexus

The choroid plexus produces approximately 80% of the CSF with the remainder formed from the brain interstitial fluid and ependymal lining of the ventricular system.

The choroid plexus is distributed throughout the ventricular system within the inner surface of each lateral ventricle and the roofs of the third and fourth ventricles. It consists of a stromal core of connective tissue and capillaries surrounded by a single layer of cuboidal epithelial cells. These choroidal epithelial cells are specifically adapted for secretion with an apical brush border containing microvilli to increase the surface area of numerous mitochondria and well-developed endoplasmic reticulum. Along with the microvilli, both primary and motile cilia are also found on the apical luminal surface. The function of these are unclear but the motile cilia appear to be involved in CSF flow and the primary cilia may have a role as osmoreceptors and/or chemoreceptors.[1] The choroidal epithelial cells are joined together by tight junctions at the apical, CSF facing, cell membrane restricting the passage of ions and molecules from blood to the CSF. This constitutes the blood–CSF barrier. However, compared to the blood-brain barrier, the blood–CSF barrier is much more permeable. The basal border of the epithelial cells rests on a basal lamina, which separates it from the highly vascular stromal core. The choroidal blood vessels, unlike those in the rest of the cerebral vasculature, have fenestrated endothelium allowing rapid transport of substrates from the blood to the choroidal epithelium for the production of CSF (Figure 3.1).[2]

Cerebrospinal Fluid Secretion

Cerebrospinal fluid is produced at a rate of 0.3–0.5 ml/min or 500–600 ml/day in the adult. Cerebrospinal fluid volume is renewed about four times a day. The total volume of CSF is about 150 ml in adults and 50 ml in the neonate, divided between the intraventricular, subarachnoid, and spinal spaces.

Cerebrospinal fluid formation involves a complex array of transporters and channels in the choroidal epithelium. It is thought to occur in two stages: by passive filtration of fluid across the highly permeable capillary endothelium and regulated secretion across the choroidal epithelium. This is an active, energy-dependent process involving a range of ion pumps and transporters. The main determinants of secretion involve:

- Na^+/K^+-ATPase actively secretes Na^+ into and K^+ out of the CSF.
- Carbonic anhydrase is essential for the passage of carbon dioxide (CO_2) that does not readily cross the epithelial cells. Carbonic anhydrase catalyses the conversion of water and CO_2 to hydrogen ions and bicarbonate:

$$H_2O + CO_2 \Leftrightarrow H_2CO_3 \Leftrightarrow H^+ + HCO_3^-$$

Sodium ion ($Na+$) is quantitatively the most important ion transported, facilitated by Na^+/K^+-ATPase, and provides the driving force for CSF secretion. The Na^+/K^+-ATPase also creates an electrochemical gradient exploited by a range of other transporters involved in CSF secretion. Different transporters are expressed at the basolateral and apical membranes. The K^+/Cl^- co-transporter is co-located with the Na^+/K^+-ATPase in the apical membrane. The supply of Cl^- is dependent upon its exchange with HCO_3^- at the basolateral membrane; a process dependent upon carbonic anhydrase. The carrier proteins of basolateral membranes exchange H^+ and HCO_3^- ions for Na^+ and Cl^- ions. It is the osmotic gradient created by the secretion of Na^+, Cl^-, and to a lesser extent HCO_3^- that drives the secretion of water. Due to its high aquaporin (AQP)-1 expression, the apical membrane has high water permeability. In contrast to this, the basolateral membrane lacks significant AQP1 expression.[3]

The choroid plexus also secretes growth factors, vitamins B_1, B_{12}, C, folate, β2-microglobulin, arginine vasopressin, and nitric oxide. Both secretion and composition of the

CSF can be regulated by autonomic and humoral signals. The choroid plexus receives cholinergic, adrenergic, and serotoninergic autonomic innervation. Aldosterone, angiotensin II, and atrial natriuretic peptide may also affect its production.[2] Pharmacological modification of CSF production can be achieved by using the carbonic anhydrase inhibitor, acetazolamide, which reduces CSF production by 50%–100%.

CEREBROSPINAL FLUID CIRCULATION

Traditional teaching describes the CSF circulating through the ventricular system into the spinal canal and subarachnoid spaces, across the arachnoid granulations and back into the blood stream. The ventricular system consists of two paired lateral ventricles and C-shaped cavities within the cerebral hemispheres communicating via the foramen of Munro with the third ventricle. From the third ventricle, the CSF drains via the aqueduct of Sylvius into the diamond-shaped fourth ventricle and from here it leaves the ventricular system via the midline foramen of Magendie and laterally via the foramina of Luschka. Cerebrospinal fluid is largely reabsorbed into the venous system in the dural sinuses via arachnoid villi and granulations with the rate of reabsorption dependent upon the pressure gradient between the subarachnoid space and the venous sinus pressure. A small proportion of CSF may return to the blood stream via arterial and neural lymphatics located in the perineural sheaths of cranial and spinal nerves. However, this notion of predominant bulk passage is now thought to be an oversimplification. Cerebrospinal fluid circulation is much more complex with the CSF contents entering the brain interstitial fluid. Flow is more likely a combination of direct bulk flow subjected to pulsatile flow that is related to the heart rate and a continuous bidirectional fluid exchange between the CSF and interstitial fluid spaces.[4] Research indicates that lymphatics may play an important role in absorption of CSF and interstitial fluid.

With aging or Alzheimer's disease an increase in CSF capacity can result in a CSF turnover reduction, compromising its ability to clear harmful metabolites such as amyloid. This can further impair CSF production and transport (Figure 3.2).

CEREBROSPINAL FLUID COMPOSITION

Although CSF concentrations are very similar to those of plasma, it is not simply an ultrafiltrate. Cl^- and Mg^{2+} concentrations are higher and K^+ and Ca^{2+} concentrations are lower than those of plasma. When in good health, the CSF is free of red blood cells and contains only a few

Table 3.1 Typical cerebrospinal fluid and plasma contents of ions

Substance (mEq/L)	CSF	Plasma
Na^+	149	148
K^+	2.9	4.3
Cl^-	130	106
HCO^{-3}	22	25
Ca^{2+}	2.1	4.8
Mg^{2+}	2.3	1.7
PO_3^{-4}	0.5	1.8

Table 3.2 Composition of normal cerebrospinal fluid

Components	Values
White cell count	<4 mm^{-3}; mainly lymphocytes (85%)
Glucose	2.8–4.2 $mmol/L^{-1}$ or 50–75 mg/100 ml (60–80% plasma level)
Protein	0.15–0.45 g/L^{-1} or 15–45 mg/100 ml
IgG	~10% of total protein

white cells; normally less than 4 cells mm^{-3} of the adult CSF. Small numbers of monocytes, lymphocytes, and in neonates, neutrophils are normal. Glucose in CSF is about 60–80% that of plasma. It contains 0.3% of plasma proteins; both protein and glucose content increase and decrease, respectively, as CSF flows from the ventricles to the subarachnoid spaces. Variations in the closely regulated composition of CSF can be used for diagnostic purposes (Tables 3.1 and 3.2).

CEREBROSPINAL FLUID DYNAMICS

The CSF space is a dynamic pressure system. In adults, CSF occupies 11% of the intracranial space with the remaining space being occupied by the brain and blood. The CSF pressure is the result of a dynamic equilibrium between CSF formation, CSF absorption, and resistance to flow. Cerebrospinal fluid pressure can be measured directly by an intraventricular catheter inserted in the lateral ventricle or via a lumbar drain. Lumbar CSF pressure is used in the assessment of pathological conditions such as hydrocephalus and idiopathic intracranial hypertension. An intraventricular catheter remains the gold standard for measurement of intracranial pressure (ICP).

In the horizontal position, ICP has physiological values ranging between 3–4 mmHg before the age of one year, and between 10–15 mmHg in adults. Higher values correspond to intracranial hypertension. The CSF pressure varies with the systolic pulse wave, respiratory cycle, abdominal pressure, jugular venous pressure, physical activity, and posture.

Intracranial pressure is derived from the circulation of blood and CSF. Any factor that increases cerebral blood flow or CSF circulation may result in a rise in ICP. The vascular component of this is difficult to express quantitatively but the circulatory CSF component may be expressed using Davson's equation.[5]

> Davson's equation: CSF circulatory component of ICP = (resistance to CSF outflow) × (CSF formation) + (pressure in sagittal sinus).

From this it can be seen how a rise in ICP can occur as a result of either an increase in the rate of CSF formation, increase in arachnoid villi outflow resistance or increase in dural sinus pressure.

The capacity of the intracranial contents to adapt to volume changes can be assessed by measuring intracranial compliance; classically done using a CSF bolus injection. Intracranial compliance is the sum of three compliances—the CSF buffering capacity, the arterial bed, and venous compliance. Compliance decreases with increasing ICP and following a head injury all three compensatory mechanisms can be quickly exhausted.

The normal ICP trace is pulsatile reflecting both the cardiac and respiratory cycles with an amplitude between 2 and 10 mmHg. The cardiac component of the waveform consists of three peaks, P1, P2, and P3 correlating with the arterial pressure waveform in each cardiac cycle. These waveforms are usually 1–4 mmHg in amplitude. The P1 wave (percussion wave) correlates with arterial pulsation transmitted via the choroid plexus to the CSF. The P2 (tidal wave) is the result of forces generated by both the arterial pulse wave and resistance from the intracranial parenchyma. The P3 (dicrotic wave) reflects closure of the aortic valve. The respiratory component of the waveform reflects the cerebral venous pulsation generated by the changes in intrathoracic pressure as a result of respiration.[5] With increasing ICP, the respiratory component decreases and eventually disappears whereas the relative amplitude of the cardiac component increases with an elevated P2 and rounding of the waveform (Figure 3.3).

As intracranial compliance decreases pathological waves appear. Lundberg described three types of cyclic CSF pressure waves A, B, and C (Table 3.3).

Given next are some of the pathological conditions with altered CSF dynamics resulting in raised ICP.

Table 3.3 Lundberg waves, variations in icp waveform

Types of ICP waves
A waves: pathological, plateau-shaped, amplitude 50–100 mmHg, last 5–20 minutes, suggestive of low brain compliance
B waves: rhythmic oscillations, amplitude <50 mmHg, occur every 1–2 minutes, seen in ventilated patients, less useful clinically, suggestive of low brain compliance
C waves: rhythmic oscillations, amplitude <20 mmHg, occur every 4–8 minutes, synchronous with spontaneous variations in blood pressure, non-pathological

HYDROCEPHALUS

Any situation with a disturbance in CSF production, circulation or absorption can result in hydrocephalus. These factors can occur independently or in combination. Clinically, hydrocephalus can be divided into communicating and non-communicating types depending upon whether the ventricular system communicates with the subarachnoid space in the basal cisterns. Examples of types of communicating hydrocephalus include meningitis, subarachnoid haemorrhage or sagittal sinus thrombosis. Non-communicating hydrocephalus can result from aqueduct stenosis, intrinsic tumours or intraventricular haemorrhage.

Normal Pressure Hydrocephalus

Normal pressure hydrocephalus is uncommon. It can occur at any age but typically occurs in the elderly. It is associated with ventriculomegaly and a triad of gait disturbance, memory loss, and urinary incontinence. Intracranial pressure may be normal but patients may have abnormal ICP pulsatility.

Idiopathic Intracranial Hypertension

Idiopathic intracranial hypertension is a diagnosis of exclusion in patients with intracranial hypertension, symptoms of raised ICP, and normal imaging. It typically occurs in young, overweight females but also in some children.

CONCLUSIONS

The CSF provides buoyancy and mechanical protection to the brain and a stable ionic environment. CSF formation involves a complex array of transporters and channels in the choroidal epithelium. It is an active, energy-dependent process. The main determinants of secretion are Na^+/K^+-ATPase and carbonic anhydrase activity. The CSF pressure is the result of a dynamic equilibrium between CSF formation, CSF absorption, and resistance to flow.

REFERENCES

1. Damkier HH, Brown PD, Praetorius J. Cerebrospinal fluid secretion by the choroid plexus. *Physiological Reviews* 2013; 93:1847–92.
2. Sakka L, Coll G, Chazal A. Anatomy and physiology of cerebrospinal fluid. *European Annals of Otorhinolaryngology, Head and Neck Diseases* 2011;128:309–16.
3. Benarroch EE. Choroid plexus-CSF system: Recent developments and clinical correlations. *Neurology* 2016; 86:286–96.
4. Brinker T, Stopa E, Morrison J, Klinge P. A new look at cerebrospinal fluid circulation. *Fluids and Barriers of the CNS* 2014;11:10.
5. Czosnyka M, Pickard JD. Monitoring and interpretation of intracranial pressure. *J Neurol Neurosurg Psychiatry* 2004;75:813–21.

4

Intracranial Pressure

A. Sherrington

ABSTRACT

Intracranial pressure (ICP) is the pressure within the cranial cavity or skull. It is determined by the volume of its contents, namely brain, blood, and cerebrospinal fluid (CSF). Basically, the contents are essentially non-compressible, therefore, an increase in volume of one may initially be compensated by a reduction in volume of another but will ultimately result in increased ICP. As ICP increases, cerebral perfusion pressure (CPP) determined by the mean arterial pressure (MAP) and ICP may become compromised. If adequate perfusion pressure is not maintained, brain tissue ischaemia may occur.

This chapter includes the components of intracranial contents and the factors which affect their volume. It also describes the Monro–Kellie doctrine and pressure–volume relationship within the intracranial cavity and the limited mechanisms for compensation that exist within this closed system. Finally, it describes the common pressure waveform patterns that are observed while monitoring ICP.

KEYWORDS

Intracranial pressure (ICP); intracranial volume; intracranial compliance; compensation; pressure waveform; Lundberg waves.

INTRODUCTION

Intracranial pressure (ICP) is the pressure within the cranial cavity or skull and thus is determined by the volume of its contents, namely the brain, blood, and cerebrospinal fluid (CSF). As these contents are essentially non-compressible, an increase in volume of one may initially be compensated by a reduction in another but will ultimately result in increased ICP. As ICP increases, the cerebral perfusion pressure (CPP), which is determined by the mean arterial pressure (MAP) and ICP, may become compromised. If adequate perfusion pressure is not maintained, it leads to the interruption of cerebral blood flow (CBF) and thus brain tissue oxygen supply. If CBF falls below critical limits (around 20 ml/100 g/minute) brain tissue ischaemia will develop and progress to irreversible brain injury. Severe intracranial hypertension is a neurological emergency and if uncontrolled will inevitably lead to brain herniation and death. It is therefore important in the practice of neurocritical care to understand the dynamic factors contributing to variation in ICP in order to apply therapies intended to manipulate these parameters and maintain adequate cerebral perfusion and oxygenation.

INTRACRANIAL CONTENTS

Brain

The brain is the single largest component of intracranial contents, weighing approximately 1400 g in an average adult, and occupying around 80% of the compartment volume. The brain consists of approximately 80% water with 80% of this being intracellular and the remaining being in the interstitial compartment (Figure 4.1).[1]

The position of the brain within the cranium is supported by relatively inelastic dural reflections of the falx cerebri sitting between the cerebral hemispheres, and the tentorium between the hemispheres and the cerebellum. In pathological states, this creates compartments of the brain across which a pressure differential may exist, which leads to distortion of brain structures. The three classically described herniation syndromes associated with increase in ICP are transtentorial (lateral or central), subfalcine, and tonsillar herniation. The posterior fossa (inferior to the tentorium) is significantly smaller than the supratentorial compartment accounting for only 20% of brain volume including the brainstem and cerebellum. The smaller capacity of the compartment and sensitivity of structures within it mean that volume expansion in the posterior fossa is frequently associated with neurological deterioration. It is also common for lesions in the posterior fossa to cause CSF outflow obstruction leading to hydrocephalus and its earlier presentation.

Pathological states that increase the volume of the brain include expanding space occupying lesions such as tumours and abscesses as well as intracranial haematoma. Cerebral oedema may also increase brain volume as a result of cell membrane failure (cytotoxic oedema), disruption of the blood–brain barrier (vasogenic oedema) or obstructed CSF outflow (interstitial oedema).

Blood

Blood moves during the arterial and venous circulation in the brain, of which approximately 150 ml constitutes 10% of the intracranial volume. Under normal circumstances, CBF is maintained at a relatively constant level by autoregulatory mechanisms. The effects of hypoxaemia and hypercarbia in increasing CBF may increase cerebral arterial volume. Similarly, pathological states affecting venous outflow such as venous sinus thrombosis or jugular vein obstruction may also increase venous blood volume. Intrathoracic pressure increases caused by coughing, straining, or other valsalva manoeuvre will also be transmitted through the venous system.

The blood within the venous sinuses is easily compressed and therefore provides capacity for compensation within the blood volume. Due to the autoregulatory mechanisms affecting arterial wall tension, the blood volume within the arterial compartment has much lower compliance than that in the venous bed.

Cerebrospinal Fluid

CSF is a specialized extracellular fluid which provides mechanical protection, a stable chemical environment and constant glucose supply. It was once believed that the brain was suspended in the CSF such that it became weightless (in accordance with Archimedes' law), but it is now understood that the volume of CSF is insufficient to have this effect. Despite this, the role of CSF stores

in maintaining ICP is significant. Production and reabsorption of CSF is continuous and in dynamic equilibrium under normal conditions. At any given time, there is around 150 ml circulating within the intracranial compartment in the ventricular and subarachnoid spaces and accounting for the final 10% of its volume. The circulatory CSF component of ICP can be described by Davson's equation:

CSF circulatory component of ICP = (resistance to CSF outflow) × (CSF formation) + (pressure in sagittal sinus)

From this it follows that if the circulation of CSF is obstructed (for example, following a head injury, subarachnoid haemorrhage, or compression of CSF pathways by a mass lesion), then hydrocephalus may develop leading to an increase in ICP.

It is clear that there is significant interaction between the three components—brain, blood, and CSF in pathological states. An increase in ICP due to brain parenchymal expansion, mass lesion or hydrocephalus will cause venous sinus compression and obstruction to venous outflow and a progressively associated increase in ICP. The resultant ischaemia may lead to cerebral oedema and further exacerbation of intracranial hypertension, and so on. In the case of a severe head injury, these events occurring concurrently may culminate in a state of severe refractory intracranial hypertension.

VOLUME AND PRESSURE

The Monro–Kellie Doctrine

The Monro–Kellie hypothesis was proposed by the Scottish anatomists Alexander Monro and his student George Kellie in their papers of 1783[2] and 1824,[3] respectively. The principles of this doctrine have underpinned the foundation of our understanding of the relationship between intracranial contents and pressure ever since. Their hypothesis states that the brain is enclosed in a rigid structure of the skull providing a fixed volume and that the brain parenchyma is essentially incompressible. If the volume of the intracranial compartment has to remain constant, the cerebral blood volume must remain constant. It follows that in order to accommodate incoming arterial blood supply there must be continuous venous outflow. This hypothesis was strongly supported by the exsanguination experiments of Abercrombie who drained dogs of their blood volume and demonstrated preservation of brain perfusion until a very late stage.

This initial understanding focused only on the brain and blood flow and neglected the contribution of CSF. It was the subsequent experiments of George Burrows[4] that demonstrated the reciprocal relationship between the volume of blood and CSF in the intracranial compartment and thus CSF volume also came to be considered as part of the Monro–Kellie doctrine. In 1902, Cushing[5] described the triad of clinical signs accompanying an increase in ICP, namely a widening pulse pressure, irregular respiration, and bradycardia. He went on to quantify the Monro–Kellie doctrine by stating that if the skull remains intact, then the sum of the volumes of the brain, CSF, and intracranial blood volume must remain constant and thus any increase in the volume of one compartment may only occur at the expense of another.

Normal Intracranial Pressure

The normal range of mean ICP in a healthy adult in a resting, horizontal position is 5–15 mmHg. With sustained pressure, an ICP of >20–25 mmHg is considered to be intracranial hypertension. Given the significant postural changes in pressure, the zero position is generally taken to be at the level of the foramen of Monro, which is approximated in clinical practice to the level of the external auditory meatus. The resting pressure is not static, rather it fluctuates in a cyclical manner with both pulse and respiration.[6] Any action resulting in a Valsalva manoeuvre will also cause a transient increase in ICP (often of around 60 mmHg), transmitted via increased pressure in the jugular and/or epidural veins. However, in healthy individuals, these fluctuations are not associated with any neurological impairment. This demonstrates that it is not so much the ambient pressure in itself which leads to impairment, but rather the damaging effects of reduced CBF and mechanical distortion syndromes of the brain parenchyma that occur as a consequence of intracranial hypertension.

Compensation and Compliance

According to the Monro–Kellie doctrine, there must be reciprocal compensation between the intracranial components. Small and transient changes in the volume of intracranial contents can be accommodated by compensatory mechanisms which exist to prevent an increase in ICP. The term compliance is often used to describe the capacity for compensation of the intracranial contents and may be defined as the change of volume (dV) per unit change of pressure (dP). In fact, the term elastance is probably more accurate to describe the intracranial relationship since this is the inverse of compliance and represents the volume-pressure response or dP/dV, i.e., the change in pressure per unit change in volume. Thus compliance decreases with rising ICP and the elastance or volume-pressure response increases.

Since both CSF and blood are in continuation with low pressure extra cranial systems, these are the components which offer the greatest compliance or buffering capacity for an increase in intracranial volume.

The initial response to an increase in volume is the displacement of CSF from the intracranial compartments through the foramen magnum into the spinal subarachnoid space, and to a lesser degree via the optic foramen to the perioptic subarachnoid space. In this way, the CSF volume acts as the first buffer against an increase in ICP. Further increases in ICP will also lead to increased CSF reabsorption and will suppress CSF production as a result of reduced choroid plexus perfusion. Patients with cerebral atrophy and increased CSF volume will exhibit enhanced buffering capacity, and therefore tolerate greater changes in brain or blood volume without significant increases in ICP. Conversely, if CSF outflow is blocked (for example in subarachnoid haemorrhage or secondary to compression along the CSF flow pathway), then buffering capacity is dramatically reduced.

The venous blood compartment offers a secondary buffer to rising ICP with external compression of the cortical and bridging veins extruding blood extracranially to reduce venous volume. Arterial compliance is lower since the muscular walls are under active control and thus arterial blood volume is only affected at a late stage. Once this occurs, it represents a haemodynamic shift that if left unchecked will lead to parenchymal ischaemia. These buffering systems can be demonstrated schematically as shown in Figure 4.2.

MRI abnormalities seen in intracranial hypertension include meningeal enhancement, engorgement of cerebral venous sinuses, and prominence of the spinal epidural venous plexus demonstrating some of these compensatory mechanisms.

Within the clinical context, it is widely recognized that the degree to which ICP is affected by a change in volume will depend on the rate of that change. Slow growing tumours such as meningiomas outside eloquent areas of the brain may present at a late stage, after fully exploiting compensatory mechanisms. In this situation, at the time of presentation, the brain may already exist within a critical region of the pressure–volume curve but the patient may have experienced few symptoms of raised ICP. In contrast to this, acutely developing space occupying lesions such as haematoma may cause a more significant increase in ICP whilst occupying a lesser volume.

Assessing Compliance

The traditional method for assessing intracranial compliance involved injecting a bolus injection of saline into the CSF. Newer methods include ICP monitoring devices which include a distensible balloon, phase-coded MRI imaging, and transcranial Doppler measurement. In clinical practice, other methods such as CO_2 reactivity may also be useful.

Intracranial Pressure Waveforms

The normal ICP waveform has three components and can provide clinically significant information about the state of intracranial compliance.

In a compliant brain, the normal ICP waveform consists of three upstrokes (P1, P2, and P3) of decreasing magnitude (Figure 4.3). As ICP increases and intracranial compliance decreases, there is an increase in the magnitude of P2.

- P1 (percussion wave) represents arterial pulsation and corresponds with the delivery of blood to the intracranial compartment. It is sharply peaked and relatively consistent in amplitude.
- P2 (tidal wave) is a reflexive wave; as the effects of P1 are transmitted back through the intracranial compartment, the size of this wave represents the degree of intracranial compliance. As ICP increases and intracranial compliance decreases, there is less absorption of P1 and the magnitude of P2 increases. When P2 is greater than P1 this serves as an indicator of increasing ICP.
- P3 (dicrotic wave) probably represents aortic valve closure in a close resemblance to the arterial pressure waveform. Any waves seen following P3 represent retrograde venous pulsation.

The classic description by Lundberg in 1960[7] refers to three periodic wave patterns of ventricular pressure fluctuations in human beings, namely:

- Lundberg A waves or 'plateau waves' describe a steep increase in ICP usually with amplitude of >50 mmHg lasting for 5–10 minutes. They are always pathological and represent a significant degree of intracranial hypertension and therefore are frequently associated with poor outcome.[8]
- Lundberg B waves are rhythmic oscillations of ICP occurring at a frequency of 0.5–2 Hz and lower amplitude of around 20 mmHg and are associated with instability in ICP.
- Lundberg C waves are more rapid oscillations at a frequency of 4–8 Hz with low amplitude and have

been documented in healthy subjects. The clinical significance of these waves is unclear but it is most likely that they represent an interaction between the cardiac and respiratory cycles.

Lundberg waves A and B can be seen in Figure 4.4.

The Intracranial Pressure–Volume Relationship

In a pure model of the pressure–volume relationship of an incompressible substance in a fixed volume container, there is a linear relationship between the two. However, despite the rigid container formed by the skull and dura, and relatively incompressible contents, the pressure-volume relationship of the intracranial cavity does not follow this model since it includes more than one parameter within a system that exhibits dynamic compensatory capacity.[9] The curve this produces (Figure 4.5) was characterized by Langfitt et al. in 1965[10] and may be described in four phases.

When the intracranial volume is low (A), capacity for compensation is high and thus the system maintains good compliance, and will tolerate an increase in volume without an increase in pressure. The curve in this region is relatively flat. As the total intracranial volume increases, the compensatory mechanisms become more limited and compliance falls such that a modest increase in volume leads to a significant increase in pressure at the inflection point of the curve (B). This tends to occur around an ICP of 20–25 mmHg. Once compensatory mechanisms have been exhausted a point is reached where any further increase in volume leads to an exponential increase in pressure (C). Eventually, the ICP reaches a point where it approximates to MAP and CPP is critically low. Beyond this point, any further increase leads to a collapse of the cerebral arterial bed and the curve reaches a final plateau (D).

Cerebral Perfusion Pressure

For the majority of organs in the human body, the outflow or zero pressure determining blood flow is coupled to atmospheric pressure. The brain is unusual in this regard, the outflow pressure determining perfusion pressure is not related to atmospheric pressure, but rather to the venous pressure in the bridging veins which can be approximated to ICP.

$$CPP = MAP - mean\ ICP$$

Whilst ICP measurement in itself has not been proven to alter the outcome following severe head injury, studies have shown both a reduction in mortality following the introduction of protocols aimed at reducing ICP and a lower mortality in those patients in whom ICP control was achieved compared to those in whom it was not.[11,12] Further studies have shown that patients who die have significantly low CPP.[13] Control of ICP and maintenance of CPP are therefore widely accepted treatment targets in many head injury management algorithms.[14,15]

CONCLUSIONS

Intracranial pressure is the pressure within the cranial cavity or skull and thus is determined by the volume of its contents. As ICP increases, CPP determined by the MAP and ICP may become compromised. If adequate perfusion pressure is not maintained, brain tissue ischaemia may develop.

REFERENCES

1. Rowland LP, Fink ME, Rubin L. *Principles of Neural Science*. 3rd ed. Leonard B, editor. Cerebrospinal fluid: blood-brain barrier, brain edema and hydrocephalus. New York: Elsevier; 1991, 1050–3.
2. Monro A. *Observations on the Structure and Functions of the Nervous System*. London: Creech and Johnson; 1783.
3. Kelly G. Appearances observed in the dissection of two individuals; death from cold and congestion of the brain. *Transcripts Medical-Surgical Society of Edinburgh* 1824;1(84).
4. Burrows G. *On Disorders of the Cerebral Circulation and on the Connection between Affections of the Brain and Diseases of the Heart*. Lea, Blanchard, editors. Philadelphia: Longman, Brown, Green, and Longmans; 1846.
5. Cushing H. Some experimental and clinical observations concerning states of increased intracranial tension. *The American Journal of the Medical Sciences* 1902;124(3): 375–4003.
6. Hamer J, Alberti E, Hoyer S, Wiedemann K. Influence of systemic and cerebral vascular factors on the cerebrospinal fluid pulse waves. *Journal of Neurosurgery* 1977;46(1): 36–45.
7. Lundberg N. Continuous recording and control of ventricular fluid pressure in neurosurgical practice. *Acta Psychiatrica Scandinavica Supplementum* 1962;21(3):489.
8. Moss E, Gibson JS, Mcdowall DG, Gibson RM. Intensive management of severe head injuries. *Anaesthesia* 1983; 38(3):214–25.
9. Löfgren J, Essen C von, Zwetnow NN. The pressure-volume curve of the cerebrospinal fluid space in dogs. *Acta Neurologica Scandinavica* 1973;49(4):557–74.
10. Langfitt TW, Weinstein JD, Kassell NF. Cerebral vasomotor paralysis produced by intracranial hypertension. *Neurology* 1965;15(7):622.
11. Lang E, Chestnut R. Intracranial pressure and cerebral perfusion pressure in severe head injury. *New Horizons* 1995;3:400–9.
12. Marchall LF, Gautille T, Klauber MR, et al. The outcome of severe closed head injury. *Journal of Neurosurgery* 1991;75(1S):S28–36.
13. Marmarou A, Anderson R, Ward L, Choi SC, Young HF. Impact of ICP stability and hypotension on outcome in patients with severe head trauma. *Journal of Neurosurgery* 1991;75(1S):S59–66.
14. Rosner MJ, Daughton S. Cerebral perfusion pressure management in head injury. *The Journal of Trauma: Injury, Infection, and Critical Care* 1990;30(8):933–41.
15. Foundation BT. American Association of Neurological Surgeons, Congress of Neurological Surgeons. Management and prognosis of severe traumatic brain injury. 3rd ed. United States: *Journal of Neurotrauma* 2007.

5

Postoperative Care of the Neurosurgical Patient

C. Gray, A. M. Benson, E. Farag, and A. K. Khanna

ABSTRACT

Postoperative monitoring of the neurosurgical patient in the intensive care unit (ICU) can be complex and challenging for even the most seasoned clinician. This is because the relationship between systemic and neurological homeostasis is complex. The aim of the neurointensivist is to prevent and detect neurological decline and maintain systemic homeostasis. This chapter provides a comprehensive review of the tenets of essential monitoring for the post-neurosurgical patient. The areas covered include basic respiratory and haemodynamic monitoring, glycaemic control, and electrolyte balance. The chapter also covers specific considerations of bedside neurological examination, brain oxygenation and intracranial pressure monitoring, electroencephalogram and neuroimaging in these patients. A review of the major post-neurosurgical complications in the ICU is also provided.

KEYWORDS

Neurosurgical; monitoring; postoperative monitoring; intensive care unit (ICU); complications.

INTRODUCTION

Postoperative neurosurgical patients are at risk of developing complications like any other postoperative surgical patient. Close systemic and neuromonitoring is useful in determining patients who are at risk of rapid clinical deterioration, as timely detection is paramount for favourable patient outcomes. The decision as to which monitors are to be used should be based on patient presentation and clinical judgement. Optimally, postoperative care should occur by experienced nursing and medical staff familiar with various monitoring modalities utilized during the postoperative period.

Postoperative Monitoring and the Need for Intensive Care Unit Admission

The primary aim of postoperative neurosurgical care is to detect and prevent neurological decline while supporting neurological and systemic homeostasis. The failure of a patient to regain preoperative status can be due to a myriad of factors, including anaesthetic, surgical, or disease-related complications. Many neurosurgical cases may not require lengthy postoperative observation; however, complicating factors such as cerebral oedema, intracranial haemorrhage, seizures, or the presence of comorbid conditions may dictate the need for intensive care.[1,2]

There is little direct evidence to support the minimum monitoring standards after specific neurosurgical procedures. Postoperative neurosurgical patients usually have at least one, if not a combination of the following abnormalities: altered consciousness, pulmonary insufficiency or loss of protective airway reflexes, risk of rapid neurological deterioration, or cardiovascular instability. Additionally, procedure length and complexity may dictate the need for close observation and frequent monitoring. Despite this agreement, there are currently no conclusive studies defining absolute criteria for ICU admission.[1,2]

As in any critical care setting, basic monitoring such as electrocardiography (ECG), pulse oximetry, and blood pressure should be used for a critically ill neurosurgical patient. In many institutions, 'multimodality monitoring', or the combined use of multiple monitors is the standard. The use of multiple tools is predicated upon the insensitivity of a clinical neurological examination to detect disease progression in a patient population where the clinical features of disease may be confounded by the effects of sedation and analgesia, or in deeply comatose patients with minimum neurological response.[1–3]

In common with all postsurgical care, airway management, safe weaning of ventilator support, control of haemodynamics, fluid and electrolyte balance, and adequate analgesia are imperative for successful neurosurgical postoperative care. Attention to each of these is critical as systemic derangements can have a profound effect on neurological outcome. Furthermore, invasive monitoring, specific to neurosurgical procedures, such as intracranial pressure (ICP) monitoring and the possible presence of lumbar drains requires specific expertise and training often only found in the ICU.[1,2]

The intensity of postoperative monitoring should be determined by the complexity of the surgical procedure and patient comorbidities. It is imperative to recognize that the information provided by one single monitor will not influence the outcome. Instead, it is how the information provided is integrated and interpreted into clinical decision-making, along with how the patient is treated, that will ultimately influence outcomes.[1,2]

POSTOPERATIVE MONITORING AND MANAGEMENT

Respiratory Monitoring and Pulmonary Complications

Hypoxia and hypercarbia have been shown to be important secondary insults in neurosurgical patients. Morbidity and mortality due to prolonged hypoxia (defined as PaO_2 <60 mmHg) is almost 50%. The arterial partial pressure of carbon dioxide ($PaCO_2$) is an important determinant of cerebral blood flow (CBF) and cerebral perfusion pressure (CPP). Both hypoxia and hypercapnia will cause cerebral vasodilation and patients with low intracranial compliance are at risk of increased ICP. As such, in addition to monitoring oxygenation, monitoring of $PaCO_2$ is generally practiced in both spontaneously breathing and mechanically ventilated patients. The change in $PaCO_2$ can be directly determined with arterial blood gas analysis or estimated with end-tidal CO_2 ($ETCO_2$).[4,5]

Although evidence is lacking, continuous intra-arterial blood pressure monitoring is common practice not only because of the need for accurate blood pressure control, but also to prevent devastating derangements in cerebral perfusion and oxygenation. There is controversy regarding the usefulness of $ETCO_2$ as a surrogate for $PaCO_2$, as there is considerable variability between the two values, as well as inconsistent $PaCO_2$–$ETCO_2$ gradient over time. It is therefore recommended that $PaCO_2$ should be monitored whenever possible.[5]

It is important to note that airway and pulmonary complications in neurosurgical patients not only increase the length of hospital stay, but also long-term morbidity.[6] In the immediate postoperative period, neurosurgical patients may need continued mechanical ventilation. Many patients may require re-intubation in the immediate postoperative period for a plethora of reasons, including but not limited to, cranial nerve dysfunction, altered airway patency, brainstem compression from oedema, haematoma or acute obstructive hydrocephalus, or mechanical airway obstruction due to oedema secondary to positioning or length of surgery. Additional factors associated with increased re-intubation risk include age above 65 years, presence of chronic obstructive pulmonary disease, higher American Society of Anesthesiologists (ASA) physical status classification, operative time greater than 3 hours, preoperative renal failure, and quadriplegia.[6]

Due to prolonged immobilization, neurosurgical patients are at high risk for development of deep vein thrombosis (DVT) or pulmonary embolism (PE). Current evidence suggests early implementation of subcutaneous heparin, although some neurosurgeons may have reservations starting early postoperative anticoagulation. As such, sequential compression devices should be considered for all patients, as these devices decrease the incidence of DVT. Optimally, it is suggested that a combination therapy consisting of both heparin and sequential compression devices be used; however, for patients at high risk for anticoagulation, sequential Doppler ultrasound for deep vein thrombosis should be considered.[7]

Postoperative neurosurgical patients are also at risk for development of neurogenic pulmonary oedema (NPE), a condition associated with high morbidity resulting in hypoxaemia, characterized by pulmonary vascular congestion, protein-rich alveolar fluid, and intra-alveolar haemorrhage. While many pathophysiological mechanisms have been proposed, the process is not well understood. Neurogenic pulmonary oedema manifests as tachycardia, tachypnea, and hypoxaemia, typically with pulmonary infiltrates on chest radiography. It may result after traumatic brain or spinal cord injury, or after other insults such as intracranial haemorrhage, intracranial hypertension, or seizure. Neurogenic pulmonary oedema is usually self-limited, and treatment is supportive, including aggressive diuresis, and maintenance of haemodynamics by using inotropes and vasopressors if warranted. Prophylaxis has not been proven, although it has been suggested that strict haemodynamic control and the blunting of catecholamine response may be beneficial in NPE prevention.[8]

Haemodynamic Monitoring and Blood Pressure Control

Hypotension, hypertension, and hypoxia are frequent insults found to be detrimental in patients with traumatic brain injury (TBI), and it is reasonable to assume that the same can be applied to postoperative neurosurgical patients. Postoperative derangements in haemodynamic status can be detected using continuous ECG and blood pressure monitoring.[4,6]

There is usually no need for invasive haemodynamic monitors such as pulmonary artery catheters or cardiac output monitors, unless they are needed to monitor pre-existing cardiac comorbidities or neurogenic pulmonary oedema. However, continuous intra-arterial blood pressure monitoring has become common as short periods of hypotension may compromise cerebral perfusion and oxygenation.[4]

Postoperative neurosurgical patients often exhibit labile blood pressure, which may result from a myriad of neurogenic, cardiogenic, or systemic causes. Systemic hypotension is a known cause of secondary neurologic injury, and if encountered, should be aggressively treated. In the immediate postoperative period, hypovolaemia largely contributes to the development of hypotension. Normovolaemia can be restored by using either isotonic or hypertonic intravenous fluids. Fluid administration can facilitate the return of adequate blood pressure, thereby reducing the risk of ischaemia and additional neurologic damage. Vasopressor medications such as norepinephrine, phenylephrine, or dopamine may be required with choice of therapy depending on the clinical circumstance and patient comorbidities.[9]

Hypertension is also common in neurosurgical patients, particularly during emergence from general anaesthesia and in the early postoperative period. The common causes of postoperative hypertension include surgical stress response, pain, central neurogenic effects either from direct injury or neurohumoral stimulation of the brainstem and/or carotid baroreceptors and increased ICP provoking a Cushing's reflex, or pre-existing hypertensive disease.[9,10]

Blood pressure must be managed in a manner that allows adequate perfusion to critical organs such as the brain and heart; however, hypertension cannot go uncontrolled

as there is an association between hypertension and intracranial haemorrhage.[9,10] Therefore, the underlying cause of hypertension should be determined and treated immediately.

Careful blood pressure regulation can be achieved with the use of any number of antihypertensive medications, including beta blockers (esmolol and labetalol), calcium channel blockers (nicardipine), angiotensin converting enzyme inhibitors (enalaprilat), or hydralazine. Although many antihypertensive medications are available, it is important to avoid nitroglycerine and sodium nitroprusside, which cause cerebral vasodilation and may increase ICP and/or disrupt cerebrovascular autoregulation.[9]

Currently, there are no absolute thresholds for blood pressure management; instead, blood pressure control depends on the individual patient, surgical procedure, comorbid conditions, and clinical situation.

Fluid, Sodium, and Glucose Management

Fluid and electrolyte homeostasis are crucial for the successful care of postoperative neurosurgical patients. Perioperative fluid management in a neurosurgical patient is challenging because of the potential presence of increased ICP, surgical bleeding, and derangements associated with neurologic injury. Disturbances in fluid and electrolyte balance may occur secondary to underlying neurological disease processes or it may be iatrogenic.[1,11]

The goal of fluid management in the postoperative period is not only to restore intravascular volume, but also to minimize the impact of fluid resuscitation on the development or exacerbation of cerebral oedema. Replacement of fluids must be done judiciously using isotonic or hypertonic fluids as administration of hypo-osmolar fluids and dextrose containing solutions cause increased brain water content and ICP. As a result, hypoosmolar fluids and dextrose containing solutions should be avoided unless dextrose is needed to treat hypoglycaemia.[12]

Depending on the clinical situation, a variety of intravenous fluids can be administered, including crystalloid, colloid, hypertonic saline, or blood products. The exception is in patients with TBI.[13] The Saline versus Albumin Fluid Evaluation (SAFE) trial compared albumin versus saline for fluid resuscitation in TBI patients. It was noted that albumin was associated with a 33.2% mortality compared to 20.4% mortality with saline.[14]

Impairment of the blood–brain barrier is inevitable following intracranial surgery. In this situation, water and electrolyte derangements may cause rapid disorientation, alterations in consciousness (as measured by the Glasgow Coma Scale [GCS]), or induce seizures. This is particularly evident with disorders of sodium balance. Disturbances in sodium are both common, and extremely deleterious, as the main determinant of movement across the blood–brain barrier is the osmotic pressure gradient produced by osmotically active solutes, including plasma sodium. When hypo- or hyper-natraemia occurs, measurement of urinary sodium, serum and urine osmolarity, and intervascular volume status should be undertaken in an effort to determine the cause and direct appropriate treatment.[11]

Similarly, glucose intolerance and hyperglycaemia are also frequent. Postoperative hyperglycaemia is expected to be a part of surgical stress response; however, it has been shown to be associated with increased morbidity and mortality in patients with spinal cord injury, subarachnoid haemorrhage, TBI, and stroke. While hyperglycaemia should be avoided, aggressive insulin protocols have not shown improvement in neurological outcomes. The Normoglycemia in Intensive Care Evaluation and Surviving Using Glucose Algorithm Regulation (NICE–SUGAR) trial studied aggressive insulin therapy versus regimens controlling glucose to less than 180 mg/dL in a mixed cohort of critically ill patients. The conclusion was that there is no benefit, but in fact, increased mortality associated with the use of intensive insulin therapy.[15]

Temperature Control

Thermoregulation is a highly complex process dependent on positive and negative feedback from nearly every tissue in the body. The hypothalamus and skin have a major role in thermal regulation and these physiologic response mechanisms have been well described.[2,16]

Intraoperative thermal dysregulation results in hypothermia as anaesthetics modulate thermoregulatory thresholds and influence responses. Cold surroundings, exposed body surfaces, cold intravenous fluid administration, and mechanical ventilation contribute to the difficulty in temperature maintenance in the operating theatre and later. Perioperative hypothermia is nearly ubiquitous with a reported incidence as high as 70%.[16]

Postoperatively, neurosurgical patients are at increased risk of systemic complications associated with low temperature such as impaired coagulation, changes in drug metabolism, myocardial events, and postoperative shivering. Postoperative shivering is not only a source of discomfort for patients but can have additional consequences as it increases ICP and intraocular pressure. It also increases systemic metabolic rate and oxygen consumption by as much as 200%.[2,16]

The management of hypothermia includes core temperature monitoring and active re-warming, including the use of forced warm air devices. Raising ambient temperature, cutaneous warming, and administration of warm intravenous fluids also helps restore normothermia. Meperidine is an effective pharmacological treatment for postoperative shivering. Other proposed medications for the treatment of shivering include clonidine, tramadol, physostigmine, and magnesium sulphate.[2,16,17]

The decrease in metabolic rate and oxygen demand induced by hypothermia has led to the hypothesis that hypothermia may be beneficial for neuroprotection and improvement in neurological outcomes. A variety of studies have been conducted in animals demonstrating the benefits of mild hypothermia; however, in human beings, the only proven benefit of hypothermia on neurological outcomes is following cardiac arrest secondary to ventricular tachycardia or fibrillation.[17]

Hyperthermia occurs less frequently intraoperatively, but can pose a problem during the postoperative course. Hyperthermia is not without consequence, and in patients with neurological disease even a slight elevation in brain temperature can be deleterious. Both cerebral blood flow and cerebral metabolic rate increase in the presence of fever. Additionally, hyperthermia causes changes in membrane stability, enzyme function, neurotransmitter release, disruption of the blood-brain barrier, cerebral oedema, and epileptiform activity. Hyperpyrexia is an independent risk factor for worse outcomes in TBI, subarachnoid haemorrhage, and stroke.[18]

In an effort to minimize neurological damage and improve outcomes, the underlying cause of hyperthermia should be determined and treatment initiated. There is no ideal treatment method; either physical cooling or pharmacological treatments are acceptable. Physical cooling can be complicated by patient discomfort as well as an elevation in the cerebral metabolic rate. The risk–benefit profile of pharmacological treatment has not been clearly established.[2,18]

Neuromonitoring

Any postoperative neurosurgical patient is at risk of developing complications. Systemic and neuromonitoring are used to facilitate the quick detection of neurological deterioration as a means to expedite treatment and minimize impact on outcomes.

Serial Clinical Neurologic Examination

Repeated clinical examination is the foundation of neurological monitoring in the postoperative setting, as clinical deterioration is usually the first sign of developing complications. Sedation, analgesics such as opioid medications, and neuromuscular blockade remain confounders for any clinical scale of consciousness, but a brief neurological assessment is usually sufficient to establish baseline neurological function and detect changes. Standardized scoring systems have been developed to facilitate repeated, consistent, quantitative reporting of neurological status. In neurosurgical patients, the two most useful scores are the GCS and the more recent Full Outline of Unresponsiveness (FOUR) score.[7,5,19]

Originally developed as a prognostic tool for patients with brain injury, the GCS is now also frequently utilized to estimate the level of consciousness in critically ill patients and has been used as a predictor of successful extubation in neurosurgical patients. However, the GCS is unable to detect subtle neurological changes, especially since the scale is confounded by endotracheal intubation and does not consider brainstem reflexes.[1,5]

The FOUR score is determined from four components: eye response, motor response, brainstem reflexes, and respiration. While it is more difficult to perform than the GCS, it has prognostic significance in a range of neurological conditions and provides better discrimination than the GCS in deeply comatose patients. The FOUR score has been demonstrated to have a higher inter-rater reliability than GCS, but experience with this novel score remains limited. Current recommendations suggest that both the GCS and FOUR score provide reliable measures of neurological state and should be routinely used to plot trends in overall clinical progress.[5,19]

Assessment for delirium is also recommended in neurocritical care patients. The Confusion Assessment Method for the ICU (CAM-ICU) and the Intensive Care Delirium Screening Checklist (ICDSC) are two validated tools utilized for delirium assessment. The ICDSC may be preferred as the score does not include changes in wakefulness and attention, signs that may be attributed to recent sedative or pain medications. The diagnosis of delirium in a neurocritical care patient may represent progression of an underlying disease or surgical complication, and prompt evaluation for a new neurological deficit should be done.[1]

Intracranial Pressure Monitoring

Intracranial pressure is defined as the pressure within the cranial vault relative to the ambient atmospheric pressure. When compensatory mechanisms which control ICP such as changes in cerebrospinal fluid (CSF) dynamics, CBF, and cerebral blood volume are exhausted, the ICP begins to increase. Normally, resting ICP is less than 10 mmHg. The absolute threshold that defines intracranial hypertension is uncertain, but generally an ICP greater than 20–25 mmHg is considered abnormal, although both higher and lower thresholds have been described.[1,5]

Several devices are used to measure ICP. Intraparenchymal monitors or intraventricular catheters are considered to be the most accurate and reliable. In addition to providing direct ICP measurement, intraventricular catheters also allow for the drainage of CSF, and as a result are the preferred modality for ICP measurement in patients with hydrocephalus. The duration of ICP measurement varies by clinical context. However, it is important to understand that one disadvantage is an increase in infection risk with longer duration of use.[5]

Current recommendations support the use of ICP monitoring in patients who are at risk of intracranial hypertension. Monitoring of ICP is routinely used as a method to direct both medical and surgical therapy. Increased ICP, especially refractory to treatment is a well-known negative predictive factor, specifically for mortality.[1]

Intracranial pressure monitoring is well established and has an excellent safety profile, but there are complications associated with its use. Two such major complications are ventriculitis and haemorrhage. Ventriculitis occurs in up to 10% of cases and the duration of catheter placement correlates with increased risk of CSF infection. Risk factors for infection include intraventricular and subarachnoid haemorrhage, cranial fracture with CSF leak, craniotomy, systemic infection, as well as catheter manipulation, leak, and drainage. Prophylactic antibiotic treatment has not been shown to reduce infection risk and the most effective method to reduce ventriculitis is the aseptic technique during catheter insertion.[5,20]

Haemorrhage is the second major complication of ICP catheter placement. Patients with coagulopathies are at greatest risk, although the overall risk remains low at only 1–2%. Nevertheless, haemorrhage can be a devastating complication that requires prompt recognition and treatment. If it is small, the haemorrhage can simply be observed, but a large haematoma will require surgical evacuation.[5]

Brain Oxygenation and Cerebral Blood Flow Monitoring

In addition to ICP catheters, invasive neuromonitoring also includes jugular venous and intraparenchymal catheters used to determine cerebral oxygenation. Depending on the circumstances, these monitors may be placed at any point in the perioperative period.

Cerebral oxygenation can be measured locally with the use of an intraparenchymal pO_2 catheter. The catheter measures pO_2 over a small surface area providing an average brain tissue oxygenation ($PbtO_2$) value for the brain around the catheter tip. When placed in normal brain tissue, $PbtO_2$ values represent global brain oxygenation. Conversely, when the catheter is placed in an injured area, the $PbtO_2$ values reflect only local brain oxygenation.[5]

Jugular venous oxygen saturation ($SjvO_2$) catheters can be percutaneously placed with the tip positioned in the jugular bulb. Differences may exist in oxygen saturation values between the internal jugular bulbs due to mixing of cerebral venous blood before the division of the sagittal sinus. Therefore, the dominant internal jugular vein should be determined and cannulated.[5]

Jugular venous oxygen saturation and brain tissue oxygenation are measures of cerebral oxygenation. Since these measures give an indication of CBF relative to cerebral metabolic requirements, $SjvO_2$ or $PbtO_2$ may be used as surrogates for cerebral perfusion. If CBF is appropriate for the brain's metabolic requirement, brain tissue oxygenation will be normal, whereas in the case of brain hypoperfusion, brain oxygenation will be reduced.[5,21]

The complications associated with $PbtO_2$ and $SjvO_2$ monitoring are similar to that of ICP monitoring, including mainly infection and haemorrhage. As these catheters tend to be smaller than the ICP catheter, the risk of haemorrhage is low. There is a risk of carotid puncture or pneumothorax when placing a jugular venous catheter, but these complications can be reduced by using ultrasound. Infection prevention is also similar to that of ICP catheters. Careful attention should be paid to the aseptic technique during placement and the duration of monitoring should be limited.[5]

Electroencephalogram

The overall incidence of seizures in postoperative neurosurgical patients is approximately 17%. Patients are particularly at high risk after TBI, evacuation of chronic subdural haematoma, subarachnoid haemorrhage, surgical procedures for abscess, intracerebral haemorrhage, and acute ischaemic stroke.[5]

Electroencephalogram supplies information about the brain's electrical activity with the goal of identifying changes in brain function that may not be apparent with clinical examination such as ischaemia or non-convulsive seizures. According to the American Clinical Neurophysiology Society consensus recommendations, continuous EEG monitoring is recommended over routine EEG monitoring to identify non-convulsive seizure in patients with persistently abnormal mental status, those with acute supratentorial brain injury, and patients with seizure risk who require pharmacological muscle relaxation.[1,5,22]

No prospective studies have demonstrated that the treatment of EEG identified neurological changes improves outcome, but there is increasing evidence that secondary neurological injuries such as seizure and ischaemia can worsen outcome. Specifically, seizure duration and delay of diagnosis are both associated with increased mortality.[5]

The use of bispectral index score (BIS) measurements has been suggested as a tool for EEG quantification. Several studies have expressed concern regarding this concept as there is wide inter- and intra-individual variability and monitor sensitivity to electrical interference. Currently, the routine use of BIS is not advised.[1]

Neuroimaging

Neuroimaging, in the strict sense, is not a monitor, but can be helpful in the setting of acute clinical deterioration to guide both diagnosis and therapy.

The risk of transporting patients to scanners is well documented, thus the benefit of information garnered from imaging must justify taking the risk involved not only in travel but also in radiation and contrast exposure. Computed tomography (CT) scanning is a standard examination procedure for patients with new focal neurologic signs or a decreased level of consciousness. Non-contrast CT is used predominantly to evaluate for acute intracranial pathology such as haemorrhage, although this technique has low sensitivity for detecting acute ischaemia. Magnetic resonance imaging (MRI) is useful in the early detection of ischaemia and allows for detailed imaging of the brain parenchyma and underlying pathology when compared to CT. There is no difference between CT and MRI imaging modalities in the diagnosis of acute cerebral haemorrhage.[5]

Positron emission tomography (PET) is the only imaging modality that provides cerebral blood flow measurements as well as measurements of cerebral oxygen and glucose metabolism.[20] Currently, there are no accepted indications for postoperative PET imaging.

POSTOPERATIVE COMPLICATIONS

Infectious Complications

The reported incidence of hospital acquired infections in the neuro-ICU is 20%–30%.[20,22] Though neurointensive care patients are associated with increased length of hospital stay, morbidity, and mortality, they are particularly susceptible to infections due to catheter and line placement, prolonged mechanical ventilation, neurosurgical procedures, acquired immune suppression secondary to steroid and/or barbiturate use, and organic brain injury.[22]

Ventilator-Associated Pneumonia

Ventilator-associated pneumonia (VAP) is defined as pneumonia that develops 48–72 hours after endotracheal intubation with an estimated prevalence of 9%–27%. Being associated with an increased duration of mechanical ventilation, increased length of ICU stay, and increased healthcare cost, VAP is the most commonly reported nosocomial infection in mechanically ventilated patients and accounts for approximately 50% of all antibiotics administered in the ICU.[20]

The causative organism often depends on the duration of mechanical ventilation. Early-onset VAP or pneumonia occurring within the first four days is usually caused by *Haemophilus influenzae*, *Streptococcus pneumoniae*, and methicillin-sensitive *Staphylococcus aureus*. After four days of endotracheal intubation, the causative pathogens are most likely multidrug-resistant organisms such as *Pseudomonas aeruginosa*, Acinetobacter, and methicillin-resistant *S. aureus* (MRSA).[20]

If there is high clinical suspicion for VAP, antibiotics should be administered empirically, as delayed antimicrobial therapy is associated with increased mortality. Definitive diagnosis can be confirmed or dismissed once the cultures return, and culture results should ultimately guide continued antibiotic therapy. Clinical response guides the duration of therapy with treatment ranging from 8–14 days.[20]

Given the high prevalence of VAP, prevention has gained increasing importance. Care bundles have been designed based upon measures that have been shown to decrease VAP. These include oral care with chlorhexidine, elevation of the head of bed to more than 30 degrees, use of subglottic suction endotracheal tubes, avoidance of re-intubation, minimization of transport out of the ICU, and the use of daily weaning trials to facilitate early extubation.[20]

Bacteraemia

Bacteraemia is the second most common hospital acquired infection in neurological ICU, with most infections associated with indwelling central venous catheters. The most frequent pathogens associated with catheter-related bacteraemia are *Staphylococcus epidermidis*, *S. aureus*,

and Enterococcus. According to the Infectious Diseases Society of America (IDSA) guidelines, a blood infection in the presence of a central venous catheter without another apparent source should be considered as catheter-related bacteraemia.[20]

Often antimicrobial therapy is initiated empirically with the choice of antibiotic depending on the severity of disease, risk factors for infection, and the likely pathogens associated with the device. It should be noted that antibiotic treatment is not recommended in situations involving positive cultures from a removed catheter but also not accompanied by clinical signs of infection, positive device cultures with negative peripheral blood cultures, and phlebitis in the absence of infection.[20]

In the setting of confirmed catheter-related bacteraemia, short- and long-term catheters should be removed, especially when the bacteraemia is associated with haemodynamic instability or sepsis, suppurative thrombophlebitis or endocarditis.[20]

Aseptic insertion technique is paramount for the prevention of catheter-related infection.[20]

Urinary Tract Infections

Urinary tract infections (UTIs) account for 22%–36% of all hospital acquired infections, with the prevalence in the ICU ranging between 8%–21%. While the majority (80%) of UTIs are attributable to indwelling urethral catheters, other risk factors include old age, female gender, severe underlying illness, diabetes mellitus, and bacterial colonization of the drainage system.

Most ICU-acquired catheter-associated UTIs (CAUTI) are monomicrobial, with *E. coli*, *P. aeruginosa*, and Enterococcus being the predominant pathogens. Less than 25% of hospitalized patients with catheter-associated bacteriuria develop symptoms of UTI.[20]

Due to the broad spectrum of infective organisms and the increased likelihood of antimicrobial resistance, a urine culture should be obtained prior to the initiation of treatment. Antimicrobial treatment should be tailored to the individual causative organism based on susceptibility data. Asymptomatic bacteriuria does not require treatment, and in fact, treatment should be avoided due to concerns of increasing antimicrobial resistance.[20]

More importantly, prevention is the key, and the most effective strategy to reduce the development of UTIs is to reduce the use of internal and external catheters. Indwelling catheters should be placed only when indicated and removed as quickly as possible.[20]

Ventriculitis

Bacterial ventriculitis (BV) is inflammation of the ventricular drainage system due to bacterial infection of the CSF. Usually, BV is observed in association with CSF shunts, and intracranial devices, such as external ventricular drainage (EVD) devices. Additional risk factors include the type of EVD, insertion technique, frequency of CSF sampling, and duration of placement, as infection risk significantly increases after five days.[22,20]

The most common pathogens responsible for CSF shunt and EVD infections are Gram-positive organisms found on the skin, such as *Staphylococcus epidermidis*, *S. aureus*, and *Propionibacterium acnes*. In TBI patients and following brain surgery, aerobic Gram-negative bacilli, including Pseudomonas are also common.[20,22]

Ventriculitis is diagnosed by both the presence of clinical symptoms and positive CSF analysis. Clinical symptoms include fever, decreased mental status, nuchal rigidity, seizure, and other signs of meningitis. A CSF analysis yields a positive Gram stain and culture, as well as increased protein, decreased glucose, and increased white blood cell count. It should be noted that a positive CSF culture in the absence of clinical signs is suggestive of contamination or colonization and does not require treatment.[20]

The diagnosis of ventriculitis can be difficult in patients who have a neurologic injury that causes inflammation and degeneration of the blood–brain barrier, as CSF may already contain blood leading to increased protein and white blood cells, as well as decreased glucose. The presence of a high lactate concentration can assist with diagnosis. In neurosurgical patients, current practice guidelines recommend the initiation of empiric antibiotics if the CSF lactate is >4.0 mmol/L, pending results of additional studies.[20]

Vancomycin and cefepime are antibiotics recommended for empiric treatment of ventriculitis post neurosurgery, as well as in the setting of CSF infection, head trauma, skull fracture, and penetrating trauma. Antibiotic therapy is guided by CSF Gram stain and culture and treatment response. The duration of therapy should be 10–14 days, but may be administered for a longer period if required. Additionally, any infected hardware should be removed, replaced, or externalized.[20]

The ventricles can serve as a source of persistent infection resulting in difficulty in ventriculitis treatment. Although specific indications remain controversial, there is a consensus that in some cases intraventricular antibiotic administration may be helpful. Particularly in post-neurosurgery patients, intraventricular antibiotics can lead to rapid CSF sterilization with a lower relapse rate. There is also agreement that intrathecal antibiotic administration is safe and effective for the treatment of infections caused by multi-drug resistant organisms. Typically, intrathecal antibiotics are indicated when there is a failure to achieve appropriate CSF drug concentrations or when CSF cultures are persistently positive, despite appropriate antibiotic dosing and source control.[20]

Post-Neurosurgery Wound Infection

Most neurosurgical operations are considered to be clean and therefore at the lowest risk for surgical site infection; however, the incidence of infection still ranges from 1%–8%, with the mortality rate as high as 14%.[20]

Superficial craniotomy wound site infections are of concern due to the potential for spread to the bone flap or meninges; however, spinal surgical infections are usually incisional or soft tissue infections. Intracranial infection is usually due to meningitis, subdural empyema, or brain abscess. Infection risk is increased with the presence of CSF leakage (usually associated with posterior fossa and transnasal surgical approaches), entry into the paranasal sinuses, and the use of external ventricular drainage devices. Additionally, patient characteristics such as extremes of age, diabetes mellitus, immunocompromise, malignancy, and the presence of remote site infection (such as pneumonia or UTIs) have all been associated with increased risk of surgical site infection.[20]

Postoperative central nervous system infection is a serious complication that requires immediate recognition and treatment. The recommended management of neurosurgical wounds involves surgical drainage for definitive source control in conjunction with antibiotic therapy. Empiric antibiotic therapy is directed by mechanism of infection, predisposing conditions, as well as antibiotic susceptibility and penetration. In most cases, the empiric antibiotic regimen will consist of vancomycin and a fourth generation cephalosporin, such as cefepime. Cultures from the infected wound site should be obtained, and ultimately, antibiotic treatment must be selected based on pathogen susceptibility. The duration of treatment is usually 3–6 weeks depending on the clinical response.[20]

Postoperative Nausea and Vomiting

Postoperative nausea and vomiting (PONV) are common following neurosurgical procedures. A major distressing and unpleasant postoperative symptom, the overall incidence of PONV is approximately 25%–30% for all surgeries, but increases to more than 50% after craniotomies. The high incidence of PONV in neurosurgical patients is attributable to the surgical site, especially procedures being performed in proximity to emetic centres in the brainstem or the structures responsible for equilibrium.[23]

While the exact aetiology of PONV remains unelucidated, research suggests multiple risk factors such as young age, female gender, nonsmoking status, and previous history of motion sickness or PONV as predisposing causes. Other risk factors include obesity, anxiety, dehydration, general vs regional anaesthesia, and use of opioids.[23,24]

In addition to causing patient distress, prolonged vomiting may cause further dehydration, acid-base imbalances, and electrolyte derangements. The physical act of retching and vomiting may result in an elevation in arterial, venous, and ICPs, potentially increasing the risk of neurologic dysfunction or intracranial haemorrhage. Non-intubated patients with depressed airway reflexes are at an increased aspiration risk.[25]

There is dearth of good quality evidence addressing the treatment of established PONV in neurosurgical patients and medications used to treat PONV are not without adverse side effects, especially when administered to the neurosurgical population. Clinicians must be careful in the selection of antiemetic medications, especially if there is an ongoing need for neurocognitive monitoring. In this context, sedating antiemetics such as anticholinergics and antihistamines are undesirable.[23,25]

Updated guidelines for the management of PONV recommend prophylaxis and treatment in an effort to improve patient satisfaction and reduce morbidity. No single medication class is fully effective in the prevention and treatment of PONV mainly because there is no medication that blocks all of the vomiting centre pathways. For this reason, combination therapy is suggested as a means of targeting the multiple receptors involved.[26]

The 5-HT3 (serotonin) receptor antagonists such as ondansetron; butyrophenones such as droperidol; and the corticosteroid dexamethasone have all been found to be equally effective in the prevention and treatment of nausea and vomiting, with each medication reducing the risk of PONV by about 25%. The 5-HT3-receptor antagonists are widely used, especially in the neurosurgical population, not only because of efficacy, but also because of lack of side effects such as somnolence and extrapyramidal symptoms. For these same reasons, droperidol has also been extensively used in postoperative neurosurgical patients. In 2001, the United States Food and Drug Administration inserted a black box warning against usage of 'large doses' of droperidol secondary to reports of QT prolongation leading to cardiac rhythm

changes. It should be noted, however, that droperidol doses used for the treatment of PONV have never been associated with fatal cardiac dysrhythmias.[23–25]

Dexamethasone is also effective as an antiemetic. The effect is attributed to the anti-inflammatory mechanism of action, which reduces the ascending impulses to the vomiting centre. While being efficacious, dexamethasone has a delayed effect, and therefore should be used only for PONV prevention and not as a rescue therapy.[23,24]

Propofol has also been found to be as effective as ondansetron and low doses can be used as a rescue treatment. Its antiemetic effect may be brief and the drug should be used with caution as the sedative effects can interfere with the neurological examination.[24]

Nonpharmacological measures such as acupuncture, acupressure, and electrical stimulation have been found to be effective in reducing nausea. Stimulation of the P6 point is thought to release endogenous β-endorphins in the CSF or stimulate a change in serotonin transmission activating serotonergic fibres. While likely not effective as a single treatment, this method may be used as a part of a multimodal approach to PONV management.[26]

Pain Control

Pain is considered the fifth vital sign, and regular evaluation and intervention is required to provide adequate pain relief. Effective postoperative pain management reduces the development of subsequent chronic pain disorders and helps to minimize other postoperative complications, particularly those related to immobility, such as development of deep vein thrombosis and atelectasis.[27]

Pain management in postoperative neurosurgical patients can be challenging. Many patients may already suffer from chronic pain making acute postoperative pain management more difficult. The mainstay of pain control is based on the World Health Organization (WHO) pain ladder. This advocates a stepwise approach to analgesia starting with non-opioid medications and escalation to stronger opioids, while also incorporating a variety of adjuvant medications. Severe surgical pain will frequently require the simultaneous initiation of all three steps of the pain ladder.[27]

Opioids remain the foundation of postoperative pain control; however, care must be taken in their administration as opioids may mask neurologic deterioration. When used in amounts just sufficient to relieve pain, opioid medications should not cause a significant increase in $PaCO_2$ and subsequent increase in ICP. Patient-controlled analgesic (PCA) devices can be used and have been found to be highly effective with minimal complication.[27]

Non-steroidal anti-inflammatory drugs (NSAIDs) are frequently utilized in a multimodal pain regimen; however, their use in neurosurgical patients remains controversial. Due to their inhibitory effect on platelet function, NSAIDs are believed to increase postoperative bleeding risk. This is of particular concern for postoperative craniotomy and spinal surgery patients; however, there is low risk of intracranial haematoma following elective supratentorial surgery in patients who have returned to their preoperative status within 6 hours after surgery. As a result, some institutions introduce the use of NSAIDs after 6 hours for any type of neurosurgical patient given that the surgery was elective, uncomplicated, and there is no preoperative history of a clotting disorder. Another concern surrounding the use of NSAID is the possible impairment of bone fusion, although there is no any direct evidence to support this in human beings.[27]

As a part of multimodal pain management, preventive analgesia is a concept that describes the reduction of postoperative pain through the use of a drug that has an effect longer than the duration of that agent. Ketamine, an N-methyl-D-aspartate (NMDA) receptor antagonist has been described as such a medication in the context of other non-neurological surgeries. However, concerns remain regarding the use of ketamine in the neurosurgical population because of its effect on increased ICP. There is some consensus that gabapentin provides a similar preventive analgesic benefit. Scalp blocks can also provide effective and lasting analgesia and may be considered for post-craniotomy pain.[27]

Overall, safe and effective pain relief is achievable in most patients, despite the diversity of neurosurgical procedures and diverse pain presentations.

POSTOPERATIVE SEIZURE PROPHYLAXIS AND TREATMENT

Every intracranial procedure is associated with a risk of seizure activity. Overall, the incidence of seizures in postoperative neurosurgical patients is around 15%–20%, with 77.5% of postoperative seizures occurring within the first 6 hours. After craniotomy, there are two major mechanisms that may contribute to the development of seizure: free radical generation, particularly from iron and thrombin from blood components that have leaked into tissue during surgery, and disturbance of the ion balance across cell membranes due to local ischaemia or hypoxia. In addition, systemic aetiologies, such as severe hypoxia/ischaemia, substance withdrawal, metabolic disturbances, and systemic infection may also contribute.[1,6,28]

Many neurosurgical patients will receive prophylactic anti-epileptic drugs (AEDs) on admission, and some at therapeutic doses, especially if the patient initially presented with seizure or there is a previous seizure history. Despite this, there is lack of evidence that AEDs prevent the onset of postoperative seizure. In patients with brain tumours, recent guidelines from the American Academy of Neurology recommend against prophylactic anti-seizure medications, and in patients who may have already been placed on such medications, it is preferable to taper off the anti-seizure medication over the week following surgical resection (6). For head trauma, the guidelines support treatment for up to one week to prevent early posttraumatic seizure. In the case of haemorrhagic stroke, the recommendation is to discontinue AEDs after one week in patients with subarachnoid haemorrhage when the cerebral aneurysm has been secured.[6,28]

If patients are already taking AEDs prior to surgery, these medications should continue to be administered in the perioperative period, including the day of surgery. In the immediate postoperative period, it is preferable to use AEDs available in parental forms due to erratic enteric absorption and the possibility of postoperative nausea and vomiting. There are several major AEDs available in an intravenous (IV) form. These IV medications should be used to substitute the oral form of the same medication or in the circumstance where an extra medication dose is needed to reach therapeutic concentrations.[28]

In patients experiencing a single postoperative generalized seizure, lorazepam, diazepam, or midazolam can be administered. Prophylaxis for a second seizure can be achieved by administration of home AEDs in patients with a history of epilepsy. Otherwise, if prior to surgery the patient has never experienced seizures phenytoin, valproate, or levetiracetam can be considered. If patients remain encephalopathic or with a new, unexplained focality in the neurological examination for longer than the expected postictal period, an urgent head CT and/or commencement of continuous EEG monitoring should be considered.[28]

In the event a patient has multiple seizures or enters into status epilepticus, the management is similar to that previously mentioned with a focus on airway, breathing, and circulation (ABC), and use of benzodiazepines as first-line AEDs. If management continues to be unsuccessful, general anaesthetics such as phenobarbital, pentobarbital or propofol may be used. These medications are especially preferred if the goal becomes burst-suppression. Pentobarbital is considered superior to phenobarbital due to shorter elimination half-life and in a meta-analysis, pentobarbital was determined to be more efficacious than either midazolam or propofol.[28]

CONCLUSIONS

The complexity of relationship between brain and other systems makes postoperative care of neurosurgical patients challenging. Proper homeostasis has to be maintained between various systems of the body and the brain. Monitoring is an essential and integral part of postoperative care for early detection of complications and timely intervention.

DISCLOSURE OF FUNDING

This study was supported by the Anaesthesiology Institute, Cleveland Clinic, Cleveland, Ohio, USA. None of the authors has a personal financial interest to report.

REFERENCES

1. Pritchard C, Radcliffe J. General principles of postoperative neurosurgical care. *Anesthesia and Intensive Care Medicine* 2014;15(6):267–72.

2. Suarez J. Outcome in neurocritical care: Advances in monitoring and treatment and effect of a specialized neurocritical care team. *Crit Care Med* 2006;34(Suppl 9): S232–38.

3. Le Roux P, Menon D, Citerio G, et al. Consensus summary statement of the international multidisciplinary consensus conference on multimodality monitoring in neurocritical care. *Intensive Care Med* 2014;40:1189–209.

4. Siegemund M, Steiner L. Postoperative care of the neurosurgical patient. *Curr Opin Anaesthesiol* 2015;28(5): 487–93.

5. Wijdicks EF, Bamlet WR, Maramattom BV, Manno EM, McClelland RL. Validation of a new coma scale: The FOUR score. *Ann Neurol* 2005;58(4):585–93.

6. Pasternak JJ, Lanier WL. Neuroanesthesiology update. *J Neurosurg Anesthesiol* 2016;28(2):93–122.

7. Collen JF, Jackson JL, Shorr AF, Moores LK. Prevention of venous thromboembolism in neurosurgery: a metaanalysis. *Chest* 2008;134(2):237–49.

8. Sedy J, Zicha J, Kunes J, Jendelova P, Sykova E. Mechanisms of neurogenic pulmonary edema development. *Physiol Res* 2008;57(4):499–506.

9. Schubert A. Cardiovascular therapy of neurosurgical patients. *Best Pract Res Clin Anaesthesiol* 2007;21(4): 483–96.

10. Basali A, Mascha EJ, Kalfas I, Schubert A. Relation between perioperative hypertension and intracranial hemorrhage after craniotomy. *Anesthesiology* 2000;93(1):48–54.

11. Fraser JF, Stieg PE. Hyponatremia in the neurosurgical patient: epidemiology, pathophysiology, diagnosis, and management. *Neurosurgery* 2006;59(2):222–9.

12. Jeremitsky E, Omert LA, Dunham CM, Wilberger J, Rodriguez A. The impact of hyperglycemia on patients with severe brain injury. *J Trauma* 2005;58(1):47–50.

13. Finfer S, Bellomo R, Boyce N, French J, Myburgh J, Norton R. A comparison of albumin and saline for fluid resuscitation in the intensive care unit. *N Engl J Med* 2004;350(22):2247–56.

14. SAFE Study Investigators; Australian and New Zealand Intensive Care Society Clinical Trials Group; Australian Red Cross Blood Service; George Institute for International Health, Myburgh J, Cooper DJ, Finfer S, et al. Saline or albumin for fluid resuscitation in patients with traumatic brain injury. *N Engl J Med* 2007;357(9):874–84.

15. Finfer S, Chittock D, Su S, et al. Intensive versus conventional glucose control in critically ill patients. *N Engl J Med* 2009;360(13):1283–97.

16. Kurz A. Thermal care in the perioperative period. *Best Pract Res Clin Anaesthesiol* 2008:22(1):39–62.

17. Varon J, Acosta P. Therapeutic hypothermia. *Chest* 2008;133(5):1267–74.

18. Lenhardt R, Grady M, Kurz A. Hyperthermia during anesthesia and intensive care unit stay. *Best Prac Res Clin Anaesthesiol* 2008;22(4):669–94.

19. Pfister D, Strebel SP, Steiner LA. Postoperative management of adult central neurosurgical patients: systemic and neuro-monitoring. *Best Pract Res Clin Anaesthesiol* 2007;21(4):449–63.

20. Rivera-Lara L, Ziai W, Nyquist P. Management of infections associated with neurocritical care. *Handbook of Clin Neurol* 2017;140:365–78.

21. Rao GS, Durga P. Changing trends in monitoring brain ischemia: from intracranial pressure to cerebral oximetry. *Curr Opin Anaesthesiol* 2011;24(5):487–94.

22. Humphreys H, Jenks PJ. Surveillance and management of ventriculitis following neurosurgery. *J Hosp Infect* 2015;89:281–6.

23. Eberhart LH, Morin AM, Kranke P, Missaghi NB, Durieux ME, Himmelseher S. Prevention and control of postoperative nausea and vomiting in post-craniotomy patients. *Best Pract Res Clin Anaesthesiol* 2007;21(4): 575–93.

24. Gan TJ, Meyer T, Apfel CC, et al. Consensus guidelines for managing postoperative nausea and vomiting. *Anesth Analg* 2003;97(1):62–71.

25. Fabling JM, Gan TJ, El-Moalem HE, Warner DS, Borel CO. A randomized, double-blinded comparison of ondansetron, droperidol, and placebo for prevention of postoperative nausea and vomiting after supratentorial craniotomy. *Anesth Analg* 2000;91(2):358–61.

26. Lai LT, Ortiz-Cardona J, Bendo AA. Perioperative pain management in the neurosurgical patient. *Anesthesiol Clin* 2012;30(2):347–67.

27. Vecht CJ, van Breemen M. Optimizing therapy of seizures in patients with brain tumors. *Neurology* 2006;67(Suppl 4):S10–S13.

28. Glantz MJ, Cole BF, Forsyth PA, et al. Practice parameter: Anticonvulsant prophylaxis in patients with newly diagnosed brain tumors. *Neurology* 2000;54:1886–93.

Part II

Clinical Monitoring

Editor: Jose I. Suarez

6

Haemodynamic Monitoring

K. Desai and J. I. Suarez

ABSTRACT

Haemodynamic monitoring is essential in any intensive care unit (ICU) and for any intensivist, including a neurointensivist, pulmonary intensivist, surgical intensivist, or cardiovascular anaesthesia intensivist. A good understanding of the basic physiology of monitored parameters and their clinical implications in terms of use for patient care has become the mainstay of our existence as intensivists. This chapter provides an overview of the current techniques and parameters available for haemodynamic monitoring including arterial blood pressure (ABP), central venous pressure, pulmonary artery and occlusion pressure, cardiac output (CO) estimation, and tissue oxygenation among others.

KEYWORDS

Haemodynamic monitoring; cardiac output (CO); arterial blood pressure (ABP); shock; oxygen delivery; resuscitation.

INTRODUCTION

Haemodynamic monitoring is essential in any intensive care unit (ICU) and has become one of the main avenues used by practitioners when caring for critically-ill patients. This is crucial for providing the best care to any ICU patient presenting with complex multiple system diseases including those admitted to the neurocritical care unit (NCCU). Therefore, it is important for intensivists to familiarize themselves with the basic physiology of monitored parameters and their clinical implications. There are multiple haemodynamic tools available. However, there are still no reliable data indicating that the best technique is in terms of its effectiveness on different patients and at the appropriate time in any given clinical setting. It is important to emphasize here that the clinical examination is always going to be the most important parameter to consider when monitoring patients in the NCCU and that haemodynamic tools should be interpreted within the context of information gained from such a clinical assessment.

Circulatory shock and systemic hypotension are medical emergencies and when sustained can result in end-organ dysfunction, tremendous morbidity, and mortality. Early resuscitation has been recommended as the goal to provide adequate oxygen delivery (DO_2) to meet the metabolic demands in such deranged physiological states and thereby reverse any existing tissue hypoperfusion.[1] Both invasive and non-invasive techniques are used to monitor these patients. This chapter provides a summary of the most relevant haemodynamic monitoring parameters and their potential application in the NCCU patient.

The chapter further discusses the following parameters that are commonly monitored in the NCCU: arterial blood pressure (ABP); central venous pressure (CVP); pulmonary artery (PA) and occlusion pressure; cardiac output (CO) estimation; and tissue oxygenation.

ARTERIAL BLOOD PRESSURE

Arterial blood pressure can be seen as a force that drives blood into the tissues. A significant decrease in its value can become life-threatening and result in various manifestations including tachycardia, oliguria, and encephalopathy. However, some NCCU patients may not experience tachycardia despite hypotension or shock due to the fact that they have been prescribed beta-blocking medications.[2] The main values derived from ABP monitoring include the systolic blood pressure (SBP), diastolic blood pressure (DBP), pulse pressure (PP), and the mean arterial pressure (MAP). Systolic blood pressure represents the pressure generated during left ventricular ejection, while DBP is the pressure generated during ventricular filling as blood is pushed from the heart to the periphery. The difference between SBP and DBP is the PP, which depends on left ventricular stroke volume, compliance of the arteries, and rate of left ventricular ejection.[1] It is important to realize that DBP is important to monitor as it reflects the vasomotor tone and contributes to coronary perfusion. Mean arterial pressure determines cerebral and peripheral organ perfusion and is calculated as follows:

$$MAP = DBP + 1/3 \ (SBP - DBP)$$

Although, pressure waveforms vary at different arterial sites, MAPs remain the same.[1,2] Arterial blood pressure is not a good measure of perfusion just by itself. For example, based on randomized controlled trials (RCTs), increasing MAP from 65 mmHg to 85 mmHg does not have any beneficial effect on renal function or metabolic measures of perfusion.[3–5]

Non-Invasive Monitoring of Arterial Blood Pressure

The most common and easy method of measuring ABP is via a sphygmomanometer.[6] This is distinct from the automated blood pressure monitors. Arterial blood pressure should be measured via the manual method (identifying the Korotkoff sounds) in an unstable patient, if there is no invasive technique available.[7,8] Sphygmomanometer ABP measurements show higher SBP and lower DBP when compared to invasive methods. This is due to summation of the pressure waves during cuff insufflation causing higher SBPs, while ischaemic vasodilation during arterial occlusion by the inflated cuff leads to lower DBPs.

Invasive Monitoring of Arterial Blood Pressure

Arterial catheterization is the optimal way of monitoring ABP in any unstable ICU patient, since it provides continuous and accurate measurement. In addition, arterial catheterization may serve as an access for arterial blood sampling for blood gas analysis and other laboratory work. The radial artery is the most commonly used site followed by the axillary artery and sometimes femoral artery if the other sites are difficult to cannulate. It is

important to stress that there is a risk of limb ischaemia if arterial catheter placement is associated with vessel rupture or dissection. In case of cardiac arrest where the radial and axillary pulse may be very feeble, it is feasible to access the femoral artery for immediate cannulation and prompt ABP monitoring.

Once ABP monitoring is started, practitioners should keep in mind that MAP reductions below 65 mmHg in a non-hypertensive patient can result in compromised organ perfusion.[1] Therefore, efforts should be invested to keep the MAP between 60 mmHg and 90 mmHg.[4] According to published guidelines, target MAP in patients with traumatic brain injury (TBI) is 90 mmHg and in patients with systemic shock is 65 mmHg.[9] Another relevant aspect is the patient's volume status. Information about the volume status can be ascertained from the ABP height during mechanical ventilation. Positive pressure ventilation leads to greater systolic variation (>10 mmHg) of ABP in hypovolaemic patients.[10–12]

Square Wave Test

Square wave test is an easy bedside test to check the dynamic response of an arterial line and accuracy of the ABP recording. It can, within a matter of a few minutes, differentiate between an over-damped and an under-damped arterial waveform. This arterial dynamic response is a function of the natural resonant frequency and damping coefficient.[10,11] The natural resonant frequency is represented by rapidity of system vibration in response to a pressure signal, and the damping coefficient is the rapidity with which the vibrations come to rest in the system.

The square wave test is performed by squeezing the fast flush valve set on the arterial line resulting in a sudden increase of about 300 mmHg pressure from the saline bag. The latter results in a waveform that rises sharply, plateaus, and drops off sharply once the flush valve is released.

CENTRAL VENOUS PRESSURE

Central venous access is primarily used for infusion of large amounts of fluids, hypertonic solutions, vasoactive medications, or for frequent blood sampling (laboratory work or monitoring of central venous oxygen saturation [$ScvO_2$]). In the past, CVP monitoring was used to assess volume status but recent literature has shown that it is a poor indicator of intravascular volume and thus is gradually falling out of use at most institutions.[1]

Central venous catheterization can be performed in the internal jugular, subclavian, and femoral veins.

Although guidelines recommend avoiding the placement of femoral central line in order to reduce the risk of catheter-related bloodstream infections, yet, there is no clear and conclusive difference in the rates of infection between the three sites.[13] Placement of central venous catheters, especially in the internal jugular and femoral veins, with ultrasound guidance makes this a very safe and almost complication-free procedure. Although placement of subclavian venous catheter is associated with complications such as pneumothorax, it may also carry the lowest risk of bloodstream infections when the three sites are compared (the difference again being statistically non-significant).[13]

Central venous pressure provides an estimation of the right ventricular preload. However, this is by no means the same as preload responsiveness and hence is not a good measure of fluid responsiveness.[3,14,15] The latter is due to the complexity of the CVP waveform and its multiple determinants (Figure 6.1).

The main factors determining CVP are blood volume, compliance of the venous system, right ventricular function, and pulmonary artery pressure (PAP).[3] Dynamic changes in CVP are observed in various clinical situations. For example, a decrease of more than 2 mmHg during inspiration could suggest volume responsiveness,[16] whereas high value recordings >12 mmHg may indicate larger mean systemic pressure, providing adequate perfusion pressure gradient to sustain venous return.[17] The normal CVP value in a non-ventilated, spontaneously breathing patient without any elevation in the intra-abdominal pressure is less than 4 mmHg. In a patient on positive pressure ventilation, the normal range is 6–12 mmHg. Central venous pressure should be measured ideally at end-expiration. Non-invasively, CVP can be measured by inspection of the jugular venous pulsation. As the patient sits supine at 45 degrees, the jugular venous distension is measured above the sternal angle.[18]

PULMONARY ARTERY AND OCCLUSION PRESSURE

HJC Swan and his colleagues invented the Swan-Ganz pulmonary artery catheter (PAC) in 1970.[19] Pulmonary artery catheter insertion has been performed routinely for almost 40 years. It helps in critical care monitoring of patients by floating a bedside balloon catheter in the PA to obtain right atrial, PA occlusion pressure, cardiac output, and mixed venous oxygen saturation. Controversy regarding the use of PAC emerged due to the lack of prospective RCTs supporting improved outcomes, lack of consensus on goals of therapy and limited ability for the clinician to interpret data accurately. It is noteworthy that

mortality benefit was seen in an early small prospective trial with its use for supranormal haemodynamics in surgical patients.[20] However, PAC insertion for goal-directed therapy in high-risk surgical patients showed no mortality benefit or hospitalization benefit, but showed a higher rate of pulmonary embolism.[21] Meta-analyses of RCTs of PAC use showed no significant change in mortality or days of hospitalization.[22] The main complications associated with PAC placement include pneumothorax, infection, embolization, arterial rupture, and cardiac arrhythmias.

Mean PAP (measured in the main PA) provides information regarding pulmonary vascular resistance (PVR). The systolic PAP is the afterload against which the right ventricle has to work.[1] The PA occlusion pressure (measured in the medium-sized PA) gives information about PVR, pulmonary oedema, intravascular volume status, left ventricle (LV) preload and performance. In addition, pulmonary hypertension can result from increase in pulmonary vasomotor tone, vascular obstruction or from LV failure. Pulmonary vascular resistance can be derived as follows:

$$PVR = \frac{Mean\ PAP - PA\ Occlusion\ Pressure}{CO}$$

Pulmonary arterial pressure monitoring can help in guiding therapies. Pulmonary hypertension due to increased PVR is responsive to inhaled nitric oxide (NO), or intravenous (IV) pulmonary vasodilators, whereas pulmonary embolism and vascular loss (emphysema) are non-responsive to such treatments. If pulmonary hypertension is associated with normal PVR, it is likely due to LV failure.[1]

Pulmonary oedema can result from elevated pulmonary capillary pressure, increased capillary permeability, or both. If pulmonary capillary pressures are higher than 20 mmHg, fluid is forcefully pushed across the pulmonary capillaries resulting in alveolar flooding. If a pre-existing or concomitant alveolar or capillary injury is present, this can occur even at lower pulmonary capillary pressures. Pulmonary artery occlusion pressure can be used to estimate pulmonary capillary pressures. If pulmonary oedema is present, capillary pressures higher than 18 mmHg suggest LV failure while lower values would indicate capillary leak.[1]

Neither absolute values of PA occlusion pressure nor their change in response to fluid challenge predict preload or volume responsiveness.[23] This is due to several reasons:

1. The relationship between PA occlusion pressure and LV end-diastolic volume (LVEDV) is curvilinear and

varies based on right ventricular volume, intrathoracic pressure, and myocardial ischaemia;

2. PA occlusion pressure provides an estimate of the LV intramural pressure but not of the distending pressure for LV filling; and

3. PA occlusion pressure does not take into account the pericardial pressures or LV diastolic compliance.

Another issue to be considered is the relationship between PA occlusion pressure and LV performance. The latter depends on factors such as preload (LVEDV), afterload (LV wall stress, which is a product of LVEDV and diastolic pressure), heart rate, and LV contractility.[1] PA occlusion pressure can be used to plot the Frank–Starling curve of PA occlusion pressure versus LV stroke work. Patients with heart failure will have PA occlusion pressure greater than 18 mmHg and a cardiac index of less than 22 L/min/m². Low PA occlusion pressure suggests hypovolaemia, whereas high values suggest volume overload.

CARDIAC OUTPUT ESTIMATION

Cardiac output is the primary determinant of tissue DO_2 and is calculated as the product of heart rate (HR) and stroke volume (SV),

$$SV = ESV - EDV$$

where ESV is the End Systolic Volume and EDV is the End Diastolic Volume.

Stroke volume is an important haemodynamic parameter to target for optimization of the haemodynamic status of a patient, as increasing HR does not necessarily result in a linear change in CO.[3]

Non-Invasive Measurement of Cardiac Output

There are currently several techniques to measure CO in a non-invasive manner including echocardiography, ultrasound, plethysmographic pressure profile analysis, and bioreactance.[1]

Echocardiography

Transthoracic echocardiogram (TTE) is used to measure aortic root flow and hence calculate CO. This involves calculation of the cross-sectional area and velocity of blood flow through this area. In addition, the left ventricular outflow tract (LVOT) diameter is measured in the parasternal long axis in systole, followed by pulse wave estimation of LVOT velocity time integral in apical

long axis or 5-chamber view.[24,25] The cardiac output can be estimated as follows:

$$CO = HR \times SV = HR \times Pi \ (LVOT \ diameter/2)^2 \times LVOT \ VTI$$

$$SV = LVOT \ area \times LVOT \ VTI$$

$$= Pi \ (LVOT \ diameter/2)^2 \times LVOT \ VTI$$

where VTI stands for velocity time integral expressed in centimetres.

Bioreactance

Electrical bioimpedance, although available for a long time now, has limited accuracy in certain situations taking into account the electrical interference.[26] The frequency modulation component of the thoracic impedance signal (i.e., bioreactance) eliminates the artefact to a great extent, thereby making accurate CO measurements.[27] Based on validation studies comparing bioreactance and PAC thermodilution CO measurements, bioreactance has good accuracy.[28] Furthermore, it can also be used in combination with fluid bolus or passive leg raising manoeuvre (PLR) to check for fluid responsiveness.

Invasive Measurement of Cardiac Output

Intensivists can also estimate CO using invasive techniques such as insertion of a PAC or via arterial pulse pressure waveform analysis.

Thermodilution Technique for Cardiac Output Estimation via Pulmonary Artery Catheter

This is a frequently used method for continuous CO estimation; however, the trend is changing now.[29] Cardiac output is measured by injecting cold fluid through the proximal port of the PAC, which lies at the level of the right atrium. This cold fluid mixes with blood in the right ventricle and the thermistor picks up the change in blood temperature. Cardiac output is inversely proportional to the area under the temperature versus time curve. A random thermal signal using an induction coil in the right ventricular region of the PAC permits estimation of CO continuously. In addition, CO measurements can also be performed via transthoracic thermodilution methods where the thermal change is measured in a central artery like the femoral artery instead of the pulmonary artery.[1] Lastly, CO via PAC also can be determined using the Fick's principle; however, this is beyond the scope of this book.

Arterial Pulse Pressure Waveform Analysis

This is a minimally invasive CO monitoring method requiring insertion of an arterial catheter and is based on the variation in pulse pressure waves. Multiple devices are available that analyse pulse pressure waveforms and the techniques that require external calibration are considered the most accurate.[30] Methods commonly employed for calibration include transthoracic lithium dilution[31] and thermodilution.[32] An increase in CO by 15% after a fluid challenge is considered to be the gold standard that reflects fluid responsiveness. If there is no response in improvement of CO or less than 15% response, inotropes should be considered due to the possibility of impaired cardiac contractility. The concepts of pulse pressure variation (PPV)[33,34] or stroke volume variation (SVV)[35,36] have been validated to detect CO changes with positive pressure ventilation and thereby identify patients who are volume responsive.[37] Volume responsiveness is defined as an increase in PPV or SVV of 15% in a patient who is on mechanical ventilation with a tidal volume of at least 8 cc/kg.[1] This is not very accurate in patients who have arrhythmias or are spontaneously breathing given the varied R–R intervals and ventricular interdependence induced left ventricular diastolic compliance changes, respectively.

Tissue Oxygenation

There is no specific normal value of CO, despite there being a range of recommended normal CO. The latter depends on the extent of physiological derangement for each individual based on the underlying pathogenesis of the disease. The optimal CO for an individual is that which keeps up with the increased metabolic demand in the abnormal state. Maintaining normal CO does not necessitate adequate tissue blood flow as the vasomotor tone will vary to keep ABP within the acceptable range.[1] Therefore, for assessing adequate tissue DO_2, oxygen saturation in venous and arterial blood needs to be studied. Pulmonary artery catheter provides mixed venous oxygen saturation (SvO_2) of the whole body, while central venous catheters provide $ScvO_2$ from the brain and the upper part of body. However, the most widely available methodology to assess gross tissue oxygenation is pulse oximetry, which provides continuous monitoring of arterial blood oxygen saturation (SaO_2), and thus reduces the need for repeated arterial blood gas analysis. The absence of arterial pulse would not allow the pulse oximetry to work and measure SaO_2. Therefore, it is also referred to as pulse ox or SpO_2.[38] SpO_2 is used to detect hypoxaemia defined as values less than 90%.[39] In addition, it is important to note that there is no additional benefit of providing supplementary oxygen, if the SpO_2 is already close to 95% given the oxyhaemoglobin dissociation curve. Hence, an SpO_2 of 95% equals a PaO_2 between 60 mmHg (SaO_2 >91%) and 160 mmHg (SaO_2 >99%). Pulse oximetry is also used for plethysmographic waveform analysis and this in turn is based on beat-to-beat changes, which helps in detecting volume responsiveness.[40,41]

Venous Oximetry, Venous Oxygen Saturation, and Central Venous Oxygen Saturation

There are some other important concepts that are applied in the ICU setting to patients with compromised DO_2. It is already discussed that DO_2 is the oxygen delivery to the entire body and can be calculated as follows:

$DO_2 = CO \times CaO_2$, where $CaO_2 = Hb \times 1.36 \times SaO_2 \times PaO_2 \times 0.0031$. In addition, oxygen consumption (VO_2) can also be derived: $VO_2 = CO \times (CaO_2 - CVO_2)$, where CaO_2 is oxygen content of arterial blood, and CVO_2 is oxygen content of venous blood. The latter also can be estimated as follows: $CVO_2 = CaO_2 - (VO_2/CO)$.

Venous oxygen saturation is an important factor determining CVO_2 and it correlates well with oxygen supply to demand ratio. Reductions in $ScvO_2$ and SvO_2 may indicate increased oxygen extraction and are typically observed in conditions of metabolic stress. However, low SvO_2 can also result from low CO, anaemia (low DO_2), exercise (high vO_2), and hypoxaemia. Reduction in SvO_2 lower than 50 per cent would suggest some degree of tissue hypoxaemia.[42] $ScvO_2$ is generally lower by 2–3 per cent when compared with SvO_2, as the lower body extracts less oxygen compared to the upper body.[43] However, septic shock results in higher $ScvO_2$ compared to SvO_2 and this reverses cardiogenic and hypovolemic shock.

CONCLUSIONS

Haemodynamic monitoring is essential in any ICU and for any intensivist, including a neurointensivist, pulmonary intensivist, surgical intensivist or cardiovascular anaesthesia intensivist. A good understanding of the basic physiology of the monitored parameters and their clinical implications in terms of use for patient care has become the mainstay of our existence as intensivists.

REFERENCES

1. Pinsky MR. Functional hemodynamic monitoring. *Crit Care Clin* 2015;31(1):89–111.

2. Wo CC, Shoemaker WC, Appel PL, et al. Unreliability of blood pressure and heart rate to evaluate cardiac output in emergency resuscitation and critical illness. *Crit Care Med* 1993;21:218–23.

3. Hollenberg SM. Hemodynamic monitoring. *Chest* 2013;143(5):1480–8.

4. LeDoux D, Astiz ME, Carpati CM, Backow EC. Effects of perfusion pressure on tissue perfusion in septic shock. *Crit Care Med* 2000;28(8):2729–32.

5. Bourgoin A, Leone M, Delmas A, Garnier F, Albanese J, Martin C. Increasing mean arterial pressure in patients with septic shock: effects on oxygen variables and renal function. *Crit Care Med* 2005;33(4):780–6.

6. Pickering TG. Principles and techniques of blood pressure measurement. *Cardiol Clin* 2002;20:207–23.

7. Cohn JN. Blood pressure measurement in shock: mechanism of inaccuracy in auscultatory and palpatory methods. *JAMA* 1967;199:118–22.

8. Karnath B. Sources of error in blood pressure measurement. *Hosp Physician* 2002;3:33–37.

9. Bratton SL, Chestnut RM, Ghajar J, et al. Guidelines for the management of severe traumatic brain injury, I:Blood pressure and oxygenation. *J Neurotrauma* 2007; 24(suppl1):S7–S13.

10. McGhee BH, Bridges EJ. Monitoring arterial blood pressure: what you may not know. *Crit Care Nurse* April 2002;22:60–79.

11. Bersten AD, Soni N. *Oh's Intensive Care Manual.* Butterworth-Heinemann: 7th ed; April 2015.

12. Newhouse BJ, Montecino R. Invasive Hemodynamic Monitoring. In: Sandberg W, Urman R, Ehrenfeld J Editors. *The MGH Textbook of Anesthetic Equipment.* Philadelphia: Elsevier (Saunders), 2011;148–59.

13. Marik PE, Flemmer M, Harrison W. The risk of catheter-related bloodstream infection with femoral venous catheters as compared to subclavian and internal jugular venous catheters: A systematic review of the literature and meta-analysis. *Crit Care Med* Aug 2012;40:2479–85.

14. Marik PE, Baram M, Vahid B. Does central venous pressure predict fluid responsiveness? A systematic review of the literature and the tale of seven mares. *Chest* 2008;134: 172–8.

15. Kumar A, Anel R, Bunnell E, et al. Pulmonary artery occlusion pressure and central venous pressure fail to predict ventricular filling volume, cardiac performance, or the response to volume infusion in normal subjects. *Crit Care Med* 2004; 32:691–9.

16. Magder SA, Georgiadis G, Cheong T. Respiratory variations in right atrial pressure predict response to fluid challenge. *J Crit Care* 1992;7:76–85.

17. Gelman S. Venous function and central venous pressure: a physiologic story. *Anesthesiology* 2008;108:735–48.

18. Constant J. Using internal jugular pulsations as a manometer for right atrial pressure measurements. *Cardiology* 2000;93:26–30.

19. Swan HJ, Ganz W, Forrester J, et al. Catheterization of the heart in man with use of a flow-directed balloon-tipped catheter. *N Engl J Med* 1970;283:447–51.

20. Shoemaker WC, Appel PL, Kram HB, Waxman K, Lee TS. Prospective trial of supranormal values of survivors as therapeutic goals in high-risk surgical patients. *Chest* 1988 Dec;94(6):1176–86.

21. Sandham JD, et al. A randomized controlled trial of the use of pulmonary artery catheters in high-risk surgical patients. *New Engl J Med* 2003 Jan;348(1):5–14.

22. Shah MR, Hasselblad V, Stevenson LW, et al. Impact of the pulmonary artery catheter in critically ill patients: meta-analysis of randomized clinical trials. *JAMA* 2005 Oct 5; 294(13):1664–70.

23. Osman D, Ridel C, Ray P, et al. Cardiac filling pressures are not appropriate to predict hemodynamic response to volume challenge. *Crit Care Med* 2007;35:64–68.

24. Shiran A, Adawi S, Ganaeem M, Asmer E. Accuracy and reproducibility of left ventricular outflow tract diameter measurement using transthoracic when compared with transesophageal echocardiography in systole and diastole. *Eur J Echocardiogr* 2009:319–24.

25. Lang RM, Badano LP, Mor-Avi V, et al. Recommendations for cardiac chamber quantification by echocardiography in adults: an update from the American Society of Echocardiography and the European Association of Cardiovascular Imaging. *J Am Soc Echocardiogr* 2015 Jan:1–39.

26. Raaijmakers e, Faes TJ, Scholten RJ, et al. A meta-analysis of three decades of validating thoracic impedance cardiography. *Crit Care Med* 1999;27:1203–13.

27. Keren H, Burkhoff D, Squara P. Evaluation of a noninvasive continuous cardiac output monitoring system based on thoracic bioreactance. *Am J Physiol* 2007;293:H583–H589.

28. Raval NY, Squara P, Cleman M, et al. Multicenter evaluation of noninvasive cardiac output measurement by bioreactance technique. *J Clin Monit Comput* 2008;22:113–19.

29. Shure D. Pulmonary-artery catheters-peace at last? *N Engl J Med* 2006;354:2273–4.

30. Opdam HI, Wan L, Bellomo R. A pilot assessment of the FloTrac cardiac output monitoring system. *Intensive Care Med* 2007;33:344–9.

31. Jonas MM, Kelly FE, Linton RA, et al. A comparison of lithium dilution cardiac output measurements made using central and antecubital venous injection of lithium chloride. *J Clin Monit Comput* 1999;15:525–8.

32. Della Rocca G, Costa MG, Pompei L, et al. Continuous and intermittent cardiac output measurement: pulmonary

artery catheter versus aortic transpulmonary technique. *Br J Anaesth* 2002;88:350–6.

33. Michard F, Chemla D, Richard C, et al. Clinical use of respiratory changes in arterial pulse pressure to monitor the hemodynamic effects of PEEP. *Am J Respir Crit Care Med* 1999;159:935–9.

34. Michard F, Boussat S, Chemla D, et al. Relation between respiratory changes in arterial pulse pressure and fluid responsiveness in septic patients with acute circulatory failure. *Am J Respir Crit Care Med* 2000;162:134–8.

35. Berkenstadt H, Margalit N, Hadani M, et al. Stroke volume variation as a predictor of fluid responsiveness in patients undergoing brain surgery. *Anesth Analg* 2001;92:984–9.

36. Reuter D, Felbinger TW, Schmidt C, et al. Stroke volume variation for assessment of cardiac responsiveness to volume loading in mechanically ventilated patients after cardiac surgery. *Intensive Care Med* 2002;28:392–8.

37. Michard F, Teboul JL. Predicting fluid responsiveness in ICU patients: a critical analysis of the evidence. *Chest* 2002;121:2000–8.

38. Wukitisch MW, Peterson MT, Tobler DR, et al. Pulse oximetry: analysis of theory, technology, and practice. *J Clin Monit* 1988;4:290–301.

39. Van de Louw A, Cracco C, Cerf C, et al. Accuracy of pulse oximetry in the intensive care unit. *Intensive Car Med* 2001;27:1606–13.

40. Cassesson M, Besnard C, Durand PG, et al. Relation between respiratory variations in pulse oximetry plethysmographic waveform amplitude and arterial pulse pressure in ventilated patients. *Crit Care* 2005;9:R562–8.

41. Natalini G, Rosano A, Taranto M, et al. Arterial versus plethysmographic dynamic indices to test responsiveness for testing fluid administration in hypotensive patients: a clinical trial. *Anesth Analg* 2006;103:1478–84.

42. Shoemaker WC, Appel PL, Kram HR. Tissue oxygen debt as a determinant of lethal and non-lethal postoperative organ failure. *Crit Care Med* 1988;16:1117–20.

43. Scheinman MM, Brown MA, Rapaport E. Critical assessment of use of central venous oxygen saturation as a mirror of mixed venous oxygen in severely ill cardiac patients. *Circulation* 1969;40:165–72.

7

Respiratory Monitoring

S. O. Kazmi and J. I. Suarez

ABSTRACT

Respiratory monitoring in the neurocritical care unit (NCCU) is paramount and close attention needs to be paid to this patient population who may need emergent airway protection in case of neurological compromise. Patients with a decreased level of consciousness as measured by the Glasgow Coma Scale (GCS) need to be monitored for imminent failure of airway protection. Special attention should be paid to patients with a neuromuscular diagnosis. These patients generally do not show signs of respiratory failure until late in the disease course when they may suddenly collapse. A forced vital capacity of less than 20 ml/kg, a negative inspiratory force of less than –30 cmH$_2$O and a positive expiratory pressure of less than 40 cmH$_2$O have been shown to be good predictors for the need of mechanical ventilation in the neurocritically ill patient. Weaning strategies should be initiated promptly.

KEYWORDS

Respiratory failure; mechanical ventilation; weaning; tracheostomy; non-invasive positive pressure ventilation.

INTRODUCTION

Over the past half century, there has been an increase in the number of intensive care units (ICUs) throughout the world. The primary reason for this increase is better management of the airway with the introduction of artificial ventilation which has subsequently led to an increase in survival. This is a crucial aspect of care for neurological and neurosurgical patients who depend on airway security to survive their disease course. Thus, respiratory monitoring in the neurocritical care unit (NCCU) is paramount and close attention needs to be paid to this patient population who may need emergent airway protection in case of neurological compromise. In this context, a recent study showed that among mechanically ventilated patients, 45% were intubated for neurological reasons comprising of coma and neuromuscular aetiologies.[1] This data also indicates the burden of disease and the need for identification and proper management of this patient population.

INDICATIONS FOR RESPIRATORY MONITORING

Every patient admitted to the NCCU needs to be monitored for respiratory compromise. Table 7.1 shows some of the most common neurological indications for close respiratory monitoring. Practitioners should monitor changes in the respiratory status of these patients and particularly of those with a low threshold for aggressive airway management. It should be considered that even though these patients are admitted to the NCCU, they may experience general causes of respiratory failure including pneumonia, pulmonary oedema, acute respiratory distress syndrome (ARDS), chronic obstructive pulmonary disease (COPD), asthma exacerbation, pneumothorax, hemothorax, flail chest syndrome, and malignancy.

Patients with a decreased level of consciousness as measured by the Glasgow Coma Scale (GCS) need to be monitored for imminent failure of airway protection. A GCS of less than 8 has been shown to increase

Table 7.1 Indications for respiratory monitoring

Decreased level of consciousness (Glasgow Coma Scale <10)
Dysarthria
Dysphagia
Increased respiratory rate
Accessory muscle use for respiration
Anxiety in a patient with intracranial or neuromuscular disorders
Elevated intracranial pressure
Severe stroke
Intracerebral haemorrhage
Subarachnoid haemorrhage
Subdural haematoma
Epidural haematoma
Severe traumatic brain injury
Seizures (status epilepticus, prolonged postictal stat, epilepsy partialis continua)
Polyneuropathy
Neuromuscular junction disorders (myasthenia gravis, Lambert-Eaton syndrome, botulism)
Myopathy
Spinal injury
Posterior fossa injury

aspiration.[2] Special attention is required for patients with a neuromuscular diagnosis as they generally show no signs of respiratory failure until late stages of the disease when they may suddenly collapse. It is important to appreciate that since there is no defect in gaseous exchange in the lungs, arterial blood gases (ABG) do not usually change in these patients. A forced vital capacity (FVC) of less than 20 ml/kg, a negative inspiratory force (NIF) of less than −30 cmH$_2$O and a positive expiratory pressure (PEP) of less than 40 cmH$_2$O have shown to be robust predictors of the need for mechanical ventilation in Guillain-Barre Syndrome patients.[3] These bedside measurements can be extrapolated to include other neuromuscular disorders such as myasthenia gravis or Lambert–Eaton syndrome in making a decision for early intubation.

RESPIRATORY PARAMETERS

Certain tools and measures can aid in management of the airway in a neurocritically ill patient. A basic respiratory examination should be conducted on every

patient being admitted to the NCCU. The respiratory rate should be evaluated for any signs of respiratory distress. Auscultation of the lungs should be performed to detect any obvious pathology (e.g., pneumothorax). Crackles and wheezes must be documented along with the patient's history for evidence of asthma or COPD. A chest X-ray should be performed in all patients as this serves not only as a baseline investigation for further examinations, but also because it has a high diagnostic efficiency.[4] Pulse oximetry should be established on every patient to give information on oxygen saturation which is easily displayed on the monitor. Arterial blood gases and venous blood gases (VBG) should be obtained daily or when any changes are made to respiratory management. A recent study showed that the VBG in conjunction with pulse oximetry can give reliable parameters compared to ABG, and can even be used when arterial access is difficult.[5]

In patients undergoing mechanical ventilation, special parameters need to be assessed on a daily basis. The fraction of inspired oxygen (FiO$_2$) should be kept at the lowest possible setting to maintain adequate oxygenation. The standard practice is to start the patient on 100% FiO$_2$ while being intubated and then lower the setting to around 40%–60% to maintain arterial oxygen saturation (SaO$_2$) >94%. The FiO$_2$ should be titrated to the patient's comfort and requirement with care to avoid hyperoxia. Studies have shown that increased oxygenation is associated with worse clinical outcomes and an increase in adverse effects.[6,7] Lung protective ventilation should be employed with lower tidal volumes of 6–8 ml/kg as this reduces mortality when compared to higher tidal volumes as evidenced by the Acute Respiratory Distress Syndrome Clinical Network (ARDS-NET) trial.[8] A positive end-expiratory pressure of 5–8 cmH$_2$O should be maintained as this reduces the rates of pneumonia and hypoxia.[9] Plateau pressures (PPlat) should be documented daily in mechanically ventilated patients aiming at values of less than 30 cmH$_2$O at all times.[10] In addition, the rapid shallow breathing index (RSBI) has been shown to be associated with failure of extubation and values of less than 105 should be obtained prior to weaning.[11] Serial RSBI's and RSBI rate have better predictive values than a single RSBI measurement in relation to extubation success and should be employed in the mechanically ventilated patient.[12] Table 7.2 summarizes the respiratory parameters that should be monitored in the NCCU setting.

Table 7.2 Respiratory parameters and their recommended values

Respiratory rate (normal range 6–20 breaths per minute)
Chest X-ray
Pulse oximetry (oxygen saturation >94%)
Arterial blood gas (PaO$_2$ >80 mmHg, PaCO$_2$ 35–45 mmHg, pH 7.35–7.45)
FiO$_2$ (30%–100%)
PEEP (5–8 cmH$_2$O)
VT (6–8 ml/kg)
Pplat <30 cmH$_2$O
RSBI <105

Abbreviations: PaO$_2$: arterial oxygen pressure; PaCO$_2$: arterial carbon dioxide pressure; FiO$_2$: inspired oxygen fraction; PEEP: positive end-expiratory pressure; Pplat: plateau pressure; RSBI: rapid shallow breathing index; VT: tidal volume.

AIRWAY MONITORING AND MANAGEMENT

In the emergency setting, practitioners must secure a proper and reliable airway, which is paramount for survival. Various tools and techniques have been developed to facilitate this process. The jaw thrust–chin lift manoeuvre allows opening of the air passages and prevents the tongue from collapsing on the airway.[13] Once this manoeuvre has been employed, adequate ventilation, also called rescue breathing, can be achieved by a simple bag mask ventilation. If bag mask ventilation is difficult, then oropharyngeal or nasopharyngeal airways can be used.[14] The laryngeal mask airway (LMA) is used commonly to maintain a patent airway as it is easy to use.[15] Alternatively, the intubating laryngeal mask airway (ILMA) can be used if endotracheal intubation is difficult. Nowadays, the use of video laryngoscopy is widespread in the NCCU and emergency room settings. This has increased the first attempt success rates compared to direct laryngoscopy.[16–19] Table 7.3 enlists some tools that can aid in securing an airway.

Special considerations should be taken into account when practitioners are faced with a difficult airway. The latter is one where bag mask ventilation is problematic or when endotracheal intubation is challenging. Certain criteria have been developed to assess a difficult airway. In the MOANS criteria, the 'M' stands for Mask for a difficult mask seal, the 'O' for Obesity and Obstruction, the 'A' for Age greater than 55, the 'N' for No teeth and the 'S' which refers to Stiff lungs or Stiff chest wall.[20] A patient meeting most or all of the MOANS criteria will prove to be difficult to ventilate using a bag mask.

Table 7.3 Tools that help secure the airway

Oropharyngeal airway
Nasopharyngeal airway
Laryngeal mask airway
Intubating laryngeal mask airway
Oesophageal-tracheal double lumen airway
Fibreoptic scope
Direct laryngoscopy
Video laryngoscopy (GlideScope, C-MAC)
Surgical airway (cricothyroidotomy, tracheostomy, retrograde airway)

Another common criteria is the LEMON criteria (Look criteria, Evaluate criteria for mouth opening and airway position, Mallampati score, airway Obstruction, and Neck mobility).[21,22] A patient meeting most or all of the LEMON criteria will be difficult to intubate.

In patients with trauma, the cervical spine should be immobilized with minimal movement of the neck to prevent spinal cord injury. In order to secure the airway with endotracheal intubation, rapid sequence induction and intubation should be used. The most common agents include intravenous lidocaine (1.5 mg/kg), opiates (fentanyl at 2–3 μg/kg, morphine, hydromorphone), etomidate (0.3 mg/kg), propofol (2 mg/kg), thiopental, rocuronium (1.2–1.4 mg/kg), vecuronium (0.1–0.2 mg/kg) or cisatracurium and ketamine (2 mg/kg).[23]

Respiratory Monitoring Using Non-Invasive Positive Pressure Ventilation

Non-invasive positive pressure ventilation (NIPPV) can be used occasionally to avoid invasive endotracheal intubation. It consists of a full face mask that can be attached to the ventilator in order to provide pressure support ventilation. If positive end expiratory pressure (PEEP) is added to pressure support then it is termed Bi-level. The inspiratory pressures and expiratory pressures can be adjusted depending on whether a high–low or low–high strategy is employed.[24,25] The use of NIPPV has been supported in certain cases of severe COPD exacerbation, acute cardiogenic pulmonary oedema, and certain immunocompromised states.[26–31]

Respiratory Monitoring in the Mechanically Ventilated Patient

In terms of guaranteeing ventilation in acute respiratory compromise, endotracheal intubation remains the best

Table 7.4 Major modes of ventilation in modern ventilators

Continuous Mandatory Ventilation (CMV)
Volume Control/Assist Control (VC/AC)
Pressure Control/Assist Control (PC/AC)
Synchronized Intermittent Mandatory Ventilation (SIMV)
Pressure Support Ventilation (PSV)

form of achieving adequate gaseous exchange. This involves placing a tube that passes from the oropharynx into the trachea. The tube is then connected to a ventilator which provides artificial breathing support in the form of positive pressure ventilation.

There are more than 100 different modes of ventilation in modern ICUs throughout the world with no one mode being clearly proven to be superior than the other. In general, these ventilators support respiration using three basic breath sequences: continuous mandatory ventilation (CMV), intermittent mandatory ventilation (IMV), and continuous spontaneous ventilation (CSV). These can be further sub-classified into different patterns depending on whether the breaths are volume controlled or pressure controlled. The main modes of ventilation in modern ventilators are listed in Table 7.4.

The major respiratory parameters that need to be monitored in the mechanically ventilated patient include the tidal volume (VT), FiO_2, respiratory rate, PEEP, Pplat, and RSBI. These parameters should be titrated based on the oxygen saturation and ABGs of the patient. FiO_2 should be maintained at the lowest possible level in order to prevent oxygen toxicity. Lung protective ventilation with low VTs (6–8 ml/kg of ideal body weight) should be implemented. RSBIs should be measured daily and efforts should be made to extubate the patient as soon as possible.

It is imperative to closely monitor the ventilator and its respective settings and changes must be made for better ventilation according to the disease process. For example, in cases of elevated intracranial pressure (ICP), transient hyperventilation can be used to promote hypocapnia, which in turn will cause vasoconstriction and lower ICP.[32] Hyperventilation should only be used as a bridge to more definitive ICP reduction since prolonged and indiscriminate hypocapnia can lead to cerebral ischaemia.[33,34]

As soon as the primary aetiology that necessitated implementation of mechanical ventilation has resolved or begun to improve, weaning from the ventilator should be instituted. For example, in neuromuscular illnesses, as there is no primary defect in ventilation but

more so in breathing mechanics, once immunotherapy has been started efforts should be made to wean the patient off the ventilator. In these cases, waiting for a long period before pursuing tracheostomy is reasonable, given a superior recovery rate.[35] In other cases such as large malignant strokes where there is a low likelihood of reasonable recovery from a respiratory standpoint, tracheostomy can be pursued earlier in order to wean off the ventilator.[36]

Standard practice includes obtaining daily chest X-rays to evaluate the lung parenchyma and identify the proper level of the endotracheal tube. The endotracheal tube should be placed roughly 4 cm above the carina.[37,38] Daily ABGs should also be obtained and depending on their values, in conjunction with the chest X-ray, changes to the ventilator settings can be made. In most institutions, respiratory therapists have protocols that can be followed to determine the optimal efficiency of mechanical ventilation.[39]

WEANING FROM MECHANICAL VENTILATION

Weaning strategies should be started from day 1 when mechanical ventilation is provided and the patient meets the prerequisites. General criteria includes an absence of hypoxaemia (PaO_2/FiO_2 >150, PO_2 >60mmHg, PEEP <5–8 cmH_2O), a mental status examination with the patient's ability to follow commands, haemodynamic stability, and an absence of acidosis.[40,41] As such, the term 'weaning' is incorrect as patients are not required to be slowly weaned off the ventilator in order to achieve extubation success. Different strategies can be employed based on physician preference and institutional protocol. Patients can be switched from CMV to lower levels of support. Another technique involves stopping continuous ventilation during which the patient is allowed to breathe spontaneously. These spontaneous breathing trials (SBT) should be carried out daily to assess for removal of the endotracheal tube. They are usually carried out for 30–120 minutes at a time. Pressure support can be added to aid in these weaning trials which range from levels of 3–13 cmH_2O. If a patient is able to tolerate the SBT and all the prerequisites are met, extubation can be planned. The patient is evaluated for a cuff leak test to assess for laryngeal oedema prior to removal of the endotracheal tube. Once the tube is removed, the patient is asked to cough and aggressive suctioning is done to prevent aspiration of secretions. Non-invasive ventilation can be utilized to help with respiratory distress after extubation. It has been shown to decrease mortality in patients who have failed a SBT.[42,43]

In patients with multiple failed attempts at weaning or disease process that does not permit weaning, a permanent form of airway needs to be established. This is because the longer the endotracheal tube remains in the airway, the higher the chance of complications. In this regard, tracheostomy is a simple procedure in which an opening is made in the trachea via the neck into which a small tube can be inserted for ventilation. Tracheostomies increase patient comfort and expedite weaning from mechanical ventilation. The optimal timing for tracheostomy is still debatable. A recent systematic review and meta-analysis of 10 randomized control trials comparing early versus late tracheostomy in acutely brain-injured patients showed a reduction in long-term mortality, ICU stay, and duration of mechanical ventilation with early tracheostomy. Although the overall rates of tracheostomy were lower in the delayed group, they showed similar long-term mortality.[44]

CONCLUSIONS

Respiratory monitoring in the NCCU is a cornerstone of good patient care. Practitioners need to be well-versed with the management of respiratory parameters and act upon the information received in the best interest of the patient. Management strategies should be tailored to the specific neurological condition of the patient. Timely intervention can reduce morbidity and mortality and increase quality of life in neurologically ill patients.

REFERENCES

1. Kübler A, Maciejewski D, Adamik B, Kaczorowska M. Mechanical ventilation in ICUs in Poland: a multi-center point-prevalence study. *Med Sci Monit* 2013;19:424–9.

2. Adnet F, Baud F. Relation between Glasgow Coma Scale and aspiration pneumonia. *Lancet* 1996;348:123–4.

3. Lawn ND, Fletcher DD, Henderson RD, Wolter TD, Wijdicks EF. Anticipating mechanical ventilation in Guillain-Barre syndrome. *Arch Neurol* 2001;58(6):893–8.

4. Palazzetti V, Gasparri E, Gambini C, et al. Chest radiography in intensive care: an irreplaceable survey? *Radiol Med* 2013 Aug;118(5):744–51.

5. Zeserson E, Goodgame B, Hess JD, et al. Correlation of venous blood gas and pulse oximetry with arterial blood gas in the undifferentiated critically ill patient. *J Intensive Care Med* 2016 Jun 9; 2018;33(3):176–81.

6. Helmerhorst HJ, Arts DL, Schultz MJ, et al. Metrics of arterial hyperoxia and associated outcomes in critical care. *Crit Care Med* 2016 Oct 19; 2017;45(2):187–95.

7. Girardis M, Busani S, Damiani E, et al. Effect of conservative vs conventional oxygen therapy on mortality among patients in an intensive care unit: The oxygen-icu randomized clinical trial. *JAMA* 2016 Oct 18;316(15):1583–9.

8. The Acute Respiratory Distress Syndrome Network. Ventilation with lower tidal volumes as compared with traditional tidal volumes for acute lung injury and the acute respiratory distress syndrome. *N Engl J Med* 2000;342:1301–8.

9. Manzano F, Fernandez-Mondejar E, Colmenero M, et al. Positive-end expiratory pressure reduces incidence of ventilator-associated pneumonia in nonhypoxemic patients. *Crit Care Med* 2008;36(8):2225–31.

10. Jaswal DS, Leung JM, Sun J, et al. Tidal volume and plateau pressure use for acute lung injury from 2000 to present: a systematic literature review. *Crit Care Med* 2014 Oct;42(10):2278–89.

11. Yang KL, Tobin MJ. A prospective study of indexes predicting the outcome of trials of weaning from mechanical ventilation. *N Engl J Med* 1991;324:1445–50.

12. Karthika M, Al Enezi FA, Pillai LV, Arabi YM. Rapid shallow breathing index. *Ann Thorac Med* 2016 Jul-Sep; 11(3):167–76.

13. Safar P, Escarraga LA, Chang F. Upper airway obstruction in the unconscious patient. *J Appl Physiol* 1959;14: 760–4.

14. Rees SG, Gabbott DA. Use of the cuffed oropharyngeal airway for manual ventilation by non-anaesthetists. *Anaesthesia* 1999;54:1089–93.

15. Benumof JL. Laryngeal mask airway and the ASA difficult airway algorithm. *Anesthesiology* 1996;84(3):686–99.

16. Malik MA, Subramaniam R, Maharaj CH, et al. Randomized controlled trial of the Pentax AWS, Glidescope, and Macintosh laryngoscopes in predicted difficult intubation. *Br J Anaesth* 2009;103(5):761–8.

17. Jungbauer A, Schumann M, Brunkhorst V, et al.: Expected difficult tracheal intubation: a prospective comparison of direct laryngoscopy and video laryngoscopy in 200 patients. *Br J Anaesth* 2009;102(4):546–50.

18. Aziz MF, Dillman D, Fu R, et al. Comparative effectiveness of the C-MAC video laryngoscope versus direct laryngoscopy in the setting of the predicted difficult airway. *Anesthesiology* 2012;116(3): 629–36.

19. Sakles JC, Patanwala AE, Mosier JM, et al. Comparison of video laryngoscopy to direct laryngoscopy for intubation of patients with difficult airway characteristics in the emergency department. *Intern Emerg Med* 2014;9(1): 93–8.

20. Walls RM, Murphy MF. *Manual of Emergency Airway Management*. 3rd ed. Philadelphia: Lippincott Williams & Wilkins; 2008.

21. Walls RM. Rapid-sequence intubation in head trauma. *Ann Emerg Med* 1993;22:1008–13.

22. Soyuncu S, Eken C, Cete Y, Bektas F, Akcimen M. Determination of difficult intubation in the ED. *Am J Emerg Med* 2009;27:905–10.

23. Bucher J, Koyfman A. Intubation of the neurologically injured patient. *J Emerg Med* 2015 Dec;49(6):920–7.

24. Brochard L, Mancebo J, Wysocki M, et al. Noninvasive ventilation for acute exacerbations of chronic obstructive pulmonary disease. *N Engl J Med* 1995;333:817–22.

25. Kramer N, Meyer TJ, Meharg J, et al. Randomized, prospective trial of noninvasive positive pressure ventilation in acute respiratory failure. *Am J Respir Crit Care Med* 1995;151:1799–806.

26. Peter JV, Moran JL, Phillips-Hughes J, Warn D. Noninvasive ventilation in acute respiratory failure: a meta-analysis update. *Crit Care Med* 2002;30:555–62.

27. Keenan SP, Sinuff T, Cook DJ, Hill N. Which patients with acute exacerbation of chronic obstructive pulmonary disease benefit from noninvasive positive pressure ventilation? A systematic review of the literature. *Ann Intern Med* 2003;138:861–70.

28. Masip J, Roque M, Sanchez B, et al. Noninvasive ventilation in acute cardiogenic pulmonary edema: systematic review and meta-analysis. *JAMA* 2005;294(24):3124–30.

29. Confalonieri M, Calderini E, Terraciano S, et al. Noninvasive ventilation for treating acute respiratory failure in AIDS patients with Pneumocystis carinii pneumonia. *Intensive Care Med* 2002;28:1233–8.

30. Conti G, Marino P, Cogliati A, et al. Noninvasive ventilation for the treatment of acute respiratory failure in patients with hematologic malignancies: a pilot study. *Intensive Care Med* 1998;24:1283–8.

31. Antonelli M, Conti G, Bufi M, et al. Noninvasive ventilation for treatment of acute respiratory failure in patients undergoing solid organ transplantation: a randomized trial. *JAMA* 2000;283:235–41.

32. Allen CH, Ward JD. An evidence-based approach to management of increased intracranial pressure. *Crit Care Clin* 1998;14:485–95.

33. Muizelaar JP, Marmarou A, Ward JD, et al. Adverse effects of prolonged hyperventilation in patients with severe head injury: a randomized clinical trial. *J Neurosurg* 1991;75:731–9.

34. Rosner MJ, Daughton S. Cerebral perfusion pressure management in head injury. *J Trauma* 1990;30(8):933–40; discussion 40.

35. Rabinstein AA, Mueller-Kronast N. Risk of extubation failure in patients with myasthenic crisis. *Neurocrit Care* 2005;3(3):213–5.

36. Julian Bösel. Airway management and mechanical ventilation in the neurocritically ill. 2013 Neurocritical Care Society Practice Update.

37. Salem MR. Verification of endotracheal tube position. *Anesthesiol Clin North America* 2001 Dec;19(4):813–39.

38. Rudraraju P, Eisen LA. Confirmation of endotracheal tube position: a narrative review. *J Intensive Care Med* 2009 Sep–Oct;24(5):283–92.

39. Chia JY, Clay AS. Effects of respiratory-therapist driven protocols on house-staff knowledge and education of mechanical ventilation. *Clin Chest Med* 2008 Jun;29(2):313–21, vii.

40. MacIntyre NR, Cook DJ, Ely EW, Jr., et al. Evidence-based guidelines for weaning and discontinuing ventilatory support: a collective task force facilitated by the American College of Chest Physicians; the American Association for Respiratory Care; and the American College of Critical Care Medicine. *Chest* 2001;120:375S–95S.

41. Hendra KP, Celli BR. Weaning from mechanical ventilation. *Int Anesthesiol Clin* 1999;37:127–43.

42. Nava S, Ambrosino N, Clini E, et al. Noninvasive mechanical ventilation in the weaning of patients with respiratory failure due to chronic obstructive pulmonary disease. A randomized, controlled trial. *Ann Intern Med* 1998;128(9):721–8.

43. Ferrer M, Esquinas A, Arancibia F, et al. Noninvasive ventilation during persistent weaning failure: a randomized controlled trial. *Am J Respir Crit Care Med* 2003;168(1):70–6.

44. McCredie VA, Alali AS, Scales DC, et al. Effect of early versus late tracheostomy or prolonged intubation in critically ill patients with acute brain injury: A systematic review and meta-analysis. *Neurocrit Care* 2016 Sep 6.

8

Intracranial Pressure Monitoring

K. Desai and J. I. Suarez

ABSTRACT

The field of neurocritical care encompasses many different goals aimed towards aggressive and optimal management of neurologically injured, sick, and complicated patients. A very important goal of neurocritical care is to manage secondary brain injury. The latter can be primarily a result of traumatic or vascular conditions. Secondary brain injuries include cerebral oedema, cerebral ischaemia, intracranial hypertension, metabolic dysfunction at the cellular level, and seizures among others, and should be recognized and managed promptly. Intracranial pressure (ICP) monitoring, despite the lack of strong scientific evidence, is a very important parameter for early recognition of these conditions and thus allows for the treatment of these derangements based on individualized protocols. This chapter discusses the pathophysiology of ICP, different ICP waveforms; assessment of ICP trends, ICP derived indices, and the various ICP monitoring devices currently in use.

KEYWORDS

Intracranial pressure (ICP); secondary brain injury; hypoxia; hypotension; cerebrovascular physiology; intracranial hypertension.

INTRODUCTION

The field of neurocritical care encompasses a wide variety of diseases affecting the brain, spinal cord, and peripheral nervous system. In addition, neurointensivists have to encounter the critical interplay between the neurological system and the rest of the organs in the body. A very important goal of neurocritical care is to manage secondary brain injury. Secondary brain injury can result from a myriad of traumatic[1] or vascular aetiologies.[2,3] Secondary brain injury consists of cerebral oedema, cerebral ischaemia, intracranial hypertension, metabolic dysfunction at the cellular level, and nonconvulsive seizures among others. Timely recognition and aggressive management of these conditions help to improve patient outcomes. Recognition requires continuous monitoring with tools that are sensitive and specific enough to be able to detect subtle changes which can then be acted upon to change the trajectory of the disease and its related complications.

The concept of a monitor (from the Latin verb *monere* = to warn) has always been a fundamental aspect of critical care.[4] More recently, multimodality neuromonitoring (MMNM), with published guidelines from the Neurocritical Care Society, is being more commonly used in neurocritical care units (NCCUs) across North America.[5] The impact of MMNM on patient outcomes is not clearly known at this time. There are multiple parameters used either in isolation or in combination to provide cerebral physiological data. These are ICP, brain tissue oxygenation ($PbtO_2$), lactate pyruvate ratio, regional cerebral blood flow, jugular venous oxygen saturation, near infra-red spectroscopy, and electroencephalography (EEG). Thus, careful monitoring of these parameters helps in individualized management of secondary brain injuries, which can be targeted and directed at the underlying patient-specific pathophysiology.

Intracranial pressure has been the most studied and validated parameter in the NCCU. Despite no level 1 recommendations regarding its use and application, ICP monitoring is currently the most commonly used modality in the NCCU. The availability of reliable ICP monitoring devices has facilitated the management of patients with suspected intracranial hypertension. The lack of ICP monitoring can lead to the indiscriminate use of induced hyperventilation and osmotic diuretics compromising cerebral blood flow (CBF), which in term may result in cerebral ischaemia.[4]

INTRACRANIAL PRESSURE: THE BASICS

Lumbar cerebrospinal fluid (CSF) pressure described by Quinke in 1891 was initially used as a surrogate for measurement of ICP. However, the possibility of induced brainstem compression through tonsillar or tentorial herniation resulted in this procedure falling out of favour soon thereafter.[6] In 1960, Lundberg described the technique of direct cannulation of the cerebral ventricular system to measure ICP.[7]

The human brain is viscoelastic in consistency and weighs approximately 1,400 grams in air. If placed on a hard surface, it would collapse under its own weight but once floating in CSF it weighs only about 50 grams. Cerebrospinal fluid shields the brain from coup contrecoup and other types of traumatic injuries. In addition, despite the brain being in a tight box and CSF in a leak-proof craniospinal axis, there is flow of CSF to other extracranial compartments allowing the lumbar-thecal sac to be distended in cases of elevated ICP as CSF is squeezed out of the intracranial compartment.[7]

The Monro–Kellie doctrine states that the total intracranial volume remains more or less constant even if there is a change in the volumes of individual compartments (i.e., brain, blood, and CSF) as illustrated in Figure 8.1.

This means that any additional space occupying entity in the intracranial compartment may result in elevated ICP and eventually herniation, brainstem compression, and brain death, if compensatory mechanisms fail. Many pathological conditions can lead to ICP elevation. There are various causes of increased ICP. An intracranial mass results in cerebral oedema (vasogenic, cytotoxic); increased CSF volume could be due to excessive production, decreased absorption or outflow obstruction and increased intracranial blood volume could be a result of vasodilatation or obstructed venous outflow. Intracranial pressure values vary with body position and the normal range of ICP in the supine position is 7–15 mmHg,[8] which on standing upright, due to hydrostatic pressure gradient becomes negative between –10 mmHg to –15 mmHg.[9] ICP is derived from the circulation of cerebral blood and CSF as follows:

$$ICP = ICP_{vascular} + ICP_{CSF}$$

The vascular component is difficult to quantify and it is derived from the pulsation of cerebral blood volume (CBV) and averaged due to its non-linear mechanisms of regulation.[10] The contributors to the vascular component include arterial blood pressure (ABP), autoregulation, and cerebral venous outflow. The CSF component can be expressed by the Davson's equation:[11]

$$ICP_{CSF} = (\text{resistance to CSF outflow}) \times (\text{CSF formation}) + (\text{pressure in the saggital sinus})$$

Intracranial pressure measurements are used to calculate the cerebral perfusion pressure (CPP).

$$CPP = MAP (\text{Mean Arterial Pressure}) - ICP$$

Cerebral perfusion pressure is the pressure gradient across the cerebrovascular bed and is an important regulator of CBF.[10] Under normal circumstances, cerebral vascular autoregulatory mechanisms are present with CPP values between 50 and 150 mmHg to keep a constant CBF. CPP of 60–70 mmHg is commonly targeted in most neurocritically ill patients irrespective of their malady. CPP is inversely proportional to ICP and is a product of CBF and cerebrovascular resistance. The above equation underlies the importance of CPP-targeted therapies rather than ICP-targeted therapies. Just lowering the ICP without taking into consideration CPP can still result in CPP values <60 mmHg, which can be detrimental in the setting of a secondary brain injury. However, overshooting CPP values >70 mmHg may be detrimental. Robertson et al. compared CPP- and ICP-oriented therapies and showed a decrease in ischaemic insults in CPP-oriented therapy (CPP >70 mmHg) but an increase in respiratory complications with no overall difference in outcome.[12]

In the setting of increased ICP, compliance allows the brain to swell only up to about 10% (Figure 8.1). Any additional swelling will compromise the autoregulatory intracranial mechanisms resulting in early signs of mass effect or herniation if prolonged.[13] Such mechanisms involve CSF and venous outflow adjustments. CSF shifts from the ventricular or subarachnoid space to the spinal compartment. However, the spinal compartment is small and not sufficient to allow the CSF shift to compensate for significant changes in intracranial volume.[14] The second compensatory mechanism involves primarily venous outflow of blood through the cerebral venous system and by changes in calibre of arteries in response to elevated ICP (Figure 8.2). Arterial pressure of carbon dioxide (PaCO_2) is the single most important regulator of arterial calibre changes. Minor compensation also occurs at the level of the arachnoid villi where the resistance to CSF absorption is reduced thus reducing the effective CSF volume. Exhaustion of compensatory reserve results in a linear increase in ICP with increase in intracranial volume. This can be best illustrated based on the pressure-volume curve shown in Figure 8.2. Intracranial compliance is defined as a change in volume for a given change in pressure and it decreases rapidly as the inflection point is passed. In patients with cerebral atrophy, the curve shifts to the right to accommodate for increase in volume.[13]

INTRACRANIAL PRESSURE WAVEFORM AND TRENDS IN MONITORING

The normal ICP waveform has several distinct peaks as shown in Figure 8.3. P1 or WP is the percussion wave thought to be produced by arterial pulsations transmitted from the choroid plexus. P2 or WT is the tidal wave, which represents cerebral compliance. P3 or WD is the dicrotic wave, which represents venous pulsations and occurs due to closure of the aortic valve. Interpretation of ICP waveform is as important as assessment of the trend of ICP values over time rather than a single number. The following patterns can be seen when ICP waveforms are monitored continuously in patients with acute cerebral injury:[10]

1. *Low and stable ICP (below 20 mmHg)*: SEEN in early periods after brain trauma before swelling evolves (Figure 8.4)
2. *High and stable ICP (above 20 mmHg)*: Seen commonly after acute head injury (Figure 8.5)
3. *Vasogenic waves*: Lundberg A and B waves (Figures 8.6 and 8.7). Lundberg A waves, also called plateau waves are seen due to sudden increases in ICP of 50–80 mmHg and may last for 5–20 minutes. These are strong indicators of failing brain compliance and reflect ongoing cerebral ischaemia. Lundberg B waves are due to ICP increase higher than 20 mmHg that last 1–2 minutes.
4. *ICP waves related to changes in arterial pressure and hyperemia* (Figure 8.8)
5. *Refractory intracranial hypertension*: If not promptly addressed, leads to death in most cases (Figure 8.9)

In addition to evaluating the values and contour of the three peaks already discussed, analysis of ICP waveform includes three other components: pulse waveform; respiratory waveform; and slow waves (Figure 8.10).[10]

Pulse waveform has multiple components where frequency is equal to the heart rate. Amplitude of the pulse waveform is most helpful in the evaluation of various indices derived from ICP (Figure 8.10). Respiratory waveform is related to the frequency of the respiratory cycle. Slow waves are not well-defined but the power of ICP slow waves of has been reported to be predictive of outcome in patients with intracranial hypertension post head injury.[15]

Intracranial Pressure Derived Indices

The absolute ICP value is used as a parameter to guide management in patients with intracranial hypertension. However, investigators have continued to define and validate various ways to improve the predictive value of ICP monitoring. One area that has been developed is that of ICP indices, mainly compensatory reserve index (RAP) and pressure reactivity index (PRx).

Compensatory reserve index is a correlation coefficient between the mean ICP and the ICP mean wave amplitude (AMP)—the RAP index [correlation coefficient (R) between AMP amplitude (A) and mean pressure (P); index of compensatory reserve]. This was first introduced as a potential indicator of neurological deterioration in traumatic brain injury (TBI) patients. It was subsequently used to characterize the pressure–volume compensatory reserve in patients with hydrocephalus. The RAP index has been shown to be a reliable measure of the compensatory reserve. The RAP close to 0 suggests good pressure-volume compensatory reserve (Figure 8.11).

The RAP close to +1 suggests low pressure–volume compensatory reserve. The RAP is +1 following head injury and cerebral oedema and any further increase in ICP results in a decrease in AMP and RAP values falling to less than 0. This suggests exhaustion of cerebral autoregulatory reserve and that the cerebral arterioles are unable to dilate any further after this point. The pulse pressure transmission thereby decreases from the arterial bed to the intracranial compartment.

Pressure reactivity index assesses cerebrovascular reactions by observing responses in relation to slow changes in ABP. In the setting of intact cerebral autoregulation and a reactive vascular bed, changes in ABP result in inverse changes in CBV and ICP. On the other hand, in situations with deranged autoregulation and impaired vascular bed reactivity, changes in ABP result in linear changes in ICP. Negative PRx values suggest a reactive vascular bed while positive PRx suggests impaired reactivity of the vascular bed. Abnormal PRx and RAP values have been found to predict poor outcomes following head injury.[16]

INTRACRANIAL PRESSURE MONITORING DEVICES

Several devices to monitor ICP are currently commercially available. The controversy still exists regarding the timing for placement of these devices, rationale to monitor ICP, and the ICP thresholds to target for management. Despite monitoring changes in ICP and utilizing CPP targeted therapies in clinical practice, there are no robust studies supporting improvement in clinical outcomes.[17–20] There are four anatomical locations for placement of ICP monitoring devices: ventricular space, brain parenchyma, subarachnoid space, and epidural space. Each of these has their own advantages and disadvantages. The choice of placement site is usually based on the clinical scenario, feasibility of placement (based on head imaging) and operator experience. Some of the common conditions mandating ICP monitoring are TBI, subarachnoid haemorrhage (SAH), stroke, encephalitis, and fulminant hepatic failure. We will describe each one of these techniques below.

Intraparenchymal Monitor

Intraparenchymal monitors are commonly used (the Camino® device is one of the commercially available ones). They are used for their reliable waveforms, easy maintenance, and simple insertion technique at the bedside. Additional monitoring probes such as the Licox® (PbtO$_2$) or Hemedex® (CBF) can be added to the Camino device. The disadvantages are inability to recalibrate once externally calibrated before placement, fragility of the fibre-optic device and inability to drain/obtain CSF. Their accuracy has been tested in comparison to ventricular catheters and studies have shown variations over a range of 2–5 mmHg. There is the possibility of monitor displacement after 5 days of monitoring and it may need to be replaced. Despite this, there is minimal under- or over-reading.

Intraventricular Monitor

Intraventricular monitors, also known as external ventricular drains (EVD), are also available as the most common devices used for ICP monitoring and CSF drainage in patients with CSF outflow obstruction resulting in acute hydrocephalus. The Codman®, Hummingbird®, and Becker® products are available in the United States. Neurosurgeons usually place these devices and nowadays they are antibiotic-coated to reduce the risk of infection. Placement of EVD and intraparenchymal monitors by neurointensivists has become frequent in some institutions across North America, and studies

have shown no difference in the risk of complications when compared to neurosurgeons.[21] Technical details regarding placement of EVDs are beyond the scope of this chapter.

There are two types of EVD monitors: fluid-coupled and air-coupled. The main advantage of fluid-coupled devices is the ability to re-zero (recalibrate) it after insertion. However, this might be cumbersome for the ICU nursing staff. The level of the transducer has to be at the tragus of the ear to get accurate ICP measurements. Changing the patients' position does not require the device to be re-zeroed. The air coupled device (Hummingbird® variety) senses pressure by utilizing a proprietary bladder filled with air. The advantages here include no need to re-zero, artefact-free readings, and high-fidelity waveforms among others. It also allows for continuous ICP monitoring and CSF drainage at the same time, which is not possible with the fluid-coupled system.

External ventricular drains are used not only for ICP monitoring but also CSF drainage for diagnostic and therapeutic purposes. In addition, EVDs act as conduits for the delivery of chemotherapeutic agents, antibiotics, and recombinant tissue plasminogen activator (rt-PA) in cases of blood clot related obstruction to CSF drainage.[22] The major disadvantages include the invasive nature of the procedure, tracking haemorrhage, infection, difficulty in placement if effaced or a massive shift in ventricles, and upward herniation in cases of posterior fossa lesions. Antibiotic prophylaxis for the short term (preferably 3 days) should be considered in patients receiving EVDs. Based on a randomized study of 228 patients, the infection rate decreased from 11% to 3% with antibiotic use, but there was emergence of methicillin-resistant *Staphylococcus aureus* and *Candida* pathogens.[23] Long-term antibiotic use can lead to *Clostridium difficile* colitis. Efforts to reduce infection include subcutaneous tunnelling of the catheter, minimal access to the catheter unless absolutely necessary, and use of antibiotic-impregnated catheters.

Weaning of EVDs is based on the ability of patients to tolerate a clamping trial. However, there is no consensus on an ideal EVD weaning approach. It has been proposed that an abnormal resorption of CSF is when 200 cc is drained at a level of 20 cm of H$_2$O. Once the CSF drainage is less than the above threshold, clamping trials are started for 24 hours. Early (within 24 hours) versus late (96 hours) weaning does not change the rate of permanent shunt placement; however, patients who had early weaning stayed fewer days in the ICU and hospital.[24] After 24 hours of successful clamping, if the patient remains asymptomatic, a repeat head imaging is suggested to evaluate ventricular size and brain parenchymal masses and shifts. If head imaging also remains unchanged, then the EVD is removed. Prolonged placement of EVD is associated with complications, the rate of ventriculitis based on one study was 3 per cent when EVD was present for more than 10 days.[25] If there is a failure to wean EVD, permanent shunts should be considered and placed promptly.

Subarachnoid Intracranial Pressure Monitor

The subarachnoid bolt is a fluid-coupled system that connects the intracranial space to an external transducer at the bedside via a saline-filled tubing. This is rarely used. The main advantages of subarachnoid bolts are that it is minimally invasive and have a low risk of infection. However, subarachnoid bolts are less accurate when compared to EVDs or intraparenchymal devices, susceptible to blockage from tissue debris and increased cerebral oedema, required frequent recalibration, and are associated with increased risk of bleeding in the subarachnoid space.

Epidural Intracranial Pressure Monitor

The Gaeltec® device is inserted into the inner table of the skull and superficial to the dura mater.[26] This was used more commonly than the intraparenchymal and EVD catheters, especially in patients with underlying coagulopathy where reversal was not possible or those with chronic liver failure. They have become obsolete now with the availability of novel reversal agents for oral anticoagulants.

CLINICAL EVIDENCE FOR INTRACRANIAL PRESSURE MONITORING AND THRESHOLDS

High ICP is related to increased disability and mortality. However, based on a Cochrane database review, the role of routine ICP monitoring in the management of acute encephalopathy is controversial.[27] Relative to normal ICP, elevated ICP is associated with a 3.5- to 6.9-fold increase in the probability of death. Elevated but reducible ICP is associated with 3- to 4-fold increases in the probability of death or a poor neurological outcome. Refractory ICP is associated with significant increase in the relative risk of death (OR >100).[28] Aggressive ICP monitoring and treatment of patients with severe TBI is associated with statistically significant improvement in outcome. The Brain Trauma Foundation has published its guidelines for the management of severe TBI incorporating recommendations for ICP monitoring and management

of intracranial hypertension in 2016.[29] These guidelines state the following:

- There are no Level I or Level IIA recommendations on ICP monitoring.
- There is Level IIB recommendation to use ICP monitoring in the management of severe TBI patients to reduce in-hospital and 2-week post-injury mortality.
- ICP should be monitored in all salvageable patients with a severe TBI (Glasgow coma scale [GCS] 3–8 after resuscitation) and an abnormal CT scan. An abnormal CT scan is one that reveals haematoma, contusions, swelling, herniation, or compressed basal cisterns.
- ICP monitoring is indicated in patients with severe TBI with a normal CT scan if two or more of following are present: Age >40 years, unilateral or bilateral motor posturing, or systolic blood pressure <90 mmHg.

The body of evidence supporting the above recommendations includes four Class 2 and one Class 1 studies. The Class 1 study worthy of mention here is the BEST TRIP Trial, which was published in 2012.[30] The latter compared outcomes of TBI patients in Bolivia/Ecuador whose treatment was informed by ICP monitoring with those whose treatment was informed by imaging and clinical exam. The results showed no difference between the groups for 6-month mortality or 6-month Glasgow Outcome Scale-Extended (GOS-E) scales. Thus, ICP monitoring was not superior to clinical assessment in TBI patients.

Based on the Brain Trauma Foundation Guidelines, fourth edition, the following recommendations were made in regards to ICP thresholds:

- There is insufficient evidence to provide Level I or Level IIA recommendation.
- There is Level IIB recommendation to treat ICP above 22 mmHg as values above this level are associated with increased mortality.
- There is Level III recommendation to support the combined use of ICP and clinical/CT brain findings in making management decisions.

Although Randomised Evaluation of Surgery with Craniectomy for Uncontrollable Elevation of Intracranial Pressure (RESCUEicp) Trial results[31] were not published at the time of release of Brain Trauma Foundation Guidelines, fourth edition, the trial showed lower ICP values (<25 mmHg) and indices in patients who received decompressive craniectomy compared to those who received medical care. The trial also showed a decrease in mortality at 6 months in TBI and refractory intracranial hypertension patients who underwent decompressive craniectomy but at the cost of higher rates of vegetative state, lower severe disability, and upper severe disability.

Without ICP monitoring, significant information, and thereby a good therapeutic target, is unavailable if outside the normal range. ICP monitoring should be used in the context of the entire clinical scenario, i.e., clinical examination and imaging findings should be combined with other measurable and validated multi-modality monitoring tools.

CONCLUSIONS

An important goal of neurocritical care is to prevent and manage secondary brain injury. Despite the lack of strong scientific evidence, ICP monitoring remains a very important parameter for early recognition of brain injury and thus facilitates early intervention and treatment of these derangements.

REFERENCES

1. Bratton SL, Chestnut RM, Ghajar J, et al. Guidelines for the management of severe traumatic brain injury. VI. Indications for intracranial pressure monitoring. *J Neurotrauma* 2007;24(Suppl 1):S37–S44.

2. Andrews PJ, Citerio G. Intracranial pressure. Part one: historical overview and basic concepts. *Intensive Care Med* 2004;30:1730–3.

3. Citerio G, Andrews PJ. Intracranial pressure. Part two: clinical applications and technology. *Intensive Care Med* 2004;30:1882–5.

4. Hemphill JC, Rabinstein AA, Samuels OB. *The Practice of Neurocritical Care by the Neurocritical Care Society*. Chapter 10 Multimodality monitoring. 2015:374–98.

5. Le Roux P, Menon DK, Citerio G, et al. Neurocritical Care Society; European Society of Intensive Care Medicine. Consensus summary statement of the International Multidisciplinary Consensus Conference on Multimodality Monitoring in Neurocritical Care: a statement for healthcare professionals from the Neurocritical Care Society and the European Society of Intensive Care Medicine. *Intensive Care Med* 2014 Sep;40(9):1189–209.

6. Ross N, Eynon CA. Intracranial pressure monitoring. *Curr Anaesth Crit Care* 2006;16:255–61.

7. Lundberg N. Continuous recording and monitoring of ventricular pressure in neurosurgical practice. *Acta Psychiatr Neurol Scand* 1960;140(Suppl):36.

8. Albeck MJ, Borgesen SE, Gjerris F, et al. Intracranial pressure and cerebrospinal fluid outflow conductance in healthy subjects. *J Neurosurg* 1991;74:597–600.

9. Chapman PH, Cosman ER, Arnold MA. The relationship between ventricular fluid pressure and body position in normal subjects and subjects with shunts: A telemetric study. *Neurosurgery* 1990;26:181–9.

10. Czosnyka M, Pickard JD. Monitoring and interpretation of intracranial pressure. *J Neurol Neurosurg Psychiatry* 2004;75:813–21.

11. Davson H, Hollingsworth G, Segal MB. The mechanism of drainage of the cerebrospinal fluid. *Brain* 1970;93: 665–78.

12. Robertson CS, Valadka AB, Hannay HJ, et al. Prevention of secondary ischemic insults after severe head injury. *Crit Care Med* 1999;27:2086–95.

13. Wijdicks EF. *The Practice of Emergency and Critical Care Neurology*. 2nd ed, Chapter 22 Increased Intracranial Pressure. 2016;250–68.

14. Ropper AH, Rockoff MA. Physiology and clinical aspects of raised intracranial pressure. In: Ropper AH, ed. *Neurological and Neurosurgical Intensive Care*. 3rd ed. New York: Raven Press; 1993:11–27.

15. Balestreri M, Czosnyka M. Intracranial hypertension: what additional information can be derived from ICP waveform after head injury? *Acta Neurochir* 2004 Feb;146(2):131–41.

16. Steiner LA, Czosnyka M, Piechnik SK, et al. Continuous monitoring of cerebrovascular pressure reactivity allows determination of optimal cerebral perfusion pressure in patients with traumatic brain injury. *Crit Care Med* 2002;30:733–8.

17. Cremer OL, van Dijk GW, van Wensen E, et al. Effect of intracranial pressure monitoring and targeted intensive care on functional outcome after severe head injury. *Crit Care Med* 2005;33:2207–13.

18. Mack WJ, King RG, Ducruet AF, et al. Intracranial pressure following aneurysmal subarachnoid hemorrhage: monitoring practices and outcome data. *Neurosurg Focus* 2003;14:e3.

19. Rosner MJ, Daughton S. Cerebral perfusion pressure management in head injury. *J Trauma* 1990;30:933–40.

20. Thees C, Scholz M, Schaller MDC, et al. Relationship between intracranial pressure and critical closing pressure in patients with neurotrauma. *Anesthesiology* 2002;96: 595–9.

21. Ehtisham A, Taylor S, Bayless L, Klein MW, Janzen JM. Placement of external ventricular drains and intracranial pressure monitors by neurointensivists. *Neurocrit Care* 2009;10(2):241–7.

22. Ziai WC, Tuhrim S, Lane K, et al. Clear III Investigators. A multicenter, randomized, double-blinded, placebo-controlled phase III study of Clot lysis Evaluation of Accelerated Resolution of Intraventricular Hemorrhage (CLEAR III). *Int J Stroke* 2014 Jun;9(4):536–42.

23. Poon WS, Ng S, Wai S. CSF antibiotic prophylaxis for neurosurgical patients with ventriculostomy: a randomized study. *Acta Neurochir Suppl* 1998;71:146–48.

24. Klopfenstein JD, Kim LJ, Feiz-Erfan I, et al. Comparison of rapid and gradual weaning from external ventricular

drainage in patients with aneurysmal subarachnoid hemorrhage: a prospective randomized trial. *J Neurosurg* 2004;100:225–9.

25. Martinez-Manas RM, Santamarta D, de Campos JM, Ferrer E. Camino intracranial pressure monitor: prospective study of accuracy and complication. *J Neurol Neurosurg Psychiatry* 2000;69:82–86.

26. Amin N, Greene-Chandos D. Intracranial pressure monitoring. In: Editors: Miller CM, Torbey MT. Neurocritical Care Monitoring. demos MEDICAL, New York, 2015:1–17.

27. Forsyth RJ, Wolny S, Rodrigues B. Routine intracranial pressure monitoring in acute coma. *Cochrane Database Syst Rev* 2010(2):CD002043.

28. Stein SC, Georgoff P, Meghan S, et al. Relationship of aggressive monitoring and treatment to improved outcomes in severe traumatic brain injury. *J Neurosurg* 2010;112:1105–12.

29. Guidelines for the management of severe traumatic brain injury, 4th ed. Sept 2016. Available from: https://www.braintrauma.org/uploads/13/06/Guidelines_for_Management_of_Severe_TBI_4th_Edition.pdf. Last accessed on 27 July 2018.

30. Chestnut RM, Temkin N, Carney N, et al. A trial of intracranial-pressure monitoring in traumatic brain injury, *N Engl J Med* 2012;367:26.

31. Hutchinson PJ, Kolias AG, Timofeev IS, et al. Trial of decompressive craniectomy for traumatic intracranial HTN. *N Engl J Med* 2016;375:12.

9

Cerebral Oxygenation

B. Butt and J. I. Suarez

ABSTRACT

Cerebral oxygenation is a balance between cerebral oxygen supply and demand, and a mismatch can lead to cerebral hypoxia or ischaemia with adverse outcomes. Currently several devices are available for the detection of cerebral hypoxia and ischaemia, each with their own advantages and disadvantages. Even though there is evidence suggesting an association between cerebral hypoxia/ischaemia and poor outcomes, it still remains to be determined whether restoring cerebral oxygenation improves outcomes. None of the monitors for cerebral oxygenation are sufficiently effective to be considered as the standard of care.

KEYWORDS

Brain tissue oxygenation; cerebral metabolism; hypoxia; oxygen delivery; oxygen consumption.

INTRODUCTION

Hypoxia is defined as a condition in which the tissues of the body do not receive sufficient oxygen supply.[1,2] It is an interruption in oxygen supply whereas ischaemia refers to the interruption of oxygen supply and impairment of blood flow.[3] Hypoxia can lead to detrimental consequences for the brain even though the brain represents only 2% of the total body weight. The brain consumes a disproportionate portion of the total body oxygen consumption because of its high cellular demand.[4] At the onset of acute hypoxia, the human body attempts to maintain adequate oxygenation but body stores of oxygen are limited. As a result, anaerobic metabolism ensues and lactic acid increases due to inadequate mitochondrial oxygenation, which, if severe, can lead to cell death. Hypoxia generates systemic changes that are meant to compensate for the lack of oxygen. For example, hypoxia is detected by the carotid body chemoreceptors, which in turn mediate a response resulting in hyperventilation. It is important to note that in patients under the influence of general anaesthesia, muscle relaxants or opioids, this response is hampered. In addition, acute hypoxia results in increased sympathetic nervous discharge, which translates into a constellation of symptoms such as shortness of breath, tachypnoea,

tachycardia, cyanosis, diaphoresis, and confusion.[5] The clinical manifestations of cerebral hypoxia and ischaemia can remain occult in sedated or unconscious patients and hence brain monitoring is helpful to detect reduced cerebral oxygenation.[6]

CEREBRAL METABOLISM AND OXYGEN CONSUMPTION

Neurons lack oxygen storage, have limited reserves of glycogen, and are dependent on adequate cerebral blood flow (CBF). Therefore, neurons are sensitive to hypoxic and ischaemic states. Increased oxygen demand or decreased oxygen supply is counteracted by increased CBF. Acute hypoxia is a potent cerebral vasodilator that results in an increase in CBF and also increases nitric oxide and adenosine which in turn further contribute to vasodilation.[5] However, there are limits to the CBF autoregulation.

In anaerobic states, the regeneration of nicotinamide adenine dinucleotide (NAD^+) from reduced NADH has to be accomplished through the conversion of pyruvate to lactate and a hydrogen ion through lactate dehydrogenase. However, this pathway is not efficient as it only yields 2 molar equivalents of adenosine-5-triphosphate (ATP) for each mole of glucose. On the other hand, approximately 30–38 moles of ATP are generated under aerobic conditions. If the hypoxic/ischaemic state is not reversed, the consequence is mitochondrial failure which increases intracellular calcium. Intracellular calcium regulates the activity of lipolytic enzymes, proteolytic enzymes, protein kinases, protein phosphatases, and gene activation and expression. Thus, an ischaemic insult results in excessive increase in intracellular calcium, which in turn leads to neuronal death. Furthermore, excessive neuronal depolarization occurs during cerebral ischaemia. Glutamate, an excitatory neurotransmitter, is released in excess after cerebral ischaemia and activates glutamate receptors. The N-methyl-D-aspartate (NMDA) and amino-3-hydroxy-5-methyl-4-isoxazolepropionate (AMP) glutamate receptors are linked to influx of calcium and the resultant cellular damage from calcium described above. In addition, reperfusion injury caused by the production of free radicals has been hypothesized to further contribute to secondary injury and delayed cell death. Increased free radical formation causes increased lipid peroxidation, protein oxidation, and deoxyribonucleic acid (DNA) damage.[7,8]

Cortical spreading depression (CSD) or spreading depolarization is another phenomenon worth mentioning. It is characterized by a wave of electrophysiological hyperactivity followed by a wave of inhibition. Cortical spreading depression is elicited from focal ischaemic injury, traumatic brain injury (TBI) and haemorrhage. It leads to depressed spontaneous cortical activity lasting anywhere from minutes to hours. CSD and depolarization waves are associated with dramatic failure of brain ion homeostasis, efflux of excitatory amino acids from nerve cells, increased energy metabolism and changes in CBF. A prospective multicenter study has shown that after controlling for other variables associated with poor prognosis, CSD in TBI patients is associated with a worse prognosis.[9,10]

The brain extracts oxygen from arterial blood at a rate sufficient to meet its metabolic requirements and leaving an oxygen-poor venous effluent. The saturation of oxygen of this venous blood is related to the cerebral metabolic rate for oxygen ($CMRO_2$) and CBF by the Fick's equation:[11]

$$CMRO_2 = CBF \times (CaO_2 - CjO_2)$$

CaO_2 represents arterial oxygen content while CjO_2 represents jugular venous oxygen content. $CaO_2 - CajO_2$ represents arteriovenous oxygen difference ($AVDO_2$) and with the above equation rearranged $AVDO_2$ is a ratio of $CMRO_2$/CBF. $AVDO_2$ in a healthy brain is in the range of 4–9 ml/dL; a higher value represents a scenario where

blood flow is low relative to metabolic requirements. Conversely, a lower value represents hyperaemia.[11]

CEREBRAL VENOUS DRAINAGE

Deoxygenated blood from the brain drains into the major venous sinuses and eventually into the sigmoid sinuses. It then drains into the internal jugular veins with the exception of the paired inferior petrosal sinuses which drain directly into the internal jugular vein. The right internal jugular vein is usually the dominant side. At the origin in the posterior jugular foramen, the internal jugular vein is dilated and this portion is known as the jugular bulb. Of note, the facial vein which is transporting extracerebral blood drains into the internal jugular vein a few centimetres below the jugular bulb. Furthermore, the caudal portion of the internal jugular vein also dilates again before joining the subclavian vein and this is known as the interior jugular bulb.[11]

CEREBRAL OXYGENATION MONITORING

There are different methods available for global and regional cerebral oxygenation monitoring. The jugular venous oxygen saturation ($SjvO_2$) monitoring assesses for global oxygenation whereas brain tissue oxygen tension ($PbtO_2$) and near-infrared spectroscopy (NIRS) based cerebral oximetry measures regional oxygenation. In addition, cerebral microdialysis (CMD) assesses local brain tissue biochemistry.

Jugular Venous Oxygen Saturation

Monitoring of $SjvO_2$ was the first bedside measure of cerebral oxygenation. It is important to recognize that $SjvO_2$ represents a global estimate of cerebral oxygenation.[12] Jugular venous oxygen saturation was initially performed by placing a needle into the jugular bulb which is approximately 1 centimetre anterior and inferior to the mastoid process. The blood was analysed from this location for oxygen saturation of haemoglobin and a reading of less than 50% was considered 'critical' as it indicated cerebral hypoxia. This technique was then used during carotid endarterectomy (CEA) or to calculate $AVDO_2$ in neurocritical care units (NCCUs).[13]

Jugular venous oxygen saturation intends to measure the balance between cerebral oxygen supply and demand. It can be measured in two ways. This can be done through intermittent blood sampling obtained from the internal jugular vein or in a continuous fashion by the insertion of an oximetry catheter into the jugular bulb.[5] The median normal value for $SjvO_2$ typically is around 62% and the normal value range lies between 55% and 75%.[14] A drop in this value would indicate increased cerebral metabolic rate, hyperthermia, pain, seizures, reduced CBF or reduced oxygen delivery from inadequate cerebral perfusion, vasoconstriction, vasospasm, arterial hypoxia, hypotension, or anaemia. Higher values of $SjvO_2$ on the other hand would indicate an increased CBF or reduced cerebral metabolic rate as in brain death, arteriovenous shunting, hypothermia, coma, intake of sedative drugs, increased cerebral perfusion pressure (CPP), vasodilation, systemic hypertension, and other causes of oxygen utilization failure.[5,11]

In a retrospective study investigating $SjvO_2$ measurements, patients were divided into two groups, one with abnormal values (i.e., less than 55% or greater than 75%), and another group with normal values.[15,16] Patients in the abnormal group had a significantly higher occurrence of intracranial hypertension. The events associated with $SjvO_2$ desaturations were hyperventilation, hypovolaemia, and anaemia.

In TBI at least, jugular venous desaturation is related to CBF reduction which in turn is often due to reduced CPP from various causes including increased intracranial pressure (ICP), cerebral vasospasm, hypotension or vasoconstriction secondary to hypocapnia.[17]

The Brain Trauma Foundation has listed level III evidence in support of maintaining $SjvO_2$ over 50%.[18] Jugular venous oxygen saturation monitoring had traditionally been utilized for cardiac surgeries, but its main utility is in the NCCU where it helps detect deficiency in cerebral perfusion after TBI and subarachnoid haemorrhage (SAH). Jugular venous oxygen saturation has also helped in the past to guide therapeutic hyperventilation. It has been shown that patients with severe TBI defined by a Glasgow Coma Scale (GCS) of less than 8, a single reading of $SjvO_2$ less than 50% lasting more than 10 minutes was associated with increased mortality.[19] Furthermore, multiple or prolonged episodes of jugular venous desaturation in addition to $SjvO_2$ values over 75% also are associated with a bleak or poor long-term prognosis post TBI.[20,21]

Elevations in $SjvO_2$ constitutes a heterogeneous group of conditions and are commonly associated with hyperaemia, but also with reduced cerebral metabolic demand, arteriovenous shunting or even cell death. In addition, $SjvO_2$ has also been studied as a possible prognostic marker in comatose survivors of cardiac arrest. Jugular venous oxygen saturation is not low in these patients except in the setting of cardiac failure when mixed venous oxygen saturation also falls. In non-survivors, a gradual increase in $SjvO_2$ as compared to mixed venous oxygen is seen over 24 hours after resuscitation. This suggests a global failure of cerebral oxygen extraction. Jugular venous oxygen saturation becoming greater than mixed venous oxygen at 24 hours is reasonably specific for increased mortality.[11]

It is important to realize the limitations that come with $SjvO_2$ measurements. First, the dominant jugular vein needs to be cannulated, which is the right side in most cases. Second, the positioning of the catheter is important to prevent mixture of blood samples with extracranial circulation. Third, there is catheter associated risks which include risk of thrombosis of the jugular vein, puncture of the carotid artery during insertion, and haematoma. Fourth, as already mentioned, $SjvO_2$ measures global cerebral ischaemia and therefore regional areas of ischaemia can be missed when using this modality.[6] Lastly, it has been shown that with a combination of positron emission tomography (PET) and $SjvO_2$ more than 13% of the brain needs to become ischaemic before the $SjvO_2$ begins to fall below the threshold of 50%.[12]

Arteriovenous oxygen difference, which is the amount of oxygen extracted by the brain from each deciliter of blood supplied to it, is obtained by sampling of jugular venous bulb blood sampling. It is important to confirm placement of the jugular venous catheter with imaging to ensure that the position of the catheter tip is in the region of the jugular bulb, which would prevent contamination of extracranial blood, namely the facial vein. Slight changes in position of the catheter tip during nursing care can lead to inaccurate sampling.[22] However, we must note that there are no trials available so far showing benefit of $SjvO_2$ directed therapy on patient outcome in the NCCU.[6]

Brain Tissue Oxygen Tension

Brain tissue oxygen tension provides local measurements of brain oxygenation in contrast to the global readings of $SjvO_2$. It represents a dynamic variable which entails interaction between cerebral oxygen delivery and demand along with tissue oxygen diffusion gradients. Moreover, $PbtO_2$ actually represents a biomarker for cellular function and not a simple monitor for hypoxia.[6] Both local cerebral and systemic variables affect the $PbtO_2$. The cerebral variables include CPP, ICP, CBF, cerebral vasospasm, and brain tissue gradients for oxygen diffusion whereas the systemic variables include PaO_2, $PaCO_2$, FiO_2, mean arterial pressures, haemoglobin level, and cardiopulmonary function.[6] It is unclear which intervention or even combination of interventions is most useful in improving $PbtO_2$.[6,23] Normal values of $PbtO_2$ have been reported to be from 35 mmHg to

50 mmHg and a value less than 15 mmHg could be considered as a marker for focal cerebral ischaemia.[2] Preliminary evidence suggests that patients managed with $PbtO_2$-guided therapy have associated improved clinical outcome after severe TBI. Among patients that received $PbtO_2$ therapy, 38.8% had an unfavourable outcome and 61.2% had a favourable outcome. Furthermore, combined ICP/CPP and $PbtO_2$ monitoring equated to a better outcome after severe TBI than ICP/CPP therapy alone.[17,24] Moreover, brain hypoxia which was defined as either $PbtO_2$ <15 mmHg or <10 mmHg was associated with worse clinical outcomes.[24] Of note, brain oxygen monitoring with $PbtO_2$ was part of the guidelines for management of severe TBI (GCS <8) in 2007.[24,25]

Brain tissue oxygen tension probes should be inserted in non-lesioned brain tissue as these are the areas that are most responsive to changes in oxygen delivery.[13,26] $PbtO_2$ monitoring is mainly used in patients with TBI and poor-grade SAH to help guide management, but it also has been used during surgery for intracranial aneurysms, arteriovenous malformations, and cerebral angiography. Guidelines from the Neurocritical Care Society recommend $PbtO_2$ monitoring in comatose patients with SAH to help identify patients at high risk of delayed cerebral ischaemia (DCI). In addition, $PbtO_2$ monitoring has also been used in determining the target $PaCO_2$ during hyperventilation as a mode to reduce intracranial hypertension because cerebral ischaemia can happen with even the modest reductions in $PaCO_2$.[12,27] Brain tissue oxygen tension monitoring has also been used in intracerebral haemorrhage (ICH) where it may help identify an optimal CPP target.[6]

There is no clear consensus on the treatment of low $PbtO_2$ at the moment. If $PbtO_2$ is less than 20 mmHg, head positioning is satisfactory and the probe is functioning, and one can consider the following manoeuvres sequentially or in parallel: increasing fraction of inspired oxygen (FiO_2); adding positive end-expiratory pressure (PEEP); endotracheal tube suctioning, physiotherapy, and obtaining a chest radiography to clear the airways and rule out parenchymal lung disease; checking haemoglobin and administering blood if anaemic; reducing ICP; reducing excessive metabolic demand through analgesics to alleviate pain; administering antipyretics if patients are febrile; and checking for seizures using electroencephalogram (EEG).[6]

It is important to realize that there are no definitive randomized controlled clinical trials suggesting the utility of $PbtO_2$-guided therapy on outcomes following severe TBI.[12] Brain tissue oxygen tension monitoring catheters are similar in size to intraparenchymal ICP monitors and are placed via bolt, burr hole or craniotomy in the subcortical white matter. The readings within the first hour are inaccurate and a run-in period is important. As already mentioned, $PbtO_2$ monitoring provides focal or local readings and the area interrogated by the probe is approximately 17 mm^2. Thus, the placement of the probe is important and should ideally be in the perilesional area where there is viable and at-risk brain tissue. Satisfactory position of the probe should be confirmed with non-contrast head computed tomography (CT) scanning.[6]

The main limitation of the $PbtO_2$ monitoring is obviously its invasiveness and thus it is usually reserved for patients with severe TBI. Another limitation is that because of the local nature of the monitoring, it may miss important pathology away from the probe location. Therefore, adequate probe positioning is very important. Furthermore, the fact that there is one hour run-in period increases the chances of missing early ischaemic/hypoxic changes.[6] Lastly, despite the low chance of intraparenchymal haemorrhage, it is relatively safe. There are currently two commercial probes available in the United States for $PbtO_2$ monitoring: Licox® probe and the Neurovent PTO®.[13] The greatest advantage of $PbtO_2$ monitoring is that it provides focal real-time monitoring of critically perfused tissue.[13,28]

Near-Infrared Spectroscopy

Tissues contain light absorbing pigments known as chromophores namely haemoglobin, myoglobin, and cytochrome oxidase, which have absorption spectra that depend on their redox state.[11] The NIRS is based on the transmission and absorption of near-infrared light (wavelength ranging from 700–950 nm) as it passes through tissue. Currently, cerebral oximetry obtained by NIRS is the only non-invasive bedside tool for cerebral oxygenation. However, the available commercial devices measure regional cerebral oxygen saturation ($rScO_2$). Near-infrared spectroscopy assesses arterial, venous, and capillary blood within the field of view so the measured $rScO_2$ values actually represent tissue oxygen saturation from all three compartments.[6] Since most of the blood in the brain is venous, NIRS oximetry gives a measure of mostly venous oxygen saturation which reflects oxygen extraction.[11] The $rScO_2$ values are affected by several variables including arterial oxygen saturation, $PaCO_2$, blood pressure, haematocrit, CBF, cerebral blood volume, and cerebral metabolic rate of oxygen ($CMRO_2$).[6]

Cerebral oximeters can be divided into two main groups namely the saturation monitors and concentration monitors. Saturation monitors measure the ratio of haemoglobin and oxyhaemoglobin without including path length in the calculation while concentration monitors measure the amount of oxyhaemoglobin and reduced haemoglobin.[13] The NIRS has been utilized during cardiac surgery, carotid surgery, and surgery with the head-up position.[6,29] Near-infrared spectroscopy has also been used to monitor cortical changes during cerebral vasospasm after SAH.[29]

Studies have investigated NIRS in patients with carotid occlusive disease. Intraoperative NIRS during CEA showed cerebral desaturation in 50% patients after internal carotid cross-clamping. Cerebral oxygen saturation has been shown to correlate with transcranial Doppler blood flow velocities, electroencephalogram readings, and clinical evidence of ischaemia. A drop in tissue oxygenation index (TOI) of more than 13% has been shown to be the threshold for ischaemia.[11] The use of NIRS to monitor TBI patients has also shown similar changes with regard to oxygenation status with other monitoring devices. Near-infrared spectroscopy was able to detect 97% of cerebral hypoperfusion events as compared with 53% detected by jugular bulb oximetry.[11]

The normal reported range of $rScO_2$ is between 60% and 75% but there is some intra-individual and inter-individual variability. Hence, NIRS-based cerebral oximetry is considered to be a trend monitor. Although there is no established $rScO_2$ ischaemic threshold, clinical studies use values less than or equal to 50% or greater than or equal to 20% from baseline as a trigger to initiate interventions to improve cerebral oxygenation.[6] Low values of $rScO_2$ have been associated with poor outcomes after acute brain injury, but the use of NIRS in brain injury has been hampered by the inability to define NIRS-derived thresholds for hypoxia or ischaemia and the lack of a gold standard against which to compare NIRS-derived variables.[12] A study of TBI patients identified an association between $rScO_2$ values below 60% for an increased amount of time and intracranial hypertension, low CPP, and mortality.[12,30]

The advantages of NIRS over other neuroimaging techniques are that NIRS is non-invasive, has high temporal and spatial resolution, and provides simultaneous measurements over multiple regions of interest. However, comparison of NIRS with $SjvO_2$ has shown that NIRS is less accurate in determining cerebral oxygenation.[17,31] A disadvantage of NIRS includes contamination of extracerebral circulation, which decreases the accuracy of measurements. Furthermore, there is a lack of standardization between commercial devices. Lastly, as mentioned before, the thresholds for cerebral hypoxia or ischaemia have not been definitely determined.[6]

Cerebral Microdialysis

Cerebral microdialysis is a bedside monitor used to analyse brain tissue biochemistry. It was introduced in the mid-1990's and is now more commonly used as a bedside monitor to identify cerebral hypoxia and ischaemia. Cerebral microdialysis is a regional monitoring technique that characterizes local tissue biochemistry. The CMD technique is based on the principle of diffusion of water soluble substances through a semipermeable membrane. The catheter, when inserted into brain tissue, is perfused with isotonic fluid within the surrounding tissue interstitium. This perfusate, such as Ringer's solution, enters the microdialysis catheter through the inlet tube, which then flows to the catheter tip and in turn is lined by a semipermeable membrane across which exchange of molecules between the interstitial and perfusion fluid takes place. This fluid then passes out via the outlet tube to a collecting chamber known as the microvial, which is then sent for analysis. Like with other modalities, the selection of the correct site for monitoring is paramount. For TBI individuals, it is recommended that the CMD catheter be located in 'at risk' pericontusional brain tissue, and if possible placement of a second catheter in 'normal' tissue as well. Cerebral microdialysis samples are usually collected at hourly intervals at the bedside and analyzed using commercially available monitors. These monitors include measurements for analysis of glucose, pyruvate, lactate, glycerol, and glutamate. As CMD is an invasive procedure, there exists the chance of insertion-related complications such as a small amount of intracerebral blood around the catheter, but these are rare.[32] Applications for CMD include TBI and SAH. Cerebral hypoxia/ischaemia causes a significant increase in lactate as described above and hence the lactate–pyruvate ratio (LPR) increases in hypoxic states. An LPR greater than 20–25 is considered a threshold for cerebral ischaemia and associated with poor outcomes in TBI.[17]

CONCLUSIONS

Cerebral oxygenation is a balance between cerebral oxygen supply and demand. There are several available devices for the detection of cerebral hypoxia and ischaemia. However, none of the monitors for cerebral oxygenation have become effective enough to become the standard of care.

REFERENCES

1. Ward DS, Karan SB, Pandit JJ. Hypoxia: developments in basic science, physiology and clinical studies. *Anaesthesia* 2011;66(Suppl 2):19–26.

2. Bullock MR, Povlishock JT. Guidelines for the management of severe traumatic brain injury. *J Neurotrauma* 2007; 24(Suppl 1):2 p preceding S1.

3. Zauner A, Daugherty WP, Bullock MR, et al. Brain oxygenation and energy metabolism: part I-biological function and pathophysiology. *Neurosurgery* 2002;51(2): 289–301; discussion 302.

4. Masamoto K, Tanishita K. Oxygen transport in brain tissue. *J Biomech Eng* 2009;131(7):074002.

5. Manninen PH, Unger ZM. Chapter 21 - Hypoxia A2. In: Prabhakar, Hemanshu, eds. *Complications in Neuroanesthesia.* 2016; Academic Press: San Diego. pp. 169–80.

6. Kirkman MA, Smith M. Brain Oxygenation Monitoring. *Anesthesiol Clin* 2016;34(3):537–56.

7. Dunn IF, et al. Principles of cerebral oxygenation and blood flow in the neurological critical care unit. *Neurocrit Care* 2006;4(1):77–82.

8. Mulvey JM, et al. Multimodality monitoring in severe traumatic brain injury: the role of brain tissue oxygenation monitoring. *Neurocrit Care* 2004;1(3):391–402.

9. Hartings JA, et al. Spreading depolarisations and outcome after traumatic brain injury: a prospective observational study. *The Lancet Neurology* 2011;10(12):1058–64.

10. Lazaridis C. Cerebral oxidative metabolism failure in traumatic brain injury: 'Brain shock'. *J Crit Care* 2017 Feb;37:230–3.

11. Ercole A, Gupta AK. Cerebral oxygenation. In: Matta BF, Menon DK, Smith M, editors. *Core Topics in Neuroanaesthesia and Neurointensive Care.* Cambridge: Cambridge University Press, 2011;72–84.

12. Smith M, Citerio G, Kofke WA. *Oxford Textbook of Neurocritical Care.* 2016: 129–40.

13. Smythe PR, Samra SK. Monitors of cerebral oxygenation. *Anesthesiol Clin North America* 2002;20(2):293–313.

14. Robertson CS, Cormio M. Cerebral metabolic management. *New Horiz* 1995;3(3):410–22.

15. Schoon P, et al. Incidence of intracranial hypertension related to jugular bulb oxygen saturation disturbances in severe traumatic brain injury patients. *Acta Neurochir Suppl* 2002;81:285–7.

16. Dutton RP, McCunn M. Traumatic brain injury. *Curr Opin Crit Care* 2003;9(6):503–9.

17. Haddad SH, Arabi YM. Critical care management of severe traumatic brain injury in adults. *Scand J Trauma Resusc Emerg Med* 2012;20:12.

18. Carney N, Totten AM, O'Reilly C, et al. Guidelines for the management of severe traumatic brain injury, 4th ed. *Neurosurgery* 2017 Jan 1;80(1):6–15.

19. Feldman Z, Robertson CS. Monitoring of cerebral hemodynamics with jugular bulb catheters. *Crit Care Clin* 1997;13(1):51–77.

20. Macmillan CS, Andrews PJ, Easton VJ. Increased jugular bulb saturation is associated with poor outcome in traumatic brain injury. *J Neurol Neurosurg Psychiatry* 2001; 70(1):101–4.

21. Cormio M, Valadka AB, Robertson CS. Elevated jugular venous oxygen saturation after severe head injury. *J Neurosurg* 1999;90(1): 9–15.

22. Pennings FA, Bouma GJ, Ince C. The assessment of determinants of cerebral oxygenation and microcirculation in cerebral blood flow: mechanisms of ischemia, diagnosis, and therapy. Springer Berlin Heidelberg: Berlin, Heidelberg. 2002;149–64.

23. Bohman LE, et al. Response of brain oxygen to therapy correlates with long-term outcome after subarachnoid hemorrhage. *Neurocrit Care* 2013;19(3):320–8.

24. Nangunoori R, et al. Brain tissue oxygen-based therapy and outcome after severe traumatic brain injury: a systematic literature review. *Neurocrit Care* 2012;17(1):131–8.

25. Brain Trauma Foundation, American Association of Neurological Surgeons, Congress of Neurological Surgeons et al. Guidelines for the management of severe traumatic brain injury. Brain oxygen monitoring and thresholds. *J Neurotrauma* 2007;24(Suppl 1):S65–70.

26. Sarrafzadeh AS, et al. Cerebral oxygenation in contusioned vs. nonlesioned brain tissue: monitoring of PtiO2 with Licox and Paratrend. *Acta Neurochir Suppl* 1998;71:186–9.

27. Rangel-Castilla L, et al. Cerebral hemodynamic effects of acute hyperoxia and hyperventilation after severe traumatic brain injury. *J Neurotrauma* 2010;27(10): 1853–63.

28. Dings J, Meixensberger J, Roosen K. Brain tissue pO2-monitoring: catheter stability and complications. *Neurol Res* 1997;19(3):241–5.

29. Ghosh A, Elwell C, Smith M. Review article: cerebral near-infrared spectroscopy in adults: a work in progress. *Anesth Analg* 2012;115(6):1373–83.

30. Dunham CM, et al. Cerebral hypoxia in severely brain-injured patients is associated with admission Glasgow Coma Scale score, computed tomographic severity, cerebral perfusion pressure, and survival. *J Trauma* 2004;56(3):482–9; discussion 489–91.

31. Lewis SB, et al. Cerebral oxygenation monitoring by near-infrared spectroscopy is not clinically useful in patients with severe closed-head injury: a comparison with jugular venous bulb oximetry. *Crit Care Med* 1996; 24(8): 1334–8.

32. Ghosh A, Smith M. Brain tissue biochemistry. *Core Topics in Neuroanaesthesia and Neurointensive Care.* In: Matta BF, Menon DK, Smith M, editors. Cambridge: Cambridge University Press, 2011;85–100.

10

Cerebral Metabolism

S. Sivakumar and J. I. Suarez

ABSTRACT

High-energy phosphates derived from aerobic metabolism of glucose contribute to a majority of cerebral metabolic needs during normal physiological states. Cerebral energy dysfunction has been identified as an important determinant of prognosis in states of acute brain injury. Monitoring of cerebral metabolism using cerebral microdialysis, positron emission tomography, and jugular bulb oximetry in these patients reveal energy dysfunction with reduced availability and utilization of glucose and an increase in utilization of alternative energy sources like lactate. Secondary injury is characterized by a cascade of cellular and molecular events consisting of ischaemic, metabolic, and immunological insults initiated by the primary event which can occur at lower thresholds in a susceptible brain. One of the goals of multimodal monitoring in neurointensive care is to detect potentially harmful pathophysiological events before they cause irreversible brain injury; therefore, research aimed at integration of data from multimodal monitoring to improve clinical outcomes are underway.

KEYWORDS

Metabolism; metabolic rate; tissue oxygen tension; metabolic crisis; mitochondria; multimodal monitoring; microdialysis.

INTRODUCTION

An understanding of normal cerebral metabolism, its relationship with cerebral blood flow (CBF), and its response to pathological derangements help in the management of patients with acute brain injury. This chapter reviews the basic principles of cerebral metabolism, the relationship between cerebral metabolism and CBF in normal physiology and in brain injury. In addition, an overview of the methods available for monitoring cerebral metabolism, their practical implications, and current literature on cerebral metabolism in acute brain injury are discussed.

CEREBRAL METABOLISM

The human brain has a high metabolic demand relative to other tissues. The brain receives about 15%–20% of the resting cardiac output and uses up to 20% of total oxygen consumption and 25% of total glucose consumption.[1] About 50% of this energy expenditure is for synaptic activity; 25% is used for maintenance of transmembrane ionic gradients and the remaining energy is spent on biosynthesis.[2] The majority of cerebral energy consumption is by the neurons with less than 10% constituting glial cells.[3] Although energy requirements of the brain are substantial, the brain lacks the ability to store fuel and has a very small reserve of metabolic substrates, thereby, requiring a constant supply of energy metabolites.[4] The energy necessary for these processes are generated from the metabolism of a number of energy substrates such as glucose, ketone bodies, lactate, glycerol, fatty acids, and amino acids. However, glucose is the preferred substrate (Table 10.1).

Principles of Brain Glucose Metabolism

Under normal physiological conditions, the brain depends on high-energy phosphates such as adenosine triphosphate (ATP) derived from the aerobic metabolism of glucose. The rate-limiting step in glucose metabolism

Table 10.1 Cerebral haemodynamic and metabolic parameters

Parameter	Formula
Ohms law for flow (Q)	$\dfrac{\text{Pressure gradient between inflow and outflow }(\Delta P)}{\text{Resistance (R)}}$
Poiseuille's law for flow (Q)	$Q = (\Pi r^4 \Delta P)/8\eta L$ r: radius; η: viscosity; L: length
Cerebral perfusion pressure (CPP)	Mean arterial pressure (MAP) − Intracranial pressure (ICP)
Cerebral Blood Flow (CBF) (ml/min) [By central volume principle]	$CBF = \dfrac{\text{Cerebral blood volume}}{\text{Mean transit time (T)}}$
Arterial oxygen content (CaO_2) (ml/dL)	$1.34 \times \text{Haemoglobin} \times SaO_2 + 0.0031 \times PaO_2$
Jugular venous oxygen content $CjvO_2$ (ml/dL)	$1.34 \times \text{Haemoglobin} \times SjvO_2 + 0.0031 \times PjvO_2$
Arteriovenous oxygen difference $AVDO_2$ (ml/dL)	CaO_2 (ml/dL) − $CjvO_2$ (ml/dL)
Oxygen extraction ratio (O_2ER) (%)	$\dfrac{AVDO_2\left(\frac{ml}{dL}\right)}{CaO_2\left(\frac{ml}{dL}\right)} \times 100\% = \dfrac{VO_2\,(\text{oxygen uptake})}{DO_2\,(\text{oxygen delivery})}$
Arteriovenous glucose difference AVDG (ml/dL)	ArtGluc (ml/dL) − JVGluc (ml/dL)
Arteriovenous lactate difference AVDL (ml/dL)	ArtLact (ml/dL) − JVLact (ml/dL)
Cerebral metabolic rate of oxygen $(CMRO_2)$ (ml/100 g/min)	$\dfrac{AVDO_2\left(\frac{ml}{dL}\right) \times CBF\left(\frac{ml}{100g}{min}\right)}{100}$
Cerebral metabolic rate of glucose CMRG (ml/100 g/min)	AVDG (ml/dL) × CBF (ml/100 g/min)/100
Cerebral metabolic rate of lactate CMRL (ml/100 g/min)	AVDL (ml/dL) × CBF (ml/100 g/min)/100
Metabolic ratio (MR)	$CMRO_2/CMRG$
Aerobic index (AI)	$AI\,(\%) = \dfrac{AVDO_2\left(\frac{\mu mol}{ml}\right)}{6 \times AVDG\left(\frac{\mu mol}{ml}\right)} \times 100\%$
Anaerobic Index (ANI)	$ANI\,(\%) = \dfrac{AVDL\left(\frac{\mu mol}{ml}\right)}{2 \times AVDG\left(\frac{\mu mol}{ml}\right)} \times 100\%$

is the entry of glucose into the cell, which is facilitated by carrier-mediated mechanisms (endothelial glucose transporter 1)[5] and by simple diffusion. Shuttling from the extracellular space into astrocytes and neurons occurs through glucose transporter 1 and glucose transporter 3, respectively.[6] Glucose is metabolized in two sequential pathways: glycolysis and oxidative phosphorylation. The complete oxidation of one molecule of glucose in the cell produces 38 moles of ATP represented by the following equation:

$$C_6H_{12}O_6 + 6O_2 + 38\ ADP + 38\ P_i \rightarrow 6CO_2 + 44H_2O + 38ATP$$

The first set of chemical reactions that occur in the cytoplasm is known as glycolysis. In this process, one molecule of glucose is converted into two molecules of pyruvic acid with a net gain of two molecules of ATP. Under anaerobic conditions, pyruvic acid is reduced to lactic acid, which may remain within the cell for metabolism or be transported back into the bloodstream. While nearly 15% of pyruvate is converted into lactate under normal physiological states, this amount can increase to partially supply energy demands. Pyruvate diffuses across cellular compartments and reaches the mitochondria, where, in the presence of oxygen, it enters the citric acid cycle (Krebs cycle). The citric acid cycle is a common pathway for oxidation of molecules and a source of building blocks for biosynthesis, generation of ATP, CO_2 and nicotinamide adenine dinucleotide (NAD). Nicotinamide adenine dinucleotide enters the electron transport chain and results in the production of ATP through oxidative phosphorylation. Oxygen is consumed as the electron acceptor allowing restoration of NAD^+. This pathway constitutes aerobic respiration. The electron transport chain is the final step in the production of ATP from NADH and flavin adenine dinucleotide ($FADH_2$) formed during glycolysis, fatty acid oxidation, and the citric acid cycle. Figure 10.1 shows a simplified diagram of aerobic respiration. During functional activation, the increase in glucose metabolism above resting levels is associated with an increase in glycolysis in astrocytes and oxidative metabolism in neurons.[7,8]

Ketones, Organic Acids, and Amino Acids

Following a period of adaptation, the brain uses alternative substrates for metabolism.[9] In the developing brain and in states of prolonged starvation, ketones (acetoacetate and β-hydroxybutyrate) are important metabolic substrates for the brain.[10] Most patients with inborn errors of ketogenesis develop normally, suggesting the role of ketones primarily as alternative sources of fuel during illness or prolonged fasting. The ability of ketones to act as an alternative fuel source explains the effectiveness of the ketogenic diet in patients with glucose transporter 1 (GLUT1) deficiency.[11] However, its effectiveness in other pathological states such as epilepsy remains unexplained. Amino and organic acids can also be metabolized within the brain. These

are minor energy substrates except during periods of metabolic stress.

Lactate

Endogenous lactate produced by aerobic glycolysis can be an important substrate for neurons.[12] This becomes significant during periods of hypoglycaemia. A glucose lactate shuttle exists between astrocytes and neurons. The astrocyte-neuron lactate shuttle hypothesis (ANLS),[13,14] suggests a major metabolic role for brain-derived lactate as a substrate for neuronal energy metabolism and that lactate contributes to maintain synaptic transmission, particularly during periods of intense activity. Lactate that is released into the extracellular space from astrocyte metabolism is subsequently consumed aerobically by neurons.[15] Increased neuronal activity leads to release of potassium, glutamate, and other neurotransmitters into the extracellular space which are then taken up by astrocytes thereby restoring the composition of the cerebral cortical microenvironment. This uptake is an energy-dependent process that requires increased astrocyte glycolysis and production of lactate.[15] The coupling of neuronal activity to astrocytic glycolysis is the principle that permits studies based on 2-deoxyglucose to reflect local brain functionality.[16]

CEREBRAL METABOLIC PARAMETERS

The coupled astrocytic-neuronal unit has implications on measurements of tissue level metabolism. An increase in neuronal activity leads to increased astrocytic glycolysis, which is measured as the cerebral metabolic rate of glucose (CMRG) and 2-deoxyglucose phosphorylation. This compensatory glycolysis does not deplete glucose from the extracellular space. The lactate produced by the astrocytes is then consumed aerobically by neurons, which is reflected by the cerebral metabolic rate of oxygen ($CMRO_2$). The lactate consumed by neurons is not reflected in arteriovenous differences of lactate as it is not derived from the blood, and will not be measured by conventional cerebral metabolic rate of lactate (CMRL) determination. Lactate, pyruvate, and lactate–pyruvate ratio (LPR) are other parameters measured using cerebral microdialysis (CMD). An elevated LPR reflects metabolic crisis (described later). Pathological correlates of cerebral microdialysate with different types of tissue injury are described in Table 10.2.

Cerebral Blood Flow Metabolism Coupling

Intrinsic mechanisms modulate local blood supply to the brain to match functional activity. This results in minimal variations in oxygen extraction fraction across the brain

Table 10.2 Types of tissue hypoxia and neuromonitoring profiles in traumatic brain injury

Type	Pathophysiology	a PET profile b Neuromonitoring profile
Ischaemia	Inadequate CBF	**a** ↓ CBF, ↓ CMRO$_2$, ↑ OEF **b** ↓ PbrO$_2$, ↑ LPR (high lactate/low pyruvate)
Low extraction	Low arterial PO$_2$ (hypoxaemic hypoxia) Low haemoglobin concentration (anaemic hypoxia) Low half-saturation tension P50 (high-affinity hypoxia)	**a** ≅ CBF, ≅ OEF, ↓ CMRO$_2$ **b** ↓ PbrO$_2$, ↑ LPR (high lactate/low pyruvate)
Shunt	Arteriovenous shunting (microvascular shunt)[*,**]	**a** ↑ CBF, ↓ OEF, ≅ ↓ CMRO$_2$ **b** ≅ PbrO$_2$, ↑ LPR (high lactate/low pyruvate)
Perfusion dysfunction	Diffusion barrier (intracellular or interstitial oedema)[$]	**a** ≅ CBF, ↓ OEF, ↓ CMRO$_2$ **b** ≅ PbrO$_2$, ↑ LPR (high lactate/low pyruvate)
Uncoupling	Mitochondrial dysfunction[$$]	**a** ↓ CMRO$_2$, ≅ CBF, ≅ ↓ OEF **b** ≅ PbrO$_2$, ↑ LPR (high lactate/normal pyruvate)
Hypermetabolic	Increased demand	**a** ↑ CBF, ↑ OEF, ≅ CMRO$_2$ **b** ↓ PbrO$_2$, ↑ LPR (high lactate/low pyruvate)

*Jespersen SN, Ostergaard L. The roles of cerebral blood flow, capillary transit time heterogeneity, and oxygen tension in brain oxygenation and metabolism. *J Cereb Blood Flow Metab* 2012;32:264–77.

**Bragin DE, Bush RC, Muller WS, Nemoto EM. High intracranial pressure effects on cerebral cortical microvascular flow in rats. *J Neurotrauma* 2011;28:775–85.

$Menon DK, Coles JP, Gupta AK, et al. Diffusion limited oxygen delivery following head injury. *Crit Care Med* 2004;32:1384–90.

$$Verweij BH, Muizelaar JP, Vinas FC, Peterson PL, Xiong Y, Lee CP. Impaired cerebral mitochondrial function after traumatic brain injury in humans. *J Neurosurg* 2000;93:815–20.

Reprinted with permission from: *Neurosurg Clin N Am.* 2016;27(4). Lazaridis C, Robertson CS. *The Role of Multimodal Invasive Monitoring in Acute Traumatic Brain Injury*, pp. 509–17, Table 1 with permission from Elsevier.

Notes: ≅: variable; CBF: cerebral blood flow; ≅: no change or in either direction; LPR: lactate/pyruvate ratio; OEF: oxygen extraction fraction; P50: oxygen half-saturation of haemoglobin; PbrO$_2$: partial brain tissue oxygen tension; PO$_2$: arterial oxygen tension.

despite regional variations in CBF and oxygen metabolism. In clinical conditions such as induced coma or hypothermia where cerebral function is depressed, CBF and CMRO$_2$ are decreased. On the other hand, hypermetabolic states (e.g., excitotoxicity and seizures) increase energy requirements with corresponding increase in CBF. This regulatory mechanism can be impaired by injury or pathological states, which can result in secondary ischaemic insults. These are described in greater detail later in this chapter.

METHODS OF MONITORING CEREBRAL METABOLISM

Cerebral Blood Flow Monitoring

Classical measurements of cerebral metabolism require measurement of global CBF and the arterial-venous difference of substrates such as oxygen, glucose, or lactate (Table 10.3). The cerebral metabolic rate of that substrate is calculated by multiplying CBF with the arterial venous difference. Quantitative determination of CBF using nitrous oxide was first described in the 1940s.[17] Imaging

Table 10.3 Cerebral blood flow thresholds

Cerebral blood flow (ml/100 g/min)	Threshold	Consequences
40–60	—	Normal
20–30	Neurologic function	Start of neurologic symptoms Altered mental status
16–20	Electrical failure	Isoelectric electroencephalogram Loss of evoked potentials
10–12	Ionic pump failure	Na$^+$ and K$^+$ pump failure Cytotoxic oedema
<10	Metabolic failure	Complete metabolic failure with gross disturbance of cellular energy homoeostasis

Reprinted with permission from: Doberstein C, Martin NA. Cerebral blood flow in clinical neurosurgery. In Youmans R, editor. *Neurological Surgery: A Comprehensive Reference Guide to the Diagnosis and Management of Neurosurgical Problems*. Philadelphia: WB Saunders; 1996. p. 521, Table 21–4 with permission from Elsevier.

techniques such as stable xenon computed tomography (CT) scanning or perfusion CT scanning can be used to provide the global CBF value to calculate the cerebral metabolic rate of substrate. While these imaging techniques can identify regional differences in blood flow, they do not provide regional information about cerebral metabolism. Positron emission tomography (PET) scanning is capable of providing regional metabolic information and has been used in the context of traumatic brain injury (TBI). A technique allowing for continuous monitoring at bedside uses thermal diffusion to measure local CBF. An intraparenchymal probe with a thermistor and temperature sensor measures the thermal gradient between the distal thermistor that is heated by 2°C and the proximal temperature sensor. This provides a quantified regional CBF measurement in ml/100 g/min.[18] A mean value of 18–25 ml/100 g/min is considered normal. Serial changes or trends rather than absolute values may better detect early neurologic deterioration, delayed cerebral ischaemia or help assess response to therapy.[19] Data showing correlation with clinical outcomes are lacking at this time.

Positron Emission Tomography quantitative measures of metabolic processes in the brain using targeted radiopharmaceuticals can be obtained using PET. These radiotracers emit positrons which undergo radioactive decay before colliding with electrons to produce 2 photons.

Positron emission tomography scanners can detect these photons (gamma rays) and reconstruct an image of spatial density that indicates functional activity and metabolic processes within the brain. Radiopharmaceuticals are usually labelled with short-lived positron emitters: Carbon-11 (^{11}C) or Fluorine-18 (^{18}F). 2-[^{18}F] fluoro-2-deoxy-D-glucose (FDG), an analogue of glucose which can be utilized to measure metabolism in the brain is the most commonly used probe. Positron emission tomography correlates in acute brain injury are shown in Tables 10.3 and 10.4.

Jugular Venous Oxygen Saturation

While several measures of metabolism provide static information, neurocritically-ill patients have rapidly changing haemodynamics which necessitate continuous monitoring of variables. Jugular venous oxygen saturation (SjvO$_2$) monitoring provides continuous information about global adequacy of CBF relative to the metabolic requirements of the brain. Jugular venous oxygen saturation monitoring has been used for the identification and treatment of secondary ischaemic insults in brain injured patients.[20] Jugular venous oxygen saturation of <50% is a threshold to avoid in order to reduce mortality and improve outcomes in patients with severe TBI.[20]

Table 10.4 Triphasic hypothesis of glucose metabolism after traumatic brain injury

Phase 1: Hypermetabolism	Phase 2: Hypometabolism	Phase 3: Normal metabolism

• Hyperglycaemia
• Abnormal brain metabolites
  – Low cerebral glucose
  – LPR increase
  – High glutamate
• Abnormal PET
  – High FDG uptake
	• Hyperglycaemia/normoglycaemia
	• Abnormal brain metabolites
	  – Normal/low cerebral glucose
	  – Normal/low LPR
	• Abnormal PET
	  – Low FDG uptake
		• Normoglycaemia
		• Unknown brain metabolites
		• Improved PET
		  – Normalization of FDG uptake

Hours to days → Days to weeks → Weeks to months		
• Control of systemic glucose • Control of ICP, oxygen, and temperature • Control of cerebral metabolic energy crisis • Control of seizures	• Optimization of systemic glucose • Control of ICP, oxygen, and temperature • Delivery of fuel and nutrition	• Rehabilitation and therapy

Reprinted with permission from: Buitrago Blanco MM, Prashant GN, Vespa PM. Cerebral Metabolism and the Role of Glucose Control in Acute Traumatic Brain Injury. *Neurosurg Clin N Am.* 2016;27:453–63, with permission from Elsevier.
Notes: Three distinct phases of glucose metabolism after TBI. An early phase of hypermetabolism (phase 1): early systemic derangement in glucose control (hyperglycaemia), increased metabolic rate of glucose locally, and/or globally (CMRG) abnormal glucose metabolism in the brain characterized by low glucose and abnormal glycolysis metabolites (hyperglycolysis) and physiological abnormalities manifested as subclinical seizures. Phase 2 is characterized by hypometabolism and consists of abnormal to normal glycaemia, normalization of extracellular LPR or decrease, and decreased CMRG at the local and global level. Phase 3 or return to physiological metabolism has scarce data. The bottom half of the table lists potential strategies to address each stage.

Partial Brain Tissue Oxygen Tension

As discussed above, $SjvO_2$ monitoring provides information at a global level, whereas a brain tissue oxygenation probe can be used to provide local measurements of tissue oxygenation ($PbtO_2$).[21,22] The device most commonly in use is the Licox® catheter (Integra Neurosciences, San Diego, CA). Diffusion of oxygen through a permeable membrane into an electrolyte solution causes depolarization at the nearby cathode starting an electrical current depending on the amount of oxygen.

Tissue oxygenation should not be viewed simplistically as a marker of tissue hypoxia, but rather as a complex measure resulting from mechanisms involved in oxygen delivery and in the utilization pathway.[23] Diringer and colleagues found no improvement in $CMRO_2$ measured using PET after normobaric hyperoxia.[24] Studies that evaluated the use of $PbtO_2$ in the management of severe TBI showed a trend towards reduced mortality among patients treated with $PbtO_2$ monitoring.[25]

Electroencephalography and Electrocorticography

Electrocorticography (ECOG) is an invasive form of electroencephalogram (EEG) monitoring that is more sensitive than surface EEG. Electrocorticography entails positioning recording grids and strips on the cortical surface of the brain intraoperatively. Electrocorticography allows for detection of self-propagating waves of neural and astrocyte depolarization known as cortical spreading depression (CSD). Cortical spreading depression waves can lead to depressed spontaneous cortical activity correlated with clinical outcomes and predict metabolic crisis, increased ICP, vasospasm, and delayed cerebral ischaemia.[26] Prolonged depolarizations can reflect neurovascular uncoupling with disturbed CBF autoregulation and correlate with a worse prognosis in TBI.[27] Periodic discharges and seizures on depth EEG have shown to correlate with metabolic crisis after TBI.[28]

Cerebral Microdialysis

Cerebral microdialysis was first described in the 1950s. A tubular-shaped membrane at the tip of the probe was used to monitor chemical events in the 1970s by Ungerstedt and Pycock at the Karolinska Institute in Stockholm in the brain tissue of animal models, and subsequently in humans.[29,30] The application of CMD was endorsed by the International Multidisciplinary Consensus Conference on Multimodality Monitoring in Neurocritical Care.[31,32] The CMA/M Dialysis system

(M Dialysis Inc, North Chelmsford, MA) is considered the gold standard in human clinical applications (Figure 10.2). The current body of evidence is insufficient to support its routine use in patients with severe TBI.[33] However, CMD has gained attention since it allows for detection of metabolic distress even in the absence of elevated ICP or cerebral ischaemia.[34]

Glycaemic Control in Critical Illness

Energy requirements during critical illness can be higher than that during normal physiological states. Insulin insufficiency, insulin resistance, stress-induced hormonal dysregulation, and increased catecholamines are some of the reasons associated with hyperglycaemia during periods of acute illness.[35] In intensive care unit (ICU) patients, modest hyperglycaemia can be associated with a substantial increase in hospital mortality rates, and glucose has been shown to have a higher independent predictive value for mortality than the Acute Physiology and Chronic Health Evaluation II (APACHE II) score.[36] Among survivors of myocardial infarction admitted to the ICU, hyperglycaemia on admission is an independent predictor of adverse outcomes and increased mortality at 6 months,[37] 1 year,[38] and 2 years.[39] Critical illness characteristics such as age, history of diabetes, cardiac surgery, and prolonged mechanical ventilation can determine glycaemic control in the ICU. Poor glycaemic control, even among non-diabetic patients results in increased insulin requirement and increased mortality.[40] These findings have fuelled research aimed at establishing optimum thresholds for glycaemic control among patients with critical illness.

A randomized trial of intensive insulin therapy (to maintain serum glucose between 80 and 110 mg/dL) among patients admitted in the surgical ICU showed significant reduction in hospital mortality over conventional treatment (insulin only if blood glucose exceeded 215 mg/dL) (4.6% vs 8.0; ARR 42%; 95% CI 22%–62%).[41] Similar thresholds for glycaemic control did not significantly reduce mortality among patients admitted to a medical ICU in a randomized trial conducted by the same team and in a meta-analysis.[42,43] The Normoglycemia in Intensive Care Evaluation and Survival Using Glucose Algorithm Regulation (NICE-SUGAR) study was a large, multicentre, randomized trial of intensive (81–108 mg/dL) vs. conventional (180 mg/dL or less) glucose control among 6,104 medical and surgical ICU patients.[44] Intensive glucose control increased mortality at 90 days (27.5% vs. 24.9%; OR for intensive control 1.14; 95% CI 1.02–1.28, p = 0.02). Severe hypoglycaemia (glucose <40 mg/dL) was significantly more frequent in the intensive control arm (6.8% vs 0.5%, p<0.001). In a randomized trial of intensive insulin therapy (to keep blood glucose between 80–110 mg/dL) vs. conventional treatment to keep levels less than 151 mg/dL among neurocritically ill patients, no differences in mortality or functional outcomes at 3 months were observed between the groups with a trend towards higher mortality in the intensive therapy group.[45]

METABOLIC AND HAEMODYNAMIC RESPONSE TO BRAIN INJURY

Concept of Primary and Secondary Injury

The pathophysiology of brain injury can be explained in terms of primary and secondary events. Primary injury occurs at the moment of impact and is considered immediate and irreversible. Some mechanisms of cell death, however, can occur over hours suggesting the possibility of reversibility.[46] Secondary injury consists of ischaemic, metabolic, and immunological insults initiated by the primary event that can occur at lower thresholds in a susceptible brain. Aetiological factors that may lead to these secondary events, which may be characterized by biochemical, cellular, and molecular phenomenon include hypotension, hypoxaemia, intracranial hypertension, oedema, or seizures.[47,48] One of the goals of multimodal monitoring in the NCCU is to detect potentially harmful pathophysiological events before they cause irreversible brain injury and potentially allow for implementation of interventions aimed at improving clinical outcomes.[49,50]

Ischaemia

Cerebral ischaemia can be focal, due to occlusion of a blood vessel or global as in a cardiac arrest. As mentioned, brain ischaemia results in failure of energy mechanisms and leads to anaerobic glycolysis. Lactate accumulation results in acidosis and reduced tissue pH which can impair autoregulatory mechanisms. The clinical metabolic consequences of different thresholds of CBF are shown in Table 10.2.

The two distinct areas of haemodynamic and metabolic functioning in focal ischaemia are the ischaemic core and penumbra. The central ischaemic core consists of brain parenchyma destined to die. The collateral area composed of viable cells with CBF between the thresholds for energy failure and complete infarction is known as the penumbra.[51] The ischaemic penumbra represents a therapeutic target for interventions aimed at restoring CBF in a time-dependent

fashion. Positron emission tomography-based studies have been used to study haemodynamics. In the presence of autoregulatory vasodilation, there is an initial decrease in the ratio of CBF to cerebral blood volume (CBV), which is followed by increased oxygen extraction in hypoperfused areas.[52] When this process fails to maintain adequate oxygen supply, $CMRO_2$ declines with an increase in cerebral lactate and the threshold for an infarct is reached.[53] Other changes include a massive release of glutamate and potassium in the extracellular space. An example of regional cerebral ischaemia with corresponding metabolic parameters in severe TBI is shown in Figure 10.3.

Traumatic Brain Injury

Traumatic brain injury is associated with altered cerebral haemodynamics and failure of autoregulation. Defective autoregulation is associated with poor outcomes. Preserved CO_2 vasoreactivity can be seen in the presence of disturbed pressure autoregulation, whereas impaired CO_2 reactivity is seen in patients with poor neurological status.[54,55] Secondary brain injury can be due to several mechanisms including the following: ischaemia; excitotoxicity; energy failure and cell death cascades; axonal injury; secondary cerebral swelling; inflammation; and regeneration.[47]

Secondary cerebral ischaemia is common after severe TBI and associated with unfavourable outcomes.[56,57] Tissue dysoxia/hypoxia with a resultant cellular energy failure underlies these mechanisms of secondary injury. The different types, causes, and neuromonitoring and metabolic profiles of tissue hypoxia are shown in Table 10.3. Data integrated from multimodal monitoring and neuroimaging are required to ascertain the underlying nature of tissue hypoxia.[58–61]

Ischaemia can be more severe in patients with intracranial haematoma and diffuse oedema.[62] Focal ischaemia can be secondary to raised ICP and compression of small arteries, or due to a diffusion barrier for oxygen secondary to oedema.[60] Early reduction in CBF can cause periods of hyperaemia where there is blood flow in excess of cellular needs and can contribute to ICP elevation.[63] Ischaemia as a cause of secondary injury has long been the target of intervention strategies in patients with TBI, with management strategies aimed at augmentation of cerebral perfusion, CBF, and oxygen delivery. In a randomized trial of either CBF targeted (CPP kept >70 mmHg, $PaCO_2$ kept at 35 mmHg) vs ICP targeted management protocol (CPP >50 mmHg, $PaCO_2$ of 25–30 mmHg) for severe TBI, the risk of

cerebral ischaemia was 2.4-fold greater among the ICP-targeted group. However, the beneficial effects were offset by a five-fold increase in the frequency of adult respiratory distress syndrome.[64]

How glucose and other sources of energy to the brain should be delivered to sustain metabolic demands after TBI is a focus of current research. Similar to that of other critical illnesses, hyperglycaemia in TBI can be a manifestation of disease severity, with evidence pointing to secondary injury from hyperglycemia.[65] Early spontaneous systemic hyperglycaemia after TBI has been shown to correlate with poor clinical outcomes.[66–68] The concept of hyperglycosis, an abnormal state of increased glucose metabolism relative to rate of oxygen use, representing a non-physiologic decoupling between oxidative metabolism and glycolysis was first defined in severe TBI using PET studies.[69] Hyperglycosis was defined as a metabolic ratio ($CMRO_2$/CMRG) of less than 0.35, and this metabolic anomaly is now referred to as cerebral metabolic energy crisis—a hallmark of cellular dysfunction after TBI. Early hyperglycolysis is a transient phenomenon, which is followed by a period of depression in cerebral glucose metabolism within days of acute injury and can last for weeks to months (Table 10.4).[70] Periods of abnormal increase in neuronal activity can manifest as cerebral metabolic crises with subclinical seizures leading to secondary injury.[28]

Cerebral metabolism following TBI is sensitive to fluctuating blood glucose levels and hence the management of glycaemic status is important. Cerebral microdialysis studies demonstrate that metabolic crises and hyperglycolytic states can result from intensive insulin therapy and tight glucose control and offers no clinical benefit in outcomes.[71–73] In patients with severe TBI, a blood glucose level between 108 mg/dL and 162 mg/dL correlated with optimal cerebral glucose levels and LPR.[74] Rather than considering the brain or serum glucose in isolation, the brain/serum glucose ratio, a reflection of glucose transport across the blood–brain barrier (BBB) may be a more sensitive marker of metabolic distress and outcomes.[75]

Among TBI patients, while persistent low levels of extracellular glucose levels in cerebral dialysate (<0.02 mmol/l at a perfusion rate of 2 ml/min) correlate with severity of injury[76] and poor neurologic outcomes at 6 months, no correlation was found with increased cerebral lactate levels or brain ischaemia.[77] This has raised the question regarding the ability of the injured brain to use lactate resulting from a hyperglycolytic state as an energy source. Further, glucose enters the hexose monophosphate shunt/pentose phosphate

pathway (PPP) during metabolic crisis, which could potentially explain the lack of lactate increase in tissue.[78] Such observations depict a deviation from the brain hyperglycosis hypothesis and postulate that lactate is considered an alternate fuel pathway for the injured brain.[79]

Cerebral tissue LPR is a marker for metabolic stress and secondary injury, which when elevated above a threshold level of 25 predicts severity of injury and indicates poor outcomes.[80–82] This elevation in LPR can occur without ischaemia and can result from astrocytic hyperglycosis.[34,83,84] The increase in glutamate release at the neuronal synapse following TBI stimulates astrocytic glycolysis and glycogenolysis may be another source of non-hypoxic lactate production to fulfil cerebral energy needs after TBI.[84] Lactate has been shown to reinforce neuronal hydroxycarboxylic acid receptor 1 (HCA1), a regulator of glucose entry into PPP during TBI which is crucial for cell repair and protection from oxidative damage, supporting the hypothesis of its role as a neuroprotective substrate.[78,85] In a pilot study among early severe TBI patients, a short (3-hour) infusion of hypertonic sodium lactate to raise serum lactate to 5 mmol/L was associated with significant increase in CMD lactate, pyruvate, and glucose with reduction in CMD glutamate and ICP suggesting that lactate can be utilized aerobically as a preferential energy substrate by the injured human brain with sparing of cerebral glucose.[86] Blood lactate is also a major precursor of glucose through gluconeogenesis. A four-fold increase of blood lactate conversion to blood glucose has been observed in TBI compared to healthy controls.[85] Knowledge of the functional status of mitochondria and presence of oxygen diffusion barriers is critical in interpreting an increased LPR; increased lactate with near normal pyruvate may indicate mitochondrial failure rather than ischaemia (Table 10.3).[87]

Metabolic Patterns in Raised Intracranial Pressure

Intracranial pressure (ICP) thresholds at which treatment should be initiated and monitoring strategy planned should be considered in the context of the type of brain injury. In diffuse brain injuries, intracranial hypertension can decrease CPP. A decrease in glucose and $PbtO_2$ is seen with increases in glutamate and lactate (Figure 10.4). Oxygen and metabolism recover as ICP returns to baseline. Jugular venous or brain tissue oxygenation probes placed in relatively normal brain are recommended. In focal brain injuries, increasing brain oedema can cause a shift of intracranial structures and brainstem herniation with relatively lower ICP levels; probes placed in the area of injury will help guide treatment strategies.

EVIDENCE FOR THERAPIES TARGETING CEREBRAL METABOLISM IN TRAUMATIC BRAIN INJURY

Hypothermia is known to preserve tissue in the setting of a metabolic challenge. Therapeutic hypothermia is used for neuroprotection after a cardiac arrest and acute coronary syndromes.[88,89] Hypothermia can be applied early and prior to raised ICP (prophylactic hypothermia) or as a treatment for refractory ICP elevation. Two recent trials in the paediatric population failed to show benefit and additionally suggested harm with prophylactic hypothermia for TBI.[90,91] A randomized trial of hypothermia (32°C to 35°C) plus standard care vs. standard care alone for intracranial hypertension refractory to stage 1 treatments among adult TBI patients within 10 days of injury resulted in worse outcomes among the hypothermia group.[92] Early (within 2.5 hours) and short-term (48 hours post injury) prophylactic hypothermia is not recommended to improve outcomes in patients with diffuse TBI.[20]

Anaesthetics, analgesics, and sedatives are the commonly used therapies in acute TBI. One of the presumed mechanisms of action of sedatives and barbiturates is the suppression of metabolism, improving coupling of CBF to metabolic demands resulting in higher brain oxygenation with lower CBF, and decreased ICP from decreased CBV. Other mechanisms include inhibition of oxygen-free radical-induced lipid peroxidation.[93,94] However, these medications can cause a paradoxical decrease in CPP which negates the benefits of decreased ICP. The Brain Trauma Foundation (BTF) guidelines do not advise barbiturate-induced burst suppression on EEG as prophylaxis against development of intracranial hypertension; however, the intervention can be considered to control elevated ICP that is refractory to maximum medical therapy and surgery.[20]

Steroids were initially used in the treatment of brain oedema secondary to tumours. Steroids restore altered vascular permeability in brain oedema and attenuate free radical production in experimental models.[95,96] In the Corticosteroid Randomization after Significant Head Injury (CRASH) trial, over 10,000 patients with TBI were randomized to 48 hours of methylprednisolone infusion or placebo. Risk of death or significant disability was higher in the steroid group; steroids are not recommended for improving outcome or reducing ICP.[97]

Brain Trauma Foundation: Recommendations for Monitoring Traumatic Brain Injury[20]

Level I: high quality, level IIA: moderate quality, and level IIB/III: low quality evidence.

I. Intracranial pressure monitoring – Level IIB

• Management of severe TBI patients using information from ICP monitoring is recommended to reduce in hospital and 2-week post-injury mortality.
• Intracranial pressure should be monitored in all salvageable patients with a TBI (GCS 3–8 after resuscitation) and an abnormal CT scan (evidence of hematomas, contusions, swelling, herniation, or compressed basal cisterns).
• ICP monitoring is indicated in patients with severe TBI with a normal CT scan in the presence of ≥2 of the following: Age >40 years, unilateral or bilateral motor posturing, or systolic blood pressure (SBP) <90 mmHg.
• Treating ICP above 22 mmHg is recommended.

II. Cerebral perfusion pressure (CPP) monitoring – Level IIB

• Management of severe TBI using guideline-based recommendations for CPP (between 60 and 70 mmHg) is recommended to reduce 2-week mortality.
• Avoid aggressive attempts to maintain CPP above 70 mmHg with fluids and pressor to reduce the risk of adult respiratory failure (Level III).

III. Advanced cerebral monitoring – Level III

• Jugular venous saturation of <50% is a threshold to avoid in order to reduce mortality and improve outcomes at 3 and 6 months post injury.

Monitoring in Aneurysmal Subarachnoid Haemorrhage

After the rupture of intracranial aneurysms, a global reduction in CBF can occur proportional to clinical severity of subarachnoid haemorrhage (SAH).[98] A reduction in $CMRO_2$ and CBV can reduce cerebral perfusion, which can be associated with a decrease in CBF.[99] Initial flow reduction is related to metabolic depression from blood or byproducts.[99] A progressive decrease in CBF during the first 14 days with subsequent increase has been reported after aneurysmal SAH.[100,101] High-grade SAH is frequently associated with vasospasm and intracranial hypertension. Vasospasm can cause cerebral ischaemia. Delayed cerebral ischaemia (DCI) and infarction are associated with morbidity after SAH. While acute reductions in serum glucose, even to levels within a normal range, has been associated with brain energy metabolic crisis and LPR elevation in poor-grade SAH patients[102], a recent study has shown that lactate and glucose can be elevated within 24 hours of SAH due to sympathetic activation, and are associated with DCI and poor outcome.[103] CSD waves on EEG can lead to depressed spontaneous cortical activity, predict metabolic crisis, increased ICP, vasospasm, and DCI. In a CMD study, brain lactate was elevated (>4 mmol/L) in SAH patients predominantly because of hyperglycolysis ($PbrO_2$ >20 mmHg, CMD pyruvate >119 μmol/L) rather than hypoxia ($PbrO_2$ <20 mmHg); this pattern was associated with good long-term recovery.[104]

CONCLUSIONS

Cerebral energy dysfunction has been identified as an important determinant of prognosis in states of acute brain injury. Secondary injury is characterized by a cascade of cellular and molecular events consisting of ischaemic, metabolic, and immunological insults initiated by the primary event which can occur at lower thresholds in a susceptible brain. One of the goals of multimodal monitoring in neurointensive care is to detect potentially harmful pathophysiological events before they cause irreversible brain injury.

REFERENCES

1. Go KG. The cerebral blood supply. Energy metabolism of the brain. In: Go KG, ed. *Cerebral Pathophysiology*. Amsterdam: Elsevier, 1991;66–172.

2. Verweij BH, Amelink GJ, Muizelaar JP. Current concepts of cerebral oxygen transport and energy metabolism after severe traumatic brain injury. *Prog Brain Res* 2007;161:111–24.

3. Siesjo BK. Cerebral circulation and metabolism. *J Neurosurg* 1984;60:883–908.

4. Guyton A. *Textbook of Medical Physiology*. Philadelphia: WB Saunders; 11th edition, 2006; 767.

5. McEwen BS, Reagan LP. Glucose transporter expression in the central nervous system: relationship to synaptic function. *Eur J Pharmacol* 2004;490:13–24.

6. Simpson IA, Carruthers A, Vannucci SJ. Supply and demand in cerebral energy metabolism: the role of nutrient transporters. *J Cereb Blood Flow Metab* 2007;27:1766–91.

7. Fox PT, Raichle ME, Mintun MA, Dence C. Nonoxidative glucose consumption during focal physiologic neural activity. *Science* 1988;241:462–4.

8. Kasischke KA, Vishwasrao HD, Fisher PJ, Zipfel WR, Webb WW. Neural activity triggers neuronal oxidative metabolism followed by astrocytic glycolysis. *Science* 2004;305:99–103.

9. McIlwain H. Metabolic adaptation in the brain. *Nature* 1970;226:803–6.

10. Hasselbalch SG, Knudsen GM, Jakobsen J, Hageman LP, Holm S, Paulson OB. Brain metabolism during short-term starvation in humans. *J Cereb Blood Flow Metab* 1994;14:125–31.

11. Morris AA. Cerebral ketone body metabolism. *J Inherit Metab Dis* 2005;28:109–21.

12. Gallagher CN, Carpenter KL, Grice P, et al. The human brain utilizes lactate via the tricarboxylic acid cycle: a 13C-labelled microdialysis and high-resolution nuclear magnetic resonance study. *Brain* 2009;132:2839–49.

13. Pellerin L, Bouzier-Sore AK, Aubert A, et al. Activity-dependent regulation of energy metabolism by astrocytes: an update. *Glia* 2007;55:1251–62.

14. Pellerin L, Pellegri G, Bittar PG, et al. Evidence supporting the existence of an activity-dependent astrocyte-neuron lactate shuttle. *Dev Neurosci* 1998;20:291–9.

15. Turner DA, Adamson DC. Neuronal-astrocyte metabolic interactions: understanding the transition into abnormal astrocytoma metabolism. *J Neuropathol Exp Neurol* 2011; 70:167–76.

16. Clarke DD SL. Regulation of cerebral metabolic rate. In: Siegel GJ, Agranoff BW, Albers RW, et al., editors. *Basic Neurochemistry: Molecular, Cellular and Medical Aspects*. 6th ed. Philadelphia: Lippincott-Raven; 1999. Available from: https://www.ncbi.nlm.nih.gov/books/NBK28194/.

17. Kety SS, Schmidt CF. The nitrous oxide method for the quantitative determination of cerebral blood flow in man: theory, procedure and normal values. *J Clin Invest* 1948;27:476–83.

18. Vajkoczy P, Roth H, Horn P, et al. Continuous monitoring of regional cerebral blood flow: experimental and clinical validation of a novel thermal diffusion microprobe. *J Neurosurg* 2000;93:265–74.

19. Vajkoczy P, Horn P, Thome C, Munch E, Schmiedek P. Regional cerebral blood flow monitoring in the diagnosis of delayed ischemia following aneurysmal subarachnoid hemorrhage. *J Neurosurg* 2003;98:1227–34.

20. Carney N, Totten AM, O'Reilly C, et al. Guidelines for the management of severe traumatic brain injury, 4th ed. *Neurosurgery*. 2016.

21. Gopinath SP, Valadka AB, Uzura M, Robertson CS. Comparison of jugular venous oxygen saturation and brain tissue PO2 as monitors of cerebral ischemia after head injury. *Crit Care Med* 1999;27:2337–45.

22. van Santbrink H, Maas AI, Avezaat CJ. Continuous monitoring of partial pressure of brain tissue oxygen in patients with severe head injury. *Neurosurgery* 1996; 38:21–31.

23. Nortje J, Gupta AK. The role of tissue oxygen monitoring in patients with acute brain injury. *Br J Anaesth* 2006;97:95–106.

24. Diringer MN, Aiyagari V, Zazulia AR, Videen TO, Powers WJ. Effect of hyperoxia on cerebral metabolic rate for oxygen measured using positron emission tomography in patients with acute severe head injury. *J Neurosurg* 2007;106:526–9.

25. Stiefel MF, Spiotta A, Gracias VH, et al. Reduced mortality rate in patients with severe traumatic brain injury treated with brain tissue oxygen monitoring. *J Neurosurg* 2005;103:805–11.

26. Dreier JP. The role of spreading depression, spreading depolarization and spreading ischemia in neurological disease. *Nat Med* 2011;17:439–47.

27. Hinzman JM, Andaluz N, Shutter LA, et al. Inverse neurovascular coupling to cortical spreading depolarizations in severe brain trauma. *Brain* 2014;137:2960–72.

28. Vespa P, Tubi M, Claassen J, et al. Metabolic crisis occurs with seizures and periodic discharges after brain trauma. *Ann Neurol* 2016;79:579–90.

29. Ungerstedt U. Microdialysis—principles and applications for studies in animals and man. *J Intern Med* 1991;230: 365–73.

30. Hillered L, Persson L, Ponten U, Ungerstedt U. Neurometabolic monitoring of the ischaemic human brain using microdialysis. *Acta Neurochir (Wien)* 1990;102:91–7.

31. Hutchinson P, O'Phelan K. Participants in the International Multidisciplinary Consensus Conference on Multimodality M. International multidisciplinary consensus conference on multimodality monitoring: cerebral metabolism. *Neurocrit Care* 2014;21(Suppl2):S148–58.

32. Le Roux P, Menon DK, Citerio G, et al. Consensus summary statement of the International Multidisciplinary Consensus Conference on Multimodality Monitoring in Neurocritical Care: a statement for healthcare professionals from the Neurocritical Care Society and the European Society of Intensive Care Medicine. *Neurocrit Care* 2014;21(Suppl2):S1–26.

33. Chamoun R, Suki D, Gopinath SP, Goodman JC, Robertson C. Role of extracellular glutamate measured by cerebral microdialysis in severe traumatic brain injury. *J Neurosurg* 2010;113:564–70.

34. Vespa P, Bergsneider M, Hattori N, et al. Metabolic crisis without brain ischemia is common after traumatic brain injury: a combined microdialysis and positron emission tomography study. *J Cereb Blood Flow Metab* 2005;25:763–74.

35. Kavanagh BP, McCowen KC. Clinical practice. Glycemic control in the ICU. *N Engl J Med* 2010;363:2540–6.

36. Krinsley JS. Association between hyperglycemia and increased hospital mortality in a heterogeneous population of critically ill patients. *Mayo Clin Proc* 2003;78:1471–8.

37. Ainla T, Baburin A, Teesalu R, Rahu M. The association between hyperglycaemia on admission and 180-day mortality in acute myocardial infarction patients with and without diabetes. *Diabet Med* 2005;22:1321–5.

38. Bolk J, van der Ploeg T, Cornel JH, Arnold AE, Sepers J, Umans VA. Impaired glucose metabolism predicts mortality after a myocardial infarction. *Int J Cardiol* 2001;79:207–14.

39. Norhammar AM, Ryden L, Malmberg K. Admission plasma glucose. Independent risk factor for long-term prognosis after myocardial infarction even in nondiabetic patients. *Diabetes Care* 1999;22:1827–31.

40. Rady MY, Johnson DJ, Patel BM, Larson JS, Helmers RA. Influence of individual characteristics on outcome of glycemic control in intensive care unit patients with or without diabetes mellitus. *Mayo Clin Proc* 2005;80:1558–67.

41. van den Berghe G, Wouters P, Weekers F, et al. Intensive insulin therapy in critically ill patients. *N Engl J Med* 2001;345:1359–67.

42. Van den Berghe G, Wilmer A, Hermans G, et al. Intensive insulin therapy in the medical ICU. *N Engl J Med* 2006;354:449–61.

43. Wiener RS, Wiener DC, Larson RJ. Benefits and risks of tight glucose control in critically ill adults: a meta-analysis. *JAMA* 2008;300:933–44.

44. Investigators N-SS, Finfer S, Chittock DR, et al. Intensive versus conventional glucose control in critically ill patients. *N Engl J Med* 2009;360:1283–97.

45. Green DM, O'Phelan KH, Bassin SL, Chang CW, Stern TS, Asai SM. Intensive versus conventional insulin therapy in critically ill neurologic patients. *Neurocrit Care* 2010;13:299–306.

46. Tisdall MM, Smith M. Multimodal monitoring in traumatic brain injury: current status and future directions. *Br J Anaesth* 2007;99:61–7.

47. Kochanek PM, Clark RS, Ruppel RA, et al. Biochemical, cellular, and molecular mechanisms in the evolution of secondary damage after severe traumatic brain injury in infants and children: Lessons learned from the bedside. *Pediatr Crit Care Med* 2000;1:4–19.

48. Chesnut RM, Marshall LF, Klauber MR, et al. The role of secondary brain injury in determining outcome from severe head injury. *J Trauma* 1993;34:216–22.

49. Fakhry SM, Trask AL, Waller MA, Watts DD, Force INT. Management of brain-injured patients by an evidence-based medicine protocol improves outcomes and decreases hospital charges. *J Trauma* 2004;56:492–9; discussion 9–500.

50. Patel HC, Menon DK, Tebbs S, Hawker R, Hutchinson PJ, Kirkpatrick PJ. Specialist neurocritical care and outcome from head injury. *Intensive Care Med* 2002;28:547–53.

51. Hakim AM. The cerebral ischemic penumbra. *Can J Neurol Sci* 1987;14:557–9.

52. Robertson CS, Contant CF, Gokaslan ZL, Narayan RK, Grossman RG. Cerebral blood flow, arteriovenous oxygen difference, and outcome in head injured patients. *J Neurol Neurosurg Psychiatry* 1992;55:594–603.

53. Baron JC, Rougemont D, Soussaline F, et al. Local interrelationships of cerebral oxygen consumption and glucose utilization in normal subjects and in ischemic stroke patients: a positron tomography study. *J Cereb Blood Flow Metab* 1984;4:140–9.

54. Dobserstein C MN. Cerebral blood flow in clinical neurosurgery. In: Winn RH, editor. *Youmans Neurological Surgery*. 5th ed. Philadelphia: WB Saunders; 2004:519–69.

55. Obrist WD, Langfitt TW, Jaggi JL, Cruz J, Gennarelli TA. Cerebral blood flow and metabolism in comatose patients with acute head injury. Relationship to intracranial hypertension. *J Neurosurg* 1984;61:241–53.

56. Bouma GJ, Muizelaar JP, Choi SC, Newlon PG, Young HF. Cerebral circulation and metabolism after severe traumatic brain injury: the elusive role of ischemia. *J Neurosurg* 1991;75:685–93.

57. Graham DI, Adams JH. Ischaemic brain damage in fatal head injuries. *Lancet* 1971;1:265–6.

58. Jespersen SN, Ostergaard L. The roles of cerebral blood flow, capillary transit time heterogeneity, and oxygen tension in brain oxygenation and metabolism. *J Cereb Blood Flow Metab* 2012;32:264–77.

59. Bragin DE, Bush RC, Muller WS, Nemoto EM. High intracranial pressure effects on cerebral cortical microvascular flow in rats. *J Neurotrauma* 2011;28:775–85.

60. Menon DK, Coles JP, Gupta AK, et al. Diffusion limited oxygen delivery following head injury. *Crit Care Med* 2004;32:1384–90.

61. Verweij BH, Muizelaar JP, Vinas FC, Peterson PL, Xiong Y, Lee CP. Impaired cerebral mitochondrial function after traumatic brain injury in humans. *J Neurosurg* 2000;93:815–20.

62. Bouma GJ, Muizelaar JP, Stringer WA, Choi SC, Fatouros P, Young HF. Ultra-early evaluation of regional cerebral blood flow in severely head-injured patients using xenon-enhanced computerized tomography. *J Neurosurg* 1992;77:360–8.

63. Fieschi C, Battistini N, Beduschi A, Boselli L, Rossanda M. Regional cerebral blood flow and intraventricular pressure in acute head injuries. *J Neurol Neurosurg Psychiatry* 1974;37:1378–88.

64. Robertson CS, Valadka AB, Hannay HJ, et al. Prevention of secondary ischemic insults after severe head injury. *Crit Care Med* 1999;27:2086–95.

65. Lam AM, Winn HR, Cullen BF, Sundling N. Hyperglycemia and neurological outcome in patients with head injury. *J Neurosurg* 1991;75:545–51.

66. Young B, Ott L, Dempsey R, Haack D, Tibbs P. Relationship between admission hyperglycemia and neurologic outcome of severely brain-injured patients. *Ann Surg* 1989;210:466–72; discussion 72–3.

67. Rovlias A, Kotsou S. The influence of hyperglycemia on neurological outcome in patients with severe head injury. *Neurosurgery* 2000;46:335–42; discussion 42–3.

68. Liu-DeRyke X, Collingridge DS, Orme J, Roller D, Zurasky J, Rhoney DH. Clinical impact of early hyperglycemia during acute phase of traumatic brain injury. *Neurocrit Care* 2009;11:151–7.

69. Bergsneider M, Hovda DA, Shalmon E, et al. Cerebral hyperglycolysis following severe traumatic brain injury in humans: a positron emission tomography study. *J Neurosurg* 1997;86:241–51.

70. Bergsneider M, Hovda DA, McArthur DL, et al. Metabolic recovery following human traumatic brain injury based on FDG-PET: time course and relationship to neurological disability. *J Head Trauma Rehabil* 2001;16:135–48.

71. Vespa P, Boonyaputthikul R, McArthur DL, et al. Intensive insulin therapy reduces microdialysis glucose values without altering glucose utilization or improving the lactate/pyruvate ratio after traumatic brain injury. *Crit Care Med* 2006;34:850–6.

72. Oddo M, Schmidt JM, Carrera E, et al. Impact of tight glycemic control on cerebral glucose metabolism after severe brain injury: a microdialysis study. *Crit Care Med* 2008;36:3233–8.

73. Vespa P, McArthur DL, Stein N, et al. Tight glycemic control increases metabolic distress in traumatic brain injury: a randomized controlled within-subjects trial. *Crit Care Med* 2012;40:1923–9.

74. Meierhans R, Bechir M, Ludwig S, et al. Brain metabolism is significantly impaired at blood glucose below 6 mM and brain glucose below 1 mM in patients with severe traumatic brain injury. *Crit Care* 2010;14:R13.

75. Kurtz P, Claassen J, Schmidt JM, et al. Reduced brain/serum glucose ratios predict cerebral metabolic distress and mortality after severe brain injury. *Neurocrit Care* 2013;19:311–9.

76. Sanchez JJ, Bidot CJ, O'Phelan K, et al. Neuromonitoring with microdialysis in severe traumatic brain injury patients. *Acta Neurochir Suppl* 2013;118:223–7.

77. Vespa PM, McArthur D, O'Phelan K, et al. Persistently low extracellular glucose correlates with poor outcome 6 months after human traumatic brain injury despite a lack of increased lactate: a microdialysis study. *J Cereb Blood Flow Metab* 2003;23:865–77.

78. Dusick JR, Glenn TC, Lee WN, et al. Increased pentose phosphate pathway flux after clinical traumatic brain injury: a [1,2-13C2]glucose labeling study in humans. *J Cereb Blood Flow Metab* 2007;27:1593–602.

79. Glenn TC, Kelly DF, Boscardin WJ, et al. Energy dysfunction as a predictor of outcome after moderate or severe head injury: indices of oxygen, glucose, and lactate metabolism. *J Cereb Blood Flow Metab* 2003;23:1239–50.

80. Stein NR, McArthur DL, Etchepare M, Vespa PM. Early cerebral metabolic crisis after TBI influences outcome

despite adequate hemodynamic resuscitation. *Neurocrit Care* 2012;17:49–57.

81. Timofeev I, Carpenter KL, Nortje J, et al. Cerebral extracellular chemistry and outcome following traumatic brain injury: a microdialysis study of 223 patients. *Brain* 2011;134:484–94.

82. Hutchinson PJ, Jalloh I, Helmy A, et al. Consensus statement from the 2014 International Microdialysis Forum. *Intensive Care Med* 2015;41:1517–28.

83. Sala N, Suys T, Zerlauth JB, et al. Cerebral extracellular lactate increase is predominantly nonischemic in patients with severe traumatic brain injury. *J Cereb Blood Flow Metab* 2013;33:1815–22.

84. Patet C, Suys T, Carteron L, Oddo M. Cerebral lactate metabolism after traumatic brain injury. *Curr Neurol Neurosci Rep* 2016;16:31.

85. Glenn TC, Martin NA, McArthur DL, et al. Endogenous nutritive support after traumatic brain injury: peripheral lactate production for glucose supply via gluconeogenesis. *J Neurotrauma* 2015;32:811–19.

86. Bouzat P, Sala N, Suys T, et al. Cerebral metabolic effects of exogenous lactate supplementation on the injured human brain. *Intensive Care Med* 2014;40:412–21.

87. Nielsen TH, Schalen W, Stahl N, Toft P, Reinstrup P, Nordstrom CH. Bedside diagnosis of mitochondrial dysfunction after malignant middle cerebral artery infarction. *Neurocrit Care* 2014;21:35–42.

88. Ibrahim K, Christoph M, Schmeinck S, et al. High rates of prasugrel and ticagrelor non-responder in patients treated with therapeutic hypothermia after cardiac arrest. *Resuscitation* 2014;85:649–56.

89. Arrich J, Holzer M, Havel C, Mullner M, Herkner H. Hypothermia for neuroprotection in adults after cardiopulmonary resuscitation. *Cochrane Database Syst Rev* 2016;2:CD004128.

90. Adelson PD, Wisniewski SR, Beca J, et al. Comparison of hypothermia and normothermia after severe traumatic brain injury in children (Cool Kids): a phase 3, randomised controlled trial. *Lancet Neurol* 2013;12:546–53.

91. Hutchison JS, Ward RE, Lacroix J, et al. Hypothermia therapy after traumatic brain injury in children. *N Engl J Med* 2008;358:2447–56.

92. Andrews PJ, Sinclair HL, Rodriguez A, et al. Hypothermia for intracranial hypertension after traumatic brain injury. *N Engl J Med* 2015;373:2403–12.

93. Roberts I, Sydenham E. Barbiturates for acute traumatic brain injury. *Cochrane Database Syst Rev* 2012;12:CD000033.

94. Bilotta F, Gelb AW, Stazi E, Titi L, Paoloni FP, Rosa G. Pharmacological perioperative brain neuroprotection: a qualitative review of randomized clinical trials. *Br J Anaesth* 2013;110(Suppl1):i113–20.

95. Maxwell RE, Long DM, French LA. The effects of glucosteroids on experimental cold-induced brain edema. Gross morphological alterations and vascular permeability changes. *J Neurosurg* 1971;34:477–87.

96. Hall ED. The neuroprotective pharmacology of methylprednisolone. *J Neurosurg* 1992;76:13–22.

97. Edwards P, Arango M, Balica L, et al. Final results of MRC CRASH, a randomised placebo-controlled trial of intravenous corticosteroid in adults with head injury-outcomes at 6 months. *Lancet* 2005;365:1957–9.

98. Kobayashi KI KT. Cerebral blood flow and metabolism in patients with ruptured aneurysms. *Acta Neurol Scand Suppl* 1979;60:292–3.

99. Fein JM. Cerebral energy metabolism after subarachnoid hemorrhage. *Stroke* 1975;6:1–8.

100. Sundt TM, Jr., Whisnant JP. Subarachnoid hemorrhage from intracranial aneurysms. Surgical management and natural history of disease. *N Engl J Med* 1978;299:116–22.

101. Meyer CH, Lowe D, Meyer M, Richardson PL, Neil-Dwyer G. Progressive change in cerebral blood flow during the first three weeks after subarachnoid hemorrhage. *Neurosurgery* 1983;12:58–76.

102. Helbok R, Schmidt JM, Kurtz P, et al. Systemic glucose and brain energy metabolism after subarachnoid hemorrhage. *Neurocrit Care* 2010;12:317–23.

103. vanDonkelaar CE, Dijkland SA, van den Bergh WM, et al. Early circulating lactate and glucose levels after aneurysmal subarachnoid hemorrhage correlate with poor outcome and delayed cerebral ischemia: a two-center cohort study. *Crit Care Med* 2016;44:966–72.

104. Oddo M, Levine JM, Frangos S, et al. Brain lactate metabolism in humans with subarachnoid hemorrhage. *Stroke* 2012;43:1418–21.

11

Electrophysiological Monitoring

S. Sivakumar and J. I. Suarez

ABSTRACT

Electrophysiological monitoring aims at characterizing neurophysiology in real time for monitoring and management of acute injuries of the central nervous system, particularly among comatose patients. The recognition of non-convulsive seizures, quantitative measures to detect regional ischaemia and recognition of electroencephalographic and evoked potential (EP) phenotypes that indicate prognosis after cardiac arrest and spinal injuries have increased the utilization of electrophysiological monitoring in intensive care.

KEYWORDS

Electroencephalogram (EEG); evoked potential (EP); status epilepticus (SE); coma.

INTRODUCTION

A close relationship between electroencephalographic activity and cerebral metabolism, a high sensitivity for early detection of hypoxic ischaemic neuronal dysfunction due to selective vulnerability of cortical layers that generate electroenchepalographic activity and its value in cerebral localization are rationales for the use of the electroencephalogram (EEG) as a monitoring tool. This is valuable in neurointensive care where clinical examination is often clouded by sedatives, coma, or disorders of primary neurological modalities. Similarly, evoked potentials (EPs) have become increasingly important to provide prognostic information and follow neurological function.

ELECTROENCEPHALOGRAPHY

Technical Aspects

The placement of EEG electrodes in the critical care unit is similar to the standard application. The International 10–20 system first formalized in 1958 is the most widely used system for placement of electrodes (see Figure 11.1).[1] The potential difference between pairs of electrodes or between an electrode and its reference point is amplified and displayed on moving paper or an oscilloscope screen.

Specific stipulations for a brain death protocol include the demonstration of no electrical activity greater than 2 microvolts at a sensitivity of 2 microvolts/mm, with a filter setting of 0.1 s or 0.3 s and 70 Hz, and at least 30 min of recording.[2]

A detailed account of the aspects of recording are beyond the scope of this chapter. A variety of montages can be recorded. Some of the challenges to continuous EEG (cEEG) monitoring include machine and personnel availability, cost, and requirements for interruption during imaging. Technical challenges unique to intensive care unit (ICU) EEG monitoring include an abundance of artefacts. Examples include excessive noise from amplifiers, environmental artefacts generated by currents from external devices, and intravenous infusions and bioelectric artefacts arising from the patient including ocular, cardiac, glossokinetic, muscle, and movement artefacts. Stimuli in encephalopathic patients (e.g., suction, examination, noise, pain) can elicit highly epileptiform patterns such as periodic discharges, rhythmic delta or unequivocally evolving electrographic seizures which can be focal or generalized. This is termed stimulus-induced periodic, rhythmic, or ictal discharges (SIRPIDs) (Figure 11.2). The duration and prominence of the pattern correlates with the duration and degree of stimulation, and the pattern can usually be reproduced with further stimulation. Although it is an electrographic finding with no obvious clinical accompaniment, some patients can have clinical seizures as well which are typically focal motor. The exact clinical, therapeutic, and prognostic significance of SIRPIDs is under investigation.

The Critical Care Monitoring Committee of the American Clinical Neurophysiology Society has proposed standardized nomenclature for rhythmic and periodic EEG patterns encountered in the ICU. The committee has attempted to develop standardized terminology for common and controversial patterns seen in critically ill patients in order to allow a scientific study, the latest version of which was released in 2012.[3] Consensus statements on indications, technical specifications, and clinical practice of cEEG in critically ill adults and children was proposed in 2015.[4,5]

INDICATIONS FOR ELECTROENCEPHALOGRAPHIC MONITORING IN THE INTENSIVE CARE UNIT

Diagnosis and Management of Seizures and Status Epilepticus

The prevalence of seizures in patients monitored with cEEG (generally for 24 hours or more) ranges from 8% in those without prior seizures and with no subtle signs of seizures, 48% after convulsive status epilepticus (SE) to more than 50% in those who are comatose in a neurological ICU.[6] Most studies of acute brain injury (traumatic brain injury [TBI], intracerebral haemorrhage [ICH], and subarachnoid haemorrhage [SAH]) show a prevalence of seizures of 15%–40%. Seizures appear to be an independent predictor of worse outcome in multiple populations. Generalized convulsive status epilepticus (GCSE) is the most obvious indication for EEG monitoring. Clinical assessment of ongoing seizures is often confounded by sedating anticonvulsants, intubation, and associated pharmacological paralysis. Up to 75% of seizures in the ICU can be non-convulsive.[7] In a series of over 550 patients who underwent cEEG

monitoring, seizures were detected in 19% of patients and were exclusively non-convulsive in 92% of them.[8] Earlier studies showed that even after the control of convulsive status epilepticus, up to 48% of patients have persistent electrographic seizures, a high proportion of which are nonconvulsive.[9] Continuous EEG monitoring allows for detection of ongoing seizures in this patient population in the absence of overt clinical signs of convulsive activity.

Once seizures are detected, EEG is essential for monitoring the effects of therapeutic interventions and in the titration of anaesthetic medications for refractory seizures. Induction of burst-suppression pattern on cEEG and titration of antiepileptic therapy for seizure control have been widely used strategies in the management of SE, with a debate on which of these strategies is superior. One study demonstrated seizure control without suppression—burst or isoelectric EEG patterns to correlate with good functional recovery among nonanoxic patients with refractory status epilepticus (RSE).[10]

Seizure duration and delay to diagnosis are variables significantly associated with increased mortality,[11] and utilization of cEEG has the potential to reduce mortality from early diagnosis and treatment. A short snapshot of the recording often fails to characterize seizure propensity. Among ICH patients, 28% of seizures were detected only after the first 24 hours of recording highlighting the role for cEEG.[12] In patients with unexplained coma or at risk for seizures based on underlying brain injury, 48 hours of EEG recording should be considered.[13] Urgent EEG is recommended in patients with SE (and RSE) that do not return to functional baseline within 60 minutes after administration of seizure medication.[14] Electroencephalographic patterns for common diagnoses in the neurointensive care unit are shown in Table 11.1.

Intracerebral and Subarachnoid Haemorrhage

In patients with ICH, seizure rates of up to 31% have been reported, more than half of which can be nonconvulsive.[12] In the same study, seizures occurred

Table 11.1 Common neurological, medical, and surgical conditions and associated electroencephalographic patterns on critical care continuous electroencephalogram

Differential diagnoses	Clinical utility and electrophysiological patterns
Epilepsy	• Confirm diagnosis of convulsive and non-convulsive seizures and identify a focal/lateralized or generalized source of ictal activity • Monitor therapy: Pharmacological induction of burst suppression or electrographic seizure control for refractory status epilepticus

(Cont'd)

Table 11.1 (*Cont'd*)

Differential diagnoses	Clinical utility and electrophysiological patterns
Infections and neurodegenerative disorders	• Among ICU patients with sepsis, absence of reactivity, delta-predominant background, periodic discharges are independent predictors of mortality • Herpes simplex encephalitis is associated with periodic lateralized epileptiform discharges (PLEDs) that are maximal in temporal region(s); PLEDs can be seen in other acute or subacute unilateral lesions • EEG is among the diagnostic criteria for Creutzfeldt–Jakob disease. EEG can evolve from diffuse slowing and frontal intermittent rhythmic delta activity (FIRDA) during the early stages to disease typical generalized periodic discharges to a reactive coma in pre-terminal stages
Cerebrovascular disease	• Ischaemia: Initially, there is subtle loss of faster frequencies (beta and alpha, sometimes sleep spindles). With further drop in flow but while ischaemia is reversible, slowing appears—first excess theta, then delta. With further decrease in flow, there is suppression of all the frequencies corresponding with infarction. This ability of EEG to detect ischaemia early is the basis for cEEG monitoring in patients at high risk for ischaemia like SAH • Acute stroke is the most common aetiology of PLEDs, although nonspecific; PLEDs tend to decrease in amplitude, frequency, and ultimately cease with time (days–weeks) • Primary brainstem injury and 'locked in' states can have a normal EEG • Haemorrhage: Nonspecific focal slowing. With intraventricular and subarachnoid haemorrhage, diffuse slowing and FIRDA can be seen; may correlate with raised intracranial pressure • All intracranial haemorrhages can be associated with epileptiform discharges, PLEDs or seizures • Subdural and epidural haemorrhages tend to produce focal slowing and attenuation (from underlying cortical dysfunction) of ipsilateral normal faster frequencies
Brain tumours	• Focal slowing, PLEDs, epileptiform discharges
Neurosurgical procedures	• Breach rhythms can be seen in skull defects, which cause a low impedance pathway for electrical activity resulting in accentuation of underlying higher frequencies. Normal underlying cerebral activity appears at a higher voltage and is sharper, which can be misinterpreted as epileptiform activity
Cerebral metabolism and metabolic disorders	• Monitoring pharmacologically induced burst suppression for reduction of cerebral metabolic rate used for neuroprotection and management of refractory intracranial hypertension
Acute encephalopathy	• Slowing of alpha rhythm, excess slowing into theta and delta rhythms, loss of alpha, loss/attenuation of sleep transients, FIRDA are non-specific patterns of encephalopathy • Triphasic waves, a subset of generalized periodic discharges, are suggestive of toxic/metabolic encephalopathy, e.g., sepsis, hepatic, renal aetiologies • Generalized periodic epileptiform discharges (GPEDs) or GPDs can be seen after status epilepticus, Hashimoto and metabolic encephalopathy
Coma	• Bilateral independent PLEDs (BIPLEDs) are seen with coma; associated with seizures during acute illness and worse outcome than unilateral PLEDs • GPDs can be seen in post anoxic coma and is associated with poor prognosis • EEG is used to guide therapy in pharmacologically induced coma
Drugs and toxins	• Benzodiazepines and barbiturates cause diffuse slowing as well as excess fast activity, primarily in beta rhythm range. At higher doses, it can cause suppression-burst followed by electrocerebral inactivity (barbiturates tends to have bursts of higher amplitude than with benzodiazepines; propofol in between these two) • High doses of any centrally acting medication can cause diffuse slowing • GPDs can be seen in medication toxicity (lithium, baclofen, ifosfamide, and cefepime)
Psychiatric disorders	• Normal or near normal EEG can be seen in psychogenic processes • Video EEG is used in the diagnosis of psychogenic non-epileptiform seizures
Prognostication	• Post-anoxic coma: GPDs, burst suppression, alpha coma and a low amplitude nonreactive record have been associated with poor neurological outcomes

more commonly in lobar haematomas (23%) than in deep haemorrhages (11%). Haematoma expansion and peri-haematoma oedema can be associated with seizures.[12] Among comatose patients with SAH, the rates of nonconvulsive status epilepticus (NCSE) exceeding 30% despite prophylactic phenytoin administration has been described.[15] Nonconvulsive status epilepticus in patients with SAH has been associated with very high mortality rates, approaching 80% to 100% in studies.[15,16] High clinical severity grade (Hunt and Hess grade IV or V), old age, and focal lesions on imaging are the risk factors for seizures. Prophylactic antiepileptic medications, however, have been associated with worse outcome after SAH.[17,18] Therefore, routine antiepileptic drug (AED) prophylaxis should be reserved for patients with high-grade SAH and patients at risk for aneurysm re-rupture. Electroencephalogram has a role in monitoring cerebral ischaemia and SAH.[19] Delayed cerebral ischaemia (DCI) is a major cause of morbidity and mortality following aneurysmal SAH.[20] The alpha-delta ratio and alpha variability on cEEG has shown detection of DCI development before ischaemic changes on computed tomography (CT) scan are apparent and before clinical deterioration.[21] After controlling for clinical and radiological findings, a poor outcome (dead or moderately to severely disabled) after SAH was associated with the absence of EEG reactivity, sleep architecture, and the presence of periodic lateralized epileptiform discharges (PLEDs), generalized periodic epileptiform discharges (GPEDs) or bilateral independent PLEDs.[22] A poor outcome was also seen in 92% of patients with NCSE in this study. Using cEEG, the seizure burden has been shown to be associated with unfavourable 3-month functional and cognitive outcomes after SAH.[23] Implementation of cEEG in SAH patients can probably improve early detection of DCI and thus impact outcomes.

Traumatic Brain Injury

Among patients with TBI, up to 33% of them undergoing routine EEG recording can have seizures.[24] Patients with contusions are at risk for persistent seizures. Despite prophylactic phenytoin, 22% of patients with TBI can have early post-traumatic seizures with more than half being nonconvulsive.[25] Nonconvulsive post-traumatic electrographic seizures have been associated with prolonged increase in ICP and cerebral metabolic crisis.[26] Seizures can also be triggered by surgical evacuation of subdural haematoma.[27] Literature supports the use of cEEG for seizure detection in TBI despite prophylactic

administration of phenytoin. Paroxysmal autonomic instability with dystonia has been associated with raised ICP and EEG can help discriminate these events from seizures.[28] With lower degrees of brain injury, EEG has a prognostic role; patterns such as burst suppression and alpha coma have often been correlated with poor prognosis.[29] All patients with TBI having unexplained and persistent altered consciousness should be monitored using EEG.[14] EEG should be used to rule out nonconvulsive seizures in patients with TBI and a GCS below 8, particularly in those with large cortical contusion/haematoma, depressed skull fracture or penetrating injury.[14]

Cerebral Ischaemia

In patients with ischaemic stroke, seizures occur in about 6%, with rates higher than 10% among those with large volume infarcts.[30,31] Mortality among acute stroke patients with SE can be as high as three times that of those without; SE is an independent predictor of poor outcomes after acute stroke.[32] Electroencephalogram can detect cerebral ischaemia at an early stage with abnormalities occurring when cerebral blood flow drops to 25 to 30 mL/100 g/minute whereas infarction occurs when CBF drops to 10 ml/100 g/min to 12 ml/100 g/min.[33] Loss of beta activity followed by slowing to theta and then delta frequency and finally flattening to a burst suppression or continuous suppression pattern are signs of ischaemia on EEG.[25] A pattern of regional attenuation without delta frequency can predict massive infarction with malignant oedema.[34] Electroencephalogram can show improvement in cerebral perfusion after induced hypertension.[35] Electroencephalogram-derived indexes (global alpha–delta ratio [ADR] and Brain Symmetry Index) are predictive of 6-month functional recovery (positive predictive values [PPV] 60%).[36]

Hypoxic Ischaemic Encephalopathy

Among patients who remain comatose after a cardiac arrest, 40% to 66% do not regain consciousness.[37] Epileptiform discharges and electrographic seizures are common cEEG findings among comatose post cardiac arrest patients and tend to be associated with poor neurologic outcomes.[38] Hypoxic ischaemic encephalopathy (HIE) following cardiac arrest can be associated with seizures in 10% to 33% of patients.[39,40] The rewarming phase after hypothermia protocol for cardiac arrest is a common time for seizures, potentially explained by discontinuation of hypothermia, sedation, paralytics which could have treated electrographic seizure activity.

Electroencephalography in Prognostication after a Cardiac Arrest

Electroencephalogram within 24 hours after a cardiac arrest has been shown to predict good or poor outcome of comatose patients. Even among patients who recover with good outcomes, EEG activity can be severely disturbed or completely absent in the first few hours after a cardiac arrest. However, in patients with good neurologic recovery, EEG reactivity improves to a certain extent within 24 hours,[41–44] with the absence of recovery within this time interval accurately predictive of poor outcome. Reactive background rhythm or continuous pattern on amplitude integrated EEG has a higher likelihood of good neurological prognosis despite the presence of seizures.[45–47] Utilizing the standardized critical care EEG terminology of the American Clinical Neurophysiology Society[3] to evaluate prospectively recorded EEGs in the Target Temperature Management (TTM) trial, 'highly malignant EEG' patterns defined by suppressed EEG background without discharges or with continuous periodic discharges and burst-suppression background with or without discharges had a 100% specificity for poor outcome after 72 hours; 'malignant EEG' pattern on the other hand defined by malignant periodic or rhythmic patterns (abundant periodic discharges; abundant rhythmic polyspike-/spike-/sharp-and-wave; unequivocal electrographic seizure), malignant background (discontinuous background; low-voltage background; reversed anterior-posterior gradient) or unreactive EEG (absence of background reactivity or only stimulus-induced discharges) had a low specificity (48%), which increased to 96% if two malignant features were present.[48]

Myoclonic SE may have worse prognosis in the setting of a cardiac arrest treated with hypothermia, when 'reticular' rather than when associated with an EEG correlate. Patients with post-anoxic NCSE, preserved brainstem reflexes, and EEG reactivity may have favourable outcomes compared to those with myoclonic post-anoxic SE, if they are treated as SE.[49] Absence of electroencephalographic activity >20–21 μV ≤72 hours after a cardiac arrest predicts poor outcomes (cerebral performance category [CPC] scale 4–5) with 0% false positive rate.[50] Clinical examination findings of absent pupillary light reflexes on day 3 and no motor response on day 3 have similar specificity rates. However, somatosensory evoked potential (SSEP) is least susceptible to toxic metabolic effects.

In a large cohort of comatose patients after a cardiac arrest monitored with cEEG, unfavourable EEG pattern at 24 hours (defined as isoelectric, low-voltage (<20 μV), or burst-suppression pattern with identical bursts) and absent SSEP at 72 hours together had a specificity of 100%, sensitivity of 50% and positive predictive value of 100% for predicting poor outcomes at 6 months (cerebral performance category of 3–5); whereas favourable EEG patterns at 12 hours (defined as normal, continuous pattern or diffuse slowing <8 Hz) were strongly associated with good outcomes.[51] Electroencephalogram beyond 24 hours had no additional predictive value. Similar results were seen in a recent paediatric population following cardiac arrest, with a background activity on cEEG within 12 hours post return of spontaneous circulation associated with good outcomes.[52]

Brain death is associated with electrocerebral silence on EEG. Absence of electrical activity when at least 30 minutes of recording is done with adherence to the minimal technical criteria for EEG recording, including 16-channel EEG instruments are required when used as an ancillary test in the diagnosis of brain death.

In recent years, multimodal outcome prediction models after cardiac arrest incorporating electrophysiology have been extensively studied. Among patients treated with therapeutic hypothermia after a cardiac arrest, the absence of electroencephalographic reactivity is an independent predictor of mortality and poor outcomes at 3 months.[45,53] In combination with clinical examination and neuron-specific enolase (NSE) levels >33 μg/ml, cEEG yields the best predictive performance for outcomes after a cardiac arrest (receiver operating characteristic [ROC] 0.89 for mortality and 0.88 for poor outcome).[53] In one study, the addition of SSEP did not improve prognostic accuracy and SSEP was not an independent predictor of outcomes.[53] Monitoring of patients after a cardiac arrest with EEG during therapeutic hypothermia is recommended within 24 hours after rewarming to rule out nonconvulsive seizures among comatose patients and as a tool to assist with prognostication of coma after a cardiac arrest.[14]

Metabolic Encephalopathy

Metabolic encephalopathy is a risk factor for seizures. While approximately 15% of patients with hepatic encephalopathy have epileptiform abnormalities, more than half develop frank electrographic seizures.[54] Moreover, sepsis is a common cause of epileptic encephalopathy. In a retrospective study among medical ICU patients, the rate of periodic discharges or electrographic seizures were more than thrice among septic patients than those without sepsis (32% vs 9%), and were independent risk factors for death or severe disability at discharge.[55] In the same study, among patients with sepsis found to have seizures, presence of coma was not associated with a significant difference in the prevalence of electrographic seizures or periodic discharges. Continuous EEG is recommended in all patients with acute brain injury with unexplained and persistent altered consciousness and among comatose ICU patients without acute primary brain condition with unexplained impairment of mental status to exclude nonconvulsive seizures, particularly in those with severe sepsis or renal/hepatic failure.[14,56]

QUANTITATIVE ELECTROENCEPHALOGRAM

A high prevalence of cEEG monitoring in the ICU makes it labour-intensive to review these studies. Quantitative EEG (QEEG) techniques have helped in this regard. Apart from seizure detection, other acute events such as ischaemia, hydrocephalus, and haemorrhage can be detected. Quantitative EEG consists of a series of instruments that depict mathematical properties of EEG over a period of time. Spectrograms or compressed spectral arrays (CSA) are the most widely used compressed data format. They consist of 3D plots with time on the X-axis, frequency on the Y-axis, and EEG power on the Z-axis. Electroencephalogram power spectral analysis trends show that the amplitude contributed to the EEG by each frequency over time. They are computed using Fast-Fourier-Transformation analysis of EEG. This is followed by amplitude assessment in each frequency band. Vertical access lists the frequency and colour provides a measure of amplitude. Measures are calculated for specific brain regions and each hemisphere can be compared to provide an 'asymmetry spectrogram' to assess amplitude differences. Fast-Fourier-Transformation power trends assess the total power in a certain band of frequencies (e.g. total alpha power) or the ratio of power in two specific frequency bands (e.g., power in alpha range vs delta range or 'alpha–delta ratio').[57,58] Transitions from faster alpha frequency to delta can be amplified or averaged over a period of time. However, artefacts can produce similar changes and CSA does not detect individual epileptiform discharges.

Amplitude integrated EEG is a quantitative tool which provides information on amplitude and variation of cerebral activity. Thickness of tracing provides information on moment to moment amplitude variability, e.g., burst suppression results in thick tracing due to alternate bursts and suppressions. The overall magnitude of tracing reflects the voltage amplitude of EEG at each period of time, e.g., amplitude increase during seizure may increase the overall magnitude of tracing.[59] Figure 11.3 shows seizures in CSA displays and Figure 11.4 shows NCSE on CSA.

Quantitative EEG provides an assessment of stroke size and severity. The rate of change in average delta power yields a correlation with volume of initial mean transit time, follow-up diffusion weighted imaging volume, and 30-day National Institutes of Health Stroke Scale (NIHSS) score.[60] Subacute delta–alpha power ratio and relative alpha power has been shown to correlate with 30 days of NIHSS.[61] Quantitative EEG is also useful in monitoring vasospasm and DCI after aneurysmal SAH. In a quantitative cEEG study among SAH patients, detection of a decrease in the ADR (alpha power/delta power) was strongly associated with DCI.[58] A decline in ADR during periods of arousal among patients with high-grade SAH is associated with DCI.[58] Another measure called alpha variability has been shown to have good sensitivity in detecting angiographic vasospasm.

ELECTROCORTICOGRAPHY

Intracranial EEG recordings can also be obtained in the ICU via subdural strips or intraparenchymal 'depth' electrodes. These electrodes can detect seizure activity that is otherwise not detected via scalp electrodes and can provide artefact-free recordings in real time and help clarify equivocal patterns.

Brazilian physiologist Leao first described the spreading depression (SD) of electrocorticographic activity in the cerebral cortex.[62] Subsequently, the large spreading negative slow voltage variation of the extracellular space that accompanies this depression was reported. A similar spreading negative slow voltage variation can occur in the cortex in response to ischaemia. Depth electrodes can also detect peri-injury depolarization (PIDs), which are related to cortical spreading depression (CSD). Cortical spreading depression is common in acute brain injury, including ischaemia, trauma, and haemorrhages with evidence suggesting that they contribute to secondary neuronal injury.[63] In large middle cerebral artery, strokes, CSD, and PID can occur with reasonably high incidence.[64]

Among patients having ICH with haematoma expansion, postoperative peri-haematomal oedema progression is associated with occurrence of isolated and clustered spreading depolarizations.[65]

Electrocorticographic studies in SAH have shown that over 70% of patients can have CSD. The occurrence of delayed ischaemic neurological deficits was time-locked to a sequence of recurrent CSD with a negative predictive value of almost 100%.[66] Thus CSD with prolonged depression periods are an early indicator of ischaemic brain injury after SAH. Waves of CSD following SAH can result in stress on the balance of brain oxygen supply and demand causing waves of brain tissue hypoxia followed by rebound hyperoxia. This biphasic pattern transitions to monophasic hypoxia once delayed neurological ischaemic deficit occurs.[67]

Prolonged depolarizations can reflect neurovascular uncoupling with disturbed flow autoregulation and correlate with worse prognosis in TBI.[68] Periodic discharges and seizures on depth EEG have shown correlation with metabolic crisis after brain trauma.[69] Among patients with acute brain injury caused by trauma, SAH or ICH, CSD, and PID are significantly associated with seizures, most of which are subclinical.[70]

EVOKED POTENTIALS IN THE INTENSIVE CARE UNIT

Among EPs, median nerve SSEP is most useful in neurocritical care. Motor EPs, visual EPs, and brainstem EPs provide an interrogation of the other pathways.

Somatosensory Evoked Potentials

The median SSEP entails peripheral electrical stimulation of the mixed median nerve. The stimulus is just strong enough to produce a muscle twitch, and is repetitively delivered at a frequency of around 5 Hz, which sends impulses up the neuro-axis via brachial plexus, posterior columns of the spinal cord, through the brainstem, into the thalamus, and finally to the cerebral cortex. This interrogates the intact connectivity of peripheral sensory nerves to cortical projections. The Erb's point potential is essential to determine if the initial stimulus was adequate in terms of voltage to be transmitted into the central nervous system, that the peripheral nerve conduction is intact, and that the velocity of conduction along peripheral nerve is normal. This measurement is of particular significance in patients treated with hypothermia, which can slow or block peripheral nerve conduction. Severe trauma can also cause peripheral nerve injuries which can affect test results. Sedative medications even at doses sufficient to induce isoelectric EEG do not cause absence of cortical N20 potentials; however, later potentials such as N35 and N70 may be suppressed.[71] Cortical lesions are likely to cause abnormal or absent potentials rather than conduction delays.[71]

Electrical signals directed upwards from the baseline are referred to as negative deflections (N), while downward deflections below baseline are positive deflections (P). The negative deflection with a 20 ms latency, designated the N20 and the positive deflection at 22ms latency,

designated the P22 are of prime clinical significance and are grouped together as N20–P22 response. The N20 is the first cortical potential generated from the primary sensory cortex and P22 from area 4 of the motor cortex. N13 is a postsynaptic cervical spinal cord potential. P14 measures subcortical generators from caudal medial lemniscus. N18 is a subcortical far-field potential generated in the brainstem and/or thalamus. In humans, there is usually a series of negative and positive deflections after the N20 (P25, N35, N70), that represent intracortical and corticothalamocortical secondary processing of stimuli referred to as middle-latency potentials, which are indirect measures of conscious response to stimulation and cognition.[72] Table 11.2 shows the interpretation of short-latency SSEP patterns. Figure 11.5 shows SSEPs.

Somatosensory evoked potentials are assessed as normal, abnormal (increased latency or reduced amplitude) or absent on either side. This provides a 6-point scale in which both hemispheres are considered. After a cardiac arrest, SSEP has utility in identifying patients with poor outcome. Bilateral absence of the N20–P22 responses during hypothermia or after rewarming in patients with hypoxic-ischaemic coma is associated with a poor prognosis and high specificity (0% false positive rate).[73] Among patients who were not treated with therapeutic hypothermia, bilateral absence of SSEP for 24–72 hours had similar predictive

Table 11.2 Clinical interpretation of median nerve somatosensory evoked potential in comatose patients with traumatic brain injury or cardiac arrest

Level	SSEP findings	Clinical correlation
0	Normal P14, normal N20	Normal
1a	Normal P14, increased P14–N20 interval, normal N20	Usually reversible subcortical dysfunction due to sedatives, metabolic disturbances, or hypothermia
1b	Absent P14, abnormal N20	Uncertain pattern
2	Normal P14, unilateral or bilateral N20 distortion	Brainstem or subcortical injury due to traumatic axonal injury or ischaemia, often reversible
3	Normal P14, unilateral or bilateral N20 absence	Irreversible cortical injury

Source: Cruccu G, Aminoff MJ, Curio G, et al. Recommendations for the clinical use of somatosensory-evoked potentials. *Neurophysiol.* 2008;119:1705–19. Permission from Elsevier.

capability for poor outcomes (CPC 4–5).[50] Normal SSEP in this clinical setting, however, has less predictive capacity.[74] Guidelines for prognostication after cardiac arrest finds strong evidence for the use of SSEP as a specific marker of poor outcome (death or persistent vegetative state) after resuscitation from cardiac arrest.[75,76] Somatosensory evoked potential should be performed 1–3 days after resuscitation. Caution should be exercised towards interpretation of SSEP performed during hypothermia, as hypothermia can slow peripheral conduction.

Somatosensory evoked potentials can assist with prognostication after severe TBI.[77] Since transient EP conduction block can result from contusion and cerebral oedema that can subsequently resolve, loss of cortical potential may not provide the same strength of evidence for irreversible cortical injury that it does with cardiac arrest.[71] Normal SSEPs (grade 1) after TBI are associated with around 57% chance of good recovery whereas bilaterally absent SSEPs (grade 6) are associated with 1% chance of functional recovery.[74] Early SSEP grades among comatose TBI patients can predict cognitive and functional outcomes.[78] Changes in median SSEP has been shown to precede a rise in ICP.[79] As with cardiac arrest, middle latency SSEP has been studied in TBI. In a recent study among 81 patients with severe TBI who underwent SSEP during the first 6 days, improved prognostic accuracy was identified for middle-latency EP when included in the predictive model.[80]

Prognostic information on recovery to ambulation, hand function, and bladder function after spinal cord injury can be obtained using SSEPs and motor EPs.[81] Evolution of tibial SSEPs can provide prognostic information.[82]

Intraoperative SSEP changes during carotid endarterectomy have a high specificity towards predicting neurological outcomes. Patients with perioperative deficits are 14 times more likely to have changes in intraoperative SSEPs.[83]

Brainstem Auditory Evoked Potentials

Brainstem auditory evoked potentials (BAEP) measure the conduction of acoustic stimuli that are presented as a series of clicks, which in turn produce potentials conducted via the acoustic nerve through the brainstem, thalamus, and cortex. Signal conduction is measured from the mastoid and scalp electrodes. Wave I represents peripheral conduction along the acoustic nerve; wave II and III reflect conduction within the medulla and pons; waves IV and V reflect conduction through the lateral lemniscus and inferior colliculus, respectively; wave VI in the medial geniculate body of thalamus and wave VII conduction to the primary auditory cortex in the superior temporal gyrus. Waves I–V are referred to as short-latency BAEP and wave VII is a middle-latency BAEP. The presence of wave I with the absence of subsequent waves is suggestive of irreversible brainstem and cortical injury.[71] Brainstem auditory evoked potentials can complement SSEP and EEG in the confirmation of brain death by demonstrating absent brainstem conduction. Caveats include the absence of waves I–VII in sensorineural hearing loss.[71] Since the brainstem is relatively resistant to hypoxic ischaemia, BAEP does not have a significant role in prognostication after cardiac arrest.

Event-Related Potentials

Event-related potentials (ERP) testing are long-latency variations of BAEP or SSEP. Although largely investigational, this tool is gaining popularity as a bedside marker of interaction with external stimuli. Commonly used ERPs include the P300, N100, N400 and mismatch negativity (MMN). Mismatch negativity is a negative deflection at 150 to 250 ms in response to processing of deviant auditory stimuli; it is obtained by subtracting ERP of standard stimulus from ERP of deviant simulus.[84] There is a growing evidence for the role of MMN in prognostication of comatose TBI and cardiac arrest patients. Bilaterally absent N20 on SSEP with absent MMN has approximately 90% specificity for death or vegetative state in patients with TBI and 100% specificity for death or vegetative state post a cardiac arrest (with or without hypothermia).[72]

CONCLUSIONS

Electroencephalography is valuable in neurointensive care where clinical examination is often clouded by sedatives, coma, or disorders of primary neurological modalities. Similarly, EPs are increasingly important to provide prognostic information and follow neurological function.

REFERENCES

1. Klem GH, Luders HO, Jasper HH, Elger C. The ten-twenty electrode system of the International Federation. The International Federation of Clinical Neurophysiology. *Electroencephalogr Clin Neurophysiol Suppl* 1999;52:3–6.

2. Wijdicks EF. Determining brain death in adults. *Neurology* 1995;45:1003–11.

3. Hirsch LJ, LaRoche SM, Gaspard N, et al. American Clinical Neurophysiology Society's Standardized Critical

Care EEG Terminology: 2012 version. *J Clin Neurophysiol* 2013;30:1–27.

4. Herman ST, Abend NS, Bleck TP, et al. Consensus statement on continuous EEG in critically ill adults and children, part I: indications. *J Clin Neurophysiol* 2015;32:87–95.

5. Herman ST, Abend NS, Bleck TP, et al. Consensus statement on continuous EEG in critically ill adults and children, part II: personnel, technical specifications, and clinical practice. *J Clin Neurophysiol* 2015;32:96–108.

6. Brenner RP. EEG in convulsive and nonconvulsive status epilepticus. *J Clin Neurophysiol* 2004;21:319–31.

7. Jordan KG. Neurophysiologic monitoring in the neuroscience intensive care unit. *Neurol Clin* 1995;13: 579–626.

8. Claassen J, Mayer SA, Kowalski RG, Emerson RG, Hirsch LJ. Detection of electrographic seizures with continuous EEG monitoring in critically ill patients. *Neurology* 2004;62:1743–8.

9. DeLorenzo RJ, Waterhouse EJ, Towne AR, et al. Persistent nonconvulsive status epilepticus after the control of convulsive status epilepticus. *Epilepsia* 1998;39:833–40.

10. Hocker SE, Britton JW, Mandrekar JN, Wijdicks EF, Rabinstein AA. Predictors of outcome in refractory status epilepticus. *JAMA Neurol* 2013;70:72–7.

11. Young GB, Jordan KG, Doig GS. An assessment of nonconvulsive seizures in the intensive care unit using continuous EEG monitoring: an investigation of variables associated with mortality. *Neurology* 1996;47:83–9.

12. Claassen J, Jette N, Chum F, et al. Electrographic seizures and periodic discharges after intracerebral hemorrhage. *Neurology* 2007;69:1356–65.

13. Hemphill JC, 3rd; Greenberg SM; Anderson CS; et al. Guidelines for the management of spontaneous intracerebral hemorrhage: a guideline for healthcare professionals from the American Heart Association/ American Stroke Association. *Stroke* 2015;46:2032–60.

14. Claassen J, Taccone FS, Horn P, et al. Recommendations on the use of EEG monitoring in critically ill patients: consensus statement from the neurointensive care section of the ESICM. *Intensive Care Med* 2013;39:1337–51.

15. Dennis LJ, Claassen J, Hirsch LJ, Emerson RG, Connolly ES, Mayer SA. Nonconvulsive status epilepticus after subarachnoid hemorrhage. *Neurosurgery* 2002;51:1136–43; discussion 44.

16. Little AS, Kerrigan JF, McDougall CG, et al. Nonconvulsive status epilepticus in patients suffering spontaneous subarachnoid hemorrhage. *J Neurosurg* 2007;106:805–11.

17. Rosengart AJ, Huo JD, Tolentino J, et al. Outcome in patients with subarachnoid hemorrhage treated with antiepileptic drugs. *J Neurosurg* 2007;107:253–60.

18. Naidech AM, Kreiter KT, Janjua N, et al. Phenytoin exposure is associated with functional and cognitive disability after subarachnoid hemorrhage. *Stroke* 2005;36:583–7.

19. Kondziella D, Friberg CK, Wellwood I, Reiffurth C, Fabricius M, Dreier JP. Continuous EEG monitoring in aneurysmal subarachnoid hemorrhage: a systematic review. *Neurocrit Care* 2015;22:450–61.

20. Koenig MA. Management of delayed cerebral ischemia after subarachnoid hemorrhage. *Continuum (Minneap Minn)* 2012;18:579–97.

21. Rots ML, van Putten MJ, Hoedemaekers CW, Horn J. Continuous EEG monitoring for early detection of delayed cerebral ischemia in subarachnoid hemorrhage: a pilot study. *Neurocrit Care* 2016;24:207–16.

22. Claassen J, Hirsch LJ, Frontera JA, et al. Prognostic significance of continuous EEG monitoring in patients with poor-grade subarachnoid hemorrhage. *Neurocrit Care* 2006;4:103–12.

23. De Marchis GM, Pugin D, Meyers E, et al. Seizure burden in subarachnoid hemorrhage associated with functional and cognitive outcome. *Neurology* 2016;86:253–60.

24. Ronne-Engstrom E, Winkler T. Continuous EEG monitoring in patients with traumatic brain injury reveals a high incidence of epileptiform activity. *Acta Neurol Scand* 2006;114:47–53.

25. Vespa PM, Nuwer MR, Nenov V, et al. Increased incidence and impact of nonconvulsive and convulsive seizures after traumatic brain injury as detected by continuous electroencephalographic monitoring. *J Neurosurg* 1999;91:750–60.

26. Vespa PM, Miller C, McArthur D, et al. Nonconvulsive electrographic seizures after traumatic brain injury result in a delayed, prolonged increase in intracranial pressure and metabolic crisis. *Crit Care Med* 2007;35:2830–6.

27. Rabinstein AA, Chung SY, Rudzinski LA, Lanzino G. Seizures after evacuation of subdural hematomas: incidence, risk factors, and functional impact. *J Neurosurg* 2010;112:455–60.

28. Blackman JA, Patrick PD, Buck ML, Rust RS, Jr. Paroxysmal autonomic instability with dystonia after brain injury. *Arch Neurol* 2004;61:321–8.

29. Synek VM. Prognostically important EEG coma patterns in diffuse anoxic and traumatic encephalopathies in adults. *J Clin Neurophysiol* 1988;5:161–74.

30. Mecarelli O, Pro S, Randi F, et al. EEG patterns and epileptic seizures in acute phase stroke. *Cerebrovasc Dis* 2011;31:191–8.

31. Reith J, Jorgensen HS, Nakayama H, Raaschou HO, Olsen TS. Seizures in acute stroke: predictors and prognostic significance. The Copenhagen Stroke Study. *Stroke* 1997;28:1585–9.

32. Malek AM, Wilson DA, Martz GU, et al. Mortality following status epilepticus in persons with and without epilepsy. *Seizure* 2016;42:7–13.

33. Astrup J, Siesjo BK, Symon L. Thresholds in cerebral ischemia—the ischemic penumbra. *Stroke* 1981;12: 723–5.

34. Jordan KG. Continuous EEG monitoring in the neuroscience intensive care unit and emergency department. *J Clin Neurophysiol* 1999;16:14–39.

35. Wood JH, Polyzoidis KS, Epstein CM, Gibby GL, Tindall GT. Quantitative EEG alterations after isovolemic-hemodilutional augmentation of cerebral perfusion in stroke patients. *Neurology* 1984;34:764–8.

36. Sheorajpanday RV, Nagels G, Weeren AJ, van Putten MJ, De Deyn PP. Quantitative EEG in ischemic stroke: correlation with functional status after 6 months. *Clin Neurophysiol* 2011;122:874–83.

37. Zandbergen EG, de Haan RJ, Stoutenbeek CP, Koelman JH, Hijdra A. Systematic review of early prediction of poor outcome in anoxic-ischaemic coma. *Lancet* 1998;352:1808–12.

38. Mani R, Schmitt SE, Mazer M, Putt ME, Gaieski DF. The frequency and timing of epileptiform activity on continuous electroencephalogram in comatose post-cardiac arrest syndrome patients treated with therapeutic hypothermia. *Resuscitation* 2012;83:840–7.

39. Rossetti AO, Logroscino G, Liaudet L, et al. Status epilepticus: an independent outcome predictor after cerebral anoxia. *Neurology* 2007;69:255–60.

40. Legriel S, Bruneel F, Sediri H, et al. Early EEG monitoring for detecting postanoxic status epilepticus during therapeutic hypothermia: a pilot study. *Neurocrit Care* 2009;11:338–44.

41. Cloostermans MC, van Meulen FB, Eertman CJ, Hom HW, van Putten MJ. Continuous electroencephalography monitoring for early prediction of neurological outcome in postanoxic patients after cardiac arrest: a prospective cohort study. *Crit Care Med* 2012;40:2867–75.

42. Tjepkema-Cloostermans MC, Hofmeijer J, Trof RJ, Blans MJ, Beishuizen A, van Putten MJ. Electroencephalogram predicts outcome in patients with postanoxic coma during mild therapeutic hypothermia. *Crit Care Med* 2015;43:159–67.

43. Tjepkema-Cloostermans MC, van Meulen FB, Meinsma G, van Putten MJ. A Cerebral Recovery Index (CRI) for early prognosis in patients after cardiac arrest. *Crit Care* 2013;17:R252.

44. Hofmeijer J, Tjepkema-Cloostermans MC, van Putten MJ. Burst-suppression with identical bursts: a distinct EEG pattern with poor outcome in postanoxic coma. *Clin Neurophysiol* 2014;125:947–54.

45. Rossetti AO, Urbano LA, Delodder F, Kaplan PW, Oddo M. Prognostic value of continuous EEG monitoring during therapeutic hypothermia after cardiac arrest. *Crit Care* 2010;14:R173.

46. Rundgren M, Rosen I, Friberg H. Amplitude-integrated EEG (aEEG) predicts outcome after cardiac arrest and induced hypothermia. *Intensive Care Med* 2006; 32:836–42.

47. Rundgren M, Westhall E, Cronberg T, Rosen I, Friberg H. Continuous amplitude-integrated electroencephalogram predicts outcome in hypothermia-treated cardiac arrest patients. *Crit Care Med* 2010;38:1838–44.

48. Westhall E, Rossetti AO, van Rootselaar AF, et al. Standardized EEG interpretation accurately predicts prognosis after cardiac arrest. *Neurology* 2016;86: 1482–90.

49. Rossetti AO, Oddo M, Liaudet L, Kaplan PW. Predictors of awakening from postanoxic status epilepticus after therapeutic hypothermia. *Neurology* 2009;72:744–9.

50. Sandroni C, Cavallaro F, Callaway CW, et al. Predictors of poor neurological outcome in adult comatose survivors of cardiac arrest: a systematic review and meta-analysis. Part 1: patients not treated with therapeutic hypothermia. *Resuscitation* 2013;84:1310–23.

51. Hofmeijer J, Beernink TM, Bosch FH, Beishuizen A, Tjepkema-Cloostermans MC, van Putten MJ. Early EEG contributes to multimodal outcome prediction of postanoxic coma. *Neurology* 2015;85:137–43.

52. Ostendorf AP, Hartman ME, Friess SH. Early electroencephalographic findings correlate with neurologic outcome in children following cardiac arrest. *Pediatr Crit Care Med* 2016;17:667–76.

53. Oddo M, Rossetti AO. Early multimodal outcome prediction after cardiac arrest in patients treated with hypothermia. *Crit Care Med* 2014;42:1340–7.

54. Ficker DM, Westmoreland BF, Sharbrough FW. Epileptiform abnormalities in hepatic encephalopathy. *J Clin Neurophysiol* 1997;14:230–4.

55. Oddo M, Carrera E, Claassen J, Mayer SA, Hirsch LJ. Continuous electroencephalography in the medical intensive care unit. *Crit Care Med* 2009;37:2051–6.

56. Claassen J, Vespa P. Participants in the International Multi-disciplinary Consensus Conference on Multimodality M. Electrophysiologic monitoring in acute brain injury. *Neurocrit Care* 2014;21(2):S129–47.

57. Labar DR, Fisch BJ, Pedley TA, Fink ME, Solomon RA. Quantitative EEG monitoring for patients with subarachnoid hemorrhage. *Electroencephalogr Clin Neurophysiol* 1991;78:325–32.

58. Claassen J, Hirsch LJ, Kreiter KT, et al. Quantitative continuous EEG for detecting delayed cerebral ischemia in patients with poor-grade subarachnoid hemorrhage. *Clin Neurophysiol* 2004;115:2699–710.

59. Maynard D, Prior PF, Scott DF. Device for continuous monitoring of cerebral activity in resuscitated patients. *Br Med J* 1969;4:545–6.

60. Finnigan SP, Rose SE, Walsh M, et al. Correlation of quantitative EEG in acute ischemic stroke with 30-day NIHSS score: comparison with diffusion and perfusion MRI. *Stroke* 2004;35:899–903.

61. Finnigan SP, Walsh M, Rose SE, Chalk JB. Quantitative EEG indices of sub-acute ischaemic stroke correlate with clinical outcomes. *Clin Neurophysiol* 2007;118:2525–32.

62. Leao AA. Further observations on the spreading depression of activity in the cerebral cortex. *J Neurophysiol* 1947;10:409–14.

63. Fabricius M, Fuhr S, Bhatia R, et al. Cortical spreading depression and peri-infarct depolarization in acutely injured human cerebral cortex. *Brain* 2006;129:778–90.

64. Dohmen C, Sakowitz OW, Fabricius M, et al. Spreading depolarizations occur in human ischemic stroke with high incidence. *Ann Neurol* 2008;63:720–8.

65. Helbok R, Schiefecker AJ, Friberg C, et al. Spreading depolarizations in patients with spontaneous intracerebral hemorrhage: Association with perihematomal edema progression. *J Cereb Blood Flow Metab* 2016.

66. Dreier JP, Woitzik J, Fabricius M, et al. Delayed ischaemic neurological deficits after subarachnoid haemorrhage are associated with clusters of spreading depolarizations. *Brain* 2006;129:3224–37.

67. Bosche B, Graf R, Ernestus RI, et al. Recurrent spreading depolarizations after subarachnoid hemorrhage decreases oxygen availability in human cerebral cortex. *Ann Neurol* 2010;67:607–17.

68. Hinzman JM, Andaluz N, Shutter LA, et al. Inverse neurovascular coupling to cortical spreading depolarizations in severe brain trauma. *Brain* 2014;137:2960–72.

69. Vespa P, Tubi M, Claassen J, et al. Metabolic crisis occurs with seizures and periodic discharges after brain trauma. *Ann Neurol* 2016;79:579–90.

70. Fabricius M, Fuhr S, Willumsen L, et al. Association of seizures with cortical spreading depression and peri-infarct depolarisations in the acutely injured human brain. *Clin Neurophysiol* 2008;119:1973–84.

71. Guerit JM, Amantini A, Amodio P, et al. Consensus on the use of neurophysiological tests in the intensive care unit (ICU): electroencephalogram (EEG), evoked potentials (EP), and electroneuromyography (ENMG). *Neurophysiol Clin* 2009;39:71–83.

72. Koenig MA, Kaplan PW. Clinical applications for EPs in the ICU. *J Clin Neurophysiol* 2015;32:472–80.

73. Sandroni C, Cavallaro F, Callaway CW, et al. Predictors of poor neurological outcome in adult comatose survivors of cardiac arrest: a systematic review and meta-analysis. Part 2: Patients treated with therapeutic hypothermia. *Resuscitation* 2013;84:1324–38.

74. Robinson LR, Micklesen PJ, Tirschwell DL, Lew HL. Predictive value of somatosensory evoked potentials for awakening from coma. *Crit Care Med* 2003;31:960–7.

75. Wijdicks EF, Hijdra A, Young GB, Bassetti CL, Wiebe S. Quality Standards Subcommittee of the American Academy of N. Practice parameter: prediction of outcome in comatose survivors after cardiopulmonary resuscitation (an evidence-based review): report of the Quality Standards Subcommittee of the American Academy of Neurology. *Neurology* 2006;67:203–10.

76. Wijdicks EF, Varelas PN, Gronseth GS, Greer DM. American Academy of N. Evidence-based guideline update: determining brain death in adults: report of the Quality Standards Subcommittee of the American Academy of Neurology. *Neurology* 2010;74:1911–8.

77. Houlden DA, Li C, Schwartz ML, Katic M. Median nerve somatosensory evoked potentials and the Glasgow Coma Scale as predictors of outcome in comatose patients with head injuries. *Neurosurgery* 1990;27:701–7; discussion 7–8.

78. Houlden DA, Taylor AB, Feinstein A, et al. Early somatosensory evoked potential grades in comatose traumatic brain injury patients predict cognitive and functional outcome. *Crit Care Med* 2010;38:167–74.

79. Amantini A, Fossi S, Grippo A, et al. Continuous EEG-SEP monitoring in severe brain injury. *Neurophysiol Clin* 2009;39:85–93.

80. Bosco E, Zanatta P, Ponzin D, et al. Prognostic value of somatosensory-evoked potentials and CT scan evaluation in acute traumatic brain injury. *J Neurosurg Anesthesiol* 2014;26:299–305.

81. Curt A, Dietz V. Electrophysiological recordings in patients with spinal cord injury: significance for predicting outcome. *Spinal Cord* 1999;37:157–65.

82. Spiess M, Schubert M, Kliesch U, group E-SS, Halder P. Evolution of tibial SSEP after traumatic spinal cord injury: baseline for clinical trials. *Clin Neurophysiol* 2008;119:1051–61.

83. Nwachuku EL, Balzer JR, Yabes JG, Habeych ME, Crammond DJ, Thirumala PD. Diagnostic value of somatosensory evoked potential changes during carotid endarterectomy: a systematic review and meta-analysis. *JAMA Neurol* 2015;72:73–80.

84. Duncan CC, Barry RJ, Connolly JF, et al. Event-related potentials in clinical research: guidelines for eliciting, recording, and quantifying mismatch negativity, P300, and N400. *Clin Neurophysiol* 2009;120:1883–908.

12

Neuroimaging

S. Thota

ABSTRACT

The use of advanced neuroimaging has become part of routine workup for patients in the intensive care unit (ICU). Computed tomography (CT) is the investigation of choice due to its ready availability and speed. Contrast-enhanced CT, CT angiography, or magnetic resonance imaging (MRI) play an ancillary role and are reserved for cases where an abnormality is identified on unenhanced CT that requires further characterization, or intracranial pathology is still suspected despite a negative head CT. In this chapter, various traumatic and nontraumatic brain emergencies commonly seen in the ICU setting are discussed. Also, interesting miscellaneous conditions where imaging plays a crucial role are briefly described.

KEYWORDS

Neuroimaging; computed tomography (CT); magnetic resonance imaging (MRI); intensive care unit (ICU); haemorrhage.

INTRODUCTION

It is often challenging to follow the clinical status of patients in the intensive care unit (ICU) as a majority of patients are sedated, paralysed, and may be intubated. The clinicians often lose the ability to carefully examine patients who may be developing life threatening neurological disorders.[1] The use of advanced neuroimaging has become a mainstay in the routine workup for any critically ill patient who is suspected to develop any acute neurological dysfunction. However, transporting critically ill patients out of the ICU is a challenge. Inadvertent loss of intravenous and arterial line in haemodynamically unstable patients may lead to serious adverse events. Therefore, any diagnostic test is warranted only if results of the test are likely to change patient management. Comatose patients with known neurological disorders may benefit from surveillance imaging of the brain even in the absence of any clinical suspicion. Computed tomography (CT) is the investigation of choice due to its availability, speed, and compatibility with accompanying life support systems. Examination performed for trauma or acute mental status changes generally do not require contrast administration.[2]

Additional studies such as contrast-enhanced CT, CT angiography (CTA), or magnetic resonance imaging (MRI) largely play an ancillary role in the ICU setting and are generally reserved for cases in which (1) an abnormality is identified on unenhanced CT that requires further characterization, or (2) intracranial pathology is still suspected despite a negative head CT.

INTENSIVE CARE UNIT PATIENTS WITH TRAUMATIC BRAIN EMERGENCIES

Computed tomography is the ideal imaging modality to evaluate for acute intracranial haemorrhage and bone fracture. Diffuse axonal injury and cortical contusion are the two most common findings in patients with trauma due to a closed head injury. A cortical contusion is an injury of the brain surface and it may be either haemorrhagic or nonhaemorrhagic. Contusions tend to involve the regions of the brain that are in close proximity with crests of bone. Anterior and basal frontal, temporal, and occipital lobes are particularly vulnerable. The term 'coup' is used for an injury that lies directly beneath the area of impact. The term 'countercoup' is used for injury that occurs remotely from the site of impact along the direct line but opposite to this site caused by acceleration effects. Haemorrhagic contusions are well-demonstrated by CT and appear as areas of increased density generally following the configuration of the gyri. Haemorrhagic contusions are surrounded by a thin halo of oedema. Computed tomography obtained 24 to 48 hours post-trauma often show contusions to be larger and more numerous than on initial CT scans.[3]

Diffuse axonal injury (DAI) results from shearing forces due to rapid deceleration. Common locations for DAI are the grey-white matter junction, the corpus callosum, and the brainstem. This is in the order of most to least common and also from least severe to most severe. Computed tomography is often normal. On MRI fluid-attenuated inversion recovery (FLAIR) scans, injuries at the grey-white matter junction are seen as small foci of abnormal high signal intensity, most commonly involving the frontal lobes. If the lesions are haemorrhagic, they are detected on T2*-weighted gradient echo scans or susceptibility weighted imaging due to the presence of deoxyhaemoglobin. The second most common presentation is a shear injury of the corpus callosum with a majority involving the splenium. Lesions of the brainstem are seen most often in the pons and dorsolateral midbrain (Figure 12.1). Brainstem lesions have poor prognosis, often with fatal outcome. Shearing injuries in patients less than 2 years of age should raise the suspicion of non-accidental trauma.[4]

The dura is strongly adherent to the inner table of the skull. An epidural haematoma is the accumulation of blood between the inner table of the skull and the dura, and is usually due to a skull fracture with laceration of a blood vessel. The fracture *per se* is of little clinical significance unless they are depressed. The most common location of epidural bleed is temporal/parietal due to laceration of the middle meningeal artery. Epidural haematoma in the posterior cranial fossa are less common and occur due to an occipital skull fracture with secondary laceration of the transverse sinus. An intervening lucid interval is noted in 50% of cases after the initial trauma with subsequent rapid deterioration. On CT, a biconvex, extra axial fluid collection is noted, which can cross the midline and tentorium with the venous sinuses displaced away from the skull. In adults, epidural haematomas do not cross the suture line, although in children and with venous bleeds, this is not true. On CT, an acute epidural haematoma will be hyperdense to brain parenchyma and may show a hypodense component due to active bleeding (Figure 12.2). On MRI, the displaced dura may be seen with the acute epidural haematoma itself having

the signal intensity characteristics of oxyhaemoglobin or deoxyhaemoglobin. Magnetic resonance imaging is more sensitive for detecting coexisting parenchymal brain injuries and the subacute stage of haemorrhage.[5]

Subdural haematomas is caused most commonly due to trauma with tearing of the bridging veins and demonstrate a convex inward border. The density and signal intensity of subdural haematomas vary with age. Acute (1–3 days) subdural haematomas are hyperattenuating relative to cerebral cortex. With the resorption of blood products, the collection becomes isodense to hypodense relative to the cerebral cortex. In the subacute phase (3 days to 3 weeks), subdural haematomas may become difficult to observe on CT when it becomes isodense to the cortex (Figure 12.3). Secondary signs, including displacement of the cortex from the inner table of the skull and sulcal effacement are helpful signs for diagnosing small isodense subdural haematomas. In the chronic phase, subdural haematomas become hypodense to the cortex. Contrast-enhanced studies can display enhancing membranes and inward displacement of enhancing vessels. On MRI, the signal intensity of blood products in the subdural space follows the temporal progression of deoxyhaemoglobin to intracellular methaemoglobin and extracellular methaemoglobin. Bilateral convexity or interhemispheric subdural haematomas in a child should raise the suspicion of non-accidental trauma.

NON-ACCIDENTAL TRAUMA

Non-accidental trauma (NAT) also known as child abuse can be caused by injuries due to direct impact or acceleration-deceleration forces secondary to shaking and is characterized by the triad of subdural haemorrhage, retinal haemorrhage, and encephalopathy. Findings include skull fractures, subdural haematoma, and contusions. The skull fracture and scalp haematoma are well visualized on a CT. Bilateral subdural haematomas of differing ages strongly support the diagnosis of NAT. Territorial infarcts and/or global hypoxic injury may also be seen. Chronic blood products, residual from prior haemorrhagic contusions are well seen on T2*-weighted scans. Imaging is vital when NAT cases require emergent neurosurgical interventions and provides critical data for the hospital child protective services, and clinicians should maintain a low threshold for performing a CT or MRI of the head in all cases of suspected abuse.

PENETRATING INJURIES

Gunshot wounds are best evaluated by CT. Bony defects at the entry site as well as extensive skull fractures and metal fragments from the bullet are well demonstrated on CT. Oedema may be extensive. Parenchymal haemorrhage and subdural haematomas are commonly seen.

INTENSIVE CARE UNIT PATIENTS WITH NONTRAUMATIC INTRACRANIAL EMERGENCIES

The imaging features of nontraumatic intracranial entities seen in ICU patients are grouped into four general categories, including (1) vascular emergencies, (2) hydrocephalus and associated conditions, (3) central nervous system (CNS) infections, and (4) miscellaneous processes, including toxic exposures and pituitary apoplexy.

Vascular Emergencies

More than two-thirds of clinically evident acute strokes are caused by cerebral ischaemia with the remaining being caused by intracranial haemorrhage. In adults, cerebral infarcts are most commonly caused by atherosclerosis with vessel occlusion due to either thrombosis or embolism. Common sites of atherosclerosis include the carotid bifurcation, distal internal carotid artery, and middle cerebral artery. Risk factors for infarction in an adult are hypertension, hypercholesterolemia, smoking, diabetes, cardiovascular disease, obesity, oral contraceptives, and cocaine. Leading causes of infarction in young patients and children include congenital and acquired heart disease and sickle cell disease.

With widespread availability of thrombolytic treatment, rapid diagnosis is now critical to optimize outcomes in patients with acute neurological deficit. The National Institute of Neurological Disorders and Stroke tissue plasminogen activator (NINDS-tPA) trial demonstrated that patients receiving intravenous (IV) tPA within 3 hours of stroke onset were 30% more likely to have little or no disability at 3 months than patients receiving placebo. The European Cooperative Acute Stroke Study III (ECASS III) trial showed that clinical outcomes are also improved in patients receiving IV tPA up to 4.5 hours after stroke onset, but there is gradually diminishing benefit with increasing time from ictus. Intra-arterial recanalization techniques including direct intra-arterial thrombolysis and use of mechanical clot retrieval devices are widely available and generally considered for patients presenting outside of the effective window of IV thrombolysis for up to 6 hours from the onset of stroke symptoms. All patients in the ICU with suspected acute ischaemic cerebral infarctions should undergo emergent cross-sectional brain imaging. The primary goal of imaging in an acute setting are (1) to identify the presence of haemorrhage (contraindication to treatment),

(2) to identify large vessel occlusion, and (3) to assess the volume of irreversibly injured brain tissue.[6]

The second step in the workup of stroke involves evaluation of cervical and intracranial arterial supply, performed with CT or MR angiography. Images are obtained of the aortic arch and vessels are traced superiorly into the third or fourth order intracranial branches to evaluate for aneurysms, stenosis, vessel occlusion, and dissections. Diagnostic 4-vessel angiography is recommended for confirmation. Magnetic resonance imaging is a study of choice if dissection is suspected, as it allows for better visualization of the lumen, wall of the vessel, and also may be used to visualize an intramural haematoma.[7]

The third step in the workup of a stroke is the perfusion study. This can be performed in CT by monitoring the first pass of the iodinated contrast agent bolus through the cerebral circulation. It involves continuous cine imaging over the same area of brain tissue to help produce a perfusion curve. Based on this information, colour-coded maps are produced which include cerebral blood volume (CBV), cerebral blood flow (CBF), and mean transit time (MTT). When evaluating the perfusion study, it is important to not only analyse each component but also to analyse them as a whole to help get an overall picture of the brain's perfusion status. In at-risk ischaemic tissue, there is elevated mean transit time with slightly decreased CBF and slightly decreased or normal CBV, which means that blood volume is maintained but it takes a longer amount of time to get to that specific portion of the brain. In contrast, infarcted tissue has elevated MTT, with decreased blood flow and volume, indicating that there is essentially no blood flow to this region. Computed tomography perfusion is routinely performed in many centres to determine the mismatch between brain with markedly reduced CBF, CBF (<12 cm^3/100 g/min) in the irreversibly infarcted core, and potentially salvageable brain tissue in areas where CBF is reduced (12–22 cm^3/100 g/min), and prolonged MTT, the ischaemic penumbra. Treatment options include thrombolysis or thrombectomy, and the decision is largely dictated by the presence and extent of an ischaemic penumbra which is the tissue at risk.

Arterial infarcts are easily recognized due to their territorial distribution and their involvement of both grey and white matter. Middle cerebral artery (MCA) supplies the lateral cerebral hemispheres with the lenticulostriate branches from the M1 segment supplying the globus pallidus, putamen, and the anterior limb of the internal capsule. More than half of ischaemic cerebral infarctions involve the MCA territory. Early CT findings of an MCA infarction include hyperdensity of the MCA trunk or its branches and parenchymal hypodensity, local brain swelling, or territorial loss of grey-white differentiation. Effacement of normally slightly hyperdense basal ganglia (disappearing basal ganglia sign) or insular cortex (the insular ribbon sign) are early findings of an acute MCA infarction (Figure 12.4). Posterior circulation strokes are caused by obstruction of the vertebral, basilar, or posterior cerebral arteries and their branches and may involve the posterior-inferior temporal lobe, medial parietal lobe, occipital lobe, and portions of the brainstem, thalamus, and internal capsule. Thrombosis of the basilar artery is potentially catastrophic with a mortality rate of 80%–90% if left untreated. On unenhanced CT, thrombus within the basilar artery may appear hyperdense and the appearance of a dense artery may proceed the development of parenchymal hypodensity. The anterior cerebral artery (ACA) supplies the anterior putamen, hypothalamus, corpus callosum, caudate nucleus, and medial surface of the cerebral hemisphere. Anterior cerebral artery infarcts are by far the least common accounting for up to 5% of ischaemic strokes. ACA strokes often result from primary vessel disease (e.g., atherosclerosis, vasculitis or vasospasm related to aneurysmal subarachnoid haemorrhage [aSAH]) rather than from emboli. ACA infarcts may also occur as a result of subfalcine herniation as the ACA becomes compressed under the falx cerebri. ACA infarctions are often seen in combination with MCA infarctions. On unenhanced CT, ACA infarcts appear hypodense involving the medial aspect of superior frontal and parietal lobes adjacent to the falx. A hyperdense ACA may also be seen in some cases indicating acute thrombus within the vessel.

Watershed infarction occurs in the boundary zones between major arterial territories and accounts for nearly 10% of ischaemic strokes. It is thought that hypoperfusion in combination with severe occlusive disease of the internal carotid arteries can cause both embolization and decreased brain perfusion, which is most pronounced at the arterial border zones resulting in watershed infarcts. Like other ischaemic infarcts, acute watershed infarcts are hypodense on CT and demonstrate high signal intensity on diffusion-weighted imaging (DWI), T2-weighted, and FLAIR sequence (Figure 12.5). Lacunar infarcts are small, deep cerebral infarcts that result from occlusion of small penetrating arteries arising from the major cerebral arteries. They are most frequently seen with hypertension and commonly involve the basal ganglia, internal capsule, thalamus, and brainstem. Pontine infarcts are most frequently unilateral, paramedian, and sharply marginated at the midline.

Magnetic resonance imaging is relatively more sensitive than CT for detection of early brain infarcts. Magnetic resonance imaging is also superior to CT for detection of lacunar infarcts and infarcts involving the posterior fossa and brainstem. Cytotoxic oedema develops in an area of ischaemia within minutes, which is seen as high signal intensity on DWI with a corresponding low apparent diffusion coefficient (ADC) (restricted diffusion) on the calculated apparent diffusion coefficient map. Impaired function of the sodium potassium pump leads to a net flow of water into the cell with cytotoxic oedema leading to restricted diffusion seen on DWI. In the early stage of a territorial infarct, there may be subtle loss of cortical sulci and a slight increased thickness of cortical grey matter that may also be visualized on T1-weighted scans. By 24 hours, vasogenic oedema is present in a majority of infarcts and seen as high signal intensity on T2-weighted scans with corresponding low signal intensity on T1-weighted scans. On CT, vasogenic oedema is seen as an area of low attenuation compared to the normal adjacent brain. Vasogenic oedema typically persists for weeks.[8]

Cerebral infarcts are staged into hyperacute (less than 6 hours), acute (less than 24 hours), subacute (more than 1 day to 1 month), and chronic (more than 1 month). Enhancement in the infarcted area can be in the form of intravascular, meningeal, and parenchymal. Intravascular enhancement can be seen in the first day and up to a week. A short segment of a single vessel, or of multiple enhancing vessels, may be seen. Meningeal enhancement usually seen from days 1 to 3, adjacent to the area of infarction, is the least common form of abnormal enhancement. Parenchymal enhancement is common during the first month but not typically seen in the first week and may persist for up to 8 weeks. Parenchymal enhancement is usually gyriform in pattern and basal ganglion infarcts usually show a ring-like pattern. Haemorrhagic transformation can be seen with ischaemic infarcts in up to 25% of cases. Deoxyhaemoglobin will be visualized on MR sequences sensitive to T2*. At a slightly later stage, methaemoglobin is seen which is well visualized on T1-weighted sequences. Petechial haemorrhage is much more common than parenchymal haematoma. Haemorrhage occurs when the ischaemic brain is reperfused as it contains vessels with damaged endothelium. Predisposing factors for haemorrhagic transformation include lysis of an embolus, opening of collaterals, and restoration of normal blood pressure following hypotension, hypertension, and anticoagulation.[9,10]

CEREBRAL VENOUS THROMBOSIS AND INFARCTION

Cerebral venous thrombosis (CVT) is a rare cause of stroke that can be difficult to recognize due to variable clinical presentation. Cerebral venous thrombosis predominantly affects young women and risk factors include oral contraceptive use, dehydration, malignancy, inflammatory bowel disease, collagen vascular disease, pregnancy, and underlying hypercoagulable state. Imaging is critical for early diagnosis and initiation of therapy. Cerebral venous thrombosis is generally classified as involving the deep or superficial venous systems, and often both are simultaneously involved.[11] On CT and MRI, imaging clues to CVT include regional oedema with or without haemorrhage, not corresponding to an arterial territory. Venous territories include symmetric deep grey and white matter (deep cerebral vein), parasagittal frontoparietal (superior sagittal sinus), and posterolateral temporal (vein of Labbe). The venous thrombus appears hyperdense on non-contrast CT. On contrast CT and CT venography the clot produces a filling defect within the veins or dural sinuses. The thrombus may be visible as uniform hyperintense or iso-intense signals on T1-weighted images filling a dural sinus. MR venography demonstrates the absence of flow-related enhancement within the involved veins. Isolated cortical vein thrombosis may be identified as serpiginous susceptibility artifact on T2* sequences (Figure 12.6).

Parenchymal Haemorrhage

In adults, parenchymal haemorrhage is commonly due to hypertension and the typical location for hypertensive haemorrhage include, in order of decreasing frequency, the basal ganglia (in particular the putamen), thalamus, pons, and cerebellar hemisphere. On CT, hyperacute bleed is of moderate density that rapidly increases further in density due to clot formation and retraction. In the subacute stage, a progressive loss in attenuation begins. By 1–4 weeks, a haematoma will be isodense to the brain and in the chronic stage, it appears hypodense to the brain. Large cerebellar haematomas may compress the brainstem or the fourth ventricle causing obstructive hydrocephalus which requires emergent surgical evacuation. It is quite common for intraparenchymal haematomas to expand within the first few hours of symptom onset, a finding that is associated with poor outcome. Therefore, any deterioration in clinical status requires emergent reimaging to determine whether the haematoma has grown. Subsequent deterioration at 24–48 hours after haemorrhage onset is often caused by worsening cerebral oedema.

On MRI, haemorrhage follows a temporal progression of changes in the signal intensity depending on the biochemical and oxidation characteristics of haemoglobin. This change in signal intensity is best seen on MRI if the field strength is of 1.5 Tesla and above. In hyperacute haemorrhage, oxyhaemoglobin demonstrates signal intensity of fluid, low on T1- and high on T2-weighted scan. Within hours (acute haemorrhage), deoxyhaemoglobin is evident as distinctive low signal intensity on T2-weighted images. Deoxyhaemoglobin can appear isointense to mildly hypointense on T1-weighted images. In subacute haemorrhage, intracellular methaemoglobin demonstrates distinctive high signal intensity on T1-weighted scan and low signal on T2-weighted scan. Later with red blood lysis, methaemoglobin becomes extracellular in location. Extracellular methaemoglobin has distinctive high signal intensity on both T1- and T2-weighted scans. In the chronic stage, methaemoglobin is converted into hemosiderin that exhibits pronounced low signal intensity on T2-weighted scans due to susceptibility effects. Central fluid with high signal on both T1- and T2-weighted scans is seen surrounded by a hemosiderin rim (Figure 12.7). A hemosiderin cleft will be left if the central fluid is resorbed. Evaluation of parenchymal haemorrhage on MR does not always follow the characteristic pattern described; factors such as dilution, clotting, and haematocrit can alter the appearance. Enhancement is not seen in acute hypertensive haemorrhages and the presence of enhancement within or adjacent to a haematoma should prompt a workup to exclude alternative diagnoses such as tumour or vascular malformation.

Subarachnoid Haemorrhage

Spontaneous subarachnoid haemorrhage (SAH) commonly occurs due to rupture of an intracranial aneurysm. Most aneurysms are saccular and occur in predictable sites in the circle of Willis, usually at vessel bifurcations. The most common locations are the anterior communicating artery (ACoA), posterior communicating artery (PCoA), MCA bifurcation, and basilar artery (5%). Unenhanced CT is the imaging modality of choice for suspected SAH with a reported sensitivity greater that 95% within the first 24 hours. As in traumatic SAH, aSAH has a typical appearance of high attenuation in the cisternal spaces. Subarachnoid haemorrhage due to aneurysmal rupture is typically diffuse, which often makes it impossible to localize the source of bleeding. In some cases, the presence of a more prominent or focal clot may suggest location of an aneurysm. Aneurysms arising at the ACoA tend to bleed into the anterior interhemispheric fissure, into the septum pellucidum, and into the frontal horns of the lateral ventricle. Middle cerebral artery aneurysms tend to involve the ipsilateral Sylvian fissure. The PCoA and basilar artery aneurysms tend to be more diffuse or localized to the basilar cisterns. Compression on the nerve by the PCoA aneurysm may result in oculomotor nerve palsy. Posterior inferior cerebellar artery aneurysm tends to bleed into the perimedullary cistern and around the brainstem. CT can be negative in patients with SAH due to either time delay between the haemorrhage and imaging or the small quantity of bleed. This is the reason for a standard for lumbar puncture to be performed after a negative head CT in patients with suspected SAH. The sensitivity of CT in SAH decreases markedly following the first few days.[12]

On MRI, the FLAIR sequence is very sensitive to changes in the CSF and even a small amount of SAH is seen as abnormal high signal intensity with the sulci. This appearance is not specific for SAH though and a similar finding can be seen in any disease process that causes subtle change in the composition of CSF such as meningitis. The administration of O_2 in an ICU patient who is often ventilated and anesthetized can cause high signal intensity of the CSF. Acute subarachnoid blood is seen as low signal intensity on T2* weighted images. SAH can also be seen as high signal intensity on T1-weighted scans due the presence of methaemoglobin. This persists for days to weeks.

Although digital subtraction angiography is considered the gold standard for detection of ruptured aneurysms, noninvasive assessment with CTA or magnetic resonance angiography (MRA) are frequently performed first. Compared to digital subtraction angiography (DSA), CTA has a reported sensitivity of 96%–98%, but the sensitivity is slightly lower for aneurysms smaller than 3 mm and aneurysms arising at the skull base or cavernous segment of ICA because of artefacts caused by the adjacent bone. Three-dimensional time-of-flight (TOF) MRA is probably slightly less sensitive than CTA for aneurysm detection (Figure 12.8). The images demonstrate a superiorly directed outpouching arising from the basilar artery terminus consistent with basilar tip aneurysm. For patients with suspected aneurysmal SAH, negative CTA or MRA should be followed up with a DSA. A total of 15%–20% of patients with spontaneous SAH will have negative results on both noninvasive and conventional angiography. Most angiographically negative cases of SAH are caused by an aetiology other than aneurysm and a minority of false negative angiogram may occur as a result of transient aneurysm thrombosis, severe vasospasm, or inadequate angiographic technique. Approximately 10% of cases of spontaneous SAH fall into the category of nonaneurysmal perimesencephalic SAH. These haemorrhages are typically confined to the perimesencephalic cisterns anterior to the brainstem.

Their aetiology is unknown, but it has been suggested that they may be caused by venous bleeding. They tend to have excellent outcomes compared to patients with aneurysmal SAH and do not appear to be at risk for rebleeding.

Intraventricular Haemorrhage

Intraventricular haemorrhage is believed to arise from tearing of the subependymal veins and is more commonly found within the lateral ventricles. It may also arise as an extension from an adjacent parenchymal haemorrhage or retrograde extension of SAH. Intraventricular haemorrhage may result in acute noncommunicating hydrocephalus secondary to clot obstructing the normal circulation of CSF. Ventricular bleed is well seen as hyperdensity on CT in an acute setting. Layering of a small amount of bleed in the dependent portion of the lateral ventricles is commonly visualized on MRI, a sign that can persist for days to weeks following haemorrhage.

MISCELLANEOUS INTRACRANIAL EMERGENCIES

Cerebral Amyloid Angiopathy

Multiple cortical and subcortical microhaemorrhages are best seen on gradient echo T2-weighted, T2*-weighted, or susceptibility-weighted MR sequences. Cerebral amyloid angiography is also a recognized cause of spontaneous convexity SAHs and superficial cortical siderosis in the elderly. Superficial cortical siderosis appears as a thin stripe of low-signal intensity in the leptomeninges and cortical surface on T2-weighted or blood sensitive sequences. This finding presumably represents hemosiderin deposition caused by prior episodes of SAH or primary bleeding in the superficial cortical layers.[13]

Cerebral Vasospasm

Vasospasm is the delayed subacute narrowing of the intracranial vasculature following SAH, usually secondary to aneurysm rupture. Angiographically evident vasospasm occurs in 60% of patients with aSAH. It accounts for half of the death in patients surviving aneurysm treatment. Vasospasm risk is related to the amount of subarachnoid and intraventricular haemorrhage. It typically occurs 4 to 20 days after SAH and is most severe at 7 to 10 days. It may involve either the proximal or distal intracranial arteries. Transcranial Doppler ultrasound detects elevated blood velocities due to vasospasm and is used to screen patients in the intensive care setting. Drawbacks include operator dependence and limited evaluation of the anterior cerebral arteries or posterior circulation. Computed tomography angiography may be used to confirm equivocal cases but may overestimate the degree of vessel narrowing (Figure 12.9). Catheter angiography is the gold standard for evaluating the severity of vessel narrowing. The stenosis is typically smoothly marginated and may occur over long segments of the vessels. The calcium channel antagonist, nimodipine is given prophylactically to reduce vasospasm-related morbidity. Induced hypervolemia and hypertension are used to maintain cerebral perfusion. When medical therapy fails, endovascular techniques with intra-arterial vasodilators and balloon angioplasty are performed.

Brain Herniation

The brain can herniate from one compartment into another due to intracranial pressure resulting from a mass, oedema, haemorrhage, or inflammatory process. The most common cause of brain herniation is trauma. It is not uncommon for several different herniations to occur concomitantly.

The most common type of brain herniation is subfalcine herniation which is caused by a supratentorial mass on one side of the interhemispheric falx that shifts the brain to the opposite side. Herniation of the brain occurs across the midline under the inferior or 'free' margin of the falx (Figure 12.10). The cingulate gyrus, anterior cerebral artery, and internal cerebral vein can be displaced to the contralateral side under the falx. The ipsilateral ventricle is usually compressed and displaced towards the midline. There can be dilatation of the contralateral lateral ventricle due to occlusion of the foramen of Monro. The herniated anterior cerebral artery can be compressed against the free margin of the falx resulting in infarction.

The second most common type of cerebral herniation is descending transtentorial herniation caused by a large hemispheric mass. This results in obliteration of the basilar cisterns and inferior displacement of the third ventricle and brainstem. Complications arising from this include compression of the posterior cerebral artery (PCA) and basilar arteries resulting in infarction, dural haemorrhages in the pons and midbrain, and compression of the oculomotor nerve (resulting in ipsilateral pupillary dilatation). Unilateral downward herniation with medial displacement of the temporal lobe over the incisura is uncal herniation. On CT, both the ipsilateral ambient cistern and lateral portion of the prepontine cistern may be widened. With increasing mass effect, the uncus and hippocampus can both herniate through the tentorial incisura.

In the posterior fossa, the cerebellum can herniate downward through the foramen magnum (tonsillar herniation) or upwards through the incisura resulting in obliteration of the quadrigeminal cistern. This can obstruct the aqueduct causing hydrocephalus. Tonsillar herniation is well visualized on magnetic resonance demonstrating inferior displacement of the cerebellar tonsils, pointing of the tonsillar tip and obliteration of cerebrospinal fluid (CSF) at the level of the foramen magnum.

Following a craniectomy, oedematous brain can herniate outward through the skull defect. This is the least common type of supratentorial brain herniation known as external herniation.

Complications of Cerebrospinal Fluid Shunts

The most frequently used type of shunt is the ventriculoperitoneal (VP) shunt, which diverts CSF from the ventricles into the peritoneal cavity. Modern VP shunts consist of three components: a proximal ventriculostomy catheter, a shunt valve to regulate CSF flow, and a distal peritoneal catheter. Shunt failure is a common complication of CSF shunting and are most often caused by a mechanical malfunction or shunt infection. Shunt malfunction usually occurs in the first 6 months following insertion and can be caused by shunt obstruction, shunt disconnection, and fracture resulting in increased intracranial pressure. The proximal ventricular catheter is the most common site of obstruction but blockage can occur at any point along the shunt. Obstruction at the distal end is typically caused by adhesions or encystment in the peritoneum. Radiological evaluation of suspected shunt malfunction includes unenhanced head CT to assess change in ventricular size or intraventricular catheter position and plain radiographs covering the entire course of the shunt to identify catheter disconnections, kinks, breaks, or distal migration. Increasing ventricular size is an indicator of an obstructive shunt malfunction; however, shunt malfunction cannot be excluded in the absence of ventricular enlargement because scarring around the ventricular walls may prohibit ventricular expansion in some patients. A less common cause of shunt failure is overshunting, which occurs when a shunt's valve is set to remove more fluid than necessary for a particular patient. Early rapid reduction in ventricular size can cause collapse of the ventricles and accumulation of extra-axial fluid such as subdural hygromas or haematomas. When the rate of CSF overdrainage is slower, patients present with shunt malfunction and small ventricles on imaging, so-called slit ventricle syndrome. Shunt infection usually occurs during the perioperative period within the first

2 months following placement and the patient presents with symptoms of meningitis and ventriculitis and shows findings of the same on imaging.[14]

Hypoxic-Ischaemic Encephalopathy

Hypoxic-ischaemic encephalopathy (HIE) results from inadequate delivery of oxygen and nutrients to the cerebrum. Severe global impairment of cerebral blood flow and oxygenation may occur in cardiac arrest, drowning, choking, etc. Mild to moderate hypoxic-ischemic events result in watershed infarcts at the confluence of the ACA, PCA, and MCA territories. Severe anoxic insults primarily affect the grey matter structures which are areas with excitatory amino acid receptors and high metabolic demand: basal ganglia, thalami, cerebral cortex (particularly sensorimotor and visual cortices), cerebellum, and hippocampi. Non-contrast CT is insensitive during the first 24 hours. After 24 hours, findings on CT include diffuse sulcal and ventricular effacement (cerebral oedema), diffuse loss of grey-white matter differentiation, and hypoattenuation of deep grey nuclei. A minority of patients may demonstrate the so-called reversal sign in which there is reversal in the normal CT densities of grey and white matter with white matter being of higher density than the cortical grey matter. The 'white cerebellum' sign may be seen in which the cerebellum and brainstem demonstrate apparent high attenuation because of the development of diffuse cerebral oedema. Magnetic resonance imaging is the best imaging modality for the diagnosis of HIE. T2 and FLAIR sequences become abnormal after 12–24 hours. Diffusion weighted imaging is the most sensitive for detecting injury within the first few hours and demonstrates restricted diffusion (Figure 12.11). Magnetic resonance spectroscopy reveals elevation in lactate and glutamine-glutamate. In 2%–3% of cases, patients with HIE may demonstrate a period of relative clinical stability or even improvement followed by acute neurological decline, usually 2–3 weeks after the initial insult. Magnetic resonance imaging performed during the period of delayed neurological decline demonstrates symmetric confluent T2 and FLAIR hyperintensity in the cerebral white matter with corresponding restricted diffusion on DWI. Majority of patients have complete or near complete recovery. The condition may rarely progress to paresis or death.[15]

Posterior Reversible Encephalopathy Syndrome

This clinico-radiologic entity is characterized by a distinct pattern of typically reversible brain oedema that primarily affects the parietal and occipital lobes. It frequently occurs in the setting of acute severe hypertension (hence previously referred to as acute hypertensive encephalopathy). Additional risk factors include eclampsia, renal disease, immunosuppressant therapy (especially cyclosporine A and tacrolimus) or high-dose multidrug antineoplastic chemotherapy, solid organ or bone marrow transplantation, and certain autoimmune diseases including lupus. Posterior reversible encephalopathy syndrome (PRES) can also occur in the setting of infection, sepsis, or shock. Women are more commonly affected than men. Posterior circulation is usually involved with FLAIR sequence MRI demonstrating bilateral symmetric abnormal high signal intensity due to vasogenic oedema in the parieto-occipital lobes. The cortex as well as subcortical white matter is involved in non-vascular distribution. Basal ganglia may be involved and in advanced disease the involvement of cerebral hemispheres may be more extensive. These areas do not demonstrate restricted diffusion (Figure 12.12). Magnetic resonance angiography in cases of PRES may show evidence of vasculopathy, demonstrated as vessel irregularity with alternate foci of vasoconstriction and vasodilatation. With appropriate treatment, the prognosis is usually excellent and most patients demonstrate complete resolution of clinical and radiographic findings. Rarely, however, PRES may progress to irreversible ischaemia and infarction.[16]

Wernicke Encephalopathy

Wernicke encephalopathy is a rare acute neurological emergency caused by thiamine (Vitamin B1) deficiency. It most commonly occurs in alcoholics but can be found in other conditions producing thiamine depletion due to severe malnutrition such as hyperemesis gravidum, starvation, anorexia nervosa, and bariatric surgery. The triad of classical clinical presentation includes ophthalmoplegia, ataxia, and confusion. The most common presentation is diminished consciousness. On FLAIR, abnormal bilateral hyperintensity can be seen in mammillary bodies around the third ventricle and in the medial thalami, tectal plate, and periaqueductal grey matter. Enhancement of mammillary bodies is a distinctive feature and may be the only abnormality.[17]

Hepatic Encephalopathy

This can be seen in patients with acute or chronic liver disease and is characterized on MR imaging by high signal intensity in the globus pallidus on T1-weighted images, which is thought to be due to manganese deposition. Similar findings can be seen with hyperalimentation.

Carbon Monoxide Poisoning

Carbon monoxide (CO) has 250 times the affinity for haemoglobin of oxygen and inhalation of CO results in impaired oxygen transport. The hallmark of CO poisoning is symmetric injury to the globus pallidus initially causing vasogenic oedema followed by gliosis and cystic encephalomalacia and then atrophy. Computed tomography in patients with acute CO poisoning demonstrates symmetric hypodensity in the basal ganglia with preferential involvement of the globus pallidi. On MR imaging, appearance is that of 'eye of the tiger'. On FLAIR sequence, the globus pallidi demonstrates central cavitation seen as low signal intensity due to fluid and peripheral gliosis seen as abnormal high signal. A small percentage of patients with CO poisoning develop a delayed leukoencephalopathy identical to that seen in patients with hypoxic-ischaemic brain injury.[18]

Osmotic Demyelination

Osmotic demyelination syndrome encompasses both pontine and extra pontine myelinosis. Previously referred to as central pontine myelinolysis, this occurs due to rapid correction of severe chronic hyponatremia and is often seen in the setting of alcoholism or malnutrition. Oligodendrocytes are very sensitive to osmotic changes leading to cerebral injury that predominantly affects the white matter. On T2-weighted imaging, abnormal symmetrical high signal is noted in the central pons with sparing of the periphery and corticospinal tracts (Figure 12.13). There is usually no enhancement or mass effect. Extrapontine myelinolysis is most commonly seen in conjunction with central pontine myelinolysis with symmetric involvement of the basal ganglia and deep white matter, especially in the external capsule. Extrapontine involvement is almost always symmetric.[19]

Pituitary Apoplexy

Pituitary adenomas are extremely common in the general population and are frequently an asymptomatic incidental finding on brain CT or MRI. In rare instances, pituitary adenomas can haemorrhage and rapidly enlarge resulting in a potentially life-threatening condition known as pituitary apoplexy. Less commonly, pituitary apoplexy is the result of pituitary infarction without a pre-existing tumour. It is characterized clinically by sudden onset of headache, bitemporal hemianopia, and pituitary malfunction with or without loss of consciousness. Computed tomography may demonstrate a haemorrhagic mass in the suprasellar cistern with enlarged sella. Magnetic resonance imaging is the imaging modality of choice in patients with suspected pituitary apoplexy. On MRI, the gland is enlarged and may be hyperintense on unenhanced T1-weighted sequences and hypointense on T2-weighted sequences indicating the presence of haemoglobin breakdown products and may demonstrate a blood/fluid level. Compression of the anterior third ventricle may cause noncommunicating hydrocephalus.[20]

INFECTIOUS AND INFLAMMATORY INTRACRANIAL CONDITIONS IN THE INTENSIVE CARE UNIT

Bacterial Meningitis and Its Complications

Even with widespread use of antibiotics, bacterial meningitis is still associated with high rates of morbidity and mortality. Imaging is not required for the evaluation or management of uncomplicated meningitis as the diagnosis is usually based on clinical examination and CSF analysis. Imaging may be requested to exclude increased intracranial pressure prior to lumbar puncture. Imaging also helps in evaluating complications of meningitis, including cerebritis, brain abscess, subdural empyema, ventriculitis, hydrocephalus, infarction or venous thrombosis. FLAIR MR images may demonstrate non-specific finding of abnormally high-signal intensity CSF in the subarachnoid space. Contrast-enhanced MRI may show focal or diffuse pial enhancement (Figure 12.14a and Figure 12.14b). Underlying source of meningitis such as infection of paranasal sinus, mastoids or middle ear should undergo prompt consultation with neurosurgery or otolaryngology.[21]

Subdural Empyema

Subdural empyema is loculated purulent collections in the subdural space. In adults, empyema is most commonly caused by the spread of parameningeal infections such as sinusitis, otitis, or as a postsurgical complication. In children, subdural empyema also commonly occurs as a complication of bacterial meningitis. Subdural collections cross coronal or lambdoid sutures distinguishing them from epidural abscess. The presence of restricted diffusion differentiates subdural empyema from subdural effusion (Figure 12.15). The differentiation of subdural empyema and sterile effusion is critical since the former often requires rapid surgical drainage.[22]

Herpes Encephalitis

Herpes encephalitis results from primary infection or reactivation of herpes simplex virus (HSV-1). This virus, which causes oral herpes, may lie dormant in the trigeminal ganglion for decades. The areas typically involved include the medial temporal lobe, inferior frontal lobe, insula, and cingulate gyrus with predilection for the cortex over the white matter. Initially unilateral, the infection can spread to similar areas on the other side of the brain. Early MRI findings include T2 and FLAIR hyperintensity, T1 hypointensity and restricted diffusion on DWI. Later findings include gyriform cortical hyperintensity on T1-weighted images and post contrast enhancement of the cortices (Figure 12.16). Other viral encephalitis, limbic encephalitis, cerebral infarction, and neoplasm are included in the differential diagnosis. Clinical presentation and the classic distribution of signal changes differentiate it from acute infarction. Herpes simplex virus crosses vascular boundaries. The paucity of mass effect, presence of restricted diffusion, and predilection for grey matter distinguish it from most neoplasms.[23]

Progressive Multifocal Leukoencephalopathy

Progressive multifocal leukoencephalopathy (PML) is a demyelinating process caused by John Cunningham (JC) polyomavirus. This virus infects or becomes active in patients with severe immunodeficiency such as acquired immunodeficiency syndrome (AIDS), lymphoproliferative or myeloproliferative disorders, immunosuppressive therapy, or congenital immunodeficiency. Recent cases of PML have occurred in patients with multiple sclerosis undergoing treatment with natalizumab. It predominantly involves white matter but some involvement of grey matter structures is present in 50% of cases. The lesions on MRI are asymmetric and nonenhancing. In the setting of recently initiated highly active retroviral therapy (HART), marginal enhancement is more common. Such patients may experience a marked clinical deterioration termed as 'immune reconstitution inflammatory syndrome' (IRIS).[24]

Toxoplasmosis

Toxoplasmosis gondii is an intracellular parasite found throughout the world and acquired through ingestion of undercooked meat or exposure to cat faeces. Cerebral toxoplasmosis is the most common CNS opportunistic infection and the cause of intracranial mass lesions in patients with AIDS. On MRI, toxoplasmosis most commonly produces lesions that are hypointense on T1-weighted and hypo- to intermediate-signal on T2-weighted images. Most lesions measure 1 to 3 cm in diameter and they generally demonstrate marked surrounding vasogenic oedema. Nodular or ring enhancement is usually seen following contrast administration. A characteristic feature is

the small eccentric enhancing nodule along the enhancing rim, the so-called target sign (Figure 12.17). The primary differential consideration in HIV-positive patients is CNS lymphoma. Haemorrhage within the lesion favours toxoplasmosis, whereas lymphoma tends to abut the ependymal surface. Thallium-201 single photon emission computed tomography (SPECT) or fluorodeoxyglucose (FDG) positron emission tomography (PET) may be useful in differentiating the two because toxoplasmosis lesions are not radiotracer avid. With appropriate antibiotic therapy, toxoplasmosis lesions generally resolve within 3–6 months.[25]

CONCLUSIONS

Advanced neuroimaging has become part of the routine workup for patients in the intensive care unit. Computed tomography is the investigation of choice. Contrast-enhanced CT, CT angiography, or magnetic resonance imaging play an ancillary role.

REFERENCES

1. Lee K, Badjatia N. Neuroimaging in medical intensive care unit: an essential complement to the clinical examination. *Journal of Intensive Care Medicine* 2009;24(6):395–6.
2. Algethamy HM, Alzawahmah M, Young GB, Mirsattari SM. Added value of MRI over CT of the brain in intensive care unit patients. *Can J Neurol Sci* 2015 Sep;42(5):324–32.
3. Hardman JM, Manoukian A. Pathology of head trauma. *Neuroimaging Clin North Am* 2002;12:175–87.
4. Ezaki Y, Tsutsumi K, Morikawa M, Nagata I. Role of diffusion-weighted magnetic resonance imaging in diffuse axonal injury. *Acta Radiol* 2006;47:733–40.
5. Kidwell CS, Wintermark M. Imaging of intracranial hemorrhage. *Lancet Neurol* 2008;7:256–67.
6. de Lucas EM, Sanchez E, Gutierrez A, et al. CT protocol for acute stroke: tips and tricks for general radiologists. *Radiographics* 2008;28:1673–87.
7. Wintermark M, Sesay M, Barbier E, et al. Comparative overview of brain perfusion imaging techniques. *J Neuroradiol* 2005;32:294–314.
8. Konstas AA, Goldmakher CV, Lee TY, Lev MH. Theoretic basis and technical implementations of CT perfusion in acute ischemic stroke. Part 1: theoretic basis. *AJNR Am J Neuroradiol* 2009;30:662–8.
9. Srinivasan A, Goyal M, Al Asri F, et al. State-of-the-art imaging of acute stroke. *Radiographics* 2006;26:S75–S95.
10. Rovira A, Grive E, Rovira A, et al. Distribution of territories and causative mechanisms of ischemic stroke. *Eur Radiol* 2005;15:416–26.
11. Bentley JN, Figueroa RE, Vender JR, et al. From presentation to follow-up: diagnosis and treatment of cerebral venous thrombosis. *Neurosurg Focus* 2009;27:E41–47.

12. Suarez JI, Tarr RW, Selman WR. Aneurysmal subarachnoid hemorrhage. *N Engl J Med* 2006;35:387–96.

13. Chao CP, Kotsenas AL, Broderick DF. Cerebral amyloid angiopathy: CT and MR imaging findings. *Radiographics* 2006;26:1517–31.

14. Chahlavi A, El-Babba SK, Luciano MG. Adult-onset hydrocephalus. *Neurosurg Clin North Am* 2001;12:753–60.

15. Huang BY, Castillo M. Hypoxic-ischemic brain injury: imaging findings from birth to adulthood. *Radiographics* 2008;28:417–39.

16. Bartynski WS. Posterior reversible encephalopathy syndrome. Part 1. Fundamental imaging and clinical features. *AJNR Am J Neuroradiol* 2008;29:1036–42.

17. Zuccoli G, Pipitone M. Neuroimaging findings in acute Wernicke's encephalopathy: Review of the literature. *AJNR Am J Neuroradiol* 2009;192:501–8.

18. O'Donnell P, Buxton PJ, Pitkin A, Jarvis LJ. The magnetic resonance imaging appearances of the brain in acute carbon monoxide poisoning. *Clin Radiol* 2000;55:273–80.

19. Howard SA, Barletta JA, Klufas RA, et al. Osmotic demyelination syndrome. *Radiographics* 2009;29: 933–8.

20. Kreutzer J, Fahlbusch R. Diagnosis and treatment of pituitary tumors. *Curr Opin Neurol* 2004;17:693–703.

21. Kanamalla US, Ibarra RA, Jinkins JR. Imaging of cranial meningitis and ventriculitis. *Neuroimaging Clin North Am* 2000;10:309–31.

22. Ferreira N, Otta G, Amaral L, de Rocha A. Imaging aspects of pyogenic infections of the central nervous system. *Topics Magn Reson Imaging* 2005;16:145–54.

23. Bulakbasi N, Kocaoglu M. Central nervous system infections of herpes virus family. *Neuroimaging Clin North Am* 2008;8:53–84.

24. Shah R, Bag AK, Chapman PR, Curé JK. Imaging manifestations of progressive multifocal leukoencephalopathy. *Clin Radiol* 2010;65(6):431–9.

25. Dunn IJ, Palmer PE. Toxoplasmosis. *Semin Roentgenol* 1998;33(1):81–5.

13

Use of Ultrasound in Neurocritical Care

F. A. Rasulo, R. Bertuetti, and N. Latronico

ABSTRACT

Transcranial ultrasound (transcranial Doppler [TCD] and transcranial colour-coded duplex [TCCD]) is a non-invasive and accessible tool for bedside monitoring of static and dynamic cerebral blood flow velocity (CBFV) in relation to cerebrovascular diseases and response to treatment. Since its introduction by Rune Aaslid in 1982 it has become an essential neuromonitoring technique not only within the neurocritical care environment but also among other settings such as the emergency room, operating room, and general hospital wards. The main fields of clinical application of transcranial ultrasound are assessment of vasospasm, non-invasive estimation of cerebral perfusion pressure (CPP) and intracranial pressure (ICP), detection of vessel stenosis, microemboli, cerebral circulatory arrest for confirmation of brain death and evaluation of cerebrovascular autoregulation and vasomotor reactivity.

The chapter gives a brief overview regarding the types of ultrasound methods and presents future insights.

KEYWORDS

Transcranial Doppler (TCD); ultrasound; cerebral perfusion pressure (CPP); intracranial pressure (ICP); cerebral blood flow velocity (CBFV); cerebral blood flow (CBF).

INTRODUCTION

A thorough ultrasound examination, whether it be with transcranial Doppler (TCD) or transcranial colour-coded duplex (TCCD), begins with a knowledge of cerebrovascular anatomy. The major cerebral arteries are contained in a vascular structure named the Circle of Willis (circulus arteriosus cerebri) (Figures 13.1a and 13.1b).

The Circle of Willis has been named after Thomas Willis. It is an anastomotic arrangement of arteries lying at the base of the brain which encloses the stalk of the pituitary gland and allows significant communications between the blood circulation of the forebrain and hindbrain (i.e., between the internal carotid and vertebrobasilar systems following obliteration of primitive embryonic connections). Most individuals have a complete Circle of Willis, however, only half of them may present with well-developed communication between each of its components.

The intracranial arteries giving shape to the Circle of Willis (internal carotid artery [ICA], middle cerebral artery [MCA], anterior cerebral artery [ACA], and posterior cerebral artery [PCA]) are of most clinical interest and the object of investigation through the use of ultrasound and Doppler technique.[1–4]

ANATOMY OF THE MAIN CEREBRAL ARTERIES

Internal Carotid Artery

The ICA is mainly responsible for blood supply to the cerebral hemisphere and the eye (Figure 13.2). The ICA enters the base of the skull through the carotid canal of the petrous temporal bone travelling medially and reaching the cavernous sinus where it forms the S-shaped curve known as the carotid siphon. The artery penetrates the dura in its supraclinoid segment: at this level it gives off its first arterial branch: the ophthalmic artery (OA), followed by the posterior communicating artery (PCoA), and the anterior choroidal artery. The ICA then branches into the ACA and the MCA.[1–3]

Anterior Cerebral Artery

The anterior cerebral artery (ACA) is composed of five segments (Figure 13.3a). The A1 segment is the most proximal and corresponds to the portion running from its origin to the junction with the anterior communicating artery (ACoA). The ACoA potentially connects the cerebral hemispheres although it is commonly hypoplastic. The distal portions of the ACA run superiorly and cannot be insonated with TCD.[1–3]

Middle Cerebral Artery

The ICA gives rise to two terminal branches: the ACA and the MCA. Of these two branches, the MCA is readily insonated during TCD examinations. It stretches across the lateral sulcus and subsequently gives off branches and supplies substrates to most of the lateral cerebral cortex. The MCA is anatomically divided in four segments, of which M1 is the most proximal segment and divides into two or three branches known as the M2 divisions (Figure 13.4). The entire M1 segment and part of the M2 divisions can be studied with TCD.

The MCA has the following four segments:

- M1 or sphenoidal segment
- M2 divisions or insular segment
- M3 or opercular segment
- M4 or terminal cortical segment[1–3]

Posterior Communicating Artery

The PCoA (Figure 13.1b) originates from the ICA and joins the PCA. Depending on whether blood supply is provided via the carotid or the vertebrobasilar systems, blood flow through the PCoA may be in either direction.[1–3]

Vertebral Arteries

The vertebral artery (VA) (Figure 13.4) is the first branch to originate from the subclavian artery. Before it enters the skull, it runs through the vertebral canal of the cervical spine (from the sixth cervical vertebra up to the atlas). The VA angles outward to enter the cranium forming a loop behind the atlas and then goes into the skull through the foramen magnum after piercing the dura mater. The posterior inferior cerebellar artery (PICA) originates near the vertebral confluence. The diameter of the two VAs are usually not equal, in fact the left may be larger than the right causing discrepancies in blood flow velocity between the VAs.[1–3]

The Basilar Arteries

The basilar artery (BA) arises due to the confluence of the two VAs and runs on the ventral surface of the pons anteriorly and superiorly until its bifurcation (midbrain level) into the posterior cerebral arteries (PCA), which joins the PCoA forming the P1 segment. Beyond the PCoA originates the P2 segment which runs posteriorly. A thorough Circle of Willis is seen in 50% of the population. A perfect configuration is present in 18%.[1–3]

PHYSICAL PRINCIPLES

Transcranial Doppler ultrasonography follows similar principles that apply to other sound producing devices. In 1842, Christian Doppler was the first to scientifically describe the principle at the base of the shift in frequency of a sound wave of energy travelling above 20,000 Hz when either the transmitter or receiver is moving relatively to the wave-propagating medium.

Doppler technology enables the estimation of blood flow within the vessel by detecting the frequency shift produced in an ultrasound wave when reflected by a moving red blood cell. In fact, when the ultrasound wave emitted by the Doppler probe is reflected, the moving erythrocytes are exposed to a change in their frequency. Such change in frequency is incremental when the red blood cells (RBCs) are moving toward the probe while it is decremental when the red blood cells are moving away.

The change between the frequency of the original and reflected signal is known as the Doppler shift. This is directly proportional to blood flow velocity as expressed below:

$$F = \frac{2 \times Ft \times V \times \cos\theta}{C}$$

where F is the Doppler shift, Ft is the frequency of the wave emitted, V is the actual velocity, C is the velocity of sound in tissue and cos θ is the cosine of the angle between the insonated vessel and the direction of the ultrasound wave[4–13]. With an increase in angle of incidence, the difference between estimated and actual velocity increases.

Thus, a better estimate of flow velocity may be obtained by reducing the angle.[14]

For penetration into the skull, the transducer receives and transmits waves regularly. Such a modality is performed with a pulsed Doppler instrument. The shift in Doppler frequency is expressed in centimetres per second since this permits the comparison of readings from instruments that operate at different emission frequencies. A frequency of about 2 MHz seems to be most suitable for TCD applications.[8,9,15,16]

The TCD utilizes pulsed wave probes with a single piezoelectric crystal, which is stimulated in an alternate manner to produce a signal and silenced to allow the reflected wave to be interpreted (Figure 13.5). In addition to the conventional TCD, TCCD allows the operator to appreciate the intracranial parenchymal and bony structures, visualize coloured sequence of the basal cerebral arteries, and place the sample volume in a specific site of the artery in question by providing 2-dimensional grayscale, real time, and colour Doppler imaging.[17,18]

The TCD curve provides important diagnostic parameters: peak systolic velocity, telediastolic velocity, mean velocity, Gosling's 'pulsatility index' (PI), and Pourcelot's 'resistance index' (RI) (Figure 13.6).

$$PI = \frac{FVs - FVd}{FVm}$$

$$RI = \frac{FVs - FVd}{FVs}$$

An invariable cross-sectional area of the vessel and an unchanged angle of insonation are the two main assumptions which rule the use of TCD and allow detected blood flow velocities to be considered as an indirect measure of cerebral blood flow (CBF). The velocity detected by the probe as a fraction of the real velocity is dependent on the cosine of the angle of red cell insonation (measured velocity = real velocity × cosine of angle of incidence). Therefore, at 0 angle the detected and true red cell velocities are equal (cosine of 0 = 1), while at 90 degrees no detection of velocity is possible. Fortunately, the anatomic limitations of transtemporal insonation of the MCA are such that signal capture is only possible at narrow angles (<30 degrees). Thus the detected velocity is a very close approximation of the true velocity (87% to 100%). Furthermore, as long as the angle of insonation is kept constant by fixing the probe in position, changes in the detected velocity closely reflect changes in the true velocity.

Interpretation of TCD values rely on the diameter of the insonated vessel. Two parameters determine the volume per minute (flow) through a portion of the vessel. These include velocity of the erythrocytes and the cross sectional area of the vessel.[8,12,19]

Therefore, for velocity to be a reliable reflection of flow, the diameter of the vessel must not vary significantly during the measurement period.[8] Arterial carbon dioxide partial pressure ($PaCO_2$), blood pressure (BP), anaesthetic agents, and vasoactive drugs largely influence the diameter of the vessels. The basal cerebral arteries, being conductance vessels, do not dilate or constrict as the vascular resistance changes. For example, it has been shown angiographically that change in $PaCO_2$, one of the most important determinants of cerebrovascular resistance, has no effect on the diameter of the basal arteries.[20,21] Moreover, CO_2 reactivity studies performed with TCD have shown values similar to those derived using conventional CBF. Similarly, changes in BP have no impact on the diameter of the proximal segments of the basal arteries. Effects of vasoactive drugs on cerebral conductance vessels are variable, in fact, while sodium nitroprusside and phenylephrine do not significantly affect the proximal segments of the MCA, significant vasodilatation at the same level occurs when nitroglycerine is administered to healthy volunteers.[20–23]

The effect of anaesthetic agents on the diameter of basal vessels remains controversial. Intravenous agents are devoid of direct cerebral vascular effects and it is accepted that these agents do not affect the diameter of the conductance vessels.[24,25]

The situation is less clear-cut with inhalational agents as most of the evidence, but not thoroughly, suggests negligible effects on the diameter of conductance vessels.[24,26] On such a basis, it is generally accepted that during steady state anaesthetic conditions, changes in CBFV can be interpreted as average corresponding changes in cortical CBF.[21–23]

EXAMINATION TECHNIQUE

As skull bone represents the principal hindrance to ultrasound penetration and insonation of the brain parenchyma, the use of low frequency of 1–2 MHz emitting transducers and the approach through specific acoustic windows are made necessary. In fact low frequencies are able to reduce the attenuation of the ultrasound wave caused by bone and acoustic windows. There are specific points in the skull where the bone is thin enough to allow ultrasounds to penetrate.[8,9,27]

The TCCD, besides the Doppler insonation of the cerebral vessels, allows a two-dimensional visualization of the cerebral basal arteries, veins, and intracranial structures (such as ventricles and cisterns). The two-dimensional visualization renders rapid and reliable results, and aids in exact localization of the Doppler sample volume, thereby reducing examination time. (Figures 13.7, 13.8, 13.9).

As the above-mentioned Doppler insonation of the cerebral basal arteries (around the Circle of Willis) (TCD) is achieved through different 'windows' found at various locations on the skull, the small size and specific localization of these 'windows' play a distinctive role in determining: (1) a restricted variability of the angle of insonation found upon sampling the cerebral blood vessels; (2) a specific spatial and relative relationship between the window, the insonated arteries, and consequently the blood flow direction; fundamental factors for the proper identification of different vessels [Figure 13.10]. The standardized identification criteria provide highly reproducible and comparable inter-laboratory results. The criteria is as follows:

For TCCD

1. Proper site: temporal, orbital, submandibular, and occipital windows
2. Probe selection: select a low frequency probe (1–2 MHz) and the transcranial profile software
3. Position of the patient: supine for temporal and orbital, lateral decubitus for submandibular and occipital
4. Position of the operator: head of the bed while stabilizing the hand using a pillow
5. Adjust gain, depth, colour scale: Use initially a 5 mm sample volume for colour Doppler and then adjust
6. Trans-temporal window (Figures 13.11a and 13.11b): identify with 2D the petrous ridge posteriorly, carotid canal (C2–C3), foramen lacerum, cerebral falx, sphenoid wing anteriorly, cerebral peduncle, and the contralateral cranial bone (Figure 13.8). Use colour Doppler (scale 25 cm/s) to identify the vessels in the following order: bidirectional 'butterfly' terminal ICA (TICA) signal (C7) in the foramen lacerum, MCA, ACA, ACoA, then move back to TICA and find the PCoA, then the PCA, proximal (P1) and distal (P2) portion around the cerebral peduncle (P)
7. Transorbital window: select a high-frequency probe (7.5–10 MHz), reduce power setting (SPTA 17 mW/cm^2 and MI 0.28) with minimal pressure on the closed eyelid. On 2D, identify the optic nerve, then with colour Doppler the ophthalmic artery, then the carotid artery genu (C6) 'butterfly' signal. Aim the probe upward to identify the supraclinoid segment (C7) and then inferiorly to identify the cavernous or parasellar segment (C7). Insonation of the ophtalmic artery and carotid genu through the transorbital window is performed with a low frequency probe, reducing the power setting to 30%.

For the insonation of the optic nerve sheath, it is used a linear high frequency probe

8. Suboccipital window: lateral decubitus position with slight neck flexion, aim the probe at the nose ridge. Identify the foramen magnum and the two VAs and distal BA
9. Submandibular window: position the probe at the angle of the mandible and direct it medially and cephalad towards the carotid canal
10. Report velocity values and refer to normal values adjusted by age

For TCD

1. Proper site: The acoustic window through which the vessel is being insonated
2. The patient and operator positions (same as for TCCD)
3. The angle of the transducer during insonation
4. The depth at which the vessel is examined and the volume of the Doppler
5. The direction of the flow with respect to the transducer and the spectral distribution
6. The response of the Doppler signal to vibration or compression manoeuvres of the carotid artery

As already mentioned, the insonation windows used for TCD examination exploit areas where the skull bones are relatively thin or where anatomical foramens allow proper penetration of the ultrasound beam (Figure 13.12). Proper insonation through adequate ultrasonic window is of absolute importance for obtaining good propagation of ultrasound signal: recent studies conducted in intraoperative settings have shown that in ideal situations among patients, only approximately 6% of the intensity of the ultrasound used reaches the brain substance. The windows commonly utilized are:

- The transtemporal window
- The transorbital window
- The suboccipital or transforaminal window
- The submandibular window[12,13,17,28,29]

The Transtemporal Window

The insonation of the basal cerebral arteries and the Circle of Willis itself takes advantage of the thinnest portion of the squamous part of the temporal bone through which the ultrasonic beam can pass (Figure 13.13). Since a certain anatomical variability of bone structure from patient to patient exists, the passage of ultrasound may be hampered by the bone thickness or osteoporosis. Good signals are easily achievable in children and young adults.

Conversely, achieving sufficient signal strength may be difficult in elderly patients. In our experience, however, approximately 5%–10% of the examined population shows impossible acoustic window. In literature, racial and gender variations have been observed, with most of the impenetrable temporal bones and smallest windows among females of black ethnic origin.

The transtemporal window allows for the examination of the terminal portion of the ICA, its bifurcation into the middle and the ACA, and the PCA (see Figures 13.14 to 13.19). The communicating arteries (either anterior or posterior) can be sampled only in specific conditions when haemodynamic compensation through the Circle of Willis is taking place.

The patient is placed on the examining table/bed in a supine position and acoustic coupling gel is applied to the temporal area (Figures 13.11a and 13.11b). The probe is placed on the temporal area: if a TCCD machine is used the sphenoid bone, the heart (or butterfly) shaped cerebral peduncles, and basal cistern will be visualized first as the landmark; by turning on the colour mode, vessels of the Circle of Willis will become appreciable and angle adjusted pulsed Doppler will allow flow velocity detection. In view of the clinical indication, visualization of the MCA should be attempted at 2 mm to 5 mm intervals from its most superficial point below the calvarium down to the bifurcation of the A1 segment of the ACA and the M1 segment of the MCA. The MCA flow is directed towards the transducer. The ACA is insonated distally to the bifurcation and a flow running away from the transducer is normally detected. The PCA is located immediately anterior to the heart-shaped cerebral peduncles and displays a flow towards the transducer in the P1 segment while the more distal P2 segment courses around the cerebral peduncles with the flow directed away from the probe (see Figure 13.10 for directions of flow in the vessels).

If a TCD machine is used, pulsed Doppler is sited at approximately 55 mm depth, small accommodations are made until the MCA is located at the anterior, posterior, or medial windows. The MCA is then followed in its course by gradually moving the Doppler sample shallower and deeper until the bifurcation with the ACA is displayed as a bidirectional (mirror-like) Doppler signal. Anatomical positioning and/or autoregulatory response may be determined accurately using common carotid compression on the ipsilateral side in a few cases. Mean, systolic, and diastolic flow velocities are captured at each site and a hard copy produced. The bifurcation of the ACA and MCA is usually found between 60 and 70 mm depth. By gradually increasing the depth and slightly

tilting the probe anteriorly and posteriorly, respectively the ACA and PCA can be insonated. Flow in the ACA is characterized for running physiologically away from the probe while the flow in the proximal segment of the posterior cerebral (P1) artery for running towards the probe. Usually, the anatomical position of the ACA is slightly superior and anterior, and the PCA is inferior and slightly posterior. At last, the sample volume is then moved back to the bifurcation and the probe shifted interiorly in order to detect a lower velocity flow (also because the carotid shows a low resistance flow) typical of the terminal ICA (Figure 13.20).[8,13,17,28–30]

The Transorbital Window

The carotid siphon, the ophthalmic artery (OA) and sometimes, cross-insonation of the contralateral half of the Circle of Willis can be directly insonated by having the ultrasound beam cross the eye bulb. The patient is advised not to wear contact lenses or close the eyelids during examination.

Prior to the examination initiation through this window in order to reduce the ultrasonic exposure of the eye, the power output of the Doppler instrument must be decreased to 10%–20%. This approach is utilized for the identification of intracranial and extracranial collateral circulation through the ophthalmic artery and for insonation of the intracanalar segment of the ICA. Additionally, cases in which insonation of the MCA and ACA through the transtemporal window is unattainable, the transorbital approach to sample the contralateral MCA and ACA is a valid and feasible option. The transorbital approach technique (Figures 13.21 and 13.22) is as follows:

1. Acoustic gel is applied over the eyelid.
2. The probe is then gently positioned over the eye, Doppler sample depth is set in the 40–50 mm range where the OA (low diastolic flow, high resistance vessel) signal should be captured and optimized. Mean flow velocity and hard copy of the ophthalmic artery are then taken.
3. By moving sample volume deeper between 55 and 70 mm the genu, parasellar, and superclinoid segments of the ICA can be detected and tracked up to the bifurcation into the MCA and ACA. Peak flow velocity, end-diastolic flow velocity and mean flow velocities are taken.
4. For performing this cross examination requires the repositioning of the probe quite laterally, and directing the beam of ultrasound medially.[8,13,17,28,30]

The Suboccipital or Transforaminal Window

The transforaminal window takes advantage of the physiological space between the atlas and base of the skull so that the ultrasound beam bypassing through the foramen magnum can directly visualize the brainstem and sample the VAs (segments V3 and V4) as well as the BA running upon the ventral face of the pons up to its bifurcation into the posterior cerebral arteries. It is also possible to sample some of the other branches of the posterior circulation (e.g., PICA).

In order to access the transforaminal window, the patient needs to be turned to one side or in the prone position or sitting and the neck flexed so that the chin touches the chest in order to access this window site. The transducer is placed over the upper neck at the base of the skull and angled cephalad (pointing towards the bridge of the nose) through the foramen magnum towards the nose. For bidimensional ultrasound Doppler studies, the reference landmark is the hypoechoic medulla. Once the colour mode is applied the typical image displayed is a V-shaped configuration representing the two VAs merging into the BA as they run upward. Flow in the VAs and BAs is directed away from the transducer and should be interrogated up to the distal end of the BA.

For Doppler flow detection, the insonation depth is initially set at 65 mm where both the right and left VAs can be tracked individually from this (deepest) point back towards the foramen magnum, moving progressively to shallower insonation depths (from 65 down to 35 mm). The angulation of the sound beam is changed acutely towards the side of the head as the depth of insonation decreases. The extradural part of the VA runs on the posterior arch of the atlas (V3 segment) with a flow towards the transducer in this segment. The BA arise distally from the union of the two VAs and its terminal tract is found at a depth of approximately 95 to 125 mm.[12,13,28] Typical insonation depths and flow velocities are shown in Figures 13.23a and 13.23b. See also Figures 13.24 and 13.25.

The Submandibular Window

The submandibular window allows assessment of the extracranial or extradural segment of the ICA. With the transducer positioned, the beam is directed slightly medially and posteriorly. The ICA is usually identified at a depth of 40–60 mm with the flow moving away from the transducer typically observed (typical insonation depths and flow velocities are shown in Figure 13.26). The submandibular approach can be used for sampling of the distal ICA in the neck region to assess mean flow velocity ratios between the MCA (insonated through the transtemporal window) and ICA, for the so-called hemispheric or Lindegaard index in patients with subarachnoid haemorrhage at risk of developing vasospasm (Figures 13.27 and 13.28).[31] In children with sickle cell disease, this analysis should include the time averaged maximum mean velocity according to the Stroke Prevention Trial in Sickle Cell Anaemia (STOP) trial criteria.[11–13,17,32–35]

Equipment Specifications: Image TCD Versus Image TCCD

Transcranial Doppler should be performed with either an ultrasound imaging scanner with Doppler capability (TCCD) using a 1 to 5 MHz transducer that can penetrate the temporal bone and foramen magnum or a non-imaging Doppler instrument (TCD or power M-mode Doppler) with 2 MHz pulsed Doppler probe. When using TCCD, the colour or spectral Doppler mode permits the exact location of intracranial vessels; colour gain should be optimized in order to obtain well-defined images. After the anatomical identification of the vessels pulsed Doppler is applied and velocities are sampled at 2 mm to 5 mm intervals with a 3 mm to 6 mm gate. The Doppler setting and manual angle accommodation should be adjusted to obtain the highest velocity in all cases. Table 13.1 illustrates criteria for vessels identification and normal Doppler reference values for flow velocities and PI.

CLINICAL APPLICATIONS

Indications for a TCD ultrasound examination in adults include:[12,17,36–40]

1. Detection and follow-up of stenosis or occlusion in a major intracranial artery in the Circle of Willis and vertebrobasilar system, including monitoring of thrombolytic therapy for acute stroke patients
2. Detection of cerebral vasculopathy
3. Diagnosis and monitoring of vasospasm in patients with spontaneous or traumatic subarachnoid haemorrhage
4. Assessment of intracranial pressure and hydrocephalus
5. Evaluation of collateral pathways of intracranial blood flow, including after surgery monitoring
6. Detection of circulating cerebral microemboli
7. Identification of right-to-left cardiac shunts (i.e., patent foramen ovale)

Table 13.1 Summary of vessel identification criteria and reference values

Artery	Window	Depth (mm)	Direction of flow (relative to the transducer)	Relation to TICA/MCA/ACA junction	Velocity (cm/sec)			PI	Response to carotid compression
					PSV	MFV	EDV		
MCA	TT	45–65	Towards	At	90–110	62±12	35–55	0.85–1.0	↓, 0
ACA/MCA bifurcation	TT	60–65	Bidirectional	At		–			↓
ACA (A1)	TT	60–75	Away	Anterosuperior	80–90	50±11	30–40	0.75–0.95	↓, 0
PCA (P1)	TT	60–75	Towards	Posteroinferior	60–80	40±10	25–33	0.78–0.97	↓, 0
PCA (P2)	TT	60–75	Away	Posteroinferior	68–70	40–55	25–33	0.78–0.97	↓, 0
TICA	TT	60–70	Towards	Inferior		30–48			↓
Ophthalmic a	TO	45–60	Towards	–	21±5	–			0
CS, Supraclinoid	TO	60–75	Away	–		47±14			0, reversed
CS, Genu	TO	60–75	Bidirectional	–	–	–	–		0, reversed
CS, Parasellar	TO	60–75	Towards	–		47±14			0, reversed
Vertebral A.	TF	65–85	Away	–	54–74	30±10	23–34	0.77–0.95	–
BA	TF	90–120	Away	–	52–66	41±10	22–31	0.78–0.94	–
ICA	SM	40–60	Away			40±10			↓

8. Assessment of cerebrovascular autoregulation and vasomotor reactivity
9. Adjunct in the confirmation of the clinical diagnosis of brain death
10. Intraoperative and periprocedural monitoring to detect cerebral embolization, thrombosis, hypoperfusion, and hyperperfusion
11. Evaluation of sickle cell disease in order to determine stroke risk
12. Assessment of arteriovenous malformations
13. Detection and follow-up of intracranial aneurysms
14. Evaluation of positional vertigo or syncope
15. Assessment of dural venous sinus patency

Table 13.2 shows a TCD ultrasonography report.

This section discusses the most common applications of TCD and TCCD within the ICU: vasospasm, intracranial hypertension, evaluation of cerebrovascular autoregulation and vasomotor reactivity, vascular occlusion and stenosis, evaluation of microemboli, patent foramen ovale (PFO) patency, and integration with multimodality monitoring.

Vasospasm

Spontaneous subarachnoid haemorrhage is frequently caused by rupture of an intracranial saccular aneurysm. It occurs with a rate of 10–28 cases per 100,000 persons per year. The overflow of blood into the subarachnoid space can cause vasospasm by inducing constriction of the muscle wall of cerebral blood vessels and if severe enough may result in cerebral ischaemia. Physiological or paraphysiological conditions that modify flow velocity are: age, haematocrit (HCT), arterial partial pressure of carbon dioxide ($PaCO_2$), and metabolic requirements. Vasospasm is a frequent complication of subarachnoid haemorrhage (SAH)[31–33,41–43] and has an incidence ranging between 30% and 70%. Vasospasm is associated with an increase in mortality by 1.5- to 3-fold during the first two weeks. Although arterial narrowing on angiography occurs in a majority of patients, actual clinical deficits develop in only 30% of patients.[44,45] The Report of the Therapeutics and Technology Assessment Subcommittee of the American Academy of Neurology, published in 2004, approved TCD/TCCD as valuable instruments for the detection and monitoring of angiographic vasospasm affecting the major basal arteries after spontaneous SAH (incidence of 21%–70%).[31] Vasospasm, in fact, by reducing the cross-sectional area of the vessel affects the mean flow velocities (MFV) by proportionally increasing them (Figure 13.28). Variation in flow velocities can be easily captured with TCD examinations so that treatment before the onset of ischaemia may be promptly started. It is obvious, but must be pointed out, that TCD mean flow velocity in such a pathological background cannot

Table 13.2   Transcranial Doppler ultrasonography report

Indication	Sensitivity, %	Specificity, %	Reference standard	Evidence/Class
Sickle cell disease	86	91	Conventional angiography	A/I
Right-to-left cardiac shunts	70–100	>95	Transesophageal echocardiography	A/II
Intracranial steno-occlusive disease			Conventional angiography	
Anterior circulation	70–90	90–95		B/II–III
Posterior circulation	50–80	80–96		B/III
Occlusion				
MCA	85–95	90–98		B/III
ICA, VA, BA	55–81	96		B/III
Extracranial ICA stenosis			Conventional angiography	
Single TCD variable	3–78	60–100		C/II–III
TCD battery	49–95	42–100		C/II–III
TCD battery and carotid duplex	89	100		C/II–III
Vasomotor reactivity testing				
≥70% extracranial ICA stenosis/occlusion			Conventional angiography, clinical outcomes	B/II–III
Carotid endarterectomy			EEG, MRI, clinical outcomes	B/II
Cerebral microembolization			Experimental model, pathology, MRI, neuropsychological tests	
General				B/II–IV
Coronary artery bypass graft surgery microembolization				B/II–III
Prosthetic heart valves				C/III
Cerebral thrombolysis			Conventional angiography, MR angiography, clinical outcome	B/II–III
Complete occlusion	50	100		
Partial occlusion	100	76		
Recanalization	91	93		
Vasospasm after spontaneous subarachnoid hemorrhage:			Conventional angiography	I–II
Intracranial ICA	25–30	83–91		
MCA	39–94	70–100		
ACA	13–71	65–100		
VA	44–100	82–88		
BA	77–100	42–79		
PCA	48–60	78–87		
Vasospasm after traumatic subarachnoid hemorrhage			Conventional angiography	I–III
Cerebral circulatory arrest and brain death	91–100	97–100	Conventional angiography, EEG, clinical outcome	II

Courtesy: Assessment. Transcranial Doppler ultrasonography Report of the Therapeutics and Technology Assessment Subcommittee of the American Academy of Neurology, May (1 of 2) 2004 *NEUROLOGY* 62.

substitute CBF measurement. Usually, first TCD is performed at day 0 in order to obtain a basal recording and subsequently from day 3 to 10. TCD examination estimates the degree of vessel narrowing and provides monitoring about spasm progression or regression. However, interpretation of TCD velocity changes over time must be always carefully accomplished. In fact, since the first tier strategies for treatment of vasospasm are medical therapies designed to restore the reduced CBF by mainly inducing arterial hypertension and since vasospasm itself indicates impaired autoregulation, such induced changes in CPP may result into further increase in TCD velocities.

Threshold velocities above which vasospasm is detected are well-defined for MCA, however, there is lack of consensus for the other vessels. With regard to the MCA, MFV between 100 and 120 cm/sec suggests a minor narrowing of the vessel calibre that cannot be detected with digital subtraction angiography (DSA). Velocities (MFV) between 120 and 200 cm/sec indicate moderate vasospasm, which corresponds to a reduction of the lumen between 25% and 50%, while mean velocities above 200 cm/sec indicate severe vasospasm with a reduction of the radius exceeding 50%.[13,14,46,47]

An isolated increase in velocity is not sufficient for the diagnosis of vasospasm. In fact, vasospasm must be differentiated from the hyperaemic state in which increased flow velocity pattern is also present but instead of being due to a reduction in the vessel lumen it is related to an increase in cerebral perfusion. The LI[35] is a useful parameter in order to distinguish between vasospasm and hyperaemia: it is easily calculated as the ratio between the MFV in the MCA and the MFV in the ICA. According to the calculated LI, the observed increased TCD velocities can be the epiphenomenon of: hyperaemia if LI is below 3; moderate vasospasm if LI ranges between 3 and 6, and severe vasospasm if LI is above 6. In support of the suspected diagnosis of vasospasm, there are other TCD parameters that must be taken into consideration, such as velocity, that is, 50% growth in daily serial examination or the presence of asymmetry in velocities of two correspondent vessels (velocity difference exceeding 50%).[46] In literature, it is found that a fairly good correlation exists between TCD studies and angiography studies for the detection of vasospasm of the BA,[22] though less so for the other arteries at the base of the skull.[49] Table 13.3 lists the factors that affect Doppler flow velocities, PI, RI, and LI.

Middle Cerebral Artery Vasospasm

The TCD has a well-documented and established value in detecting MCA vasospasm.[31–35,41–43,48] The TCD sensitivity and specificity in detecting vasospasm ranges from 38% to 91% and from 94% to 100%, respectively. Reliability of TCD in detecting MCA vasospasm has been proved by comparing Doppler measured MFV with the presence and degree of vasospasm detected by DSA. Vora et al.[41] found that only low or very high MCA MFVs (i.e., <120 or ≥200 cm/sec) reliably predicted the absence or presence of clinically significant angiographic vasospasm (moderate or severe vasospasm: MCA MFV ≥120 cm/sec, the sensitivity of TCD for detecting moderate or severe MCA vasospasm was 88% and the specificity was 72%, whereas for MCA MFV ≥200 cm/sec, the sensitivity of TCD for detecting moderate or severe MCA vasospasm was 27% and the specificity was 98%). Intermediate velocities, which were observed in approximately one-half of the patients of the mentioned study, were not dependable and should be interpreted with caution. Interestingly, in the same study, all patients with MCA MFV 160–199 cm/sec and right-to-left MFV difference >40 cm/sec showed significant vasospasm.

Similarly, Burch et al.[50] observed that TCD has sensitivity of 43% and specificity of 93.7% for detecting moderate or severe vasospasm (lumen reduction >50%) when MCA MFV cut-off was set at 120 cm/sec. When the diagnostic criterion was instead shifted to 130 cm/sec, specificities raised to 100% for TICA and 96% for MCA and also positive predictive values performed well showing 100% and 87%, respectively. On such basis, these authors concluded that TCD accurately detects TICA and MCA vasospasm when MFVs are at least 130 cm/sec. Another factor to be taken into consideration when evaluating the presence of vasospasm is the relative day-to-day increase in MFV: an MFV increase of 50 cm/sec or more during the first 24-hour period is indicative of a high risk of delayed cerebral ischaemia due to vasospasm.[34,35,48]

As already mentioned, increased blood flow velocities (BFV) may not necessarily denote arterial narrowing (cerebral vasospasm may not be differentiated from cerebral hyperemia); so to account for this diagnostic shortcoming of TCD, calculation of LI is necessary (Figure 13.29). MCA vasospasm detection is influenced by multiple factors: incorrect vessel identification (TICA, PCA), increased collateral flow, hyperemia/hyperperfusion, proximal haemodynamic injury (cervical ICA stenosis

Table 13.3 Factors affecting Doppler flow velocities, pulsatility and resistance index and lindegard ratio

Transcranial Doppler flow velocity	Pulsatility index, resistance index
Increase	Increase
Vasospasm	Raised ICP
Hyperaemia	Hydrocephalus
Loss of autoregulation	Brain death
$\uparrow$ PaCO$_2$	Intracranial artery occlusion
Intracranial arterial stenosis	Bacterial meningitis
Increasing age	Decrease
Hyperdynamic circulation	Vasospasm
Volatile anaesthetic agents	Arteriovenous malformation
Sickle cell anaemia	Rewarming following hypothermia
Arteriovenous malformation	Hyperaemia
Bacterial meningitis	
Pre-eclampsia	**Lindegaard ratio**
Decrease	Increase
Hypotension	Vasospasm
$\downarrow$ CBF	Decrease
Brain death	Hyperaemia
Raised ICP	
$\downarrow$ PaCO$_2$	
$\uparrow$ angle of insonation	
Pregnancy	
Anaesthetic Induction agents (except ketamine)	
Hypothermia	
Fulminant hepatic failure	

or occlusion), operator inexperience, and anomalous vessel course.

Anterior Cerebral Artery Vasospasm

The capability of TCD to detect anterior cerebral artery vasospasm is not so well established yet. Aaslid and co-authors reckoned that BFV in ACAs matched poorly with residual lumen diameter. Later studies, although applying different cut-off values (120–140 cm/sec) for the detection of vasospasm, confirm a rather low sensitivity (13%–71%) and an acceptable specificity (65%–100%) for detection of ACA vasospasm using TCD. Limits of TCD in the identification of ACA vasospasm can partially be explained by the presence of collateral flow (flow diversion into the contralateral ACA through the Acomm) and by the technical difficulty in detecting the more distal A2 segment (pericallosal artery)

due to a poor angle of isonation through the temporal window.[31,49,51]

Internal Carotid Artery Vasospasm

Literature provides with only a few studies examining accuracy of TCD in detecting ICA vasospasm.[27,39] Burch et al.[50] evaluated the sensitivity and specificity of TCD at different MFV cut offs and they found that when a MFV of at least 90 cm/sec was used to indicate TICA vasospasm, the sensitivity and specificity were 25% and 93%, respectively. By increasing the MFV cut-off at 130 cm/sec, specificities were 100% for TICA and 96% for MCA, while positive predictive values were 100% (TICA) and 87% (MCA). According to their results these authors conclude that TCD accurately detects TICA and MCA vasospasm when flow velocities are at least 130 cm/sec. As well as for other vessels, diagnosis of TCD ICA vasospasm is affected by various factors such as increased collateral flow, hyperemia/hyperperfusion, and anatomical circumstances (angle of insonation >30 degrees).

Vertebral and Basilar Arteries Vasospasm

In literature an MFV ≥60 cm/sec is described as indicative of both VA and BA vasospasm.[17,52–54] The sensitivity seen in literature is around 44% and specificity 87.5% for VAs while the sensitivity is about 76.9% and specificity 79.3% for the BAs. If the cut-off is raised to ≥80 cm/sec (VA) and ≥95 cm/sec (BA), all false-positive results are discounted and specificity and positive predictive value become 100%. Despite TCD and TCCD seeming to be highly specific (100%) for VA and BA vasospasm when flow velocities are ≥80 and ≥95 cm/sec, respectively, these results appear to be inconclusive suggesting that TCD criteria for BA vasospasm have not been entirely agreed yet. In order to improve the distinction between BA vasospasm and vertebrobasilar hyperemia while enhancing the accuracy and reliability of TCD in the diagnosis of BA vasospasm, Soustiel et al.[55] formulated the correspondent Lindegaard ratio for the posterior cerebral circulation: BA/extracranial vertebral artery (eVA) ratio. A BA/eVA ratio >2.5 with BA velocity higher than 85 cm/sec showed a 86% sensitivity and 97% specificity for BA narrowing of more than 25%. A ratio >3.0 together with BA velocities higher than 85 cm/sec was 92% sensitive and 97% specific for BA narrowing of more than 50%, and the specificity rises up to 100% with MFV >95 cm/sec. VB vasospasm detection can be negatively affected by multiple factors which include severe bilateral PCA vasospasm, increased collateral flow, hyperperfusion, and anatomical variations (horizontal course of VA, and tortuous course of BA).

Complete TCD Examination with Lindegaard Ratio Determination

Although TCD identification of MCA vasospasm is most accurate, an insonation protocol studying all basilar vessels demonstrates greater diagnostic impact than sole MCA isonation. In fact, it has been proved that serial assessments of relative increase in mean flow velocities are more reliable than conventional absolute values in the diagnostic process of the vasospasm; moreover, correction for hyperemia-induced flow velocity changes (Lindegaard ratio) further improves TCD predictive value for vasospasm.[8,32,33,35,48]

Distal Vasospasm Ascertainment

In a small percentage of cases, vasospasm can be limited to the distal vascular system: distal vasospasm is often not detected by TCD. Its occurrence can be anticipated by distal distribution of blood on post-haemorrhage head CT. In some circumstances, reduced flow in the M2 segment can be detected on TCD suggestive of distal narrowing. Fortunately, isolated distal vasospasm is a rare entity:[49] newer CT angiography bolus techniques offer better depiction of the distal vasculature and CBF-based methods such as xenon CT or SPECT are useful in endorsing the diagnosis.

Cerebrovascular Autoregulation

Cerebral autoregulation (CA) is a physiological function of local brain circulation whose purpose is to maintain CBF constant despite changes in cerebral perfusion pressure (CPP).

Although clinical evaluation of CA is not so easily accomplished in all conditions, there is growing evidence proving that its assessment can give useful prognostic information in many diseases. As a matter of fact, dysfunction of CA has been observed in traumatic brain injury (TBI),[56] stroke,[57] carotid disease,[58] and in syncope (although there is still uncertainty about its pathophysiological role in this setting.[59] Cerebral autoregulation derangement is associated with an increased risk of developing ischaemia and cerebral oedema. There are two main types of CA:

1. *Vasomotor reactivity*: It is the response of the cerebral circle to changes in $PaCO_2$ and PaO_2. Cerebrovascular regulation can be estimated by fluctuation in BFV in response to blood pressure and arterial carbon dioxide tension changes. Therefore, variation (related to $PaCO_2$ and mean arterial pressure [MAP]) in BFV is a reasonable indicator of cerebral circulation autoregulation. Autoregulatory changes in BFV associated with $PaCO_2$ is CO_2 reactivity; in the range of $PaCO_2$ between 20 and 60 mmHg CBF changes by approximately 3%/mmHg change in $PaCO_2$.[60,61]

2. *Pressure type regulation*: It preserves CBF from potential CPP changes, as long as the variations are within the pressure range of 50 mmHg and 150 mmHg; pressure regulation can be further subdivided into dynamic regulation involving a rapid accommodating response of the vasomotor tone against rapid changes in arterial pressure or its pulsatile nature and static autoregulation, involving a rapid response to slow changes in average arterial pressure,[62] and MAP.

The dynamic component of CA can be assessed through the registration of changes in BFV induced by sudden controlled pharmacologically/mechanically induced episodes of hypertension and hypotension. In literature various methods of assessment of the dynamic component of autoregulation are described. Aaslid himself dedicated part of his research to this field and devised a method for assessing dynamic CA known as the 'cuff test.'[63] During this test transient blood pressure drops are provoked using thigh-cuff manoeuvres: thigh cuffs are placed on each thigh and tightened from 20 to 50 mmHg above the PAS for 2–3 min and then quickly released. The dynamic rate of regulation (dROR) whose normal value is above 40% is then calculated from the rate of change in cerebrovascular resistance (MAP/MFV in MCA) over blood pressure variation, which basically indicates how quickly the velocity of cerebral flow returns to its starting level after the hypotensive stimulus. However, potential complications related to the manipulation of systemic arterial pressure in critically ill patients represent a limit to the cuff test application. The transient hyperaemic response test (THRT) is another effective but safe test for assessing dynamic CA.[64,65] This test is based on the compensatory vasodilatation of the arterioles occurring after a brief external compression of the common carotid artery. The test involves measuring systolic flow velocity in the MCA at basal conditions first, then the ipsilateral common carotid is compressed for 10 sec causing a consensual reduction in CPP. Intact autoregulation reacts to temporary reduction in CPP with vasodilatation, increase in arterial conductance, and consequent conservation of CBF, so as the carotid compression is relieved, a transient increase in BFV (in the MCA) is observed as CPP acts on a dilated vascular bed. Transient hyperaemic response ratio (THRR) can then be calculated as the ratio between the velocity of systolic flow during the hyperaemic phase (two cycles after the compression release excluding the very first cycle) and the velocity of basic systolic flow (five cycles before compression). Range of normality for THRR is described (between 1.105 and 1.29, average [95% confidence interval (CI)] 1.2 [1.17–1.24]), THRR is more reliable as a qualitative autoregulation indicator. There is no consensus on how long the compression phase should be to get the maximum hyperaemic response. Some authors suggest 5 sec[64] whereas the others consider 10 sec[66]; whilst, as far as the strength of the compression is concerned it needs to be sufficient to cause a reduction in cerebral flow of at least 40%.[60] See Figures 13.30 and 13.31.

Static autoregulation refers to the evaluation of the autoregulatory plateau over a small range of arterial pressure change. Using TCD, MCA MFV is measured under normal physiological conditions and then repeated, once a steady state has been reached, following a 20–30 mmHg increase in mean arterial pressure induced by a hypertensive agent. The index of autoregulation is calculated as the percent change in the CVR (calculated as mean arterial pressure/BFV) per percent change in the MAP. Regarding dynamic study and continuous monitoring of cerebral autoregulatory function, no index has yet found a place as gold standard. The 'mean flow velocity index' (Mx index) describes the correlation (coefficient) between CPP and TCD detected mean flow velocity in the MCA: a positive correlation means that blood flow is pressure dependent indicating a deranged autoregulation, while a negative correlation is observed when autoregulatory function is preserved.[67] See Figures 13.32 and 13.33.

Dysfunction of the autoregulatory function can be seen in various types of brain injuries such as TBI, aSAH, and intracerebral haemorrhage. Absent autoregulation warrants careful management of systemic arterial pressure as the brain may be more prone to ischaemic/hyperaemic events. In subjects affected by ICA stenosis, impairment of autoregulation can be a marker of elevated risk of stroke, and therefore it could be employed to guide treatment towards revascularization.

Transcranial Doppler and 'effective downstream pressure'

In the 1950s, Burton described the concept of critical closing pressure (CCP)[68] as the minimum transmural pressure (MAP – ICP) in which blood flow ceases and the vessel collapses. Research in this field has given neuroscience so far precious and new insights about the possible mechanism underlying the cerebrovascular dynamics and ICP interactions, nevertheless, it has not yet found a place in clinical practice because its application is quite cumbersome and some results are not yet conclusive.

Critical closing pressure is an expression of the vasomotor tone.[69] Classically, cerebral effective downstream pressure (EDP) is believed to be determined by ICP, however, this is true only if vasomotor tone is not taken into account. The EDP indicates the value of arterial blood pressure (ABP) at which CBF approaches zero; at such a point of equilibrium, transmural pressure is equal to the ratio between the wall tension, which is given by the vasomotor tone and the radius of the vessel. So, according to the 'CPP theory' either reduction in arterial pressure, an increase in ICP or vasomotor tone can alter the balance between transmural pressure and wall tension leading to the collapse of the vessel. The difference between MAP and EDP is effective CPP (eCPP), which the CBF depends on. EDP values can be found calculating a rate of linear regression, by analysing the beat-to-beat relationship between pressure and CBFV. Once linear regression rate is produced, MAP value corresponding to zero flow (EDP) can be extrapolated. Variations in $PaCO_2$ have the opposite effect on ICP and CCP. Traditionally, CPP has always been calculated as the difference between MAP and ICP, although it is also likely that real CPP is not determined by intracranial pressure but rather by CCP. However, there is no evidence to suggest that the concept of eCPP is superior to that of CPP in terms of outcome.[63–71]

Intracranial Hypertension

Intracranial hypertension (ICH) is the most feared complication in brain injury;[72–74] when it occurs timely diagnosis and close clinical monitoring in order to prompt appropriate and early interventions are mandatory. The main stand of ICH management is ICP and CPP monitoring.

Pathophysiologically, intracranial pressure (ICP) presents at least four components driven by different mechanisms.

1. *Arterial blood inflow and volume of arterial blood*: The plateau wave of ICP is the most frequent manifestation of intracranial hypertension related to arterial vasodilatation and increase of arterial blood volume.
2. *Venous blood outflow*: Obstructions to the outflow of blood eventually lead to elevation of ICP as an increase of the whole cerebral blood volume (i.e., venous compression resulting from incorrect head position or venous thrombosis).
3. *Compliance and efficiency of cerebrospinal fluid (CSF) circulation*: Commonly observed in 'acute hydrocephalus' after brain injury or SAH. In neurocritical care, impairment of CSF circulation and a consequent rise in endoventricular pressure is commonly treated with extraventricular drainage positioning.
4. *Increase in brain volume (oedema) or space occupying lesions* (i.e., contusion, haematoma, tumour): Osmotherapy or surgical decompression is commonly used to eradicate this component.[75]

In clinical practice, monitoring absolute value of ICP as a number is not enough; it is also important to recognize the mechanism underlying the observed ICH and, given that, plan for appropriate treatment measures to control the different components. Presently, the gold standard for continuous ICP monitoring is invasive measurement through insertion of a catheter within the brain ventricles (EVD) connected to an external pressure transducer.[76,77] However, this method may be cumbersome, not always available, and accompanied by an elevated complication rate due mostly to infection, haemorrhage, and catheter obstruction.[78–81] Brain intraparenchymal catheters, despite being safer, still require an invasive procedure and cannot be recalibrated once inserted, rendering the measurements prone to imprecision due to zero drift.[46,82,83]

Although ICP can guide patient management in neurocritical care units, it is not commonly available in many non-specific settings outside this environment because it needs the presence of trained personnel for the costs, the associated risk to the patient (infections, brain tissue lesions, and haemorrhage), a broad range of diseases like in patients with risk of coagulopathy, as well as in other conditions in which invasive monitoring is not considered or outweighed by the risks of the procedure have prevented ICP monitoring. Nevertheless, since the knowledge of ICP can be critical for the successful management of patients in many sub-critical conditions, non-invasive estimation of ICP (nICP) may find a role when indications for invasive ICP monitoring are not met and when it is not immediately available or even contraindicated.

Many alternatives to invasive ICP measurement have been studied. Although some techniques seem to have potential as screening methods for ICH, none have found a valid place within daily clinical practice.[5,47,84,85]

Methods for nICP described in literature include: TCD through detection of CBF velocity indices; optic nerve sheath diameter assessment (ONSD); venous ophthalmodynamometry; ultrasound-guided eyeball compression; skull vibrations; brain tissue resonance or transcranial time of flight; otoacoustic emissions; tympanic membrane displacement (TMD); recordings of visual evoked potentials; and magnetic resonance imaging (MRI) to estimate intracranial compliance.

These techniques, however, are better suited for time-to-time measurement of instant value of ICP rather than continuous monitoring. Disclosed absolute accuracies (95% CI for prediction of ICP) are reported as follows: 9–16 mmHg for methods based on TCD waveforms; 20 mmHg and 9 mmHg for transcranial time of flight; 15–20 mmHg for TMD and otoacoustic emissions; 5–10 mmHg for ONSD; 3–5 mmHg for ophthalmodynamometry. Among these methods, TCD provides worthy information on the basis that CBFV has been shown to correlate with ICP.[6,7,86–89]

Doppler Derived CPP and ICP

Variations in ICP affect BFV in major cerebral vessels. Cerebral vessels surrounded by the brain parenchyma enclosed in the skull represent an example of Starling resistor: in fact vessels are subjected to an external pressure (ICP) and to an internal pressure represented by the ABP, plus intrinsic properties of the arterial walls such as active tension of the vessel wall and arterial wall compliance. All these variables fall into the equation describing the behaviour of CBFV.

On such a basis, TCD waveform analysis has been investigated as an estimator of nICP; more specifically when the ICP rises—but also in arterial hypotension and hypocapnia—a fall in diastolic CBFV (FVd), a peaked waveform, and an increase in PI are typically observed.[86,87] TCD-derived nICP methods rely on approximate semi-quantitative relationships between cerebrovascular dynamics and ICP. They can be classified into three categories: (1) methods based on the calculation of non-invasive CPP (nCPP); (2) methods based on the TCD-derived PI; and (3) methods based on mathematical models. Reported accuracy of these methods inter- and intra-categories shows significant variability though they are derived from the same principle.

At the base of TCD derived methods is the concept that compliant MCA has walls that can be deflected by transmural pressure (equivalent to CPP) and modulated according to the pulsatile waveform of CBFV, it behaves as a 'biological' pressure transducer. Nevertheless, transmission of this 'transducer', its linearity, stability in time, and calibration coefficients are unknown—and these factors mainly justify the limited accuracy of TCD-based methods. The absolute error may be compensated for by the ability to monitor dynamics of variations in nICP and also because TCD monitoring can easily be repeated in the bedside.[78]

Existing non-invasive ICP methods based on TCD waveform analysis display different CIs for prediction of ICP in TBI patients. The Gosling PI, first introduced in the 1970s has been for many years the most commonly used formula, and is denoted as:

$$PI = \frac{FVs - FVd}{FVm}$$

This index is based on the change that take place in the TCD waveform when the intracranial haemodynamic modifies.[19] Diastolic flow velocity is more affected by ICP increase compared with the systolic flow velocity. This behaviour results in an increased pulse peak between the diastole and the systole and hence in the PI and RI. Since PI and RI are ratios derived from the difference between the systolic and diastolic velocities, they are not affected by angle of intonation which, as physics teaches, has a great impact on measured flow velocity values. PI reliability in assessing ICP has been tested by different authors: Behrens et al.,[90] by performing lumbar infusion studies, demonstrated that PI does not accurately correlate with invasive ICP (measured by means of an intraparenchymal probe). The 95% prediction interval (i.e., the prediction interval for a single PI value) was on the order of ± 25 mmHg, indicating that a certain PI value cannot determine the corresponding ICP with an acceptable clinical precision. Similarly, Zweifel et al.,[88] prospectively analysed data from 762 recorded daily sessions (arterial blood pressure, ICP, and TCD MCA velocities and PI were recorded) and found that the correlation between PI and ICP was 0.31 (P<0.001) and the 95% prediction interval of ICP values for a given PI was more than ± 15 mmHg. The same authors performed a receiver operating curve (ROC) analysis showing that the predictive value of PI can indeed be relatively high with AUC values exceeding 0.75 but only for highly elevated ICP (>35 mmHg) and low CPP values (<55 mmHg). Therefore, as they conclude, PI is certainly not a reliable diagnostic tool in detecting critical clinical thresholds (ICP >20 mmHg, CPP <60 mmHg). Bellner et al.[87] found that the ICP value predicted from the PI by means of a derived formula (ICP = 10.972 × PI–1.284) was within ± 4.2 mmHg of the real ICP, with a 95% confidence interval in the ICP range of 5–40 mmHg.

Different formulae and mathematical approaches have been proposed for ICP and CPP estimation. As a matter of fact, many TCD methods for noninvasive ICP testing were originally intended for evaluating nCPP and incorporate in their formulae the ABP as well as the CBFV waveform. The first to propose this approach was Aaslid et al.,[5,6] who presented a formula for the estimation of CPP based on spectral PI (SPI) and the first harmonic component of the ABP which was demonstrated to be quite sensitive to the variation of CPP, but limited in accuracy.[91]

Czosnyka et al.[7] proposed a new non-PI-related formula for estimation of CPP and therefore ICP (CPP = ABP × FVd/FVm + 14) and proved that the absolute difference between real CPP and nCPP so calculated was less than 10 mmHg in 89% of measurements and less than 13 mmHg in 92% of measurements in their study. The same group of authors, in a further study, reinforced the previous results (correlation between eCPP and measured CPP was r = 0.73; p<10^6), concluded that the method shows a high positive predictive power (94%) for detecting low CPP (<60 mmHg) and also demonstrated that this formula is superior to the formula originally suggested by Aaslid for calculation of CPP. Concerning ICP, in the same study, an error in estimating ICP by less than 10 mmHg was achieved in 68% of the measurements and less than 5 mmHg in only 39% of the measurements. It follows then that the noninvasive estimation of CPP suffers from the same degree of inaccuracy as the noninvasive assessment of ICP, but since ICP is a much smaller number than CPP, a 10 mmHg error is unsatisfactory in estimating ICP, whereas this degree of error seems to be fairly low for CPP estimation.[92]

More recently Faisal et al.[93] suggested a new model-based estimation of ICP from the beat-to-beat analysis of CBFV (MCA) and arterial pressure. These authors created a mathematical algorithm for estimation of ICP simplifying the cerebrovascular physiology to a circuit-model representation. They then compared the beat-to-beat ICP estimation they obtained with invasive ICP in a pool of 37 continuously monitored patients suffering from TBI and obtained a mean error of 1.6 mmHg with a SD error of 7.6 mmHg, SD error dropped to 5.9 in 20 patients who had bilateral CBF velocity recordings. Correlation coefficient nICP and ICP was determined to be 0.9 and using a nICP of 20 mmHg as the threshold, they obtained a sensitivity of 83% and a specificity of 70% for detection of ICH.

More recently, Schmidt and colleagues,[75] applying a mathematical 'black-box' model to assess nICP from CBFV and ABP described a maximum 95% CI for ICP prediction of 12.8 mmHg. With paediatric patients, the absolute value of TCD-derived PI was found to be an unreliable noninvasive estimator for ICP in TBI. Correlation with ICP in this population was 0.36 (p = 0.04), much weaker than the correlation found by Bellner and colleagues in adults (R = 0.938; p<0.0001).

Optic Nerve Sheath Diameter (ONSD)

The sheath enclosing the optic nerve is in direct continuity with the dura mater and the CSF-containing subarachnoid space of the brain and, since the ONS is distensible, CSF pressure variations influence the volume of ONSD, particularly in the anterior, retrobulbar compartment, about 3 mm behind the globe.

Increased ICP, no matter what the cause may be, is transmitted to the subarachnoid compartment of the nerve causing enlargement of the ONS and thereby enlargement of the ONSD (Figure 13.34).[37] It is described in scientific literature as a linear relationship between perioptic CSF pressure and ICP, in fact ONSD increases almost directly

with ICP,[94] as during osmotic therapy or following CO_2 variations.[95–97] Ultrasonographic measurement of the ONSD is an extensively studied technique for noninvasive assessment of elevated ICP because of its portability, noninvasiveness, and reproducibility. The measurements are being performed using a 7.5–10.5 MHz probe, gently placed over the upper temporal eyelid.[98] The frequency chosen should be the highest that will allow visualization of the optic nerve and sheath. It is imaged as a hypoechoic structure extending from the retina posteriorly. The optic nerve sheath is subtly more echogenic and surrounds the nerve.

The US-based ONSD measurements have been compared with ICP invasively measured in order to find cut-offs and accuracy. Ultrasound of the ONS appears to be superior to CT or MR morphological changes such as size of ventricle, basilar cistern, sulci, degree of transfalcine herniation, and gray/white matter differentiation.[99–103] The cut-off value for normal ICP (ICP ≤20 mmHg) assessed with ONSD ranges from 4.8–6 mm. In literature, several studies describe high accuracy, good correlation coefficient with gold standard, and good sensitivity and specificity for this method.[104] In adult patients presenting radiological evidence of increased ICP ONSD ranges from 4.84–6.4 mm while in patients with no such radiological findings ONSD ranges from 3.49–4.94, corroborating good sensitivity and specificity of the method.

The US-acquired ONSD has been studied in the paediatric population as well in different clinical scenarios associated with ICH, such as acute hydrocephalus, intracranial lesions, and liver failure. Children, in fact, show different cut-offs for elevated ICP with respect to adults: the established upper limit of normality for elder children is 4.5 mm, and 4.0 mm for infants aged less than 1 year. These cut-points display a rather good sensitivity (83%) despite a specificity (38%) for predicting increased ICP. Although this technique (median intra-observer variation 0.1 mm with 5th and 95th centile values of 0 and 4 mm) does not seem to be accurate enough to be used as a replacement for invasive ICP measurement, it has good sensitivity in recognizing increased ICP.[101,102] See Figures 13.35a and 13.35b.

Brain Midline Shift

Brain midline shift (MLS) is a life-threatening condition that calls for expeditious diagnosis and treatment. In 1977, Becker et al. noted a twofold increase in mortality when the MLS exceeded 1 cm (53% versus 25%).[107] Recently, a MLS above 0.5 cm as evidenced on primary

CT is related to predict poor neurological outcome with a positive predictive potential of 78%, however, poor outcomes were evident in only 14% of cases without MLS on CT scan.[105–111] In a vast cohort of TBI patients it has been demonstrated that MLS >0.5 cm and a compression of the third ventricle are both major predictors of mortality within 15 days after trauma. Also in ischaemic or haemorrhagic stroke, mass effect associated with MLS is of great prognositic value and brings forward important clinical decisions.[112–114] As it follows, early detection of a MLS in neurosurgical ICU patients is very important because it allows the implementation of an appropriate treatment plan (North American recommendations from 2006 indicate surgical evacuation if MLS >0.5 cm in the presence of severe TBI, extradural, subdural or intracerebral haematoma). Although the gold standard for detection of MLS is the head CT, there are situations in which taking critical ICU patients to radiology for serial CT scan can be of significant risk both in terms of morbidity and mortality. In such situations, it could be useful to monitor the progression of the MLS with a noninvasive, portable method such as the ultrasound.

In 1996, Seidel et al. described a simple method to determine the MLS with sonography which seemed to correlate well with findings on CT.[38,39,115,116] Due to its noninvasive character and suitability for bedside application, TCCD can be used in the acute phase of stroke and for repeated monitoring at short intervals even in critically ill patients.

Ultrasound MLS (US-MLS) detection technique exploits ultrasonography of the brain parenchymal structures through the temporal acoustic bone window access by using a microconvex low frequency transducer (the same used TCCD). Measurements of the US-MLS begins with the identification of specific reference structures within the brain: (1) ipsilateral and contralateral bone table and (2) the third ventricle, identified as a double hyperechogenic image over the midbrain. The distance between the external bone table and the centre of the third ventricle is then measured bilaterally (Figure 13.36). The difference between the left and right measures (A and B) divided by two is used to calculate the US-MLS.

$$US\text{-}MLS = (B - A)/2.$$

As mentioned, CT scan represents the gold standard technique for measurement of MLS (CT-MLS); US-MLS compared to the gold standard determination

shows a positive correlation (Figure 13.37) with CT-MLS and a tendency to slightly underestimate the measure, a good specificity (84.8% [95% CI = 68.1 to 94.8%]) and sensitivity (84.2% [95% CI = 60.4 to 96.4%]), with positive likelihood ratio of 5.56 when the cut-off value is set at 0.35 cm (area under the ROC curve = 0.86 (95% CI = 0.74 to 0.94%) (Figure 13.38).[105]

TCD of Venous Sinuses

According to the Monro–Kellie doctrine, cerebral compliance firmly relies on the compressibility of the low-pressure venous or capacitance segment of the vascular bed; in fact when ICP raises venous blood volume is reduced as a first line compensatory mechanism of the system. On this basis it has been theorized that a relationship between venous blood flow (VBF) and elevated ICP exists. Venous TCD finds its application in diagnosis and follow-up of cerebral venous thrombosis, stroke, and head trauma. Serial studies assessing TCD flow velocities in the basal vein of Rosenthal and the straight sinus explored the relationship between ICP and gPI derived from VBF velocities (VBFV) (maximal VBFV – minimal VBFV)/ mean VBFV); as a result, linear relationship between mean ICP and maximal VBFV in the basal vein of Rosenthal (r = 0.645; P = 0.002) and in the straight sinus has been observed (r = 0.928; P = 0.0003). One of the limits of the technique is that the insonation of the basal vein of Rosenthal is only achievable in 88% and the straight sinus in 72% of the patients.[97,117,118]

Cerebral Circulatory Arrest

Irreversible cessation of all functions of the entire brain characterises brain death.[119] In most cases, and depending on the relative law in different countries, clinical criteria are usually deemed sufficient to ascertain a diagnosis of brain death; nevertheless, some specific clinical situations demand for further confirmatory tests. Such circumstances are: ongoing pharmacological sedation of patients, facial trauma so that brainstem reflexes cannot be assessed, previous or ethical or legal controversies, pre-existing alterations in pupillary shape and diameter and chronic obstructive pulmonary disease (COPD) that normally have elevated $PaCO_2$ levels. Despite providing little information about the brainstem activity and being influenced by sedatives, the most frequently employed confirmatory test is the EEG.

In order to confirm brain death and arrest of cerebral circulation DSA represents the gold standard, however, it is an invasive procedure that necessitates the transfer of the patient to the angiography suite. Assessment of the CBF can be carried out through the use of TCD as well. TCD, as already mentioned, is a simple, noninvasive repeatable test that can be performed at the patient's bedside. The cessation of brain circulation is caused by increased ICP which induces initial reduction in the diastolic flow velocity. As ICP rises and its value equals the diastolic arterial pressure, diastolic flow velocity becomes zero; further ICP increments determine a phenomenon called reverberating (or oscillating) flow displayed by the reappearence of a diastolic flow but in the opposite direction, and which indicates a retrograde flow during the diastolic phase of the cardiac cycle. Finally, brief systolic spikes followed by the complete disappearance of the Doppler signal are observed when the arrest of CBF takes place. These four TCD patterns describe the typical progression seen during brain death. A reverberating flow and systolic spikes are considered conclusive of cerebral circle arrest (Figures 13.39a and 13.39b).

Nevertheless, when there is no TCD signal whatsoever in any of the vessels at the base of the cranium, in order to consider such a finding as indicative of brain death, the accessibility of the acoustic window must be confirmed with a previous examination showing the presence of TCD signal of flow. Otherwise, other tests need to be undertaken to confirm the diagnosis of brain death. To exclude temporary arrest because of hypotension, systolic arterial pressure must not fall below 70 mmHg. At the same time flow patterns have to be monitored during two previous examinations at least 30 minutes apart. The reported TCD sensitivity and specificity for the diagnosis of brain death are respectively 96.5% and 100%. It is also important to stress that the central nervous system sedative drugs do not influence the diagnosis of brain death with TCD.[12,120,132]

Cerebrovascular Stenosis

The detection of carotid siphon (CS) stenosis using TCD was first reported in 1986 by Spencer and Whisler. Diagnostic criteria employed were very similar to those already used for carotid bifurcation disease. Since then, many authors have implemented the technique to other brain arteries in order to perform a rapid vascular screening in stroke patients. In fact, normal TCD findings in stroke patients have considerable clinical impact.

Definition of Stenosis with TCD

Typical TCD/TCCD features of segmental stenosis of basal cerebral arteries are: (1) disturbed flow (spectral broadening and reinforced systolic and low-frequency echo components); (2) incremented flow velocity; and (3) covibration phenomena (vibration of vessel wall and surrounding soft tissue).

With regard to flow velocity, there is still a lack of agreement about whether the PSV (>120–160 cm/sec) or the mean systolic velocity (>80–120 cm/sec) should be used as a threshold value.

In literature a sensitivity of 100% and a specificity of 97.9%, as well as positive and negative predictive values of 88.8% and 94.9% is described when using a MFV cut-off value of 100 cm/sec to identify intracranial stenosis of 50% or more. Studies assessing the vertebrobasilar system report fair sensitivity (80%) and very good specificity (97%) in detecting stenosis of at least 50% when using a PSV of 115–120 cm/sec or more.

Besides the flow velocity that best correlates with angiographic stenosis, most authors agree that also symmetry in flow velocity is a very useful data during TCD evaluation of a suspected vessel stenosis. In fact, in comparison with the contralateral vessel segment, a relative increase in PSV of more than 30% is suspicious for haemodynamically significant stenosis, and a relative increase of more than 50% indicates a definite ICA stenosis (Figures 13.40 and 13.41).[44,45,121–123]

Definition of Occlusion with TCD

Basal cerebral artery occlusion can be ascertained through the use of TCD when the following signs are seen: (1) absence of arterial signals at the expected depth, if using TCCD neither the visualization or the Doppler signs are perceivable; (2) presence of signals in vessels that communicate with the occluded artery (as a confirmation of an adequate acoustic window); and (3) increased or inverted flow in communicating vessels indicating compensatory circles. For example, occlusion of the MCA is diagnosed from the lack of an MCA flow signal in the presence of concomitant flow signals from other vessels (i.e., the PCA, the ACA, or the distal CS). In terms of reliability in detection of intracranial vessel occlusions TCD has 83% sensitivity almost 94% specificity with an overall accuracy of 91.6%.[124–128]

After initial assessment, repeated or continuous TCD monitoring allows clinicians to follow up the evolution of the occlusion and to assess for possible recanalization in the vessel whether that might occur spontaneously or induced by fibrinolysis. Moreover some studies suggest that Doppler ultrasound itself may play a role in facilitating the lysis of the thrombus in patients treated with rt-PA (higher level of recanalization). Concerning the follow-up of arterial canalization in ischaemic stroke patients, Demchuk and colleagues, following as an example the angiography-based Thrombolysis in Myocardial Infarction criteria used by cardiologists have suggested a similar classification in order to monitor the MCA during and after initiation of thrombolysis. Thrombolysis in Brain Ischaemia criteria provide a scale ranging from 0 (MCA occlusion) to 5 (normal MCA) that through the application of TCD-based criteria allows the monitoring of the MCA status during and after thrombolysis (Figure 13.42).[129–131]

Detection of Microemboli and Patent Foramen Ovale

Paradoxical embolism through the PFO is a possible cause of stroke in young patients. TCD allows the identification of a right-to-left cardiac shunt with almost 100% concordance using a transoesophageal cardiac echography through the detection of microemboli in the cerebral arteries after injection of contrast medium. Specifically, the technique is based on the injection of 9 ml of physiological solution mixed with 1 ml of air through a three-port tap into one of the large forearm veins. If there is a right-to-left shunt, gaseous microemboli are seen 5–15 seconds after the injection as 'interference' in the normal Doppler flow pattern (hyperintensity thromboembolic signal) of MCA (Figures 13.43 and 13.44). If the result of the basic test is negative, the sensitivity of the test can be improved by performing it while the patient is asked to perform a Valsalva manoeuvre. By doing so, the increased pressure in the right heart drives the passage of microemboli even through tinier shunts. Caution might be posed for extracardiac shunt (e.g., intrapulmonary) as responsible for false positives.[12,17,119]

CONCLUSIONS

Monitoring TCD/TCCD is a precious diagnostic tool for the neurointensivist: it is noninvasive, portable, easily repeatable, and low in cost. However, it is not perfect: there are some limitations due to operator dependence and suboptimal sensitivity for detecting distal vasospasm. TCD and TCCD show greatest value in detecting MCA vasospasm, although, when a TCD exam is performed in order to detect vasospasm, the entire cerebral arterial circle should be examined and Lindegard ratio should be calculated in order to rectify for hyperemia-induced flow velocity changes. In addition, trending and day-to-day comparisons of blood flow velocities are critical in identifying vasospasm.

REFERENCES

1. Patestas MA, Garther LP. *A Textbook of Neuroanatomy.* Chapter 8: Vascular supply of the central nervous system. Blackwell Publishing, 2006:p.99–117.
2. Rhoton AL. *Cranial Anatomy and Surgical Approaches.* Philadelphia: Lippincott Williams & Wilkin, 2003.
3. Grand W, Hopkins LN. *Variations in Clinical Anatomy. Vasculature of the Brain and Cranial Base.* New York: Thieme, 1999:p.43–213.
4. Krabbe Hartkamp MJ, van der Grond J, de Leeuw FE, et al. Circle of Willis: morphologic variation on three dimensional time-to-flight MR angiograms. *Radiology* 1998;207(1):103–11.
5. Klingelhofer J, Conrad B, Benecke R, et al. Evaluation of intracranial pressure from transcranial Doppler studies in cerebral disease. *J Neural* 1988;235(3):159–62.
6. Aaslid R, Lundar T, Lindegaard KF, et al. Estimation of cerebral perfusion pressure from arterial blood pressure and transcranial Doppler recordings. In: Miller JD, Teasdale GM, Rowan JO, editors. *Intracranial Pressure VI.* Berlin: Springer, 1986:p.226–32.
7. Czosnyka M, Matta BF, Smielewski P, et al. Cerebral perfusion pressure in headinjured patients: a noninvasive assessment using transcranial Doppler ultrasonography. *J Neurosurg* 1998;88:802–8.
8. Aaslid R, Markwalder TM, Nornes H. Noninvasive transcranial Doppler ultrasound recording of flow velocity in basal cerebral arteries. *J Neurosurg* 1982;57:769–74.
9. McCartney JP, Thomas-Lukes KM, Gomez CR. *Handbook of Transcranial Doppler.* New York, USA: Springer, 1997:p.6–34.
10. Aaslid R. The Doppler principle applied to measurement of blood flow velocities in cerebral arteries. In: Aaslid R, ed. *Transcranial Doppler Sonography.* Vienna: Springer-Verlag, 1986:p. 22–38.
11. Manno EM. Transcranial Doppler ultrasonography in the neurocritical care unit. *Crit Care Clin* 1997;13:79–104.
12. Rasulo FA, De Peri E, Lavinio A. Transcranial Doppler ultrasonography in intensive care. *Eur J Anaesthesiol* 2008;25(Suppl 42):167–73.
13. Hayden White, Balasubramanian Venkatesh. Applications of transcranial Doppler in the ICU: a review. *Intensive Care Med* 2006;32:981–94.
14. Eicke BM, Tegeler CH, Dalley G, et al. Angle correction in transcranial Doppler sonography. *J Neuroimaging* 1994;4:29–33.
15. Grolimund, P. Transmission of ultrasound through the temporal bone. In: Aaslid R ed. *Transcranial Doppler Sonography.* New York: Springer-Verlag, 1986:p.10–21.
16. Babikian VL, Feldmann E, Wechsler LR, et al. Transcranial Doppler ultrasonography: year 2000 update. *J Neuroimaging* 2000;10:101–15.
17. Rigamonti A, Chen R, Mariappan R. Chapter 13: Basic transesophageal and critical care ultrasound. In: Denault A,

Vegas A, Lamarche L, et al. *Critical Care Examination of the Nervous System*. CRC Press, 2017:p.229–48.

18. Bartels E, Flugel KA. Transcranial color–coded Doppler ultrasound—a new procedure for routine diagnosis of cerebrovascular diseases? *Vasa Suppl* 1992;35:16–20.

19. Gosling RG, King DH. Arterial assessment by Doppler-shift ultrasound. *Proc R Soc Med* 1974;67:p.447–9.

20. Huber P, Handa J. Effect of contrast material, hypercapnia, hyperventilation, hypertonic glucose and papaverine don the diameter of the cerebral arteries-angiographic determination in man. *Invest Radiol* 1967;2:17–33.

21. Lam AM, Newell DW. Intraoperative use of transcranial doppler sonography. *Neurosurgery Clinics of North America* 1996;7:709–22.

22. Bishop CCR, Powell S, Rutt D, et al. Transcranial Doppler measurement of the middle cerebral flow velocity: A validation study. *Stroke* 1986;17:913–15.

23. Dahal A, Russell, Nyberg-Hansen R. A comparison of regional cerebral blood flow and middle cerebral artery blood flow velocities: Simultaneous measurements in healthy subjects. *J Cereb Blood Flow Metab* 1992;12:1049–54.

24. Bisonotte B, Leon JE. Cerbrovascular stability during isoflurane anesthesia in children. *Can J Anesth* 1992;39:128–34.

25. Eng CC, Lam AM, Mayberg TS, et al. Influence of propofol and propofol–nitrous oxide anaesthesia on cerebral blood flow velocity and carbon dioxide reactivity in humans. *Anesthesiology* 1992;77:872–9.

26. Gupta S, Heath K, Matta BF. Effect of incremental doses of sevofluorane on cerebral pressure autoregulation in humans. *Br J Anaesth* 1997;79:469–72.

27. Tegeler C, Ratanakorn D. Physics and principles. In: Babikian V, Wechsler L eds. *Physics and Principles*. Woburn, Butterworth-Heinemann, 1999:p.3–13.

28. Nabavi D, Martin G, Ritter A, et al. Ultrasound assessment of the intracranial arteries. In: Pellerito J, et al. *Introduction to Vascular Ultrasonography*. Saunders, Philadelphia: Elsevier, 2012.

29. Aaslid R. Transcranial Doppler examination techniques. In: Aaslid R. *Transcranial Doppler Sonography*. New York: Springer Verlag, 1986; p.39–59.

30. Krejza J, Mariak Z, Melhem ER, Bert RJ. A guide to the identification of major cerebral arteries with transcranial color Doppler sonography. *AJR* 2000;174:1297–303.

31. Aaslid R, Huber P, Nornes H. Evaluation of cerebrovascular spasm with transcranial Doppler ultrasound. *J Neurosurg* 1984;60:37–41.

32. Laumer R, Steinmeier R, Gonner F, et al. Cerebral hemodynamics in subarachnoid hemorrhage evaluated by transcranial Doppler sonography. Part 1. Reliability of flow velocities in clinical management. *Neurosurgery* 1993;33:1–8.

33. Steinmeier R, Laumer R, Bondar I, et al. Cerebral hemodynamics in subarachnoid hemorrhage evaluated by transcranial Doppler sonography. Part 2. Pulsatility indices: normal reference values and characteristics in subarachnoid hemorrhage. *Neurosurgery* 1993;33:10–18.

34. Grosset DG, Straiton J, McDonald I, et al. Use of transcranial Doppler sonography to predict development of a delayed ischemic deficit after subarachnoid hemorrhage. *J Neurosurg* 1993;78:183–7.

35. Lindegaard KF. The role of transcranial Doppler in the management of patients with subarachnoid haemorrhage: a review. *Acta Neurochir* 1999;72:59–71.

36. Sloan MA, Alexandrov AV, Tegeler CH, et al. Assessment: transcranial Doppler ultrasonography: report of the Therapeutics and Technology Assessment Subcommittee of the American Academy of Neurology. *Neurology* 2004;62:1468–81.

37. Hansen HC, Helmke K. The subarachnoid space surrounding the optic nerves. An ultrasound study of the optic nerve sheath. *Surg Radiol Anat* 1996;18:323–8.

38. Seidel G, Gerriets T, Kaps M, Missler U. Dislocation of the third ventricle due to space–occupying stroke evaluated by transcranial duplex sonography. *J Neuroimaging* 1996;6:227–30.

39. Stolz E, Gerriets T, Fiss I, Babacan SS, Seidel G, Kaps M. Comparison of transcranial color-coded duplex sonography and cranial CT measurements for determining third ventricle midline shift in space–occupying stroke. *AJNR Am J Neuroradiol* 1999;20:1567–71.

40. Moppett IK, Mahajan RP. Transcranial Doppler ultrasonography in anaesthesia and intensive care. *Br J Anaesth* 2004;93:710–24.

41. Vora YY, Suarez–Almazor M, Steinke DE, et al. Role of transcranial Doppler monitoring in the diagnosis of cerebral vasospasm after subarachnoid hemorrhage. *Neurosurgery* 1999;44:1237–47.

42. Sloan MA, Haley Jr EC, Kassell NF, et al. Sensitivity and specificity of transcranial Doppler ultrasonography in the diagnosis of vasospasm following subarachnoid hemorrhage. *Neurology* 1989;39:1514–18.

43. Lysakowski C, Walder B, Costanza MC, et al. Transcranial Doppler versus angiography in patients with vasospasm due to a ruptured cerebral aneurysm: a systematic review. *Stroke* 2001;32:2292–8.

44. Rorick MB, Nichols FT, Adams RJ. Transcranial Doppler correlation with angiography in detection of intracranial stenosis. *Stroke* 1994;25:1931–4.

45. de Bray JM, Joseph PA, Jeanvoine H, et al. Transcranial Doppler evaluation of middle cerebral artery stenosis. *J Ultrasound Med* 1988;7:611–6.

46. Bratton SL, Chesnut RM, Ghajar J, et al. Guidelines for the management of severe traumatic brain injury. VII. Intracranial pressure monitoring technology. *J Neurotrauma* 2007;24(1):S45–54.

47. Klingelhofer J, Conrad B, Benecke R, et al. Evaluation of intracranial pressure from transcranial Doppler studies in cerebral disease. *J Neurol* 1988;235:159–62.

48. Grosset DG, Straiton J, du Trevou M, et al. Prediction of symptomatic vasospasm after subarachnoid hemorrhage by rapidly increasing transcranial Doppler velocity and cerebral blood flow changes. *Stroke* 1992;23:674–9.

49. Lennihan L, Petty GW, Fink E, et al. Transcranial Doppler detection of anterior cerebral artery vasospasm. *J Neurol Neurosurg Psychiatry* 1993;56:906–9.

50. Burch CM, Wozniak MA, Sloan MA, et al. Detection of intracranial internal carotid artery and middle cerebral artery vasospasm following subarachnoid hemorrhage. *J Neuroimaging* 1996;6:8–15.

51. Wozniak MA, Sloan MA, Rothman MI, et al. Detection of vasospasm by transcranial Doppler sonography. The challenges of the anterior and posterior cerebral arteries. *J Neuroimaging* 1996;6:87–93.

52. Sloan MA, Burch CM, Wozniak MA, et al. Transcranial Doppler detection of vertebrobasilar vasospasm following subarachnoid hemorrhage. *Stroke* 1994;25:2187–97.

53. Sviri GE, Ghodke B, Britz GW, et al. Transcranial Doppler grading criteria for basilar artery vasospasm. *Neurosurgery* 2006;59(2):360–6.

54. Soustiel JF, Shik V, Shreiber R, Tavor Y, Goldsher D. Basilar vasospasm diagnosis: investigation of a modified 'Lindegaard index' based on imaging studies and blood velocity measurements of the basilar artery *Stroke* 2002;33(1):72–77.

55. Ursino M, Giulioni M, Lodi CA. Relationships among cerebral perfusion pressure, autoregulation, and transcranial Doppler waveform: a modeling study. *J Neurosurg* 1998;89:255–66.

56. Puppo C, López L, Caragna E, Biestro A. One-minute dynamic cerebral autoregulation in severe head injury patients and its comparison with static autoregulation. A transcranial Doppler study *Neurocritical Care* 2008;8(3):344–52.

57. Aries MJH, Elting JW, de Keyser J, et al. Cerebral autoregulation in stroke: a review of transcranial Doppler studies *Stroke* 2010;41(11):2697–704.

58. Reinhard JW, Roth M, Muller T, Czosnyka M, Timmer J, Hetzel A. Cerebral autoregulation in carotid artery occlusive disease assessed from spontaneous blood pressure fluctuations by the correlation coefficient index *Stroke* 2003;34(9):2138–44.

59. Panerai RB. Transcranial Doppler for evaluation of cerebral autoregulation. *Clinical Autonomic Research* 2009;19(4):197–211.

60. Stocchetti N, Maas AI, Chieregato A, van der Plas AA. Hyperventilation in head injury: a review. *Chest* 2005;127:1812–27.

61. Maeda H, Matsumoto M, Handa N, et al. Reactivity of cerebral blood flow to carbon dioxide in hypertensive patients: evaluation by the transcranial Doppler method. *J Hypertens* 1994;12:191–7.

62. Lang EW, Diehl R, Mehdorn M. Cerebral autoregulation testing after subarachnoid hemorrhage: the phase relationship between arterial blood pressure and cerebral blood flow velocity. *Critical Care Med* 2001;29:158–63.

63. Aaslid R, Lindegaard KF, Sorteberg W, Nornes H. Cerebral autoregulation dynamics in humans. *Stroke* 1989;20(1):45–52.

64. Giller GA. A bedside test for cerebral autoregulation using transcranial Doppler ultrasound. *Acta Neurochirurgica* 1991;108:7–14.

65. Smielewsky P, Czosnyka M, Kirkpatrik P, et al. Evaluation of the transient hyperemic response test in head injured patients. *J Nerurosurg* 1997;86:773–8.

66. Cavill G, Simpson EJ, Mahajan RP. Factor affecting assessment of cerebral autoregulation using the transient hyperaemic response test. *Br J Anesth* 1998;81:317–21.

67. Czosnyka M, Kirkpatrik P, Pickard JD. Multimodal monitoring and assessment of cerebral haemodynamic reserve after severe head injury. *Cerebrovasc Brain Metab Rev* 1996;8:273–95.

68. Burton AC. On the physical equilibrium of small blood vessels. *Am J Physiol* 1951;164:319–29.

69. Richards HK, Czosnyka M, Pickard JD. Assessment of critical closing pressure in the cerebral circulation as a measure of cerebrovascular tone. *Acta Neurochir* 1999;141:1221–7, discussion 1226–7.

70. Weyland A, Buhre W, Grund S, et al. Cerebrovascular tone rather than intracranial pressure determines the effective downstream pressure of the cerebral circulation in the absence of intracranial hypertension. *J Neurosurg Anesthesiol* 2000;12:210–16.

71. Thees C, Scholz M, Schaller MDC, et al. Relationship between intracranial pressure and critical closing pressure in patients with neurotrauma. *Anesthesiology* 2002;96:595–99.

72. Muizelaar JP, Marmarou A, DeSalles AA, et al. Cerebral blood flow and metabolism in severely head injured children. Part 1: relationship with GCS score, outcome, ICP and PVI. *J Neurosurg* 1989;71:63–71.

73. Güiza F, Depreitere B, Piper I, et al. Visualizing the pressure and time burden of intracranial hypertension in adult and paediatric traumatic brain injury. *Intensive Care Med* 2015;41(6):1067–76.

74. Zoerle T, Lombardo A, Colombo A, et al. Intracranial pressure after subarachnoid hemorrhage. *Crit Care Med* 2015;43(1):168–76.

75. Cardim D, Robba C, Donnelly J, et al. Prospective study on noninvasive assessment of intracranial pressure in traumatic brain-injured patients: Comparison of four methods. *Journal of Neurotrauma* 2016;33:792–802.

76. Smith M. Monitoring intracranial pressure in traumatic brain injury. *Anesth Analg* 2008;106(1):240–8.

77. Bhatia A, Gupta AK. Neuromonitoring in the intensive care unit. I. Intracranial pressure and cerebral blood flow monitoring. *Intensive Care Med* 2007;33(7):1263–71.

78. Beer R, Lackner P, Pfausler B, et al. Nosocomial ventriculitis and meningitis in neurocritical care patients. *J Neurol* 2008;255(11):1617–24.

79. Lozier AP, Sciacca RR, Romagnoli MF, et al. Ventriculostomy-related infections: a critical review of the literature. *Neurosurgery* 2008;62(2):688–700.

80. Binz DD, Toussaint LG, Friedman JA. Hemorrhagic complications of ventriculostomy placement: a meta-analysis. *Neurocrit Care* 2009;10(2):253–6.

81. Gardner PA, Engh J, Atteberry D, et al. Hemorrhage rates after external ventricular drain placement: clinical article. *J Neurosurg* 2009;110(5):1021–5.

82. Gelabert-Gonzalez M, Ginesta-Galan V, Sernamito Garcıa R, et al. The Camino intracranial pressure device in clinical practice. Assessment in a 1000 cases. *Acta Neurochir* 2006;148(4):435–41.

83. Piper I, Barnes A, Smith D, et al. The Camino intracranial pressure sensor: is it optimal technology? An internal audit with a review of current intracranial pressure monitoring technologies. *Neurosurgery* 2001;49(5):1158–64.

84. Kristiansson H, Nissborg E, et al. Measuring elevated intracranial pressure through noninvasive methods: a review of the literature. *J Neurosurg Anesthesiol* 2013;25:372–85.

85. Raboel PH, Bartek J, Andresen M, et al. Intracranial pressure monitoring: invasive versus non-invasive methods—a review. *Crit Care Res Pract* 2012;2012:950393.

86. Bellner J, Romner B, Reinstrup P, et al. Transcranial Doppler sonography pulsatility index (PI) reflects intracranial pressure (ICP). *Surg Neurol* 2004;62:45–51. Discussion 51.

87. Voulgaris SG, Partheni M, Kaliora H, et al. Early cerebral monitoring using the transcranial Doppler pulsatility index in patients with severe brain trauma. *Med Sci Monit* 2005;11(2):49–52.

88. Zweifel C, Czosnyka M, Carrera E, et al. Reliability of the blood flow velocity pulsatility index for assessment of intracranial and cerebral perfusion pressures in head-injured patients. *Neurosurgery* 2012;71:853–61.

89. Schmidt EA, Czosnyka M, Matta BF, et al. Non-invasive cerebral perfusion pressure (nCPP): evaluation of the monitoring methodology in head-injured patients. *Acta Neurochir Suppl* 2000;76:451–2.

90. Behrens A, Lenfeldt N, Ambarki K, Malm J, Eklund A, Koskinen LO. Transcranial Doppler pulsatility index: not an accurate method to assess intracranial pressure. *Neurosurgery* 2010;66(6):1050–7.

91. Czosnyka M, Kirkpatrick P, Guazzo E, et al. Can TCD pulsatility indices be used for a non invasive assessment of cerebral perfusion pressure in head injured patients? In: Naagai H, Kamiya K, Ishii S, editors. *Intracranial Pressure IX*. Tokyo: Springer; 1994;p.149.

92. Schmidt EA, Czosnyka M, Gooskens I, et al. Preliminary experience of the estimation of cerebral perfusion pressure using transcranial Doppler ultrasonography. *J Neurol Neurosurg Psychiatr* 2001;70:198–204.

93. Kashif FM, Verghese GC, Novak V, et al. Model-based noninvasive estimation of intracranial pressure from cerebral blood flow velocity and arterial pressure. *Sci Transl Med* 2012;4(129):129ra44.

94. Hansen HC, Helmke K. Validation of the optic nerve sheath response to changing cerebrospinal fluid pressure: ultrasound findings during intrathecal infusion tests. *J Neurosurg* 1997;87(1):34–40.

95. Launey Y, Nesseler N, Le MP, Malledant Y, Seguin P. Effect of osmotherapy on optic nerve sheath diameter in patients with increased intracranial pressure. *J Neurotrauma* 2014;31(10):984–8.

96. Kim JY, Min HG, Ha SI, Jeong HW, Seo H, Kim JU. Dynamic optic nerve sheath diameter responses to short-term hyperventilation measured with sonography in patients under general anesthesia. *Korean J Anesthesiol* 2014;67(4):240–5.

97. Robba C, Bacigaluppi S, Cardim D, Donnelly J, Bertuccio A, Czosnyka M. Non-invasive assessment of intracranial pressure. *Acta Neurol Scand* 2016;134(1):4–21.

98. Shah S, Kimberly H, Marill K, et al. Ultrasound techniques to measure the optic nerve sheath: is a specialized probe necessary? *Med Sci Monit* 2009;15(5):MT63–8.

99. Tayal VS, Neulander M, Norton HJ, Foster T, Saunders T, Blaivas M. Emergency department sonographic measurement of optic nerve sheath diameter to detect findings of increased intracranial pressure in adult head injury patients. *Ann Emerg Med* 2007;49 (4):508–14.

100. Karakitsos D, Soldatos T, Gouliamos A, et al. Transorbital sonographic monitoring of optic nerve diameter in patients with severe brain injury. *Transplant Proc* 2006;38(10):3700–6.

101. Malayeri AA, Bavarian S, Mehdizadeh M. Sonographic evaluation of optic nerve diameter in children with raised intracranial pressure. *J Ultrasound Med* 2005;24(2):143–7.

102. Girisgin AS, Kalkan E, Kocak S, Cander B, Gul M, Semiz M. The role of optic nerve ultrasonography in the diagnosis of elevated intracranial pressure. *Emerg Med J* 2007;24(4):251–4.

103. Sekhon MS, Griesdale DE, Robba C, et al. Optic nerve sheath diameter on computed tomography is correlated with simultaneously measured intracranial pressure in patients with severe traumatic brain injury. *Intensive Care Med* 2014;40(9):1267–74.

104. Strumwasser A, Kwan RO, Yeung L, et al. Sonographic optic nerve sheath diameter as an estimate of intracranial pressure in adult trauma. *J Surg Res* 2011;170(2):265–71.

105. Motuel J, Biette I, Srairi M, et al. Assessment of brain midline shift using sonography in neurosurgical ICU patients. *Critical Care* 2014;18:676.

106. Becker DP, Miller JD, Ward JD, Greenberg RP, Young HF, Sakalas R. The outcome from severe head injury with early diagnosis and intensive management. *J Neurosurg* 1977;47:491–502.

107. Vollmer G, Torner JC, Jane JA, et al. Age and outcome following traumatic coma: why do older patients fare worse? *J Neurosurg* 1991;75:S37–S49.

108. Quattrocchi KB, Prasad P, Willits NH, Wagner FC Jr. Quantification of midline shift as a predictor of

poor outcome following head injury. *Surg Neurology* 1991;35:183–8.

109. Young B, Rapp RP, Norton JA, Haack D, Tibbs PA, Bean JR. Early prediction of outcome in head–injured patients. *J Neurosurg* 1981;54:300–3.

110. Ross DA, Olsen WL, Ross AM, Andrews BT, Pitts LH. Brain shift, level of consciousness, and restoration of consciousness in patients with acute intracranial hematoma. *J Neurosurg* 1989;71:498–502.

111. Lobato RD, Rivas JJ, Gomez PA, et al. Head–injured patients who talk and deteriorate into coma. Analysis of 211 cases studied with computerized tomography. *J Neurosurg* 1991;75:256–61.

112. Perel P, Arango M, Clayton T, et al. Predicting outcome after traumatic brain injury: practical prognostic models based on large cohort of international patients. *Br Med J* 2008;336:425–9.

113. Ropper AH. Lateral displacement of the brain and level of consciousness in patients with an acute hemispheral mass. *New Engl J Med* 1986;314:953–8.

114. Pullicino PM, Alexandrov AV, Shelton JA, Alexandrova NA, Smurawska LT, Norris JW. Mass effect and death from severe acute stroke. *Neurology* 1997;49:1090–5.

115. Bertram M, Khoja W, Ringleb P, Schwab S. Transcranial colour-coded sonography for the bedside evaluation of mass effect after stroke. *Eur J Neurol* 2000;7:639–46.

116. Tang SC, Huang SJ, Jeng JS, Yip PK. Third ventricle midline shift due to spontaneous supratentorial intracerebral hemorrhage evaluated by transcranial color–coded sonography. *J Ultrasound Med* 2006;25:203–9.

117. Schoser BG, Riemenschneider N, Hansen HC. The impact of raised intracranial pressure on cerebral venous hemodynamics: a prospective venous transcranial Doppler ultrasonography study. *J Neurosurg* 1999;91:744–9.

118. Schreiber SJ, Stolz E, Valdueza JM. Transcranial ultrasonography of cerebral veins and sinuses. *Eur J Ultrasound* 2002;16:59–72.

119. Droste DW, Lakemeier S, Wichter T, et al. Optimizing the technique of contrast transcranial Doppler ultrasound in the detection of right–to–left shunts. *Stroke* 2002;33:221–6.

120. Ropper AH, Kehne SM, Wechsler L. Transcranial Doppler in brain death. *Neurology* 1987;37:1733–5.

121. Schwarze JJ, Babikian V, DeWitt LD, et al. Longitudinal monitoring of intracranial arterial stenoses with transcranial Doppler ultrasonography. *J Neuroimaging* 1994;4:182–7.

122. Wilterdink JL, Feldmann E, Furie KL, et al. Transcranial Doppler ultrasound battery reliably identifies severe internal carotid artery stenosis. *Stroke* 1997;28:133–6.

123. Koch S, Romano JG, Park H, Amir M, Forteza AM. Ultrasound velocity criteria for vertebral origin stenosis. *J Neuroimaging* 2009;19(3):242–5.

124. Zanette EM, Fieschi C, Bozzao L, et al. Comparison of cerebral angiography and transcranial Doppler sonography in acute stroke. *Stroke* 1989;20:899–903.

125. Camerlingo M, Casto L, Censori B, et al. Transcranial Doppler in acute ischemic stroke of the middle cerebral artery territories. *Acta Neurol Scand* 1993;88:108–11.

126. Kushner MJ, Zanette EM, Bastianello S, et al. Transcranial Doppler in acute hemispheric brain infarction. *Neurology* 1991;41:109–13.

127. Toni D, Fiorelli M, Zanette EM, et al. Early spontaneous improvement and deterioration of ischemic stroke patients. A serial study with transcranial Doppler ultrasonography. *Stroke* 1998; 29:1144–8.

128. Demchuk AM, Christou I, Wein TH, et al. Accuracy and criteria for localizing arterial occlusion with transcranial Doppler. *J Neuroimaging* 2000;10:1–12.

129. Burgin WS, Malkoff M, Felberg RA, et al. Transcranial Doppler ultrasound criteria for recanalization after thrombolysis for middle cerebral artery stroke. *Stroke* 2000;31:1128–32.

130. Eggers J, Koch B, Meyer K, et al. Effect of ultrasound on thrombolysis of middle cerebral artery occlusion. *Ann Neurol* 2003;53:797–800.

131. Demchuk AM, Scott Burgin W, Christou I, et al. Thrombolysis in Brain Ischemia (TIBI) transcranial Doppler flow grades predict clinical severity, early recovery, and mortality in patients treated with intravenous tissue plasminogen activator. *Stroke* 2001;1:89–93.

132. Wijdicks EF. The diagnosis of brain death. *N Engl J Med* 2001;344:1215–21.

Part III

Pharmacological Care

Editor: Gretchen M. Brophy

14

Sedation and Analgesia

K. Chester and K. Greene

ABSTRACT

Sedatives and analgesics may be the most widely used agents in the neurointensive care population. Sedation and analgesia must be used judiciously in neurocritically ill patients since these agents could impair the provider's ability to obtain accurate neurological examination results. Sedatives and analgesics vary significantly in their pharmacokinetic and pharmacodynamic properties, mechanisms of action, dosing, and adverse effect profiles. As with all medications, monitoring should focus on identifying adverse drug effects while ensuring patient comfort with adequate levels of sedation and analgesia. A working knowledge of sedatives and analgesics and their unique characteristics is imperative for customizing a safe and effective analgosedative regimen for each patient that is also cost-effective.

KEYWORDS

Sedation; analgesia; neurocritical care; ketamine; propofol; dexmedetomidine; midazolam; lorazepam.

INTRODUCTION

Sedatives as a class are some of the most widely used agents in the neurointensive care population. While sedatives may be used for various indications including alcohol withdrawal or burst suppression for status epilepticus and elevated intracranial pressure (ICP), the focus of this section will be non-procedural intensive care unit (ICU) sedation with a goal of optimizing the adult patient's comfort primarily during mechanical ventilation. Sedation in general must be used judiciously in neurocritically ill patients since sedatives make an accurate neurological examination difficult or impossible. In addition, acute changes in the neurological status could become hard to detect in the presence of sedation.[1]

Sedative agents vary significantly in their pharmacokinetic properties, mechanisms of action, dosing, and adverse effect profiles. A working knowledge of sedatives is important for customizing drug selection and patient monitoring. Like with all medications, monitoring should focus on safety and efficacy. Safety monitoring involves identifying adverse drug effects while monitoring patients for efficacy ensuring adequate sedation

without over- or under-sedation. Over-sedation can lead to prolonged mechanical ventilation and increased length of stay while under-sedation may result in ventilator dyssynchrony, patient recall of unpleasant events, vital sign instability, or increased oxygen consumption.[2]

Sedative monitoring can be accomplished through observational assessment using one of two validated sedation scales recommended by the Pain, Agitation, and Delirium (PAD) Guidelines published by the Society of Critical Care Medicine: the Richmond Agitation-Sedation Scale (RASS) and the Riker Sedation-Agitation Scale (SAS)[3] (see Table 14.1). These scales were initially validated in medical and surgical ICU populations; however, a study of the feasibility and reliability of sedative scales in neurocritical care patients demonstrated that sedation monitoring with RASS was accomplished by nurses and physicians with excellent inter-rater reliability.[4] In addition, a recent review of sedative monitoring concluded that the RASS and SAS are valid and useful tools for neurocritical care patients.[1]

In addition to observational assessment, neurophysiological monitoring such as bispectral

Table 14.1 Riker sedation-agitation scale

Score	Rating	Description
7	Dangerously agitated	Pulling at endotracheal tube (ETT), trying to remove catheters, climbing over bedrail, striking at staff, thrashing side-to-side
6	Very agitated	Requiring restraint and frequent verbal reminding of limits, biting ETT
5	Agitated	Anxious or physically agitated, calms to verbal instructions
4	Calm and cooperative	Calm, easily arousable, follows commands
3	Sedated	Difficult to arouse but awakens to verbal stimuli or gentle shaking, follows simple commands but drifts off again
2	Very sedated	Arouses to physical stimuli but does not communicate or follow commands, may move spontaneously
1	Unarousable	Minimal or no response to noxious stimuli, does not communicate or follow commands

Reprinted with permission from: Riker RR, Picard JT, Fraser GL. Prospective evaluation of the Sedation-Agitation Scale for adult critically ill patients. *Crit Care Med* 1999;27(7):1325–9.

index (BIS) monitoring may occasionally be used in neurocritically ill patients, primarily those requiring deep sedation, such as in the setting of neuromuscular blockade when observational assessment scales such as RASS become invalid. The BIS has been validated in the neurocritical care population.[5] This type of monitoring provides a near continuous assessment of the patient's level of sedation with a score of 0 to 100 derived from encephalographic monitoring with proprietary software. A BIS value of 60 has a high sensitivity of detecting drug-induced unconsciousness while a BIS value of >97 indicates the patient is awake and unsedated.[6] Evidence supporting the routine use of BIS monitoring for routine ICU sedation is lacking and some agents such as ketamine may confound BIS value interpretation.[7]

According to the most recent PAD guidelines, sedative medications for routine ICU sedation should be titrated to maintain light rather than a deep level of sedation in adult ICU patients unless clinically contraindicated. Clinical contraindications to light sedation in neurocritically ill patients may include refractory ICP management, shivering, deep sedation for paralysis, or in the management of status epilepticus. Both light levels of sedation and the choice of sedative are associated with improved clinical outcomes.[3] Intensive care protocols that require decrease in sedative doses or daily sedation interruption have demonstrated a reduction in ventilator days, ICU stay, and total sedative doses.[1]

SEDATIVE STRATEGIES

The need to revise routine sedative strategies in the ICU was addressed in the recent guidelines which emphasized avoiding deep sedation whenever possible. When patients

are agitated, pain and other causes of agitation should always be assessed and addressed before initiating or increasing sedative medications. The common causes of agitation are enlisted in Table 14.2. Many patients can maintain a calm and cooperative demeanour without the need for traditional sedative infusion by administering either analgesic bolus doses or an analgesic infusion with an agent such as fentanyl. Eliminating the need for a true sedative agent increases the accuracy of neurological examination and reduces the patient's risk of experiencing adverse effects as a result of the medication.[8]

When the need for a traditional sedative such as benzodiazepines or propofol arises, the minimum effective dose should be targeted and used in combination with analgesia. A combination of sedation and analgesia takes advantage of the synergistic properties by reducing the effective doses of both agents used to obtain the desired level of sedation. Older patients may respond more profoundly to sedatives due to diminished renal or hepatic function and also changes in volume of distribution.

Table 14.2 Common causes of agitation in the intensive care unit common causes of agitation

Causes
Pain
Delirium
Hypoxemia
Hypoglycaemia
Hypotension
Drug or alcohol withdrawal

Source: Barr J, Fraser GL, Puntillo K, et al. Clinical practice guidelines for the management of pain, agitation, and delirium in adult patients in the intensive care unit. *Crit Care Med* 2013;41(1):263–306.

Table 14.3 Factors that influence choice of sedatives

Factors
• Cause of agitation • Baseline neurological function • Haemodynamic variables • Presence of pain • Level of sedation required – deep versus light sedation • Organ function

Source: Barr J, Fraser GL, Puntillo K, et al. Clinical practice guidelines for the management of pain, agitation, and delirium in adult patients in the intensive care unit. *Crit Care Med* 2013;41(1):263–306.

Lower starting doses should be considered in this patient population as well as patients with organ dysfunction that could impair drug clearance.[1,8] The choice of the sedative agent should depend on several factors that are enlisted in Table 14.3.

Sedative agents can be broadly classified as benzodiazepines or non-benzodiazepines based on their chemical structure. While benzodiazepine infusions were once commonplace for routine ICU sedation, their use is being replaced by non-benzodiazepine agents such as propofol or dexmedetomidine which carry less risk for the development of delirium. In the neurocritical care unit, non-benzodiazepine agents are preferred due to their shorter half-life and awakening times in the setting of a patient population that requires frequent neurological examination.

The ideal sedative agent would have a rapid onset, short duration of action independent of organ function, be free of adverse effects, and have no drug interactions. Unfortunately, a sedative with all of these properties does not exist; therefore, knowledge of the available agents and their properties is paramount in customizing a safe and effective sedative regimen for each patient that is also cost-effective. The properties and pharmacology of sedative agents that are considered for sedation of brain-injured patients are given in Tables 14.4 and 14.5.

Table 14.4 Sedatives used in the neurocritical care unit

Class/Drug	Sedation/ Analgesia	MOA	Adverse effects	Pearls
Benzodiazepine Sedatives				
Midazolam	+++/0	GABA receptor agonist	Prolonged sedation, hypotension	Lipophilic; prolonged duration in patients with renal insufficiency or with high doses
Lorazepam	+++/0	GABA receptor agonist	Prolonged sedation, hypotension	Risk of propylene glycol toxicity with high doses
Non-benzodiazepine Sedatives				
Propofol	+++/0		Hypotension, bradycardia, PRIS, hypertriglyceridaemia, pancreatitis	Highly lipophilic; duration prolonged with longer duration infusions; injection site pain
Dexmedetomidine	++/+	Alpha$_2$ receptor agonist	Hypotension, bradycardia, transient hypertension (with LD), dry mouth, atrial fibrillation	Highly hydrophilic but able to readily cross BBB; Does not cause respiratory depression but may cause loss of oropharyngeal muscle tone
Ketamine	+++/++	NMDA receptor antagonist	Hypotension or hypertension, tachycardia	Highly lipophilic; Preserves airway reflexes; Higher incidences of hypertension and tachycardia with larger doses given over <60 s; emergence reactions; hypotension in catecholamine-depleted patients

Abbreviations: BBB: blood–brain barrier; GABA: gamma-aminobutyric acid; LD: loading dose; MOA: mechanism of action; PRIS: propofol-related infusion syndrome; NMDA: N-methyl-d-aspartate; 0: none.
Sources: (1) Brophy GM, Human T, Shutter L. Emergency neurological life support: Pharmacotherapy. *Neurocrit Care* 2015; 23(2):S48–68. (2) Barr J FG, Puntillo K, Ely EW, Gelinas C, Dasta JF. Clinical practice guidelines for the management of pain, agitation, and delirium in adult patients in the intensive care unit. *Crit Care Med* 2013; 263–306. (3) Erstad BL, Patanwala AE. Ketamine for analgosedation in critically ill patients. *J Crit Care* 2016;35:145–9. (4) Li A, Yuen VM, Goulay-Dufay S, Kwok PC. Pharmacokinetics and pharmacodynamics of dexmedetomidine. *Drug Dev Ind Pharm* 2016;42(12):1917–27.

Table 14.5   Pharmacology of sedatives for routine intensive care unit sedation of neurocritically ill patients

Drug	Onset (min)	Elimination half-life	Active metabolite(s)	Usual LD (IV)	Usual maintenance dosing (IV)	CYP enzyme interactions	Metabolic pathway
Midazolam	2–5	3–11 hr	Yes	0.01–0.05 mg/kg	2–8 mg/hr	Yes – 3A4	Hepatic – active metabolite (1–hydroxymethylmidazolam) cleared renally
Lorazepam	5–20	8–15 hr	No	0.02–0.04 mg/kg	1–4 mg/hr	No	Hepatic glucuronidation
Propofol	1–2	4–7 hr; may be up to 1–3 days with prolonged infusions (>10 days)	No	1–1.5 mg/kg – caution in patients with risk of hypotension	5–50 mcg/kg/min	Yes – 2B6, 2C9, 2C19, 3A4 but appear to be clinically insignificant	Hepatic conjugation
Dexmedetomidine	15 min; 5–10 min if LD is administered	1.8–3.1 hr	No	1 mcg/kg over at least 10 min – avoid in haemodynamically unstable patients. Loading doses are not routinely necessary	0.2–1.5 mcg/kg/hr	Yes – 2A6 but shown to be clinically irrelevant	Hepatic – glucuronidation and oxidation
Ketamine	0.5	300 min	Yes – norketamine with 1/3 potency of parent compound	0.1–0.5 mg/kg over at least 1 minute	0.05–0.4 mg/kg/hr	Yes – CYP2C9 and 3A4	Hepatic – hydroxylation and N–demethylation

Abbreviations: BBB: Blood–brain barrier; PRIS: Propofol-related infusion syndrome.

Sources: (1) Brophy GM, Human T, Shutter L. Emergency neurological life support: Pharmacotherapy. *Neurocrit Care* 2015;23(2):S48–68. (2) Barr J FG, Puntillo K, Ely EW, Gelinas C, Dasta JF. Clinical practice guidelines for the management of pain, agitation, and delirium in adult patients in the intensive care unit. *Crit Care Med* 2013:263–306. (3) Erstad BL, Patanwala AE. Ketamine for analgosedation in critically ill patients. *J Crit Care* 2016;35:145–49.

4. Li A, Yuen VM, Goulay-Dufay S, Kwok PC. Pharmacokinetics and pharmacodynamics of dexmedetomidine. *Drug Dev Ind Pharm* 2016; 42(12):1917–27.

It is important to consider that patients may become dependent on sedatives. Dependency is determined by the dose and duration of therapy. It is recommended to monitor for withdrawal symptoms and wean sedation by no more than 25% daily. This strategy also applies to opioid analgesic infusions.[8] If withdrawal symptoms develop during weaning, the amount and frequency of titrations should be reduced.

SEDATIVE AGENTS

Benzodiazepines

Benzodiazepines are a class of structurally related compounds that exert their effects by activating the gamma-aminobutyric acid (GABA$_A$) chloride channel, an inhibitory channel in the central nervous system. Benzodiazepines are known to have sedative, anxiolytic, amnestic, hypnotic, and anticonvulsant properties.[3] While there are several agents in this class, midazolam and lorazepam have been the primary benzodiazepines used for continuous intravenous infusion and bolus administration for sedation of mechanically ventilated patients. Midazolam has a short onset of action, but over time can accumulate in adipose tissue resulting in a prolonged duration of action unless daily sedation interruptions and careful down-titration strategies are used.[1] In addition, midazolam is converted in the body to an active metabolite that is cleared renally. Patients with renal impairment may experience prolonged sedation due to the effects of midazolam's active metabolite. Unlike midazolam, lorazepam is cleared hepatically through glucuronidation. High doses of lorazepam can lead to anion gap metabolic acidosis due to accumulation of the propylene glycol found in the lorazepam injectable formulation.

Historically, benzodiazepines have always played a significant role in the management of ICU sedation of mechanically ventilated patients. Their use in this setting has more recently diminished due to growing evidence that benzodiazepine use is associated with the development of delirium in critically ill patients.[3] When compared to most non-benzodiazepine sedatives, both midazolam and lorazepam have longer half-lives necessitating longer waiting for an accurate neurological examination. In addition, benzodiazepines can cause vasodilation yielding hypotension. Most studies suggest that the haemodynamic instability is comparable to dexmedetomidine or propofol;[1] however, a more recent study suggests that the instability may be less than dexmedetomidine.[9]

Non-Benzodiazepines

Propofol

Like benzodiazepines, propofol is also thought to have activity at the GABA$_A$ receptor though this agent is structurally unrelated to the benzodiazepine class. Being highly lipophilic in nature, propofol readily crosses the blood–brain barrier to its site of action. It is manufactured as a lipid formulation that provides relevant caloric intake which should be considered in the patient's nutritional regimen. Propofol has a rapid onset of action and short duration of action making it an appealing sedative for brain injured patients. With prolonged infusions, propofol, like midazolam, can accumulate in adipose tissue yielding a longer than predicted duration of action.

Propofol-related infusion syndrome (PRIS) is an uncommon adverse effect associated with high mortality. This condition is characterized by bradycardia, dyslipidaemia, metabolic acidosis, and rhabdomyolysis. Proposed risk factors include young age, administration of exogenous catecholamines, and cumulative dosage of propofol.[10] An infusion rate limit of 5 mg/kg/hr with vigilance is recommended in the most recent guidelines for brain trauma.[11] Triglycerides should be monitored at least weekly with higher doses and prolonged infusions. Occasionally, patients may have green urine discolouration; however, this effect is benign and therapy should be continued. Propofol is associated with a high incidence of hypotension, up to 30%.[1] In a retrospective study comparing dexmedetomidine and propofol across two academic medical centres, there was no difference in the incidence of hypotension (23% vs 26%, p = 0.52) or bradycardia (8.6% vs 5.5%, p = 0.28) between the agents.[12] Predictors of severe hypotension with propofol in neurocritical care patients include baseline mean arterial pressure (MAP) 60–70 mmHg and the need for renal replacement therapy.[13]

Dexmedetomidine

Dexmedetomidine has recently gained popularity as a sedative for neurocritically ill patients, though high quality evidence for its use in this patient population is lacking. Dexmedetomidine is a highly selective, central-acting, alpha-2 agonist. When alpha-2 receptors are activated, neuronal activity is suppressed and norepinephrine release is inhibited.[14] Like propofol, this agent has a rapid onset and short duration of action making it appealing for patients in need of frequent neurological assessments. Its use for sedation in neurocritically ill patients has grown with the emergence of evidence demonstrating a lower incidence of delirium compared to benzodiazepines.[9] Dexmedetomidine is unique in that it has no respiratory depressant effects making this agent a consideration for agitated patients during the peri-extubational period. In addition, dexmedetomidine lowers the shivering threshold and may be included in anti-shivering protocols in neurointensive care units.

In addition, dexmedetomidine has mild analgesic properties though it is not recommended for use as a single analgesic agent. A retrospective analysis of dexmedetomidine in neurologically ill patients demonstrated that this patient population may require high doses of dexmedetomidine to achieve the desired levels of sedation and wean off adjunctive sedatives or analgesics. Starting doses in this study population were higher than Food and Drug Administration (FDA) approvals and ranged from 0.4 to 1 mcg/kg/min to achieve the desired levels of sedation. These doses appeared to be safe.[15]

Dexmedetomidine is associated with a high incidence of hypotension and bradycardia that is more profound with bolus doses.[15] Other adverse effects that may be seen are dry mouth and atrial fibrillation.

Ketamine

Ketamine is classified as a dissociative agent that inhibits N-methyl-d-aspartate (NMDA) receptors but also has activity at opioid and GABA receptors, thereby imparting its analgesic and sedative properties.[16] This sedative is highly lipophilic, yielding a high volume of distribution. As a result, ketamine has the potential to accumulate in adipose tissue, a particular concern in obese patients.[16] Ketamine is known to cause psychotomimetic effects. Up to 30% of patients will experience hallucinations and psychosis, known as emergence reactions, during recovery from ketamine.[17] In general, it is recommended to avoid the use of ketamine in patients with a history of psychosis or drug withdrawal that could cause or precipitate psychotic reactions. In contrast to other sedatives, ketamine has the potential to increase heart rate and blood pressure through its sympathomimetic effects. It should be avoided in patients with a history of ischaemic cardiac disease or cardiac conditions that could be aggravated by ischaemia. Hypotension could occur in catecholamine depleted patients.[16,18] While there has been a concern for increased ICP with ketamine administration, more recent literature suggests no substantial adverse effects in brain-injured patients. Overall, use of ketamine for neurocritically ill patients is primarily limited to the management of refractory status epilepticus and is not routinely used for general ICU sedation due to paucity of

data in this setting and the availability of alternate sedative agents.

Barbiturates

Continuous infusion barbiturates such as thiopental and pentobarbital have limited use as sedatives in neurocritically ill patients due to their undesirable adverse effect profiles which include immunosuppression, hypotension, and bradycardia. Barbiturate use is primarily reserved for refractory ICP management and status epilepticus due to their effects on cerebral metabolic and electrical activity.[1]

ANALGESIA

Like sedation, analgesia remains to be the cornerstone of ICU practices to control discomfort, agitation, and delirium, facilitate mechanical ventilation and procedures, and to blunt catecholamine activity. Analgesia has been proven beneficial in the management of various disease states, specifically within the neurologically injured population where it is used for effective treatment of elevated ICP, management of paroxysmal sympathetic hyperactivity, abortive therapy for shivering during targeted temperature modulation, and in patients suffering from drug withdrawal. While there is a valid use for analgesia, utilization of these agents continues to pose challenges for neuro-specific patients. Contrary to the benefits of optimizing patient comfort, the goal to select appropriate analgesic strategies necessary for the critically ill state parallels the goal to maintain the ability to perform a neurological examination. Consequently, analgosedation must be delicately balanced.

Impact, Contributions, and Neuro-Specific Information

Pain is iatrogenic or generally associated with an underlying disease process and a major component of a number of conditions and illnesses amongst the neurocritical care population. Pain and inadequate management of pain contributes to unnecessary ICU suffering. Pain has been reported in the majority of the critically ill population irrespective of their indication for intensive care. Over 30% of patients report pain at rest,[19] and approximately 80% of patients report pain needs not met during their ICU stay.[20]

Pain in neurocritically ill patients, particularly those undergoing neurosurgical procedures, has been previously described as trivial; however, more recently awareness of pain contributions to the brain-injured patients has increased.

It has been found that this population often experiences more intense pain than previously recognized.[21] Tables 14.6 and 14.7 show the spectrum of neuro-related illnesses

Table 14.6 Spectrum of diseases encompassing pain within the neurologic population

Disease	Pain		
	Neurogenic	**Neuropathic**	**Central**
Anterior spinal artery infarct	+	+++	+++
Arteriovenous malformation (AVM)	+	+	+
Beçhet's syndrome (BS)	?	—	—
Eclampsia	+	+	
Encephalopathies	+	+	+
Encephalitis	+	+	+
Epileptic syndromes	—	+	+
Gullain-Barré syndrome (GBS)	—	+	—
Headache syndromes	+++	+++	+
Meningitis	+	+	—
Multiple sclerosis (MS)	+	+++	+++
Myasthenia gravis (MG)–post thymectomy	+++	—	—
POEMS syndrome	+++	+	—
Postoperative	+++	+++	+
Paraneoplastic disease	+	+	?
Poliomyelitis	+	+++	+
Prion disease	?	?	+
Root avulsion	+++	+++	+++
Sinus venous thrombosis (SVT)	+	+	—
Spinal cord injury (SCI)	+++	+++	+++
Subarachnoid haemorrhage (SAH)	+++	+++	—
Stroke	+	+	+
Syringomyelia	+	+++	+
Tetanus	+++	?	?
Traumatic Brain Injury (TBI)	+++	+++	+
Tumour	+	+	+
Vasculitis	+	+++	+

Note: '?' represents unknown.
Reprinted with permission from: Petzold A, Girbes A. Pain Management in Neurocritical Care. *Neurocrit Care* 2013;19:232–56.

and their respective types of pain contributions and for categories of pain according to neurosurgical or related procedures.

Reports indicate that neurosurgical patients experience moderate to severe pain within the first 48 hours of the ICU stay, specifically immediately within the 12-hour postoperative period.[22–24] Surprisingly, in an international analgesic audit of 173 neurocritically ill patients with diagnoses associated with moderate to severe pain, only 43% received pain relieving medications from two or more drug classes while approximate 33% received one medication or did not receive any medication at all.[25] Consequently, unrelieved pain will have both psychosocial and physical effects on patients. The impact is multidimensional and negatively affects the immune, cardiovascular, pulmonary system as well as has systemic effects on hypercoagulability, catabolism, and myocardial oxygen consumption.[26,27]

Iatrogenic contributions to ICU painful stimuli are often due to mundane routine aspects of the care of a critically ill patient and commonly involves procedures including nasogastric tube insertions, mobilization and turning of patients, indwelling catheters, and chest tube removal.[28] Types of pain specific to these patients include neurogenic, neuropathic, and central pain; the latter which primarily involves damage or dysfunction to the central nervous system including the brain, brainstem, and spinal cord. Central pain is primarily due to thalamic insults and tends to be one of the most challenging types of pain to manage. Moreover, central pain can be induced and aggravated by urinary retention, constipation, infectious aetiologies, and muscle spasms in addition to cutaneous, visceral, auditory, and visual input.[29]

Recognition and Monitoring

Causes of pain within the ICU are subjective and also multifaceted leading to self-reporting of pain as the gold standard for assessment.[30] As with many general ICU patients, and specifically, neurocritical care patients, an altered state of consciousness, sedative therapies, and the presence of mechanical ventilation often prevents recognition of pain. When a patient with preserved motor function is not able to self-report pain, additional validated tools such as the Behavioural Pain Scale (BPS) and the Critical-Care Pain Observation Tool (CPOT) are recommended as reliable pain monitoring tools at the bedside. These scales along with the Nonverbal Pain Scale (NVPS) have been studied in the neurocritical care population.[31–33] Yet, endorsement of measurement techniques for such scales should be approached with

Table 14.7 Categories of pain according to neurosurgical or related procedures

Severe pain	Moderate pain	Mild pain
Complex cervical, thoracic, lumbar spinal surgery	Craniotomy, cranioplasty	Increased intracranial pressure (ICP) bolt insertion
Cervical or lumbar laminectomy/laminoplasty	Posterior fossa craniectomy	Burr hole biopsy
Foramen magnum decompression	Transsphenoidalhypophysectomy	Trigeminal thermocoagulation
Sacral nerve stimulator	V/P shunt insertion and revision	Drainage of a chronic subdural hematoma
	Anterior cervical decompression	Carpal tunnel decompression
	Lumbar microdiscectomy	Ulnar nerve transposition
	Spinal cord stimulator	Muscle biopsy
	Deep brain stimulator	
	Carotid endarterectomy	

Reprinted with permission from: Petzold A, Girbes A. Pain Management in Neurocritical Care. *Neurocrit Care* 2013;19:232.

caution as brain injured patients with loss of consciousness have failed to demonstrate similar responses to pain as general ICU patients, warranting additional studies in this specific population.[34]

Interestingly, a survey done in the United States including 42 centres of Neurocritical Care Society members working in neurocritical care ICUs reported that the BPS and CPOT are utilized less than 40% of the time.[35] The Nociception Scale (NCS) is the only scale that has been validated to assess nociceptive pain in a minimally conscious or vegetative state or for patients with severe head trauma.[36,37]

Historically, vital signs such as increased heart rate, blood pressure, and respiratory rate have been utilized as indicators of pain. It is undeniable that vital sign changes may occur when pain is evoked or when other stressors may occur; however, attention is necessary to avoid the use of vital signs as a sole indicator for pain assessment. Vital sign parameters have shown inconsistencies in procedures or exposures that may or may not be pain provoking. The patients' self-report of pain has also been noted to be discrepant with vital sign increases.[31,38] Overall, pain assessments have been associated with improved outcomes, specifically related to ventilator weaning and should be performed routinely in all critically ill patients. Of note, the use of neuromuscular blocking agents obviates any type of pain assessment. Essentially, vital signs may be used an indicator to prompt performance of an assessment when a patient is unable to self-report.

Management

The overall goals for all critically ill patients as it relates to analgesia and sedation have changed to devote more focus to early mobilization, necessitating improvements in pain control with the utilization of minimal sedation. Consequently, initiation of analgesia is a baseline management strategy often employed prior to sedative therapy and is recommended by recent guidelines not only for the control of pain itself but also for anxiety and agitation as a result of pain in the ICU. Recent guidelines have contributed to the current practice management in neurocritically ill adults; however, specific recommendations for this population are lacking. Nevertheless, prior to the management of all patients, causes of pain should be appropriately evaluated and treated. Attention should be given to appropriate selection of both non-pharmacologic and pharmacologic therapies.

Non-pharmacological and adjuvant neurocritical care interventions for managing pain include but are not limited to the following measures:[3,27]

- Ensuring that the patient is properly positioned for comfort and their respective injury
- Minimizing irritating physical stimulants (disposition of ventilator tubing, loosening of tight bandages)
- Application of heat or cold packs and eye covers
- Massages and physiotherapy
- Optimal nursing care and moral support

Optimal analgesia for a neurologically injured patient would be an agent with quick onset, short duration of action, and minimal sedating properties. Selection of the ideal analgesic agent is multifactorial and often dependent upon medication availability, the dosage form required for the patient, disease state inducing pain, pain severity, medication metabolism, adverse effect profile, and physiological effects on cerebral haemodynamics. To date, there is no literature encompassing the effectiveness of various analgesics and references to guide a particular therapy in the neurologically critically ill patient.

Pharmacological agents commonly used for analgesia in neurocritical care patients are opioids, acetaminophen, nonsteroidal anti-inflammatory drugs (NSAIDs), anti-epileptics, tricyclic antidepressants, and alpha$_2$ adrenergic agents. Steroids are frequently used in many neurocritical care paradigms responsible for vasogenic oedema including metastatic neoplasms, and inflammatory processes (e.g., meningitis, cerebral abscess, encephalitis) that may be advantageous in reducing pain. Short courses of steroids have also been used in the management of headache associated with subarachnoid hemorrhage. Medications that may be useful for acute treatment of central pain include neuropathic agents (e.g., amitriptyline, gabapentin), propofol, and lidocaine. Table 14.8 lists pharmacological analgesic agents utilized for pain management.

According to the 2013 PAD guidelines for critically ill patients, intravenous (IV) opioid analgesics should be considered as the first line for non-neuropathic related pain with the addition of non-opioid agents (such as IV, oral, or rectal acetaminophen[39–42] or IV ketamine[43,44]) being utilized adjunctively when safely appropriate for the following reasons: (1) to minimize the IV opioid requirement or potentially eliminate its need, and (2) to reduce the incidence and severity of adverse effects associated with opioids.[3]

Despite the use of acetaminophen and NSAID for pain control, we neither have prospective or outcomes data for their analgesic effects within the ICU. A recent retrospective study comparing oral versus IV acetaminophen in patients with neurological illnesses identified pain relief at 30 minutes post dose with the IV formulation; however, there was no difference in pain relief at 3 hours when compared to oral therapy.[45] For neuropathic contributions to pain, gabapentin and carbamazepine are the first line agents for management. Evidence supports that these agents are superior to the sole use of an opioid analgesic for this spectrum of pain.[46,47]

TYPES OF PHARMACOLOGICAL AGENTS

Opioid Analgesics

Opioids interact with a variety of receptors and the analgesic effects being primarily mediated by effects on μ- and κ-receptors, the latter of which is responsible for the sedative properties of the medications. Fentanyl, hydromorphone, and morphine are the most commonly used agents within the ICU setting. Fentanyl is a highly lipid soluble analgesic that maintains popularity in the critical care setting secondary to its ability to be administered IV as well as its lack of histamine release related properties which makes it most suitable for haemodynamically unstable patients.[48] Additionally, its high first pass metabolism to inactive metabolites permits use in patients with hepatic or renal insufficiency. Fentanyl also lacks major vasodilatory properties in contrast to morphine that undergoes glucuronidation to produce an active metabolite (3- and 6-glucuronide morphine) which accumulates in patients with renal insufficiency. The metabolite is assumed to possess 2–8 times potency greater than the parent compound[3,27,49–52] Remifentanil is a selective μ-agonist primarily utilized for anaesthesia induction and maintenance (versus postoperative or long-term analgesia) owing to its ultra-rapid onset and extremely short half-life that is independent of infusion duration. Remifentanil also possesses a unique blood and tissue metabolism by nonspecific plasma esterases, eliminating the concern for use in patients with both renal and hepatic disease.[53]

Adverse effects of opioid analgesics include tolerance, intestinal dysmotility, central nervous system depressant effects resulting in respiratory depression, and hypotension. Haemodynamic instability is more common in those who are volume depleted. There is no tolerance associated with gastrointestinal side effects and all critically ill patients should receive some form of routine stimulant laxatives to minimize or prevent constipation or gastric ileus.

Non-Opioid Analgesics

Anticonvulsants

Anticonvulsants, including carbamazepine have demonstrated efficacy in the treatment of many syndromes associated with neuropathic pain including diabetic neuropathy, multiple sclerosis, neuralgias, and Guillain-Barre syndrome. Although the precise mechanisms of action remains poorly understood, gabapentin decreases sensitivity in the neurons of the dorsal horn located in the brain and spinal cord. While offering anti-inflammatory and analgesic benefits, both carbamazepine and gabapentin can reduce analgesic consumption but should not be used for acute management of pain.[47,54] The major side effects include ataxia, dizziness, drowsiness, nausea, and vomiting.

Acetaminophen

Acetaminophen is attractive as a mild analgesic and for adjunctive therapy with opioids. Acetaminophen is thought to reduce opioid requirements by approximately 20–30%. It remains an attractive adjunct analgesic due to its favourable adverse effect profile compared to opioids (i.e., gastrointestinal bleeding, renal failure).[55] Hepatotoxicity is a serious dose-related adverse effect with the incidence being higher in those receiving exceedingly high doses, particularly greater than 4 g/day. The IV formulation rapidly penetrates the CSF which likely makes it responsible for its relatively quick onset (15 versus

Table 14.8 Analgesics used in the neurointensive care unit

Class/Drug	Sedation/ Analgesia	MOA	Adverse events	Pearls
Opioid				
Morphine	+/+++	Mu receptor agonist	Respiratory depression, gastric dysmotility, and hallucinations, histamine release can precipitate itching and hypotension	Active metabolites, morphine-3 and 6-glucoronide, accumulate in renal failure Accumulation and prolonged sedation in obese patients Metabolism occurs through CYP450 isoenzyme 3A4
Hydromorphone	+/+++	Mu receptor agonist	Respiratory depression, gastric dysmotility, nausea, hypotension	7 to 11 times more potent than morphine Longer duration than morphine
Fentanyl	+/+++	Mu receptor agonist	Respiratory depression, muscle rigidity (high doses), gastric dysmotility, hypotension	Rapid onset Preferred for haemodynamically unstable Some degree of accumulation with prolonged infusions
Remifentanil	+/+++	Mu receptor agonist	Nausea, respiratory depression, Muscle rigidity (high doses), gastric dysmotility, hypotension, bradycardia	Rapid onset Postoperative analgesia should be provided prior to discontinuation in the postoperative setting due to rapid clearance Metabolism through plasma esterase can result in renal or hepatic insufficiency Dose reduction necessary in obese patient (dose on IBW)
Non-opioids				
Acetaminophen	0/++	Inhibit synthesis of prostaglandins in CNS and peripherally block pain impulse generation	Liver failure	Available PO and IV Undergoes glucuronidation, sulphonation, and oxidation via cytochrome P450 (CYP2E1) enzyme Should not exceed >4 grams per day due to increased risk of hepatic injury
Ibuprofen	0/++	Reversibly inhibits cyclooxygenase-1 and 2 enzymes (COX1 and COX2)	Fluid retention, GI bleeding, renal failure	Available PO and IV
Ketorolac	0/+++	Reversibly inhibits cyclooxygenase-1 and 2 enzymes (COX1 and COX2)	Gastrointestinal bleeding, renal failure, fluid retention	Available intravenously Use not recommended beyond 5 days due to increased risk of gastrointestinal bleeding

Alpha₂ Agonist				
Clonidine	+/+	Alpha₂ receptor agonist (pre- and post-synaptic)	Dry mouth, bradycardia, hypotension, rebound hypotension	α_2:α_1 activity 220:1 Has sedative and mild pain relieving properties
Dexmedetomidine	++/++	Alpha₂ receptor agonist (pre- and post-synaptic)	Dry mouth, bradycardia, hypotension, adrenal suppression, atrial fibrillation, rebound hypotension with prolonged administration	Greater specificity for alpha₂ receptor (α_2:α_1 activity 1620:1) Reduce dose in hepatic insufficiency (~50%) Has analgesic properties that are opioid sparing, but not routinely used alone as an analgesic Hypotension and bradycardia are common IV loading doses can cause haemodynamic instability Has sedative and mild pain relieving properties
Other				
Gabapentin	+/++	Bind to the α2δ subunit on the calcium channel	Somnolence, dizziness, nausea and visual disturbances	Beneficial for neuropathic pain Requires renal adjustment
Ketamine	+++/++	Antagonism of NMDA receptors, Mu, kappa, and delta receptor agonist	Emergence delirium Psychotropic effects Tachycardia hypersalivation	Highly lipophilic Preserves airway reflexes In usual doses, lacks cardiac depressant effects Higher incidences of HTN and tachycardia with larger doses given over <60 s Hypotension in catecholamine-depleted patients
Lidocaine	0/+++	Blocks sodium channels, G-protein coupled receptors, and NMDA receptors	Mild: numbness and tingling in fingers, toes, and around the mouth; metallic taste; tinnitus Severe: seizures, psychosis, cardiovascular collapse	Has anti-inflammatory properties Contraindicated in first and second degree heart conduction blocks; potential cardiovascular instability with clonidine and beta-blockers Mild side effects occur as an early warning of lidocaine toxicity. Avoid serum levels >5 mcg/ml

Abbreviations: CNS: central nervous system; COX: cyclooxygenase; IBW: ideal body weight; IV: intravenous; MOA: mechanism of action; NMDA: N-methyl-d-aspartate; PO: oral.

Sources: (1) Mirski MA, Hemstreet MK. Critical care sedation for neuroscience patients. *J Neurol Sci* 2007; 261(1–2):16–34. (2) Ehieli E, Yalamuri S, Brudney CS, Pyati S. Analgesia in the surgical intensive care unit. *Postgrad Med J* 2016. (3) O'Neil CK, Hanlon JT, Marcum ZA. Adverse effects of analgesics commonly used by older adults with osteoarthritis: focus on non-opioid and opioid analgesics. *Am J Geriatr Pharmacother* 2012;10(6):331–42.

45 minutes) compared to oral or rectal formulations. This characteristic also makes it attractive for postoperative pain management.[56,57]

NSAIDs

Nonsteroidal anti-inflammatory medications and cyclooxygenase (COX) inhibitors provide anti-inflammatory effects and may be used adjunctively in pain management in selected neurocritical care patients. Unfortunately, general use is limited by the oral route of administration in addition to adverse effects such as increased risk of bleeding secondary to platelet inhibition and potential risk for renal insufficiency. These agents should also be avoided specifically in intracranial pathologies involving alterations in blood haemostasis (e.g. subarachnoid haemorrhage, intracerebral haemorrhage) and for patients who may be candidates for elective decompressive craniotomies.

Alpha₂ Agonist

Dexmedetomidine and clonidine possess multidimensional analgesic activity through a variety of mechanisms interacting through noradrenergic pathways in addition to peripheral, supraspinal, and spinal cord activity.[58] Dexmedetomidine is approved by the FDA for adult sedation via continuous infusion and should not be used as a primary analgesic agent.[59] Clonidine is used for allodynia, a common central mediated type of pain associated with syndromes such as paroxysmal sympathetic activity.[60]

Ketamine and Lidocaine

Unlike opioids, ketamine lacks respiratory depressant effects at analgesic doses but can increase both heart rate and blood pressure. Ketamine is generally administered as a bolus dose when prescribed for pain and may be preferred in the setting of haemodynamic instability when pain management is required. Emergence reactions are a common adverse effect. Lidocaine has both analgesic and anti-inflammatory properties. Like ketamine, it has been shown to significantly reduce pain intensity and opioid consumption after surgery. [61] It can be administered as a transdermal patch applied to the affected regions and is useful for neuropathic pain. Avoid high doses of lidocaine due to risk of toxic central nervous system side effects that include respiratory depression, seizures, and psychiatric symptoms.[62]

CONCLUSIONS

The sedative and analgesic agents available for use in neurocritically ill patients have unique pharmacokinetic, pharmacodynamic, and adverse effect profiles. The need for frequent neurologic assessments precludes the use of long-acting agents for routine ICU analgosedation in this patient population. Pain should always be treated first prior to treating agitation. When pain management or sedation is necessary, shorter acting agents are generally preferred except in circumstances where deep sedation may be required such as in the setting of ICP management. A working knowledge of sedatives and analgesics and their unique characteristics is imperative for customizing a safe and effective analgosedative regimen for each patient that is also cost-effective. In addition to implementing daily sedation interruptions and/or weaning protocols, close sedative and analgesic monitoring for adverse drug effects, depth of sedation, and patient comfort should be the routine practice in neurocritical care units.

REFERENCES

1. Seder DB, Jagoda A, Riggs B. Emergency neurological life support: airway, ventilation, and sedation. *Neurocrit Care* 2015; 23(2):S5–22.
2. Olson DM, Thoyre SM, Peterson ED, Graffagnino C. A randomized evaluation of bispectral index-augmented sedation assessment in neurological patients. *Neurocrit Care* 2009;11(1):20–27.
3. Devlin JW, Skrobik Y, Gélinas C, et al. Clinical practice guidelines for the prevention and management of pain, agitation/sedation, delirium, immobility, and sleep disruption in adult patients in the ICU. *Crit Care Med* 2018;46(9):e825–e873.
4. Yu A, Teitelbaum J, Scott J, et al. Evaluating pain, sedation, and delirium in the neurologically critically ill-feasibility and reliability of standardized tools: a multi-institutional study. *Crit Care Med* 2013;41(8):2002–7.
5. Deogaonkar A, Gupta R, DeGeorgia M, et al. Bispectral index monitoring correlates with sedation scales in brain-injured patients. *Crit Care Med* 2004;32(12):2403–6.
6. Bard JW. The BIS monitor: a review and technology assessment. *AANA J* 2001;69(6):477–83.
7. Sengupta S, Ghosh S, Rudra A, Kumar P, Maitra G, Das T. Effect of ketamine on bispectral index during propofol-fentanyl anesthesia: a randomized controlled study. *Middle East J Anaesthesiol* 2011;21(3):391–5.
8. Brophy GM, Human T, Shutter L. Emergency neurological life support: pharmacotherapy. *Neurocrit Care* 2015;23(2):S48–68.
9. Jakob SM, Ruokonen E, Grounds RM, et al. Dexmedetomidine vs midazolam or propofol for sedation during prolonged mechanical ventilation: two randomized controlled trials. *JAMA* 2012;307(11):1151–60.
10. Mijzen EJ, Jacobs B, Aslan A, Rodgers MG. Propofol infusion syndrome heralded by ECG changes. *Neurocrit Care* 2012;17(2):260–4.

11. Bratton SL, Chestnut RM, Ghajar J, et al. Guidelines for the management of severe traumatic brain injury. XI. Anesthetics, analgesics, and sedatives. *J Neurotrauma* 2007;24(1):S71–6.

12. Erdman MJ, Doepker BA, Gerlach AT, Phillips GS, Elijovich L, Jones GM. A comparison of severe hemodynamic disturbances between dexmedetomidine and propofol for sedation in neurocritical care patients. *Crit Care Med* 2014;42(7):1696–702.

13. Jones GM, Doepker BA, Erdman MJ, Kimmons LA, Elijovich L. Predictors of severe hypotension in neurocritical care patients sedated with propofol. *Neurocrit Care* 2014;20(2):270–6.

14. Tran A, Blinder H, Hutton B, English S. Alpha-2 agonists for sedation in mechanically ventilated neurocritical care patients: a systematic review protocol. *Syst Rev* 2016;5(1):154.

15. Grof TM, Bledsoe KA. Evaluating the use of dexmedetomidine in neurocritical care patients. *Neurocrit Care* 2010;12(3):356–61.

16. Erstad BL, Patanwala AE. Ketamine for analgosedation in critically ill patients. *J Crit Care* 2016;35:145–9.

17. Green SM, Li J. Ketamine in adults: what emergency physicians need to know about patient selection and emergence reactions. *Acad Emerg Med* 2000;7(3):278–81.

18. Lippmann M, Appel PL, Mok MS, Shoemaker WC. Sequential cardiorespiratory patterns of anesthetic induction with ketamine in critically ill patients. *Crit Care Med* 1983;11(9):730–4.

19. Chanques G, Sebbane M, Barbotte E, Viel E, Eledjam JJ, Jaber S. A prospective study of pain at rest: incidence and characteristics of an unrecognized symptom in surgical and trauma versus medical intensive care unit patients. *Anesthesiology* 2007;107(5):858–60.

20. Erstad BL, Puntillo K, Gilbert HC, et al. Pain management principles in the critically ill. *Chest* 2009;135(4):1075–86.

21. Gottschalk A. Craniotomy pain: trying to do better. *Anesth Analg* 2009;109(5):1379–81.

22. Flexman AM, Ng JL, Gelb AW. Acute and chronic pain following craniotomy. *Curr Opin Anaesthesiol* 2010;23(5):551–7.

23. Mordhorst C, Latz B, Kerz T, et al. Prospective assessment of postoperative pain after craniotomy. *J Neurosurg Anesthesiol* 2010; 22(3):202–6.

24. Thibault M, Girard F, Moumdjian R, Chouinard P, Boudreault D, Ruel M. Craniotomy site influences postoperative pain following neurosurgical procedures: a retrospective study. *Can J Anaesth* 2007;54(7):544–8.

25. Zeiler FA, AlSubaie F, Zeiler K, Bernard F, Skrobik Y. Analgesia in neurocritical care: an international survey and practice audit. *Crit Care Med* 2016;44(5):973–80.

26. Shannon K, Bucknall T. Pain assessment in critical care: what have we learnt from research. *Intensive Crit Care Nurs* 2003;19(3):154–62.

27. Jacobi J, Fraser GL, Coursin DB, et al. Clinical practice guidelines for the sustained use of sedatives and analgesics in the critically ill adult. *Crit Care Med* 2002;30(1):119–41.

28. Puntillo KA, White C, Morris AB, Perdue ST, Stanik-Hutt J, Thompson CL, et al. Patients' perceptions and responses to procedural pain: results from Thunder Project II. *Am J Crit Care* 2001;10(4):238–51.

29. Foix C, Chavany J, Levy M. Syndrome pseudo-thalamique d'origine pariétale. Lesio de l'artère du sillon interparietale. *CR Soc Neurol* 1927;35:68–78.

30. Loeser JD, Treede RD. The Kyoto protocol of IASP basic pain terminology. *Pain* 2008;137(3):473–7.

31. Payen JF, Bru O, Bosson JL, et al. Assessing pain in critically ill sedated patients by using a behavioral pain scale. *Crit Care Med* 2001;29(12):2258–63.

32. Gélinas C, Fillion L, Puntillo KA, Viens C, Fortier M. Validation of the critical-care pain observation tool in adult patients. *Am J Crit Care* 2006;15(4):420–7.

33. Gélinas C, Klein K, Naidech AM, Skrobik Y. Pain, sedation, and delirium management in the neurocritically ill: lessons learned from recent research. *Semin Respir Crit Care Med* 2013;34(2):236–43.

34. Gélinas C, Arbour C. Behavioral and physiologic indicators during a nociceptive procedure in conscious and unconscious mechanically ventilated adults: similar or different? *J Crit Care* 2009;24(4):628.e617–27.

35. Yu A, Teitelbaum J, Skrobik Y. Evaluating pain, sedation, and delirium in the neurologically critically ill. 64th Annual Meeting of the American Academy of Neurology (AAN). New Orleans, LA 2012.

36. Schnakers C, Chatelle C, Vanhaudenhuyse A, et al. The Nociception Coma Scale: a new tool to assess nociception in disorders of consciousness. *Pain* 2010;148(2):215–19.

37. Boly M, Faymonville ME, Schnakers C, et al. Perception of pain in the minimally conscious state with PET activation: an observational study. *Lancet Neurol* 2008;7(11):1013–20.

38. Siffleet J, Young J, Nikoletti S, Shaw T. Patients' self-report of procedural pain in the intensive care unit. *J Clin Nurs* 2007;16(11):2142–8.

39. Pettersson PH, Jakobsson J, Owall A. Intravenous acetaminophen reduced the use of opioids compared with oral administration after coronary artery bypass grafting. *J Cardiothorac Vasc Anesth* 2005;19(3):306–9.

40. Candiotti KA, Bergese SD, Viscusi ER, Singla SK, Royal MA, Singla NK. Safety of multiple-dose intravenous acetaminophen in adult inpatients. *Pain Med* 2010;11(12):1841–8.

41. Rapanos T, Murphy P, Szalai JP, Burlacoff L, Lam-McCulloch J, Kay J. Rectal indomethacin reduces postoperative pain and morphine use after cardiac surgery. *Can J Anaesth* 1999;46(8):725–30.

42. Hynninen MS, Cheng DC, Hossain I, et al. Non-steroidal anti-inflammatory drugs in treatment of postoperative pain after cardiac surgery. *Can J Anaesth* 2000;47(12):1182–7.

43. Schmittner MD, Vajkoczy SL, Horn P, et al. Effects of fentanyl and S(+)-ketamine on cerebral hemodynamics, gastrointestinal motility, and need of vasopressors in patients with intracranial pathologies: a pilot study. *J Neurosurg Anesthesiol* 2007;19(4):257–62.

44. Guillou N, Tanguy M, Seguin P, Branger B, Campion JP, Mallédant Y. The effects of small-dose ketamine on morphine consumption in surgical intensive care unit patients after major abdominal surgery. *Anesth Analg* 2003;97(3):843–7.

45. Nichols DC, Nadpara PA, Taylor PD, Brophy GM. Intravenous versus oral acetaminophen for pain control in neurocritical care patients. *Neurocrit Care* 2016;25(3): 400–6.

46. Pandey CK, Bose N, Garg G, et al. Gabapentin for the treatment of pain in guillain-barré syndrome: a double-blinded, placebo-controlled, crossover study. *Anesth Analg* 2002;95(6):1719–23, table of contents.

47. Pandey CK, Raza M, Tripathi M, Navkar DV, Kumar A, Singh UK. The comparative evaluation of gabapentin and carbamazepine for pain management in Guillain-Barré syndrome patients in the intensive care unit. *Anesth Analg* 2005;101(1):220–5.

48. Shapiro BA, Warren J, Egol AB, et al. Practice parameters for intravenous analgesia and sedation for adult patients in the intensive care unit: an executive summary. Society of Critical Care Medicine. *Crit Care Med* 1995;23(9): 1596–600.

49. Lötsch J, Geisslinger G. Morphine-6-glucuronide: an analgesic of the future? *Clin Pharmacokinet* 2001;40(7): 485–99.

50. Buetler TM, Wilder-Smith OH, Wilder-Smith CH, Aebi S, Cerny T, Brenneisen R. Analgesic action of i.v. morphine-6-glucuronide in healthy volunteers. *Br J Anaesth* 2000;84(1):97–9.

51. Mazoit JX, Butscher K, Samii K. Morphine in postoperative patients: pharmacokinetics and pharmacodynamics of metabolites. *Anesth Analg* 2007;105(1):70–8.

52. Wagner BK, O'Hara DA. Pharmacokinetics and pharmacodynamics of sedatives and analgesics in the treatment of agitated critically ill patients. *Clin Pharmacokinet* 1997;33(6):426–53.

53. Muellejans B, López A, Cross MH, Bonome C, Morrison L, Kirkham AJ. Remifentanil versus fentanyl for analgesia based sedation to provide patient comfort in the intensive care unit: a randomized, double-blind controlled trial [ISRCTN43755713]. *Crit Care* 2004;8(1): R1–R11.

54. Egerod I, Jensen MB, Herling SF, Welling KL. Effect of an analgo-sedation protocol for neurointensive patients: a two-phase interventional non-randomized pilot study. *Crit Care* 2010;14(2):R71.

55. McNicol ED, Tzortzopoulou A, Cepeda MS, Francia MB, Farhat T, Schumann R. Single-dose intravenous paracetamol or propacetamol for prevention or treatment of postoperative pain: a systematic review and meta-analysis. *Br J Anaesth* 2011;106(6): 764–75.

56. Bertolini A, Ferrari A, Ottani A, Guerzoni S, Tacchi R, Leone S. Paracetamol: new vistas of an old drug. *CNS Drug Rev* 2006;12(3-4):250–75.

57. Jahr JS, Lee VK. Intravenous acetaminophen. *Anesthesiol Clin* 2010;28(4):619–45.

58. Ehieli E, Yalamuri S, Brudney CS, Pyati S. Analgesia in the surgical intensive care unit. *Postgrad Med J* 2017;93(1095):38–45.

59. Szumita PM, Baroletti SA, Anger KE, Wechsler ME. Sedation and analgesia in the intensive care unit: evaluating the role of dexmedetomidine. *Am J Health Syst Pharm* 2007;64(1):37–44.

60. Rabinstein AA, Benarroch EE. Treatment of paroxysmal sympathetic hyperactivity. *Curr Treat Options Neurol* 2008;10(2):151–7.

61. McCarthy GC, Megalla SA, Habib AS. Impact of intravenous lidocaine infusion on postoperative analgesia and recovery from surgery: a systematic review of randomized controlled trials. *Drugs* 2010;70(9):1149–63.

62. Collinsworth KA, Kalman SM, Harrison DC. The clinical pharmacology of lidocaine as an antiarrhythmic drug. *Circulation* 1974;50(6):1217–30.

15

Osmotherapy Agents

C. C. May, K. S. Smetana, and A. M. Cook

ABSTRACT

Osmotherapy agents (mannitol and hypertonic saline [HTS]) are typically first line pharmacotherapy options for patients with elevated intracranial pressure (ICP). These agents are ideally used as rapid bolus infusions in order to maximize the change in serum osmolarity, modulation of cerebral blood volume (CBV), and improvement in blood rheology. Various administration considerations are important for the bedside clinician when infusing mannitol and HTS including the risk of phlebitis, electrolyte and intravascular volume fluctuations, and changes in renal function. Clinical trials and meta-analyses show little difference in neurological outcomes between mannitol and HTS, though HTS may be more effective at reducing ICP.

KEYWORDS

Mannitol; sodium chloride; intracranial pressure (ICP); osmolarity; hypertonic; rheology; traumatic brain injury (TBI); neurocritical care.

INTRODUCTION

Elevations in intracranial pressure (ICP) in patients with traumatic brain injury (TBI), stroke, meningitis, brain tumour, or other central nervous system (CNS) pathologies are associated with poor outcomes. The pathogenesis of elevated ICP varies depending on the initial insult, but typically occurs due to a combination of hyperaemia, cytotoxic cellular swelling, extravasation of fluid into the CNS interstitial space, and vasogenic oedema.[1] Non-pharmacologic measures such as elevation of the head of the bed or acute hyperventilation may mitigate elevations in ICP but do not have a sustained and consistent effect. The use of hyperosmolar solutions (termed osmotherapy) to modulate CNS/brain water and dynamics of CNS blood flow has long been a primary pharmacological strategy to reduce ICP, dating back to the 1930s with the use of urea. The beneficial effects of osmotherapy agents on ICP, cerebral blood flow (CBF), and blood viscosity are widely accepted as a result of many mechanistic studies performed in humans and animal models.[2–4] Mannitol and HTS solutions are the mainstay for osmotherapy in contemporary practice. Each agent has subtle differences and advantages for use.

PHYSIOCHEMICAL PROPERTIES

The physiochemical properties of mannitol and HTS are summarized in Table 15.1. Both of them are small molecules that distribute primarily in the intravascular blood volume and minimally in the intracellular space. The kidneys are the primary means of maintaining sodium homeostasis through active and passive reabsorption of sodium and chloride ions within the nephrons. In contrast, mannitol is typically removed in the kidney via glomerular filtration and minimal reabsorption occurs. This is the basis for the osmotic diuretic effect of mannitol.

Mannitol 20% solution for injection is the most commonly used formulation of mannitol for treatment of elevated ICP. This concentration is the best balance between high osmolarity and solubility at room temperature. When mannitol is exposed to low ambient temperatures, the solution may crystallize and should not be infused. If crystals are present when administering mannitol packaged in a vial, the vial may be gently warmed to re-dissolve the crystals, either in a warm water bath or with gentle manual rolling. Alternatively, when utilizing mannitol bags, if crystals are present, the solution

Table 15.1 Summary of characteristics of various osmotherapy agents

	Mannitol 20%	**3% Sodium chloride**	**7.5% Sodium chloride**	**23.4% Sodium chloride**	**8.4% Sodium bicarbonate**
Molecular weight (kDa)	182	58.44	58.44	58.44	84
pH	4.5–7	4.5–7	4.5–7	4.5–7	7–8.5
Elimination	Glomerular filtration limited reabsorption	Renal/sodium transporters and glomerular filtration	Renal/sodium transporters and glomerular filtration	Renal/sodium transporters and glomerular filtration	Renal/sodium transporters and glomerular filtration
Osmolality (mOsm/L)	1,098	1,027	2,566	8,008	2,002
Dose*	0.25–1.6 gm/kg	1.25–5 ml/kg	0.5–2ml/kg	20–30 ml	0.5–2 ml/kg
Equi-osmolar dose	0.5 gm/kg	2.5 ml/kg	1 ml/kg	0.3 ml/kg (or 30 ml)	1 ml/kg
Infusion site	Central preferred	Central preferred	Central preferred IO also studied (maximum 500 ml)	Central	Central preferred
Administration considerations	Use 0.22 micron in-line filter	Medication safety measures due to concentrated electrolyte	Medication safety measures due to concentrated electrolyte	Medication safety measures due to concentrated electrolyte	Compatibility limitations
Adverse effects	Phlebitis Hypovolemia Rebound/ withdrawal	Phlebitis Hyperchloremic acidosis Hypernatremia Hypervolemia	Phlebitis Hyperchloremic acidosis Hypernatremia Hypervolemia	Phlebitis Hyperchloremic acidosis Hypernatremia Hypervolemia	Phlebitis Metabolic alkalosis Hypernatremia Hypervolemia

*Infusion rate should be over 5–20 minutes.

should be heated using a dry-heat cabinet with overwrap intact. Due to the potential for crystallization, infusion of mannitol at 20% or greater should include a 0.22 micron in-line filter.

'Normal saline' (0.9% NaCl) is a commonly used replacement fluid in intensive care units (ICU) which contains 9 g/L of sodium or 154 mEq/L of both sodium and chloride ions. Although 'normal saline' is a misnomer, given its supraphysiological composition of NaCl, any solution which contains a concentration higher than 0.9% is considered a HTS solution.[5–7] Commonly used preparations include 3%, 5%, 7.5%, 14.6%, and 23.4% (Table 15.1). Hypertonic saline solutions exhibit excellent solubility and no risk of crystallization at room temperature, so similar precautions with infusion administration are not necessary.

MECHANISM OF ACTION

The primary advantage of utilizing osmotherapy agents is their rapid onset of action. Barry and colleagues described increased plasma volume expansion within minutes after administration of 20% mannitol[8] (Figure 15.1). Increased plasma volume has been linked to enhancing cardiac output (CO) and mean arterial pressure (MAP) after mannitol infusion.[2,9] Additionally, there is an immediate decrease in haematocrit and increase in red blood cell deformability leading to an overall reduction in viscosity; this subsequently improves CBF through cerebral microvasculature.[3,10] With intact autoregulation, the lower viscosity, enhanced CBF, and cerebral oxygen delivery leads to vasoconstriction, thus keeping CBF constant but decreasing cerebral blood volume with a resulting decrease in ICP.[11,12] This mechanism is thought to be the more immediate of the two, reducing ICP within 5 minutes and the effect is thought to last about 2 hours.[3,4] Similar data supports this mechanism of action with HTS. One study demonstrated that when 7.5% sodium chloride is administered over two minutes, the observed sodium concentration peaks at 152 mEq/L, suggesting that the extravascular compartment expands promptly through intracellular loss of water.[13] If cerebral autoregulation is intact, venoconstriction occurs due to acute plasma expansion resulting in reduced venous blood acutely reducing ICP. This compensatory mechanism wanes over 20–30 minutes allowing time for the osmolar gradient to form and sustain ICP control. The redistribution of water to increase plasma volume occurs in a stepwise fashion; first from red blood cells (RBCs) and endothelium followed by the interstitium and tissue cells.[14] This results in three important physiological alterations which may result in improved CBF due to reduced vascular resistance: reduced RBC diameter, increased endothelial lumen size, and haemodilution. Additionally, HTS acts as an arteriolar vasodilator due to the direct relaxant effect on smooth muscle counteracting vasospasm and increasing CBF.[13,15,16]

The osmotic effect of mannitol appears to begin within 15 minutes and peak effects are seen between 30 and 120 minutes.[7,17,18] The duration of the osmotic effect has been documented to last for 1 to 6 hours and is variable based on the clinical condition and renal elimination of mannitol.[17,19] Wisner et al. assessed brain water content after induction of haemorrhagic shock in mechanically brain injured rats, comparing 6.5% HTS to lactated Ringer's (LR). Hypertonic saline was found to reduce the brain water content in the uninjured hemisphere with no effect on the injured area.[20] Once the osmotic gradient is established, water moves across the blood–brain barrier (BBB) into the vascular compartment and ICP decreases by reducing brain water content causing reduction in perilesional oedema.[11,21,22] The transport of solutes across the BBB is a selective process which is dependent upon the osmotic reflection coefficient (RQ). Neither mannitol nor sodium chloride freely diffuses across an intact BBB, allowing for a gradient to be established between the plasma and brain. The RQ for mannitol is 0.9, which can potentially lead to rebound cerebral oedema, sodium chloride has a RQ of 1 indicating almost complete exclusion from an intact BBB.[23–25] Therefore, the potential for mannitol to diffuse or be taken up into the brain is slightly higher than HTS in situations where the BBB is not intact.

In addition to haemodynamic and cerebrovascular alterations, HTS may aid in attenuation of secondary injury through direct and indirect mechanisms. Hypertonic saline has been shown to alter the inflammatory cascade seen after brain injury through reduced leukocyte migration and adherence to brain cells.[26] Hypertonic saline also aids in the restoration of normal cell polarity through correction of electrolyte imbalances resulting in an intracellular shift of cerebral osmolytes (amino acids such as glutamate, polyhydric alcohols, and methyl amines), which can propagate secondary injury.[15,27] Lastly, HTS may have inherent antioxidant properties further mitigating the inflammatory process.

The use of HTS resulted in significant reductions in both reactive oxygen species and nitric oxide compared to mannitol.[28]

INDICATION AND INITIATION OF TREATMENT

Although osmotherapy is commonly used 'when ICP is elevated', there are specific recommendations and instances where use of osmotherapy is optimal. Ideally, osmotherapy agents are administered when the patient has elevated ICP (or clinical signs and symptoms), rather than prophylactically. The response to osmotherapy may be influenced by the cumulative dose, as experience with mannitol suggests that larger doses are required with prolonged use.[29] These points suggest that prophylactic administration of mannitol or administration outside of acute elevations in ICP may reduce the response expected during future ICP control.

Mannitol has been the mainstay in therapy to reduce acute ICP elevations associated with TBI. Interestingly, the specific recommendation to use mannitol for intracranial hypertension after TBI was removed from the most recent TBI guidelines, though no suitable alternatives are posited.[30,31] Conventionally, an ICP >20 mmHg is the threshold for osmotherapy initiation, though the most recent recommendations suggest a threshold of >22 mmHg.[31] Osmotherapy appears to have greater response in patients with higher ICPs.[17,32] Patients who have no ICP monitoring, but are at high likelihood of having elevated ICP based on imaging and clinical examination are also likely to benefit from acute osmotherapy. Cruz and colleagues evaluated patients presenting with acute subdural haematoma (SDH) randomized to receive high dose (up to 1.4 g/kg) versus conventional dose (up to 0.7 g/kg) mannitol prior to surgical intervention.[33] Clinical outcomes and postoperative severe brain swelling after acute SDH treatment were significantly better for patients who were in the high-dose treatment group compared with the conventional dose group (p<0.01 and p<0.03, respectively). This study underscores the importance of prompt treatment of elevated ICP and the use of effective/aggressive doses as a temporizing measure.

Another common utilization of mannitol is in the operating room. Due to the tumour size, brain oedema, or increased ICP, brain relaxation is required prior to an intracranial operation. The practice of administering mannitol in the operating room contributes to decreased brain volume and ICP, and allows the neurosurgeon the best access to the operating site, while avoiding excessive pressure under the surgical retractors. Mannitol in intravenous bolus doses ranging from 0.25 to 1.5 g/kg

Table 15.2 Hypertonic saline (3% NaCl) protocol[a]

Serum sodium	<130 mEq	130–135 mEq	136–140 mEq	>140 mEq
3% HTS rate[b,c]	Increase by 20 ml/hr	Increase by 10 ml/hr	No change	Hold infusion, follow sliding scale with q6h serum sodium checks

[a] Initiate protocol with scheduled NaCl tabs 3 g PO/NGT every 6 hours, 3% HTS infusion at 20 ml/hr IV, and obtain serum sodium levels every 6 hours; [b] Max rate is 80 ml/hr;
[c] If on hold initiate a rate that correlates with serum sodium levels.
Adapted from: Woo C, Rao VA, Sheridan W, et al. Performance characteristics of a sliding-scale hypertonic saline infusion protocol for the treatment of acute neurologic hyponatremia. *Neurocrit Care* 11(2):228–34.

have been utilized.[34] Seo et al. completed a dose finding study in patients undergoing supratentorial brain tumour resection and found that brain relaxation increased as the dose of mannitol increased; however, imbalances in serum electrolytes increased with high-dose mannitol (1.5 g/kg) and the authors recommended no more than 1 g/kg of mannitol during an operation.[35]

Similar data exists for most indications of HTS at equi-osmolar doses to mannitol. Hypertonic saline lends the added advantage of preventing and treating cerebral oedema associated with hyponatremia, though data is conflicting on the overall benefit of maintaining mild hypernatremia to have sustained ICP lowering effects.[36,37] Continuous HTS infusions to maintain mild hypernatremia may reduce excursions of ICP elevations.[38] In addition, dosing algorithms of HTS have been used to maintain mild hypernatremia in the context of elevated ICP[39] (Table 15.2).

DOSING AND ADMINISTRATION

The overriding principle of osmotherapy agent dosing includes the use of high osmolar loads over a short period. Historically, mannitol was administered as a continuous infusion under the premise that continuous osmolar withdrawal of brain water may maximize the therapeutic effect. In fact, this tends to be a less efficient way to infuse mannitol and now the contemporary practice is to infuse mannitol (and HTS) as a rapid IV bolus. With a rapid infusion (<20 minutes), initial plasma expansion is maximized, which potentiates cerebral venoconstriction response. Numerous studies confirm the safety of rapid infusion, though hypotension may be more frequent as the infusion time decreases.[32,33,40] One report noted that clinically important hypotension was most likely to occur when larger osmotic loads were given over a short period of time (<5 minutes) leading to a reduction in peripheral vascular resistance.[41] To prevent hypotension, slower infusions of 10–20 minutes are recommended and have been shown to successfully reduce ICP.[33,40–42]

Patients who have compromised cardiac function or those who have met their capacity to increase cardiac output (CO) may be at especially high risk for hypotension with rapid infusion.

The use of moderate to high doses of osmotherapy creates an acute shift in osmolarity in the serum, potentiating a 'dehydration' response. When evaluating studies that report dose-response data, mannitol doses less than 0.5 g/kg appear to have reduced efficacy and duration of action.[17,32] Several studies demonstrate a more significant reduction in ICP and more durable response when using mannitol doses ranging from 0.5 g/kg to 2.5 g/kg.[17,32,33] However, higher initial doses may be necessary when the ICP is exceedingly high or when herniation is imminent.[29] Analogous osmolar loads have been studied with HTS, including sodium bicarbonate[43] (Table 15.1).

The site of infusion is one factor that may cause practitioners to select one agent over the other. The use of hyperosmolar solutions through peripheral veins has the potential to cause significant phlebitis (which begets the moniker for HTS, 'hot salt'). The osmolarity threshold for peripheral administration is controversial as most of the data available are focused on continuous infusion of hyperosmolar solutions, rather than intermittent bolus dosing. Traditionally, the optimal osmolarity of a peripheral infusion is <900 mOsm/L, though studies with peripheral parenteral nutrition suggest an osmolarity of up to 1,100 mOsm/L as tolerable.[44,45] The concern of phlebitis may not be solely due to the osmolarity of a solution. One study found that, compared to total volume and osmolarity, the osmolarity infusion rate (number of milliOsmoles infused per hour) correlated well with phlebitis rates (r=0.95). The phlebitis rate of the group which received 84 mOsm/hr was 4% at 48 hours and increased to 14% after 14 days.[46] This osmolarity infusion rate would be comparable to receiving 3% HTS at a rate of 80 ml/hr. Infusion rates of 3% HTS as high as 75 ml/hr are potentially safe via peripheral administration, but further studies are warranted to assess the safety of this infusion.[47] Ideally, mannitol and HTS solutions (≥3%) should be administered through a central line when possible, though clinicians should not hesitate to infuse these agents peripherally in emergent situations.

MONITORING THERAPY AND ADVERSE EFFECTS

Osmotherapy agents are associated with several adverse effects including nephrotoxicity (particularly mannitol), hypernatremia (HTS), electrolyte abnormalities (both), and a rebound/withdrawal effect (mannitol, Table 15.1). Screening for many of these potential problems is easily accomplished by routine laboratory monitoring.

Mannitol-induced acute renal failure (ARF) is a well-described adverse effect.[48–53] The incidence of mannitol-induced ARF in patients with tumour, ischaemic stroke, intracranial haemorrhage (ICH), subarachnoid haemorrhage (SAH), subdural haematoma, and TBI has been reported at rates ranging from 11.8%–76%, with varying definitions of ARF leading to a majority of the variability.[54,55] Although this adverse effect has been well-reported, the mechanism by which this occurs is not well understood. Potential mechanisms as to how mannitol causes ARF include histological alterations consisting of proximal and distal tubular cells vacuolization ('osmotic nephrosis'), increased sodium delivery to the macula densa which may trigger an intense tubuloglomerular feedback response reducing glomerular filtration and afferent arteriolar renal vasoconstriction.[49,50,56–58] Despite the variety of possible mechanisms, mannitol-induced ARF is usually transient and reversible with cessation of mannitol.[48–50,56] The predisposing factors for ARF include advanced age, history of hypertension, sepsis, hypovolemia, hypotension, concomitant nephrotoxic agents, or pre-existing renal disease.[42,52,54,55,59]

The use of serum osmolarity as a threshold for safety after mannitol administration has been advocated for many years. Some guidelines recommend reducing the dose or holding mannitol therapy when the serum osmolarity is greater than 310 to 320 mOsm/kg due to the potential risk of renal failure.[42,55,60] Other guidelines and reports offer no specific recommendations on how to monitor mannitol therapy as data to support this recommendation are scant.[30,31] In fact, serum osmolarity does not appear to correlate well with the development of renal failure based on studies of neurocritical care and TBI patients.[54]

The calculation of an osmole gap (OG) should be used as a surrogate for mannitol serum concentrations given that ARF appears to be aggravated if mannitol accumulates because of incomplete clearance.[61] Osmole gap is the difference between the measured serum osmolality (mOsml/kg) and the calculated serum

osmolarity (mOsm/L). An OG <20 mOsm/kg appears to be the most reliable indicator for mannitol clearance (and thus reduced risk of nephrotoxicity); however, various reports of mannitol-nephrotoxicity case series suggest that the risk of developing ARF is highest when OG exceeds 60–75 mOsm/kg and the occurrence of ARF with an OG <55 mOsm/kg is rare.[59,62–64] Clinicians have several equations available to estimate serum osmolarity, though formulas that do not require magnesium and calcium are preferred as they may be more cost-efficient, reducing the need for extra laboratory data.[61]

In addition to serum osmolarity, serum sodium is imperative to evaluate when treating patients with elevated ICP and using osmotherapy. One of the primary concerns with the use of HTS is the risk for osmotic demyelination syndrome (ODS) which can result from a rapid rise in serum sodium. Guideline recommendations for the treatment of hyponatremia suggest checking serum sodium concentrations every four hours with the infusion of 3% HTS or equivalent,[65] though this frequency may be excessive for patients with sodium concentrations within the normal range. Mannitol has variable effects on serum sodium concentrations. Hypernatremia can develop after inadequate volume resuscitation in the setting of free water loss caused by mannitol osmotic diuresis.[66,67] Conversely, acute hyponatremia may occur after mannitol administration. A reduction in serum sodium is seen immediately after mannitol infusion and begins to return to baseline about 180 minutes after drug administration.[35]

Other laboratory parameters that should be evaluated at least daily in patients receiving osmotherapy are serum chloride, potassium, and creatinine. Hyperchloremia is well-associated with metabolic acidosis, which is typically benign in the acute phases of illness. Balancing the chloride/bicarbonate concentrations in the serum may be more significant if ventilator weaning is possible to ensure balanced acid-base status. The use of mixed chloride/acetate solution is one method of reducing the amount of chloride given while still giving hypertonic doses of sodium (Table 15.3). Hyperchloremia has also been associated with renal dysfunction, although this has not been specifically described in the neurocritical care population after HTS use.[68] However, hypernatremia (Na >155 mEq/L) was found to be an independent risk factor for the development of acute kidney injury across various neurological injuries.[69] Mannitol also has variable effects on potassium. Intracellular potassium may passively move out of the cell in response to cellular dehydration leading to clinically relevant hyperkalaemia.[70] Conversely, mannitol may cause hypokalaemia resulting from osmotic diuresis.

Table 15.3 Examples of formulas for compounding balanced hypertonic sodium solutions

	2% NaCl/Acetate	3% NaCl/Acetate
Sodium chloride 4 mEq/ml	88 mEq (22 ml)	128 mEq (32 ml)
Sodium acetate 2 mEq/ml	60 mEq (30 ml)	92 mEq (46 ml)
Sterile water	448 ml	422 ml

Although debated, there is a theoretical risk of a phenomenon called rebound ICP associated with mannitol administration. The rebound phenomenon has been hypothesized to be due to interstitial and intracellular accumulation of mannitol in the brain, producing a reversed osmotic gradient between the blood and interstitial space in the brain causing water to be drawn back into the brain. Mannitol accumulation may occur in areas of disrupted BBB or in the setting of glioma and meningioma. This effect may be more significant after repeat doses and in oedematous white matter.[23–25] Therefore, the most likely mechanism of mannitol accumulation is the existence of a disrupted BBB surrounding injured or peri-tumoural brain tissue. The magnitude of rebound ICP and relative contributions of mannitol accumulation and increase in brain water remain unclear. However, the avoidance of long-term mannitol administration or utilizing CSF osmolarity measurements may prevent theoretical rebound effect. Clinicians should be wary of the potential for rebound effects of mannitol after prolonged consistent mannitol use (>2–3 days) or in patients with suspected BBB disruption.

CLINICAL EFFICACY

With the similarities in mechanisms of action between mannitol and HTS, it is of little surprise that the clinical efficacy appears to also be similar. Clinical trials evaluating mannitol or HTS have generally suggested that various osmotherapy agents are similarly effective at lowering elevated ICP (Table 15.1). Several studies in the early stages of using HTS either compared similar volumes of infusion (but not equi-osmolar doses) of mannitol and HTS or combined HTS with hetastarch to potentiate the volume expansion effect.[71–73] Two of these studies suggested that HTS plus hetastarch had a greater impact on ICP reduction than mannitol. However, hetastarch is not combined with HTS in contemporary practice due to the potential for bleeding and renal dysfunction. Two more recent studies comparing equi-osmolar doses of the two osmotherapy options also suggest that HTS has

greater impact on ICP reduction or ICP burden.[74,75] Three separate meta-analyses have been performed to combine all the small clinical studies to evaluate the overall treatment effect. Mortazavi et al. evaluated studies that compared HTS to mannitol or other therapies (normal saline in one trial) and concluded that HTS was less likely to exhibit treatment failure or diminished response compared to mannitol (OR 0.36, 95% confidence interval 0.19–0.68, p = 0.002).[76] The meta-analysis by Kamel et al. suggested that there was no difference in quantitative reduction in ICP between therapies, but treatment success was more likely with HTS (RR 1.16, 95% confidence interval 1.00–1.33, p = 0.046).[77] The meta-analysis by Li et al. suggested that HTS was superior to mannitol for ICP reduction at 60 and 120 minutes after the dose.[78] Given the importance of timing when treating acutely elevated ICP, it seems reasonable to advocate that both osmotherapy agents should be used interchangeably. However, clinicians may elect to make HTS more readily available in patient care units that commonly treat patients with elevated ICP in order to make HTS the agent of choice.

CONCLUSIONS

Osmotherapy agents form the first line of pharmacotherapy options for patients with raised ICP. These agents are ideally used to maximize the change in serum osmolarity, modulation of cerebral blood volume, and improvement in blood rheology. Various administration considerations are important for the bedside clinician when infusing mannitol and HTS including the risk of phlebitis, electrolyte and intravascular volume fluctuations, and changes in renal function. There is little difference in neurological outcomes between mannitol and HTS, though HTS may be more effective at reducing ICP.

REFERENCES

1. Xi G, Keep RF, Hoff JT. Pathophysiology of brain edema formation. *Neurosurgery Clinics of North America* 2002;13(3):371–83.
2. Mendelow AD, Teasdale GM, Russell T, et al. Effect of mannitol on cerebral blood flow and cerebral perfusion pressure in human head injury. *J Neurosurg* 1985;63(1):43–8.
3. Muizelaar JP, Wei EP, Kontos HA, et al. Mannitol causes compensatory cerebral vasoconstriction and vasodilation in response to blood viscosity changes. *J Neurosurg* 1983;59(5):822–8.
4. Muizelaar JP, van der Poel HG, Li ZC, et al. Pial arteriolar vessel diameter and CO2 reactivity during prolonged hyperventilation in the rabbit. *J Neurosurg* 1988;69(6):923–7.

5. Jha S, Prabhu D. Is normal saline really 'normal'? *International Journal of Critical Illness and Injury Science* 2013;3(2):161.

6. Reddy S, Weinberg L, Young P. Crystalloid fluid therapy. *Critical Care* 2016;20:59.

7. Hypertonic saline. *Mosby's Dictionary of Medicine*. MO: Mosby/Elsevier, 2009;879.

8. Barry KG, Berman AR. Mannitol infusion. III. The acute effect of the intravenous infusion of mannitol on blood and plasma volumes. *N Engl J Med* 1961;264:1085–8.

9. Rosner MJ, Coley I. Cerebral perfusion pressure: a hemodynamic mechanism of mannitol and the postmannitol hemogram. *Neurosurgery* 1987;21(2):147–56.

10. Burke AM, Quest DO, Chien S, et al. The effects of mannitol on blood viscosity. *J Neurosurg* 1981;55(4):550–3.

11. Donato T, Shapira Y, Artru A, et al. Effect of mannitol on cerebrospinal fluid dynamics and brain tissue edema. *Anesth Analg* 1994;78(1):58–66.

12. Muizelaar JP, Wei EP, Kontos HA, et al. Cerebral blood flow is regulated by changes in blood pressure and in blood viscosity alike. *Stroke* 1986;17(1):44–8.

13. Rocha-e-Silva M, Poli de Figueiredo LF. Small volume hypertonic resuscitation of circulatory shock. *Clinics (Sao Paulo)* 2005;60(2):159–72.

14. Mazzoni MC, Borgström P, Arfors KE, et al. Dynamic fluid redistribution in hyperosmotic resuscitation of hypovolemic hemorrhage. *Am J Physiol* 1988;255(3 Pt 2): H629–37.

15. Doyle JA, Davis DP, Hoyt DB. The use of hypertonic saline in the treatment of traumatic brain injury. *J Trauma* 2001;50(2):367–83.

16. Walsh JC, Zhuang J, Shackford SR. A comparison of hypertonic to isotonic fluid in the resuscitation of brain injury and hemorrhagic shock. *J Surg Res* 1991; 50(3):284–92.

17. Sorani MD, Morabito D, Rosenthal G, et al. Characterizing the dose-response relationship between mannitol and intracranial pressure in traumatic brain injury patients using a high-frequency physiological data collection system. *J Neurotrauma* 2008;25(4):291–8.

18. Sorani MD, Manley GT. Dose-response relationship of mannitol and intracranial pressure: a metaanalysis. *J Neurosurg* 2008;108(1):80–7.

19. Brown FD, Johns L, Jafar JJ, et al. Detailed monitoring of the effects of mannitol following experimental head injury. *J Neurosurg* 1979;50(4):423–32.

20. Wisner DH, Schuster L, Quinn C. Hypertonic saline resuscitation of head injury: effects on cerebral water content. *J Trauma* 1990;30(1):75–8.

21. Cascino T, Baglivo J, Conti J, et al. Quantitative CT assessment of furosemide- and mannitol-induced changes in brain water content. *Neurology* 1983;33(7): 898–903.

22. Bell BA, Smith MA, Kean DM, et al. Brain water measured by magnetic resonance imaging. Correlation with direct estimation and changes after mannitol and dexamethasone. *Lancet* 1987;1(8524):66–9.

23. Palma L, Bruni G, Fiaschi AI, et al. Passage of mannitol into the brain around gliomas: a potential cause of rebound phenomenon. A study on 21 patients. *J Neurosurg Sci* 2006; 50(3):63–6.

24. Kaufmann AM, Cardoso ER. Aggravation of vasogenic cerebral edema by multiple-dose mannitol. *J Neurosurg* 1992;77(4):584–9.

25. Sankar T, Assina R, Karis JP, et al. Neurosurgical implications of mannitol accumulation within a meningioma and its peritumoral region demonstrated by magnetic resonance spectroscopy: case report. *J Neurosurg* 2008;108(5):1010–13.

26. Hartl R, Medary MB, Ruge M, et al. Hypertonic/hyperoncotic saline attenuates microcirculatory disturbances after traumatic brain injury. *J Trauma* 1997; 42(Suppl 5):S41–7.

27. Enriquez P, Bullock R. Molecular and cellular mechanisms in the pathophysiology of severe head injury. *Curr Pharm Des* 2004;10(18):2131–43.

28. Mojtahedzadeh M, Ahmadi A, Mahmoodpoor A, et al. Hypertonic saline solution reduces the oxidative stress responses in traumatic brain injury patients. *J Res Med Sci* 2014;19(9):867–74.

29. McGraw CP, Alexander Jr. E, Howard G. Effect of dose and dose schedule on the response of intracranial pressure to mannitol. *Surg Neurol* 1978;10(2):127–30.

30. Brain Trauma Foundation; American Association of Neurological Surgeons; Congress of Neurological Surgeons et al. Guidelines for the management of severe traumatic brain injury. II. Hyperosmolar therapy. *J Neurotrauma* 2007;24(Suppl 1):S14–20.

31. Carney N, Totten AM, O'Reilly C, Ullman JS, Hawryluk GW, Bell MJ, et al. Guidelines for the management of severe traumatic brain injury. 4th ed. *Neurosurgery* 2017 1;80(1):6–15.

32. James HE. Methodology for the control of intracranial pressure with hypertonic mannitol. *Acta Neurochir (Wien)* 1980;51(3–4):161–72.

33. Cruz J, Minoja G, Okuchi K, et al. Successful use of the new high-dose mannitol treatment in patients with Glasgow Coma Scale scores of 3 and bilateral abnormal pupillary widening: a randomized trial. *J Neurosurg* 2004; 100(3):376–83.

34. Quentin C, Charbonneau S, Moumdjian R, et al. A comparison of two doses of mannitol on brain relaxation during supratentorial brain tumor craniotomy: a randomized trial. *Anesth Analg* 2013;116(4):862–8.

35. Seo H, Kim E, Jung H, et al. A prospective randomized trial of the optimal dose of mannitol for intraoperative brain relaxation in patients undergoing craniotomy for supratentorial brain tumor resection. *J Neurosurg* 2016:1–8.

36. Wells DL, Swanson JM, Wood GC, et al. The relationship between serum sodium and intracranial pressure when

using hypertonic saline to target mild hypernatremia in patients with head trauma. *Crit Care* 2012;16(5):R193.

37. Human T, Cook AM, Anger B, et al. Treatment of hyponatremia in patients with acute neurological injury. *Neurocrit Care* 2017; 27(2):242–8.

38. Simma B, Burger R, Falk M, et al. A prospective, randomized, and controlled study of fluid management in children with severe head injury: lactated Ringer's solution versus hypertonic saline. *Crit Care Med* 1998;26(7):1265–70.

39. Woo CH, Rao VA, Sheridan W, et al. Performance characteristics of a sliding-scale hypertonic saline infusion protocol for the treatment of acute neurologic hyponatremia. *Neurocrit Care* 2009;11(2):228–34.

40. James HE, Langfitt TW, Kumar VS, et al. Treatment of intracranial hypertension. Analysis of 105 consecutive, continuous recordings of intracranial pressure. *Acta Neurochir (Wien)* 1977;36(3–4):189–200.

41. Cote CJ, Greenhow DE, Marshall BE. The hypotensive response to rapid intravenous administration of hypertonic solutions in man and in the rabbit. *Anesthesiology* 1979;50(1):30–35.

42. Procaccio F, Stocchetti N, Citerio G, et al. Guidelines for the treatment of adults with severe head trauma (part II). Criteria for medical treatment. *J Neurosurg Sci* 2000;44(1):11–8.

43. Bourdeaux C, Brown J. Sodium bicarbonate lowers intracranial pressure after traumatic brain injury. *Neurocrit Care* 2010;13(1):24–8.

44. Boullata JI, Gilbert K, Sacks G, et al. A.S.P.E.N. clinical guidelines: parenteral nutrition ordering, order review, compounding, labeling, and dispensing. *J Parenter Enteral Nutr* 2014;38(3):334–77.

45. Le A, Patel S. Extravasation of noncytotoxic drugs: a review of the literature. *Ann Pharmacother* 2014;48(7):870–86.

46. Timmer JG, Schipper HG. Peripheral venous nutrition: the equal relevance of volume load and osmolarity in relation to phlebitis. *Clin Nutr* 1991;0(2):71–5.

47. Jones GM, Bode L, Riha H, et al. Safety of continuous peripheral infusion of 3% sodium chloride solution in neurocritical care patients. *Am J Crit Care* 2016;26(1):37–42.

48. Weaver A, Sica DA. Mannitol-induced acute renal failure. *Nephron* 1987;45(3):233–5.

49. Dorman HR, Sondheimer JH, Cadnapaphornchai P. Mannitol-induced acute renal failure. *Medicine (Baltimore)* 1990;69(3):153–9.

50. Goldwasser P, Fotino S. Acute renal failure following massive mannitol infusion. Appropriate response of tubuloglomerular feedback? *Arch Intern Med* 1984; 144(11):22141–6.

51. Rello J, Triginer C, Sánchez JM, et al. Acute renal failure following massive mannitol infusion. *Nephron* 1989;53(4):377–8.

52. Perez-Perez AJ, Pazos B, Sobrado J, et al. Acute renal failure following massive mannitol infusion. *Am J Nephrol* 2002;22(5–6):573–5.

53. Horgan KJ, Ottaviano YL, Watson AJ. Acute renal failure due to mannitol intoxication. *Am J Nephrol* 1989; 9(2):106–9.

54. GondimFde A, Aiyagari V, Shackleford A, et al. Osmolality not predictive of mannitol-induced acute renal insufficiency. *J Neurosurg* 2005;103(3):444–7.

55. Dziedzic T, Szczudlik A, Klimkowicz A, et al. Is mannitol safe for patients with intracerebral hemorrhages? Renal considerations. *Clin Neurol Neurosurg* 2003;105(2):87–9.

56. Whelan TV, Bacon ME, Madden M, et al. Acute renal failure associated with mannitol intoxication. Report of a case. *Arch Intern Med* 1984;144(10):2053–5.

57. Temes SP, Lilien OM, Chamberlain W. A direct vasoconstrictor effect of mannitol on the renal artery. *Surg Gynecol Obstet* 1975;141(2):223–6.

58. Lilien CM. The paradoxical reaction of renal vasculature to mannitol. *Invest Urol* 1973;10(5):346–53.

59. Gadallah MF, Lynn M, Work J. Case report: mannitol nephrotoxicity syndrome: role of hemodialysis and postulate of mechanisms. *Am J Med Sci* 1995;309(4):219–22.

60. Torre-Healy A, Marko NF, Weil RJ. Hyperosmolar therapy for intracranial hypertension. *Neurocrit Care* 2012;17(1):117–30.

61. Garcia-Morales EJ, Cariappa R, Parvin CA, et al. Osmole gap in neurologic-neurosurgical intensive care unit: Its normal value, calculation, and relationship with mannitol serum concentrations. *Crit Care Med* 2004;32(4): 986–91.

62. Rabetoy GM, Fredericks MR, Hostettler CF. Where the kidney is concerned, how much mannitol is too much? *Ann Pharmacother* 1993;27(1):25–8.

63. Visweswaran P, Massin EK, Dubose Jr. TD. Mannitol-induced acute renal failure. *J Am Soc Nephrol* 1997; 8(6):1028–33.

64. van Hengel P, Nikken JJ, de Jong GM, et al. Mannitol-induced acute renal failure. *Neth J Med* 1997;50(1):21–4.

65. Verbalis JG, Goldsmith SR, Greenberg A, et al. Hyponatremia treatment guidelines 2007: expert panel recommendations. *Am J Med* 2007;120(11)(Suppl 1): S1–21.

66. Gipstein RM, Boyle JD. Hypernatremia complicating prolonged mannitol diuresis. *N Engl J Med* 1965;272: 1116–7.

67. Stuart FP, Torres E, Fletcher R, et al. Effects of single, repeated and massive mannitol infusion in the dog: structural and functional changes in kidney and brain. *Ann Surg* 1970;172(2):190–204.

68. Yunos NM, Bellomo R, Hegarty C, et al. Association between a chloride-liberal vs chloride-restrictive intravenous fluid administration strategy and kidney injury in critically ill adults. *JAMA* 2012;308(15):1566–72.

69. Michael J Erdman HR, Lauren Bode, Jason Chang, Morgan Jones G. Predictors of acute kidney injury in neurocritical care patients receiving continuous hypertonic saline. *The Neurohospitalist* 2017;7(1):9–14.

70. Ropper AH. Hyperosmolar therapy for raised intracranial pressure. *N Engl J Med* 2012;367(8):746–52.

71. Vialet R, Albanèse J, Thomachot L, et al. Isovolume hypertonic solutes (sodium chloride or mannitol) in the treatment of refractory posttraumatic intracranial hypertension: 2 ml/kg 7.5% saline is more effective than 2 ml/kg 20% mannitol. *Critical Care Medicine* 2003;31(6):1683–7.

72. Bentsen G, Breivik H, Lundar T, et al. Hypertonic saline (7.2%) in 6% hydroxyethyl starch reduces intracranial pressure and improves hemodynamics in a placebo-controlled study involving stable patients with subarachnoid hemorrhage. *Crit Care Med* 2006;34(12):2912–7.

73. Harutjunyan L, Holz C, Rieger A, et al. Efficiency of 7.2% hypertonic saline hydroxyethyl starch 200/0.5 versus mannitol 15% in the treatment of increased intracranial pressure in neurosurgical patients — a randomized clinical trial [ISRCTN62699180]. *Crit Care* 2005;9(5):R530–40.

74. Oddo M, Levine JM, Frangos S, et al. Effect of mannitol and hypertonic saline on cerebral oxygenation in patients with severe traumatic brain injury and refractory intracranial hypertension. *J Neurol Neurosurg Psychiatry* 2009;80(8): 916–20.

75. Mangat HS, Chiu YL, Gerber LM, et al. Hypertonic saline reduces cumulative and daily intracranial pressure burdens after severe traumatic brain injury. *J Neurosurg* 2015;122(1):202–10.

76. Mortazavi MM, Romeo AK, Deep A, et al. Hypertonic saline for treating raised intracranial pressure: literature review with meta-analysis. *J Neurosurg* 2012;116(1): 210–21.

77. Kamel H, Navi BB, Nakagawa K, et al. Hypertonic saline versus mannitol for the treatment of elevated intracranial pressure: a meta-analysis of randomized clinical trials. *Crit Care Med* 2011;39(3):554–9.

78. Li M, Chen T, Chen SD, et al. Comparison of equimolar doses of mannitol and hypertonic saline for the treatment of elevated intracranial pressure after traumatic brain injury: a systematic review and meta-analysis. *Medicine (Baltimore)* 2015;94(17):e736.

16

Vasoactive Drugs

A. Castle and K. Owusu

ABSTRACT

Blood pressure (BP) management is a key component of care for the neurocritically ill patient. Both hypertension and hypotension can cause or exacerbate neurologic injury. Achievement of patient and disease-specific BP goals may improve the likelihood of a good outcome. However, this can be particularly difficult in patients with an acute brain injury. For example, when neurologic disorders are associated with autonomic dysfunction, haemodynamic instability may be difficult to control and patients may respond to vasoactive medications differently. This chapter describes the commonly used medications to decrease or augment blood pressure in neurocritically ill patients. Knowledge of the appropriate use, dosing, and effects of vasoactive drugs is essential for all neurocritical care practitioners.

KEYWORDS

Vasoactive; vasopressor; hypotension; hypertension; paroxysmal sympathetic hyperactivity (PSH); perfusion.

INTRODUCTION

Vasoactive agents are used in neurocritical care for haemodynamic augmentation and to correct hypertension. In this setting, vasoactive pharmacotherapy may be utilized to optimize end-organ perfusion and provide adequate oxygenation to vital organs. In addition to fluid augmentation that facilitates restoration of tissue perfusion in certain shock states, they are often used in neurocritical care to induce hypertension even in the absence of clinical hypotension. For example, vasoactive agents have a critical role in increasing blood pressure (BP) during neurological emergencies including stroke, traumatic brain injury (TBI), spinal cord injury (SCI), and post carotid endarterectomy in the setting of defective vascular autoregulation. Vasoactive drug therapies have direct and indirect effects on cerebral blood flow (CBF). Careful thought must therefore be given to patient-specific traits when selecting vasoactive agents. In this chapter, we will compare the various available vasoactive drug therapies and highlight their role in therapy in the setting of various neurologic disorders.

BLOOD PRESSURE MANAGEMENT IN ACUTE NEUROLOGIC EMERGENCIES

Arterial hypotension and hypertension can be observed in the setting of acute ischaemic stroke (AIS). Blood pressure spontaneously decreases during the acute phase of ischaemic stroke, typically immediately after the onset of symptoms.[1] An extreme decrease in BP is detrimental to the ischaemic brain as it causes a further decrease in brain perfusion and subsequently exacerbates ischaemic injury.[1,2] Hypertension is typically more common and arterial hypotension may suggest other causes including arrhythmia, ischaemia, and aortic dissection, or shock.[2] Hypothetically, moderate arterial hypertension may improve cerebral perfusion of the ischaemic brain. However, significant arterial hypertension may also exacerbate oedema of the ischaemic brain and subsequent haemorrhagic transformation.[2] While the optimal BP range is unclear, a systolic blood pressure (SBP) range of 121–200 mmHg and a diastolic blood pressure (DBP) range of 81–110 mmHg has been suggested, while considering stroke subtype and other patient-specific factors including comorbid conditions.[2–4]

Several antihypertensive agents have been evaluated in the context of neurologic injury. In the setting of ischaemic stroke, The Evaluation of Acute Candesartan Cilexetil Therapy in Stroke Survivors (ACCESS) trial assessed the efficacy of an angiotensin converting enzyme inhibitor (ACE-I) candesartan in acute SBP reduction (10%–15%) within 24 hours of randomization.[5] In comparison to placebo, there were no differences in the primary endpoint assessed by functional dependency, however, there was a reduction in the secondary endpoint of 12-month mortality favouring the candesartan arm.[5] Similarly, several other clinical trials evaluating the potential benefits of angiotensin-mediated antihypertensive agents in the setting of AIS have found no difference in clinical endpoints in comparison to placebo.[6–8] More recently in 2014, a *Journal of the American Medical Association* publication assessed the effects of immediate BP reduction on death and major disability using several antihypertensive agents including ACE-I, calcium channel blockers (CCB), and diuretics.[9] While reductions in BP between the arms were achieved within 24 hours, there were no differences between the primary combined endpoint of death or dependency rate at 14 days or hospital discharge when an antihypertensive agent was initiated within 24 hours of randomization.[9]

The acute treatment of hypertension in the setting of neurologic injury is often accomplished with intravenous agents including nicardipine, labetalol, nitroprusside, and clevidipine. A 2008 comparison of nicardipine and labetalol for acute hypertension management in AIS revealed similar tolerability between both agents and a smoother BP control in patients who received nicardipine in comparison to labetalol.[10] Patients with AIS who are eligible for acute reperfusion therapy with elevated BP exceeding the threshold of 185/110 mmHg are recommended to receive either agent.[2] Afterload reducing agents including hydralazine and enalaprilat are reasonable considerations and sodium nitroprusside may be considered if BP is not controlled with the use of the aforementioned agents or if diastolic BP exceeds 140 mmHg.[2] Along with hydralazine and enalaprilat, sodium nitroprusside is less desirable due to associated prolonged antihypertensive effect and unpredictable blood pressure response.[11,12] Clevidipine, a short-acting dihydropyridine calcium channel antagonist, is an attractive agent for acute hypertension management due to its rapid onset and offset of effect.[13] Table 16.1 compares the parenteral antihypertensive agents used commonly in the setting of neurologic injury.

COMPARISON OF VASOPRESSORS IN NEUROLOGIC INJURY

A major cerebral artery occlusion leading to acute ischaemic stroke produces a core infarction surrounded by salvageable penumbra. The vulnerable areas beyond the core of the infarct continue to receive low blood flow and maintain viability through collateral circulation. Facilitating blood flow with vasoactive agents may have clinical utility in optimizing end-organ perfusion and the provision of adequate oxygen delivery to the penumbra. Little is known about the role of induced hypertension in the setting of large vessel occlusion in AIS. To date, only a single randomized trial has assessed the effects of induced BP elevation on function and perfusion in AIS.[14] In this trial, 15 patients were randomized 2:1 to pharmacologically induced BP elevation or conventional management. Induced hypertension was achieved with continuous intravenous infusion (CIV) of phenylephrine for 24 hours and midodrine, fludrocortisone, and sodium chloride (NaCl) tablets were initiated thereafter to facilitate wean of injectable phenylephrine while maintaining goal mean arterial pressure (MAP). Patients in the intervention group had less severe neurological deficit at day 3 and at 6–8 weeks than the control group.[14]

Acute changes in BP in the setting of TBI lead to significant effects on cerebral blood flow due to impaired autoregulatory mechanisms.[15] When BP or MAP targets are not achieved with the administration of fluids during TBI, vasopressors are recommended.[15] Norepinephrine is a reasonable selection and dopamine should be avoided due to concerns of cerebral vasodilation and increase in intracranial pressure (ICP).[16] A 2011 publication in *Neurocritical Care*, assessing the effects of vasopressors on haemodynamic augmentation after severe TBI in adult patients, concluded that patients who received phenylephrine had higher MAP and cerebral perfusion pressure (CPP) compared to patients who received dopamine and norepinephrine, respectively.[17] Due to its pure alpha-agonistic activity, phenylephrine should be considered in patients with TBI who exhibit tachycardia.

Compared to other types of shock, there is limited literature comparing the available vasoactive drug therapies in neurogenic shock. In this setting, norepinephrine, dopamine, and phenylephrine have all been shown to improve CBF.[18] A direct comparison of cerebrovascular effects between norepinephrine and dopamine administration concluded that norepinephrine led to predictable increases in cerebral flow velocities estimated with transcranial

Table 16.1 Comparison of commonly used parenteral antihypertensive agents in neurocritical care

Class	Agents	Half-life	Duration of action	Comments
Angiotensin converting enzyme (ACE) inhibitors	Enalaprilat	35 hr	12–24 hr	Unpredictable response dependent on plasma volume and plasma renin activity
Beta blockers	Esmolol	9 min	30 min	Cardioselective
	Labetalol	5.5 hr	16–18 hr	Less antihypertensive efficacy compared to nicardipine. May cause bronchospasm and heart block. Avoid in patients with CHF or heart block
Calcium-channel antagonists	Clevidipine	1–5 min	5 hr	Contraindicated in severe aortic stenosis due to risk of severe hypotension. Formulated in lipid-emulsion (contraindicated in patients with soy or egg allergies as well as disordered lipid metabolism)
	Nicardipine	45 min	<8 hr	Associated with decreased oxygen saturation (possible pulmonary shunting)
Nitrates	Nitroglycerine	1–4 min	5–10 min	Greater extent of venodilation > arteriolar dilation. Clinical utility in patients with concomitant myocardial ischaemia. May cause headache and reflex tachycardia
	Nitroprusside	2 min Thiocyanate (3 days; prolonged in renal failure)	10 min	Vasodilatory effects may lead to an increase in ICP. Metabolized to cyanide, possibly leading to the development of cyanide or thiocyanate toxicity. May lead to dose-related decrease in coronary, renal, and cerebral perfusion
Vasodilator	Hydralazine	3–7 hr	2–4 hr	Little or no effect on venous circulation. May cause reflex tachycardia

Abbreviations: h: hours; min: minutes; CHF: congestive heart failure.

Sources: (1) Liu-DeRyke X, Janisse J, Coplin WM, et al. A comparison of nicardipine and labetalol for acute hypertension management following stroke. *Neurocrit Care* 2008;9:167–76. (2) Hirschl MM, Binder M, Bur A, et al. Clinical evaluation of different doses of intravenous enalaprilat in patients with hypertensive crises. *Arch Intern Med* 1995;155(20):2217. (3) Peacock WF, Varon J, Baumann B, et al. CLUE: a randomized comparative effectiveness trial of IV nicardipine versus labetalol use in the emergency department. *Crit Care* 2011;15(3):R157. (4) Shultz V. Clinical pharmacokinetics of nitroprusside, cyanide, thiosulphate and thiocynate. *Clin Pharmacokinet* 1984;9(3):239.

Doppler. Changes in cerebral flow velocities with the administration of dopamine, however, appeared to be unpredictable and inconsistent.[19] In the setting of acute SCI, there is an increased risk of hypotension due to haemodynamic instability secondary to neurogenic shock and autonomic dysreflexia.[20] Hypotension may lead to impaired spinal cord healing due to decreased delivery of nutrients to the site.[20] Therefore, a MAP goal between 85 and 90 mmHg has been advocated for the first seven days following acute cervical SCI.[21] A recent retrospective study evaluating medical and surgical management strategies after SCI identified dopamine as the commonly used vasopressor (48.0%) followed by phenylephrine (45%), norepinephrine (5.0%), epinephrine (1.5%), and vasopressin (0.5%). There was

an independent association with dopamine (OR 8.97; p<0.001) and phenylephrine (OR, 5.92, p=0.004) use and cardiovascular side effects including ventricular tachycardia, atrial fibrillation, and bradycardia.[22]

The enteral vasopressors such as midodrine have been utilized to facilitate continuous IV vasopressor administration in neurocritical care.[14] Desglymidodrine, an active metabolite of midodrine demonstrates selective alpha-1 agonistic activity and causes predominantly peripheral vasoconstriction since there are few alpha-1 receptors in the brain.[23] Droxidopa, a synthetic catecholamine-like amino acid that is converted into norepinephrine is a new potential therapy approved by the Food and Drug Administration (FDA) for orthostatic dizziness, and light-headedness in patients with neurogenic

Table 16.2 Comparison of commonly used vasopressors in neurocritical care

Vasopressor	Receptor binding				Dosing ranges	Side effects
	α–1	β–1	β–2	DA		
Dobutamine	+	+++++	+++	NA	2–20 mcg/kg/min	Hypotension, ventricular arrhythmias, cardiac ischaemia
Dopamine	+++	++++	++	+++++	1–20 mcg/kg/min	Ventricular arrhythmias, cardiac ischaemia, tissue ischaemia/gangrene (with high doses or with extravasation)
Epinephrine	+++++	++++	+++	NA	0.05–2 mcg/kg/min	Severe hypertension leading to cerebrovascular haemorrhage, ventricular arrhythmias, cardiac ischaemia
Norepinephrine	+++++	+++	++	NA	0.05–2 mcg/kg/min	Tachycardia, decreased intestinal perfusion, peripheral (digital) ischaemia
Phenylephrine	+++++	0	0	NA	0.5–9 mcg/kg/min	Reflex bradycardia, severe peripheral and visceral vasoconstriction
Vasopressin	V_2: Renal fluid reabsorption V_1: Peripheral vasoconstriction				0.04 units/min	Rebound hypotension with discontinuation, coronary ischaemia (associated with doses >0.03 units/min)

Abbreviations: NA = Not applicable; DA = Dopaminergic receptor. 29)
Sources: (1) Overgaard CB, Dzavík V. Inotropes and vasopressors. *Circulation* 2008;118:1047–56. (2) Durrant JC, Hinson HE. Rescue therapy for refractory vasospasm after subarachnoid hemorrhage. *Curr Neurol Neurosci Rep* 2015;15(2):521. (3) Levy ML, Rabb CH, Zelman V, Giannotta SL. Cardiac performance enhancement from dobutamine in patients refractory to hypervolemic therapy for cerebral vasospasm. *J Neurosurg* 1993;79:494–9.

orthostatic hypotension.[24] Droxidopa demonstrated a reduction in IV vasoactive drug requirements and improved MAP in a patient with vasoplegic syndrome who was not responsive to midodrine.[25] The commonly reported side effects of droxidopa include headache, dizziness, and nausea[26] (Table 16.2).

AUTONOMIC DYSFUNCTION IN ACQUIRED BRAIN INJURY

Paroxysmal sympathetic hyperactivity (PSH) is associated with various types of neurologic injury including TBI (79.4%), hypoxic brain injury (9.7%), and stroke (5.4%).[27,28] While this condition was described decades ago, a lack of standardization regarding diagnostic criteria and characterization of this syndrome persist. Published literature has described the condition as PSH, paroxysmal autonomic instability with dystonia (PAID), sympathetic storming, diencephalic seizures, or dysautonomia. More recent literature suggests PSH as the most appropriate nomenclature.[29] Reported rates of PSH have ranged from 8%[30] to 33%[31] in patients with TBI. Clinical manifestations of PSH generally include hypertension, hyperthermia, tachycardia, tachypnea, diaphoresis, and extensor posturing.[31] It is important to note that not all symptoms are present in each patient and symptoms often vary in severity. Symptoms of PSH occur in a cyclic

fashion, often occurring one to three times per day. In order to be considered as PSH, the syndrome must also include the following features as defined by the PSH-Assessment Measure (PSH-AM):[29]

- Clinical features occur simultaneously
- Episodes are paroxysmal in nature
- Sympathetic over-reactivity to normally non-painful stimuli
- Features persist ≥3 consecutive days
- Features persist ≥2 weeks post brain injury
- Features persist despite treatment of alternative differential diagnoses
- Medication administered to decrease sympathetic features
- ≥2 episodes daily
- Absence of parasympathetic features during episodes
- Absence of other presumed cause of features
- Antecedent acquired brain injury

The exact pathophysiology of PSH symptomatology is unknown, however, it has been attributed to a loss of cortical and subcortical control leading to a 'release phenomenon' at the level of the upper brainstem and diencephalon.[32] Boeve et al. propose that activation or disinhibition of central sympathoexcitatory regions is responsible for the sympathetic hyperactivity in PSH.[33] Thermoregulatory changes during PSH episodes have

Table 16.3 Management of paroxysmal sympathetic hyperactivity

Agent	Mechanism of action	Dose	Half-life (hours)	Peak action	Comments
Bromocriptine	Dopamine D_2 agonist	1.25 mg PO BID titrate to 10–40 mg	7	1.6 hr	Avoid use in patients with uncontrolled hypertension. May lower seizure threshold
Baclofen	$GABA_B$ agonist	5 mg TID titrate up to 80 mg/day IT administration up to 450 mcg/day reported	PO: 5 IT: 1.5	PO: Variable (hours) IT: 0.5–1 hr	IT administration titrated to patient response. Avoid abrupt discontinuation of baclofen, which may induce rigidity, fever, dystonia, or seizures
Clonidine	α-2 adrenergic agonist	0.1–0.3 mg TID PO	12–16	2–5 hr	May cause rebound hypertension with first dose or abrupt withdrawal
Dantrolene	Direct skeletal muscle relaxation by interference with calcium ion release from sarcoplasmic reticulum	0.25–2 mg/kg IV q 6–12 hours	5–9	30 min	May induce hepatotoxicity. Monitor baseline and frequent liver function tests during therapy
Benzodiazepines	GABA receptor modulator	5–10 mg IV [diazepam] 2–4 mg IV/PO [lorazepam] 1–2 mg IV [midazolam]	48 12 3	1 min 5 min (IV); 2 hr (PO) 3–5 min	Preferred in cases of severe spells with dystonia. Useful in recovering patients with a substantial component of anxiety
Dexmedetomidine	α-2 adrenergic agonist	0.2 mcg/kg/hr, titrated up to 0.7 mcg/kg/hr	2.5	5–10 min	
Gabapentin	Binds to α-delta subunit of v-gated calcium channels	300–900 mg/day titrate up to 3600–4800 mg/day	6	2–4 hr	Well tolerated for long-term use
Morphine	Mu opioid receptor agonist	2–8mg IV	2	30 min	The most useful abortive drug therapy
Propranolol	Non-selective β-blocker	20–60 mg by mouth (PO) q. 4–6 hours	3–5	90 min	β-1 selective agents are not useful in PSH

Abbreviations: BID: twice daily; h: hours; IT: intrathecally; IV: intravenously; min: minute; mg: milligrams; PO = orally; q: every; TID: three times daily; v-gated: voltage-gated.

Sources: (1) Rabinstein AA. Paroxysmal sympathetic hyperactivity in the neurological intensive care unit. *Neurol Res* 2007;29(7):680–2. (2) Blackman JA, Patrick PD, Buck ML, Rust RS, Jr. Paroxysmal autonomic instability with dystonia after brain injury. *Arch Neurol* 2004;61(3):321–8. (3) Rabinstein AA, Benarroch EE. Treatment of paroxysmal sympathetic hyperactivity. *Curr Treat Options Neurol* 2008;10(2):151–7.

been explained by both dysfunction in the hypothalamus and hypermetabolic changes that occur during sustained muscular contractions.[34] The rigidity associated with PSH may be explained by lesions in the midbrain which would block normal inhibitory signals to pontine or vestibular nuclei.[34]

Pharmacological Management of Paroxysmal Sympathetic Hyperactivity

Several drug therapies have been demonstrated to improve symptoms in patients with PSH (Table 16.3), however, the optimal treatment strategy for PSH is unknown. Pharmacotherapy should therefore be targeted at clinical symptoms aligning with patient-specific factors. Opioid analgesics have been shown to demonstrate a positive effect on PSH symptoms possibly due to the presence of opioid receptors in the brain cardiovascular nuclei, the heart, and blood vessels.[35] Pharmacological treatment for PSH typically includes a combination of preventative and abortive medication to control a patient's symptoms. Agents such as propranolol, clonidine, bromocriptine, gabapentin, and baclofen are most often used as preventative therapy, whereas drugs like morphine, dexmedetomidine, diazepam, lorazepam, midazolam, dantrolene, and baclofen intrathecally are used in the abortion of active episodes of autonomic hyperactivity. It is reasonable to begin tapering down medications once dysautonomic symptoms have been controlled for several days to weeks depending on the severity of dysautonomia.[31] Common side effects of opioids such as morphine may be desirable in PSH including hypotension, respiratory depression, and bradycardia which can counterbalance PSH symptoms. Additionally, the analgesic effects of opioids can combat the pain as a trigger for storming episodes. The utility of non-selective β blockers in the prevention of PSH episodes is not surprising as many of the syndrome's signs are associated with excessive sympathetic activity. Propranolol and labetalol have been found to be particularly useful while β-1 selective agents such as metoprolol have not shown clinical activity in mitigating autonomic dysregulation.[36] Clonidine is particularly helpful in managing the BP, heart rate, and agitation that may be associated with this syndrome. Alternatively, dexmedetomidine has also been shown to be an effective agent in this setting.[37] Symptoms of PSH such as dystonia, hyperpyrexia, and posturing can resemble neuroleptic malignant syndrome, a syndrome associated with the use of dopamine antagonists or withdrawal of dopamine agonists.[34] Consequently, clinicians have used bromocriptine, a dopamine D_2 receptor agonist, to treat PSH with good clinical response in some cases.[34] Benzodiazepines, such as lorazepam, midazolam, and diazepam are beneficial because of their anxiolytic, sedative, and muscle relaxant effects.[34] Baclofen has shown some clinical efficacy in a few cases of refractory PSH.[38,39] Gabapentin is a voltage-gated calcium channel modulator that may be useful in the recovery phase for patients with mild PSH or subacute brain injury.[40] A case series also provides evidence that gabapentin may be tried in the acute phase of refractory PSH.[41]

CONCLUSIONS

Management of BP remains a key component of care in neurocritically ill patients. The occurrence of both, hypertension and hypotension can result in neurological injury. They may also exacerbate existing injuries. Proper management of pressures may improve the likelihood of good outcome in these patients, especially those with acute brain injury.

REFERENCES

1. Ahmed N, Näsman P, Wahlgren NG. Effect of intravenous nimodipine on blood pressure and outcome after acute stroke. *Stroke* 2000;31:1250–5.
2. Jauch EC, Saver JL, Adams HP, et al. Guidelines for the early management of patients with acute ischemic stroke. A guideline for healthcare professionals from the American Heart Association/American Stroke Association. 2013;44:870–947.
3. Castillo J, Leira R, García MM, et al. Blood pressure decrease during the acute phase of ischemic stroke is associated with brain injury and poor stroke outcome. *Stroke* 2004;35:520–6.
4. Leonardi-Bee J, Bath PM, Phillips SJ, Sandercock PA. IST Collaborative Group. Blood pressure and clinical outcomes in the International Stroke Trial. *Stroke* 2002;33:1315–20.
5. Schrader J, Lüders S, Kulschewski A, et al. Acute candesartan cilexetil therapy in stroke survivors study group. The ACCESS Study: evaluation of acute candesartan cilexetil therapy in stroke survivors. *Stroke* 2003;34:1699–703.
6. Diener HC, Sacco RL, Yusuf S, et al. Effects of aspirin plus extended-release dipyridamole versus clopidogrel and telmisartan on disability and cognitive function after recurrent stroke in patients with ischaemic stroke in the Prevention Regimen for Effectively Avoiding Second Strokes (PRoFESS) trial: a double-blind, active and placebo-controlled study. *Lancet Neurol* 2008;7:875–84.
7. Bath PM, Martin RH, Palesch Y, et al. Effect of telmisartan on functional outcome, recurrence, and blood pressure in patients with acute mild ischemic stroke: a PRoFESS subgroup analysis. *Stroke* 2009;40:3541–6.
8. Sandset EC, Bath PM, Boysen G, et al. The angiotensin-receptor blocker candesartan for treatment of acute stroke (SCAST): a randomised, placebo-controlled, double-blind trial. *Lancet* 2011;377:741–50.
9. He J, Zhang Y, Xu T, et al. Effects of immediate blood pressure reduction on death and major disability in patients with acute ischemic stroke: the CATIS randomized clinical trial. *JAMA* 2014;311:479–89.
10. Liu-DeRyke X, Janisse J, Coplin WM, et al. A comparison of nicardipine and labetalol for acute hypertension management following stroke. *Neurocrit Care* 2008;9:167–76.
11. Halpern NA, Goldberg M, Neely C, et al. Postoperative hypertension: a multicenter, prospective, randomized comparison between intravenous nicardipine and sodium nitroprusside. *Crit Care Med* 1992;20(12):1637–43.
12. O'Malley K, Segal JL, Israili ZH, et al. Duration of hydralazine action in hypertension. *Clin Pharmacol Ther* 1975;18(5 Pt 1):581–6.

13. Erickson AL, DeGrado JR, Fanikos JR. Clevidipine: a short-acting intravenous dihydropyridine calcium channel blocker for the management of hypertension. *Pharmacotherapy* 2010;30(5):515–28.

14. Hillis AE, Ulatowski JA, Barker PB, et al. A pilot randomized trial of induced blood pressure elevation: effects on function and focal perfusion in acute and subacute stroke. *Cerebrovasc Dis* 2003;16:236–46.

15. Carney N, Totten AM, O'Reilly C, et al. Guidelines for the management of severe traumatic brain injury. 4th ed. 2016 [cited 2016 Dec 20]. Available from: https://braintrauma.org/coma/guidelines.

16. Ract C, Vigue B. Comparison of the cerebral effects of dopamine and norepinephrine in severe head injury patients. *Intensive Care Med* 2001;27:101–6.

17. Sookplung P, Siriussawakul A, Malakouti A, Sharma D, Wang J, Souter MJ, Chesnut RM, Vavilala MS. Vasopressor use and effect on blood pressure after severe adult traumatic brain injury. *Neurocrit Care* 2011;15(1):46–54.

18. Francoeur CL, Mayer SA. Management of delayed cerebral ischemia after subarachnoid hemorrhage. *Critical Care* 2016; 20:777.

19. Steiner LA, Johnston AJ, Czosnyka M, et al. Direct comparison of cerebrovascular effects of norepinephrine and dopamine in head-injured patients. *Crit Care Med* 2004;32(4):1049–54.

20. Readdy WJ, Dhall SS. Vasopressor administration in spinal cord injury: should we apply a universal standard to all injury patterns? *Neural Regen Res* 2016;11(3):420–1.

21. Ryken TC, Hurlbert RJ, Hadley MN, et al. The acute cardiopulmonary management of patients with cervical spinal cord injuries. *Neurosurgery* 2013;72(2):84–92.

22. Inoue T, Manley GT, Patel N, Whetstone WD. Medical and surgical management after spinal cord injury: vasopressor usage, early surgeries, and complications. *J Neurotrauma* 2014;31:284–91.

23. Bevan JA, Duckworth J, Laher I, et al. Sympathetic control of cerebral arteries: Specialization in receptor type, reserve, affinity, and distribution. *FASEB J* 1987;1:193–8.

24. Goldenberg MM. Pharmaceutical Approval Update. *Pharmacy and Therapeutics* 2014;39(5):337–44.

25. Zundel TM, Boettcher BT, Feih JT, et al. Use of oral droxidopa to improve arterial pressure and reduce vasoactive drug requirements during persistent vasoplegic syndrome after cardiac transplantation. *J Cardiothorac Vasc Anesth* 2016;30(6):1624–6.

26. Overgaard CB, Dzavík V. Inotropes and vasopressors. *Circulation* 2008;118:1047–56.

27. Penfield W, Jasper H. Autonomic seizures. In: Penfield W, Jasper H, eds. *Epilepsy and the functional anatomy of the human brain*. London: J & A Churchill Ltd, 1954; pp. 412–37.

28. Perkes I, Baguley IJ, Nott MT, Menon DK. A review of paroxysmal sympathetic hyperactivity after acquired brain injury. *Ann Neurol* 2010 Aug;68(2):126–35.

29. Baguley IJ, Perkes IE, Fernandez-Ortega JF, et al. Paroxysmal sympathetic hyperactivity after acquired brain injury: Consensus on conceptual definition, nomenclature, and diagnostic criteria. *J Neurotrauma* 2014;31(17):1515–20.

30. Baguley IJ, Slewa-Younan S, Heriseanu RE, Nott MT, Mudaliar Y, Nayyar V. The incidence of dysautonomia and its relationship with autonomic arousal following traumatic brain injury. *Brain Inj* 2007;21(11):1175–81.

31. Rabinstein AA. Paroxysmal sympathetic hyperactivity in the neurological intensive care unit. *Neurol Res* 2007;29(7):680–2.

32. Bullard DE. Diencephalic seizures: Responsiveness to bromocriptine and morphine. *Ann Neurol* 1987;21(6):609–11.

33. Boeve BF, Wijdicks EF, Benarroch EE, Schmidt KD. Paroxysmal sympathetic storms ('diencephalic seizures') after severe diffuse axonal head injury. *Mayo Clin Proc* 1998;73(2):148–52.

34. Blackman JA, Patrick PD, Buck ML, Rust RS, Jr. Paroxysmal autonomic instability with dystonia after brain injury. *Arch Neurol* 2004;61(3):321–8.

35. Siren A-L, Feuerstein G. The opioid system in circulatory control. *News Physiol Sci* 1992;7:26–30.

36. Do D, Sheen VL, Bromfield E. Treatment of paroxysmal sympathetic storm with labetalol. *J Neurol Neurosurg Psychiatry* 2000;69(6):832–3.

37. Goddeau RP, Jr, Silverman SB, Sims JR. Dexmedetomidine for the treatment of paroxysmal autonomic instability with dystonia. *Neurocrit Care* 2007;7(3):217–20.

38. Cuny E, Richer E, Castel JP. Dysautonomia syndrome in the acute recovery phase after traumatic brain injury: Relief with intrathecal baclofen therapy. *Brain Inj* 2001;15(10):917–25.

39. Becker R, Benes L, Sure U, Hellwig D, Bertalanffy H. Intrathecal baclofen alleviates autonomic dysfunction in severe brain injury. *J Clin Neurosci* 2000;7(4):316–9.

40. Rabinstein AA, Benarroch EE. Treatment of paroxysmal sympathetic hyperactivity. *Curr Treat Options Neurol* 2008;10(2):151–7.

41. Baguley IJ, Heriseanu RE, Gurka JA, Nordenbo A, Cameron ID. Gabapentin in the management of dysautonomia following severe traumatic brain injury: A case series. *J Neurol Neurosurg Psychiatry* 2007;78(5):539–41.

17

Anticonvulsants

J. J. Mucksavage and E. P. Tesoro

ABSTRACT

Seizures are complications seen in critically ill patients that can lead to significant morbidity and mortality. Status epilepticus (SE) is a neurological emergency requiring rapid control of electrographic and physical seizures. The recommended first-line agent is an intravenous benzodiazepine followed by administration of an anticonvulsant if the aetiology of the seizures cannot be identified and treated. Refractory seizure activity may necessitate the addition of continuous infusions of anaesthetics. The treatment of seizures may be complicated in critically ill patients due to cardiopulmonary instability, hepatic and/or renal dysfunction, and the potential for drug interactions. Careful monitoring is necessary to prevent adverse drug reactions as well as to ensure treatment efficacy.

KEYWORDS

Anticonvulsants; seizures; critically ill; benzodiazepines; status epilepticus (SE); phenytoin; propofol.

INTRODUCTION

Seizures are a common complication in critically ill patients and are associated with significant morbidity and mortality.[1,2] Status epilepticus (SE), defined as unremitting seizures for at least five minutes or multiple seizures between which no return to baseline is observed, is a medical emergency and must be treated in an organized and timely manner in order to optimize patient outcomes.[3–5] Proper medication selection and timely administration are essential for rapid control of both physical and electrographic signs of seizures. Various guidelines have been published on the diagnosis and treatment of SE.[6–8] This chapter focuses on the pharmacotherapy of commonly used agents in SE. Information regarding dosing, administration, and side effect monitoring of anticonvulsants in the intensive care unit (ICU) are provided in this chapter.

Several considerations must be taken when using anticonvulsants in critically ill patients. Intravenous (IV) therapy is often used since oral access may be limited or contraindicated due to trauma, surgery, dysphagia, nausea, vomiting, or ileus. Patients admitted to the ICU may have varying degrees of hepatic and renal dysfunction which

can affect metabolism and excretion of medications.[9] Cardiorespiratory effects of certain anticonvulsants merit close monitoring of blood pressure and respiratory rate. Intubation and mechanical ventilation are sometimes necessary to allow delivery of high doses of anticonvulsants to attain seizure control. Critically ill patients may also be given multiple medications that increase the risk of drug interactions. As a result of the complexities encountered in these patients, frequent monitoring is required to help guide selection of agents and adjust dosing to ensure efficacy and minimize adverse events.

BENZODIAZEPINES

Intravenous benzodiazepines are the emergent (first-line) drugs given to patients in SE because of their rapid ability to arrest seizure activity.[6] The most commonly used agents are midazolam, lorazepam, and diazepam (Table 17.1). Both lorazepam and diazepam are highly lipophilic and require propylene glycol to maintain solubility for parenteral use. Midazolam is more hydrophilic, but converts to a more lipophilic moiety in the body. The excipient propylene glycol can cause hypotension when given intravenously making midazolam

Table 17.1 Benzodiazepines used for the initial treatment of status epilepticus

Drug	Dose	Maximum dose	Comments
Diazepam	0.15–0.2 mg/kg IV 0.2–0.5 mg/kg PR	IV: 10 mg (may repeat once in non-intubated patients) PR: 20 mg	Propylene glycol diluent; highly lipophilic – may require more frequent re-dosing
Midazolam	10 mg (wt. >40 kg) IV/IM 5 mg (wt. 13–40 kg) IV/IM		May give intranasal or buccally
Lorazepam	0.1 mg/kg/dose	4 mg (may repeat once in non-intubated patients)	Propylene glycol diluent – dilute 1:1 with normal saline

a more reasonable choice in patients who have unstable blood pressures. Both diazepam and lorazepam can be diluted 1:1 with parenteral 0.9% sodium chloride to minimize the hypotensive and irritant effects of propylene glycol before administering via a peripheral vein. The maximum rate of administration for both these agents should not be exceeded in order to avoid hypotension and phlebitis. Intravascular volume status should be optimized with appropriate maintenance fluids followed by parenteral vasopressors, if needed. The IV route of administration is preferred for patients in SE since this results in quick attainment of therapeutic serum levels. However, for those clinical situations where parenteral access is limited or not available, midazolam may be given intramuscularly[10] (avoid in coagulopathic or anticoagulated patients) and diazepam may be given rectally as a gel formulation[11] (avoid in patients with ongoing diarrhoea). Midazolam has also been given via the intranasal and buccal routes, primarily in children in whom obtaining IV access may be challenging.[12] Intramuscular (IM) dosing of diazepam and lorazepam may not be optimal due to the potential for erratic absorption and delays in onset when compared to the IV route. Intraosseous devices may also be used to administer parenteral anticonvulsants, particularly in patients in whom obtaining vascular access may be difficult (e.g., infants/children, and extensive trauma). Benzodiazepines used during the initial management of SE are given in Table 17.1.

There are no major differences between the three benzodiazepine agents in terms of seizure control, although lorazepam seems to be the preferred agent in most clinical settings.[13] This may be due to its longer duration of action compared to diazepam and midazolam. Although diazepam is more lipophilic than lorazepam resulting in rapid entry into the brain, it also quickly redistributes to other fatty tissues over time. This can result in loss of seizure control from decreased concentrations in the central nervous system (CNS). Pharmacokinetically, frequent re-dosing of diazepam to maintain seizure control may be

required when compared to lorazepam. When repeated benzodiazepine dosing occurs, it is important to monitor respiratory function and intubate the patient if indicated. Patients who are on chronic benzodiazepine therapy can develop tolerance and may require higher doses to achieve cessation of seizure activity.

For patients with significant hepatic dysfunction, caution should be taken with lorazepam as it is inactivated in the liver. The duration of effect may be prolonged in these patients after repeated administration due to poor metabolism. Patients with renal failure should not receive midazolam as its active metabolites are renally eliminated and can accumulate over time, increasing the risk of over-sedation. This is especially true for continuous infusions of midazolam often seen in cases of refractory SE.[14] Table 17.2 lists the pharmacokinetic properties of some commonly used anticonvulsants.

Benzodiazepines are thought to act on the inhibitory gamma (γ) aminobutyric acid (GABA) receptors in the brain to promote seizure cessation.[15] Prolonged seizure activity is associated with changes in the GABA-receptor making them less responsive to agonist-simulation over time.[16] Thus, it is imperative that benzodiazepines be given as soon as SE is recognized in order to avoid this refractory period from developing. Unremitting seizure activity beyond 30 minutes is associated with neuronal injury which may become permanent.[17] Once seizures are stopped with benzodiazepines, anticonvulsant therapy is typically initiated for continued control of seizures unless a specific underlying aetiology is identified and treated (e.g., hypoglycaemia).

ANTICONVULSANTS

In the setting of SE, anticonvulsants are typically initiated concurrently or immediately after benzodiazepine therapy.[6] Although anticonvulsants are effective in treating seizures, their infusion times and onset of action are not as fast as the benzodiazepines. The IV administration rates of

Table 17.2 Pharmacokinetic profiles of common medications used for seizures

Drug	$T_{1/2}$	Volume of distribution (V_d)	Protein binding	Metabolism	Elimination
Diazepam	48 hours	0.8–1 L/kg	95%–99%	Hepatic (active metabolites)	Renal (not dialyzable)
Lorazepam	12 hours	1.3 L/kg	85%–91%	Hepatic (inactive metabolites)	Renal
Midazolam	1.8–6.4 hours	1–2.5 L/kg	95%	Hepatic (active metabolites)	Renal
Fos/phenytoin	Variable due to saturable kinetics (dependent on serum concentration)	0.5–1 L/kg	90%	Hepatic (saturable via CYP2C9, CYP2C19; inactive metabolites)	Biliary/renal
Valproate sodium	6–17 hours	0.14–0.23 L/kg	90%	Hepatic	Renal (removed by high-flux HD)
Phenobarbital	1.5–5 days	0.5–1 L/kg	20%–60%	Hepatic	21% renally eliminated (removed by haemodialysis)
Carbamazepine	12–17 hours	0.8–2 L/kg	76%	Hepatic (active metabolites; induces own metabolism ~3–5 weeks)	72% renally eliminated (removed by HD)
Levetiracetam	6–8 hours	0.7 L/kg	<10%	Minimally hepatic	Renally (50% removed by haemodialysis)
Lacosamide	13 hours	0.6 L/kg	<15%	Hepatic (inactive metabolites)	95% renally eliminated (~50% removed by haemodialysis)
Brivaracetam	9 hours	0.5 L/kg	20%	Hepatic (inactive metabolites)	>95% renally eliminated
Topiramate	21 hours	0.6–0.8 L/kg	15%–41%	Minimally hepatic	Renal (dialyzable)

some anticonvulsants are limited by the potential for serious adverse reactions (e.g., hypotension, respiratory depression). This relegates their use for urgent or second-line treatment. Intravenous loading doses are commonly used to attain therapeutic serum levels quickly, but infusion-related side effects and total volume limit their rate of administration and thus their overall onset of activity. It is important to initiate proper maintenance doses after loading doses in order to maintain serum levels and seizure control. Typical maintenance doses are started 8–12 hours after a loading dose. Table 17.3 contains dosing information for commonly used anticonvulsants that are used in the ICU.

Phenytoin is a commonly used anticonvulsant agent in the setting of SE. Loading doses are typically given at 20 mg/kg and infused no faster than 50 mg/min due to the presence of the propylene glycol diluent. For non-emergent cases, phenytoin can be infused at lower rates (10–25 mg/min) to decrease the risk of hypotension or phlebitis. Phenytoin is only compatible in 0.9% sodium chloride and precipitation can occur if mixed in other solutions (drugs should always be inspected for particulate matter before administration). Cardiac monitoring is recommended during phenytoin infusion to help quickly identify arrhythmias. Extravasation of phenytoin into the soft tissues can result in severe pain, local necrosis, and extensive tissue damage (purple glove syndrome).[18] Routine visual inspection of the injection site and avoiding the use of more distal access sites (e.g., hand veins) can minimize this adverse event. Oral loading with phenytoin in the setting of SE is not recommended, although it may be an option in non-emergent cases to correct a subtherapeutic serum level.

Table 17.3 Anticonvulsants used to treat seizures and status epilepticus

Drug	Loading dose	Maintenance dose	Therapeutic serum levels
Phenytoin	15–20 mg/kg IV (max rate: 50 mg/min)	4–6 mg/kg/day IV/PO divided q12hr–q8hr	10–20 mcg/ml (total) or 1–2 mcg/ml (free)
Fos/phenytoin (pro-drug of phenytoin)	15–20 mg PE/kg IV/IM (max rate: 150 mg PE/min)	4–6 mg PE/kg/day IV/IM/PO divided q12hr–q8hr	Monitored as phenytoin
Valproic acid	20–40 mg/kg IV (additional 20 mg/kg dose if needed); rate: 3–6 mg/kg/min	30–60 mg/kg/day IV divided q12hr–q8hr	50–100 mcg/ml
Phenobarbital	10–20 mg/kg IV (max rate: 100 mg/min)	1–3 mg/kg/day	15–40 mcg/ml
Carbamazepine	8 mg/kg PO (given as suspension or tablets; not appropriate in status epilepticus)	1200 mg/day divided BID/TID	4–12 mcg/ml
Levetiracetam	60 mg/kg (max dose: 4500 mg)	500–1500 mg IV/PO q12hr	Not established
Lacosamide	N/A	100–200 mg IV/PO q12hr	Not established
Brivaracetam	N/A	50–100 mg IV/PO q12hr	Not established
Topiramate	200–400 mg	300–1600 mg/day PO q12hr–q6hr	Not established

Abbreviations: q12hr: every 12 hours; q8hr: every 8 hours; PO: per oral; BID: bis in die; TID: ter in die.

In an attempt to minimize the intolerance seen with phenytoin administration, a phosphorylated IV pro-drug was developed. Fosphenytoin (dosed in milligrams of phenytoin equivalents or mgPE) is more water-soluble and does not require propylene glycol in its formulation. It is stable in 0.9% sodium chloride, dextrose solutions, and lactated Ringer's solution. It may also be infused three times as fast as phenytoin (150 mgPE/min) in emergent cases with less hypotension and arrhythmias (cardiac monitoring is still recommended). Once in the bloodstream, it is readily converted to phenytoin with a conversion half-life of 10–15 minutes. Paraesthesias around the mouth and groin are commonly reported, especially with larger doses and high infusion rates. Fosphenytoin can also be given as an IM injection during instances where IV access is unobtainable. The volume of a loading dose given by this route can be around 20–30 ml, but these doses have been shown to get readily absorbed despite the large volumes. An alternative approach would be to divide the main dose into two smaller doses. If serum levels are desired after loading doses, they should be collected two hours after an IV load and four hours after an IM load. Routine serum level measurements should be performed prior to maintenance doses to reflect the lowest concentration during the dosing interval.

Patients with epilepsy who are non-compliant or who miss several maintenance doses may go into SE due to a decrease in serum levels below the recommended therapeutic range. In order to quickly reach therapeutic serum levels, smaller 'mini' loading doses are given and can be calculated using a simplified relationship between the starting concentration, the patient's weight, and the drug's volume of distribution (Vd):

Dose in mg = (pt. weight in kg × Vd in L/kg) × (desired concentration in mg/L – starting concentration in mg/L)

This equation is commonly used to estimate parenteral loading doses for phenytoin/fosphenytoin, but can also be applied theoretically to phenobarbital and valproic acid (using their respective values for Vd). Phenobarbital is particularly sedating and higher loading doses can cause significant respiratory depression requiring endotracheal intubation.

Valproic acid (or valproate sodium in the IV form) is a broad-spectrum anticonvulsant that has been used to treat various types of SE. Structurally different than the aromatic anticonvulsants (i.e., phenytoin and phenobarbital), valproic acid has multiple mechanisms of action including activity at sodium and calcium channels as well as modulation of GABA.[15] Compared to other IV agents used for SE, it has minimal effects on blood pressure and respiratory rate. It may be preferred in critically ill patients that are haemodynamically unstable and not mechanically ventilated, or intolerant to other agents. Doses of 40 mg/kg have reported to result in serum concentrations at the higher end of the therapeutic range.[19] Caution must be exercised in patients receiving carbapenems and valproic acid concomitantly. This combination can result in drastic decreases in valproic acid concentrations, leaving patients at risk for breakthrough seizures.[20] If such a combination occurs, a change in antibiotics guided by microbiological data or a change to another anticonvulsant agent is warranted.

Levetiracetam is an anticonvulsant that has grown in popularity due to its tolerability and predictable pharmacokinetics. While its use in SE has been documented, no evidence exists to suggest its superiority over any other agent. Similar to valproic acid, it has minimal effects on blood pressure and respiratory rate making it an ideal agent to use in ICU patients with haemodynamic compromise. It is not associated with multiple drug interactions seen with many of the traditional agents since it does not have extensive hepatic metabolism or significant protein binding. Loading doses are reported to be well tolerated with minimal cardiorespiratory effects. Increased clearance of levetiracetam has been reported in patients with traumatic brain injury (TBI) and subarachnoid haemorrhage (SAH),[21] possibly resulting in subtherapeutic levels and suboptimal seizure control.

Both carbamazepine and topiramate are only available as oral preparations in the United States. Carbamazepine is not commonly used in SE but can be continued in patients with a history of epilepsy. Serum sodium levels should be monitored as hyponatraemia is a well-documented side effect. Topiramate has been used in acute SE cases but caution should be used in patients with metabolic acidosis as this drug inhibits carbonic anhydrase. Lacosamide and brivaracetam are the more recently developed anticonvulsants that have IV and enteral preparations, minimal drug interactions, and predictable pharmacokinetic profiles making them attractive agents in critically ill patients. While reports have found lacosamide to be relatively safe and effective in critically ill patients,[22,23] data on the use of brivaracetam in the ICU is still emerging.

Continuous Infusion Anticonvulsants

In addition to midazolam infusions described previously, barbiturates (specifically thiopental or its metabolite pentobarbital), propofol, and ketamine are used as infusions in the management of refractory SE. Generally due to the adverse effect profile and intensive monitoring required, these agents are considered only after other treatment strategies have failed.[6,7] Endotracheal intubation, a high level of cardiac monitoring and close neurological monitoring are required for safe administration. Additionally, continuous electroencephalography (EEG) monitoring is necessary to monitor efficacy. However, currently there is no consensus regarding the optimal goal waveform or duration of infusion therapy before weaning anaesthetic agents.[6,24] These decisions are best left to experienced neurologists familiar with these treatment strategies.

Of all the available anaesthetic infusions for the management of seizures, the barbiturates are the oldest drugs available. Barbiturates are thought to exert their anticonvulsive effects by stimulating the GABA-alpha receptor.[25] While thiopental has been used worldwide, its metabolite pentobarbital is used more commonly in the United States. Both drugs are initiated with a bolus dose and therapy is maintained with a continuous infusion. Table 17.4 provides the common dosing recommendations. The onset of action of these agents is quick when administered as an IV bolus dose and effects can occur within one minute. The anaesthetic effects are limited by redistribution of these compounds in the body. The redistribution of barbiturates contributes to elevations in serum concentrations resulting in a half-life that can approach days.[25] This creates an undesirable potential for lingering sedative effects. Other adverse effects commonly encountered during infusion therapy include hypotension, hypothermia, and immunosuppression.[25] During infusion therapy with barbiturates, vasopressors may be required to maintain adequate blood pressure and perfusion to vital organs. Careful consideration should be made with loading doses as propylene glycol is present in pentobarbital formulations leading to hypotension. In addition to the immune and cardiovascular effects discussed, ileus has also been reported necessitating alternative routes for nutrition and drug administration.[26,27]

Similar to barbiturates, propofol is thought to exert its anaesthetic activity by affecting the GABA-alpha receptor. Propofol is administered via a loading dose and maintenance therapy is provided by continuous infusion (Table 17.4). Clinicians should use caution when administering propofol as a bolus dose because of significant hypotension. Hypotension has also been reported with continuous infusions at anaesthetic doses requiring vasopressor therapy. Other cardiac effects including bradyarrhythmias have also been documented. In contrast to the prolonged sedative effects seen with barbiturate therapy, propofol has a short-half life and patients are easily awakened after short interruptions in therapy. However, during more prolonged infusions,

Table 17.4 Anaesthetic agents used for status epilepticus in mechanically ventilated patients

Drug	Dose	Comments
Midazolam	0.2 mg/kg IV at 2 mg/min, then 0.05–2 mg/kg/hr	• tachyphylaxis common • avoid in patients with renal failure
Propofol	1–2 mg/kg IV load, then 20 mcg/kg/min (titrate up to 300 mcg/kg/min)	• associated with hypotension (especially loading doses) • prolonged doses (>48 hours) and high doses (>80 mcg/kg/min) may lead to PRIS • provides 1 kcal/mL (adjust nutritional intake as needed)
Pentobarbital	10–15 mg/kg IV (max rate: 50 mg/min), then 0.5–5 mg/kg/hr	• associated with respiratory depression, ileus, decreased cardiac function/hypotension • do NOT confuse with phenobarbital
Thiopental	2–7 mg/kg IV (max rate: 50 mg/min), then 0.5–5 mg/kg/hr	• hepatically metabolized to pentobarbital • associated with respiratory depression, ileus, decreased cardiac function/hypotension
Ketamine	1.5 mg/kg IV (may repeat every 3–5 minutes), then 0.3–10 mg/kg/hr	• associated with hypertension, intracranial pressure elevations, hallucination, and neurotoxicity • NMDA antagonist

accumulation into adipose tissue can occur increasing the time needed to awaken the patient.

Propofol is formulated as a 10% lipid emulsion and contributes to total caloric intake. As such, adjustments should be made in nutritional regimen to avoid overfeeding. Triglyceride levels can also be monitored to evaluate the impact of lipid infusions and the risk of pancreatitis.[28]

One of the most worrisome risks of anaesthetic doses of propofol for seizure management is the propofol-related infusion syndrome (PRIS). This syndrome is characterized by refractory severe metabolic acidosis, bradycardia, hyperkalaemia, electrocardiography (ECG) changes, lipaemia, rhabdomyolysis, renal failure, and cardiac failure.[29] Treatment options for this condition are limited and early recognition and prompt discontinuation of propofol is critical. Unfortunately, this condition is not readily recognized and commonly leads to death. Some of the risk factors for developing PRIS include decreased oxygen delivery to tissues, serious neurological injury and/or sepsis, and high doses of one or more of the following classes of drugs: vasoconstrictors, steroids, and inotropes. Infusion doses of greater than 5 mg/kg/hr for more than 48 hours have been associated with PRIS. However, PRIS has also been reported during anaesthesia cases using high-dose therapy for short durations of time. The risk of PRIS should be considered prior to initiating propofol and careful monitoring for the signs during therapy is paramount to use this agent for seizure management.

Recently there has been a resurgence in the clinical use of ketamine. The concept of 'pharmacoresistance' describes a proposed mechanism for the development of refractory and super-refractory SE.[30] As SE continues over time, it becomes increasingly difficult to treat, and drugs like the benzodiazepines lose their effectiveness. Therefore, therapeutic targets other than the GABA-alpha receptor have been explored. Ketamine is one such agent which works by having an agonist role on the GABA-alpha receptor, but more importantly and differently than the previously discussed agents, it antagonizes the N-methyl-D-aspartate (NMDA) receptor.[25] Antagonism at the NMDA receptor has been shown to potentially benefit patients in refractory or super refractory SE.[31]

The evidence for using ketamine is currently limited and controlled trials are lacking.[32] Based on the available literature, ketamine is dosed as an initial bolus and then administered as a continuous infusion (Table 17.4). Evidence suggests that ketamine should be used with benzodiazepines to avoid neurotoxicity and potentiate efficacy.[33] The onset of action is considered to be rapid due to ketamine's ability to quickly cross into the brain. Unlike propofol and barbiturates, hypotension is less likely to be encountered and caution should be exercised when being used in hypertensive patients. Some notable toxicities include psychiatric adverse effects, sialorrhoea, and tachyarrhythmias. Historically, ketamine was associated with elevations in intracranial pressure, but more recent data is challenging the commonly held assumption.[34,35]

Non-Parenteral Administration

All the anticonvulsants have enteral formulations available for maintenance doses (fosphenytoin can be converted to phenytoin), but some consideration must be taken to ensure appropriate administration in critically ill patients with temporary or permanent feeding tubes. Extended-release or sustained-release formulations should not be crushed or opened for administration via an enteral feeding tube. Immediate-release tablets, liquids, or suspensions are more appropriate for this route.[36] Although most anticonvulsants have simple 1:1 conversions from IV to oral routes, phenytoin and valproic acid have different salt formulations that may require small adjustments when switching formulations. This has considerable consequences for phenytoin where its nonlinear kinetics can result in greater than expected changes in serum concentrations after small changes in dose. Interactions with enteral nutrition have been reported with both phenytoin and carbamazepine, and recommendations are to separate doses from tube feedings, typically by one hour on either side (enteral feeding rates must be adjusted accordingly to avoid underfeeding).[37,38]

Additional considerations in ICU patients include the presence of hypotension, hypovolaemia, and/or vasopressor use which can all minimize blood flow to the gastrointestinal (GI) tract and may affect drug absorption. Any change in GI motility may also affect the onset or duration of effect. Diarrhoea can increase transit time limiting the extent of absorption while an ileus may delay or prevent absorption. Nausea and vomiting are the common side effects of anticonvulsants and should be evaluated if encountered after initiating oral therapy.

MONITORING

Patients receiving parenteral anticonvulsants (particularly loading doses) should be on cardiac monitoring for blood pressure and heart rate due to side effects like hypotension and arrhythmias. Initial laboratory monitoring should evaluate renal and hepatic function as well as baseline serum anticonvulsant levels if appropriate. Among the anticonvulsants, phenytoin, phenobarbital, valproic acid, and carbamazepine have serum level assays for therapeutic drug monitoring. Ideally, serum levels should be drawn right before scheduled doses (i.e., trough) in order to reflect the lowest concentration during the dosing interval. For patients with low albumin and receiving highly protein bound drugs (e.g. phenytoin), a free serum concentration should be measured to account for changes in protein binding. The free concentration is pharmacologically active, but laboratory tests for these levels may not be readily available. As a result, equations have been developed specifically for phenytoin to estimate free concentrations from a measured total level. However, there is some controversy as to the accuracy of these prediction models.[39] The original Sheiner–Tozer[40] equation uses total phenytoin levels and adjusts for albumin:

$$C_{corrected} = C_{actual}/[(0.2 \times albumin) + 0.1]$$

A modified factor is used if patients have renal dysfunction:[41]

$$C_{corrected} = C_{actual}/[(0.1 \times albumin) + 0.1]$$

Changes in maintenance doses should not be made before steady state is achieved, typically after 3–5 half-lives have passed, to avoid inadvertent accumulation of drug and resulting toxicity.

Additional monitoring parameters for other anticonvulsants used in the ICU include baseline amylase/lipase and platelet count for valproic acid (pancreatitis, thrombocytopenia), sodium levels for carbamazepine (syndrome of inappropriate antidiuretic hormone), and serum bicarbonate for topiramate (metabolic acidosis). Electrocardiography should be performed on patients receiving lacosamide (conduction abnormalities), IV fos/phenytoin (arrhythmias), or propofol (PRIS).

Several anticonvulsants are strong inducers or inhibitors of the cytochrome (CYP) P450 system and can have significant interactions with drugs that are substrates of these enzymes. Phenytoin is a strong inducer of CYP3A4 as well as being a substrate of CYP2C9 and CYP2C19. Phenobarbital is an inducing agent affecting CYP2C9 and CYP3A4 (decreased concentration of substrates) while valproic acid is a significant enzyme inhibitor of CYP3A4 and CYP2D6 (increased concentration of substrates). In general, effects of enzyme inhibitors can occur more quickly than effects of inducers which are limited by rates of hepatic enzyme production.[42] Medication lists should be reviewed for drug interactions in all ICU patients, especially those receiving multiple anticonvulsant agents.

CONCLUSIONS

Anticonvulsants are commonly used in the ICU, mostly in the management of SE or the treatment of epilepsy. Complicating the use of anticonvulsants for these indications, critically ill patients may have derangements in renal and hepatic function that affect drug disposition and require frequent clinical and laboratory monitoring. Careful consideration should be made when dosing and administering these agents, and appropriate dose adjustments should be made based on the patient's clinical parameters. In addition, drug interactions and adverse effect profile should be evaluated when selecting anticonvulsant medications. The most appropriate route of administration and administration rates should be chosen carefully to improve efficacy and minimize any associated risks. While the use of anticonvulsants in an ICU setting is challenging, implementing a comprehensive approach to drug management may optimize outcomes and eliminate unnecessary adverse events.

REFERENCES

1. Legriel S, Mourvillier B, Bele N, et al. Outcomes in 140 critically ill patients with status epilepticus. *Intensive Care Med* 2008;34:476–80.

2. Legriel S. Functional outcome after convulsive status epilepticus. *Critical Care Med* 2010;38:2295–303.

3. Chen JWY, Wasterlain CG. Status epilepticus: pathophysiology and management in adults. *Lancet Neurol* 2006;5(3):246–56.

4. Meldrum BS. The revised operational definition of generalised tonic-clonic (TC) status epilepticus in adults. *Epilepsia* 1999;40:123–4.

5. Trinka E, Cock H, Hesdorffer D, et al. A definition and classification of status epilepticus–Report of the ILAE task force on classification of status epilepticus. *Epilepsia* 2015;56(10):1515–23.

6. Brophy GM, Bell R, Claassen J, et al. Neurocritical Care Society Status Epilepticus Guideline Writing Committee. Guidelines for the evaluation and management of status epilepticus. *Neurocrit Care* 2012;17(1):3–23.

7. Glauser T, Shinnar S, Gloss D, et al. Evidence-based guideline: Treatment of convulsive status epilepticus in children and adults: Report of the guideline committee of the American Epilepsy Society. *Epilepsy Curr* 2016;16(1):48–61.

8. Prasad M, Krishnan PR, Sequeira R, Al-Roomi K. Anticonvulsant therapy for status epilepticus. *Cochrane Database Syst Rev* 2014;10(9):CD003723.

9. Boucher BA, Wood GC, Swanson JM. Pharmacokinetic changes in critical illness. *Crit Care Clin* 2006;22(2):255–71.

10. Silbergleit R, Durkalski V, Lowenstein D, et al. NETT Investigators. Intramuscular versus intravenous therapy for prehospital status epilepticus. *N Engl J Med* 2012;366(7):591–600.

11. Fitzgerald BJ, Okos AJ, Miller JW. Treatment of out-of-hospital status epilepticus with diazepam rectal gel. *Seizure* 2003;12(1):52–5.

12. Jain P, Sharma S, Dua T, Barbui C, Das RR, Aneja S. Efficacy and safety of anti-epileptic drugs in patients with active convulsive seizures when no IV access is available: Systematic review and meta-analysis. *Epilepsy Res* 2016;122:47–55.

13. Riviello JJ Jr, Claassen J, LaRoche SM, et al. Neurocritical Care Society Status Epilepticus Guideline Writing Committee. Treatment of status epilepticus: an international survey of experts. *Neurocrit Care* 2013;18(2):193–200.

14. Ulvi H, Yoldas T, Müngen B, Yigiter R. Continuous infusion of midazolam in the treatment of refractory generalized convulsive status epilepticus. *Neurol Sci* 2002;23(4):177–82.

15. Rogawski MA, Löscher W. The neurobiology of antiepileptic drugs. *Nat Rev Neurosci* 2004;5(7):553–64.

16. Niquet J, Baldwin R, Suchomelova L, et al. Benzodiazepine-refractory status epilepticus: pathophysiology and principles of treatment. *Ann N Y Acad Sci* 2016;1378(1):166–73.

17. Wasterlain CG, Fujikawa DG, Penix L, Sankar R. Pathophysiological mechanisms of brain damage from status epilepticus. *Epilepsia* 1993;34(Suppl 1):S37–53.

18. Garbovsky LA, Drumheller BC, Perrone J. Purple glove syndrome after phenytoin or fosphenytoin administration: review of reported cases and recommendations for prevention. *J Med Toxicol* 2015;11(4):445–59.

19. Uberall MA, Trollmann R, Wunsiedler U, Wenzel D. Intravenous valproate in pediatric epilepsy patients with refractory status epilepticus. *Neurology* 2000;54(11):2188–9.

20. Park MK, Lim KS, Kim TE, et al. Reduced valproic acid serum concentrations due to drug interactions with carbapenem antibiotics: overview of 6 cases. *Ther Drug Monit* 2012;34(5):599–603.

21. Cook AM, Arora S, Davis J, Pittman T. Augmented renal clearance of vancomycin and levetiracetam in a traumatic brain injury patient. *Neurocrit Care* 2013;19:210–4.

22. Cherry S, Judd L, Muniz JC, Elzawahry H, LaRoche S. Safety and efficacy of lacosamide in the intensive care unit. *Neurocrit Care* 2012;16(2):294–8.

23. Ramsay RE, Sabharwal V, Khan F, et al. Safety & pK of IV loading dose of lacosamide in the ICU. *Epilepsy Behav* 2015;49:340–2.

24. Rossetti AO, Milligan TA, Vulliémoz S, Michaelides C, Bertschi M, Lee JW. A randomized trial for the treatment of refractory status epilepticus. *Neurocrit Care* 2011;14(1):4–10.

25. Cuero MR, Varelas PN. Super-refractory status epilepticus. *Curr Neurol Neurosci Rep* 2015;15(11):74.

26. Cereda C, Berger MM, Rossetti AO. Bowel ischemia: a rare complication of thiopental treatment for status epilepticus. *Neurocrit Care* 2009;10(3):355–8.

27. Chin K, Ng S, Kwek T. Thiopentone barbiturate coma: a review of outcomes and complications. *Can J Anaesth* 2006;53(Suppl 1):26098.

28. Devlin JW, Lau AK, Tanios MA. Propofol-associated hypertriglyceridemia and pancreatitis in the intensive care unit: an analysis of frequency and risk factors. *Pharmacother* 2005;25(10):1348–52.

29. Kam PC, Cardone D. Propofol infusion syndrome. *Anaesthesia* 2007;62(7):690–701.

30. Wasterlain CG, Liu H, Naylor DE, et al. Molecular basis of self-sustaining seizures and pharmacoresistance during status epilepticus: The receptor trafficking hypothesis revisited. *Epilepsia* 2009;50(Suppl 12):16–18.

31. Wasterlain CG, Naylor DE, Liu H, Niquet J, Baldwin R. Trafficking of NMDA receptors during status epilepticus: therapeutic implications. *Epilepsia* 2013;54(Suppl 6):78–80.

32. Fang Y, Wang X. Ketamine for the treatment of refractory status epilepticus. *Seizure* 2015;30:14–20.

33. Rossetti AO, Lowenstein DH. Management of refractory status epilepticus. *Lancet Neurol* 2011;10(10):922–30.

34. Zeiler FA, Teitelbaum J, West M, Gillman LM. The ketamine effect on intracranial pressure in nontraumatic neurological illness. *J Crit Care* 2014;29(6):1096–106.

35. Gaspard N, Foreman B, Judd LM, et al. Intravenous ketamine for the treatment of refractory status epilepticus: a retrospective multicenter study. *Epilepsia* 2013;54(8): 1498–503.

36. Williams NT. Medication administration through enteral feeding tubes. *Am J Health Syst Pharm* 2008;65(24): 2347–57.

37. Au Yeung SC, Ensom MH. Phenytoin and enteral feedings: does evidence support an interaction? *Ann Pharmacother* 2000;34(7–8):896–905.

38. Bass J, Miles MV, Tennison MB, Holcombe BJ, Thorn MD. Effects of enteral tube feeding on the absorption and pharmacokinetic profile of carbamazepine suspension. *Epilepsia* 1989;30(3):364–9.

39. Kiang TK, Ensom MH. A comprehensive review on the predictive performance of the Sheiner-Tozer and derivative equations for the correction of phenytoin concentrations. *Ann Pharmacother* 2016;50(4):311–25.

40. Sheiner LB, Tozer TN. Clinical pharmacokinetics: The use of plasma concentrations of drugs. In: Melmon KL, Morrelli HF, eds. *Clinical Pharmacology: Basic Principles in Therapeutics*. New York: Macmillan;1978:p.71–109.

41. Tozer TN, Winter ME. Chapter 25: Phenytoin. In: Evans WE, Schentag JJ, Jusko WJ, eds. *Applied Pharmacokinetics*. 3rd ed. Vancouver, WA: Applied Therapeutics; 1992:1–44.

42. Brodie MJ, Mintzer S, Pack AM, Gidal BE, Vecht CJ, Schmidt D. Enzyme induction with antiepileptic drugs: cause for concern? *Epilepsia* 2013;54(1):11–27.

18

Corticosteroids

B. D. Bissell and C. Morrison

ABSTRACT

Inflammation is a common complication of cerebral injury that results in a neurotoxic cascade and eventual tissue oedema. Corticosteroids play a role in the treatment of several neurological critical care diagnoses through mitigation of this inflammatory process. Dosing recommendations and steroid selection are dependent on the underlying pathophysiology, but all indications must consider potential neurological side effects with steroid use. This chapter provides a review of the evidence supporting the use of both glucocorticoids and mineralocorticoids in common neurological disease processes.

KEYWORDS

Corticosteroids; adverse drug events; hyponatraemia; meningitis; acute spinal cord injury (aSCI); vasogenic oedema.

INTRODUCTION

Corticosteroids play a crucial role in the management of several neurological disorders in the critical care setting. Inflammation is a common complication of cerebral injury that initiates a neurotoxic cascade and eventually leads to tissue oedema.[1] Corticosteroid activity can be divided into two classifications based on the physiological actions, including mineralocorticoid and glucocorticoid activity. Mineralocorticoid effects are primarily the regulation of electrolytes, whereas the result of predominantly glucocorticoid administration is diverse. Metabolic, cardiovascular, pulmonary, and immune function can all be altered with the use of glucocorticoids. Glucocorticoid presence is essential for brain development and survival; however, elevated concentrations are associated with neuronal damage.[2] Most relevant, these corticosteroids have the ability to reduce oedema through a protective effect on the blood–brain barrier (BBB) and a decrease in cerebrospinal fluid (CSF) concentrations.[3] Table 18.1 depicts the various types of corticosteroids and their physiological activity.

NEUROLOGICAL CONSIDERATIONS WITH STEROID USE

Several important considerations should be made with the use of steroids in a critically ill neurologic patient, including potential adverse drug events.[4] Adverse events observed with corticosteroid use typically correlate with the dose and duration of exposure. It is important to note that since glucocorticoids have a direct catabolic effect on skeletal muscle, myopathy can occur.[5] The inhibition of insulin-like growth factor–I that has been demonstrated in the critically ill can additionally result in actual apoptosis of the muscle.[6] Myopathy can occur between weeks and months with steroid use, with one study of brain tumour patients reporting two-thirds of the population experiencing muscle weakness after 3–4 months of therapy.[7] With regard to dosage, 40–60 mg per day of prednisone can induce a clinically significant weakness within two weeks of treatment.[8]

Another adverse event associated with steroid use is cognitive changes and transition to delirium. While the exact mechanism is unclear, a link between neuronal

Table 18.1 Relative potency of corticosteroids

Corticosteroid	Glucocorticoid activity	Mineralocorticoid activity	Glucocorticoid dose conversion (mg)	Duration (hours)
Cortisol	1	1	–	–
Aldosterone	0.3	200–1000	–	–
Hydrocortisone	1	1	20	8–12
Cortisone	0.8	0.8	25	8–12
Prednisone	4	0.8	5	12–36
Methylprednisolone	5	0.5	4	12–36
Dexamethasone	30	0	0.75	36–54
Fludrocortisone	15	150	–	24–36

activation of dopaminergic and cholinergic systems and high corticosteroids levels may be possible.[9] In a population treated with systemic corticosteroids for a median duration of 15 days for acute lung injury, a significant increase in delirium rates was found.[10] High-dose methylprednisolone used in optic neuritis and multiple sclerosis was shown to significantly decrease long-term memory recall, however, an effect on short-term memory was not seen.[11] Mood disturbances can present a challenge in those presenting with gliomas, irradiation, or increased intracranial pressure as discrimination between such manifestations and steroid effects cannot be made frequently.[4]

Hence, some of the common adverse effects with the use of steroids are myopathy, visual blurring, tremors, behavioural changes, insomnia, reduced taste and smell, and cerebral atrophy. There may be uncommon adverse effects too, such as psychosis, hallucinations, hiccups, dementia, seizures, dependency, epidural lipomatosis, and neuropathy.[4]

Hyponatraemia

Hyponatraemia, a serum sodium less than 135 mmol/L, is an electrolyte imbalance frequently encountered in the neurological intensive care unit (ICU) and commonly seen in the presence of subarachnoid haemorrhage (SAH) or traumatic brain injury (TBI). Cerebral salt wasting syndrome (CSWS) and the syndrome of inappropriate secretion of antidiuretic hormone (SIADH) are the primary causes of hyponatraemia. An inappropriate release of arginine vasopressin (AVP) is seen in SIADH leading to water retention and pressure-natriuresis with secondary release of natriuretic peptides. An excessive release of natriuretic peptides is found with CSWS leading to primary natriuresis and volume depletion with a secondary increase in the renin–angiotensin system and AVP production.[12] Controversy exists regarding

the prevalence of CSWS in relation to SIADH as well as the clinical significance in differentiation of the diagnoses and clinical diagnostics.[13] Nevertheless, the use of fludrocortisone has been reported for management of hyponatraemia secondary to suspected CSWS. Fludrocortisone stimulates the reabsorption of sodium and water in the distal tubule through its interaction with mineralocorticoid receptors.

In a randomized controlled trial of 30 patients with SAH, fludrocortisone 0.3 mg daily significantly reduced urinary sodium excretion and urine volume, preventing a shift in serum sodium.[14] Another study of 46 patients with SAH showed prevention in delayed cerebral ischaemia and reduction in natriuresis. In a case series of paediatric patients and a case report of one adult, fludrocortisone reversed a negative sodium balance, allowing for normal serum sodium.[15,16] Doses reported range from 0.1 mg two to three times daily with a duration between 4 and 125 days, however, most authors suggest continuation until normalization of sodium concentrations, roughly for 3–5 days.[17]

Meningitis

Meningitis is an inflammatory process of the meninges resulting in alterations in the BBB and neuronal integrity. Corticosteroids have been used in order to diminish neurological complications associated with severe oedema and pressure that can ensue. Corticosteroids have been demonstrated to decrease CSF concentrations of cytokines and inflammation of the brain and blood vessels.[18]

Corticosteroids have been most commonly studied for meningitis of bacterial origin. Since the addition of adjunctive dexamethasone to the guideline recommendations, a decline in overall mortality has been observed.[19] A meta-analysis of 4,121 total patients showed a significant reduction in hearing loss and neurological sequelae.[20] While a decrease in mortality was seen, this was only significant in the subgroup of patients with *Streptococcus pneumoniae* as a causative organism. Adverse events were not altered with the use of corticosteroids, with the exception of a higher incidence of recurrent fever. Of note, the benefit of corticosteroids was seen only in resource-rich countries. Dexamethasone 0.4–0.6 mg/kg/day divided into four doses or 10 mg IV every six hours is the most commonly cited regimen, however, the Infectious Diseases Society of America guidelines recommend 0.15 mg/kg in infants and children every 6 hours for four days before or concurrent with the first dose of antibiotics.[21] Timing has historically been considered a crucial factor with the use of steroids in order to blunt the cytokine release which occurs with initial bacterial killing. Conversely, no effect was demonstrated in regards to the timing of corticosteroid treatment relative to antibiotic therapy in subgroups monitored in the aforementioned meta-analysis.[20] One important pharmacokinetic alteration is worth noting. In adult human studies, dexamethasone has demonstrated variable effects on vancomycin concentrations within the CSF. In one study of 11 patients, dexamethasone increased the risk of vancomycin therapeutic failure and need for alternative treatment, however, in another trial of 14 individuals CSF levels of vancomycin when administered via continuous infusion were not reduced. Close monitoring is recommended when vancomycin and corticosteroids

are used concomitantly for the treatment of bacterial meningitis.[22,23] Based on this data, BBB penetration of other large molecules similar to vancomycin may also be impaired with concomitant steroid use and result in therapeutic failures.

One major randomized controlled trial (RCT) exists evaluating the use of dexamethasone as adjunctive therapy in HIV-associated cryptococcal meningitis. This study was prematurely halted for safety after the enrolment of 451 patients. Patients in this study were given six weeks of corticosteroids in addition to combination antifungal therapy. The use of dexamethasone failed to decrease mortality and was associated with significantly higher rates of grade 3 or 4 infection, renal events, and cardiac events. Steroid utilization was also associated with increased disability at 10 weeks (25% vs 13%, p<0.001).[24] Guidelines do not recommend the use of steroids in cryptococcal meningitis unless immune response inflammatory syndrome is present.[25]

A recent meta-analysis of nine trials evaluated dexamethasone compared to control for tuberculous meningitis. Corticosteroid use was associated with decreased mortality, significant up to two years from patient enrolment. While disabling deficits were also less common in those treated with dexamethasone, this difference was not statistically significant and the quality of evidence was low. Steroid dose regimens from included studies are shown in Table 18.2.[26]

Table 18.2 Studies evaluating steroid treatment of tuberculosis meningitis in adults

Trial	Patient population	Steroid regimen	Endpoints
O'Toole[27]	23 Indian paediatric and adult patients with moderately advanced or severe disease	Dexamethasone 9 mg IV daily for 7 days, 6 mg IV daily for 7 days, 3 mg IV daily for 7 days, then 1.5 mg IV daily for 7 days	• Decreased day 4 CSF pressure • Decreased day 14, 21, and 28 CSF leukocyte counts • Decreased day 14 and 21 CSF protein counts
Girgis[28]	280 Egyptian paediatric and adult patients	Dexamethasone 12 mg IM daily for 21 days, then tapered over 21 days	• Decreased mortality • Decreased neurologic complications and permanent sequelae
Kumarvelu[29]	47 adult Indian patients with mild, moderate, and severe disease	Dexamethasone 16 mg IV daily for 7 days 8 mg PO daily for 21 days	• Non-significant decrease in sequelae • Non-significant improvement in mental function and daily activities
Chotmongkol[30]	59 adult Thailand HIV-negative patients with eosinophilic meningitis	Prednisolone 60 mg daily for 7 days, 45 mg daily for 7 days, 30 mg daily for 7 days, 20 mg daily for 7 days, then 10 mg daily for 7 days	• Non-significant increase in mortality • Non-significant increase in disabling neurologic deficit

Lardizabal[31]	58 adult Philippine patients with stage II and III disease	Dexamethasone (IV for 5 days, then oral) 16 mg daily for 21 days, 12 mg daily for 5 days, 8 mg daily for 5 days, then 4 mg daily for 5 days		• Non-significant decrease in mortality • Non-significant decrease in disabling neurologic deficit
Thwaites[32]	545 adult Vietnam patients with or without HIV infection	Grade II and III disease: Dexamethasone 0.4 mg/kg IV daily for 7 days, 0.3 mg/kg IV daily for 7 days, 0.2 mg/kg IV daily for 7 days, 0.1 mg/kg IV daily for 7 days, then 4 mg oral daily, followed by decrease of 1 mg every 7 days	Grade I disease: Dexamethasone 0.3 mg/kg IV daily for 7 days, 0.2 mg/kg IV daily for 7 days, 0.1 mg/kg oral daily for 7 days, then 3 mg oral daily followed by decrease of 1 mg every 7 days	• Decreased mortality • Non-significant increase in proportion of severely disabled patients
Prasad[26]	87 adult Indian patients	Dexamethasone 0.15 mg/kg up to 4 mg every 6 hours for 21 days, then tapered		• Non-significant decrease in mortality • Non-significant increase in disabling neurological deficit
Malhotra[33]	97 Indian HIV-negative patients	Dexamethasone 0.4 mg/kg IV daily for 7 days, 0.3 mg/kg IV daily for 7 days, 0.2 mg/kg IV daily for 7 days, then 0.1 mg/kg IV daily for 7 days Methylprednisolone IV 1 g daily for 5 days if >50 kg		• Non-significant decrease in death or disability • Non-significant increase in disabling neurological deficit

Notes: IV = intravenous; IM = intramuscular.

The use of corticosteroids for parasitic meningitis has also been evaluated. In a study of 110 patients with eosinophilic meningitis, the use of prednisolone 60 mg divided into three doses per day for two weeks decreased the time to headache resolution and frequency of headache at the end of treatment period. Corticosteroid use also decreased the need for repeat lumbar puncture and overall analgesic requirements.[34]

Acute Spinal Cord Injury

The use of glucocorticoids in the treatment of acute spinal cord injury (aSCI) is based on the clinical benefit from an anti-inflammatory effect and proposed inhibition of lipid peroxidation. Methylprednisolone likely has a more potent maximal antioxidant effect than other glucocorticoids, so the proposed mechanism of action may be important in clinical treatment decisions.[35] The use of corticosteroids in aSCI or traumatic spinal cord injury (tSCI) has been under debate for the past three decades since the publication of the second National Acute Spinal Cord Injury Study (NASCIS II) in 1990.[36] The three different studies evaluating the use of methylprednisolone in aSCI by NASCIS are listed in Table 18.3.[35] In a questionnaire survey study that was published on the use of methylprednisolone in the treatment of aSCI, the percentage of surgeons who used steroids in 2006 versus 2013 went from 89% down to 56%.[37] A study looking at the use of the NASCIS II methylprednisolone regimen in aSCI concluded that this regimen did not improve motor score recovery and had significantly higher rate of complications.[38] One of the major complications of high dose steroid use is the incidence of gastrointestinal bleeding. A single centre, case-controlled study reported a 2.77% incidence of gastrointestinal bleeding in patients who received steroids versus no events in those who did not. Of note, 33.3% of the patients that incurred gastrointestinal bleeding died.[39] Additional evidence exists showing that high-dose steroids are associated with harmful side effects, including death.[40] The off-label dosing of methylprednisolone for aSCI is 30 mg/kg intravenously over 15 minutes followed in 45 minutes by a continuous infusion of 5.4 mg/kg/hr times 23 hours within 8 hours of injury in most drug references. In the 2013 Guidelines for the Management of Acute Cervical Spine and Spinal Cord Injury, the level 1 recommendation is against the use of methylprednisolone in these patients.[40]

Table 18.3   Studies evaluating the use of methylprednisolone in aSCI by NASCIS

Study (year published)	Population	Study groups	Results
NASCIS I (1984, 1985)	• Open and closed acute SCI within 48 hr of injury • Age ≥13 yo • No severe comorbidity	• Methylprednisolone 1000 mg bolus, then 250 mg q6hr × 10d • Methylprednisolone 100 mg bolus, then 25 mg q6hr × 10d	• No statistically significant difference in motor or sensory function between groups
NASCIS II (1990, 1991)	• Predominantly closed acute SCI within 12 hr of injury • Age ≥13 yo • No life-threatening comorbidity • No maintenance steroids • No gunshot wounds	• Methylprednisolone 30 mg/kg, then 5.4 mg/kg per hour × 23 hr • Naloxone 5.4 mg/kg, then 4 mg/kg per hr × 23 hr • Placebo	• No statistically significant differences in motor or sensory function between groups • In the subgroup treated within 8 hr • Methylprednisolone group had 5.2-point greater motor recovery than placebo (P = 0.03) • In this subgroup, differences for pinprick and light touch were not statistically significant • Methylprednisolone and naloxone groups starting treatment at >8 hr after injury had impaired motor function recovery, but this finding was not statistically significant
NASCIS III (1997, 1998)	• aSCI within 8 hr of injury • Age ≥13 yo • No serious comorbidity • No maintenance MP • No gunshot wounds	• Methylprednisolone 20–40 mg/kg, then either • Methylprednisolone 5.4 mg/kg per hr × 23 hr • MP 5.4 mg/kg per hr × 48 hr • Tirilazad 2.5 mg/kg q6hr × 48 hr	• No statistically significant differences in motor or sensation recovery • No statistically significant differences in FIM improvement • Among those starting treatment >3 hr after injury, the 48 hr infusion group had a 5.3-point greater improvement in motor score (P = 0.053) • No statistically significant differences in sensation recovery in those treated >3 hr after injury

Clinicians considering methylprednisolone therapy for aSCI should be aware that methylprednisolone is not Food and Drug Administration (FDA) approved for this indication.[40]

Vasogenic Oedema

Vasogenic oedema is defined as the extracellular accumulation of fluid resulting from disruption of the BBB and extravasations of serum proteins, while cytotoxic oedema is defined as the accumulation of intracellular fluid causing cell swelling. Increases in brain volume and intracranial pressure can result from vasogenic oedema. The use of dexamethasone has been shown to counteract the inflammatory complex caused by cytokines and chemokines that result in BBB disruption and vasogenic oedema.[41] Steroids are recommended to provide temporary symptomatic relief of symptoms associated with increased intracranial pressure and oedema secondary to brain tumours.[42] Glucocorticoid use during the perioperative period for reducing peritumoural oedema has been proven efficacious.[43] Patients with headaches have been shown to respond better than patients with focal neurological deficits.[43] With regard to the effects of pre-surgery glucocorticoid treatment on intracranial pressure monitoring and improvement in symptoms the therapy needs to be in place for 24 to 48 hours to see improvement.[43] The dosing regimen for dexamethasone for cerebral oedema is an intravenous bolus of 10 to 20 mg followed by 4 mg every 6 hours. This regimen should be tapered off after maximum response is achieved over a week to two weeks. Response to dexamethasone has shown to be dose-dependent which may allow for the use of lower doses in patients with less severe cerebral oedema.[43]

CONCLUSIONS

Corticosteroids have an important role in the management of neurologic critical care conditions. They alleviate the inflammatory process and bring about beneficial effects. However, the dose and selection of steroids depends on the underlying pathology. At the same time, one must consider potential neurologic side effects with steroid use.

REFERENCES

1. Gomes JA, Stevens RD, Lewin JJ 3rd, Mirski MA, Bhardwaj A. Glucocorticoid therapy in neurologic critical care. *Crit Care Med* 2005;33(6):1214–24.

2. Sapolsky RM, Pulsinelli WA. Glucocorticoids potentiate ischemic injury to neurons: Therapeutic implications. *Science* 1985;229:1397–1400.

3. Anderson DC, Cranford RE. Glucocorticoids in ischemic stroke. *Stroke* 1979;10:68–71.

4. Dietrich J, Rao K, Pastorino S, Kesari S. Corticosteroids in brain cancer patients: benefits and pitfalls. *Expert Rev Clin Pharmacol* 2011;4(2):233–42.

5. Konagaya M, Bernard PA, Max SR. Blockade of glucocorticoid receptor binding and inhibition of dexamethasone-induced muscle atrophy in the rat by RU38486, a potent glucocorticoid antagonist. *Endocrinology* 1986;119(1):375–80.

6. Singleton JR, Baker BL, Thorburn A. Dexamethasone inhibits insulin-like growth factor signaling and potentiates myoblast apoptosis. *Endocrinology* 2000;141(8):2945–50.

7. Dropcho EJ, Soong SJ. Steroid-induced weakness in patients with primary brain tumors. *Neurology* 1991;41(8):1235–9.

8. Bowyer SL, LaMothe MP, Hollister JR. Steroid myopathy: incidence and detection in a population with asthma. *J Allergy Clin Immunol* 1985;76(2 Pt 1):234–42.

9. Gilad G, Rabey J, Gilad V. Presynaptic effects of glucocorticoids on dopaminergic and cholinergic synaptosomes. Implications for rapid endocrine-neural interactions in stress. *Life Sci* 1987;40(25):2401–8.

10. Schreiber MP, Colantuoni E, Bienvenu OJ, et al. Corticosteroids and transition to delirium in patients with acute lung injury. *Crit Care Med* 2014;42(6):1480–6.

11. Brunner R, Schaefer D, Hess K, Parzer P, Resch F, Schwab S. Effect of corticosteroids on short-term and long-term memory. *Neurology* 2005;64(2):335–7.

12. Moritz ML. Syndrome of inappropriate antidiuresis and cerebral salt wasting syndrome: are they different and does it matter? *Pediatr Nephrol* 2012;27(5):689–93.

13. Maesaka JK, Imbriano L, Mattana J, Gallagher D, Bade N, Sharif S. Differentiating SIADH from cerebral/renal salt wasting: failure of the volume approach and need for a new approach to hyponatremia. *J Clin Med* 2014;3(4):1373–85.

14. Mori T, Katayama Y, Kawamata T, Hirayama T. Improved efficiency of hypervolemic therapy with inhibition of natriuresis by fludrocortisone in patients with aneurysmal subarachnoid hemorrhage. *J Neurosurg* 1999;91(6):947–52.

15. Lee P, Jones GR, Center JR. Successful treatment of adult cerebral salt wasting with fludrocortisone. *Arch Intern Med* 2008;168(3):325–6.

16. Taplin CE, Cowell CT, Silink M, Ambler GR. Fludrocortisone therapy in cerebral salt wasting. *Pediatrics* 2006;118(6):e1904–e1908.

17. Yee AH, Burns JD, Wijdicks EF. Cerebral salt wasting: pathophysiology, diagnosis, and treatment. *Neurosurg Clin N Am* 2010;21(2):339–52.

18. Lutsar I, Friedland IR, Jafri HS, et al. Factors influencing the anti-inflammatory effect of dexamethasone therapy in experimental pneumococcal meningitis. *J Antimicrob Chemother* 2003;52(4):651–5.

19. Castelblanco RL, Lee M, Hasbun R. Epidemiology of bacterial meningitis in the USA from 1997 to 2010: a population-based observational study. *Lancet Infect Dis* 2014;14(9):813–9.

20. Brouwer MC, McIntyre P, Prasad K, van de Beek D. Corticosteroids for acute bacterial meningitis. *Cochrane Database Syst Rev* 2015;(9):CD004405.

21. Tunkel AR, Hartman BJ, Kaplan SL, et al. Practice guidelines for the management of bacterial meningitis. *Clin Infect Dis* 2004;39(9):1267–84.

22. Viladrich PF, Gudiol F, Liñares J, et al. Evaluation of vancomycin for therapy of adult pneumococcal meningitis. *Antimicrob Agents Chemother* 1991;35(12):2467–72.

23. Ricard JD, Wolff M, Lacherade JC, et al. Levels of vancomycin in cerebrospinal fluid of adult patients receiving adjunctive corticosteroids to treat pneumococcal meningitis: a prospective multicenter observational study. *Clin Infect Dis* 2007;44(2):250–5.

24. Beardsley J, Wolbers M, Kibengo FM, et al. Dexamethasone in HIV-associated cryptococcal meningitis. *N Engl J Med* 2016;374(6):542–54.

25. Panel on Opportunistic Infections in HIV-Infected Adults and Adolescents. Guidelines for the prevention and treatment of opportunistic infections in HIV-infected adults and adolescents: recommendations from the Centers for Disease Control and Prevention, the National Institutes of Health, and the HIV Medicine Association of the Infectious Diseases Society of America. [cited 2016 November 15]. Available from: http://aidsinfo.nih.gov/contentfiles/lvguidelines/adult_oi.pdf.

26. Prasad K, Singh MB, Ryan H. Corticosteroids for managing tuberculous meningitis. *Cochrane Database Syst Rev* 2016;28(4):CD002244.

27. O'Toole RD, Thornton GF, Mukherjee MK, Nath RL. Dexamethasone in tuberculous meningitis. Relationship of cerebrospinal fluid effects to therapeutic efficacy. *Ann Intern Med* 1969;70(1):39–48.

28. Girgis NI, Farid Z, Kilpatrick ME, Sultan Y, Mikhail IA. Dexamethasone adjunctive treatment for tuberculous meningitis. *Pediatr Infect Dis J* 1991;10(3):179–83.

29. Kumarvelu S, Prasad K, Khosla A, Behari M, Ahuja GK. Randomized controlled trial of dexamethasone in tuberculous meningitis. *Tubercle and Lung Disease* 1994;75(3):203–7.

30. Chotmongkol V, Jitpimolmard S, Thavornpitak Y. Corticosteroid in tuberculous meningitis. *J Med Assoc Thai* 1996;79(2):83–90.

31. Lardizabal DV, Roxas AA. Dexamethasone as adjunctive therapy in adult patients with probable TB meningitis stage II and stage III: An open randomised controlled trial. *Philippines Journal of Neurology* 1998;4:4–10.

32. Thwaites GE, Nguyen DB, Nguyen HD, et al. Dexamethasone for the treatment of tuberculous meningitis in adolescents and adults. *N Engl J Med* 2004;351(17):1741–51.

33. Malhotra HS, Garg RK, Singh MK, Agarwal A, Verma R. Corticosteroids (dexamethasone versus intravenous methylprednisolone) in patients with tuberculous

meningitis. *Ann Trop Med Parasitol* 2009;103(7): 625–34.

34. Chotmongkol V, Sawanyawisuth K, Thavornpitak Y. Corticosteroid treatment of eosinophilic meningitis. *Clin Infect Dis* 2000;31(3):660–2.

35. Breslin K, Agrawal D. The Use of Methylprednisolone in Acute Spinal Cord Injury: A Review of the Evidence, Controversies, and Recommendations. *Pediatr Emer Care* 2012;28: 1238–48.

36. Bracken MB, Shepard MJ, Collins WF, et al. A randomized, controlled trial of methylprednisoloneor naloxone in the treatment of acute spinal-cord injury. Results of the Second National Acute Spinal Cord Injury Study. *N Engl J Med* 1990;322:1405–11.

37. Schroeder GD, et al. Survey of cervical spine research society members on the use of high-dose steroids foracute spinal cord injuries. *Spine* 2014;39:971–7.

38. Evanview N, et al. Methylprednisolone for the treatment of patients with acute spinal cord injuries: a propensity score-matched cohort study from a Canadian multi-center spinal cord injury registry. *J Neurotrauma* 2015;32:1674–83.

39. Kahn MF, et al. The effect of steroids on the incidence of gastrointestinal hemorrhage after spinal cord injury: a case–controlled study. *Spinal Cord* 2014;52:58–60.

40. Hurlbert RJ, et al. Pharmacological therapy for acute spinal cord injury. *Neurosurgery* 2103;72:93–105.

41. Michinaga S, Koyama Y. Pathogenesis of brain edema and investigation into anti-edema drugs. *Int J Mol Sci* 2015;16:9949–75.

42. Ryken TC, et al. The role of steroids in the management of brain metastases: a systematic review and evidence-based clinical practice guideline. *J Neurooncol* 2010;96: 103–14.

43. Bebawy JF. Perioperative steroids for peritumoral intracranial edema: A review of mechanisms, efficacy, and side effects. *J Neurosurg Anesthesiol* 2012;24:173–77.

19

Anticoagulants

C. Der-Nigoghossian and K. Berger

ABSTRACT

This chapter discusses the pharmacology and monitoring of parenteral and oral anticoagulants, antiplatelets and fibrinolytics in neurocritically ill patients. The risk of antithrombotics in this patient population is substantial and careful assessment of the risks and benefits is needed. Management of bleeding complications including reversal strategies tailored to each antithrombotic agent is described. Neurocritically ill patients have unique needs and cautious evaluation of the need for holding and restarting antithrombotics after an intracranial haemorrhage (ICH) is essential.

KEYWORDS

Venous thromboembolism (VTE); anticoagulants; fibrinolytics; antiplatelets; antithrombotic reversal; heparin-induced thrombocytopenia; bleeding.

INTRODUCTION

Neurocritically ill patients are at high risk for venous thromboembolism (VTE) with an incidence of asymptomatic deep vein thrombosis (DVT) of 20% in patients with intracranial haemorrhage (ICH), subarachnoid haemorrhage (SAH), and ischaemic stroke. In addition, pulmonary embolism is the third leading cause of death in patients with traumatic brain injury (TBI).[1] However, anticoagulants are not benign in this patient population and have been associated with a higher rate of mortality and prolonged bleeding in intracerebral haemorrhage.[2] Patients with large hemispheric ischaemic strokes are also at a high risk for haemorrhagic conversion with the concomitant use of anticoagulation.[3] Therefore, prevention and treatment of VTE can be challenging in these patients, especially in the presence of ICH. Careful evaluation of patient specific factors and timing of neurosurgical procedures is essential when initiating antithrombotic therapy in these patients.[1,4]

CHARACTERISTICS OF ANTITHROMBOTIC AGENTS

Parenteral Anticoagulants

Parenteral anticoagulants are those that are administered by routes other than the oral route. Unfractionated heparin (UFH) works by binding to antithrombin and converting it from a slow to very rapid inhibitor of several clotting factors including IXa, Xa, XIIa, and thrombin (IIa). Long heparin chains can also catalyse the inactivation of thrombin by forming a bridge between antithrombin and thrombin.[5] Low molecular weight heparins (LMWHs) are derived from UFH and are shorter chains of polysaccharides. Their main mechanism of anticoagulation is similar to UFH, potentiating antithrombin-mediated inhibition of coagulation factors. Most LMWHs are too short to bridge between antithrombin and thrombin. Low molecular weight heparins have an anti-Xa to anti-IIa ratio of 2:1 to 4:1 compared to a 1:1 ratio for UFH. Fondaparinux is a synthetic antithrombin-binding pentasaccharide. It selectively inhibits factor Xa activity, but does not inactivate IIa and does not affect platelet function. Unfractionated heparin binds to plasma proteins, which can reduce its anticoagulant activity. Low molecular weight heparins have less binding to plasma proteins compared to UFH resulting in higher bioavailability and more predictable anticoagulation response when given subcutaneously. Low molecular weight heparins are renally eliminated and have a prolonged elimination half-life in patients with renal dysfunction (Table 19.1). Fondaparinux is primarily eliminated unchanged in the kidneys and is contraindicated

Table 19.1 Parenteral anticoagulants

	UFH	Enoxaparin	Dalteparin	Fondaparinux	Argatroban	Bivalirudin
Indication and dosing						
Treatment	80 units/kg IV bolus; then 18 units/kg/hr	1 mg/kg subcutaneous every 12 hr or 1.5 mg/kg subcutaneous once daily	200 units/kg once daily or 100 units twice daily	<50 kg: 5 mg 50–100 kg: 7.5 mg >100 kg: 10 mg subcutaneous once daily	1–2 mcg/kg/min Start at 0.2 mcg/kg/min in critically ill patients with MODS	0.75 mg/kg IV bolus; then 1.75 mg/kg/hr
Prophylaxis of DVT/PE	5,000 units subcutaneous every 8 to 12 hr	40 mg subcutaneous once daily or 30 mg subcutaneous twice daily	2,500–5,000 units subcutaneous once daily	2.5 mg subcutaneous once daily	N/A	N/A
Pharmacokinetics						
Metabolism/ Elimination	Hepatic and reticulo-endothelial	Hepatic/Renal (40%)	Renal (20%)	Renal	Hepatobiliary	Plasma proteolysis (80%)/Renal (20%)
Half-life	30–90 min	3–6 hr	2–5 hr	17–21 hr	39–51 min	25 min
Dose adjustment in renal impairment	No	Yes	Yes	CI if CrCl <30 ml/min	No	Yes
Dose adjustment in hepatic impairment	No	No	No	No	Yes	No
Monitoring	aPTT, anti-Xa	Anti-Xa	Anti-Xa	Anti-Xa	aPTT	aPTT
Pre-surgery interruption	IV infusion: 4–6 hr Subcutaneous: 8–12 hr	12 hr (prophylaxis) 24 hr (treatment)	24 hr	2–4 days	3–4 hr	2–3 hr

Abbreviations: UFH: unfractionated heparin; aPTT: activated partial thromboplastin time; N/A: not applicable; MODS: multiple organ dysfunction; CI: contraindicated.

Sources: (1) Kearon C, Akl E, Ornelas J, et al. Antithrombotic therapy for VTE disease. Chest guideline and expert panel report. Chest 2016;149: 315–52. (2) Garcia DA, Baglin TP, Weitz JI, et al. Parenteral anticoagulants: antithrombotic therapy and prevention of thrombosis, 9th ed: American College of Chest Physicians evidence-based clinical practice guidelines. Chest 2012;141:e24S–e43S. (3) Baharoglu MI, Cordonnier C, Salman RA, et al. Platelet transfusion versus standard care after acute stroke due to spontaneous cerebral haemorrhage associated with antiplatelet therapy (PATCH): a randomised, open-label, phase 3 trial. Lancet 2016;387:2605–13. (4) Hemphill JC, Greenberg SM, Anderson CS, et al. Guidelines for the management of spontaneous intracerebral hemorrhage. Stroke 2015;46:2032–60. (5) Douketis JD, Spyropoulos AC, Spencer FA, et al. Perioperative management of antithrombotic therapy. Antithrombotic therapy and prevention of thrombosis. 9th ed. American College of Chest Physicians evidence-based clinical practice guidelines. Chest 2012;141:e326s–e350s. (6) Horlocker TT, et al. Regional anesthesia in the patient receiving antithrombotic or thrombolytic therapy. American Society of Regional Anesthesia and Pain Medicine evidence-based guidelines. 3rd ed. Reg Anesth Pain Med 2010;35:64–101.

in patients with severe renal function impairment because of an increased bleeding risk. Therefore, in patients with renal insufficiency requiring therapeutic anticoagulation, the use of UFH over LMWHs or fondaparinux is recommended. Contrary to UFH, LMWH and fondaparinux; the direct thrombin inhibitors do not require a plasma cofactor to exert their antithrombotic effect. These include bivalirudin, desirudin, and argatroban, which inhibit both circulating and clot-bound thrombin.[5]

Oral Anticoagulants

Oral anticoagulants are used to prevent the occurrence or increase of unwanted blood clots. Warfarin, a vitamin

K antagonist, inhibits the enzymes responsible for the activation of vitamin K and hinders the synthesis of vitamin K-dependent coagulation factors II, VII, IX, and X as well as proteins C and S. Dabigatran, rivaroxaban, apixaban, and edoxaban are oral anticoagulants that directly inhibit specific coagulation factors. Dabigatran etexilate is a prodrug hydrolysed to its active moiety by plasma and hepatic esterases. It specifically and reversibly inhibits both free and fibrin-bound thrombin. Rivaroxaban, apixaban, and edoxaban are direct factor Xa inhibitors that inhibit both free and fibrin-bound Xa. These agents provide multiple benefits over warfarin including fixed dosing, no requirement for routine anticoagulation monitoring, and a rapid onset of action eliminating the need for bridging with parenteral anticoagulation. They have been associated with a lower incidence of haemorrhagic stroke than warfarin in patients with atrial fibrillation. It is important to note that direct oral anticoagulants (DOACs) have not been studied in critically ill patients. Direct oral anticoagulants have less drug-drug interactions than warfarin and a more predictable pharmacodynamic and pharmacokinetic profile. However, clinically relevant interactions still occur with these agents through the cytochrome P3A4 (CYP3A4) and P-gP pathways. Strong inducers including carbamazepine, phenobarbital, and phenytoin will reduce circulating levels of the DOACs and the combination should be avoided.[6] Other factors to address including enteral access, renal function, and the need for procedures or surgeries are listed in Table 19.2.

Fibrinolytics

Fibrinolytics are proteolytic enzymes that activate the conversion of plasminogen to plasmin. These agents play a fundamental role in the management of ischaemic stroke, high-risk pulmonary embolism, and ST elevation myocardial infarction (STEMI).[7,8] Although alteplase is selective to fibrin bound plasminogen, it can also bind to other circulating proteins including fibrinogen, which can lead to bleeding. The dose of alteplase for the treatment of acute ischaemic stroke (AIS) is 0.9 mg/kg intravenous (IV) (maximum 90 mg) over 1 hour with 10% of the dose given as an IV bolus over 1 minute.[7] When alteplase is used for the treatment of pulmonary embolism it is administered as a flat, non-weight-based dose of 50–100 mg over 1–2 hours.

Tenecteplase is a fibrinolytic agent variant of alteplase that is genetically engineered to have slower plasma clearance, higher specificity for fibrin and high resistance to plasminogen-activator inhibitor-1 (PAI-1).[8] It is used for the treatment of STEMI but is contraindicated in patients with an ischaemic stroke in the previous three

months, previous ICH, active internal bleeding, and acute bleeding diathesis.[4,8]

Intra-arterial thrombolysis (IAT) is also used for the management of ischaemic stroke presenting with large vessel occlusions. The use of IAT has been reported with urokinase, prourokinase, streptokinase, alteplase, and reteplase. The type and dosing of IAT have not been standardized and are usually institution-specific.[9]

Antiplatelets

Antiplatelet agents are used for the treatment and prevention of stent thrombosis, myocardial infarction and cerebrovascular accidents (Table 19.3). Aspirin inhibits thromboxane A_2-mediated platelet activation and aggregation. Although aspirin has a half-life of 15–20 minutes, it irreversibly binds to platelets for the life of the platelet. Thus, its antiplatelet effects are maintained even after cessation of aspirin. Dipyridamole is a phosphodiesterase inhibitor that causes intraplatelet accumulation of cyclic adenosine monophosphate (AMP) and platelet inhibition.[10] $P2Y_{12}$ receptor inhibitors include clopidogrel, prasugrel, ticagrelor, and cangrelor (currently, the only parenteral $P2Y_{12}$ agent available). These agents inhibit adenosine diphosphate (ADP)-mediated platelet aggregation to prevent a conformational change of glycoprotein (GP) IIb/IIIa receptor. Pharmacogenomics variance in the *ABCB1* gene as well as CYP2C9 and CYP2C19 enzyme function can cause reduced or increased conversion of clopidogrel to its active metabolite. Therefore, interpatient variability presents a major limitation of clopidogrel. Prasugrel has a more rapid onset of action and predictable antiplatelet effect than clopidogrel. However, it is not recommended in patients with a history of stroke or transient ischaemic attack (TIA), >75 years old or <60 kg due to an increased risk of bleeding that outweighs its benefit.[10,11]

Abciximab, eptifibatide, and tirofiban are parenteral antiplatelets that inhibit GP IIb/IIIa receptors preventing platelet binding to fibrinogen and platelet aggregation. Abciximab is a murine monoclonal antibody that has a prolonged platelet-bound half-life which accounts for its prolonged platelet inhibition. Tirofiban and eptifibatide reversibly inhibit platelets and will produce restoration of platelet function within 6–8 hours of discontinuation. The latter two agents are renally eliminated and require dose adjustment in renal impairment.[12] Intra-arterial administration of tirofiban, eptifibatide, and abciximab has been shown to be safe and effective for the treatment of thromboembolism encountered during aneurysmal coil embolization.[13]

Table 19.2 Oral anticoagulants

	Rivaroxaban	Apixaban	Edoxaban	Dabigatran	Warfarin
FDA-approved indications and dosing					
Treatment of DVT/PE	15 mg PO twice daily for 21 days; then 20 mg daily	10 mg PO twice daily for 7 days; then 5 mg PO twice daily	After 5–10 days of parenteral anticoagulation: 60 mg PO once daily

30 mg once daily if: CrCl 15–50 ml/min, <60 kg, or use of P–gp inhibitors | After 5–10 days of parenteral anticoagulation: 150 mg twice daily

CrCl ≤30 ml/min Use not recommended | Individualized dosing Can start at 2–5 mg PO once daily |
| Prevention of stroke and systemic embolism in atrial fibrillation | 20 mg PO daily CrCl 15–50 ml/min 15 mg PO daily CrCl <15 ml/min not recommended | 5 mg PO twice daily

2.5 mg PO twice daily if ≥2 of: >80 yo; <60 kg; SCr >1.5 mg/dL | CrCl 50–95 ml/min 60 mg PO daily CrCl 15–50 ml/min 30 mg PO daily | 150 mg PO twice daily CrCl 15–30 ml/min 75 mg PO twice daily CrCl <15 ml/min not recommended | |
Prophylaxis of DVT/PE (post hip or knee replacement)	10 mg PO daily CrCl <30 ml/min not recommended	2.5 mg PO twice daily	Not FDA-approved	110 mg once 1–4 hours after surgery, followed by 220 mg once daily	N/A
Pharmacokinetics					
Half-life	7–13 hr	12 hr	10–14 hr	12–14 hr (prolonged in renal impairment)	40 hr
Elimination	Renal (36%); Fecal (7%)	Renal (25%); Fecal (75%)	Renal (50%)	Renal (80%)	Renal (92%)
Drug interactions	Strong dual inhibitors/ inducers of CYP3A4 and P-gP	Strong dual inhibitors/inducers of CYP3A4 and P-gP	Potent P-gP inducers and inhibitors	Potent P-gP inducers and inhibitors	CYP 2C9, 3A4, 1A2
Tube feeding administration	Yes NG No NJ (absorption is reduced by 30%)	Yes	No	No	Yes
Pre-surgery interruption	24 hr	24–48 hr	24 hr	1–2 days CrCl ≤30 ml/min: 3–5 days	Variable (5–7 days)

Abbreviations: PO: Per os; CrCl: Creatinine clearance; FDA: Food and Drug Administration; P-gP: P-glycoprotein; CYP: Cytochrome P; NG: nasogastric; NJ: Nasojejunal.

Sources: (1) Adcock DM, Gosselin R. Direct oral anticoagulants (DOACs) in the laboratory: 2015 review. *Thromb Res* 2015;136:7–12. (2) Baharoglu MI, Cordonnier C, Salman RA, et al. Platelet transfusion versus standard care after acute stroke due to spontaneous cerebral haemorrhage associated with antiplatelet therapy (PATCH): a randomised, open-label, phase 3 trial. *Lancet* 2016;387:2605–13. (3) Hemphill JC, Greenberg SM, Anderson CS, et al. Guidelines for the management of spontaneous intracerebral hemorrhage. *Stroke* 2015;46:2032–60. (4) Douketis JD, Spyropoulos AC, Spencer FA, et al. Perioperative management of antithrombotic therapy. Antithrombotic therapy and prevention of thrombosis. 9th ed. American College of Chest Physicians evidence-based clinical practice guidelines. *Chest* 2012;141:e326s–e350s. (5) Horlocker TT, et al. Regional anesthesia in the patient receiving antithrombotic or thrombolytic therapy. American Society of Regional Anesthesia and Pain Medicine evidence-based guidelines. *Reg Anesth Pain Med* 2010;35:64–101.

Table 19.3 Antiplatelet agents

	Aspirin	Dipyridamole	Clopidogrel	Prasugrel	Ticagrelor	Cangrelor	Abciximab	Tirofiban	Eptifibatide	Cilostazol
Maintenance dose	81–325 mg once daily	75–100 mg 4 times/day (Dipyridamole SR 200 mg/ASA 25mg twice daily)	75 mg once daily	10 mg once daily	90 mg twice daily	4 mcg/kg/min	0.125 mcg/kg/min (max 10 mcg/kg/min)	0.15 mcg/kg/min	2 mcg/kg/min (max 15 mg/hr)	100 mg twice daily
Pro-drug	No	No	Yes	Yes	No	No	No	No	No	No
Route	Oral	Oral	Oral	Oral	Oral	IV	IV	IV	IV	Oral
Onset	30 min	30 min	2 hr	30–60 min	30–60 min	Immediate	10 min	Immediate	Immediate	3 hr
Duration of effect post-discontinuation	7 days	24 hr	5 days	7 days	3 days	30–60 min	8–15 days	3–4 hr	4 hr	2 days
Platelet inhibition	Irreversible	Reversible	Irreversible	Irreversible	Reversible	Reversible	Mainly irreversible	Reversible	Reversible	Reversible
% Platelet inhibition	20	–	40	70	95	>90	>80	>80	>80	–

Abbreviation: IV: intravenous.

Sources: (1) Hall R, Mazer CD. Antiplatelet drugs: a review of their pharmacology and management in the perioperative period. *Anesth Analg* 2011;112:292–318. (2) Wallentin L. P2Y(12) inhibitors: differences in properties and mechanisms of action and potential consequences for clinical use. *Eur Heart J* 2009 Aug;30(16):1964–77. (3) Baron TH, Kamath PS, McBane RD. Management of antithrombotic therapy in patients undergoing invasive procedures. *N Engl J Med* 2013;368:2113–24.

THERAPEUTIC MONITORING

The activated partial thromboplastin time (aPTT) is the most widely used test for monitoring anticoagulation with continuous infusions of UFH. A therapeutic range of 1.5 to 2.5 times the normal control value for the aPTT has been recommended although not evaluated in a randomized control trial.[14] Due to inter-laboratory variability, institution-specific therapeutic ranges are established. The aPTT should be measured every 6 hours after initiation or dosage changes and this correlates with steady state concentrations of UFH.[5] Some patients can have heparin resistance that presents with a diminished response to UFH. This might be caused by several mechanisms including high levels of heparin binding proteins, increased heparin clearance, and antithrombin deficiency. Patients who require very high doses of heparin (>35,000 units/day) should have their heparin dose adjusted based on the anti-Xa levels. Antithrombin concentrate can also be administered to patients with antithrombin deficiency (antithrombin activity level ≤60%) to potentiate the effect of UFH.[15] Since LMWHs have a more predictable anticoagulant response than UFH, routine laboratory monitoring is not recommended. Peak anti-Xa levels (target range 0.6–1.0 units/ml and >1 unit/ml for once daily and twice daily dosing, respectively) measured four hours after the third dose are recommended when used at therapeutic doses in patients with obesity, pregnancy, and renal insufficiency.[5]

The intravenous direct thrombin inhibitors are also monitored with aPTT; however, the dose-response is not linear and aPTT can plateau with higher doses. All direct thrombin inhibitors may elevate prothrombin time (PT)/international normalized ratio (INR) levels to variable extents. Argatroban has the largest effect on the INR.[5] The activated clotting time (ACT) is used to monitor the anticoagulant effect of heparin and direct thrombin inhibitor during cardiac and vascular surgeries.[16]

Due to a narrow therapeutic window, frequent monitoring of PT and INR is recommended with warfarin therapy. In addition, genetic factors including variations in proteins CYP2C9 and VKORC1 have been associated with interpatient dose-response variability. Although routine laboratory monitoring is not required for DOACs, some clinical scenarios may still warrant assessment of the degree of anticoagulation. Routine coagulation screening assays, including PT and aPTT are not reliable measures of the anticoagulant effect of the DOACs. The dilute thrombin time (dTT), ecarin clotting time (ECT), and specific chromogenic anti-Xa assays are suitable methods to measure anticoagulation with DOACs. However, to date these tests lack Food and Drug Administration (FDA) approved calibrators and validated therapeutic plasma concentrations.[17]

Multiple point-of-care platelet function tests are available for the assessment of antiplatelet medications. VerifyNow® is designed to assess platelet response to major antiplatelet agents including aspirin, $P2Y_{12}$ inhibitors, and GPIIb/IIIa antagonists. Platelet function analyser (PFA-100®) provides a rapid and sensitive assessment of platelet adhesion and aggregation.[18]

Thromboelastography (TEG®) and thromboelastometry (ROTEM®) are viscoelastic haemostatic assays that measure the properties of whole blood clot formation. These point-of-care tests are becoming increasingly important in the operating room and trauma settings to assess the need for specific blood product administration. Their use in patients who are receiving anticoagulants other than heparin has not been validated.

USE OF ANTITHROMBOTIC AGENTS IN SPECIAL POPULATIONS

Obesity

Therapeutic anti-Xa levels can be achieved in obese patients receiving therapeutic dosing of LMWHs based on the actual body weight.[19] However, standard fixed dosing of LMWHs for thromboprophylaxis in these patients has been shown to be suboptimal. Data suggest that weight-based dosing of 0.5 mg/kg subcutaneously once or twice daily or a fixed high dose of 40 mg twice daily results in peak anti-Xa levels within the recommended range for thromboprophylaxis in patients with a BMI ≥40 kg/m². It is important to note that only the studies evaluating fixed high dose of 40 mg twice daily were powered to assess bleeding and thrombosis rates.[20]

Similar to LMWHs, standard dosing of UFH 5,000 units every 8 to 12 hours may be suboptimal in obese patients. High dose UFH 7,500 units subcutaneously every 8 hours in neurocritical care patients >100 kg was not associated with an increased risk of bleeding or lower incidence of VTE compared to 5,000 units every 8 hours.[21] There is no prospective data evaluating the use of high-dose UFH, so the dosing in these patients is mainly based on clinicians' judgement. Standard dosing of DOACs is recommended in patients with a BMI ≤40 kg/m² and weight of ≤120 kg. Subgroup analyses of obese patients in the DOAC trials suggest that these agents are effective and safe in this patient population. Limited data is available in patients with a BMI >40 kg/m² or >120 kg.[22]

Pregnancy

Unfractionated heparin and LMWHs are the anticoagulants of choice in pregnancy and are FDA pregnancy category C and B, respectively. Due to their large molecular size, these agents do not cross the placenta and are not associated with teratogenic or bleeding complications in the foetus. Warfarin should not be used during pregnancy since it crosses the placenta and can cause foetal haemorrhage, central nervous system abnormalities and embryopathy. Direct oral anticoagulants have not been studied in pregnancy and cannot be recommended in this patient population at this time.[4,5]

Cancer

Venous thromboembolism is a frequent complication of critically ill patients with brain tumours. Warfarin therapy in cancer patients can be challenging due to potential drug interactions with chemotherapy. In addition, randomized trials suggest that long-term therapy with LMWHs for VTE disease in this patient population significantly reduce the rate of recurrent VTE without increasing bleeding risks compared to warfarin. Therefore, guidelines suggest the use of LMWH or UFH over warfarin and DOACs in patients with cancer-associated thrombosis.[4]

MANAGEMENT OF ANTITHROMBOTIC COMPLICATIONS

Heparin-Induced Thrombocytopenia

Heparin-induced thrombocytopenia (HIT) is an uncommon but fatal condition that can lead to myocardial infarction, skin necrosis, stroke, and VTE. It is an immunoglobulin-mediated response to heparin molecules leading to platelet activation and thrombin generation. The 4T score is a clinical scoring system useful to evaluate the probability of HIT and is associated with a high negative predictive value. Points are assigned for a relative platelet decrease of at least 50%, an onset between 5 and 10 days after heparin exposure, and new thrombosis or skin necrosis at the injection site. Two laboratory tests are useful for the diagnosis of HIT. The enzyme-linked immunoabsorbent assay (ELISA) evaluates the presence of antibodies to heparin-platelet factor 4 (PF4) complex. The optical density correlates with the concentration of HIT antibodies in the patient sample. It has a high sensitivity but a low to moderate specificity. Two functional assays, the heparin-induced platelet aggregation (HIPA) and C_{14} serotonin release assay (SRA) have a high specificity and

sensitivity of >95% for the diagnosis of HIT. These assays test the ability of HIT antibodies from patients' serum to activate platelets from healthy volunteers. Due to the risk of false positive results, the ELISA test should only be sent in patients with an intermediate or high probability of HIT based on the 4T score. Patients with a positive ELISA test should have a follow-up functional assay (the SRA test) sent to confirm the diagnosis. While awaiting the laboratory results, all forms of heparin should be immediately discontinued and treatment of HIT should be initiated with an intravenous direct thrombin inhibitor such as argatroban or bivalirudin. In patients who are considered to be at high bleeding risk and cannot be anticoagulated, prophylaxis with fondaparinux may be considered. Warfarin is not recommended in the early stages of HIT due to a paradoxical microvascular thrombosis which can cause venous limb gangrene and skin necrosis. Warfarin can be initiated upon resolution of thrombocytopenia.[5,23]

Bleeding

The most common major adverse reaction associated with anticoagulants, antiplatelets, and fibrinolytics is bleeding. While minor bleeding such as epistaxis can be managed by reducing or holding a dose, patients with major bleeding or those requiring urgent surgery or procedures will require reversal of their antithrombotic agent. The need for reversal depends not only on the severity of the bleed, but also on the pharmacokinetic properties of the anticoagulant, the patient's renal and hepatic function, and the time since the last dose of the anticoagulant. The potential benefits of reversal in these cases should outweigh the thromboembolic risks associated with many of the available reversal agents. Just as supratherapeutic anticoagulation can result in clinical bleeding, unnecessary reversal may result in thromboembolic events without additional haemostasis benefits. The factors that should be considered as part of the risk assessment include the severity of bleed, indication for anticoagulation, and previous thrombosis history or thrombotic risk factors. A patient who presents with a life-threatening ICH will likely receive a different reversal regimen than someone with minor oozing through an IV site. Also, more caution might be employed when reversing a patient who is being anticoagulated for a mechanical valve than for stroke prevention in atrial fibrillation. All of these factors must be taken into consideration when determining a reversal strategy.

Of note, there are different types of pharmacological reversals. In some cases, a targeted reversal agent or antidote can be administered to directly reverse the effects of the anticoagulant. An example of this is the monoclonal antibody idarucizumab which binds to dabigatran and neutralizes its anticoagulant effect. Other drugs such as antiplatelet and fibrinolytic agents do not have targeted antidotes. Administration of a 'reversal' agent in these cases provides normalization of anticoagulation markers and possible haemostasis, but does not reverse the effects of the drug. For example, when the 4F-PCC Kcentra® is used for the reversal of apixaban, it does not directly reverse the effects of apixaban. However, the concentrated factors aid haemostasis in the presence of an anticoagulant. Recommendations for the reversal of antithrombotic agents are listed in Table 19.4.

Reversal Strategies for Parenteral Anticoagulants

Reversal strategies for parenteral anticoagulant agents differ based on mechanisms of action and pharmacokinetic profile. Unfractionated heparin has a short half-life and minor bleeding can sometimes be resolved just by holding the infusion; however, LMWHs have a longer half-life and require additional intervention. When urgent reversal is required, protamine may be considered for both anticoagulants. Protamine is a cationic peptide molecule derived from salmon sperm that binds to and rapidly neutralizes heparin.[24] Due to its lack of effect on anti-factor Xa, protamine only partially reverses LMWHs and is not indicated for the reversal of fondaparinux.[25] Unfortunately, protamine itself has anticoagulant properties, thus, it is imperative that protamine is dosed correctly based on the amount of recent heparin exposure.[26] Overestimation of heparin exposure can lead to overdosing of protamine and paradoxical increases in ACT and even bleeding.[27] In addition, clinicians should monitor for rebleeding due to a rebound effect that can occur hours after protamine administration. Protamine is associated with several serious adverse effects including pulmonary hypertension, systemic hypotension, and allergic reactions. The risk of hypertension is increased with high doses and rapid administration of protamine.[24,26]

Reversal Strategies for Oral Anticoagulants

Warfarin

Although vitamin K is the antidote for warfarin, its onset of action is delayed by 6–12 hours limiting its use as monotherapy for urgent reversal. Providing exogenous factors in the form of fresh frozen plasma (FFP) or concentrated factors (e.g., 4 factor prothrombin complex concentrates [4F-PCC]) provides an immediate haemostatic agent, but should be co-administered with vitamin K to allow the liver to start making endogenous factors and prevent rebound anticoagulation after factor consumption. Intravenous vitamin K has a faster onset than the oral formulation and is recommended for acute reversal. Subcutaneous and IM administration routes are not recommended due to their variable absorption and risk of haematoma formation, respectively.[28] The ICH related to vitamin K antagonists (INCH) trial found that 30 units/kg of 4F-PCC was superior to 20 ml/kg of FFP, with 67% of patients in the PCC group vs 9% in the FFP group reaching an INR of <1.2 within 3 hours.[29] Although guidelines recommend the administration of either 3F- or 4F-PCC, the 4F-PCC, KCentra® is the only FDA-approved PCC for the reversal of warfarin. (NCS reversal guidelines – Frontera).[30]

Dabigatran

Life-threatening bleeds caused by dabigatran, an irreversible oral direct thrombin inhibitor, were historically treated with concentrated factors such as 3F- or 4F-PCC and aPCC.[31] Recently, idarucizumab was approved for the reversal of dabigatran, changing the management approach of dabigatran reversal. Idarucizumab is a monoclonal antibody that binds to dabigatran with 350 times higher affinity than that of dabigatran to thrombin. Idarucizumab is specific to dabigatran and cannot be used to reverse the other direct thrombin inhibitors (argatroban and bivalirudin).[32] The recommended 5 g dose of idarucizumab does not depend on the dose of dabigatran or severity of bleed. Although idarucizumab rapidly normalized thrombin time and ECT in an interim analysis of 90 patients from the Reversal Effects of Idarucizumab on Active Dabigatran (RE-VERSE-AD) trial, the median time to cessation of bleed was 11.4 hours in the 35 evaluable bleeding patients. The study used radiographic criteria rather than onset of haemostasis to determine cessation of bleed and this may have resulted in longer reported time to haemostasis in many patients.[32] Some clinicians suggest that adjunctive treatment with haemostatic agents such as 3F- or 4F-PCC or aPCC may still be warranted in patients whose bleeding remains uncontrolled after administration of idarucizumab.[30] Dabigatran's primarily renal mode of elimination and low protein binding make haemodialysis a potential adjunctive therapy in bleeding patients, particularly those who present with renal failure.[33,34] Administration of vitamin K is not necessary for dabigatran-related bleeds since dabigatran directly inhibits thrombin unlike warfarin which indirectly inhibits vitamin K-dependent clotting factors.

Table 19.4 Reversal of antithrombotic agents

Reversal agent		Mechanism	Anticoagulant that it reverses	Common dose	Comments
Phytonadione (Vitamin K)		Essential co-factor for production of factors II, VII, IX, and X	Warfarin	5–10 mg IV	Delayed onset necessitates use with plasma or concentrated factors for urgent reversal Avoid rapid administration
Desmopressin		Vasopressin analogue; acts on extrarenal V2 receptors to stimulate release of vWF and fVIII	Antiplatelets (i.e., aspirin, clopidogrel, ticagrelor) (?)GIIb/IIIa inhibitors	0.3–0.4 mcg/kg IV	Limited data on efficacy in non-uremic bleeding
Idarucizumab		Monoclonal antibody that binds to dabigatran	Dabigatran	5 g IV	Possible rebound
Andexanet alfa		Recombinant Factor Xa acts as a decoy to factor Xa inhibitors	Apixaban Rivaroxaban (?)Edoxaban (?)Enoxaparin (?)Fondaparinux	400–800 mg IV bolus, followed by 4–8 mg/min infusion x2 hours	Rebound effect (anti-Xa levels increase after cessation of drip) Dose dependent on anticoagulant reversed, timing since last dose of anticoagulant, and dose of anticoagulant
Protamine		Binds to heparin to form a stable complex, neutralizing its anticoagulant activity	UFH LMWHs (i.e.; enoxaparin)	20–50 mg IV (based on heparin exposure)	1 mg protamine sulphate/ 100 units of heparin received in the previous 2.5 hours Only partially reverses LMWHs Protamine itself has anticoagulant properties and can affect aPTT
Concentrated factors	rFVIIa	Factor VIIa	Warfarin Dabigatran Rivaroxaban Apixaban (?)Edoxaban (?)Fondaparinux¶	1–5 mg IV¥	Not a true antidote, but provides haemostasis with concentrated factor replacement Amount of factors varies from vial with PCCs
	3F-PCC	Factors II, IX, X		25–50 units/kg IV (Max: 100 kg)£	
	4F-PCC	Factors II, VII, IX, X			
	4F-aPCC	Factors II, VIIa, IX, X			
Anti-fibrinolytics	Aminocaproic acid	Inhibit binding of plasmin to fibrin	Fibrinolytics (i.e., alteplase)	1–10 g IV bolus, followed by 1–2 g/hour*	Use limited to case reports TXA 10x more potent than aminocaproic acid Dose adjustment for renal impairment Risk of seizures with high dose TXA
	Tranexamic acid (TXA)			1 g IV bolus, followed by additional 1 g bolus 8 hours after first dose*	

UFH: unfractionated heparin; LMWH: low molecular weight heparin; rFVIIa: recombinant activated factor VII; PCC: prothrombin complex concentrate; DDAVP: 1-deamino-8-D-arginine vasopressin; (?): unknown.

¥Doses of 15–180 mcg/kg have been studied.

¶rFVIIa has been administered for fondaparinux reversal in case reports.

£Two randomized controlled trials of Kcentra vs plasma, used a maximum weight of 100 kg.

*Doses of antifibrinolytics vary based on indication; TXA based on CRASH-2 trial dosing.

Sources: (1) Khadzhynov D, Wagner F, Formella S, et al. Effective elimination of dabigatran by haemodialysis. A phase I single-centre study in patients with end-stage renal disease. *Thromb Haemost* 2013;109:596–605. (2) CRASH-2 trial collaborators. Effects of tranexamic acid on deathvascular occlusive events, and blood transfusion in trauma patients with significant haemorrhage (CRASH-2): a randomised, placebo-controlled trial. *Lancet* 2010;376:23.

Apixaban, rivaroxaban, and edoxaban

Like dabigatran, the oral Xa inhibitors apixaban, rivaroxaban, and edoxaban were also considered irreversible and treatment recommendations mostly included concentrated factors for haemostasis.[30] Andexanet alfa is a recombinant protein that acts as a factor Xa decoy, binding to the Xa inhibitors and neutralizing their anticoagulant effect. Due to its mechanism of action, andexanet can theoretically be used for the reversal of all factor Xa inhibitors and is also being studied for the reversal of enoxaparin (an indirect IIa and Xa inhibitor).[35] The andexanet bolus and two-hour infusion dosing depends on the Xa inhibitor that is reversed, the dose of the Xa inhibitor, and the time since last dose. The Andexanet Alfa, a Novel Antidote to the Anticoagulation Effects of FXA Inhibitors (ANNEXA-4) study showed that anti-factor Xa levels rapidly diminished following the andexanet bolus; however, a rebound effect was seen after cessation of the two-hour infusion. Despite this, 79% of patients had excellent or good haemostasis 12 hours after the andexanet infusion.[35] The effect of andexanet rebound on clinical outcomes requires further exploration. Unlike dabigatran, there is no role for haemodialysis in the elimination of the Xa inhibitors because they are highly protein bound (apixaban and rivaroxaban) or have been studied and failed to demonstrate significant removal by haemodialysis (edoxaban).[36] Similar to dabigatran, adjunctive vitamin K is not necessary for Xa inhibitor-related bleeds since they directly inhibit factor Xa.

Reversal Strategies for Fibrinolytics

Antifibrinolytics inhibit the conversion of plasminogen to plasmin preventing the breakdown of fibrin into fibrin degradation products. The nomenclature ('antifibrinolytics') makes these agents seem like an intuitive choice for the reversal of fibrinolytics (e.g., alteplase). Unfortunately, no prospective trial has assessed the benefit of antifibrinolytics for the reversal of fibrinolytic-associated bleeds and only a handful of published case reports have reported a benefit from their use for this indication.[37,38] Nonetheless, many institutional guidelines recommend the administration of an antifibrinolytic such as aminocaproic acid or tranexamic acid for bleeding due to fibrinolytic therapy. An alternative to antifibrinolytics in this setting is the administration of cryoprecipitate which provides exogenous fibrinogen. This may be the more appropriate management approach as it provides the needed substrate that has been depleted by alteplase.[30] Clinicians may empirically administer cryoprecipitate to patients with fibrinolytic-associated life-threatening bleeds, such as a clinically significant haemorrhagic conversion after an ischaemic stroke, as it may be impractical to wait for fibrinogen laboratory results.

Reversal Strategies for Antiplatelet Agents

Antiplatelet-associated bleeds may be difficult to manage because the pharmacodynamic effects of antiplatelets may extend past the pharmacokinetic half-life of the drug. While there is no reversal agent for antiplatelet drugs, desmopressin (1-deamino-8-D-arginine vasopressin, DDAVP), a vasopressin analogue, is often administered to bleeding patients or those reversed for emergent surgeries.[30] The DDAVP binds to extra-renal V2 receptors to stimulate endothelial release of von Willebrand factor and factor VIII. While in vivo this agent increases platelet adhesion, there are no prospective, placebo-controlled studies to support a clinical benefit of DDAVP in patients with ICH. Platelets are also often administered to patients receiving antiplatelet agents. Although conditionally recommended in the ICH reversal guidelines for those requiring surgical intervention,[30] the recent Platelet Transfusion Versus Standard Care After Acute Stroke due to Spontaneous Cerebral Haemorrhage Associated with Antiplatelet Therapy (PATCH) trial showed worse outcomes, including higher odds of a shift towards death or dependence at three months in patients who received platelets for ICH as compared to patients who did not receive platelets.[39] Thus, there does not seem to be a role for routine pharmacologic therapy (DDAVP) or blood products (platelets) for patients with antiplatelet-associated ICH who are not undergoing surgery. Additionally, haemodialysis is not an option for antiplatelet agent removal in bleeding patients. Clopidogrel, prasugrel, and ticagrelor (or their active metabolites) are all highly protein bound and not amenable to dialysis. Although there is data supporting haemodialysis for aspirin overdoses, the benefits of dialysis in these cases is for the management of acid/base abnormalities. The bleeding effects of aspirin will last for the platelet lifespan despite removal by dialysis.

HOLDING AND RESTARTING ANTICOAGULATION

Holding Venous Thromboembolism Prophylaxis for Elective/Scheduled Surgical Procedures

Most neurocritical care patients will require chemical VTE prophylaxis during their intensive care unit (ICU) stay.[1] Even when ordered in a timely manner, prophylaxis is often held for neurosurgical procedures, percutaneous endoscopic gastrostomy (PEG) tube placement, tracheostomy, and other procedures or surgical interventions. Moreover, pharmacologic prophylaxis is often inappropriately held after these procedures. Protocols with specific dosing recommendations as well as criteria for holding and time to restarting therapy should be developed in collaboration between neurosurgery and the ICU team as well as other surgical teams who frequently do procedures in the neurointensive care unit (i.e., general surgery for PEG/tracheostomy). Nurses should be educated on restarting prophylaxis when it is safe to do so. If patients refuse prophylaxis, nurses should inform the prescribing practitioner so that the patient can be counselled on the importance of therapy. Simple communication measures, education, and implementation of an algorithm can increase compliance to pharmacologic VTE prophylaxis.

Restarting Anticoagulation After Bleeding

Neurocritically ill patients who are admitted for an ICH or emergent neurosurgical procedure will require cessation and reversal of their anticoagulant therapy.[30]

There is no definitive data to support an optimal time for resumption of anticoagulant therapy and clinicians should carefully weigh the risks of bleeding with resumption against the risk of clotting from withholding therapy. Guidelines suggest that avoidance of oral anticoagulation for at least four weeks in patients without mechanical heart valves may decrease the risk of ICH recurrence, but that aspirin therapy can probably be started within days.[40] As the duration of time from the initial bleed increases, holding anticoagulation should be continually reassessed. Some clinicians may feel more comfortable restarting anticoagulation with an IV heparin infusion instead of direct oral anticoagulants due to their longer half-lives, lack of reversal agents, and inability to quantitatively monitor their level of anticoagulation. Heparin has a short duration and can be easily stopped or reversed if needed. If a patient's bleed remains stable on full dose anticoagulation, the heparin drip may be transitioned to a longer acting oral agent. Patients are often transitioned between oral and parenteral anticoagulants throughout their hospitalization (Table 19.5).

Table 19.5 Transitioning between anticoagulants

From this anticoagulant	To this anticoagulant	Recommendation		
Heparin	Enoxaparin	Start within 0–2 hours of discontinuation of heparin		
	Fondaparinux			
	DOAC	Start upon discontinuation of heparin		
Enoxaparin	Heparin	Prophylactic to prophylactic dosing: Start at next dosing interval of enoxaparin	Anticoagulation to anticoagulation dosing: Start at next dosing interval of enoxaparin	Prophylactic dosing of enoxaparin to anticoagulation dosing of new agent: Start new anticoagulant irrespective of last enoxaparin dose
	Fondaparinux			
	DOAC			
Argatroban	Heparin, enoxaparin	Start within 2 hours of discontinuation of argatroban (may be longer in hepatic insufficiency)		
	Fondaparinux			
	DOAC			
	Warfarin	Initiate warfarin while on argatroban (continue overlap x5 days); Argatroban elevates INR: When INR >4, hold argatroban and re-check INR in 4 hours; if therapeutic, discontinue argatroban		
Bivalirudin	Heparin, enoxaparin	Start within 2 hours of discontinuation of bivalirudin (may be longer in renal insufficiency)		
	Fondaparinux			
	DOAC			
	Warfarin	Initiate warfarin while on bivalirudin (continue overlap x5 days); Bivalirudin elevates the INR (less so than argatroban): When INR >2, hold bivalirudin and re-check INR in 4 hours, if therapeutic, discontinue bivalirudin		

(Cont'd)

Table 19.5 (*Cont'd*)

From this anticoagulant	To this anticoagulant	Recommendation		
Fondaparinux	Heparin, enoxaparin	Prophylactic to prophylactic dosing: Start at next dosing interval of fondaparinux	Anticoagulation to anticoagulation dosing: Start at next dosing interval of fondaparinux	Prophylactic dosing of fondaparinux to anticoagulation dosing of new agent: Start new anticoagulant irrespective of last fondaparinux dose
	DOAC			
DOAC	Heparin, enoxaparin	Start at next dosing interval of DOAC that is being discontinued (except if prophylactic doses of DOAC used)		
	Fondaparinux			
	Argatroban, bivalirudin			
	DOAC			
	Warfarin	Specific to individual DOAC		
Warfarin	Heparin, enoxaparin	Initiate when INR <2–3		
	Fondaparinux			
	Argatroban, bivalirudin			
	DOAC	Initiate when INR <2–3 (specific INR start points for each DOAC)		

Sources: (1) Douketis JD, Spyropoulos AC, Spencer FA, et al. Perioperative management of antithrombotic therapy. Antithrombotic therapy and prevention of thrombosis. 9th ed. American College of Chest Physicians evidence-based clinical practice guidelines. *Chest* 2012;141:e326s–e350s. (2) Horlocker TT, et al. Regional anesthesia in the patient receiving antithrombotic or thrombolytic therapy. American Society of Regional Anesthesia and Pain Medicine evidence-based guidelines. *Reg Anesth Pain Med* 2010;35:64–101. (3) Baron TH, Kamath PS, McBane RD. Management of antithrombotic therapy in patients undergoing invasive procedures. *N Engl J Med* 2013;368:2113–24.

CONCLUSIONS

There is a growing armamentarium of available antithrombotic agents with different pharmacological mechanisms of action and pharmacokinetic properties. The newer direct acting oral anticoagulants exhibit less inter-patient variability, easy dosing strategies, and low chances of ICH, but are more difficult to monitor and reverse. The most common major adverse event associated with antithrombotics is bleeding and new reversal agents allow clinicians to tailor reversal strategies. Enteral access, renal function, administration of enteral feeds, drug interactions, need for ongoing procedures or surgeries, and timing from drug administration and acute bleed are all important factors that should be considered prior to initiation or continuation of antithrombotic agents in neurocritically ill patients.

REFERENCES

1. Nyquist P, Bautista C, Jichici D, et al. Prophylaxis of venous thrombosis in neurocritical care patients: an evidence-based guideline: a statement for healthcare professionals from the neurocritical care society. *Neurocrit Care* 2016;24:47–60.
2. Rosand J, Eckman MH, Knudsen KA, Singer DE, Greenberg SM. The effect of warfarin and intensity of anticoagulation on outcome of intracerebral hemorrhage. *Arch Intern Med* 2004;164:880–4.
3. Hart RG, Lock-Wood KI, Hakim AM, et al. Immediate anticoagulation of embolic stroke: Brain hemorrhage and management options. *Stroke* 1984;15:779–89.
4. Kearon C, Akl E, Ornelas J, et al. Antithrombotic therapy for VTE disease. Chest guideline and expert panel report. *Chest* 2016;149:315–52.
5. Garcia DA, Baglin TP, Weitz JI, et al. Parenteral anticoagulants: antithrombotic therapy and prevention of thrombosis, 9th ed: American College of Chest Physicians evidence-based clinical practice guidelines. *Chest* 2012;141:e24S–e43S.
6. Soff GA. A new generation of oral direct anticoagulants. *Arterioscler Thromb Vasc Biol.* 2012;32:569–74.
7. National Institute of Neurological Disorders and Stroke rt-PA Stroke Study Group. Tissue plasminogen activator for acute ischemic stroke. *N Engl J Med* 1995;333(24):1581–7.
8. Jaff MR, McMurtry S, Stephen L, et al. Management of massive and submassive pulmonary embolism, iliofemoral deep vein thrombosis, and chronic thromboembolic pulmonary hypertension: a scientific statement from the American Heart Association. *Circulation* 2011;123:1788–830.
9. Mattle HP. Intravenous or intra-arterial thrombolysis? It's time to find the right approach for the right patient. *Stroke* 2007;38:2038–40.

10. Hall R, Mazer CD. Antiplatelet drugs: a review of their pharmacology and management in the perioperative period. *Anesth Analg* 2011;112:292–318.

11. Wallentin L. P2Y(12) inhibitors: differences in properties and mechanisms of action and potential consequences for clinical use. *Eur Heart J* 2009;30(16):1964–77.

12. Schror K, Weber AA. Comparative pharmacology of GP IIb/IIIa antagonists. *J Thromb Thrombolysis* 2003;15:71–80.

13. Brinjikji W, McDonald JS, Kallmes DF. Rescue treatment of thromboembolic complications during endovascular treatment of cerebral aneurysms. *Stroke* 2013;44:1343–7.

14. Basu D, Gallus A, Hirsh J, Cade J. A prospective study of the value of monitoring heparin treatment with the activated partial thromboplastin time. *N Engl J Med* 1972;287:324–7.

15. Finley A, Greenberg C. Review article: heparin sensitivity and resistance: management during cardiopulmonary bypass. *Anesth Analg* 2013;1210–22.

16. Saw J, Bajzer C, Casserly IP, et al. Evaluating the optimal activated clotting time during carotid artery stenting. *Am J Cardiol* 2006;97:1657–60.

17. Adcock DM, Gosselin R. Direct oral anticoagulants (DOACs) in the laboratory: 2015 review. *Thromb Res* 2015;136:7–12.

18. Bonello L, Tantry US, Marcucci R, et al. Consensus and future directions on the definition of high on-treatment platelet reactivity to adenosine diphosphate. *J Am Coll Cardiol* 2010;56:913–33.

19. Becker RC, Spencer FA, Gibson M, et al. TIMI 11A Investigators. Influence of patient characteristics and renal function on factor Xa inhibition pharmacokinetics and pharmacodynamics after enoxaparin administration in non-ST-segment elevation acute coronary syndromes. *Am Heart J* 2002;143:753–9.

20. Vandiver JW, Ritz LI, Lalama JT. Chemical prophylaxis to prevent venous thromboembolism in morbid obesity: literature review and dosing recommendations. *J Thromb Thrombolysis* 2016;41:475–81.

21. Samuel S, Iluonakhamhe EK, Adair E, et al. High dose subcutaneous unfractionated heparin for prevention of venous thromboembolism in overweight neurocritical care patients. *J Thromb Thrombolysis* 2015;40:302–7.

22. Martin K, Beyer-Westendorf J, Davidson BL, et al. Use of the direct oral anticoagulants in obese patients: guidance from the SSC of the ISTH. *J Thromb Haemost* 2016;14:1308–13.

23. Greinacher A. Heparin-induced thrombocytopenia. *N Engl J Med* 2015;373:252–61.

24. Horrow JC. Protamine: a review of its toxicity. *Anesth Analg* 1985;64:348–61.

25. Crowther MA, Berry LR, Monagle PT, Chan AK. Mechanisms responsible for the failure of protamine to inactive low-molecular-weight heparin. *Br J Haematol* 2002;116:178–86.

26. Sokolowska E, Kalaska B, Miklosz J, Mogielnicki A. The toxicology of heparin reversal with protamine: past, present and future. *Expert Opin Drug Metab Toxicol* 2016;12:897–909.

27. Mochizuki T, Olson PJ, Szlam F, et al. Protamine reversal of heparin affects platelet aggregation and activated clotting time after cardiopulmonary bypass. *Anesth Analg* 1998;87:781–5.

28. Holbrook A, Schulman S, Witt DM, et al. Evidence-based management of anticoagulant therapy: Antithrombotic Therapy and Prevention of Thrombosis. 9th ed. American College of Chest Physicians Evidence-Based Clinical Practice Guidelines. *Chest* 2012;141(Suppl 2):e152S–84S.

29. Steiner T, Poli S, Griebe M, et al. Fresh frozen plasma versus prothrombin complex concentrate in patients with intracranial haemorrhage related to vitamin K antagonists (INCH): a randomised trial. *Lancet Neurol* 2016;15:566–73.

30. Frontera JA, Lewin JJ 3rd, Rabinstein AA, et al. Guideline for reversal of antithrombotics in intracranial hemorrhage: a statement for healthcare professionals from the neurocritical care society and society of critical medicine. *Neurocrit Care* 2016;24:6–46.

31. Grottke O, Aisenberg J, Bernstein R, et al. Efficacy of prothrombin complex concentrates for the emergency reversal of dabigatran-induced anticoagulation. *Crit Care* 2016;20:115.

32. Pollack CV Jr, Reilly PA, Eikelboom J, et al. Idarucizumab for dabigatran reversal. *N Engl J Med* 2015;373:511–20.

33. Stangier J, Rathgen K, Stahle H, Mazur D. Influence of renal impairment on the pharmacokinetics and pharmacodynamics of oral dabigatran etexilate: an open-label, parallel-group, single-centre study. *Clin Pharmacokinet* 2010;49:259–68.

34. Khadzhynov D, Wagner F, Formella S, et al. Effective elimination of dabigatran by haemodialysis. A phase I single-centre study in patients with end-stage renal disease. *Thromb Haemost* 2013;109:596–605.

35. Connolly SJ, Milling TJ Jr, Eikelboom JW, et al. Andexanet alfa for acute major bleeding associated with factor Xa inhibitors. *N Engl J Med* 2016;375:1131–41.

36. Parasrampuria DA, Marbury T, Matsushima N, et al. Pharmacokinetics, safety, and tolerability of edoxaban in end-stage renal disease subjects undergoing haemodialysis. *Thromb Haemost* 2015;113:719–27.

37. Yaghi S, Beohme AK, Dibu J, et al. Treatment and outcome of thrombolysis-related hemorrhage: a multicenter retrospective study. *JAMA Neurol* 2015;72:1451–7.

38. Goldstein JN, Marrero M, Masrur S, et al. Management of thrombolysis-associated symptomatic intracerebral hemorrhage. *Arch Neurol* 2010;67:965–9.

39. Baharoglu MI, Cordonnier C, Salman RA, et al. Platelet transfusion versus standard care after acute stroke due to spontaneous cerebral haemorrhage associated with antiplatelet therapy (PATCH): a randomised, open-label, phase 3 trial. *Lancet* 2016;387:2605–13.

40. Hemphill JC, Greenberg SM, Anderson CS, et al. Guidelines for the management of spontaneous intracerebral hemorrhage. *Stroke* 2015;46:2032–60.

20

Muscle Relaxants

T. Human

ABSTRACT

For many years, neuromuscular blocking agents (NMBAs) and skeletal muscle relaxants have been used in neurocritical care. Considerations of the pharmacology, pharmacokinetics, drug interactions, and adverse effects in the acute neurologically injured patient needs to be understood in order to choose the most appropriate agent.

KEYWORDS

Neuromuscular blocking agents (NMBAs); skeletal muscle relaxants; baclofen withdrawal.

INTRODUCTION

For many years, neuromuscular blocking agents (NMBAs) have been used in neurocritical care for indications including tracheal intubation, ventilator synchrony, malignant intracranial hypertension, refractory shivering or tetany. Considerations of the pharmacology, pharmacokinetics, drug interactions, and adverse effects in the acute neurologically injured patient needs to be understood in order to choose the most appropriate agent.

MECHANISM OF ACTION OF NEUROMUSCULAR BLOCKING AGENTS

Neuromuscular blocking agents exhibit their effect through interruption of the signal transmission at the neuromuscular junction and are categorized as either depolarizing or non-depolarizing agents (Table 20.1). The only commercially available depolarizing NMBA, succinylcholine, works by mimicking the action of acetylcholine (ACh) at the nicotinic cholinergic receptor.[1] Receptor binding causes sodium and calcium cellular influx, ultimately resulting in membrane depolarization and then contraction. With succinylcholine, the initial depolarization may be seen clinically as fasciculations notably in the hands, feet, and face occurring within 30–60 seconds after administration.[2] This is followed by paralysis that lasts for 5–10 minutes. In order to prevent fasciculations, some providers administer a small dose of a non-depolarizing NMBA approximately three minutes prior to the succinylcholine bolus.[2,3] The non-depolarizing NMBA occupies a sufficient number of receptors to prevent widespread depolarization from succinylcholine channel activation. The short duration of effect of succinylcholine is secondary to its rapid metabolism by plasma pseudocholinesterases and should be used only for short procedures such as tracheal intubation, and is not indicated for prolonged use in the intensive care unit (ICU). These are specified in Table 20.2.

Non-depolarizing NMBAs are competitive antagonists at nicotinic receptors preventing Ach from binding to the receptor with resultant neuromuscular blockade.[1] Non-depolarizing NMBAs can be further classified based on their chemical structure, aminosteroid (pancuronium, vecuronium, rocuronium) or benzyl-isoquinolinium (atracurium, cisatracurium, doxacurium, mivacurium). Additionally, non-depolarizing agents differ in their onset, duration of activity (short, intermediate, long-acting), pharmacokinetic and adverse effect profiles, and cost, all of which should be considered when choosing the best NMBA for the patient. These have been discussed in detail in the following sections.

Table 20.1 Classification and pharmacology of neuromuscular blocking agents

	Pancuronium	**Vecuronium**	**Rocuronium**	**Atracurium**	**Cisatracurium**	**Succinylcholine**
Potency	Long acting	Intermediate	Intermediate	Intermediate	Intermediate	Short
Type*	A	A	A	B	B	D
Time to max blockade (min)	2–3	3–4	1–2	3–5	2–3	<1
Duration of action (min)	90–100	35–45	30	20–35	40–60	5–10

*A: aminosteroid, B: benzylisoquinolinium, D: depolarizing agent.
Sources: (1) Fisher DM. Clinical pharmacology of neuromuscular blocking agents. *Am J Health Syst Pharm*. 1999;56:S4–9. (2) Murray MJ, DeBlock H, Erstad B, et al. Clinical practice guidelines for sustained neuromuscular blockade in the adult critically ill patient. *Critical Care Medicine*. 2016;44:2079–103.

Table 20.2 Common continuous infusion dosing of neuromuscular blocking agents

Drug	**Bolus dosing**		**Continuous infusion**	
	Dosing	**Duration (single dose)**	**Maintenance infusion**	**Drip increment**
Pancuronium	0.05–0.1 mg/kg	90–100 min	1–2 mcg/kg/min	0.25 mcg/kg/min
Vecuronium	0.05–0.1 mg/kg	35–45 min	0.5–1.5 mcg/kg/min	0.25 mcg/kg/min
Rocuronium	0.6–1.2 mg/kg	30 min	10–12 mcg/kg/min	0.1 mg/kg/min
Cisatracurium	0.1–0.2 mg/kg	40–60 min	2–5 mcg/kg/min	2 mcg/kg/min

INDICATIONS FOR NEUROMUSCULAR BLOCKING AGENTS

The following indications may be observed for NMBAs:

- Tracheal Intubation
- Facilitate Mechanical Ventilation
- Decrease Oxygen Consumption
- Prevent or Treat Elevated Airway Pressures
- Malignant Intracranial Pressure
- Pathologic Tetany
- Refractory Shivering
- Therapeutic Hypothermia

Acute Respiratory Distress Syndrome[4]

Three multicentre randomized trials assessed the role of NMBA in patients with acute respiratory distress syndrome (ARDS) with an overarching positive result. Along with low tidal volume ventilation modes in patients with ARDS, a 48-hour infusion of cisatracurium improved oxygenation, decreased the risk of barotrauma, reduced 28-day and in-hospital mortality, and importantly did not increase the risk for ICU-acquired weakness.[5–7] The mechanism of these benefits are not fully understood, however, the theory is that the NMBA prevents ventilator asynchrony, elevated airway pressures, and worsening lung injury. Therefore, dose strategies for both continuous infusions and bolus dosing for plateau airway pressures exceeding 30–35 cm H_2O may be considered.

Traumatic Brain Injury

In patients with traumatic brain injury (TBI), NMBA are commonly considered for rapid sequence intubation, mechanical ventilator synchrony, attenuation of intracranial pressure (ICP) surges that may accompany tracheal suctioning, and for the management of malignant intracranial hypertension. The controversy as to whether bolus administration of NMBAs cause ICP elevations during rapid sequence intubation (RSI) can be addressed with the evaluation of these small studies. Two studies suggest that ICP elevations occurred after succinylcholine administration and one found a reduction in ICP after atracurium.[2,8,9] No other study observed changes in ICP after NMBA administration and therefore should be considered relatively safe for RSI. Caution should be considered in patients that may be sensitive to the vagolytic (pancuronium, rocuronium) or histamine-releasing (atracurium) effects and alternative agents (vecuronium) should be considered in such patients. Additionally, non-depolarizing agents may be considered safer when compared to succinylcholine.

Traumatic brain injury is an independent risk factor for acute lung injury and ventilation may be challenging in this population. Avoidance of ventilator asynchrony by administering NMBA may decrease the risk of barotrauma and prevent ICP spikes due to increased intra-thoracic pressures and reduced jugular venous return. Neuromuscular blocking agents may also reduce oxygen (O_2)

consumption by reducing energy expenditure.[4,10] The risks and benefits of administering NMBAs for mechanical ventilation synchrony has not been evaluated systematically in the TBI population, however, the benefits appear to outweigh the risks at this time, as long as adverse effects are monitored and closely managed.

Several small studies in TBI patients with ICP concerns have shown that doses of NMBAs given prior to suctioning are effective in mitigating cough and changes in ICP and cerebral perfusion pressure (CPP) during tracheal suctions.[9,11,12] These studies are small, observational, and report physiological outcomes that may have little impact on larger more significant outcomes. However, it seems to be reasonable to recommend small doses of NMBAs in patients with malignant ICPs prior to tracheal suctioning to prevent detrimental elevations in ICP.

Two retrospective studies addressed the question as to whether NMBAs should be used to manage elevated ICPs in the TBI population. Hsiang et al. reviewed 514 patients from the National Coma Data Bank and found that early paralysis, continued for at least 12 hours in patients with severe TBI, did not improve outcomes but increased the risk of pneumonia, prolonged ICU length of stay, and resulted in a higher proportion of survivors with severe disability compared to patients that received NMBAs for less than six hours.[13] Even after controlling for age, admission Glasgow Coma Scale (GCS), head computed tomography (CT) results, hypotension, and single-versus multiple-system trauma, these results continued to remain significant. A similar retrospective study found no difference in mortality or length of stay between patients that received NMBA versus those that did not. The authors did however find in a post hoc analysis, a correlation between continuous infusion of NMBAs and the length of time that ICP was greater than 20 mmHg (13.5 hours vs 6.5 hours; p<0.5).[14] The results from these studies do not fully guide us on the utility of NMBAs for treatment of elevated ICP but should give us an insight into the potential risks of using continuous infusion of NMBAs in this population.

TARGETED TEMPERATURE MANAGEMENT

Elevated body temperatures (fever or hyperthermia) in patients with acute neurologic injury has been shown to be associated with prolonged ICU length of stay and worse neurocognitive outcomes.[15] Temperature management, both mild hypothermia and normothermia, are common treatment modalities for patients in the neurointensive care unit. Shivering is a common physiological response recognized among patients treated with targeted

temperature management (TTM) and its effect are often robust and temperature goals cannot be accomplished. In these cases shivering must be controlled in order to reach the target temperature. Neuromuscular blocking agents have been identified as a potential treatment option for shiver mitigation in patients undergoing TTM that have failed other pharmacological therapies. Retrospective studies with pancuronium, vecuronium, atracurium, and cisatracurium in combination with sedation have been shown to be effective in the prevention of shivering during the initiation of TTM and improved time to target temperature.[16–19] Studies further suggest that patients who receive NMBAs for TTM after cardiac arrest may have better prognosis than those who do not.[15,16] These results must be further considered however in that the selection bias for patients receiving NMBAs may in fact be the true confounder improving outcomes. Patients who shiver while undergoing TTM after cardiac arrest have a better prognosis than those who do not shiver, regardless of NMBA administration. Furthermore, no study has yet demonstrated superiority of NMBA therapy over sedation or opioids for shiver treatment or prevention with respect to time to target, neurological recovery, or mortality.

Careful consideration of the paralytic dosing must be made in patients undergoing TTM as hypothermia has been shown to impair renal, hepatic, and enzymatic elimination of drugs, including NMBAs.[20–23] Several studies have shown an increase in NMBA serum concentrations as the core temperature is reduced to 34 degrees Celsius as well as an almost doubling of the duration of action.[24,25] Additionally, monitoring with peripheral nerve stimulation (PNS) may not be as useful during TTM as there is a recognized reduction in muscle twitch response when core temperatures are reduced regardless of the presence of a NMBA.[26,27]

Taking into consideration the long-term effects of NMBA administration, including prolonged paralysis due to higher than expected serum concentrations and the loss of accuracy of monitoring during TTM, the recommendation would be to use NMBAs after all other non-pharmacological and pharmacological options have been exhausted.

MONITORING NEUROMUSCULAR BLOCKING AGENTS

Patients receiving long-term neuromuscular blockade should be monitored both clinically (ventilator synchrony/ asynchrony, agitation) and by PNS whenever possible to help ensure efficacy and avoid toxicity. Peripheral nerve stimulators are used to deliver four stimuli, referred to as the train of four (TOF). As the dose of NMBAs is increased the number of twitches the patient displays reduces, indicating a higher level of neuromuscular junction blockade. Choosing a TOF goal of 1 of 4 twitches will allow minimization of the NMBA administered and reduce the risk of toxicity. Studies conflict as to whether PNS monitoring actually reduces the dose of NMBA and improves recovery time but it is generally recommended along with the clinical assessment.[28] Several factors can attribute to loss of accuracy of the TOF, including but not limited to loss of adhesive on the electrode, incorrect electrode placement, peripheral oedema, and hypotension. Additionally, PNS may be unreliable and misleading in patients treated with TTM.[21,26,27] Therefore, caution should be exercised when using PNS in the setting of hypothermia.

ADVERSE EFFECTS

Neuromuscular blocking agents may cause the following drug-related adverse reactions:

- Hypersensitivity reactions, including anaphylaxis
- Cardiac arrest
- Cardiac arrhythmias
- Malignant hyperthermia
- Hypertension or hypotension
- Hyperkalaemia
- Prolonged respiratory depression
- Jaw rigidity
- Rhabdomyolysis
- Myalgias
- Skeletal muscle weakness

Cardiac Problems

All NMBAs have concern for adverse effects due to their potential cross-reactivity with muscarinic receptors, potential for histamine release, and vagolytic activity.[1,4] Pancuronium exhibits significant affinity for muscarinic receptor blockade and carries an increased concern for tachycardia. Histamine release, which is a direct action of NMBA on mast cells, results in flushing, bronchospasm, hypotension, and tachycardia and is predominately seen with agents in the benzylisoquinolinium group. Histamine release can be attenuated by slow administration over 1–5 minutes or by pre-treatment with an H$_1$- and H$_2$- receptor antagonist. Vagolytic actions are most prominent with pancuronium and rocuronium with resultant mild, dose-dependent tachycardia, and hypertension. Vagolytic activity is seen

most commonly among the aminosteroid agents and consideration should be taken when deciding which agent to use in patients with coronary artery disease and/ or those with cardiovascular collapse.

Hyperkalaemia

Of particular concern are patients receiving succinylcholine that have either been identified as having hyperkalaemia or a known risk for an exaggerated response from the muscle fasciculations and subsequent extracellular potassium release. Patients in the neurointensive care unit are often at risk and include patients with upper and lower motor neuron lesions, including spinal cord injury, stroke, Guillain-Barre syndrome, muscular dystrophy, muscle denervation, muscle immobilization, severe head injury, trauma, burn injury, and Clostridial infections. Patients admitted with cerebral pathology for more than 16 days have also been shown to be at increased risk for hyperkalaemia after succinylcholine administration.[29] During such conditions, immature ACh receptor ion channels become more sensitive to succinylcholine and remain sensitive for up to six months. Therefore, all patients should be evaluated for current and pre-existing (within the last six months) risk factors prior to administration of succinylcholine. This effect is generally seen within five minutes of the dose administered and may be life-threatening due to the risk of cardiac arrhythmias.

ICU-Acquired Weakness

The aetiology of ICU-acquired weakness remains controversial and can be classified as critical illness polyneuropathy, myopathy, or neuromyopathy and is characterized by electromyographical changes, myonecrosis with elevated creatinine phosphokinase concentrations, and acute paresis.[4] Despite a paucity in data, proposed risk factors include high-dose corticosteroids, hyperglycaemia, amount of sedation administered, and NMBA use.[30,31] Two recent trials in ARDS patients that received 48 hours of cisatricurium did not identify NMBA use as a risk factor associated with ICU-acquired weakness.[5–7,32] This however needs to be further investigated with other NMBAs and in other patient populations in the ICU including TBI, stroke, and sepsis.

Neurotoxic Metabolite

Laudanosine is a metabolite of cisatracurium and atracurium that is produced as a result of Hoffman elimination.[33] Although NMBAs are hydrophilic compounds that do not typically cross the blood–brain barrier (BBB), in the setting of acute neurologic injury, disruption of this barrier may occur and put the patient at increased risk for neurotoxicity. Accumulation of laudanosine has been shown to increase the risk for seizures being reported most commonly with cisatracurium.

Tachyphylaxis

Tachyphylaxis is thought to be the result of increased protein binding or ACh receptor upregulation in response to pharmacologic denervation. It is clinically described as a diminished or failed response to an agent after administration for at least 72 hours.[4] Rapid and high dose escalation is required to achieve the same clinical results. These higher infusion rates can put the patients at increased risk for toxicity and increase drug cost.

ADDITIONAL CONSIDERATIONS

Sedation and Analgesia

Clinicians must remember that NMBAs have no sedative, amnestic, or analgesic properties and should only be used in patients that are adequately sedated and receiving analgesia.[4,34] It is imperative that deep sedation and analgesia be initiated prior to initiation of the NMBA and continued evaluation must occur for the duration of NMBA use. At this time there is no single monitoring tool that adequately assesses sedation during NMBA use and therefore clinical signs and symptoms of distress (vital signs) must be a critical part of the hourly physical examination.

Deep Vein Thrombosis

Immobility achieved by NMBA paralysis increases venous stasis and increases the incidence of deep vein thrombosis (DVT). A recent study reported that the use of NMBAs was the strongest predictor for the development of DVTs in the ICU.[4] Mechanical and pharmacological strategies to prevent DVT have been successful in significantly reducing the incidence.

Corneal Abrasions

Neuromuscular blocking agents impair ocular protective mechanisms and put the cornea at risk for developing ulceration, infections, and scarring.[4] Scheduled eye lubricant applications along with a closed-chamber eye protection (swim goggles) appears to effectively reduce negative corneal sequelae.

Bowel Motility

Patients receiving NMBAs are at risk of constipation due to immobility and concurrent opioid administration.[4] Patients receiving continuous infusions of NMBA should also receive a laxative regimen to prevent gastrointestinal complications.

PHARMACOKINETICS/PHARMACODYNAMICS

Acute neurologically injured patients have several factors that may affect the pharmacokinetic and pharmacodynamic profile of NMBAs. A lack of understanding or recognition of these factors may result in loss of efficacy or added toxicity (Tables 20.3 and 20.4).

DRUG INTERACTIONS

Drug interactions may alter the duration of activity of NMBAs through several mechanisms including competition at the receptor site, reduced or increased clearance or metabolism, disruption of ion channels, and up- or down-regulation of ACh release or sensitivity. Understanding the effect of drug interactions on NMBA

Table 20.3 Pharmacokinetics of neuromuscular blocking agents

Drug	Pancuronium	Vecuronium	Rocuronium	Cisatracurium
Elimination	80% renal 10–20% hepatic	40% biliary 35% renal	40% biliary 30% renal	Hofmann degradation
Renal failure	↑ effect	↑ effect	Mild ↑ effect	No
Hepatic failure	Mild ↑ effect	Mild ↑ effect	Mod ↑ effect	No
Active metabolites	Yes	Yes	No	No
Histamine release hypotension	No	No	No	No
Vagal block tachycardia	Yes	No	Yes (at higher doses)	No
Ganglionic block hypotension	No	No	No	No

Note: ↑ indicates increase.

is important to allow maximal effect while minimizing and avoiding toxicity (Table 20.5).

REVERSAL OF NEUROMUSCULAR BLOCKING AGENTS

Ideally patients who receive a NMBA should be allowed to spontaneously recover from paralysis, however, there are rare instances where rapid reversal may be required. Anticholinesterase reversal agents (neostigmine, edrophonium, pyridostigmine)[35] are only effective for non-depolarizing blockers and increase ACh at the neuromuscular junction. Concomitant use of antimuscarinic agents (glycopyrrolate, atropine) may be considered to counteract the effects of ACh at the muscarinic sites (bradycardia, increased secretions, bronchoconstriction). Recognition that muscular weakness may continue even after administration of an

Table 20.4 Conditions affecting pharmacokinetics of neuromuscular blocking agents

Condition	Interaction	Effect on NMBA
Hypothermia	Alters sensitivity and pH of neuromuscular junction, reduces ACh mobilization, reduces muscle contractility, reduces hepatic and renal clearance, alters volume of distribution	Prolongs duration of NMBA
Hypokalemia	Augments blockade of nondepolarizing agents	Enhances NMBA activity
Elevated Mg^+	Inhibits Ca^+ channels in the presynaptic terminal and inhibits postjunctional potentials	Prolongs duration of NMBA
Elevated Ca^+	Ca^+ triggers ACh release	Reduces NMBA sensitivity and decrease duration of NMBA
Respiratory and metabolic acidosis	Unknown	Enhances effect of NMBA
Respiratory and metabolic alkalosis	Unknown	Reversal agents may work more slowly

Table 20.5 Common drug interactions with neuromuscular blocking agents

Drug	Interaction	Effect
Antibiotics (Aminoglycoside, tetracycline, clindamycin, vancomycin)	Reduces prejunctional ACh release, decreases postjunctional receptor sensitivity to ACh, blocks ACh receptors or disrupts ion channels	Prolongs duration of NMBA
Carbamazepine	Competes for ACh receptor	Causes NMBA resistance
Corticosteroids[*]	May decrease sensitivity of endplate to ACh	Prolongs duration of NMBA
Cyclosporin	May inhibit NMBA metabolism	Prolongs duration of NMBA
Inhaled anaesthetics (enflurane, isoflurane)	Reduces postjunctional receptor sensitivity to ACh	Prolongs duration of NMBA
Lithium	Activates K^+ channel presynaptically	Prolongs duration of NMBA
Magnesium	Competes with Ca^+ presynaptically	Prolongs duration of NMBA
Phenytoin[**]	Up-regulation of ACh receptors	Causes NMBA resistance
Theophylline	Unknown	Causes NMBA resistance

*(1) Fischer JR, Baer RK. Acute myopathy associated with combined use of corticosteroids and neuromuscular blocking agents. *Ann Pharmacother* 1996;30:1437–45. (2) Campkin NT, Hood JR, Feldman SA. Resistance to decamethonium neuromuscular block after prior administration of vecuronium. *Anesth Analg* 1993;77:78–80. (3) Kindler CH, Verotta D, Gray AT, Gropper MA, Yost CS. Additive inhibition of nicotinic acetylcholine receptors by corticosteroids and the neuromuscular blocking drug vecuronium. *Anesthesiology* 2000;92:821–32.
**(1) Richard A, Girard F, Girard DC, et al. Cisatracurium-induced neuromuscular blockade is affected by chronic phenytoin or carbamazepine treatment in neurosurgical patients. *Anesth Analg* 2005;100:538–44. (2) Koenig HM, Hoffman WE. The effect of anticonvulsant therapy on two doses of rocuronium-induced neuromuscular blockade. *J Neurosurg Anesthesiol* 1999;11:86–9. (3) Koenig MH, Edwards LT. Cisatracurium-induced neuromuscular blockade in anticonvulsant treated neurosurgical patients. *J Neurosurg Anesthesiol* 2000;12:314–8.

anticholinesterase reversal agent and monitoring for respiratory distress needs to be of utmost concern.

Sugammadex is a selective relaxant-binding agent that only reverses aminosteroid agents (rocuronium> vecuronium) by encapsulating them at the motor end-plate and preventing their ability to inhibit ACh receptors. This rapid reversal agent may allow for the use of steroidal agents for RSI in cases where succinylcholine is contraindicated and prolonged paralysis for even 20–30 minutes is undesired.[35,36]

SPECIAL PATIENT POPULATIONS

Myasthenia Gravis

Myasthenia gravis is a condition characterized by antibodies targeting nicotinic receptors, thereby reducing the number of functional nicotinic receptors.[4,37] Patients with myasthenia gravis may have impaired neuromuscular transmission and a higher sensitivity to the effects of nondepolarizing NBMAs specifically. Patients often require a reduced dose of an NMBA to achieve the desired degree of neuromuscular blockade.[38] Sensitivity is widely variable and each therapy should be individualized for NMBA effect. Initiation of therapy should begin with reduced doses and increased as needed according to the indication for NMBA.

Brain Death

The physical examination is an integral part of brain death determination and is difficult, if not impossible to perform in a patient receiving NMBAs.[39] Due to the legal definitions and the inherent impossibility of performing an adequate neurological examination when NMBA are administered, their continued use in this scenario cannot be justified. The patients TOF must be 4/4 as measured using PNS at the maximum current before a neurological examination for brain death is performed.

SPASTICITY IN THE NEUROINTENSIVE CARE

Skeletal muscle relaxants are a heterogeneous group of medications commonly used to treat spasticity from upper motor neuron syndromes (multiple sclerosis, spinal cord injury, TBI, cerebral palsy, and post-stroke syndrome) and muscular pain or spasms from peripheral musculoskeletal conditions (fibromyalgia, tension headaches, myofascial pain syndrome, mechanical back or neck pain). Although these agents are commonly administered in the neurointensive care setting, they are generally not recommended as first line. There is a paucity of data

comparing skeletal muscles relaxants to one another and no high-quality evidence supports their use. No agent has been shown to be better than another, and all of them have adverse effects, particularly sedation. Concerns about possible abuse and interaction with other drugs, especially if increased sedation is a risk, further limit their use. Muscle relaxants should generally be chosen based on adverse effect profile, tolerability, drug interactions, and cost (Table 20.6).

BACLOFEN WITHDRAWAL

Baclofen, a gamma-aminobutyric acid (GABA) analog that has inhibitory effects on spinal cord reflexes, is currently the leading agent prescribed to treat spasticity.[40] Baclofen reduces the excitability of motor neurons by inhibiting the release of excitatory neurotransmitters at the presynaptic area. In high concentrations in the cerebrospinal fluid (CSF), baclofen can also work post-synaptically, antagonizing the activity of the excitatory neurotransmitters and enhancing its effect.[41] Because of its low liposolubility and inability to efficiently cross the blood-brain barrier, high drug concentrations within the CSF are difficult to achieve with oral baclofen. Therefore, intrathecal baclofen provides an effective treatment for spasticity that is not sufficiently managed by oral baclofen.

The intrathecal pump is surgically implanted in the subcutaneous tissue of the anterior abdominal wall and the drug is delivered via a tunnelled catheter into the lumbar subarachanoid space. The pump delivers approximately 100–2000 mcg/day of baclofen and can be titrated to the desired clinical response. Long-term intrathecal baclofen causes down-regulation of $GABA_B$ receptors in the central nervous system (CNS) and spinal cord, which may cause decreased sensitivity and tolerance to baclofen over time.[41] Abrupt intrathecal withdrawal, from an empty drug reservoir, catheter displacement, pump malfunction, or programming errors can result in a predominance of excitatory effects that are associated with CNS hyperexcitability.[42] Mild symptoms include spasticity, pruritus, confusion, and anxiety.[40] More severe, life-threatening symptoms include hyperthermia, myoclonus, seizures, rhabdomyolysis, disseminated intravascular coagulation, multisystem organ failure, cardiac arrest, coma, and even death have been documented in literature.[43–47] Baclofen withdrawal with severe life-threatening symptoms is considered a medical emergency and requires treatment in the neurointensive care unit. Symptoms often mimic severe sepsis and withdrawal should always be considered if any

Table 20.6 Skeletal muscle relaxants

Drug	Mechanism of action	Common adverse effects	Clinical pearls
Baclofen	Blocks pre- and post-synaptic GABA$_B$ receptors	Drowsiness, dizziness, headache, constipation, insomnia Rare seizures Low blood pressure Respiratory depression	• As effective as Diazepam but with less sedation • Low oral absorption • Intathecal 1000× more potent than oral
Carisoprodol	Centrally acting skeletal muscle relaxant; action is not completely understood but may be related to its sedative action	Dizziness, drowsiness, headache Rare idiosyncratic reactions (mental status changes, transient quadriplegia, and temporary loss of vision) after first dose	• Caution with abrupt withdrawal due to dependence potential • Possible respiratory depression when combined with benzodiazepines, codeine or its derivatives, or other muscle relaxants • Contraindicated in acute intermittent porphyria
Cyclobenzaprine	Cyclobenzaprine acts on the locus coeruleus causing increased norepinephrine release, potentially through the gamma fibres which innervate and inhibit the alpha motor neurons in the ventral horn of the spinal cord	Anticholinergic effect (drowsiness, dry mouth, urinary retention, increased intraocular pressure) Rare arrhythmias, seizures, myocardial infarction	• Long elimination half-life • Avoid in older patients and in patients with glaucoma • Possible drug interaction with CYP450 inhibitors • Seizures reported with concomitant use of tramadol • Caution in arrhythmias, recent myocardial infarction, or congestive heart failure
Dantrolene	Reduce Ca$^+$ release from skeletal muscle sarcoplasmic reticulum	Sedation, muscle weakness, hepatitis	• Primary drug used for the treatment/prevention of malignant hyperthermia
Diazepam	Central GABA$_A$ antagonist	Dizziness, drowsiness, confusion	• Long elimination half-life; avoid in older patients and in patients with hepatic impairment • Possible drug interaction with CYP450 inhibitors • Complete blood count and liver function tests indicated for prolonged use
Gabapentin	GABA inhibitor and Ca$^+$ voltage gated channel activity but unclear of the full activity	Sedation, fatigue, peripheral oedema	• Appears to work for neuropathic pain but may have added musculoskeletal benefit in combination with other agents
Methocarbamol	Unknown	Black, brown, or green urine possible Possible exacerbation of myasthenia gravis symptoms	• Possible respiratory depression when combined with benzodiazepines, codeine or its derivatives, or other muscle relaxants
Tizanidine	Central α-2 receptor agonist	Dose-related hypotension, sedation Rare hepatotoxicity, withdrawal hypertension	• Caution with CYP1A2 inhibitors, central nervous system depressants, or alcohol • Decreased effectiveness with oral contraceptives

Sources: (1) See S, Ginzburg R. Choosing a skeletal muscle relaxant. *Am Fam Physician* 2008;78:365–70. (2) Beebe FA, Barkin RL, Barkin S. A clinical and pharmacologic review of skeletal muscle relaxants for musculoskeletal conditions. *Am J Ther* 2005;12:151–71.

of the above symptoms are present in a patient with an intrathecal baclofen pump.

Baclofen replacement is the desired treatment and intrathecal administration essential in patients with severe, life-threatening withdrawal symptoms. High doses of oral baclofen (up to 80 mg three times daily) may be effective in mitigating mild symptoms of withdrawal, however, failure is often reported especially in cases where the intrathecal doses are high.[44] Intrathecal baclofen boluses can be administered via lumbar puncture or external lumbar catheter. Intrathecal replacement bolus doses should be based on the total expected daily dose prescribed, length of time since baclofen was discontinued, and the severity of withdrawal symptoms. Replacement doses generally range from 50 to 200 mcg with activity lasting 2–8 hours after administration. In patients with severe symptoms, a more continuous solution may be necessary to ensure ongoing administration of baclofen occurs until a permanent resolution is reached (infected pump replaced, catheter unkinked). In these particular cases, baclofen can be administered continuously via a lumbar drain with an external drug delivery device.

Benzodiazepines, including lorazepam, diazepam, and midazolam are common adjuvant therapies in controlling spasticity, hyperthermia, and seizures during withdrawal as they activate central receptors and $GABA_A$ receptors of the spinal cord via a different mechanism. During a planned removal of an intrathecal pump due to infection or other causes, premedication with high doses of benzodiazepines and augmented oral baclofen may be helpful to prevent withdrawal. No specific dosing recommendations are published, however, rapid titration is generally required and admission to a neurointensive care unit is generally warranted.

Although less data exists, alternative agents to consider may be propofol, cyproheptadine, dantrolene, and tizanidine. These agents are typically administered in combination with oral baclofen and benzodiazepines and their use as monotherapy should be discouraged or used with caution. Baclofen withdrawal syndrome is a potentially life-threatening complication of intrathecal baclofen and early recognition of the syndrome, reinstitution of baclofen and adjunctive high-dose benzodiazepines, and proper intensive care management are mainstays for the management.

CONCLUSIONS

Skeletal muscle relaxants are commonly used in neurocritical are to treat spasticity from upper motor neuron syndromes and muscular pain or spasms from peripheral musculoskeletal conditions. Caution should be used when administering these agents due to concerns for excessive drowsiness, drug interactions, and limited data to support their use.

REFERENCES

1. Fisher DM. Clinical pharmacology of neuromuscular blocking agents. *Am J Health Syst Pharm* 1999;56:S4–9.
2. Minton MD, Grosslight K, Stirt JA, Bedford RF. Increases in intracranial pressure from succinylcholine: prevention by prior nondepolarizing blockade. *Anesthesiology* 1986; 65:165–9.
3. Stollings JL, Diedrich DA, Oyen LJ, Brown DR. Rapid-sequence intubation: a review of the process and considerations when choosing medications. *Ann Pharmacother* 2014;48:62–76.
4. Murray MJ, DeBlock H, Erstad B, et al. Clinical practice guidelines for sustained neuromuscular blockade in the adult critically ill patient. *Critical Care Medicine* 2016; 44:2079–103.
5. Forel JM, Roch A, Marin V, et al. Neuromuscular blocking agents decrease inflammatory response in patients presenting with acute respiratory distress syndrome. *Crit Care Med* 2006;34:2749–57.
6. Papazian L, Forel JM, Gacouin A, et al. Neuromuscular blockers in early acute respiratory distress syndrome. *N Engl J Med* 2010;363:1107–16.
7. Gainnier M, Roch A, Forel JM, et al. Effect of neuromuscular blocking agents on gas exchange in patients presenting with acute respiratory distress syndrome. *Crit Care Med* 2004;32:113–9.
8. Kovarik WD, Mayberg TS, Lam AM, Mathisen TL, Winn HR. Succinylcholine does not change intracranial pressure, cerebral blood flow velocity, or the electroencephalogram in patients with neurologic injury. *Anesth Analg* 1994; 78:469–73.
9. Werba A, Klezl M, Schramm W, et al. The level of neuromuscular block needed to suppress diaphragmatic movement during tracheal suction in patients with raised intracranial pressure: a study with vecuronium and atracurium. *Anaesthesia* 1993;48:301–3.
10. McCall M, Jeejeebhoy K, Pencharz P, Moulton R. Effect of neuromuscular blockade on energy expenditure in patients with severe head injury. *J Parenter Enteral Nutr* 2003;27:27–35.
11. Kerr ME, Sereika SM, Orndoff P, et al. Effect of neuromuscular blockers and opiates on the cerebrovascular response to endotracheal suctioning in adults with severe head injuries. *Am J Crit Care* 1998;7:205–17.
12. Kerwin AJ, Croce MA, Timmons SD, Maxwell RA, Malhotra AK, Fabian TC. Effects of fiberoptic bronchoscopy on intracranial pressure in patients with brain injury: a prospective clinical study. *J Trauma* 2000;48:878–82; discussion 82–3.

13. Hsiang JK, Chesnut RM, Crisp CB, Klauber MR, Blunt BA, Marshall LF. Early, routine paralysis for intracranial pressure control in severe head injury: is it necessary? *Crit Care Med* 1994;22:1471–6.

14. Juul N, Morris GF, Marshall SB, Marshall LF. Neuromuscular blocking agents in neurointensive care. *Acta Neurochir Suppl* 2000;76:467–70.

15. Nolan JP, Morley PT, Hoek TL, Hickey RW. Advancement Life support Task Force of the International Liaison committee on R. Therapeutic hypothermia after cardiac arrest. An advisory statement by the Advancement Life support Task Force of the International Liaison committee on Resuscitation. *Resuscitation* 2003;57:231–5.

16. Bernard SA, Gray TW, Buist MD, et al. Treatment of comatose survivors of out-of-hospital cardiac arrest with induced hypothermia. *N Engl J Med* 2002;346:557–63.

17. Hypothermia after Cardiac Arrest Study G. Mild therapeutic hypothermia to improve the neurologic outcome after cardiac arrest. *N Engl J Med* 2002;346:549–56.

18. Sladen RN, Berend JZ, Fassero JS, Zehnder EB. Comparison of vecuronium and meperidine on the clinical and metabolic effects of shivering after hypothermic cardiopulmonary bypass. *J Cardiothorac Vasc Anesth* 1995;9:147–53.

19. Cruise C, MacKinnon J, Tough J, Houston P. Comparison of meperidine and pancuronium for the treatment of shivering after cardiac surgery. *Can J Anaesth* 1992;39:563–8.

20. Smeulers NJ, Wierda JM, van den Broek L, Gallandat Huet RC, Hennis PJ. Effects of hypothermic cardiopulmonary bypass on the pharmacodynamics and pharmacokinetics of rocuronium. *J Cardiothorac Vasc Anesth* 1995;9:700–5.

21. Heier T, Caldwell JE. Impact of hypothermia on the response to neuromuscular blocking drugs. *Anesthesiology* 2006;104:1070–80.

22. Heier T, Caldwell JE, Sessler DI, Miller RD. Mild intraoperative hypothermia increases duration of action and spontaneous recovery of vecuronium blockade during nitrous oxide-isoflurane anesthesia in humans. *Anesthesiology* 1991;74:815–9.

23. Diefenbach C, Abel M, Buzello W. Greater neuromuscular blocking potency of atracurium during hypothermic than during normothermic cardiopulmonary bypass. *Anesth Analg* 1992;75:675–8.

24. Denny NM, Kneeshaw JD. Vecuronium and atracurium infusions during hypothermic cardiopulmonary bypass. *Anaesthesia* 1986;41:919–22.

25. Beaufort AM, Wierda JM, Belopavlovic M, Nederveen PJ, Kleef UW, Agoston S. The influence of hypothermia (surface cooling) on the time-course of action and on the pharmacokinetics of rocuronium in humans. *Eur J Anaesthesiol Suppl* 1995;11:95–106.

26. Ricker K, Hertel G, Stodieck G. Increased voltage of the muscle action potential of normal subjects after local cooling. *J Neurol* 1977;216:33–8.

27. Bigland-Ritchie B, Thomas CK, Rice CL, Howarth JV, Woods JJ. Muscle temperature, contractile speed, and motoneuron firing rates during human voluntary contractions. *J Appl Physiol* (1985) 1992;73:2457–61.

28. Rudis MI, Sikora CA, Angus E, et al. A prospective, randomized, controlled evaluation of peripheral nerve stimulation versus standard clinical dosing of neuromuscular blocking agents in critically ill patients. *Crit Care Med* 1997;25:575–83.

29. Blanie A, Ract C, Leblanc PE, et al. The limits of succinylcholine for critically ill patients. *Anesth Analg* 2012;115:873–9.

30. Fischer JR, Baer RK. Acute myopathy associated with combined use of corticosteroids and neuromuscular blocking agents. *Ann Pharmacother* 1996;30:1437–45.

31. Campkin NT, Hood JR, Feldman SA. Resistance to decamethonium neuromuscular block after prior administration of vecuronium. *Anesth Analg* 1993;77:78–80.

32. Richard A, Girard F, Girard DC, et al. Cisatracurium-induced neuromuscular blockade is affected by chronic phenytoin or carbamazepine treatment in neurosurgical patients. *Anesth Analg* 2005;100:538–44.

33. Latronico N, Shehu I, Seghelini E. Neuromuscular sequelae of critical illness. *Curr Opin Crit Care* 2005;11:381–90.

34. Jacobi J, Fraser GL, Coursin DB, et al. Clinical practice guidelines for the sustained use of sedatives and analgesics in the critically ill adult. *Crit Care Med* 2002;30:119–41.

35. Abad-Gurumeta A, Ripolles-Melchor J, Casans-Frances R, et al. A systematic review of sugammadex vs neostigmine for reversal of neuromuscular blockade. *Anaesthesia* 2015;70:1441–52.

36. Nicholson WT, Sprung J, Jankowski CJ. Sugammadex: a novel agent for the reversal of neuromuscular blockade. *Pharmacotherapy* 2007;27:1181–8.

37. Fambrough DM, Drachman DB, Satyamurti S. Neuromuscular junction in myasthenia gravis: decreased acetylcholine receptors. *Science* 1973;182:293–5.

38. Tripathi M, Kaushik S, Dubey P. The effect of use of pyridostigmine and requirement of vecuronium in patients with myasthenia gravis. *Journal of Postgraduate Medicine* 2003;49:311–4; discussion 4–5.

39. Wijdicks EF, Varelas PN, Gronseth GS, Greer DM. American Academy of N. Evidence-based guideline update: determining brain death in adults: report of the Quality Standards Subcommittee of the American Academy of Neurology. *Neurology* 2010;74:1911–8.

40. Coffey RJ, Edgar TS, Francisco GE, et al. Abrupt withdrawal from intrathecal baclofen: recognition and management of a potentially life-threatening syndrome. *Arch Phys Med Rehabil* 2002;83:735–41.

41. Kroin JS, Bianchi GD, Penn RD. Intrathecal baclofen down-regulates GABAB receptors in the rat substantia gelatinosa. *J Neurosurg* 1993;79:544–9.

42. Al-Khodairy AT, Vuagnat H, Uebelhart D. Symptoms of recurrent intrathecal baclofen withdrawal resulting from drug delivery failure: a case report. *Am J Phys Med Rehabil* 1999;78:272–7.

43. Green LB, Nelson VS. Death after acute withdrawal of intrathecal baclofen: case report and literature review. *Arch Phys Med Rehabil* 1999;80:1600–4.

44. Greenberg MI, Hendrickson RG. Baclofen withdrawal following removal of an intrathecal baclofen pump despite oral baclofen replacement. *J Toxicol Clin Toxicol* 2003;41:83–5.

45. Sampathkumar P, Scanlon PD, Plevak DJ. Baclofen withdrawal presenting as multiorgan system failure. *Anesth Analg* 1998;87:562–3.

46. Reeves RK, Stolp-Smith KA, Christopherson MW. Hyperthermia, rhabdomyolysis, and disseminated intravascular coagulation associated with baclofen pump catheter failure. *Arch Phys Med Rehabil* 1998;79:353–6.

47. Meinck HM, Tronnier V, Rieke K, Wirtz CR, Flugel D, Schwab S. Intrathecal baclofen treatment for stiff-man syndrome: pump failure may be fatal. *Neurology* 1994;44:2209–10.

21

Antibiotics

J. M. Makii and M. K. Zielke

ABSTRACT

Antibiotics are a common pharmacological therapy in the neurointensive care unit. This chapter reviews the mechanism of action, spectrum of activity, and common adverse effects associated with a variety of antibiotic therapies typically encountered in the neurointensive care unit. The pharmacodynamic and pharmacokinetic properties including absorption, distribution, metabolism, and excretion pathways will also be reviewed. Special consideration will be placed on the role of these agents in central nervous system (CNS) infections.

KEYWORDS

Antibiotic therapy; anti-infective; anti-fungal; infection; anti-microbial.

INTRODUCTION

Infections are a common nemesis in neurointensive care that can carry fatal consequences if not appropriately treated in a timely manner. The interaction between the host and infecting pathogen determine the most optimal course of treatment based on a number of considerations. Crucial to the treatment of any infection is identification of the pathogen, including the pathogens antimicrobial susceptibility, as well as consideration of host-specific factors. These factors include age, hepatic and renal function, prior anti-infective use, documented adverse effects from previous anti-infective use, and site of infection. In order for anti-infective therapy to be effective, an appropriate concentration to inhibit pathogen growth or ideally kill the infecting pathogen needs to be achieved in the infected tissue.[1]

For central nervous system (CNS) infections antimicrobials need to cross the blood–brain barrier (BBB) effectively to be successful. The pharmacokinetic properties that determine CNS penetration of a drug include degree of ionization, lipid solubility, molecular weight, and protein binding. Ideal agents would possess a low degree of ionization at physiologic pH (acidity), high lipid solubility, a low molecular weight, and low protein binding. Additionally, in cases of more severe

CNS infections oftentimes with drug-resistant pathogens, intraventricular or intrathecal medication administration may be needed.[2] Summaries of the most common antibiotics and anti-infective agents used in the treatment of neurointensive care infections are detailed in this section (see Table 21.1).

BETA-LACTAM ANTIBIOTICS

Almost one century ago, Alexander Fleming published his findings on the inhibitory nature of the penicillium mould on Staphylococci species.[3] This finding not only led to being awarded the Nobel Prize in Physiology or Medicine in 1945, but also paved the way for advancement of antimicrobial research for years to come. In the United States, there are now over 20 classes of antimicrobials available for use which exceeds over 100 individual agents.[4] This number will surely continue to grow with the desire to combat antimicrobial resistance.

Beta-lactam antibiotics are a commonly utilized group of antimicrobials and include all penicillins, cephalosporins, and carbapenems. They are characterized by a beta-lactam ring, which largely contributes to their antibacterial activity. The mechanism of action for all beta-lactam antibiotics is binding of the antibiotic to penicillin-binding proteins which prevent peptidoglycan

Table 21.1 Summary of antimicrobial spectrum of activity and select pharmacokinetic parameters

Antimicrobial	Spectrum of activity	CNS penetration (AUC_{CSF}/AUC_S)[*]	Renal adjustment[#] (Y/N)	Hepatic adjustment[#] (Y/N)	Bactericidal vs bacteriostatic[#]
Penicillins					
Natural penicillins	Streptococci spp. Staphylococci spp. (MSSA) Neisseria spp. Anaerobes	0.05	Y	N	Bactericidal
Penicillinase-resistant penicillins	Streptococcus spp. Staphylococcus spp. (MSSA) Neisseria spp.	0.20	N	N	Bactericidal
Aminopenicillins	Streptococcus spp. Staphylococcus spp. (MSSA) Neisseria spp. *Enterococcus faecalis*	0.13	Y	N	Bactericidal
Antipseudomonal penicillins	Streptococcus spp. Staphylococcus spp. (MSSA) *Pseudomonas aeruginosa* Gram-negative organisms	0.32	Y	N	Bactericidal
B-lactamase inhibitor combinations	Streptococcus spp. Staphylococcus spp. (MSSA) *P. aeruginosa* (piperacillin/tazobactam) *Acinetobacter baumannii* (sulbactam component of ampicillin/sulbactam) Anaerobes Gram-negative organisms	0.30	Y	N	Bactericidal
Cephalosporins					
First generation	Streptococci spp. Staphylococci spp. (MSSA) Moderate enteric gram-negative	0.04	Y	N	Bactericidal
Second generation	Streptococci spp. Staphylococci spp. (MSSA) Good enteric gram-negative *Neisseria* Anaerobes (cephamycins)	0.03	Y	N	Bactericidal
Third generation	Moderate streptococci spp. Moderate staphylococci spp. (MSSA) Enteric gram-negative *P. aeruginosa* (ceftazidime)	0.20	Y (N: ceftriaxone)	N	Bactericidal
Fourth generation	Streptococci spp. Staphylococci spp. (MSSA) Enteric gram-negative *P. aeruginosa*	0.31	Y	N	Bactericidal
Fifth generation	*Staphylococci* spp. (MSSA/MRSA)	0.14	Y	N	Bactericidal

Carbapenems					
Meropenem Doripenem Imipenem-Cilastatin Ertapenem	Streptococci spp. Staphylococci spp. (MSSA) Enteric gram-negative *P. aeruginosa* (excluding ertapenem) ESBL producing organisms AmpC producing organisms	0.40	Y	N	Bactericidal
Monobactam					
Aztreonam	Gram-negative organisms *P. aeruginosa*	0.05–0.40	Y	N	Bactericidal
Glycopeptides					
Vancomycin	*Staphylococcus aureus* (MSSA/MRSA) Coagulase-negative *Staphylococcus* *Enterococcus* spp. Clostridium spp.	0.30	Y	N	Bactericidal
Lipopeptide					
Daptomycin	*Staphylococcus aureus* (MSSA/MRSA) Enterococcus spp.	0.05	Y	N	Bactericidal
Oxazolidinones					
Linezolid Tedizolid	*Staphylococcus aureus* (MSSA/MRSA) Coagulase-negative *Staphylococcus* *Enterococcus* spp. Nocardia spp. Streptococci spp.	0.70	N	N	Bacteriostatic
Fluoroquinolones					
Levofloxacin Moxifloxacin Ciprofloxacin	*Streptococcus pneumonia* (excluding ciprofloxacin) Enterobacteriaceae *P. aeruginosa* (excluding moxifloxacin) Anaerobes (moxifloxacin)	0.70–0.90	Y (N: moxifloxacin)	N	Bactericidal
Aminoglycosides					
Gentamicin Tobramycin Amikacin	Acinetobacter spp. Enterobacteriaceae *P. aeruginosa*	0–0.30	Y	N	Bactericidal
Macrolides					
Erythromycin Clarithromycin Azithromycin	*H. influenzae* *M. catarrhalis* *Legionella* spp. *M. pneumoniae*	0.20	N (Y: clarithromycin)	N	Bacteriostatic

(Cont'd)

Table 21.1 *(Cont'd)*

Antimicrobial	Spectrum of activity	CNS penetration $(AUC_{CSF}/AUC_S)^{[*]}$	Renal adjustment[#] (Y/N)	Hepatic adjustment[#] (Y/N)	Bactericidal vs. bacteriostatic[#]
		Miscellaneous			
Metronidazole	Bacteroides spp. Parabacteroides spp. *Clostridium difficile* Microaerophilic bacteria Protozoa	0.87	N	N	Bactericidal
Trimethoprim-Sulfamethoxazole	Many gram-positive and gram-negative organisms *Stenotrophomonas maltophilia* *Listeria monocytogenes* *Pneumocystis jirovecii*	0.50/0.40	Y	N	Bacteriostatic
Rifamycins	*M. tuberculosis* Staphylococcus spp.	0.20	N	N	Bactericidal
Colistimethate sodium	*P. aeruginosa* *A. baumannii* Carbapenem-resistant Enterobacteriaceae	–	Y	N	Bacteriostatic

*(1) Nau R, Sorgel F, Eiffert H. Penetration of drugs through the blood-cerebrospinal fluid/blood-brain barrier for treatment of central nervous system infections. *Clinical Microbiology Reviews* 2010;23(4):858–83. (2) Gilbert D, Chambers H, Eliopoulos G, Saag M. *The Sanford Guide to Antimicrobial Therapy*. 44th ed. Sperryville: Antimicrobial Therapy Inc., 2014; p. 86. (3) Saravolatz LD, Stein GE, Johnson LB. Ceftaroline: A novel cephalosporin with activity against methicillin-resistant *Staphylococcus aureus*. *Clin Infect Dis* 2011;52(9):1156–63.
#Bennett JE, Dolin R, Blaser MJ. *Mandell, Douglas, and Bennett's Principles and Practice of Infectious Diseases*. Updated 8th ed. Philadelphia: Saunders, an imprint of Elsevier Inc, 2015.

synthesis, ultimately inhibiting cell wall synthesis. This class of antimicrobials is considered bactericidal.[5]

Penicillins

Penicillins can be divided into five different subclasses; natural penicillins (penicillin V and penicillin G), penicillinase-resistant penicillins (methicillin, nafcillin, and oxacillin), aminopenicillins (ampicillin and amoxicillin), antipseudomonal penicillins (piperacillin), and lastly beta-lactamase inhibitor combinations (amoxicillin/clavulanic acid, ampicillin/sulbactam, piperacillin/tazobactam).[5]

The antimicrobials within the penicillin class of beta-lactam antibiotics have similar pharmacokinetic and pharmacodynamic effects. Most antibiotics in this class have good distribution into the lung, kidneys, and muscle, however, poor distribution into the eye, cerebral spinal fluid, and brain without the presence of inflammation. Most penicillins are renally eliminated with the exception of the penicillinase-resistant penicillins, and therefore

need to be dose-adjusted in renal disease. Adverse events associated with penicillins include hypersensitivity reactions (rash, hives, and anaphylaxis) and interstitial nephritis.[5]

The spectrum of activity of these antimicrobials is dependent on the sub-class of penicillins being discussed. Natural penicillins have good coverage for Streptococcus spp., susceptible Staphylococcus spp., Neisseria spp., and anaerobes, however, have poor or no coverage against Enterococcus spp., methicillin-resistant *Staphylococcus aureus* (MRSA), and gram-negative organisms. The anti-staphylococcal penicillins expand coverage against Staphylococcus and Streptococcus species that developed resistance to penicillin, with continued coverage against Neisseria species. The aminopenicillins have similar coverage as the earlier generation penicillins with the addition of activity against *Enterococcus faecalis*. The remaining two classes of penicillins, the antipseudomonal penicillins and the beta-lactamase inhibitor combinations have an extended spectrum of activity compared to the other penicillins. As the name suggests, the antipseudomonal penicillins have activity against *Pseudomonas aeruginosa*, however, piperacillin is not used as an independent agent in the United States. It is always in combination with the beta-lactamase inhibitor, tazobactam. The addition of the beta-lactamase inhibitor prevents hydrolysis of the parent compound by Class A beta-lactamases, which restores the activity of parent compound. The beta-lactamase inhibitor combinations have good coverage against Streptococcus spp., susceptible Staphylococcus spp., gram-negative organisms, *P. aeruginosa* (piperacillin/tazobactam), *Acinetobacter baumannii* (sulbactam component of ampicillin/sulbactam), and anaerobes.[5]

Cephalosporins

The first cephalosporin was derived from *Cephalosporium acremonium* which was identified by Brotzu in 1948. The cephalosporin class of beta-lactams extends the spectrum of activity against gram-negative organisms as compared to the penicillin class of antibiotics due to the changes in the chemical structure with the addition of the 7-aminocephalosporanic acid to the beta-lactam ring. This change also protects the compound from hydrolysis by penicillinases.[6]

Cephalosporins are sub-divided into five generations. The key difference between these generations are the changes in antimicrobial coverage. First generation cephalosporins (cephalexin, cefazolin, cefadroxil) have good activity against gram-positive organisms such as Streptococci spp. and methicillin-susceptible *Staphylococcus aureus* (MSSA) with moderate activity against enteric gram-negative organisms. The second generation cephalosporins (cefuroxime, cefprozil) and cephamycins (cefoxitin, cefotetan) broaden the gram-negative coverage of the cephalosporin class with good activity against *H. influenzae* and Neisseria spp. while maintaining good coverage against Streptococci spp. and MSSA. Unique to the cephamycins, is the activity against anaerobic bacteria such as Bacteroides spp. Progression to the third generation (ceftriaxone, ceftazidime, cefotaxime, cefixime, cefdinir, cefpodoxime, ceftibuten) improves coverage against enteric gram-negative organisms but activity against gram-positive bacteria is reduced. Ceftazidime has broader coverage as compared to other third generation cephalosporins due to its activity against *P. aeruginosa*. The fourth generation is considered the broadest of all cephalosporins due to its improved enteric gram-negative coverage, including *P. aeruginosa*, as well as good activity against gram-positive organisms. No cephalosporins have activity against MRSA or Enterococcus spp. with the exception of the

fifth generation. Ceftaroline is the first cephalosporin to have activity against MRSA and ampicillin-susceptible *Enterococcus faecalis*. It maintains activity against Streptococci spp. as well as other Staphylococcus spp., however, has minimal activity against gram-negative organisms and no activity against *P. aeruginosa*.[6]

In order to counter inactivation of susceptible cephalosporins by extended spectrum beta-lactamases, combination cephalosporin with beta-lactamase inhibitors are being developed. Current combinations available for use in the United States include ceftolozane/tazobactam and ceftazidime/avibactam. The addition of the beta-lactamase inhibitor restores the activity of the parent cephalosporin specifically against Class A, C, and D beta-lactamases.[6]

The earlier generation cephalosporins have decreased penetration into the CNS, however, the later generations, such as ceftriaxone and cefepime, have improved penetration in the CNS making them ideal agents for the treatment of meningitis.[6,7] The majority of cephalosporins are renally eliminated and thus require adjustment in dosing for patients with renal insufficiency. The exception is ceftriaxone, which is excreted by way of the biliary system. Cephalosporins are typically well tolerated with a limited side effect profile. Due to the similar structure of penicillins, there is a potential for cross-reactivity in patients with reported penicillin allergies. The incidence of cross-reactivity is much less than what was once thought, with reactions occurring in less than 1% of patients.[6]

Carbapenems

The last sub-group within the beta-lactam class are the carbapenems. This group includes meropenem, doripenem, ertapenem, and imipenem. Cilastatin is formulated in combination with imipenem to prevent degradation in the renal tubules.[8] These medications not only have broader activity when compared to penicillins and cephalosporins but are also stable against beta-lactamases, specifically extended-spectrum beta-lactamases (ESBLs) and AmpC-producing organisms.[9] In addition to enhanced activity against beta-lactamases, carbapenems have good activity against gram-negative organisms including *P. aeruginosa* (excluding ertapenem), gram-positive bacteria, and anaerobes.[8,9]

Carbapenems distribute extensively into most tissues, making them a good choice for CNS infections. Like most other beta-lactams, carbapenems are renally eliminated and therefore require dose adjustment in kidney disease.[8] Carbapenem antibiotics are well-tolerated, however, may increase risks for the development of seizures. This is important to consider when treating patients with epilepsy who are prescribed valproic acid derivatives, as carbapenems significantly reduce serum levels of these antiepileptic medications.[8]

MONOBACTAM ANTIBIOTICS

Monobactam antibiotics differ from beta-lactams in chemical structure where in place of the bicyclic beta-lactam ring, there is a monocyclic ring.[8] The only monobactam available for use in the United States at this time is aztreonam. Like beta-lactam antibiotics, aztreonam is bactericidal and casts its antimicrobial effects by binding to penicillin-binding proteins, which prevents transpeptidation and ultimately cell wall synthesis. Aztreonam is highly effective against gram-negative organisms, including *P. aeruginosa*, however, offers no activity against gram-positive organisms or anaerobes.[8] Aztreonam offers moderate protection against beta-lactamase production, however, this excludes ESBLs, AmpC, and *Klebsiella pneumoniae* carbapenemase (KPC) beta-lactamases.[8] Due to the different chemical structure as compared to beta-lactams, aztreonam has little to no cross-reactivity and is well tolerated in penicillin allergic patients. Aztreonam has good penetration into most bodily tissues, including the lungs and CSF.[8] Similar to previously discussed antibiotics, aztreonam is renally eliminated and therefore must be adjusted in renal impairment.[8]

GLYCOPEPTIDES

The most commonly utilized glycopeptide in the United States is vancomycin. Vancomycin was initially derived from *Streptococcus orientalis* in the early 1950s to battle the development of penicillin-resistant and ultimately MRSA.[3,10] Vancomycin has broad gram-positive coverage, including MRSA, Enterococcus spp., and Clostridium spp. but no gram-negative activity. Vancomycin exhibits its bactericidal effect by binding to D-alanyl-D-alanine, which prevents cell wall synthesis.[11] A commonly noted adverse event associated with vancomycin use is the development of 'red man syndrome'. Red man syndrome is characterized by the development of flushing, hypotension, and tachycardia and is attributed to the rate of vancomycin infusion. Additionally, there is a concern for both ototoxicity and nephrotoxicity with the use of vancomycin.[11]

The microbial killing potential of vancomycin is best assessed using the (area under the curve [AUC]/ minimum inhibitory concentration [MIC]) ratio with a goal greater than or equal to 400, however, calculation

of the AUC is not practical in everyday practice, therefore trough values have been correlated to the AUC for clinical use.[10] Severe disease states including endocarditis, meningitis, pneumonia, osteomyelitis, bacteraemia, etc. require a goal trough between 15–20 mcg/ml. Less severe infections such as skin and soft tissue infections, a lower trough goal (10–15 mcg/ml) may be adequate.[10]

Vancomycin penetrates well into the kidney, cardiac muscle, and lung with limited penetration into the CNS.[10] Inflammation of the meninges during meningitis improves the distribution of vancomycin into the tissue. Vancomycin is not absorbed systemically when orally administered, however, the oral formulation is utilized for the treatment of *Clostridium difficile* colitis due to the local effects of the medication.[10] Lastly, vancomycin is renally eliminated and may cause nephrotoxicity, therefore, dose adjustment is required for patients with decreased renal function.[10]

LIPOPEPTIDE

Daptomycin is the only lipopeptide antimicrobial currently approved for use in the United States. Daptomycin exhibits its antimicrobial effect by targeting the cell membrane of gram-positive organisms leading to depolarization of the membrane and ultimately inhibition of ribonucleic acid (RNA) and deoxyribonucleic acid (DNA) synthesis.[11] Daptomycin has good activity against MRSA, MSSA, and Enterococcus spp., especially those isolates with increased resistance to glycopeptides.[11] Daptomycin has no activity against gram-negative organisms.

Daptomycin has a small volume of distribution suggesting minimal penetration into tissues throughout the body, including the CNS with uninflamed meninges.[11] Daptomycin becomes inactivated by pulmonary surfactants, therefore, is not an effective treatment for pneumonia. Daptomycin is renally eliminated necessitating dose adjustment in renal failure.[11] Daptomycin is relatively well tolerated, however, it is recommended to obtain a baseline creatinine phosphokinase (CPK), and monitor CPK weekly due to early reports of rhabdomyolysis associated with daptomycin use.[11]

FLUOROQUINOLONES

Fluoroquinolones are highly utilized in clinical practice secondary to their broad spectrum of activity, relative tolerability, and bioavailability. The commonly used fluoroquinolones include levofloxacin, moxifloxacin, and ciprofloxacin. Fluoroquinolones have extensive activity against gram-negative organisms including Enterobacteriaceae.[12] Both ciprofloxacin and levofloxacin have coverage against *P. aeruginosa*. Moxifloxacin and levofloxacin are designated respiratory fluoroquinolones due to their activity against *Streptococcus pneumoniae* and atypical organisms. Additionally, moxifloxacin has good coverage against anaerobic organisms.[12] Fluoroquinolones exert their bactericidal activity by inhibiting bacterial topoisomerase II (DNA-gyrase), thus preventing DNA replication and transcription.[12]

Fluoroquinolones have 100% oral bioavailability compared to the intravenous formulation. It is important to note that oral administration with concomitant enteral feedings will decrease absorption of the medication; therefore, it is recommended to hold enteral feeds around the administration time of fluoroquinolone.[12] Fluoroquinolones have a very large volume of distribution exceeding adequate concentrations in the kidney (ciprofloxacin and levofloxacin), lung, abdomen, and prostate. Cerebrospinal fluid (CSF) penetration may be limited secondary to active transport systems.[12] The majority of fluoroquinolones are renally eliminated, with the exception of moxifloxacin, and therefore require dose adjustment in renal failure.[12]

Due to the potential overuse of fluoroquinolones, there has been increasing rates of resistance with common community and hospital-acquired organisms including *E. coli, K. pneumoniae,* and *P. aeruginosa.*[12] Therefore, appropriate use of fluoroquinolones requires close monitoring.

Fluoroquinolones are associated with a series of different adverse events. The United States Food and Drug Administration (FDA) recently released a statement suggesting that fluoroquinolones should be reserved for more serious infections in which alternative options are not available secondary to the risk of tendonitis and tendon rupture.[13] Additional adverse events associated with fluoroquinolone use include *C. difficile* infections, lowering of the seizure threshold, and QTc prolongation.[12] Although these antimicrobials have a broad spectrum of activity and large volume of distribution, their use is limited by increasing resistance patterns as well as side effects.

AMINOGLYCOSIDES

Aminoglycosides have been an important antibiotic since the discovery of streptomycin in the 1940s from soil cultures of Streptomyces spp. The aminoglycosides produced from Streptomyces spp. (ending in -mycin) and Micromonospora spp. (ending in -micin) share similar physical, chemical, and pharmacological properties.[14] They display concentration-dependent killing and post-antibiotic effects against susceptible organisms by binding to the 16S ribosomal RNA. Aside from regional and individual hospital differences, most aerobic and facultative gram-negative bacilli, including Acinetobacter spp., Enterobacteriaceae, and *P. aeruginosa* are susceptible to gentamicin, tobramycin, and amikacin within the United States.[14] When administered concomitantly with beta-lactams, the net effect of the aminoglycoside combination can be additive to or synergistic against infections caused by aerobic gram-negative bacilli or aerobic gram-positive cocci.

The aminoglycosides possess low protein binding potential (<10%) and are highly hydrophilic and thus distribute into the vascular and interstitial spaces of most tissues. The volume of distribution is similar to the extracellular fluid compartment (~0.3 L/kg).[15] Adequate concentrations can be achieved in most body fluids, but transmission is poor into bronchial secretions and CSF where aerosolized and intraventricular routes are utilized to optimize therapy, respectively. Aminoglycosides are primarily eliminated unchanged in the urine. The most significant adverse reactions to aminoglycosides are nephrotoxicity, which is reversible with cessation of the drug, and ototoxicity, which is usually irreversible and can manifest as cochlear or vestibular toxicity.[14]

OXAZOLIDINONES

The oxazolidinones in their current form have only been around since the turn of the century. Linezolid was the first compound approved by the FDA in 2000 for use in the treatment of a variety of infections caused by gram-positive pathogens. Oxazolidinones work by inhibiting protein synthesis, that is binding the ribosomal RNA of the 50S subunit, ultimately inhibiting the formation of the 70S initiation complex needed for the bacterial translation process.[16] Linezolid has activity against many gram-positive organisms including coagulase-negative Staphylococci, *Enterococcus faecium*, and *Enterococcus faecalis* (vancomycin-susceptible and vancomycin-resistant strains), *Staphylococcus aureus* (methicillin-susceptible and methicillin-resistant strains), many Nocardia strains, and Streptococci spp. While usually bacteriostatic when administered concomitantly with gentamicin, linezolid exhibits bactericidal activity against Streptococci.

When given orally, absorption is rapid and bioavailability is nearly 100% with serum concentrations at or higher than the MIC90 for target pathogens throughout the dosing interval. Linezolid has low protein binding (~31% to plasma proteins) and penetration into a variety of tissues at high concentrations enough to treat most infections in CSF, pulmonary fluid, alveolar cells, pancreatic secretions, and bone.[17] Linezolid undergoes hepatic metabolism via oxidation of the morpholine ring into two inactive metabolites (aminoethoxyacetic acid and hydroxyethyl glycine) and has minimal cytochrome P-450 enzyme interaction. Urinary excretion accounts for over 80% of the drug elimination, with about 30% of the unchanged drug excreted renally. Faecal elimination of the two major metabolites accounts for the remaining excretion. There is no dose adjustment recommended for hepatic or renal impairment. Metabolites can be cleared via dialysis methods, with dosing recommended following intermittent dialysis sessions. Linezolid is also removed by continuous renal replacement therapy, but no dose adjustments are recommended.

Linezolid is well-tolerated with gastrointestinal reactions (e.g., diarrhoea, nausea, vomiting) occurring in up to 10% of patients. Notable adverse drug reactions include reversible myelosuppression, neuropathies, and lactic acidosis. Additionally, linezolid is a reversible, non-selective monoamine oxidase inhibitor and should be used with caution in patients on concomitant serotonergic agents.[18]

MACROLIDES

Macrolide antibiotics have been around since the early 1950s when erythromycin was derived from a strain of *Saccharopolyspora erythraea* (formerly known as *Streptomyces erythraeus*) found in a soil sample from the Philippines. The antibiotics in this class work by binding to the 50S ribosomal subunit to inhibit RNA-dependent protein synthesis.[19] Erythromycin is poorly soluble in water, rapidly inactivated by gastric acid, and has inconsistent oral absorption. Oral preparations by pharmaceutical manufacturers are resistant to destruction by gastric acid and have improved absorption. Azithromycin and clarithromycin were developed to improve on the shortcomings of erythromycin. They possess a greater spectrum of activity, have improved oral absorption and gastrointestinal tolerability, and longer half-lives than erythromycin. Erythromycin has activity against a broad range of gram-positive and gram-negative organisms. Clarithromycin has greater activity against gram-positive pathogens compared to azithromycin, which has decreased activity against gram-positive organisms. Conversely, azithromycin has greater activity against gram-negative organisms than erythromycin or clarithromycin, especially *H. influenza* and *M. catarrhalis*.[19] Clindamycin (a lincomycin derivative) is biologically similar to the macrolides but chemically unrelated. It has a spectrum of activity similar to erythromycin but with less gram-negative activity. Additionally, clindamycin has significantly greater activity against anaerobes than erythromycin.

As previously discussed, erythromycin requires pharmaceutical manipulation into various salt forms to increase bioavailability when given orally. Clarithromycin has good oral bioavailability (~50%) compared to azithromycin (~37%). Clindamycin has excellent bioavailability (90%). Both clarithromycin and azithromycin have wide distribution into tissues and can achieve tissue concentrations several-fold higher than serum, particularly in the pulmonary sections and lungs. Clindamycin has good penetration into bone and is actively transported into polymorphonuclear leukocytes and macrophages. All macrolides and clindamycin have poor CSF penetration.[19] The macrolides and clindamycin are metabolized hepatically and exhibit minimal renal excretion. Dose adjustments are only recommended for clarithromycin in patients with renal impairment (creatinine clearance [CrCl] <30 ml/min). Erythromycin, azithromycin, and clindamycin do not require dose adjustment in renal or hepatic insufficiency. These agents are also not removed by renal replacement therapies.[19] Aside from gastrointestinal side effects, the most notable adverse drug effect of macrolides include QT-interval prolongation.

MISCELLANEOUS AGENTS

Metronidazole

Metronidazole is a synthetic nitroimidazole antibiotic first synthesized in the early 1950s. The spectrum of activity of metronidazole and other nitroimidazoles is dependent on activation of the drug in susceptible organisms once it is passively diffused into the organism. This class of anti-infectives function as prodrugs and requires activation in the bacterial cytoplasm or organelles of protozoa.[20] The mechanism of action requires four phases; entry into the bacterial cell, reduction of the nitro group, cytotoxic effect of the reduced product, and release of end products that are inactive. The redox intermediate is thought to be the key step resulting in microorganism cell death by metronidazole.[21]

Metronidazole and related nitroimidazoles have activity against a variety of anaerobic bacteria, microaerophilic bacteria, and protozoa. Many gram-negative anaerobes are susceptible such as the Bacteroides and Parabacteroides species.[22] Metronidazole is not recommended for empiric treatment of facultative anaerobes due to its variable susceptibilities and increasing resistance.[23] Gram-positive anaerobes such as Clostridia spp. remain susceptible to metronidazole, but a few isolates of *Clostridium difficile* have shown decreased susceptibility to metronidazole.[24–26] Nitroimidazoles are also active against several protozoa including Giardia, *Entamoeba histolytica*, and *Dientamoeba fragilis*. Non-spore-forming, gram-positive anaerobic bacteria remain a significant and important void in the anaerobic spectrum of metronidazole due to intrinsic resistance to the drug. These isolates include Actinomyces, Bifidobacterium, Lactobacillus, and Propionibacterium.[24]

Oral metronidazole is rapidly absorbed with bioavailability approaching 100% and peak serum levels being attained within 1–2 hours after oral administration.[27] Metronidazole is a lipophilic molecule with low protein binding and a moderate to large volume of distribution owing to its extensive distribution into a variety of tissues at concentrations similar to that of serum.[20] The drug undergoes oxidation as the primary step for drug elimination from the body with 6%–18% of active unchanged drug recovered in the urine. Five major metabolites are formed via oxidation, glucuronidation, and metabolism through the cytochrome P450 system and excreted in the faeces and urine. Patients with moderate to severe hepatic disease should have their dose reduced by 50%.[22] Also, patients with end-stage renal disease (CrCl <10 ml/min) can have accumulation of the active metabolite. Metronidazole and its metabolites are removed by various renal replacement therapies, but renal dose adjustment is not recommended due to a poor understanding of metronidazole metabolite accumulation.[21]

Metronidazole is generally well-tolerated. Adverse effects are typically dose-dependent, mild, and reversible; with nausea, diarrhoea, dry mouth, and metallogeusia. Central nervous system toxicities can be severe and may include ataxia, encephalopathy, seizures, and aseptic meningitis. These toxicities have developed with prolonged therapy, but have resolved with discontinuation of metronidazole.[22]

Folic Acid Antagonist

One of the earliest antimicrobial compounds in clinical use, the sulphonamides, have been used as antimicrobials since the early 1930s. The parent sulphanilamide compound was improved to remove side effects and expand the spectrum of activity. In the late 1960s, trimethoprim was added to potentiate sulphonamide activity and clinically establish its important role in infectious disease treatments. The combination of trimethoprim-sulfamethoxazole

(TMP-SMX) exerts a synergistic antimicrobial effect. The sulphonamide inhibits microbial folic acid synthesis by mimicking para-aminobenzoic acid (PABA), which is ultimately required for production of dihydrofolic acid. Trimethoprim inhibits dihydrofolate reductase, thereby blocking the production of tetrahydrofolic acid, and ultimately folic acid.[28] In combination, two DNA precursor components are inhibited resulting in a bacteriostatic inhibition of bacterial growth.

The sulphonamides have activity against a broad spectrum of both gram-positive and gram-negative organisms in a wide array of infections. Notable infections or pathogens often treated with TMP-SMX include urinary, respiratory, or gastrointestinal tract infections, skin and soft tissue infections, sexually transmitted diseases, infections caused by Nocardia spp., *Pneumocystis jirovecii*, *Stenotrophomonas maltophilia*, *Listeria monocytogenes*, *Plasmodium falciparum*, *Toxoplasma gondii*, Acanthamoeba, and many others. Trimethoprim-sulfamethoxazole is readily absorbed from the gastrointestinal tract and gets distributed widely throughout the body including the CSF, lung secretions, urine, human breast milk, and seminal fluid.[29] Trimethoprim-sulfamethoxazole is metabolized via the CYP2C9 and CYP3A4 hepatic enzyme system and also inhibits CYP2C9 (TMP-SMX) and CYP2C8 (TMP). Trimethoprim-sulfamethoxazole is excreted in the urine as metabolites and unchanged drug.[30] The drug is removed by haemodialysis and patients with renal insufficiency require dose adjustments. Trimethoprim-sulfamethoxazole can cause a variety of adverse drug reactions, more commonly gastrointenstinal disturbances such nausea, vomiting, and diarrhoea. Toxic epidermal necrolysis and Stevens-Johnson syndrome have occurred (<1%).[31] Drug-induced hyperkalaemia can occur typically in combination with an angiotensin converting enzyme inhibitor, angiotensin receptor blocker, or a potassium-sparing diuretic. Additionally, drug-induced thrombocytopenia can manifest from impaired folate usage.

Rifamycins

The rifamycin class (rifampin, rifabutin, rifapentine) of antimicrobials have very precise indications for use. These indications include treatment of mycobacterial infections as well as inhibition of Staphylococcal biofilm production.[32] Rifamycins are bactericidal and inhibit RNA synthesis by binding to the beta subunit of DNA-dependent RNA polymerase.[32] Although these agents were initially effective independently, they rapidly developed resistance and are now used in combination with other treatments.

Of the rifamycins, rifampin is likely to be the most commonly used. It is widely distributed and highly lipophilic, thus penetrating well into most tissues including the CSF.[32] Rifampin primarily undergoes hepatic metabolism and therefore does not require dose adjustment in renal insufficiency. It is important to note that rifampin has many drug interactions due to its induction of the CYP3A4 enzyme. Significant interactions include anticoagulants, antiretrovirals, immunosuppressants, and others.[32] It is important to thoroughly evaluate all potential drug interactions when initiating this therapy.

Polymyxins

The polymyxins were discovered in 1947 and were largely not used until the 1980s due to the availability of alternative less toxic agents. The two agents available include polymyxin B and polymyxin E (colistimethate sodium [CMS]). It is important to note the specific formulation of CMS used as this often leads to dosing confusion (1 million IU = 80 mg of colistimethate = 30 mg 'colistin base activity').[33] Due to the emergence of antimicrobial resistance, the polymyxins have had a resurgence of use in severe gram-negative infections. Polymyxins work by penetration and disruption of the outer cell membrane of bacteria by competitive displacement of divalent cations.[34] The polymyxins have activity against many gram-negative organisms, most notably multidrug resistant *P. aeruginosa* and *A. baumannii*, and carbapenem-resistant Enterobacteriaceae. Polymyxins are not absorbed orally and only utilized via the oral route for gut decontamination, which is not available in the United States. Colistimethate sodium distributes widely into tissue, except that it has poor distribution into the biliary tract, CSF, joint and pleural fluid. Only about 30% of the inactive prodrug, CMS, is hydrolyzed into colistin (active drug), and a small fraction

of CMS is found unchanged in urine.[34] The most notable adverse effect of CMS is dose-related nephrotoxicity, which is reversible upon drug discontinuation. Due to its poor CNS penetration, CMS has been administered via the intraventricular and intrathecal routes in severe gram-negative CNS infections.[34]

ANTIVIRALS

There are a multitude of antivirals available for use in the United States, however, for the purposes if this chapter, the authors will be focusing on acyclovir use for the treatment of CNS infections.

The Infectious Diseases Society of America (IDSA) guidelines recommend that patients with suspected viral encephalitis must be empirically treated with acyclovir until final culture data is available. The majority of viruses causing encephalitis tend to be treated with supportive care, with the exception of herpes virus, varicella zoster virus, and cytomegalovirus.[35] Early initiation of acyclovir (within two days of presentation) has proven benefit on patient prognosis with herpes simplex encephalitis, thus giving support to empiric treatment.[36]

Acyclovir through a series of mechanisms is converted to acyclovir triphosphate which inhibits binding of deoxyguanosine triphosphate to DNA polymerase, thus preventing DNA synthesis and viral replication.[37] It has activity against both herpes simplex viruses and varicella zoster virus. It distributes widely into the tissues including the brain, kidneys, lungs, and CSF.[37] It is primarily excreted through the kidneys and therefore requires adjustment in renal dysfunction.[37] A severe adverse effect associated with the use of acyclovir is the development of renal failure secondary to precipitation of the drug in the renal tubules. It is important to maintain adequate hydration to minimize the risk of acyclovir crystal formation[38] (see Table 21.2).

Table 21.2 Summary of antiviral spectrum of activity and select pharmacokinetic parameters

Antimicrobial	Spectrum of activity	CNS penetration (AUC_{CSF}/AUC_S)[*]	Renal adjustment[#] (Y/N)	Hepatic adjustment[#] (Y/N)
Acyclovir	Herpes virus Varicella Zoster Virus	0.31	Y	N

*(1) Nau R, Sorgel F, Eiffert H. Penetration of drugs through the blood-cerebrospinal fluid/blood-brain barrier for treatment of central nervous system infections. *Clinical Microbiology Reviews* 2010;23(4):858–83. (2) Gilbert D, Chambers H, Eliopoulos G, Saag M. *The Sanford Guide to Antimicrobial Therapy*. 44th ed. Sperryville: Antimicrobial Therapy Inc., 2014; p. 86. (3) Saravolatz LD, Stein GE, Johnson LB. Ceftaroline: A novel cephalosporin with activity against methicillin-resistant *Staphylococcus aureus*. *Clin Infect Dis* 2011;52(9):1156–63.
#Bennett JE, Dolin R, Blaser MJ. *Mandell, Douglas, and Bennett's Principles and Practice of Infectious Diseases*. Updated 8th ed. Philadelphia: Saunders, an imprint of Elsevier Inc, 2015.

ANTIFUNGALS

There are three main classes of antifungals; azole antifungals, echinocandins, and the polyene antifungal. Historically, the most frequently utilized class of antifungals were the azoles, however, with increasing resistance, the other classes have become more highly utilized.

Azoles

The azole antifungals include fluconazole, voriconazole, posaconazole, itraconazole, and isavuconazole. Azole antifungals exhibit their effect by inhibiting the cytochrome P-450 enzyme, lanosterol 14-alpha-demethylase, thus decreasing ergosterol synthesis which is a necessary component for cell membrane production.[39] Of all of the azole antifungals, fluconazole tends to be the most versatile azole and therefore will be discussed moving forward.

Fluconazole has good activity against most Candida spp. Exceptions include *Candida krusei, Candida glabrata, Candida norvegensis,* and *Candida inconspicua,* which are intrinsically resistant to most azole antifungals.[39] Fluconazole has a large volume of distribution and penetrates well into the CNS. Fluconazole is eliminated by the kidneys, so in cases of renal impairment dose adjustments are required.[39] Azole antifungals have many drug interactions due to their activity on cytochrome P-450 enzymes. It is important for the practitioner to thoroughly evaluate potential drug interactions when initiating azole antifungals. Notable interactions include warfarin, calcineurin inhibitors, antiretrovirals, and antiepileptics.[39]

Echinocandins

The echinocandin class of antifungals include caspofungin, micafungin, and anidulafungin. They work by inhibiting the synthesis of B(1,3)-D-glucan, an essential component of fungal cell walls which leads to cellular lysis.[39]

The three enchinocandins have similar spectrum of activity, covering most Candida spp. with decreased efficacy only seen in *Candida parapsilosis* and *Candida guilliermondii.*[39] The echinocandins also have decent activity against *Aspergillus* spp.[40] They have volumes of distribution that are similar to that of total body water limiting penetration into the CSF.[39] This class of antifungals is not renally eliminated, and therefore does not require renal dose adjustment. Clearance of caspofungin may be impaired in patients with hepatic insufficiency, and therefore dose reduction is recommended.[39] The echinocandins are generally well-tolerated and have minimal drug interactions.

Polyene Antifungal

Amphotericin-B is the only polyene antifungal currently available for use in the United States. Amphotericin-B exerts its activity by binding to ergosterol, thus altering cell membrane permeability.[39]

There are four formulations available, amphotericin-B deoxycholate and three lipid related formulations, amphotericin-B colloidal dispersion, amphotericin-B lipid complex, and liposomal amphotericin-B. The conventional formulation, amphotericin-B deoxycholate, is associated with significant side effects, including renal toxicity secondary to direct vasoconstriction on renal arterioles, electrolyte wasting, and infusion-related reactions.[39] In order to combat the side effects of conventional amphotericin-B, the liposomal associated formulations were developed which have significantly lower concentration in the kidneys, decreasing the risk of nephrotoxicity.[39]

It is important to recognize that the dosing between the formulations differ significantly. Amphotericin-B deoxycholate is typically dosed 0.3 mg/kg/day to 1 mg/kg/day, whereas the lipid related formulations are dosed 3 mg/kg/day to 5 mg/kg/day.[39] This poses the risk of potential medication errors secondary to the fact that deoxycholate is one-tenth the dose of lipid formulations. Although different formulations of amphotericin-B display varying pharmacokinetics, it should be noted that all formulations minimally penetrate into the meninges or CSF, making it difficult to treat CNS infections with intravenous therapy.[39] Amphotericin-B has activity against most fungi, however, there is substantial resistance that has been reported to *Candida lusitaniae*[39] (see Table 21.3).

Table 21.3 Summary of antifungal spectrum of activity and select pharmacokinetic parameters

Antimicrobial	Spectrum of activity	CNS penetration $(AUC_{CSF}/AUC_S)^{[*]}$	Renal adjustment[#] (Y/N)	Hepatic adjustment[#] (Y/N)	Fungicidal vs fungistatic[@]
Azoles	Candida spp. (except *C. krusei, C. glabrata*)	0.80	Y	N	Fungistatic

(Cont'd)

Table 21.3 (*Cont'd*)

Antimicrobial	Spectrum of activity	CNS penetration (AUC_{CSF}/AUC_S) [*]	Renal adjustment [#] (Y/N)	Hepatic adjustment [#] (Y/N)	Fungicidal vs fungistatic [@]
Echinocandins	Candida spp. (except *C. parapsilosis, C. guilliermondii*) Aspergillus spp.	–	N	Y	Fungicidal
Polyene antifungal	Candida spp. (except *C. lusitaniae*) Aspergillus spp.	–	N	N	Fungicidal

*(1) Nau R, Sorgel F, Eiffert H. Penetration of drugs through the blood-cerebrospinal fluid/blood-brain barrier for treatment of central nervous system infections. *Clinical Microbiology Reviews* 2010;23(4):858–83. (2) Gilbert D, Chambers H, Eliopoulos G, Saag M. *The Sanford Guide to Antimicrobial Therapy*. 44th ed. Sperryville: Antimicrobial Therapy Inc., 2014; p. 86. (3) Saravolatz LD, Stein GE, Johnson LB. Ceftaroline: A novel cephalosporin with activity against methicillin-resistant *Staphylococcus aureus*. *Clin Infect Dis* 2011;52(9):1156–11.

#Bennett JE, Dolin R, Blaser MJ. *Mandell, Douglas, and Bennett's Principles and Practice of Infectious Diseases*. Updated 8th ed. Philadelphia: Saunders, an imprint of Elsevier Inc, 2015.

@Venisse N, Gregoire N, Marliat M, Couet W. Mechanism-based pharmacokinetic-pharmacodynamic models of in vitro fungistatic and fungicidal effects against *Candida albicans*. *Antimicrob Agents Chemother* 2008;52(3):937–43.

CONCLUSIONS

This chapter and the associated tables provide an overview of the most common agents that may be utilized to treat infections that occur in the neurointensive care unit. The focus of this chapter is interpretation and application of pharmacokinetic parameters of medication and pharmacodynamic qualities of patients. Understanding these properties will optimize appropriate treatment of infections, especially those of the CNS.

REFERENCES

1. Eliopoulos GM, Moellering RC. Principles of anti-infective therapy. In: Bennett JE, Dolin R, and Blaser MJ eds, *Mandell, Douglas, and Bennett's Principles and Practice of Infectious Diseases*. Updated 8th ed. Philadelphia: Saunders, an imprint of Elsevier Inc, 2015:224–34.
2. Tunkel AR. Approach to the patient with central nervous system infection. In: Bennett JE, Dolin R, and Blaser MJ eds, *Mandell, Douglas, and Bennett's Principles and Practice of Infectious Diseases*. Updated 8th ed. Philadelphia: Saunders, an imprint of Elsevier Inc, 2015: 1091–6.
3. Fleming A. On the antibacterial action of cultures of a penicillium, with special reference to their use in the isolation of B. influenzæ. *Br J Exp Pathol* 1929;10(3):226–36.
4. Bennett JE, Dolin R, Blaser MJ. *Mandell, Douglas, and Bennett's Principles and Practice of Infectious Diseases*. Updated 8th ed. Philadelphia: Saunders, an imprint of Elsevier Inc, 2015.
5. Doi Y, Chambers HF. Penicillins and β-Lactamase Inhibitors. In: Bennett JE, Dolin R, and Blaser MJ eds, *Mandell, Douglas, and Bennett's Principles and Practice of Infectious Diseases*. Updated 8th ed. Philadelphia: Saunders, an imprint of Elsevier Inc, 2015:263–77.
6. Craig WA, Andes DR. Cephalosporins. In: Bennett JE, Dolin R, and Blaser MJ eds, *Mandell, Douglas, and Bennett's Principles and Practice of Infectious Diseases*. Updated 8th ed. Philadelphia: Saunders, an imprint of Elsevier Inc, 2015: 278–92.
7. Tunkel AR, Hartman BJ, Kaplan SL, et al. Practice guidelines for the management of bacterial meningitis. *Clin Infect Dis* 39;2004:1267–84.
8. Doi Y, Chambers HF. Other β-lactam antibiotics. In: Bennett JE, Dolin R, and Blaser MJ eds, *Mandell, Douglas, and Bennett's Principles and Practice of Infectious Diseases*. Updated 8th ed. Philadelphia: Saunders, an imprint of Elsevier Inc, 2015:293–7.
9. Petri WA. Penicillins, cephalosporins, and other β-lactam antibiotics. *Goodman and Gilman's The Pharmacological Basis of Therapeutics*. 12th ed. Laurence Brunton; New York: McGraw Hill; 2011.
10. Levine DP. Vancomycin: a history. *Clin Infect Dis* 2006 Jan 1;42(1):S5–12.
11. Murray BE, Arias CA, Nannini EC. Glycopeptides (vancomycin and teicoplanin), streptogramins (quinupristin-dalfopristin), lipopeptides (daptomycin), and lipoglycopeptides (telavancin). In: Bennett JE, Dolin R, and Blaser MJ eds, *Mandell, Douglas, and Bennett's Principles and Practice of Infectious Diseases*. Updated 8th ed. Philadelphia: Saunders, an imprint of Elsevier Inc; 2015:377–400.
12. Hooper DC, Stahilevitz J. Quinolones. In: Bennett JE, Dolin R, and Blaser MJ eds, *Mandell, Douglas, and Bennett's Principles and Practice of Infectious Diseases*. Updated 8th ed. Philadelphia: Saunders, an imprint of Elsevier Inc; 2015:419–39.

13. FDA Drug Safety Communications. FDA Drug Safety Communication: FDA updates warnings for oral and injectable fluoroquinolone antibiotics due to disabling side effects. [cited 2016]. Available from: http://www.fda.gov/downloads/Drugs/DrugSafety/UCM513019.pdf.

14. Leggett JE. Aminoglycosides. In: Bennett JE, Dolin R, and Blaser MJ eds, *Mandell, Douglas, and Bennett's Principles and Practice of Infectious Diseases*. Updated 8th ed. Philadelphia: Saunders, an imprint of Elsevier Inc; 2015:310–21.

15. Bailey DN, Briggs JR. Gentamicin and tobramycin binding to human serum in vitro. *J Anal Toxicol* 2004;28: 187–9.

16. Cox HL, Donowitz GR. Linezolid and other oxazolidinones. In: Bennett JE, Dolin R, and Blaser MJ eds, *Mandell, Douglas, and Bennett's Principles and Practice of Infectious Diseases*. Updated 8th ed. Philadelphia: Saunders, an imprint of Elsevier Inc, 2015:406–09.

17. Di Paolo A, Malacarne P, Guidotti E, et al. Pharmacological issues of linezolid: an updated critical review. *Clin Pharmacokinet* 2010; 49:439–47.

18. Narita M, Tsuji BT, Yu VL. Linezolid-associated peripheral and optic neuropathy, lactic acidosis, and serotonin syndrome. *Pharmacotherapy* 2007;27:1189–97.

19. Sivapalasingam S, Steigbiegel NH. Macrolides, clindamycin, and ketolides. In: Bennett JE, Dolin R, and Blaser MJ eds, *Mandell, Douglas, and Bennett's Principles and Practice of Infectious Diseases*. Updated 8th ed. Philadelphia: Saunders, an imprint of Elsevier Inc; 2015:358–76.

20. Lofmark S, Edlund C, Nord CE. Metronidazole is still the drug of choice for treatment of anaerobic infections. *Clin Infect Dis* 2010;50(suppl 1):S16–S23.

21. Soares GM, Figueiredo LC, Faveri M, et al. Mechanisms of action of systemic antibiotics used in periodontal treatment and mechanisms of bacterial resistance to these drugs. *J Appl Oral Sci* 2012;20(3):295–309.

22. Nagel JL, Aronoff DM. Metronidazole. In: Bennett JE, Dolin R, and Blaser MJ eds, *Mandell, Douglas, and Bennett's Principles and Practice of Infectious Diseases*. Updated 8th ed. Philadelphia: Saunders, an imprint of Elsevier Inc, 2015:350–7.

23. MiendjeDeyi VY, Bontems P, Vanderpas J, et al. Multicenter survey of routine determinations of resistance of *Helicobacter pylori* to antimicrobials over the last 20 years (1990 to 2009) in Belgium. *J Clin Microbiol* 2011;49(6):2200–09.

24. Baines SD, O'Connor R, Freeman J, et al. Emergence of reduced susceptibility to metronidazole in Clostridium difficile. *J Antimicrob Chemother* 2008;62(5):1046–52.

25. Lynch T, Chong P, Zhang J, et al. Characterization of a stable, metronidazole-resistant Clostridium difficile clinical isolate. *PLoS ONE* 2013;8(1):e537–57.

26. Moura I, Spigaglia P, Barbanti F, Mastrantonio P. Analysis of metronidazole susceptibility in different Clostridium difficile PCR ribotypes. *J Antimicrob Chemother* 2013; 68(2):362–5.

27. Lau AH, Lam NP, Piscitelli SC, et al. Clinical pharmacokinetics of metronidazole and other nitroimidazole anti-infectives. *Clin Pharmacokinet* 1992; 23(5):328–64.

28. Matthews DA, Bolin JT, Burridge JM, Filman DJ, Volz KW, Kraut J. Dihydrofolate reductase. *J Biol Chem* 1985;260:392–9.

29. Pater RB, Welling PG. Clinical pharmacokinetics of co-trimoxazole (trimethoprim/sulfamethoxazole). *Clin Pharmacokinet* 1980;5:405–23.

30. Zinner S, Mayer K. Sulfonamides and Trimethoprim. In: Bennett JE, Dolin R, and Blaser MJ eds, *Mandell, Douglas, and Bennett's Principles and Practice of Infectious Diseases*. Updated 8th ed. Philadelphia: Saunders, an imprint of Elsevier Inc, 2015:410–18.

31. Mittmann N, Knowles SR, Koo M, et al. Incidence of toxic epidermal necrolysis and Stevens-Johnson syndrome in an HIV cohort: an observational, retrospective case series study. *Am J Clin Dermatol* 2012;13:49–54.

32. Maslow MJ, Portal-Celhay C. Rifamycins. *Mandell, Douglas, and Bennett's Principles and Practice of Infectious Diseases*. Updated 8th ed. Philadelphia: Saunders, an imprint of Elsevier Inc; 2015:339–49.

33. Li J, Nation RL. Defining the dosage units for colistin methane sulfonate: urgent need for international harmonization. *Antimicrob Agents Chemother* 2006;50:4231–2.

34. Kaye KS, Pogue JM, Kaye D. Polymixins (Polymixin B and Colistin). In: Bennett JE, Dolin R, and Blaser MJ eds, *Mandell, Douglas, and Bennett's Principles and Practice of Infectious Diseases*. Updated 8th ed. Philadelphia: Saunders, an imprint of Elsevier Inc; 2015:401–5.

35. Tunkel AR, Glaser CA, Bloch KC, et al. The management of encephalitis: clinical practice guidelines by the Infectious Diseases Society of America. *Clin Infect Dis* 2008;47:303–27.

36. Raschilas F, Wolff M, Delatour F, et al. Outcome of and prognostic factors for herpes simplex encephalitis in adult patients: results of a multicenter study. *Clin Infect Dis* 2002;35(3):254–60.

37. Aoki F. Antivirals against herpes viruses. In: Bennett JE, Dolin R, and Blaser MJ eds, *Mandell, Douglas, and Bennett's Principles and Practice of Infectious Diseases*. Updated 8th ed. Philadelphia: Saunders, an imprint of Elsevier Inc; 2015:546–62.

38. Perazella MA. Crystal-induced acute renal failure. *Am J Med* 1999;106(4):459–65.

39. Rex JH, Stevens DA. Drugs active against fungi. Pneumocystis and Microsporidia. In: Bennett JE, Dolin R, and Blaser MJ eds, *Mandell, Douglas, and Bennett's Principles and Practice of Infectious Diseases*. 8th ed. Philadelphia: Saunders, an imprint of Elsevier Inc; 2015:479–94.

40. Nau R, Sorgel F, Eiffert H. Penetration of drugs through the blood-cerebrospinal fluid/blood–brain barrier for treatment of central nervous system infections. *Clinical Microbiology Reviews* 2010;23(4):858–83.

Part IV

Fluids and Dyselectrolytemia

Editor: Concezione Tommasino

22

Fluid Management

C. Tommasino

ABSTRACT

Fluid management in critically ill, brain-damaged patients is part of the routine neurointensive care, and is aimed at correcting fluid deficit, maintaining intravascular volume, providing adequate brain tissue perfusion and oxygenation, and minimizing secondary brain insults. Fluids should be considered like any other drug with indications, contraindications, and side effects. It is important to identify which compartment is depleted since specific losses should be replaced with appropriate fluids. Balanced plasma-adapted crystalloids should be used for fluid replacement, such as urinary output and insensible losses; while colloids are indicated for volume replacement. Fluids that reduce osmolality should be avoided, especially in patients whose baseline osmolality has been increased by hyperosmolar fluids. Glucose containing solutions should be used only in premature and newborns to prevent hypoglycaemia, and should be used with caution in patients with normal glucose metabolism. A practical approach to fluid management in these patients should include appropriate administration of maintenance fluid volumes, choosing fluid solutions based on their composition and osmolality, and relevant haemodynamic monitoring.

KEYWORDS

Fluid; crystalloid; colloid; hypertonic saline; mannitol; glycocalyx; blood–brain barrier (BBB); brain insult.

INTRODUCTION

Fluid management in patients with brain pathology is a component of routine neurointensive care. It aims at correcting fluid deficit, maintaining intravascular volume, and providing adequate brain tissue perfusion and oxygenation, and minimizing secondary brain damage. Brain perfusion may be impaired by primary neurologic conditions and by conditions that affect circulating blood volume, such as fluid deficit, and this impairment is frequently associated with poor patient outcome.[1] Although hypovolaemia can concur to secondary brain damage, recent studies have indicated a potential hazard of volume overload on the brain through the side effects on the endothelial glycocalyx and on cardiovascular and respiratory systems. Thus, rational fluid management strategy should aim at maintaining normovolaemia, replacing actual losses with the appropriate fluids and avoiding unnecessary fluid overload.

Infusing fluid represents a therapeutic measure and fluids should be considered like any other drug with indications, contraindications, and side effects. Both the amount and composition of the fluids infused are pertinent to understand their effects on the brain. Every therapeutic intervention should have a logical basis and, when feasible, an evidence-based indication. It is essential to recognize which compartment is depleted since specific losses should be restored with appropriate fluid, and physiological understanding is the only key to guide rational therapeutic decisions.[2]

Physiology

Total body water (TBW) varies with age: it is 70%–75% in full term babies; 65%–75% in young children, and 60% in adolescents and adults. Approximately two-thirds of the TBW is stored intracellularly in the intracellular fluid (ICF) compartment, and one-third forms the extracellular fluid (ECF) compartment, which consists mostly of interstitial space (80%) and blood plasma (20%). Transcellular fluids, such as intra-ocular, cerebrospinal, and gastrointestinal fluid, belonging to the ECF, are not instantly available for equilibration with the other fluid compartments.

The major factors that control the physiologic fluid movement between the intravascular and extravascular spaces are the transcapillary hydrostatic gradient, the osmotic and oncotic gradients, and the relative permeability of vascular barriers that separate these spaces. In 1896, Ernest Starling, a British physiologist, introduced a model describing the forces driving water across vascular membranes. According to this classic model, fluid movement is proportional to the hydrostatic pressure gradient minus the colloid oncotic pressure (COP) gradient across a vessel wall.[3] A sufficient COP within the intravascular space and a low extravascular COP are required to produce a physiologically active inward-directed force in order to contrast the hydrostatic pressure gradient. Animal studies, however, have demonstrated that the vascular barrier also works if the oncotic pressure outside the endothelial cell line equals the intravascular COP.

The Starling model has been integrated into a revised version, which takes into consideration the endothelial glycocalyx, a thin layer of proteins and enzymes that maintains vascular integrity and regulates the permeability of microvascular circulation. The glycocalyx plays a central role in the function of the vascular barrier, and this has led to a new concept of capillary fluid movement and, hence, intravascular fluid administration.[4] The glycocalyx is semi-permeable with respect to anionic macromolecules, such as albumin and other plasma proteins. While water and ions can freely cross the glycocalyx, colloids are withheld in the healthy vasculature by this structure. In agreement to present knowledge, the inward-directed oncotic force maintaining the vascular compartment in equilibrium develops solely at the endothelial surface layer, and is independent from interstitial COP.

GLYCOCALYX AND THE CRITICALLY ILL PATIENT

The integrity of the endothelial glycocalyx plays a major role for maintaining tissue fluid homeostasis, fluid shifting, and volume effects of different solutions used for fluid therapy. The glycocalyx is a fragile structure and is compromised/disrupted in several pathological conditions which can frequently occur in critically ill paediatric patients, such as systemic inflammatory states and sepsis, acute hyperglycaemia, surgery, and trauma. Furthermore, the endothelial glycocalyx can be impaired by excessive

volume loading (iatrogenic hypervolaemia).[5] Great care is required when choosing fluid therapy (type and amount) in septic neurocritical paediatric patients who need large amounts of fluid to stabilize cardiac preload.

CAPILLARY CHARACTERISTICS AND FUNCTION OF THE VASCULAR BARRIER

The prevalent capillary type has a continuous basement membrane and a single layer of endothelial cells joined by junctions that are punctuated by breaks. These intercellular clefts are the primary channels for transcapillary fluid flow. The endothelial glycocalyx layer covers fenestrations and intercellular clefts and has a thickness of up to 100 nm. Water and electrolytes cross the vascular endothelial barrier easily through the glycocalyx, and then the intercellular clefts or through fenestrations in the more specialized capillaries.

In the capillaries of the brain and spinal cord, endothelial cell membranes are tightly opposed by zona occludens tight junctions with few breaks (blood–brain barrier [BBB]), resulting in very small effective pore sizes of barely 1 nm.[6] Water flux across the BBB is facilitated via preformed specialized channels, the aquaporins, and the BBB is relatively impermeable to many small polar solutes (Na^+, K^+, Cl^-). The BBB restricts entry of unwanted substances circulating in the blood and prevents loss of required substances, while providing the entry of the metabolic substrates necessary for the brain cells. The BBB behaves as a semipermeable membrane that permits only water to move freely between the interstitial space and vasculature, mainly according to osmotic gradients. The water permeability of the BBB is much lower than that of peripheral capillaries, but still sufficiently large that even very small osmotic gradients could drive net water movement into the brain. The permeability to small ions is very low and the intravenous administration of hypotonic fluids which decrease plasma osmolality can easily be responsible for the increase in brain water content that is brain oedema.[7]

To summarize, according to the revised Starling model, the forces that explain fluid movement through the BBB are the transendothelial pressure difference, the osmotic gradient, and the plasma–subglycocalyx COP difference, while the interstitial COP is not a direct determinant of transcapillary flow.

Osmolarity and Osmolality

Osmolarity (mOsm/L) and osmolality (mOsm/kg) are determined by the total number of 'dissolved particles' in a solution, regardless of their size. Osmolarity

Table 22.1 Calculated plasma osmolarity

Calculated Osmolarity	$2 \times [Na^+] + (BUN\ mg/dL \div 2.8) + (glucose\ mg/dL \div 18)$
Effective Osmolarity*	$2 \times [Na^+] + (glucose\ mg/dL \div 18)$
Plasma osmolality is primarily determined by the concentration of sodium salts with minor contributions from glucose and blood urea nitrogen (BUN).	

*BUN is lipid soluble, equilibrates across the cell membranes, and does not contribute to fluid distribution; can be omitted from calculation. The most important factor is serum sodium concentration (Na^+).

measures the concentration of osmotically active particles per litre of solution, and is calculated by adding the milliequivalent (mEq) concentrations of the ions in the solution. Osmolality describes the molar number of osmotically active particles per kilogram of solvent and is directly measured. Calculated versus measured osmolality is relevant in neurosurgical patients. For crystalloid solutions, osmolality can differ from osmolarity, in case particles are not totally dissociated. For example, commercial Ringer's lactate solution has a calculated osmolarity of approximately 275 mOsm/L but a measured osmolality of approximately 254 mOsm/kg, indicating incomplete dissociation.[3] Plasma osmolality varies between 280 and 290 mOsm/kg, and if the technology to measure osmolality is not available, osmolarity

can be calculated from serum sodium (Na^+), blood urea nitrogen (BUN), and glucose (Table 22.1). The calculation, however, introduces a bias, overestimating osmolarity in the lower ranges and underestimating it in the higher ranges.

Colloid Oncotic Pressure

Colloid oncotic pressure is the osmotic pressure produced by large molecules (e.g., albumin, hetastarch). It is directly measured and the normal plasma value is about 20 mmHg (~1 mOsm/kg).

FLUIDS FOR INTRAVENOUS ADMINISTRATION

Fluids suitable for intravenous use, crystalloid and colloid solutions, are categorized on the basis of osmolality, oncotic pressure, and dextrose content.

Crystalloids

Crystalloids are solutions of inorganic ions and small organic molecules dissolved in water that do not contain high-molecular-weight compounds and have an oncotic pressure of zero (Table 22.2). They are inexpensive, require no special compatibility testing, and have a very low incidence of adverse reactions and no religious objections to their use. Crystalloids can be hypo-osmolar, isosmolar, or hyperosmolar with respect to plasma.

Table 22.2 Composition of commonly used intravenous fluids: crystalloids

Fluids	Osmolarity (mOsm/L)	Na+	Cl+	K+	Ca2+	Mg+	Dextrose	Lactate/Acetate
		mEq/L					g/L	
5% Dextrose in H2O (D5W)	277						50	
5% Dextrose in 0.45% NaCl	405	77	77				50	
5% Dextrose in 0.9 NaCl	561	154	154				50	
5% Dextrose in Ringer's solution	525	130	109	4	3		50	
Ringer's solution	309	147	156	4	4–4.5			
Ringer's lactate solution	274	130	109	4	3			28/–
5% Dextrose in Ringer's lactate solution	525	130	109	4	3		50	28/–
PlasmaLyte	298	140	98	5		3		–/27
Hartmann's solution	278	131	111	5	4			29/–
0.45% NaCl	154	77	77					
0.9% NaCl (normal saline, NS)	308	154	154					
3.0% NaCl	1026	513	513					
20% Mannitol	1098							

Osmolarity: calculated value (osmol = mg ÷ molecular weight × 10 × valence).
The composition of the solutions can vary slightly depending on the manufacturer.

Crystalloids with ionic composition close to plasma may be referred to as 'balanced' or 'physiologic', and can be used for fluid replacement, such as urinary output and insensible losses.

Hypo-Osmolar Crystalloids

Hypo-osmolar crystalloids reduce plasma osmolality, cause brain oedema even in an entirely normal brain, and increase ICP. Hypo-osmolar crystalloids (0.45% NaCl) should not be used in patients with brain pathology, and 5% dextrose (D5W) is basically 'free' water (as the sugar is readily metabolized). Hypo-osmolar fluids cause water shifts to the brain because the BBB is water permeable, both when it is intact or disrupted.[7] Hypo-osmolar solutions should only be considered if the goal is to achieve a positive free-water balance.

Isosmolar Crystalloids

Isosmolar crystalloids have an osmolarity of about 300 mOsm/L, and do not change plasma osmolality. Potassium, calcium, and lactate may be added to more closely replicate the ionic makeup of plasma (Table 22.2). Ringer's lactate solution is slightly hypotonic (measured osmolality about 254 mOsm/kg) in relation to the plasma, can decrease serum osmolality, and increase brain water content and ICP, mostly when large amounts are infused. Small volumes of Ringer's lactate are unlikely to be detrimental. If large volumes are needed, a change to a more isotonic fluid such as normal saline (NS, 0.9% NaCl) is probably advisable taking into account that rapid infusion of large volumes of NS can induce a dose-dependent dilutional–hyperchloraemic acidosis. Ringer's lactate solution and PlasmaLyte contain bicarbonate precursors (lactate and acetate in the liver result in the production of an equivalent amount of bicarbonate).

Hyperosmolar Crystalloids

Hyperosmolar crystalloid solutions can be made hyperosmolar by the inclusion of electrolytes (e.g., Na^+ and Cl^-, as in hypertonic saline (HS) and low molecular weight solutes such as in mannitol (Table 22.2). Osmotic therapy is a cornerstone in the management of intracranial hypertension. Its effectiveness depends on the integrity of the BBB, the reflection coefficient of the osmotic agent, and the osmotic gradient created. The ability of these solutions to lower ICP and reduce mass effect is explained by a reduction in brain water content, since HS and mannitol establish an osmotic gradient between blood and brain in the presence of a relatively intact BBB.

Mannitol

Mannitol is a cornerstone in the management of raised ICP in paediatric and adult patients, and is recommended by both the Brain Trauma Foundation and the European Brain Injury Consortium. The recommended dose of mannitol is 0.25 to 1 g/kg, using the smallest possible effective dose infused over 10 to 15 minutes.[8] Mannitol increases osmolality, and a serum osmolality >320 mOsm/kg is associated with adverse renal and central nervous system effects. The osmotic diuresis may lead to hypotension, especially in hypovolaemic patients, and, although controversial, the accumulation of mannitol in cerebral tissue can reverse the brain–blood gradient with exacerbation of oedema and increased ICP.

Hypertonic Saline

Hypertonic saline is efficacious in controlling intracranial hypertension after severe brain damage. Generally, a 3% solution is used, although concentrations up to 23.4% have been reported.[9] In acute resuscitation from haemorrhagic shock in patients with multiple trauma and head injury, HS quickly restores circulating volume, and decreases ICP through brain water reduction in the uninjured brain.

Hypertonic saline has been used electively to reduce elevated ICP unresponsive to mannitol treatment. Hypertonic saline is potentially more effective because the BBB permeability to Na^+ is low, and the reflection coefficient (selectivity of the BBB to a particular substance) of NaCl is more than that of mannitol. Moreover, HS solutions result in volume expansion, improved cardiac output and regional blood flow, and provide beneficial immunomodulation. Adverse effects after HS administration can include renal failure, coagulopathy, hyperkalaemia, pulmonary oedema, and central pontine myelinolysis. The evidence for renal failure, coagulopathy, pulmonary oedema, and hyperkalaemia is tenuous, and small clinical trials have shown no evidence of demyelination disorders in the paediatric patient. The sodium load may be a concern in patients with neurologic injury and/or at risk for seizures.

Glucose-Containing Solutions

Apart from premature and small newborn infants, who are prone to hypoglycaemia and may require glucose-containing intravenous fluids, these solutions are avoided in all patients with brain pathology and normal glucose metabolism because they can potentially exacerbate ischaemic damage and cerebral oedema. Several studies of glucose homoeostasis infer that serum glucose control may limit secondary neurological damage, although there is currently no evidence to support 'tight' glycaemic control and conventional glycaemic targets following traumatic brain injury is suggested.[10] Solid evidence indicates that hyperglycaemia exacerbates neurological damage, and the infusion of 5%–10% dextrose in the paediatric critically ill population leads invariably to hyperglycaemia, which is associated with worse outcome.[11] Furthermore, urinary loss of glucose causes osmotic diuresis with secondary dehydration and electrolyte abnormalities. Studies with low dextrose Ringer's lactate solutions in paediatric patients have shown that low dextrose concentration (1 or 0.9%) prevents hypoglycaemia and is associated with blood glucose concentrations in the normal range.[12] Given the potential impact of both hyperglycaemia and hypoglycaemia on the brain,[11] in neurocritical care, frequent evaluation of blood glucose concentrations is mandatory.

Glucose Control and Enteral/Parenteral Nutrition

Patients with brain damage, especially head trauma, have increased requirement of nutritional support. With practically equivalent quantities of supply, the mode of nutrient administration (enteral or parenteral nutrition) has no effect on neurologic outcome, notwithstanding potential advantages of enteral nutrition (decreased risk of hyperglycaemia, lower risk of infection, prevention of bacterial translocation from the gastrointestinal tract). In the critically ill brain-damaged patient glycaemic control during nutrition is critical, which can be easily achieved with judicious use of insulin and glucose-containing fluids to minimize hyperglycaemia and avoid hypoglycaemia, especially during parenteral nutrition.

Colloid Solutions

Colloid solutions possess an oncotic pressure almost identical to that of plasma, and are indicated for volume replacement. The colloids currently available include natural colloids (human albumin solutions) and semisynthetic colloids (dextrans, gelatins, hydroxyethyl starches [HES]). Colloids expand the intravascular space (IVS) through their COP and molecular weight (MW); the higher the oncotic pressure and MW, the greater the initial volume increment of the IVS. The duration of this volume effect, however, is limited by the plasma half-life, which depends on colloid MW and organ elimination (mainly by the kidneys). Thus different colloids have different duration of volume effects.

Albumin

Albumin is the most frequently used plasma expansion agent and has been considered the gold standard for maintenance of COP, especially in the paediatric population. The safety of albumin in patients with brain pathology has been recently questioned, since head trauma patients resuscitated with albumin had a higher mortality rate compared to saline.[13] It needs to be underlined, however, that the albumin preparation used in the Saline versus Albumin Fluid Evaluation (SAFE) study (5% solution) was a severely hypoosmotic solution (260 mOsm/L), and the SAFE study mainly confirms that hypoosmotic solutions are harmful in patients with brain injury, rather than evaluating the colloid compound itself.[14]

Synthetic Colloids

The cost and decreased availability of albumin have led some European countries to choose synthetic colloids. The Association of Paediatric Anaesthetists of Great Britain and Ireland encourage the use of gelatins, and the Association of French Speaking Pediatric Anesthetists members from France frequently use hetastarch solutions, whereas in the United States, albumin remains the first choice colloid.[15] Each synthetic colloid has individual physicochemical characteristics that determine their possible efficacy and adverse effects.

Gelatin

Gelatin products are derived from bovine collagen and are prepared as poly-dispersive solutions through multiple chemical modifications. They have a low MW and the duration of volume expansion is modest, which requires repeated infusions to maintain adequate circulating volume. The effect on the coagulation system is limited to dilution of coagulation factors, platelets, and red blood cells, and is well-tolerated in terms of renal function. Disadvantages of gelatins include a high anaphylactoid potential, which is the highest among all synthetic colloids.

Hydroxyethyl Starch

Hydroxyethyl starch solutions originate from amylopectin, a highly branched polymer of glucose, and are the first synthetic colloids with a configuration similar to albumin. Available preparations are characterized by their concentration, molar substitution, and MW (Table 22.3). Higher MW and extensive molar substitution attain

Table 22.3 Colloids: hydroxyethyl starch solutions

	HES 670/0.75	HES 450/0.7	HES 130/0.4
Availability	US	Europe/US	Europe/US
Concentration %	6	6	6
Volume effect (hr)	5–6	5–6	2–3
Molecular weight (kD)	670	450	130
Molecular substitution (MS)	0.75	0.7	0.4
C2/C6 ratio	4:1	4:1	9:1
Na^+	143	140	154
Cl^-	124	118	154
Oncotic pressure (mmHg)	25–30	25–30	36

slower elimination that affects both coagulation and renal function. The third-generation HES solutions with a molar substitution of around 0.4 (tetrastarches) have less influence on coagulation and renal function and are approved for use in children with a maximal daily dose of 50 ml/kg. Since side effects of HES are dose-dependent, moderate doses of 10–20 ml/kg are considered very safe, compared to the maximum dose, which may drive critical haemodilution, dilutional coagulopathy, or iatrogenic hypervolaemia.

MONITORING INTRAVENOUS FLUID THERAPY

Conscious patients, including neonates, small infants, and children are able to maintain normal blood pressure for long periods of time through vasoconstriction, even in the presence of large fluid deficits or in shock conditions. Hypovolaemia can easily be insufficient to sustain cerebral perfusion and oxygenation, and should be avoided, especially in the presence of acute brain injuries.[1] In critically ill children, some or all of the regulatory mechanisms are suppressed so that hypotension frequently indicates reduced blood volume. Volume status monitoring allows tailoring fluid treatment in individual patients. Monitoring standard parameters such as heart rate, arterial blood pressure, urine output, refilling time, and skin temperature may be insufficient in the neurocritical patient, and other parameters should be used to estimate the volume status. For appropriate fluid management, volume status monitoring should be able to evidentiate hypovolaemia and avoid iatrogenic hypervolaemia,[16] which may have a major impact on mortality, especially in critically ill paediatric patients,

such as it occurs in adults.[17] Monitoring may include invasive or less invasive methods, which are becoming more popular, easy to use, and less expensive. Vena cava distensibility is described as a reliable dynamic indicator of volume status and low central venous pressure. Dynamic haemodynamic measures (e.g., pulse pressure variation), abnormal respiratory-synchronous invasive blood pressure curve, or pulse oximetry signal variations (i.e., perfusion or plethismographic variability index) may indicate low filling pressures even in young children. Hypovolaemia and reduced oxygen delivery can be suspected in the presence of metabolic acidosis and increasing lactate concentrations. Central venous oxygen saturation ($ScvO_2$) is a particularly rapid indicator of peripheral organ and tissue utilization of oxygen delivery.

FLUID STRATEGY

In order to prescribe the proper fluid therapy, it is important to identify which compartment is depleted because specific losses should be replaced with appropriate fluids. As a general rule, isosmolar crystalloids should be given at a rate sufficient to replace urinary output and insensible losses (e.g., skin and lungs), and colloids should be used to replace blood loss and maintain normovolaemia. Available data indicate that intravascular volume replacement and expansion will have no effect on cerebral oedema, as long as normal serum osmolality is maintained and true volume overload (which affects the glycocalyx) is avoided. Fluids that reduce osmolality should be proscribed, especially in patients whose baseline osmolality has been increased by hyperosmolar fluids (mannitol, HS).

Hypovolaemia is the most common cause of circulatory failure and can lead to critical tissue perfusion. Colloids may be used to rapidly treat or prevent hypovolaemia with the advantage of markedly reducing the total volume of administered infusion. Table 22.4 illustrates the intravascular volume expansion obtained with different types of fluids. Volume replacement with crystalloid solutions with the aim to maintain the haematocrit at approximately 33%, is calculated on a 3:1 ratio (crystalloids to blood loss) because of the larger distribution space of

Table 22.4 Intravascular volume increase after fluid administration

Fluid infused	Intravascular volume increase
1 L Isotonic Crystalloid	~ 250 ml
1 L 5% Albumin	~ 500 ml
1 L Hetastarch	~ 750–800 ml

the crystalloids. If large volumes are needed, combination of isotonic crystalloids and colloids may be the best choice in order to avoid volume overload.

CHOICE OF FLUID AND IATROGENIC HYPONATRAEMIA IN CHILDREN

The historic approach of infusing hypotonic fluids in children,[2] results in a high incidence of hospital-acquired hyponatraemia, which increases brain water content even in the normal brain. The number of brain cells decreases with age, and children have a larger brain to intracranial volume ratio compared to adults, with less room for brain expansion, which explains the frequent occurrence of intracranial hypertension in case of brain oedema. Furthermore, animal studies in prepubertal rats and newborn dogs have demonstrated a limited ability to extrude sodium from the brain and, as a consequence, a greater vulnerability to hyponatraemia.[18] While profound hyponatraemia results in seizure activity, coma and death, even moderate hyponatraemia is suspected to cause subclinical neuronal damage. Recent studies have demonstrated that hypotonic solutions exacerbate the tendency to develop dilutional hyponatraemia, while isotonic saline solutions are protective.[19] Although there is still a debate on the ideal solution to infuse in children,[20] it is essential to individualize the fluid treatment and monitor sodium concentration in every child receiving fluids. Large amounts of normal saline may contribute to metabolic acidosis, and this can be avoided using solutions with a more plasma-adapted composition. Ringer's lactate is frequently used in children as it is a balanced solution with a physiologic amount of base calcium and potassium. It must be emphasized, however, that because of the low sodium level (130 mEq/L) Ringer's lactate can result in hyponatraemia. A more suitably available balanced solution to use would be Plasmalyte (sodium concentration 140 mEq/L) (Table 22.2).

NEED FOR MORE APPROPRIATE CRYSTALLOID SOLUTIONS

A recent European Consensus Statement indicates that the appropriate crystalloid solution for children should have osmolarity and sodium content close to the physiological range in order to avoid hyponatraemia; an addition of 1%–2.5% glucose in order to avoid hypoglycaemia, lipolysis or hyperglycaemia; and should also include metabolic anions (i.e., acetate, lactate, or malate) as bicarbonate precursors, to avoid acid-base balance disturbances (i.e., hyperchloraemic acidosis).

Currently, such solutions are not commercially available in many European countries and authorisation for such a solution is highly recommended because it will improve the safety and effectiveness of perioperative fluid therapy in children.[20]

CONCLUSIONS

Fluid management may affect clinical outcome in patients with brain pathology. Awareness of potential harms arise from both hypo/hypervolaemia and/or use of hypotonic fluids. More recent studies point out that in critically ill brain-injured patients hypervolaemia may be detrimental because of altering endothelial glycocalyx and affecting fluid movement across the BBB. Literature supports the use of isotonic, balanced, plasma-adapted solutions to avoid dilutional and hyperchloraemic acidosis, to reduce the risk of hyponatraemia, especially when large amounts of fluids are needed, and to avoid disturbances of acid-base physiology. Glucose containing solutions should be used with caution in critically ill brain-injured patients. Although the general aim of fluid management is to maintain normovolaemia using isotonic fluids, volume status monitoring should be pursued in order to minimize secondary brain insults. A practical approach to fluid management in these patients should include: appropriate administration of maintenance fluid volumes choosing fluid solutions based on their composition and osmolarity; and relevant haemodynamic monitoring.

REFERENCES

1. Clifton GL, Miller ER, Choi SC, Levin HS. Fluid thresholds and outcome from severe brain injury. *Crit Care Med* 2002;30:739–45.
2. Holliday M, Segar W. Reducing errors in fluid therapy management. *Pediatrics* 2003;111:424–5.
3. Tommasino C, Picozzi V. Volume and electrolyte management. *Best Pract Res Clin Anaesthesiol* 2007;21:497–516.
4. Chappell D, Jacob M. Role of the glycocalix in fluid management: Small things matter. *Best Pract Res Clin Anaesthesiol* 2014;28:227–34.
5. Chappell D, Bruegger D, Potzel J, et al. Hypervolemia increases release of atrial natriuretic peptide and shedding of the endothelial glycocalyx. *Critical Care* 2014;18:538.
6. Woodcock TE, Woodcock TM. Revised Starling equation and the glycocalyx model of transvascular fluid exchange: an improved paradigm for prescribing intravenous fluid therapy. *Br J Anaesth* 2012;108:384–94.
7. Tommasino C, Moore S, Todd MM. Cerebral effects of isovolemic hemodilution with crystalloid or colloid solutions. *Crit Care Med* 1988;16:862–8.

8. Marshall LF, Smith RW, Rauscher LA, Shapiro HM. Mannitol dose requirements in brain-injured patients. *J Neurosurg* 1978 Feb;48(2):169–72.

9. Suarez JI, Qureshi AI, Bhardwaj A, et al. Treatment of refractory intracranial hypertension with 23.4% saline. *Crit Care Med* 1998 Jun;26(6):1118–22.

10. Plummer MP, Notkina N, Timofeev I, Hutchinson PJ, Finnis ME, Gupta AK. Cerebral metabolic effects of strict versus conventional glycaemic targets following severe traumatic brain injury. *Crit Care* 2018;22(1):16.

11. van den Heuvel I, Vlasselaers D. Clinical benefits of tight glycaemic control: Focus on the paediatric patient. *Best Pract Res Clin Anaesthesiol* 2009;23:441–8.

12. Berleur MP, Dahan A, Murat I, Hazebroucq G. Perioperative infusions in paediatric patients: rationale for using Ringer–lactate solution with low dextrose concentration. *J Clin Pharm Ther* 2003;28:31–40.

13. Myburgh J, Cooper DJ, Finfer S, et al. Saline or albumin for fluid resuscitation in patients with traumatic brain injury. *N Engl J Med* 2007;357:874–84.

14. Van Aken HK, Kampmeier TG, Ertmer C, Westphal M. Fluid resuscitation in patients with traumatic brain injury: what is a SAFE approach? *Curr Opin Anaesthesiol* 2012; 25:563–5.

15. Saudan S. Is the use of colloids for fluid replacement harmless in children? *Curr Opin Anaesthesiol* 2010;23:363–7.

16. Carcillo JA, Fields Al. Clinical practice parameters for hemodynamic support of pediatric and neonatal patients in septic shock. *Crit Care Med* 2002;30:1365–78.

17. Mascia L, Sakr Y, Pasero D, Payen D, Reinhart K, Vincent JL. Sepsis occurrence in acutely ill patients I. Extracranial complications in patients with acute brain injury: a post-hoc analysis of the SOAP study. *Intensive Care Med* 2008;34:720–7.

18. Arieff AI. Postoperative hyponatraemic encephalopathy following elective surgery in children. *Paediatr Anaesth* 1998;8:1–4.

19. Neville KA, Sandeman DJ, Rubinstein A, et al. Prevention of hyponatremia during maintenance intravenous fluid administration: a prospective randomized study of fluid type versus fluid rate. *J Pediatr* 2010;156:313–19.

20. Sumpelmann R, Becke K, Crean P Johr M, et al. European consensus statement for intraoperative fluid therapy in children. *Eur J Anaesthesiol* 2011;28:637–9.

23

Dyselectrolytemias: Water and Electrolyte Management

C. Tommasino

ABSTRACT

Dyselectrolytemias are common in hospitalized patients and dysnatraemias (hypo/hypernatraemia) are among the most common electrolyte abnormalities. Dysnatraemias can be the result of the underlying brain pathology and/or the surgical treatment (diabetes insipidus [DI], cerebral salt wasting syndrome [CSWS], and syndrome of inappropriate antidiuretic hormone secretion [SIADH]). A serious complication of dysnatraemias is brain injury, which can occasionally result in death or permanent neurological damage.

In most cases, dyselectrolytemias can result from improper fluid management (hospital-acquired hyponatraemia, hypomagnesaemia, and hypocalcaemia). The main factor contributing to hyponatraemic encephalopathy, especially in children, is the routine use of hypotonic fluids in patients with impaired ability to excrete free water because of volume depletion, pulmonary and central nervous system diseases, or postoperative state. Iatrogenic hyponatraemia can be easily avoided by using balanced isotonic electrolyte solutions. Early diagnosis and treatment of water and electrolyte imbalance are pivotal to prevent the potential adverse effects of these disorders on the central nervous system (CNS).

KEYWORDS

Dyselectrolytemia; hyponatraemia; hypernatraemia; hypomagnesaemia; syndrome of inappropriate antidiuretic hormone secretion (SIADH); diabetes insipidus (DI); cerebral salt wasting syndrome (CSWS); water balance.

INTRODUCTION

Abnormalities of water and electrolyte balance are common in neurocritical care patients and a structured approach is required to provide appropriate diagnosis and treatment to avoid life-threatening or disabling effects. These abnormalities can be as a result of the underlying brain pathology and/or surgical treatment (diabetes insipidus [DI], cerebral salt wasting syndrome [CSWS], and syndrome of inappropriate antidiuretic hormone secretion [SIADH]) or can be iatrogenic, mostly due inappropriate fluid management (hyponatraemia, hypomagnesaemia, and hypocalcaemia).

REGULATION OF WATER HOMOEOSTASIS

Normal cellular function requires normal plasma osmolality, which is maintained by water homoeostasis, and is tightly regulated by the elaborate interaction between antidiuretic hormone (ADH) and the thirst mechanism. Water balance indicates a state of equilibrium, in which fluid intake equals fluid losses in the gastrointestinal tract, urine, sweat, and other secretions. The mechanisms controlling water balance under normal physiological conditions are summarized in Figure 23.1, which considers a condition of increased plasma osmolality.

As a result of osmoreceptor stimulation in the hypothalamus, ADH is quickly released and binds to receptors in the distal renal tubules and collecting ducts (V2 receptors) leading to expression of water channels (aquaporins) and water reabsorption from the urine into the systemic circulation. At the same time, the thirst centre stimulation in the brain promotes water intake.

As a consequence, plasma water increases secondary to reduction of water excretion (ADH-mediated) and increased water intake (thirst-mediated) with final normalization of plasma osmolality. Regulation of this homoeostatic process is so precise that plasma osmolality rarely varies by more than 2%, once access to water is unrestricted.[1]

In critically ill patients, and neurosurgical patients in particular, water and electrolyte imbalances can be related to either overproduction of ADH with excess water retention and SIADH, or underproduction of ADH, driving excess water loss and DI. Furthermore, water and electrolyte disturbances could be the effects of inappropriate fluid management.[2]

DYSELECTROLYTAEMIAS

Sodium Disorders

Sodium is the main cation in the extracellular fluid compartment; it is critical for the electrochemical gradient responsible for cellular function and is the major determinant of extracellular fluid volume. Plasma sodium reflects the relative proportions of sodium and water, and not the absolute amount of sodium in the body.

The normal value of plasma sodium is 135–45 mEq/L.[3]

Hyponatraemia

Hyponatraemia occurs when plasma sodium is under 135 mEq/L; if plasma sodium is under 130 mEq/L, hyponatraemia is *severe*. When the decrease in plasma sodium from normal to <130 mEq/L occurs in less than 48 hours, the clinical condition is termed *severe acute* hyponatraemia.

Hyponatraemia is the most frequent dyselectrolytemia in hospitalized patients resulting from too much water or too little sodium in the extracellular fluid. Hyponatraemia is rarely caused by sodium depletion and generally indicates extended extracellular fluid volume.

Hyponatraemia can increase brain water content (that is cerebral oedema), and neurointensive care patients are more prone to develop hyponatraemia-related clinical symptoms because of their brain pathology, intracranial hypertension, or surgery. Moreover, in paediatric patients the intracranial space is smaller than adults because at around 6 years of age their brains have the adult size whereas their skulls reach the final adult dimensions at 16 years of age. This explains why children have a higher risk of developing symptomatic hyponatraemia and tend to develop hyponatraemic encephalopathy at higher plasma sodium concentrations.[4] The symptoms of hyponatraemia are quite variable, the only consistent

symptoms being headache, nausea, vomiting, and weakness. In the neurocritical care setting, the clinical manifestations of hyponatraemia are difficult to recognize because the presentingfeatures are nonspecific, and in the neurosurgical patient can be confused with other conditions. As cerebral oedema worsens, signs and symptoms of hyponatraemic encephalopathy may manifest; patients can manifest behavioural changes (disorientation, agitation) and impaired response to verbal and tactile stimuli. Progressive cerebral swelling may result in seizures, focal neurological deficits, raised intracranial pressure, transtentorial herniation, coma, respiratory arrest, and, ultimately, death. The symptoms do not progress always in the same way since advanced symptoms can present suddenly.

In neurocritical care patients, the SIADH and CSWS are two potential causes of hyponatraemia.[5]

Syndrome of inappropriate antidiuretic hormone secretion

In the absence of either hypovolaemia or hyperosmolality, SIADH arises secondary to excessive ADH secretion, inducing water retention by increased water permeability in the renal collecting ducts.[6] Syndrome of inappropriate antidiuretic hormone secretion can present during several illnesses, especially in the central nervous system (CNS) or pulmonary disorders, during malignancies and with specific medications.

Disorders of CNS frequently associated with SIADH include infection, haemorrhage, head trauma, neoplasm, vasculitis or thrombosis. Syndrome of inappropriate antidiuretic hormone secretion is characterized by hyponatraemia, hypo-osmolarity, oliguria, and inappropriately high urine osmolarity, while the volume status is normal. The majority of ADH-retained water remains in the cellular compartment, explaining why patients lack signs of intravascular volume expansion. Hyponatraemia from SIADH is especially harmful in children with encephalitis, as even mild hyponatraemia (sodium <135 mEq/L) has been linked to neurological deterioration and herniation.[7] Before the diagnosis of SIADH, exclusion of other diseases such as heart, liver, and kidney dysfunctions, adrenal insufficiency (low plasma cortisol level = 10–16 mcg/dL), and hypothyroidism is mandatory. In the postoperative period, however, ADH secretion is potentially elevated in all patients, whether appropriate or not. Many factors in this setting can concur to a nonosmotic ADH secretion: pain, stress, anxiety, nausea and vomiting, and use of narcotics that constitute nonosmotic stimuli for ADH release.[8]

Cerebral salt wasting syndrome

It is a relatively uncommon cause of hyponatraemia in patients with neurologic diseases. It is characterized by hypovolaemic hyponatraemia, secondary to marked diuresis and natriuresis (negative sodium balance: Na^+ loss in urine $>Na^+$ intake/day). The exact mechanism for CSWS remains unclear, the cause probably relates to decreased sympathetic outflow to the kidney and amplification of the circulating natriuretic peptide, particularly brain natriuretic peptide.[9] Cerebral salt wasting syndrome can be accompanied by dramatic diuresis, natriuresis, and contraction of blood volume. The incidence of CSWS in paediatric neurosurgical patients is not well determined and no study has defined the potential risk factors for the development process of CSWS. Small reports illustrate cases of CSWS in paediatric neurosurgical patients, but the current literature is a mixture of aetiologies, including tumour, head injury, hydrocephalus, and postoperative stroke.[10] Determining the volume status in hyponatraemic patients is the key point to discriminate between SIADH and CSWS (Table 23.1). Invasive haemodynamic monitoring and/or more sophisticated non-invasive techniques should be used to correctly assess intravascular volume status in all patients. In children the hydration state can be assessed rather well by simple clinical examinations (e.g., capillary refill time [sternum, forehead], skin turgor, fontanelles), however, volume depletion in many cases is subclinical and difficult to assess based only on clinical symptoms and physical examinations, measurements of blood pressure, or pulse rate according to posture change.

Table 23.1 Principal features distinguishing syndrome of inappropriate antidiuretic hormone secretion and cerebral salt wasting syndrome

	SIADH	CSWS
Plasma sodium	⇩	⇩
Plasma osmolality	⇩	⇩
Volaemia	=	⇩
Plasma urea	⇩	⇧
Urinary output	⇩	⇧
Urine sodium*	<20 mEq/L	>40 mEq/L
Treatment	Fluid restriction Vaptans (?)	Fluid replacement (0.9% saline)

*no gold standard cut-off value of urinary sodium excretion to distinguish between the two syndromes.

Notes: = represents no change; downward arrows represent decrease; upward arrows represent increase; ? represents unknown.

Management of Hyponatraemia

Rapid diagnosis and appropriate treatment of hyponatraemia can avoid morbidity and mortality, especially in neurocritical care settings. Sodium deficit can be calculated with the following formula:

$$[(normal\ Na^+\ (mEq/L) - (measured\ Na^+\ (mEq/L)] \times TBW\ (L)$$

Use 135 mEq/L as normal Na^+; estimate TBW (total body water) as 0.6 L/kg × body weight (kg).

The suitable treatment of hyponatraemia depends on the underlying cause and facilitation of a precise diagnosis. It may be appropriate to compare plasma sodium changes over time with changes in blood urea, blood pressure, and calculate the hourly fluid balance. Falling plasma sodium concentration, in a patient who is euvolaemic and has a falling blood urea and low urine output suggests a diagnosis of SIADH. If hyponatraemia coincides with a progressive increase in urine volume, a fall in blood pressure, and a rise in blood urea (no diuretic therapy), the diagnosis of CSWS should be considered (see Table 23.1). The correction of hyponatraemia must consider the rate of its development and the associated symptoms. In general, a 0.5 mEq/L increase in serum sodium per hour with a maximum total increase of 10–12 mEq/L in 24 hours is recommended. A too rapid correction of hyponatraemia may represent a risk factor for developing cerebral demyelination, causing severe neurological damage.[11]

Discriminating between SIADH and CSWS is of utmost importance, since the proper treatment for each disease is different (Table 23.1). Syndrome of inappropriate antidiuretic hormone secretion is caused by excess of renal water reabsorption through inappropriate ADH secretion, and the patient tends to be euvolaemic or, rarely, slightly hypervolaemic. Fluid restriction is recommended as the first line of treatment for hospitalized patients with SIADH, in both the United States recommendations and European guidelines.[12,13] In patients with SIADH, when hyponatraemia is severe (<110 to 115 mEq/L), the administration of hypertonic saline (HS) and furosemide might be appropriate. Vasopressin receptor antagonists (vaptans) have emerged as a new class of drugs for the treatment of SIADH. Vaptans (mostly V2 receptor antagonists) block the effects of elevated ADH and promote aquaresis, the electrolyte-sparing excretion of water, resulting in the correction of serum sodium.[14] Data supporting the use of vaptans for SIADH in neurosurgical patients is scarce and more evidence is needed in paediatric patients.[15]

Cerebral salt wasting syndrome is caused by natriuresis causing negative sodium balance and volume depletion; the patient is hypovolaemic and the mainstay of treatment is intravenous (IV) replacement of water and sodium, and 0.9% sodium chloride is frequently used as the initial fluid. In the postoperative period among patients with brain tumour, CSWS needs to be corrected quickly with volume expansion and salt resuscitation in order to prevent hyponatraemic seizures. Cerebral salt wasting syndrome is always self-limiting and intense fluid treatment is essential only for a few days.[16]

Management of Acute Hyponatraemic Encephalopathy

Acute hyponatraemic encephalopathy is a medical urgency and requires immediate treatment. In patients with acute symptomatic hyponatraemia, a bolus of hypertonic solution such as sodium chloride 2.7% solution (Na^+ = 462 mmol/L) at 2 ml/kg (up to a maximum of 100 ml) should be given over 10 to 15 minutes to quickly restore the plasma sodium concentration, providing frequent electrolyte analysis.[17,18] If symptoms persist, the bolus can be repeated. Life-threatening complications secondary to acute hyponatraemic encephalopathy should never be managed with fluid restriction alone.[19]

Hypernatraemia

Hypernatraemia is defined when plasma sodium is greater than 145 mEq/L; it is a common electrolyte disorder in neurosurgical patients undergoing surgery in the pituitary and hypothalamic areas.

In general, hypernatraemia is frequently linked to volume depletion (water deficit), more than due to increased serum sodium concentration. In every case, hypernatraemia indicates increased osmolality and always causes cellular dehydration. Brain cell shrinkage secondary to hypernatraemia can cause vascular rupture, with intracranial bleeding, subarachnoid haemorrhage (SAH), and the resultant morbidity may be severe or even life-threatening. Free water deficit can be calculated according to the following formula:

$$[(\text{measured } Na^+ \text{ (mEq/L)} \div \text{desired } Na^+ \text{ (mEq/L)}) \times \text{TBW (L)}] - \text{TBW (L)}$$

Use 145 mEq/L as desired Na^+; estimate TBW as 0.6 L/kg × body weight (kg).

Diabetes Insipidus

Central DI arises from a deficiency of ADH due to a hypothalamic-pituitary disorder, which leads to polyuria, polydipsia, and electrolyte and haemodynamic derangements that are secondary to excessive fluid loss. Polyuria (defined in children as urine output >4 ml/kg/hr and in neonates >6 ml/kg/hr) and polydypsia defined as water intake of more than 2 L/m²/day (or more than 5 L/day) are essential features of DI. The production of large volumes of dilute urine results in progressive dehydration and hypernatraemia occurs subsequently. The hallmarks of central DI include polyuria, urine osmolality inappropriately low (<350 mmol/kg) relative to serum osmolality (>305 mmol/kg; above normal because of water loss), and hypernatraemia (>145 mmol/L). A urine-specific gravity of less than 1.002 with increasing serum sodium suggests DI.[14] Diabetes insipidus is frequent in the acute phase of neurosurgical procedures (pituitary and craniopharyngioma surgery), is usually transient in nature, and is much more common after surgical removal of craniopharyngiomas (frequent in children) than after removal of pituitary adenomas. Diabetes insipidus also presents in other conditions including SAH, head trauma, bacterial meningitis or encephalitis involving the base of the brain, phenytoin use, and alcohol intoxication. Patients with severe intracranial hypertension or in brain death commonly develop DI. Awareness of thirst in ill patients may be diminished or absent and they can develop severe hypernatraemia, which only occurs when fluid replacement is insufficient to restore water loss.

In the postoperative period, DI usually presents within two days after surgery, with sudden onset of hypotonic polyuria and, in conscious patients, thirst. In a majority of the cases DI resolves by the third postoperative day, and in only a few cases becomes persistent. A triphasic response is infrequently observed. The first phase is characterized by transient (0.5–2 days) DI owing to axonal damage and/or oedema interfering with ADH secretion. This is followed by an antidiuretic phase, lasting 10–14 days due to unregulated release of ADH. Finally, the third phase of permanent DI occurs when more than 90% of ADH secreting neurons have been destroyed.[20]

Management

The aim of DI treatment is to re-establish normonatraemia using accurate balancing of intake and output to avoid fluid overload. The water deficit is replaced over 24 to 48 hours and hypernatraemia should not be reduced by more than 1 to 2 mEq/L/hr, as rapid reduction may cause harm to the patient such as cerebral oedema, seizures, or permanent brain damage. This timing allows redistribution of the replacement fluid, preventing fluid overload. At the beginning of treatment 0.9% sodium chloride should be used to prevent the sodium level dropping too quickly and the rate of sodium fall should be closely monitored. In case of worsening or unresponsive hypernatraemia during 48 hours, the use of hypotonic solution should be considered, in the form of 0.45% NaCl and free water, with appropriate K$^+$ supplementation.[17] In very young infants and neonates, treatment strategy can rely on fluids alone. Older children and adults with DI are treated with an infusion of aqueous vasopressin and judicious fluid administration (fluid that matches urine output and estimated insensible losses) to avoid fluid overload.

Intravenous aqueous vasopressin (desmopressin) at a dose of 0.5 mU/kg/hr is infused and titrated (0.5–10 mU/kg/hr) every 10 minutes to keep the urine output at less than 2 ml/kg/hr. At the same time, hypotonic fluids should be administered to slowly reduce the hypernatraemia and maintain plasma sodium concentration in the normal range. During treatment, it is necessary to evaluate plasma potassium concentration and treat possible hypokalaemia, which can cause renal resistance to desmopressin therapy. This approach requires hourly monitoring of serum electrolytes and urine output, and the patient should be treated in the neurocritical care setting. It is recommended to switch to fluids by mouth as soon as possible, since oral fluid intake facilitates urinary loss replacement and maintenance of normonatraemia.[21]

Desmopressin is administered to replace the endogenous ADH, which is in insufficient quantity because of reduced pituitary secretion or hypothalamic production. During desmopressin treatment, plasma Na$^+$ concentration should be continuously monitored. Even if rare, DI could proceed to SIADH, with the development of hyponatraemia, and in this context the use of desmopressin will further reduce plasma sodium concentration.

IATROGENIC DYSELECTROLYTAEMIAS

Maintenance Fluid Therapy and Iatrogenic Hyponatraemia

Maintenance fluid therapy represents the volume of fluids and amount of electrolytes needed to replace insensible and urinary losses. Calculation of maintenance fluids for infants and children has long been based on the landmark work of Holliday and Segar, based on energy expenditure in children.[22] Unfortunately, in the same paper, the authors suggested the use of a hypotonic solution with very low sodium content.[22] While there is no logical basis for using hypotonic fluids, except in conditions of free-water deficit, hypernatraemia or ongoing free-water losses, even today in common practice is to administer hypotonic fluid for hydration to paediatric patients.

Hypotonic fluids should never be used in the perioperative period, especially if the patient has a plasma sodium in the low–normal or distinctly hyponatraemic range (<135 mEq/L).[17]

Many studies in children have reported severe hyponatraemic encephalopathy related, totally or partly, to the use of hypotonic solutions and recent data demonstrate that isotonic fluid is safer than hypotonic fluid in terms of risk of hyponatraemia.[23] Meta-analyses of studies on hypotonic versus isotonic fluids for fluid maintenance in hospitalized children have concluded that the use of hypotonic maintenance fluid raises the risk of hyponatraemia.[24,25]

Intravenous fluids should be utilized with the same care as any other medicine, especially with respect to fluid composition and the volume given. The goal of maintenance fluids is not to restore volume deficit, but rather to replace urinary and insensible losses, and children should receive isotonic fluids that contain sodium in the range of 131–154 mEq/L.[26]

Table 23.2 indicates routine maintenance IV fluid rates for children and young people using the Holliday–Segar formula, which should be used only as a starting point. Maintenance fluid needs should be individualized based on the clinical status of the patient, taking into consideration the underlying pathology and timing of fluid management.[17,26] In patients with relevant fluid deficit or excess, the infusion rate should be adapted to the actual requirement, whenever possible. Fluid composition is extremely important in all patients, especially in the neurointensive care setting, where a variety of clinical conditions represent non-osmotic triggers for ADH secretion (respiratory disorders, CNS infection, postoperative states, head injury, vomiting, pyrexia, pain, stress, drugs such as narcotics, etc.) putting the patients at risk of hospital-acquired hyponatraemia, since ADH produces an increase in water retention relative to sodium.[1,2,4–8] In order to reduce the fluid overload, children with increased ADH may benefit from either restricting fluids to 50%–80% of the routine maintenance needed, or reducing fluids calculated on the basis of insensible losses of 300–400 ml/m^2/24 hours plus urinary output.[17]

Iatrogenic hyponatraemia can be avoided using balanced isotonic electrolyte solutions, monitoring the

Table 23.2 Maintenance fluid requirements in children

Child weight (kg)	Calories (kcal/kg)	Fluid (ml/kg/day)*
3–10 kg	100 kcal/kg	100 ml/kg/day or 4 ml/kg/hr *e.g., 8 kg child 800 ml or 768 ml*
10–20 kg	1000 kcal + 100 kcal for every 2 kg >10	1000 ml + 50 ml for every 1 kg >10 or 40 ml/hr + 2 ml/kg/hr for each kg >10 *e.g., 15 kg child 1000 + 250 = 1250 ml or 960 + 240 = 1200 ml*
>20 kg	1500 kcal + 100 kcal for every 5 kg >20	1500 ml + 20 ml for each kg >20 or 60 ml/hr + 1 ml/kg/hr for each kg >20 kg *e.g., 25 kg child 1500 + 100 = 1600 ml 1440 + 120 = 1560 ml*

Maintenance fluids in children with body weight >40 Kg = 1500 ml/m² body surface area.

Maximal volume over 24 hr period: males 2500 ml; female 2000 ml.

*To avoid excess of fluids (in conditions with increased ADH secretion): restrict fluids to 50%–80% of the maintenance needed; or reduce fluids, calculated on the basis of insensible losses of 300 to 400 ml/m²/24 hours + urinary output.

Sources: (1) Cerdà-Esteve M, Cuadrado-Godia E, Chillaron JJ, et al. Cerebral salt wasting syndrome: review. *Eur J Intern Med* 2008;19: 249–54. (2) Mishra G, Chandrashekhar SR. Management of diabetes insipidus in children. *Indian J Endocrinol Metab* 2011;15 (Suppl 3):S180–7.

fluid balance (including oral intake) as accurately as possible, and monitoring the plasma sodium concentration regularly.[17] When measuring serial plasma sodium over time, the same sampling techniques (capillary or venous blood) and measurement method should be used in order to prevent misleading information. Administering fluid-like plasma composition in maintenance fluid therapy is the most physiological approach to prevent hospital-acquired hyponatraemia. Furthermore, balanced isotonic electrolyte solutions with 1% glucose, which mimics the composition of ECF more closely (Table 23.3), will be available in many European countries in the near future.[26]

Patients with the following risk factors should receive only isotonic solutions:

- Plasma sodium at the lower normal reference range (≤135 mEq/L)
- Intravascular volume depletion
- Hypotension

Table 23.3 Composition of extracellular fluid and balanced electrolyte solution with 1% glucose

Cations (mEq/L)	ECF*	BES with 1% glucose
Na⁺	142	140
K⁺	4.5	4
Ca²⁺	2.5	2
Mg²⁺	1.25	2
Anions (mM/L)		
Cl⁻	103	118
HCO₃⁻	24	–
Acetate	–	30
Lactate	1.5	–
Glucose	2.78–5	55.5
Theoretical osmolarity (mOsm/kg)	291	296

Abbreviations: extracellular fluid (ECF); balanced electrolyte solution (BES).

*The composition of ECF is similar across all age groups.

Source: Sümpelmann R, Becke K, Brenner S, et al. Perioperative intravenous fluid therapy in children: guidelines from the Association of the Scientific Medical Societies in Germany. *Paediatr Anaesth* 2017;27:10–18.

- CNS infection
- Head injury
- Bronchiolitis, pneumonia
- Sepsis
- Perioperative and postoperative period
- Excessive gastric or diarrhoeal losses
- Salt wasting syndrome
- Chronic conditions such as diabetes or pituitary deficits
- Replacement of ongoing losses

Potassium Disorders

Potassium ions (K⁺) are necessary for the function of all living cells and influence multiple physiological processes. Potassium is the major intracellular cation with its content in the plasma tightly controlled, and it is reabsorbed in the kidney to maintain serum potassium concentration within narrow limits.

The normal value of plasma potassium is 3.5–5.5 mEq/L. Critical levels are <3.0 or >6.0 mEq/L.[3]

Hypokalaemia

Hypokalaemia is generally defined as a serum K⁺ level of less than 3.5 mEq/L. Plasma K⁺ below 2.5 mEq/L indicates a severe deficiency of potassium. Hypokalaemia is potentially life-threatening and may be iatrogenically acquired by inadequate IV fluid replacement. Hypokalaemia symptoms are non-specific and are mainly related to muscular or cardiac function, with weakness and fatigue, muscle cramps and pain; palpitation and/ or electrocardiographic (ECG) changes (ST depression, T-wave flattening, and U waves). Severe hypokalaemia may manifest as bradycardia with cardiovascular collapse. Every 1 mEq/L decrease in serum K^+ corresponds to a deficit of potassium of around 200–400 mEq.

Normal plasma level of magnesium is required for appropriate K^+ reabsorption in the kidney. When potassium level is in the 2.5–3.5 mEq/L range, patients may receive only oral potassium. If the level is less than 2.5 mEq/L, K^+ should be given intravenously, with continuous ECG monitoring, and serial measurement of K^+ levels. Potassium is irritant when infused in peripheral veins and a maximum of 10 mEq/hr may be given; higher dosages such as 20 mEq/hr should be given through central venous access. For life-threatening arrhythmia, a maximum of 40 mEq/hr may be given via a central line with cardiac monitoring.

Hyperkalaemia

Hyperkalaemia is defined as a serum K^+ concentration greater than 5.5 mEq/L. It can result from decreased excretion (renal failure) because of a shift from the intracellular to extracellular space (metabolic acidosis) and may be iatrogenic (blood transfusion). Symptoms are nonspecific and predominantly related to muscular or cardiac function. Electrocardiography findings usually correlate with the K^+ level, but life-threatening arrhythmias can occur without warning, at almost any level of hyperkalaemia.

Electrocardiography conduction abnormalities include peaked T waves, prolonged PR and QRS intervals, sine waves, ventricular fibrillation, and asystole. The aggressiveness of therapy is mostly related to the rapidity of hyperkalaemia development and the absolute level of hyperkalaemia.

Hyperkalaemia can be a medical emergency. Levels higher than 7 mEq/L can drive harmful haemodynamics and neurologic consequences, while levels exceeding 8 mEq/L can produce respiratory or cardiac arrest and can readily be fatal.

All sources of exogenous potassium should be immediately discontinued and, unless ECG changes are present, blood test should be repeated before treating the hyperkalaemia. Treatment of severe hyperkalaemia consists of immediate stabilization of the myocardial cell membrane (calcium chloride or gluconate); enhancement of cellular uptake of potassium (bicarbonate, dextrose and insulin, salbutamol or albuterol); and enhancement of total body potassium elimination (furosemide).[27] Emergent haemodialysis is sometimes necessary to treat severe symptomatic life-threatening hyperkalaemia that is resistant to drug therapy, particularly in patients without adequate renal function.

Hyperkalaemia and Transfusion

Transfusion of large volumes of blood, especially blood older than 10–14 days, is the major cause of hyperkalaemia in all patients. It is caused by leakage of red blood cells (RBCs) during storage and can induce serious arrhythmias and death. The rise of serum potassium in children is fast due to small blood volume. In order to reduce the risk of hyperkalaemia, many blood banks have policies to issue blood before the end of day 5 following donation (and within 24 hours of irradiation) for neonates and infants who will require massive transfusions.

Intravenous sodium bicarbonate 1 mmol/kg, and calcium chloride 20 mg/kg, or calcium gluconate 60 mg/kg may be used to treat hyperkalaemia causing arrhythmias. Use of IV dextrose/insulin, hyperventilation, and sympathomimetics can be useful.[28]

Magnesium Disorders

Magnesium plays a major role in overall cell functions, including DNA and protein synthesis, glucose and fat metabolism, oxidative phosphorylation, neuromuscular excitability, and enzyme activity. Magnesium ion is essential for normal cardiac electrophysiologic activity. Most of total body magnesium is intracellular (99%) and the kidney is the major regulator of total body magnesium homoeostasis.

Normal values of plasma magnesium are 1.8–2.3 mg/dL (0.74–0.94 mEq/L).[3]

Hypomagnesaemia

Hypomagnesaemia is defined as a plasma magnesium level of less than 1.8 mg/dL (<0.74 mEq/L). A deficiency of magnesium in the blood may result from inadequate intake, intracellular shift (treatment of diabetic ketoacidosis), gastrointestinal loss (chronic diarrhoea, malabsorption, vomiting, and nasogastric suction), rapid blood transfusion (citrate toxicity), or more frequently, increased urinary losses.[29]

Hypomagnesaemia may be asymptomatic. Symptoms usually occur when magnesium concentration is below 1.2 mg/dL (0.49 mEq/L). Hypomagnesaemia often coexists

Table 23.4 Electrolyte maintenance requirements in paediatric patients: preterm, term, children, and adolescents

	Preterm	Term/Children	Adolescent
Na⁺	3–4.5 mEq/kg/day	2–4 mEq/kg/day	60–100 mEq/day
Cl⁻	2–3 mEq/kg/day	2–4 mEq/kg/day	60–150 mEq/day
K⁺	2–3 mEq/kg/day	2–4 mEq/kg/day	70–150 mEq/day
Ca²⁺	3–4.5 mEq/kg/day	Term 0.5–3 mEq/kg/day Children 1–2.5 mEq/kg/day	10–30 mEq/day
Phosphorus	1.5–2.5 mEq/kg/day	0.5–2 mEq/kg/day	10–40 mEq/day
Mg²⁺	0.35–0.6 mEq/kg/day	Term 0.25–1 mEq/kg/day Children 0.25–0.5 mEq/kg/day	10–30 mEq/day

with other dyselectrolytemias, such as hypocalcaemia or hypokalaemia. Manifestations of magnesium deficiency are mostly cardiovascular and neuromuscular, and include muscle weakness, tetany, spasms, or cramps, and generalized seizures, as may be seen with hypocalcaemia. The most life-threatening cardiovascular effect of hypomagnesaemia are dysrhythmias (torsades de pointes and ventricular tachycardia).

Mild to moderate deficiency of magnesium (1.2–1.7 mg/dL) should be treated with diet or oral magnesium supplements. Symptomatic patients should receive 3–4 g (24–32 mEq) of IV magnesium sulphate slowly over 12–24 hours, and the dose can be repeated to maintain serum magnesium level above 1.2 mg/dL. Life-threatening arrhythmias are treated with 1–2 g of magnesium sulphate solution administered IV over a 5-minute period.[30]

Calcium Disorders

Calcium is the most abundant mineral element in the body. Hypocalcaemia may increase central as well as peripheral neural excitability and can lead to tetany, convulsive seizures, and cardiovascular effects (disturbances of the electrical rhythm). Hypercalcaemia can be associated with tubulointerstitial nephropathy, anorexia, nausea, ECG disturbances, and a spectrum of neurological changes from headache to coma.

Normal values of plasma calcium are 4.3–5.2 mEq/L (8.8–10.7 mg/dL or 2.2–2.6 mmol/L).[3]

Hypocalcaemia and Transfusion

Calcium is essential for the successful initiation of the coagulation cascade. The citrate present in stored blood is a chelating agent and, therefore chelates calcium, prevents clot formation, and produces hypocalcaemia. The degree of hypocalcaemia depends on the rate of transfusion and the state of liver function. Hypocalcaemia may be more frequent with administration of fresh frozen plasma, since it exhibits a higher concentration of citrates per unit of volume. Citrate toxicity, leading to hypocalcaemia, will manifest in the infant as hypotension, hypomagnesaemia, tetany, and arrhythmias.

Hypocalcaemia may be treated by administering calcium fluoride 5–10 mg/kg IV or calcium gluconate 15–30 mg/kg IV. If the blood loss is continuous and prolonged, IV infusion of calcium chloride at the rate of 10 mg/kg/hr may be used.

Table 23.4 summarizes the electrolyte maintenance requirements in paediatric patients.

CONCLUSIONS

Electrolyte disturbances are common in neurologic patients and sodium disturbances are among the most common electrolyte abnormalities. Dyselectrolytaemias can occasionally result in death or permanent neurological damage. Similarly excess of fluids in the body can also be dangerous. Early diagnosis and treatment of water and electrolyte imbalance are fundamental to prevent the undesirable effects of these disorders on the central nervous system.

REFERENCES

1. Robertson GL, Aycinena P, Zerbe RL. Neurogenic disorders of osmoregulation. *Am J Med* 1982;72:339–53.
2. National Patient Safety Agency, National Health Service. Reducing the risk of hyponatraemia when administering intravenous infusions to children. 2007. London, England. Available from: http://www.npsa.nhs.uk.
3. Rose BD, Post TW. *Clinical physiology of acid-base and electrolyte disorders.* New York: McGraw-Hill, 2001.
4. Arieff AI, Ayus JC, Fraser CL. Hyponatraemia and death or permanent brain damage in healthy children. *BMJ* 1992;304:1218–22.

5. Williams CN, Riva-Cambrin J, Bratton SL. Etiology of postoperative hyponatremia following pediatric intracranial tumor surgery. *J Neurosurg Pediatr* 2016;17:303–9.

6. Albanese A, Hindmarsh P, Stanhope R. Management of hyponatremia in patients with acute cerebral insults. *Arch Dis Child* 2001;85:246–51.

7. McJunkin JE, de los Reyes EC, Irazuzta JE, et al. La Crosse encephalitis in children. *N Engl J Med* 2001;344:801–7.

8. Halberthal M, Halperin M, Bohn D. Acute hyponatremia in children admitted to hospital: retrospective analysis of factors contributing to its development and resolution. *BMJ* 2001;322:780–2.

9. Yee AH, Burns JD, Wijdicks EF. Cerebral salt wasting: pathophysiology, diagnosis, and treatment. *Neurosurg Clin N Am* 2010;21:339–52.

10. Hardesty DA, Kilbaugh TJ, Phillip BS. Cerebral Salt Wasting Syndrome in post-operative pediatric brain tumor patients. *Neurocrit Care* 2012;17:382–7.

11. Moritz ML, Ayus JC. Preventing neurological complications from dysnatremias in children. *Pediatr Nephrol* 2005; 20:1687–700.

12. Verbalis JG, Goldsmith SR, Greenberg A, et al. Diagnosis, evaluation, and treatment of hyponatremia: expert panel recommendations. *Am J Med* 2013;126:S1–42.

13. Spasovski G, Vanholder R, Allolio B, et al. Clinical practice guideline on diagnosis and treatment of hyponatraemia. *Eur J Endocrinol* 2014;25:1–47.

14. Tommasino C, Picozzi V. Volume and electrolyte management. *Best Pract Res Clin Anaesthesiol* 2007;21:497–516.

15. Schrier RW, Gross P, Gheorghiade M, et al. Tolvaptan, a selective oral vasopressin V2-receptor antagonist, for hyponatremia. *N Engl J Med* 2006;355:2099–112.

16. Cerdà-Esteve M, Cuadrado-Godia E, Chillaron JJ, et al. Cerebral salt wasting syndrome: review. *Eur J Intern Med* 2008;19:249–54.

17. National Institute for Health and Care Excellence. Intravenous fluid therapy in children and young people in hospital. NICE guidelines [NG29] 2015.

18. Haycock GB. Hyponatraemia: diagnosis and management. *Arch Dis Child Educ Pract Ed* 2006;91:ep37–41.

19. Moritz ML, Ayus JC. The pathophysiology and treatment of hyponatraemic encephalopathy: an update. *Nephrol Dial Transplant* 2003;18:2486–91.

20. Barzilay Z, Smoekh E. Diabetes insipidus in severely brain damaged children. *J Med* 1987;19:47–53.

21. Mishra G, Chandrashekhar SR. Management of diabetes insipidus in children. *Indian J Endocrinol Metab* 2011;15 (Suppl 3):S180–7.

22. Holliday MA, Segar WE. The maintenance need for water in parenteral fluid therapy. *Pediatrics* 1957;19:823–32.

23. McNab S, Duke T, South M, et al. 140 mmol/L of sodium versus 77 mmol/L of sodium in maintenance intravenous fluid therapy for children in hospital (PIMS): a randomised controlled double-blind trial. *Lancet* 2015 Mar 28;385(9974):1190–7.

24. Wang J, Xu E, Xiao Y. Isotonic versus hypotonic maintenance IV fluids in hospitalized children: a meta-analysis. *Pediatrics* 2014;133:105–13.

25. Foster BA, Tom D, Hill V. Hypotonic versus isotonic fluids in hospitalized children: a systematic review and meta-analysis. *J Pediatr* 2014;165:163–9.

26. Sümpelmann R, Becke K, Brenner S, et al. Perioperative intravenous fluid therapy in children: guidelines from the Association of the Scientific Medical Societies in Germany. *Paediatr Anaesth* 2017;27:10–18.

27. Chime NO, Luo X, McNamara L, Nishisaki A, Hunt EA. A survey demonstrating lack of consensus on the sequence of medications for treatment of hyperkalaemia among pediatric critical care providers. *Pediatr Crit Care Med* 2015 Jun;16(5):404–9.

28. Barcelona SL, Thompson AA, Coté CJ. Intraoperative pediatric blood transfusion therapy: a review of common issues. Part II: transfusion therapy, special considerations, and reduction of allogenic blood transfusions. *Paediatr Anaesth* 2005;15(10):814–30.

29. Augus ZS. Hypomagnesaemia. *J Am Soc Nephrol* 1999;10:1616–22.

30. Noronha JL, Matuschak GM. Magnesium in critical illness: metabolism, assessment, and treatment. *Intensive Care Med* 2002;28(6):667–79.

Part V

Neurological Care

Editor: Abhijit Lele

24

Altered Mental Status

M. R. Hallman and A. M. Joffe

ABSTRACT

Clinicians frequently encounter patients with altered mental status (AMS). The list of potential aetiologies is vast. An understanding of normal arousal and cognition as well as common patterns of abnormal presentation is critical to the diagnostic process. This chapter provides a framework for identifying the specific components of altered mental status and describes commonly encountered conditions. Conditions that primarily affect arousal and alertness are distinguished from those that affect the content and coherence of thought. A suggested diagnostic approach to patients with altered mental status is presented.

KEYWORDS

Altered mental status (AMS); coma; obtunded; delirium; confusion.

INTRODUCTION

Altered mental status (AMS) is a broad and non-specific term that describes a variety of common and non-specific findings. Between 4%–10% of patients presenting to the hospital carry the diagnosis.[1] Despite the availability of a variety of classification and diagnostic frameworks, the lexicon remains inconsistent and potentially confusing. This chapter divides AMS into two general categories: (1) arousal disorders and (2) confusional states. This system is more intuitive if one considers states of arousal as the level of consciousness and confusion as the content of consciousness.

AROUSAL AND ALERTNESS

The Normal State

In the normal state of arousal an individual is aware of self and their environment. Additionally, they should interact with their environment in a cogent manner. While the daily circadian rhythms and variations in the degree of internal and external stimuli will cause periods of lesser and greater attention throughout the day—even sleep, the normal state is defined by the ability of the individual to be brought rapidly back to a state of full attention in response to appropriate stimuli.

The neural pathways that govern arousal and alertness are complex. It is likely that they are more complex than our current understanding suggests. For the purposes of describing and understanding common clinical presentations of altered arousal, however, a basic model based upon decades old experimental findings remains comprehensive and accurate. The work of Bremer, Moruzzi, Magoun, and the Scheibels led to conceptualization of a reticular activating system (RAS).[2–4] The reticular formation has historically been thought of as an anatomically inconspicuous group of neurons located in the paramedian upper brainstem tegmentum and lower diencephalon that receive the ascending innervation from the spinothalamic and trigeminothalamic tracts, and then project these signals widely throughout the cortex for further processing. Numerous neurotransmitters have been implicated in the control of alertness including glutamine, acetylcholine, dopamine, norepinephrine, serotonin, orexin, and histamine.[5] The incoming information is modulated by descending projections from the cortex to the reticular formation. Not only does the reticular formation serve as a relay station for incoming sensory information, but proper functioning is necessary to maintain arousal. Insults that affect the function of any component of the RAS pathway may lead to alterations in consciousness. Recent experiments utilizing advanced imaging techniques such as high angular resolution diffusion imaging (HARDI) seek to more precisely define the connections and pathways that are necessary for arousal and awareness.[6,7] For more detailed discussion about the neurobiology of arousal, the reader is referred to *Bradley's Neurology in Clinical Practice*, 6th ed. and *Plum and Posner's Diagnosis of Stupor and Coma*, 4th ed.[5,8]

The Continuum of Altered Arousal

The terms drowsiness, somnolence, stupor, obtundation, semi-coma, and coma are commonly used to describe states of decreased arousal. Table 24.1 lists characteristic findings of the stages of progressively decreasing arousal. From a practical standpoint, this is indeed a continuum and there is often overlap as patients move from one stage to another. Clinically, the descriptors can be helpful in directing diagnostic efforts as well as monitoring the progression of disease in a patient whose condition is changing.

There are many possible ways to categorize the pathologies, which may result in AMS, but perhaps the most clinically useful categorization broadly divides the pathologies into two categories. In the first class are those disorders affecting cerebral cellular function through mechanical means such as blunt or penetrating trauma, shear injury, hydrocephalus, or haemorrhage. The second class includes disorders impacting cellular function through non-mechanical means, which is broadly subdivided into toxic and metabolic disorders.

Toxic and Metabolic Disorders

This category is a diverse group of systemic disorders that cause derangements of normal cellular chemistry and function. The overall clinical presentation may vary, and an altered sensorium may be one manifestation. Based on widely cited work of Plum and Posner, nearly two-thirds of patients admitted to the hospital with coma of uncertain aetiology were ultimately diagnosed with a toxic or metabolic aetiology.[8] Of these, just under half were related to toxins of some sort.

Toxic disorders are those derangements caused by the presence of an exogenous substance such as alcohol, anaesthetic agents, or carbon monoxide. Metabolic disorders are those where the amount of an important endogenous substance or homoeostatic process is altered. These include disorders such as hyponatraemia, hypothermia, and hypoglycaemia. The list of potential toxins and metabolic disorders that may be causing AMS is extensive. The most common aetiologies are listed in Table 24.2. The reader is also referred to the excellent review by Edlow et al. for a more comprehensive list of potential aetiologies.[9] The first step in creating a differential diagnosis is the performance of a comprehensive history and physical examination. However, laboratory studies and radiologic imaging are almost always required to correctly identify the underlying disorders. Diagnosis and treatment of all the potential toxic and metabolic disorders is beyond the scope of this text, and the reader is referred to *Harrison's Principles of Internal Medicine* for additional reading regarding the diagnosis of management of specific derangements.[10]

It is important to note that the patient's presentation may be due to an aetiology from more than one category

Table 24.1 Characteristic findings in states of decreased consciousness

Level of arousal	Characteristic findings
Drowsiness or somnolence	• Indistinguishable from light sleep • Arousal improves in response to verbal or light tactile stimuli • Arousal may be maintained for a short duration of time following stimulation • Confusion and inattentiveness present, but improves with arousal
Stupor	• Responsive only to deep and repeated stimuli • Arousal is not maintained without repeated stimuli • Restlessness and stereotyped motor activity are common
Obtundation or 'Semi-coma'	• No meaningful or purposeful response to external stimuli or internal needs • Pupillary, corneal and pharyngeal reflexes often maintained
Coma	• No meaningful or purposeful response to external stimuli or internal needs • Diminished or absent pupillary, corneal, and pharyngeal reflexes

Adapted from: Ropper AH, Samuels MA, Klein J. *Adams and Victor's Principles of Neurology*. 10th ed. New York: McGraw-Hill Education Medical; 2014.

Table 24.2 Common aetiologies of coma and altered mental status

Toxins	Metabolic derangements	Mechanical insults
Uraemia	Hypoxaemia	Penetrating trauma
Ammonia (NH₃)	Hypercapnia	Shear injury
Anaesthetic agents	Hyponatraemia	Hydrocephalus
Opioids	Hypernatraemia	Tumour
Dissociative agents	Hypoglycaemia	Cerebral abscess
Alcohols	Hyperosmolarity	Haemorrhage
Antiepileptic agents	Hyperthermia	Ischaemic stroke
Antidepressants	Hypothermia	Cerebral oedema
	Hypothyroidism	
	Low thiamine level	
	Seizure	
	Infection	

simultaneously. For example, a patient who suffers from anoxic encephalopathy due to a cardiac arrest may also develop cerebral oedema and intracranial hypertension. Individuals who are under the influence of alcohol may also have low thiamine levels. In addition, it is likely that any toxic or metabolic derangement of sufficient severity to result in AMS is likely enough to precipitate a mechanical fall, which could result in traumatic brain injury. Thus, while the broad diagnostic categorization proposed is a useful paradigm at the time of initial patient contact, it is not infallible.

Structural Disorders

While any structural disorder has the potential to cause AMS, there are discrete anatomical locations that must necessarily be affected to result in a state of coma. Focal injuries to the upper brainstem and diencephalon, which disrupt the ascending axis of the RAS, may be sufficient to cause coma. Cortical injuries may also result in coma, but generally require involvement of both hemispheres, i.e., unilateral cerebral injuries alone are typically insufficient to cause coma although it has been suggested that occasionally significant left hemispheric injury alone can cause coma.[11] The potential sites where mechanical injuries can cause coma include the mid brain, brainstem, diencephalon, hypothalamic region, and bilateral cortex.[12] It is important to note that mechanical lesions may initially affect an area distant to these critical areas, but through the development of mass effect, pressure may still be applied to these areas. Plum and Posner's series found that of the one-third of comas attributed to structural causes, approximately two-thirds of these

were related to supratentorial lesions and one-third to infratentorial lesions.[8] Intraparenchymal and subdural haemorrhages accounted for most of the supratentorial lesions while brainstem infarcts predominated below the tentorium.

Coma Mimics

The Persistent Vegetative State

The persistent vegetative state (PVS) was first described in 1972.[13] In 1994, a multi-society task force published a consensus definition describing this clinical condition as complete unawareness of self and environment, partial or complete preservation of hypothalamic and brainstem automatic functions and preserved sleep–wake cycles.[14] It has been suggested that historical terms used to describe this same clinical scenario such as *neocortical death* and the *apallic syndrome* should be retired. The vegetative state generally develops as part of the natural progression of coma. It may start within days to weeks following the initial onset of deep coma and may be associated with eye opening, roving eye movement, respiratory variations, and other automatism such as swallowing, grimacing, grunting, and moaning. However, there are no consistent, purposeful movements or behaviours. This may only be evident following prolonged observation and repeated testing, and it is common for lay persons to mistakenly believe that a patient in a PVS is responsive. Table 24.3 compares the PVS to other conditions than may mimic coma. In cases where the underlying pathology is related to traumatic injury, the vegetative state is termed persistent after a period of 12 months. In cases of non-traumatic dysfunction, persistence for 3 months is sufficient to make the diagnosis.

Minimally Conscious State

In many ways, the minimally conscious state (MCS) is different from the vegetative state only by the severity of impairment. Minimally conscious state differs most notably from the vegetative state in that patients with MCS, while still severely impaired, are able to repeatedly and reproducibly follow simple commands, respond appropriately to yes/no questions (either verbally or through gestures), display appropriate emotional responses such as smiling and crying in response to stimuli, reach for and hold objects, and track objects with their eyes.[15] It is somewhat intuitive that because MCS is less severe than PVS, recovery is often more complete, but it should also be noted that persistent severe disability is likely in nearly all cases.[16,17]

Table 24.3 Conditions that mimic coma

Condition	Self-awareness	Sleep-wake cycle	Motor function	Experience of pain and suffering
Coma	No	No	No purposeful movement	No
Persistent Vegetative State	No	Normal	No purposeful movement	No
Minimally Conscious State	Yes	Normal	Reproducibly follow simple commands	Yes
Locked-in Syndrome	Yes	Normal	Quadriplegia and pseudobulbar palsy; vertical eye movement and blinking preserved	Yes
Akinetic Mutism	Yes	Normal	Minimal movement	Yes
Catatonia	Variable	Normal	Often displays active resistance	Variable

Adapted from: The Multi-Society Task Force on PVS. Medical aspects of the persistent vegetative state (1). *N Engl J Med* 1994;330:1499–508.

Locked-in Syndrome

It is critical that the locked-in syndrome be distinguished from states of coma and persistent vegetation because underlying, patients remain fully conscious and sensate. The syndrome is typically a result of basilar artery occlusions causing ventral pontine infarcts, although tumours, tetrodotoxin, encephalitis, swine flu, and measles have also been implicated.[18] Due to the predilection for affecting corticobulbar and corticospinal tracts, the patient is clinically quadriplegic and unable to move facial muscles aside from raising the eyelids and vertical eye movement. However, the somatosensory tracts and RAS neurons responsible for arousal remain intact leading to what is sometimes referred to as a de-efferented state. With proper medical care and support it is possible for patients to live long lives and communicate with those around them. The diagnosis is typically made based on the classical physical examination findings just mentioned in combination with neuroimaging showing lesions in the appropriate areas.

Akinetic Mutism

In akinetic mutism, patients remain alert and vigilant, but are unable to speak or move. On closer examination, they may be able to speak short syllables in hushed tones or produce faintly perceptible movements. However, it is often difficult to distinguish the diagnosis from other forms of reduced movement. In the case of akinetic mutism, there is usually an exogenous causal factor such as a stroke, mass, or toxin that disrupts frontal-subcortical circuits and prevents the transmission of movement signals.[19]

Catatonia

Catatonia is characterized by an awake patient who typically lies motionless and mute and does not react to internal or external stimuli. In this way, it is very much similar to akinetic mutism and the two entities may be confused. However, a structural lesion is typically lacking in catatonia. When actively moved by an examiner, the limbs often exhibit a waxy flexibility and occasionally active resistance. Repetitive simple movements and repetitive vocalization have been described as well. While once thought to be a subtype of schizophrenia, catatonia is now recognized to occur with a variety of psychiatric and medical diseases including severe psychosis or depression. Oftentimes it is impossible to diagnose the underlying disorder until the catatonia is treated.[20]

Non-Convulsive Seizures

Non-convulsive seizure (NCS) and non-convulsive status epilepticus (NCSE) are increasingly recognized as an important consideration among differential causes of AMS. Recent reports including patients presenting with undifferentiated AMS to an emergency department suggests that one in twenty will have electroencephalography (EEG)-proven NCS or NCSE as the cause of the clinical presentation. Among hospitalized patients, the incidence of NCSE in those without any clinical signs of seizure has been reported to be 8%–18%.[21,22] Given how often it is implicated, seizure is an important diagnostic consideration in all patients presenting with AMS. It is intuitive that increased monitoring duration with EEG should increase detection, and this is borne out by observational data indicating that more than 24 hours of monitoring is often required to detect seizures.[23]

Brain Death

In order to arrive at a diagnosis of brain death, very specific criteria must be met. Diagnostic criteria were first proposed by the Harvard committee in 1968.[24]

Subsequently, the criteria were revised in 1995 and again in 2010.[25,26] Common to all iterations of these guidelines are the requirement for (1) an injury or insult deemed sufficient to cause complete and irreversible disruption of all cortical and brainstem functions, and (2) the absence of confounding or potentially reversible factors. While these criteria have a broad consensus, the manner by which they are confirmed is more contentious, often guided by local policies, procedures, and legislation. As brain death is legally synonymous with clinical death in most jurisdictions, great care must be taken in diagnosis and documentation.

APPROACH TO THE PATIENT WITH ALTERED MENTAL STATUS

The diagnostic and therapeutic approach to patients with AMS is both simple and complex. In the most rudimentary sense, it is an approach aimed first at rapid stabilization and correction of reversible, life-threatening disturbances, and then a more detailed investigation of aetiologies subsequent to initial stabilization. A suggested approach is summarized in Figure 24.1. For a more detailed review, the reader is referred to the emergency neurological life support guidelines.[27]

The initial approach should always begin by evaluating and ensuring the stability of airway, breathing, and circulation (ABCs). Further focused history and physical examination including vital signs will often yield useful information. Focal examination findings such as a unilateral dilated and unreactive pupil, stereotyped posturing or other asymmetric findings might focus further workup towards structural intracerebral lesions. In this situation, the importance of rapid diagnostic imaging increases. The preferred initial neurodiagnostic test is a cranial computed tomography (CT) scan. In patients without any localizing examination findings, toxic or metabolic disorders become much more likely. As they are relatively common, easily treatable, and the treatments are relatively benign, empiric correction of hypoglycaemia and opioid intoxication with glucose and naloxone is recommended. Serum chemistries and blood gas analysis with co-oximetry to identify electrolyte disturbances, hepatic failure, renal failure, dyshaemoglobinemias, and hypercapnia, and an extended toxicology screen should also be obtained when initial corrective measures do not rapidly improve mental status. A complete blood count should also be obtained as it can help identify infectious aetiologies such as meningitis, encephalitis, and abscesses. Additional diagnostics such as lumbar puncture, EEG, magnetic resonance imaging (MRI) and serum levels of thiamine, B12, thyroid hormones, alcohol levels, and serum osmole level may be useful in the correct clinical setting or when an aetiology is otherwise not identified.

CONFUSIONAL STATES

Delirium

Delirium is characterized by the acute (hours to days) onset of waxing and waning levels of consciousness, inattention, disturbed perception, and cognition. Three subtypes of delirium are recognized. Hyperactive delirium presents as a state of excessive or distorted cognition, which may include hallucinations, delusions, agitation, and restlessness. Some literature refers to hyperactive delirium as intensive care unit (ICU) psychosis, but this should not be confused with the psychosis that can accompany chronic psychiatric conditions such as schizophrenia or depression. In contrast, hypoactive delirium presents with symptoms associated with diminished cognition, including lethargy, behavioural withdrawal, and impaired motor skills. Acute encephalopathy is an alternative term sometimes used to describe hypoactive delirium. Patients who display features of both are diagnosed with a mixed subtype. In contrast to a number of commonly encountered diseases, which present with AMS, such as alcohol withdrawal or hepatic encephalopathy, no single pathophysiological mechanism has yet been identified to fully explain all possible presentations. The underlying pathophysiology and presentation are further muddied in the critically ill neurologically injured patient due to the primary reason for their admission to intensive care. Reported risk factors for the development of delirium while in the ICU are listed in Tables 24.4 and 24.5.

Due to the fluctuating nature of delirium, regular surveillance must be performed in order to not miss the diagnosis. Routine evaluations will optimally be coordinated with sedation breaks to distinguish pharmacology (medication-induced delirium) from other pathology. Objective delirium assessments have been validated for use in the ICU, such as the Confusion Assessment Method for the ICU (CAM-ICU) and the Intensive Care Delirium Screening Checklist (ICDSC).[28,29] Both tools are reliable.[30] Although not originally studied in the neurologically injured, their use is still recommended.[31]

Treatment of ICU delirium begins with the treatment of the patient's underlying illness that precipitated the need for intensive care. Deliriogenic medications should be discontinued or reduced in dose and frequency as much as possible. Providing adequate analgesia, not necessarily from the opiate classes, interventions to

Table 24.4 Risk factors for intensive care unit delirium

Patient factors	Acute illness factors	Treatment factors
Alcohol/Tobacco *Use or withdrawal*	Sepsis	Impaired sleep/noisy environments
Increased Age *Age greater than 65 years*	Fever	Medications (see Table 24.5)
Depression	Shock	Foley catheters
Dementia	Anaemia	Gastric tubes
	Respiratory disease *Hypercarbia or hypoxaemia*	Immobility
	Myocardial dysfunction	Sensory deprivation *Hearing aids, glasses, dentures*
	Electrolyte Abnormalities *Hyponatraemia, azotemia, hypocalcaemia, metabolic acidosis*	Faecal or Urinary Retention

Note: A number of mnemonics to aid clinicians in identifying the risk factors and aetiology of ICU delirium are available at http://www.icudelirium.org/terminology.html.

Table 24.5 Medications commonly associated with intensive care unit delirium

Prescription drugs	Non-prescription drugs
• Benzodiazepines	• Diphenhydramine
• Barbiturates	• Mandrake
• Narcotics	• Henbane
• Antiparkinson agents	• Jimson weed
• Antihistamines	• Belladonna extract
• H_2 blockers	• Valerian
• Scopolamine	• Loperamide
• Fluoroquinolones	
• Tricyclic antidepressants	
• Lithium	
• Digitalis	
• Beta Blockers	
• Muscle relaxants	
• Steroids	

promote reorientation and natural sleep, physical and occupational therapy, and interaction with familiar family and caregivers should be emphasized.

Pharmacological therapy for delirium is controversial with the weight of evidence in favour of no benefit. However, careful use of antipsychotics may be used as a sedative adjunct when psychomotor agitation becomes dangerous to the patient while other measures are being taken. Cholinergic agents, statins, and steroids are also without benefit and should be avoided for this purpose. For patients otherwise requiring continuous sedation, dexmedetomidine may be the preferred drug. Its potential benefit must be weighed against the risk of hypotension and bradycardia.

CONCLUSIONS

Many disorders can result in an AMS. An appropriate clinical response to patients presenting in this way requires an understanding of the underlying physiology and anatomy of normal consciousness and arousal as well as a systematic and comprehensive approach to diagnosis and treatment.

REFERENCES

1. Kanich W, Brady WJ, Huff JS, et al. Altered mental status: evaluation and etiology in the ED. *Am J Emerg Med* 2002;20:613–7.
2. Scheibel AB. On detailed connections of the medullary and pontine reticular formation. *Anat Rec* 1951;109.
3. Bremer F. L'activitécerebralé au cours du sommeil et de la narcose. Contribution à l'étude du mécanisme du sommeil. *Bull Acad Roy Med Belg* 1937;4:68–86.
4. Moruzzi G, Magoun HW. Brain stem reticular formation and activation of the EEG. *Electroencephalogr Clin Neurophysiol* 1949;1:455–73.
5. Daroff RB, Bradley WG. *Bradley's Neurology in Clinical Practice*. 6th ed. In: Robert B. Daroff, et al. eds. PA: Philadelphia, Elsevier/Saunders 2012;102.
6. Edlow BL, Haynes RL, Takahashi E, et al. Disconnection of the ascending arousal system in traumatic coma. *J Neuropathol Exp Neurol* 2013;72:505–23.

7. Edlow BL, Takahashi E, Wu O, et al. Neuroanatomic connectivity of the human ascending arousal system critical to consciousness and its disorders. *J Neuropathol Exp Neurol* 2012;71:531–46.

8. Posner JB, Plum F. *Plum and Posner's Diagnosis of Stupor and Coma*. 4th ed. New York: Oxford, Oxford University Press; 2007.

9. Edlow JA, Rabinstein A, Traub SJ, Wijdicks EF. Diagnosis of reversible causes of coma. *Lancet* 2014;384:2064–76.

10. Kasper DL. *Harrison's Principles of Internal Medicine*. 19th ed. In: Dennis L. Kasper, William Ellery Channing, eds. New York: McGraw Hill Education, 2015.

11. Young GB. Coma. *Ann N Y Acad Sci* 2009;1157:32–47.

12. Waxman SG. *Clinical Neuroanatomy*. 27th ed. New York: McGraw-Hill Education/Medical, 2013.

13. Jennett B, Plum F. Persistent vegetative state after brain damage. A syndrome in search of a name. *Lancet* 1972; 1:734–7.

14. The Multi-Society Task Force on PVS. Medical aspects of the persistent vegetative state (1). *N Engl J Med* 1994; 330:1499–508.

15. Giacino JT, Ashwal S, Childs N, et al. The minimally conscious state: definition and diagnostic criteria. *Neurology* 2002;58:349–53.

16. Estraneo A, Moretta P, Loreto V, Lanzillo B, Santoro L, Trojano L. Late recovery after traumatic, anoxic, or hemorrhagic long-lasting vegetative state. *Neurology* 2010; 75:239–45.

17. Luaute J, Maucort-Boulch D, Tell L, et al. Long-term outcomes of chronic minimally conscious and vegetative states. *Neurology* 2010;75:246–52.

18. Patterson JR, Grabois M. Locked-in syndrome: a review of 139 cases. *Stroke* 1986;17:758–64.

19. Mega MS, Cohenour RC. Akinetic mutism: disconnection of frontal-subcortical circuits. *Neuropsychiatry Neuropsychol Behav Neurol* 1997;10:254–9.

20. Rasmussen SA, Mazurek MF, Rosebush PI. Catatonia: Our current understanding of its diagnosis, treatment and pathophysiology. *World J Psychiatry* 2016;6:391–8.

21. Towne AR, Waterhouse EJ, Boggs JG, et al. Prevalence of nonconvulsive status epilepticus in comatose patients. *Neurology* 2000;54:340–5.

22. Pandian JD, Cascino GD, So EL, Manno E, Fulgham JR. Digital video-electroencephalographic monitoring in the neurological-neurosurgical intensive care unit: clinical features and outcome. *Arch Neurol* 2004;61: 1090–4.

23. Claassen J, Mayer SA, Kowalski RG, Emerson RG, Hirsch LJ. Detection of electrographic seizures with continuous EEG monitoring in critically ill patients. *Neurology* 2004;62:1743–8.

24. Beecher HK. Ethical problems created by the hopelessly unconscious patient. *N Engl J Med* 1968;278:1425–30.

25. Wijdicks EF, Varelas PN, Gronseth GS, Greer DM. American Academy of N. Evidence-based guideline update: determining brain death in adults: report of the Quality Standards Subcommittee of the American Academy of Neurology. *Neurology* 2010;74:1911–18.

26. Practice parameters for determining brain death in adults (summary statement). The Quality Standards Subcommittee of the American Academy of Neurology. *Neurology* 1995;45:1012–14.

27. Stevens RD, Cadena RS, Pineda J. Emergency neurological life support: Approach to the patient with coma. *Neurocrit Care* 2015;23(Suppl 2):S69–75.

28. Ely EW, Inouye SK, Bernard GR, et al. Delirium in mechanically ventilated patients: validity and reliability of the confusion assessment method for the intensive care unit (CAM-ICU). *JAMA* 2001;286:2703–10.

29. Bergeron N, Dubois MJ, Dumont M, Dial S, Skrobik Y. Intensive care delirium screening checklist: evaluation of a new screening tool. *Intensive Care Med* 2001;27: 859–64.

30. Plaschke K, von Haken R, Scholz M, et al. Comparison of the confusion assessment method for the intensive care unit (CAM-ICU) with the Intensive Care Delirium Screening Checklist (ICDSC) for delirium in critical care patients gives high agreement rate(s). *Intensive Care Med* 2008;34:431–6.

31. Riker RR, Fugate JE. Participants in the International Multi-disciplinary Consensus Conference on Multimodality M. Clinical monitoring scales in acute brain injury: assessment of coma, pain, agitation, and delirium. *Neurocrit Care* 2014;21(Suppl 2):S27–37.

25

Intracranial Hypertension

S. M. Khorsand and K. H. Kevin Luk

ABSTRACT

Intracranial hypertension (IH) is a neurological emergency with high morbidity and mortality requiring prompt diagnosis and treatment. The aetiologies of IH include trauma, neoplasm, arterial and venous hypertension, and hydrocephalus. Although aetiologies vary, the common pathway of IH results in cerebral ischaemia and eventually infarction. Initial signs and symptoms of IH include headache, decreased level of consciousness, cranial palsies, which can progress to coma, Cushing's triad, and death. Treatment of IH involves a stepwise, tiered approach, which involves physical, pharmacological, and surgical modalities.

KEYWORDS

Intracranial pressure; intracranial hypertension (IH); Monro–Kellie doctrine; cerebral perfusion pressure; mannitol; hypertonic saline; external ventricular drain; decompressive craniectomy; decompressive craniectomy (DECRA); Randomised Evaluation of Surgery with Craniectomy for Uncontrollable Elevation of Intracranial Pressure (RESCUEicp).

INTRODUCTION

Intracranial pressure (ICP) is defined as the pressure inside the cranial vault. The normal value is 7–15 mmHg. Intracranial hypertension (IH) represents an abnormal increase in ICP due to the disturbance of the homoeostasis inside the cranial vault. The usual cut-off for IH is 20–25 mmHg.[1] Cerebral perfusion pressure (CPP) is defined as the difference between the mean arterial pressure (MAP) and ICP or central venous pressure (CVP), whichever is higher.[1] With intact autoregulation, cerebral blood flow (CBF) is constant between 50 and 150 mmHg (Figure 25.1).

In the neurocritical care setting, IH commonly presents as a neurological emergency as a result of devastating intracranial injuries similar to the case scenario. However, in an outpatient setting, IH can also present in a subacute or chronic manner. Intracranial hypertension is the manifestation of the underlying pathology inside the cranial vault. Although initial treatment focuses on controlling and relieving the IH, definitive treatment is often necessary to address the causative pathology. While significant advances have been made in recognition and early treatment of IH, it continues to be a significant contributor to the morbidity and mortality of patients with multi-system trauma.[2]

THE MONRO–KELLIE DOCTRINE

The Monro–Kellie doctrine describe the pressure-volume relationship between ICP and intracranial contents, which include brain tissue, cerebrospinal fluid (CSF), arterial blood, and venous blood.[3–5] The underlying hypothesis is that the cranium is incompressible and the cranial vault has a finite volume. The pressure equilibrium of the cranial vault is maintained at the normal level by interaction of its contents, such that an increase in volume in a component must be compensated by reduction of volumes of the other components. Cerebrospinal fluid is the major buffer of volume changes in the cranial vault and venous blood plays a minor role in volume shift.

CEREBROSPINAL FLUID DYNAMICS

Cerebrospinal fluid is produced by the choroid plexus in the ventricular system through an ultrafiltration process.

Approximately 500 ml of CSF is produced daily and the total CSF volume is approximately 150 to 200 ml in an adult, with 25–40 ml in the ventricles. Cerebrospinal fluid circulates through the ventricles and down into the spinal subarachnoid space. It is eventually reabsorbed by the arachnoid granulation into the venous system. An increase in intracranial content can be compensated initially by shifting the CSF towards the spinal subarachnoid space without disturbing the ICP.[6]

AETIOLOGIES OF INTRACRANIAL HYPERTENSION

As stated previously, IH is the final common pathway of various intracranial pathologies. The common causes of IH are as follows:

- Mass effect
- Generalized cerebral oedema
- Disturbance of CSF flow dynamics
- Venous hypertension
- Hypertensive emergency
- Idiopathic

The most common cause of IH is traumatic brain injury (TBI), which is associated with significant morbidity and mortality.[2] Traumatic brain injury can be categorized into two distinct, yet interrelated phases. Primary injury is the consequence of initial trauma resulting in mechanical forces on the skull and brain tissue, which can produce skull fracture, disruption of vascular structures with intracranial haematoma, and shearing and compression of neuronal, glial, and vascular tissues resulting in haemorrhagic brain contusions. Thus, epidural haemorrhage, subdural haematoma, subarachnoid haemorrhage (SAH), intraparenchymal haemorrhage, and cerebral contusion can exert mass effect and result in raised ICP and obstructive hydrocephalus. Secondary injury is the consequence of progressive pathological insults to the neurons in the penumbral region starting immediately after the initial TBI. This results in astrocytosis and neuronal swelling, relative hypoperfusion, perturbation of cellular calcium homoeostasis, increased free radical generation and lipid peroxidation, mitochondrial dysfunction, inflammation, glutaminergic excitotoxicity, cellular necrosis, apoptosis, and axonal degeneration. Systemic insults such as hypotension, hypoxaemia, hypoglycaemia, hyperglycaemia, hypocapnoea, and hypercapnoea are major contributors of secondary injury. In addition to ischaemia-hypoxia, reperfusion hyperaemia appears to play a role in secondary injury. Cerebral oedema and raised ICP can result secondary to breakdown of the blood–brain barrier (BBB) and loss of cerebral autoregulation.[7–9]

Neoplasms, both primary and metastatic, can result in IH. Benign tumours rarely cause IH unless they reach a critical size or the location of tumour impedes CSF flow (e.g., a pineal gland tumour blocking the Sylvian aqueduct). However, malignant neoplasms cause breakdown of the BBB and angiogenesis, which can readily result in IH due to mass effect, vasogenic oedema, and blockage of CSF flow.

Disturbance of CSF flow dynamics can result in hydrocephalus, which can be further classified as communicating and obstructive based on the aetiology. As discussed previously, CSF flow is crucial in buffering the change of intracranial volume to maintain pressure homoeostasis. Therefore, hydrocephalus can result in IH. Obstructive hydrocephalus is usually as a result of intraventricular haemorrhage or mass effect due to intracranial haematoma or neoplasms. Subarachnoid haemorrhage results in irritation of the arachnoid granulation and decreases CSF reabsorption. In rare circumstances, such as cryptococcal meningitis and subarachnoid haemorrhage, overproduction of CSF can result in communicating hydrocephalus and raised ICP.

Venous hypertension[10] can cause raised ICP via two mechanisms: (1) the impendence of venous drainage from the dural sinuses can slow down CSF reabsorption; (2) the CPP is reduced resulting in cellular hypoxia and cerebral oedema. The most common intracerebral cause of venous hypertension is dural venous sinus thrombosis. It can occur as a result of direct trauma to the dural venous sinuses. Spontaneous cases are usually associated with an underlying hypercoagulable state (e.g., systemic lupus erythematosus, Factor V Leiden), and/or oral contraceptive use.[11] Similarly, occlusion or thrombosis of the internal jugular veins and superior vena cava can also result in raised ICP. The most common extracranial cause of venous hypertension is decompensated congestive heart failure resulting in volume overload and central venous distention.

During hypertensive emergency, there is a severe elevation of the systemic blood pressure, which results in an increase in CPP and hyperaemia. In addition, extreme blood pressures can also result in the breakdown of the BBB resulting in cerebral oedema and hypertensive encephalopathy.[12] In addition, generalized cerebral oedema is a common presentation of ischaemic-anoxic encephalopathy, and fulminant hepatic failure.

The underlying cause of idiopathic IH (pseudotumour cerebri) is not known but there is a female predisposition and is found to be more common in obese patients of childbearing age. Headaches and progressive loss of visual acuity are the most common symptoms. Papilloedema can be seen on funduscopic examination. Importantly, there is an absence of localized neurologic findings and or other causes of increased ICP. Therapeutic lumbar puncture with CSF drainage resulting in symptomatic improvement is diagnostic for the condition. Treatment includes carbonic anhydrase inhibitor to decrease CSF production, weight loss, and endovenous stenting.[13]

PATHOPHYSIOLOGY OF INTRACRANIAL HYPERTENSION

Small and/or gradual increase in intracranial content may not result in IH. The volume change is accommodated by displacement of CSF from the ventricles to the spinal subarachnoid space. In addition, the volume increase is buffered partially by shifting of venous blood and flexibility of the tentorium and falx cerebri. However, as the intracranial volume continues to increase, the ability of the cranial vault to accommodate additional volume without changing the pressure (i.e., intracranial compliance) decreases. The inflection point appears to be around 20 to 30 mmHg, where after 30 mmHg, a small volume change will result in a marked elevation of ICP.[14]

Severe IH, when accompanied by a unilateral space-occupying lesion can result in cerebral herniation syndromes. The signs and symptoms of specific syndromes will be discussed further in the next section. Therefore, physical examination findings can help the clinician to locate the mass or lesion. In addition to direct distortion of and damage to cerebral macroarchitecture, IH results in reduced CPP in the areas that are not initially injured. This can result in global hypoperfusion and cellular hypoxia. In response to the decreasing CPP, the body reacts by raising the systemic blood pressure and dilating the intracerebral blood vessel to improve CBF. However, this perpetuates a vicious cycle of increasing intracranial volume and further worsening of ICP.

Ultimately, IH results in global cerebral ischaemia and infarction. Death usually results from cessation of brainstem function and subsequent cardiopulmonary arrest. Even in the cases where IH was reversed promptly and treated aggressively, it still carries a significant morbidity and mortality in the TBI population. Early observational studies have linked sustained ICP greater than 20–25 mmHg and MAP less than 80 mmHg to poor long-term functional outcomes.[15,16] However, in a landmark randomized controlled trial of ICP monitoring in addition to imaging and clinician examination, patients who received ICP monitoring did not show improved mortality or functional outcome when compared to

the control group.[17] The current indication for ICP monitoring will be discussed in a separate chapter.

SIGNS AND SYMPTOMS

In general, patients with raised ICP present with signs and symptoms of confusion, decreased level of consciousness, headache, vomiting, and cranial nerve palsies. Symptoms can potentially progress rapidly where patients display signs of herniation including coma, abnormal breathing, and motor posturing. Patients with impending herniation can present with the Cushing's Triad: (1) increased systolic and pulse pressure; (2) bradycardia; and (3) irregular respiration.[18]

Irregular respiratory patterns can occur as a result of compression of the pons and medulla, where the respiratory centre is located. Table 25.1 summarizes the different types of abnormal breathing patterns:[19]

Patients presenting with certain herniation syndromes would present with specific signs and symptoms (Table 25.2), which allow for localization of the lesion:[20]

- Uncal herniation is usually caused by a mass over the temporal lobe. This can result in downward herniation of the uncus, which is the innermost part of the temporal lobe through the tentorium into the brainstem, especially the midbrain. It can lead to compression of the oculomotor nerve (cranial nerve [CN] III), which can result in a dilated and fixed ipsilateral pupil, progressing to a downward and outward gaze. Pupillary change is often accompanied by contralateral motor posturing due to compression of the motor fibres as they descend from the motor cortex prior to decussation.
- Central transtentorial herniation happens when there is diffuse cerebral oedema or acute hydrocephalus, which causes compression of the bilateral temporal lobes and diencephalon. These structures herniate through a notch in the tentorium cerebelli. If left untreated, this is often fatal due to disruption the vital brainstem function. Patients often present with fixed and small pupils, coma, bilateral motor posturing, and/or loss of brainstem reflexes.
- Subfalcine/cingulate herniation is the most common form of herniation syndrome. It happens when mass effect is exerted in the frontotemporal area of the cortex resulting in a shift of the cingulate gyrus to the contralateral hemisphere under the falx cerebri. It can result in contralateral hydrocephalus due to obstruction of the foramen of Monro. Clinically, the patient can present with a depressed level of consciousness and asymmetric motor posturing with the contralateral side worse than the ipsilateral side.

Table 25.1 Abnormal breathing patterns associated with brain injury

Breathing pattern	Diagram	Description	Location of lesion
Cheyne-Stokes		Gradually increasing tidal volume until it peaks, then decreases to a pause	Basal Ganglia
Apneustic		Prolonged inspiration followed by prolonged expiration that is commonly mistaken as apnoea	Rostral Pons
Ataxic		Irregular rate and tidal volume with irregular pauses	Caudal Pons
Biot's		Regular and deep inspiration followed by apnoea or pauses	Medulla

- Cerebellar/tonsillar herniation occurs as a result of downward movement of the cerebellar tonsil into the foramen magnum due to increased ICP. This can result in compression of the lower brainstem and upper cervical spinal cord. Patients can present with sudden loss of consciousness, respiratory compromise, and haemodynamic instability.

Table 25.2 Cerebral herniation syndromes and associated causes and symptoms

Type	Causes	Clinical signs
Uncal	Temporal lobe mass	Ipsilateral CN III palsy Contralateral motor posturing
Central Transtentorial	Diffuse cerebral oedema Acute hydrocephalus	Coma Bilateral motor posturing Loss of brainstem reflexes
Subfalcine	Frontotemporal convexity mass	Coma Asymmetric motor posturing (contralateral > ipsilateral)
Cerebellar	Cerebellar mass	Sudden loss of consciousness Bilateral motor posturing

TREATMENT AND MANAGEMENT ALGORITHM OF INTRACRANIAL HYPERTENSION

Rapid treatment of IH is critical and should not be delayed for imaging examinations. All treatment efforts attempt to either optimize CPP in an effort to maintain CBF or to decrease cerebral metabolic rate of oxygen consumption ($CMRO_2$). Initial management begins at the bedside and is performed in concert with pharmacological intervention and early neurosurgical consultation.

An effort should be made to maintain the patient in a neutral midline cervical position. This will maximize venous blood return via the jugular veins. At the same time, elevating the head of the bed to achieve Fowler's position (defined as 90°) or semi-Fowler's (30°–45°) will decrease CVP to further allow for maximal venous blood return. This must be balanced against potential decreases in MAP in Fowler's position, as the hypotensive IH patient will have severely impaired CPP as stated previously.[16]

Transient hyperventilation to achieve low-grade hypocapnoea may be attempted with a goal $PaCO_2$ of 25–30 mmHg. However, caution must be urged as resultant cerebral vasoconstriction will eventually lead to rebound brain tissue ischaemia.[21] Indeed, patients treated with moderate prophylactic hyperventilation had worse outcomes and thus we advocate for its use as a temporizing measure.[22]

Fever is incredibly common in neurologically injured critically ill patients with incidence of nearly 50%.[23] Normothermia and prevention of fever has been shown to reduce ICP in TBI patients and also reduces secondary injury. Conventional external cooling mechanisms and antipyretics as well as invasive intravascular cooling catheters have been studied.[24] Though early studies and animal models demonstrated protective benefits of hypothermia in TBI, the Eurotherm 3235 trial[25] failed to demonstrate any benefits of therapeutic hypothermia in TBI patients compared to standard care. Meta-analysis[26] has shown no difference in outcome between previously studied moderate hypothermia, maintenance of normothermia and avoidance of pyrexia. Hypothermia is not without complications. There is increased risk of pneumonia and coagulopathy as well as hyperglycaemia and bradycardia.[27] Thus, we advocate for a normothermia approach.

Pharmacological interventions make up the vast majority of non-surgical options for the IH patient. Hyperosmolar therapy aims at reducing intracranial water content by drawing out brain tissue water. Mannitol, an osmotic diuretic, may be used in doses of 0.25–1.00 g/kg in boluses and repeated serially.[28] Care must be taken in the haemodynamically unstable polytrauma patient (or other hypotensive patient) as these patients will become profoundly hypotensive with loss of intravascular volume resulting from subsequent brisk diuresis. Furthermore, in a TBI patient without an intact BBB, there is a theoretical risk that mannitol will deposit extravascularly resulting in rebound IH.[29]

Another effective hyperosmolar intervention is hypertonic saline (HTS) 23.4% in a 30 ml bolus infused over 15 minutes.[30,31] This is usually better tolerated in haemodynamically unstable patients and in a recent systematic review, HTS resulted in lesser ICP treatment failure compared to mannitol.[28] It is caustic and should be administered via a central line. In both mannitol and HTS administration, serum osmolarity must be monitored frequently.

In patients with malignant tumours, corticosteroids such as dexamethasone may be an effective treatment for IH due to resultant vasogenic oedema. However, this is the only instance in which IH should be treated with corticosteroids. MRC CRASH 1 (Medical Research Council Corticosteroid randomisation after significant head injury)[32] was an international double-blind randomized placebo-controlled trial in brain-injured patients, which looked at the early administration of corticosteroids. The trial was terminated early because it demonstrated increased risk of death or severe disability in the corticosteroid-treated group. The current Brain Trauma Foundation (BTF) guidelines for TBI management[33] recommends against corticosteroid administration in TBI patients.

Furosemide has been used as an adjuvant to hyperosmolar therapy though its mechanism is not entirely clear. It is believed to work by decreasing CVP in addition to its loop diuretic properties in decreasing ICP. It has been studied in animals in combination with HTS as well as mannitol and has been shown in animal models to reduce brain tissue water more than with either hyperosmolar agents [34,35]

Optimization of sedation and analgesia is important in the IH patient, as this will decrease $CMRO_2$ and CBF. Short-acting agents are ideal to allow for accurate assessment of the neurological examination with the goal of weaning sedation as soon as intracranial compliance improves and IH resolves. Care must be taken in uptitrating sedation as this may decrease MAP and thus impair CPP. The utility of artificially raising CPP with the use vasopressors has not been studied, though it is practiced at some centres. The current BTF TBI guidelines recommend maintaining CPP of 60–70 mmHg and targeting a systolic blood pressure (SBP) of greater than 100 mmHg (age 50–69 years) or 110 mmHg (age 15–49 years or >70 years).[33]

The goal of IH treatment is to optimize oxygenated CBF to an injured brain. In some instances, paralysis may aid this goal in cases of increased peripheral tissue oxygen extraction. Paralysis in the form of a continuous drip of a non-depolarizing neuromuscular blocking agent (NMBA) may decrease high tissue oxygen extraction and in combination with appropriate levels of sedation will additionally prevent instances of coughing or Valsalva, which may increase CVP and thus decrease CPP. It should be noted that a large systematic review found clinical equipoise for the use of NMBAs in effectively treating IH. Furthermore, the inability to perform serial neurological reassessments is a significant drawback of paralytic use in IH and thus we recommend this only after positioning, hyperosmolar therapy, and sedation have been optimized with persistent IH.

In the comatose patient with IH, it is important to rule out subclinical seizures or frank status epilepticus. Seizures lead to not only increased ICP but also increased $CMRO_2$ and peripheral tissue oxygen extraction from skeletal muscle contracture. An electroencephalogram (EEG) should be obtained in TBI patients in instances of persistent coma not explained by injury pattern with low threshold to treat with antiepileptic drugs (AEDs) in the presence of seizures. There is some evidence that some AEDs worsen long-term neurological outcomes in TBI patients, so prophylaxis is not routinely recommended.[36,37]

Barbiturates are the last resort in the pharmacological treatment of refractory IH. Barbiturates are γ-aminobutyric acid A (GABA$_A$) receptor agonists and include pentobarbital, thiopental, and methohexital. High-dose barbiturates are effective at treating elevated ICP but can be associated with hypotension. Barbiturates decreased the ICP by decreasing CMRO$_2$ and CBF by inducing cerebral electrical silence; that is, an isoelectric EEG. Their use has not been shown to have any impact on clinical outcome including mortality.[38,39]

Lastly, acetazolamide is specific for the treatment of idiopathic IH (IIH). A carbonic anhydrase inhibitor, which reduces CSF production, it has been shown to be most effective in patients who present with at least moderate papilloedema and can improve IIH symptoms including visual field testing, neck pain, tinnitus, and vertigo.[40]

SURGICAL INTERVENTION

As previously stated, early neurosurgical consultation is essential, and if the patient is at an institution without in-house neurosurgeons, the transfer process should be initiated immediately. Cerebrospinal diversion is the most basic level of procedural intervention, which is typically accomplished with an external ventricular drain (EVD). An EVD is a multi-orifice catheter that is inserted into the lateral ventricle (usually the largest of the two ventricles) via a burr hole operation, which can be done at the bedside or in the operating room depending on the institution. This catheter is then connected to pressure tubing, a transducer, and a collection chamber. This has the added benefit of being both a monitor and therapy, as it can monitor the ICP as well as divert CSF. The typical risks include infection, catheter tract haematoma, accidental over-drainage of CSF, and brain tissue damage. It is used in a variety of clinical situations leading to IH, including hydrocephalus, subarachnoid haemorrhage, tumours causing mass effect, and many more. Further discussion of the indications and timing of EVD insertion is discussed at length in Chapter 62, 'External Ventricular Drainage Systems'.

Decompressive unilateral frontotemporoparietal (FTP) craniectomy for evacuation of a mass-occupying lesion is well established and potentially life-saving in TBI. However, the use of decompressive bifrontal craniectomy in diffuse cerebral oedema from TBI is controversial, and many studies have sought to understand whether the lowered ICPs achieved through craniectomy result in improved long-term neurologic outcomes. The most recent of these studies showed decreased ICPs and shorter ICU length of stay with a bifrontotemporoparietal decompressive craniectomy (DECRA) over standard care,

however, the intervention arm was felt to have less acute patients. The study design also used a relatively low cut-off for defining refractory IH.[41]

The Randomised Evaluation of Surgery with Craniectomy for Uncontrollable Elevation of Intracranial Pressure (RESCUEicp) study published in September 2016 in the *New England Journal of Medicine* was a randomized controlled trial of DECRA (bifrontal or unilateral FTP) versus standard care.[42] The surgical arm patients had slightly more diffuse oedema versus mass effect injuries and had less hypoxaemia, hypotension, and drug and alcohol abuse though with the exception that in the latter this did not reach statistical significance. The outcomes from this study demonstrated significant mortality benefit to decompression, however, there was higher disability in the surgical arm, driving home points made in the earlier DECRA study: decompression leads to higher survival in a persistent vegetative state.[41]

We propose the algorithm given in Figure 25.2 for IH management in a stepwise approach. Early neurosurgical consultation for decompression and/or CSF diversion is paramount and should be undertaken in tandem with medical management of IH. Optimizing a neutral cervical position with the head of bed elevated can be initiated at the bedside even before pharmacological intervention arrives. In an intubated patient with a protected airway, sedation should be optimized with careful titration to preserve the ability to reassess the neurological examination; paralysis can also be considered. Cerebral perfusion pressure should be optimized to provide oxygenated blood flow to the brain. Hyperosmolar therapy can be initiated at any time but attention must be paid to volume status, especially in the polytrauma TBI patient. Hypothermia can then be considered to decrease CMRO$_2$. Lastly, barbiturate therapy to decrease CMRO$_2$ can be attempted as a last resort given the lack of mortality benefit.

CONCLUSIONS

Intracranial hypertension is the final common pathway for multiple intracranial pathologies. The condition carries significant morbidity and mortality and is related to the rate of ICP increase as well the duration of IH. Initial treatment is focussed on relieving ICP by shifting the intracranial contents, reducing cerebral metabolic rate, tight control of arterial blood pressure, and surgical decompression. However, definitive treatment requires addressing the underlying cause such as removal of haematoma, resection of neoplasms, or CSF shunting procedures. Recent studies on ICP monitoring and medical/surgical treatment algorithms of IH provide a framework for neurocritical care specialists to manage the condition. However, further efforts are required to improve the understanding of the condition so that individualized, optimal care can be delivered to patients with IH.

REFERENCES

1. Hemphill J, III, Smith WS, Gress DR. Neurologic critical care, including hypoxic-ischemic encephalopathy, and subarachnoid hemorrhage. In: Kasper D, Fauci A, Hauser S, Longo D, Jameson J, Loscalzo J, eds. *Harrison's Principles of Internal Medicine*. 19th ed. New York: McGraw-Hill; 2015. [accessed 2016 July 14]. Available from: http://accessmedicine.mhmedical.com/content.aspx?bookid=1130&Sectionid=79746087.

2. Rubiano AM, Carney N, Chesnut RM, Puyana JC. Global neurotrauma research challenges and opportunities. *Nature* 2015;527(7578):S193–S197.

3. Monro A. *Observations on the Structure and Functions of the Nervous System*. Edinburgh: Creech & Johnson. 1823.

4. Kellie G. Appearances observed in the dissection of two individuals; death from cold and congestion of the brain. *Trans Med Chir Soc (Edinb)*. 1824;1:84–169.

5. Mokri B. The Monro-Kellie hypothesis: applications in CSF volume depletion. *Neurology* 2001;56(12):1746–8.

6. Ropper AH, Samuels MA, Klein JP. Chapter 30. Disturbances of cerebrospinal fluid, including hydrocephalus, pseudotumor cerebri, and low-pressure syndromes. In: Ropper AH, Samuels MA, Klein JP, eds. *Adams & Victor's Principles of Neurology*. 10th ed. New York: McGraw-Hill; 2014. [cited 2016 July 23]. http://accessmedicine.mhmedical.com/content.aspx?bookid=690&Sectionid=50910881.

7. Armao D, Bouldin T. Pathology of the Nervous System. In: Reisner HM, eds. *Pathology: A Modern Case Study*. New York: McGraw-Hill; 2015. [cited 2016 July 31]. Available from: http://accessmedicine.mhmedical.com/content.aspx?bookid=1569&Sectionid=95972060.

8. Kinoshita K. Traumatic brain injury: pathophysiology for neurocritical care. *J Intensive Care* 2016;4:29.

9. Maas AIR, Stocchetti N, Bullock R. Moderate and severe traumatic brain injury in adults. *Lancet Neurol* 2008; 7(8):724–41.

10. Wilson MH. Monro-Kellie 2.0. The dynamic vascular and venous pathophysiological components of intracranial pressure. *J Cereb Blood Flow Metab* 2016;36(8):1338–50.

11. Bousser MG, Ferro JM. Cerebral venous thrombosis: An update. *Lancet Neurol* 2007;6(2):162–70.

12. Manning L, Robinson TG, Anderson CS. Control of blood pressure in hypertensive neurological emergencies. *Curr Hypertens Rep* 2014;16(6):436.

13. Kosmorsky GS. Idiopathic intracranial hypertension: Pseudotumor cerebri. *Headache* 2014;54(2):389–93.

14. Langfitt TW, Weinstein JD, Kassel NF. Cerebral vasomotor paralysis produced by intracranial hypertension. *Neurology* 1965;15(7):622–41.

15. Saul TG, Ducker TB. Effect of intracranial pressure monitoring and aggressive treatment on mortality in severe head injury. *J Neurosurg* 1982;56(4):498–503.

16. Marmarou A, Anderson RL, Ward JD, et al. Impact of ICP instability and hypotension on outcome in patients with severe head trauma. *J Neurosurg* 1992; 75(1s):S59–S66.

17. Chesnut RM, Temkin N, Carney N, et al. The Global Neurotrauma Research Group. A trial of intracranial-pressure monitoring in traumatic brain injury. *N Engl J Med* 2012;367(26):2471–81.

18. Humphries RL. Chapter 22. Head Injuries. In: Stone C, Humphries RL. eds. Current *Diagnosis & Treatment Emergency Medicine*. 7th ed. New York: McGraw-Hill; 2011. [cited 2016 July 28]. Available from: http://accessmedicine.mhmedical.com/content.aspx?bookid=385&Sectionid=40357237.

19. Bolton CF, Chen R, Wijdicks EFM, Zifko UA. Chapter 3: Clinical Observations of Disordered Breathing. In: *Neurology of Breathing*. PA, Philadelphia: Butterworth-Heinemann; 2004.

20. Kemp WL, Burns DK, Brown TG. Chapter 11. Neuropathology. In: Kemp WL, Burns DK, Brown TG, eds. *Pathology: The Big Picture*. New York, NY: McGraw-Hill;2008. [cited 2016 December 31]. Available from: http://accessmedicine.mhmedical.com/content.aspx?bookid=499&Sectionid=41568294.

21. Imberti R, Bellinzona G, Langer M. Cerebral tissue PO2 and SjvO2 changes during moderate hyperventilation in patients with severe traumatic brain injury. *J Neurosurg* 2002; 96(1):97–102.

22. Muizelaar JP, Marmarou A, Ward JD, et al. Adverse effects of prolonged hyperventilation in patients with severe head injury: a randomized clinical trial. *J Neurosurg* 1991;75:731–9.

23. Kilpatrick M, Lowry D, Firlik A. Hypothermia in the neurosurgical intensive care unit. *Neurosurgery* 2000; 47(4):850–6.

24. Puccio AM, Fischer MR, Jankowitz BT, et al. Induced normothermia attenuates intracranial hypertension and reduces fever burden after severe traumatic brain injury. *Neurocrit Care* 2009;11:82.

25. Andrews PJD, Sinclair HL, Rodriguez A, et al. The Eurotherm 3235 Trial Collaborators. Hypothermia for intracranial hypertension after traumatic brain injury. *N Engl J Med* 2015;373(25):2403–12.

26. Crompton EM, Lubomirova I, Cotlarciuc I, Han TS, Sharma SD, Sharma P. Meta-analysis of therapeutic hypothermia for traumatic brain injury in adult and pediatric patients. *Crit Care Med* 2016 Dec 9. [Epub ahead of print].

27. Polderman K. Mechanisms of action, physiological effects, and complications of hypothermia. *Crit Care Med* 2009; 37(7):186–202.

28. Burgess S, Abu-Laban RB, Slavik RS, Vu EN, Zed PJ. A systematic review of randomized controlled trials comparing hypertonic sodium solutions and mannitol for traumatic brain injury: Implications for emergency department management. *Ann Pharmacother* 2016;50(4): 291–300.

29. McManus ML, Soriano SG. Rebound swelling of astroglioma cells exposed to hypertonic mannitol. *Anesthesiology* 1998;88:1586–91.

30. Kerwin AJ, Schinco MA, Tepas JJ 3rd, Renfro WH, Vitarbo EA, Muehlberger M. The use of 23.4% hypertonic saline for the management of elevated intracranial pressure in patients with severe traumatic brain injury: a pilot study. *J Trauma* 2009;67(2):277–82.

31. Mangat HS, Chiu YL, Gerber LM, Alimi M, Ghajar J, Härtl R. Hypertonic saline reduces cumulative and daily intracranial pressure burdens after severe traumatic brain injury. *J Neurosurg* 2015;122(1):202–10.

32. Edwards P, Arango M, Balica L, et al. CRASH trial collaborators. Final results of MRC CRASH, a randomised placebo-controlled trial of intravenous corticosteroid in adults with head injury-outcomes at 6 months. *Lancet* 2005; 365(9475):1957–9.

33. Carney N, Totten AM, O'Reilly C, et al. Guidelines for the management of severe traumatic brain injury. 4th Ed. Brain Trauma Foundation 2016. [cited 2016 October 1]. Available from: https://braintrauma.org/uploads/13/06/Guidelines_for_Management_of_Severe_TBI_4th_Edition.pdf.

34. Wang LC, Papangelous A. Comparison of equivolume equiosmolar solutions of mannitol and hypertonic saline with or without furosemide on brain water content in normal rats. *Anesthesiology* 2013;118(4):903–13.

35. Thenuwara K, Todd MM, Brian JE Jr. Effect of mannitol and furosemide on plasma osmolality and brain water. *Anesthesiology* 2002;96(2):416–21.

36. Temkin NR, Dikmen SS, Wilensky AJ, Keihm J, Chabal S, Winn HR. A randomized, double-blind study of phenytoin for the prevention of posttraumatic seizures. *N Engl J Med* 1990;323:497–502.

37. Torbic H, Forni AA, Anger KE. Use of antiepileptics for seizure prophylaxis after traumatic brain injury. *Am J Health-System Pharm* 2013;70(9):759–66.

38. Majdan M, Mauritz W, Wilbacher I, Brazinova A, Rusnak M, Leitgeb J. Barbiturates use and its effects in patients with severe traumatic brain injury in five European countries. *J Neurotrauma* 2013;30(1):23–29.

39. Roberts I, Sydenham E. Barbiturates for acute traumatic brain injury. *Cochrane Database of Systematic Reviews* 2012, Issue 12. Art. No.: CD000033.

40. Wall M. Update on idiopathic intracranial hypertension. *Neurologic Clin* 2017;35(1):45–47.

41. Cooper DJ, Rosenfeld JV, Murray L. Decompressive craniectomy in diffuse traumatic brain injury. *N Engl J Med* 2011;364:1493–502.

42. Hutchinson PJ, Kolias AG, Timofeev IS. Trial of decompressive craniectomy for traumatic intracranial hypertension. *N Engl J Med* 2016;375:1119–30.

26

Cerebral Oedema

A. Lele and P. Sundararajan

ABSTRACT

Cerebral oedema is a common presenting pathology in various neurological emergencies due to a primary brain insult. There is a disruption of the normal cerebral physiology leading to rearrangement of the brain parenchymal water mass. The classification of cerebral oedema is based on different pathological processes contributing to oedema formation. The increase in brain tissue volume and intracranial pressure (ICP) manifests as sudden or gradual progressive decline in the level of consciousness, headache, nausea, non-projectile vomiting, etc. The use of serial neuroimaging such as computed tomography (CT) and magnetic resonance imaging (MRI) are critical in diagnosing cerebral oedema. Clinical management depends on a tiered approach starting with simple medical management like positioning and osmotherapy to surgical management. This chapter discusses the relevant basics of cerebral physiology, classification, clinical management, diagnostic tests, as well as medical and surgical management of cerebral oedema.

KEYWORDS

Cerebral oedema; hypertonic saline; mannitol; steroids; vasogenic; cytotoxic; intracranial hypertension (IH); aquaporin; craniectomy.

INTRODUCTION

Cerebral oedema is a common presenting pathology in various neurological emergencies such as acute ischaemic and haemorrhagic stroke, traumatic brain injury (TBI) and cerebral tumours. The consequences of cerebral oedema such as elevated intracranial pressure (ICP) and the compromised cerebral blood flow (CBF) can prove to be lethal.[1]

The pathophysiologies of cerebral oedema are diverse and so are the treatment options. This chapter presents an evidence-based update on pathophysiology, diagnosis, and management of cerebral oedema.

Definition of Cerebral Oedema

Cerebral oedema refers to the excessive and pathological accumulation of fluid within tissues.[2]

REVIEW OF CEREBRAL PHYSIOLOGY

A discussion of cerebral oedema is incomplete without a review of relevant cerebral physiology. Cerebral homoeostatic milieu depends on energy dependent processes such as sodium-potassium (Na^+–K^+) adenosine triphosphate (ATP) pump, which helps prevent the influx of sodium and water into the cells. With sodium staying extracellular, the osmotic gradient is maintained to prevent water from accumulating intracellularly. Disruption of this Na^+–K^+ pump is pathognomonic of ischaemic cerebral oedema.

Aquaporin-4 (AQP4), a water channel in the brain is also thought to be important in the pathogenesis of cerebral oedema associated with ischaemia.[3] Aquaporin-4 is abundant in the brain and spinal cord with a highly polarized distribution, abundantly expressed in astrocyte end-feet that surrounds the capillaries.[4] An overexpression of AQP4 is noted in reactive astrocytes after cerebral injury[5] and is associated with oedema formation in the acute phase of injury.[6] Aquaporin-4 via activation of P2 purinergic receptors in astrocytes also initiates downstream astrocytic Ca^{2+} signaling which potentially exacerbates brain oedema.[7]

In the build-up phase, AQP4 overexpression may result in the swelling and death of astrocytes and activation of microglia, which could be the main contributor to the blood–brain barrier (BBB) disruption that leads to plasma protein leakage and extravascular fluid accumulation.[1]

The BBB is composed of endothelial cells connected by tight junctions with extremely high electrical resistance and is highly selective in separating the circulating blood from the brain extracellular fluid. The outermost layer of the BBB at all levels of the vasculature, including capillaries comprises of astrocyte end-feet,[8] a domain that is enriched in transporters and channels involved with brain interstitial fluid (ISF) homoeostasis.[9] This barrier allows passive diffusion as well as selective transport of glucose and amino acids, and prevents entry of potential neurotoxins by active transport. The BBB is present along all capillaries in the brain, except in locations such as the roof of the third and fourth ventricle, and the pineal gland.

Disruption of BBB occurs in various neurological disorders, and is crucial in the development of vasogenic cerebral oedema.

A major receptor of vascular endothelial growth factor (VEGF) VEGFR2, is an important mediator of vascular permeability. It is overexpressed in endothelial cells, astrocytes, neuronal stomata, and processes adjacent to the damage after brain injury.[10] Studies demonstrate that VEGFR2 increases with increasing BBB permeability during the acute phase of cerebral oedema induced by various injuries.[10,11]

TYPES OF CEREBRAL OEDEMA

Cerebral oedema can be classified based on pathological processes contributing to oedema formation. The different types of cerebral oedema are summarized in Table 26.1.

Table 26.1 Classification of cerebral oedema

Pathophysiological classification
• Cytotoxic cerebral oedema (ionic oedema, cellular oedema, oncosis, necrotic volume increase)

• Vasogenic cerebral oedema
  – Cerebral tumour associated cerebral oedema
  – Hydrostatic cerebral oedema
  – High altitude cerebral oedema (HACE)

• Hydrocephalic (interstitial) cerebral oedema
• Global cerebral oedema (aneurysmal subarachnoid haemorrhage)
Anatomic classification
• Focal/localized cerebral oedema
• Global cerebral oedema

Cytotoxic Cerebral Oedema

Cytotoxic oedema is also referred to as 'ischaemic oedema' or 'cellular oedema'. It typically involves the grey and white matter, and pathophysiologically the BBB is intact. Cytotoxic oedema is seen in ischaemic or hypoxic brain injury, water intoxication, and Reye's syndrome. It does not involve the addition of new water mass to the brain as it simply represents a rearrangement of parenchymal water mass. It is an important initial step in the formation of cerebral oedema and swelling, as it generates the driving force for influx of ionic and vasogenic oedema, which do cause swelling.[9]

In normal physiological conditions, cellular influx of osmolites may occur due to primary active transport or secondary active transport. Primary active transport requires a continuous supply of ATP to provide energy for 'pumps' such as the Na^+/K^+-ATPase and Ca^{2+}-ATPase. Secondary active transport harnesses the potential energy stored in transmembrane ionic gradients previously generated through primary active transport. Examples of secondary active transporters include ion channels and co-transporters such as the $Na^+/K^+/Cl^-$ co-transporter (NKCC1) and the Na^+/Ca^{2+} exchanger. Following many types of central nervous system (CNS) injury, intracellular ATP becomes depleted and thus, mechanisms that are independent of intracellular ATP, like secondary active transport, are more likely to be relevant for the formation of ionic oedema.[9]

Ischaemic injury disrupts energy-dependent intracellular pumps such as selective and non-selective channels. Of the selective channels, sodium-potassium ATP pump is affected due to ischaemic injury leading to influx of sodium and water, which gives rise to intracellular oedema. Cellular swelling has been demonstrated to occur within 30 minutes after experimental middle cerebral artery occlusion, and is shown to persist for up to 24 hours after reperfusion.[12]

Due to their involvement in potassium and glutamate clearance, astrocytes are more prone to swelling than the neurons. Aquaporin-4 and AQP-8 are also thought to play roles in the pathophysiology of cytotoxic cerebral oedema.[6,13] After focal brain ischaemia, AQP4 is observed to lose polarized localization to astrocytic end-feet, which is associated with the loss of the astrocyte end-foot anchorage protein β-dystroglycan (DG). Furthermore, agrin-deficient mice lack polarized localization of both β-DG and AQP4 at astrocytic end-feet and do not develop cytotoxic oedema after ischaemia.[14]

Non-selective channels implicated in cytotoxic oedema typically affect the penumbra of the ischaemic core. These include acid-sensing ion channel (ASIC), sulphonylurea receptor 1 (SUR1), regulated non-selective cation (NC) (Ca-ATP) channel, transient receptor potential (TRP) channel, NKCC channel, N-methyl-D-aspartate (NMDA) receptor channel, and the AQP channel.[15]

Vasogenic Cerebral Oedema

Vasogenic cerebral oedema occurs primarily due to increased permeability of the BBB, and is typically extracellular involving mostly white matter.

As the transendothelial permeability increases, extravasation of water and plasma proteins such as albumin and IgG into the brain interstitial compartment occurs. Unlike haemorrhage, capillary structural integrity is maintained during vasogenic oedema such that the passage of erythrocytes is prohibited. Therefore, vasogenic oedema is best viewed as a cell-free blood ultra-filtrate, i.e., plasma.[16,17]

The BBB disruption has been implicated in a variety of different neurological emergencies, arterial hypertension, trauma, brain tumours, and inflammatory conditions such as meningitis or brain abscess, intracerebral haemorrhage, and may also confound cytotoxic oedema in acute ischaemic stroke.[12] This type of oedema has usually been seen in the late stages of cerebral ischaemia, further inducing focal CBF reduction, cell necrosis, and apoptosis.[18]

Peritumoural vasogenic oedema as seen in patients with meningioma is thought to depend on AQP4 expression and this expression seems independent of grade of tumour, tumour volume, or cell count.[19] While, in patients with glioma, AQP4 expression is higher than normal brain tissue, and the associated cerebral oedema is thought to be affected by osmotic pressure and hypoxia, with expression proportional to the grade of glioma.[18,20]

Cellular mechanisms implicated in the development of vasogenic cerebral oedema include disruption of calcium signaling, actin-polymerization dependent endothelial cell rounding, uncoupling of tight junctions, and enzymatic degradation of the basement membrane.[12]

The role of vascular endothelial growth factor (VEGF) in vasogenic cerebral oedema has received significant attention in the last decade. Reportedly 1000 times as potent as histamine, VEGF has been implicated in tumourigenesis and neovascularization.[21] Upregulation of VEGF increases vascular permeability promoting oedema formation.[12]

Vascular endothelial growth factor has been the target of therapies aimed at reduction of reperfusion injury.[22]

Several other metabolites implicated in cerebral tumour associated cerebral oedema include arachidonic acid metabolites, nitric oxide, leukotriene C4, serotonin, thromboxanes, and platelet-activation factor.[21]

Subtypes of vasogenic cerebral oedema include hydrostatic cerebral oedema seen in malignant hypertension and high altitude cerebral oedema (HACE).

Hydrocephalic (Interstitial) Cerebral Oedema

This type occurs in obstructive hydrocephalus, and is due to transependymal flow of cerebrospinal fluid (CSF) causing CSF to penetrate the brain. Here the CSF contains no protein, as opposed to vasogenic oedema, which is rich in proteins. Transependymal oedema describes an increase in periventricular interstitial fluid due to a failure of the ependymal lining of the ventricular wall, common in obstructive or communicating hydrocephalus.[23]

GLOBAL CEREBRAL OEDEMA IN PATIENTS WITH SUBARACHNOID HAEMORRHAGE

It has been postulated that subarachnoid haemorrhage (SAH) causes transient global ischaemia, which causes cell membrane dysfunction, contributing to cytotoxic oedema, as well as apoptotic breakdown of BBB leading to vasogenic oedema, thus causing global cerebral oedema (GCE). Delayed GCE has been associated with the use of vasopressors to augment cerebral perfusion pressure in the face of vasospasm.[24] Research on SAH patients shows that AQP4 is up-regulated in astrocytic processes with loss of polarization[25] and an increase in AQP4 levels is observed as early as 6 hours after SAH and sustained for 72 hours when observed in animal models.[26]

Factors associated with GCE after SAH include loss of consciousness at the ictus and a high Hunt and Hess score.[27] Delayed GCE was predicted by aneurysm size greater than 10 mm, loss of consciousness at the ictus and increased SAH sum scores.[27]

CEREBRAL OEDEMA IN COMMONLY ENCOUNTERED NEUROLOGICAL EMERGENCIES
Cerebral Oedema in Ischaemic Stroke

Ischaemic stroke is complicated by cerebral oedema, as the necrotic brain tissue at the stroke core undergoes cellular oedema. Ischaemic cerebrovascular disease is mainly caused by thrombosis, embolism, and focal hypoperfusion, all of which can lead to a reduction or interruption in CBF that affects neurological function. Ischaemic brain oedema is initially cytotoxic because of disturbances in cell membrane followed by vasogenic oedema which sets in due to the increased permeability of the BBB.[28]

Pathologic Basis

In stroke, the molecular cascade initiated by cerebral ischaemia includes the loss of membrane ionic pumps and cell swelling. Secondary formation of free radicals and proteases disrupts brain-cell membranes causing irreversible damage.[29]

Due to loss of membrane transporters, there is an influx of sodium and water into the necrotic cell causing cytotoxic oedema. Confounding this may be the disruption of the BBB and vasogenic oedema.[12] Cerebral oedema usually begins to develop soon after the onset of ischaemia and peaks at 24–96 hours. Usually this is confined to the ischaemic region and does not appreciably affect the adjacent brain. But when it progresses, it compresses brain regions adjacent to the ischaemic zone causing neurological worsening.[30]

Malignant cerebral and cerebellar oedema contribute to high stroke related mortality.

Cerebral Oedema in Traumatic Brain Injury

Contusional necrosis associated changes in osmolality of the contused brain attract water, and may contribute to the development of cerebral oedema in patients with TBI.[28]

A biphasic profile encompassing both vasogenic and cytotoxic components has emerged. With the aid of novel magnetic resonance imaging (MRI) techniques, vasogenic oedema as indicated by increased water diffusion distance has been demonstrated to occur in the first few hours after TBI followed by cytotoxic oedema that developed more slowly over the next few days and persisted up to a few weeks.[31]

CLINICAL MANIFESTATIONS OF CEREBRAL OEDEMA

Cerebral oedema manifests clinically due to in part by its influential relationship on intracranial volume, and disruption of the equilibrium between brain parenchymal CSF and cerebral blood volume. Expansion of brain parenchymal volume seen in ischaemic, haemorrhagic stroke, brain tumours, and inflammatory conditions causes an increase in compartmental pressure, thus affecting the level of consciousness.

In the supratentorial compartment this is often manifested by sudden or gradual progressive decline in the level of consciousness, headache, nausea, and non-projectile vomiting. Focal motor and sensory deficits are often correlated to the size of cerebral oedema in addition to the primary pathology.

In the infratentorial compartment, symptoms may rather be abrupt and commonly involve loss of consciousness.

Malignant cerebral oedema is reserved for severe cerebral oedema that leads to intracranial hypertension (ICH), causing significantly high mortality and morbidity despite aggressive medical and surgical treatment.

DIAGNOSTIC TESTS FOR CEREBRAL OEDEMA

While the CT scan is an extremely sensitive test to recognize intracranial haemorrhage, the diagnosis of cytotoxic oedema after acute ischaemic stroke is typically visible 12–24 hours after stroke onset (Figures 26.1 and 26.2).

T2 weighted abnormalities are more sensitive and visible within a few hours on MRI using fluid attenuated inversion recuperation (FLAIR) sequences (Figures 26.3, 26.4, and 26.5). Although the exact mechanism of diffusion restriction is largely unknown, it is thought to indicate cytotoxic cerebral oedema and may supersede T2 changes.[32]

Perihaematomal oedema seen in patients with intracerebral haemorrhage suggesting iron content are seen as T2 hypo-intensity on MRI.[33]

Computed tomography (CT) and MRI scans often reveal complications associated with cerebral oedema, such as midline shift of the septum pellucidum and pineal gland, effacement of cisterns, and hydrocephalus. Ischaemic areas secondary to compression of anterior or posterior cerebral arteries may be visible on CT or MRI.

Basic differences between cytotoxic and vasogenic cerebral oedema on CT and MRI imaging are summarized in Table 26.2.

TARGETED THERAPIES FOR MANAGEMENT OF CEREBRAL OEDEMA

Therapies aimed at creation of an osmotic gradient between the intracellular and extracellular compartments facilitate removal of water from the intracellular space or maintain sodium in the extracellular space. Osmotherapy is a commonly used adjuvant therapy in clinical patients with cerebral oedema. Osmotic dehydrating agents including mannitol and hypertonic saline (HTS) are widely used to relieve cerebral oedema.[34]

These therapies form the cornerstone of management of cerebral oedema across various grades of severity. The choice of one form of therapy, e.g., mannitol versus HTS, is in part dependent upon availability, understanding,

Table 26.2 Imaging characteristics of cerebral oedema

	Cytotoxic oedema	Vasogenic oedema
CT scan		
Involvement	Grey and white matter	White matter (finger-like projections)
Grey–white matter differentiation	Disrupted	Maintained
MRI		
Abnormality	No T1 or T2 changes	T1 hypointense and T2 hyperintense FLAIR signals
Diffusion	Restriction	No restriction

severity of illness, contraindications, and availability of central venous access.

There are two main groups of agents used in treatment of cerebral oedema, as the next two sections detail.

Osmotic Diuretics

Mannitol has been prescribed for treatment of cerebral oedema and ICH for many decades. An osmotic diuretic, mannitol, a polyol (sugar alcohol) exerts its effect via two mechanisms. Mannitol establishes an osmotic gradient between plasma and the brain, thus drawing water from the extracellular space into the vascular compartment. This causes an increase in CBF, a decrease in blood viscosity, improvement in cerebral oxygenation and decrease in ICP. Due its lower molecular weight of 182, it is freely filtered through the renal tubules accounting for its diuretic action. It also acts as a free radical scavenger. Mannitol cannot cross the BBB and an intact BBB is a prerequisite for mannitol's osmotic action.

The ICP effect of mannitol is dose-dependent with higher doses providing more lasting reduction in ICP. Intracranial pressure changes peak at 30–45 minutes after mannitol infusion and lasts for around six hours. The diuretic effect peaks at around 60–90 minutes, and isotonic fluid administration is warranted to maintain euvolemia. Mannitol is available for clinical use as a sterile solution of 10% and 20% in a 500 ml pre-mixed solution in water containing 50 and 100 g of mannitol, respectively. Current recommendations suggest 0.25–1 gm/kg mannitol to be given by intravenous (IV) infusion over 20–30 min.[35] Administration of mannitol requires an in-line filter, and is prone to precipitation due to crystal formation, and may require warming to dissolve crystals before administration.

Repeated usage leads to decreased efficacy of the drug due to constant accumulation of mannitol in the injured brain leading to the osmotic pressure gradient inside and outside the BBB to be reversed, thus exacerbating cerebral oedema.[36–39] Animal studies with 20% mannitol show that its intracellular accumulation is most pronounced at 18 hours.[40]

If repeat dosing of mannitol is prescribed, it is prudent to trend osmolar gap (measured osmolality – calculated osmolality) every 4–6 hours and safe continuation is warranted if the osmolar gap is kept under 20 mOsm/kg. For patients with osmolar gap greater than 20 mOsm/kg, reduction in dose and frequency of mannitol or switching to HTS is recommended. If mannitol is used in situations of BBB breakdown, 'rebound' cerebral oedema can ensue due to accumulation of mannitol in the brain parenchyma. Other side effects of mannitol include volume overload, coagulopathy, and electrolyte abnormalities, particularly hypernatraemia and hyperchloremic metabolic acidosis, and delayed hypovolaemia secondary to its diuretic effect. Caution must be exerted in patients with compensated congestive heart failure, as these patients may not tolerate mannitol well, and may need administration of a diuretic such as furosemide to augment the effect of mannitol.

Extravasation of mannitol can cause immediate pain, erythema and swelling, skin and subcutaneous ulceration, and subfascial extravasation can lead to compartment syndrome.

A 2007 Cochrane collaboration review concluded that the use of mannitol is effective in reversing acute brain swelling[41] and is the mainstay of initial cerebral oedema treatment.

Hypertonic Saline

Hypertonic saline is an alternative for management of cerebral oedema and based on current evidence has evolved to become the drug of choice in the management of cerebral herniation.[42] Hypertonic saline for clinical use are of varied concentrations. A concentration of 2% or 3% saline is usually used for continuous infusion and 23.4% reserved for bolus administration. Use of 23.4% HTS in the treatment of ICH is safe and feasible.[42] Typically administered as an IV push over 10–15 minutes, it requires a dedicated central venous access catheter. It is a hyperosmolar solution (7987 mOsm/L) which contributes to reduction in the brain water content by its osmotic effects. Hypertonic saline increases rheological properties of blood by reducing blood viscosity leading to an improvement in CBF and cerebral oxygenation.

This causes autoregulatory vasoconstriction, thereby reducing ICP. The improvement in circulation seen during HTS use is also due to arteriolar smooth muscle relaxation. A variety of other beneficial effects of HTS therapy include its vasoregulatory, immunomodulatory, and neurochemical effects,[39] and its role in reduction of CSF production.

Hypertonic saline removes free water from the intracellular to the extracellular space by establishing an osmotic pressure gradient and lowering the peripheral vascular resistance.[38] It reduces cerebral oedema by many non-osmotic molecular mechanisms. It down-regulates the expression of AQP4 in astrocytes in peri-ischaemic hemispheric tissue thus decreasing cerebral oedema[40] and has also been shown to have neuroprotective effects by preventing neuronal apoptosis.

Cerebral oedema affected regions commonly show an increase in Na^+ ions.[43] In ischaemic cerebral tissue, the NKCC1 activation plays an important role in increasing the concentration of Na^+ ions.[44–46]

The VEGF effects on the BBB junction are VEGFR2-dependent. In the acute phase of cerebral oedema, increase in VEGFR2 increases the BBB permeability and the inhibition of VEGF–VEGFR2 axis leads to a reduction of cerebral oedema.[10,11,47]

In animal studies it has been suggested that HTS alleviates cerebral oedema through inhibition of the NKCC1 co-transporter, which is mediated by attenuation of TNF-alpha and IL-beta stimulation on NKCC1,[48] and possibly downregulation of AQP4.[49] After a cardiac arrest, the use of 7.5% saline for resuscitation was shown to ameliorate cerebral oedema via the perivascular AQP4 pool attenuating the BBB.[50]

Animal studies have shown an increase in the expression of VEGF, VEGFR2 mRNA and protein 6 hours after middle cerebral artery occlusion (MCAO) peaking at 12 hours. When compared with the ischaemia group, groups given 10% HTS demonstrated lower VEGF, VEGFR2 mRNA, and protein expression correlating with reduced BBB permeability. Zonula occludens (ZO)-1 and claudin-5 are the main components of the tight junction protecting the integrity of VEGF that could down-regulate ZO-1, and claudin-5 leading to the disruption of BBB. This study also showed that HTS could reduce cerebral oedema via inhibition of VEGF and VEGFR2-mediated tight junction disruption.[51]

Animal data also suggests that 10% HTS is more effective in alleviating cerebral oedema than an equal volume of 20% mannitol as it establishes a higher osmotic gradient across the BBB.[52] In both paediatric and adult TBI, HTS has been used effectively to reduce elevated ICP

which is refractory to mannitol administration. Clinically, hypertonic is used either as a bolus or continuous infusion. In the latter, the solution is used to target a sodium between 145–155 mEq/L.[53] While there are no systematic studies regarding optimal sodium targets in patients with cerebral oedema,[54] HTS 23.4% has been safely used to reverse transtentorial herniation in patients with renal failure.[55]

Steroids

Steroids, especially dexamethasone has been the cornerstone therapy for brain tumour-related oedema for both glial and non-glial tumours. It is thought to reduce expression of VEGF and interfered with its interaction with target endothelial cells.[21]

In patients with cerebral metastases, approximately 70% of patients symptomatically improve after starting steroids. Dexamethasone is the drug of choice as it has a long half-life, low mineralocorticoid activity, and a relatively low tendency to induce psychosis.[56] Brain tumour related oedema results from opening of the interendothelial tight junctions, an increased permeability of the BBB leading to the flow of fluid into the extracellular space of the brain[57] and also due to increased endothelial pinocytosis and endothelial fenestrations.[58]

Studies show that corticosteroids produce their anti-oedema effect by reducing the permeability of tumour capillaries.[58–60] Corticosteroids decrease endothelial permeability by directly transcripting genes and mediating nontranscriptional regulation of other signaling cascades and upregulating of the tight junction components in endothelial cells[61] and partly by causing dephosphorylation of occludin and another tight junction component, ZO-1.[58]

Other mechanisms by which corticosteroids contribute to the reduction in oedema are by inducing repression of nuclear factor (NF)-κB causing inhibition of cytokine-induced barrier breakdown and expression of cell adhesion molecules[62] and by decreasing the capillary permeability by nontranscriptional regulation mechanisms that involve rearrangement and tight binding of vascular endothelial (V_E)-cadherin to the cytoskeleton.[63]

Initial reduction of intracranial pressure occurs within 24 hours, but consistent reduction is noted 2–4 days after initial dosing.[64,65] Administration of steroids 1–2 days prior to an elective surgical procedure has the potential to reduce oedema formation and improve clinical condition by the time of craniotomy.[66]

Recommendation for patients with symptomatic metastatic brain disease suggests initiation of dexamethasone at a dose of 4–8 mg/24 hours. If patients exhibit severe symptoms consistent with increased ICP, then higher doses such as ≥16 mg/24 hours should be considered.

Steroid use can lead to an array of serious side effects depending on the dosage and duration of use. Among the common side effects of steroids, gastrointestinal complications, steroid myopathy, *Pneumocystis jerovecii* pneumonitis (PJP) and osteoporosis are of concern in brain tumour patients. Most complications resolve after cessation of steroid use, but some side effects may persist such as osteoporosis and cataract formation.

PRECLINICAL DATA ON THERAPEUTIC STRATEGIES IN THE MANAGEMENT OF CEREBRAL OEDEMA

The non-selective channels offer promising therapeutic interventions. Acid-sensing ion channel has been a target of amiloride and tarantula toxin. Glibenclamide has been studied in vitro and in vivo rat models for ischaemic stroke targeting the SUR-1-regulated NC channel, and has shown to reduce oncotic cell death.[48] Capsaicin and rimonabant have shown promising neuroprotective effects that are in part due to their effect on transient receptor potential cation channel subfamily V member 1 (TRPV1) channel.[67,68] Bumetanide administered via microdialysis reduced brain oedema in the rat focal ischaemic model targeting the NKCC channel.[69]

Aquaporin-targetted inhibitors have emerged in preclinical models as novel therapies to reduce cerebral oedema.[70]

Levetiracetam in a percussion model of TBI has been shown to down-regulate AQP4 and AQP4 m-RNA expression leading to reduction in brain water content and brain oedema.[71] Oestrogen or progesterone via their alteration of AQP4 and interleukin (IL)-6 have shown to reduce brain oedema in TBI animal model.[72] Subarachnoid haemorrhage associated increase in expression of AQP4 in rat brain SAH model was shown to be inhibited by propofol.[73] Curcumin has been shown to attenuate brain oedema at 3 days' post ICH in mice model via inhibition of the AQP4 and AQP9 expression.[74]

Bevacizumab is a humanized monoclonal IgG1 antibody that binds to and inhibits the biological activity of human VEGF temporarily to normalize tumour vessels, improving the delivery of cytotoxic drugs and oxygen to the tumour, and enhancing the efficacy of chemotherapy and radiation.[75] It is the first antiangiogenic therapy that has been approved by the Food and Drug Administration (FDA) for treatment of recurrent glioblastoma.[76]

EMERGING THERAPEUTICS IN THE MANAGEMENT OF CEREBRAL OEDEMA

In a recently published randomized, double-blind, placebo-controlled phase 2 trial, Glyburide Advantage in Malignant Edema and Stroke (GAMES); Sheth et al.[77] demonstrated safety of IV glyburide in patients with large hemispheric stroke at risk for cerebral oedema. The study was stopped due to funding reasons after enrollment of 86 patients (41, drug-arm, 36, placebo-arm) and failed to achieve any primary or secondary endpoints, which were modified Rankin Score (mRS) at 90 days, and decompressive craniectomy or death by day 14, change in ipsilateral hemispheric swelling, and change in lesional swelling at 72–96 hours. There was reduction in midline shift of the brain from baseline to 72–96 hours, 30-day all-cause mortality, and less change in ipsilateral hemispheric swelling for patients without decompressive craniectomy. Reduction in levels of matrix metalloproteinase 9 (MMP-9) were observed in patients exposed to IV glyburide.[77]

NEUROSURGICAL INTERVENTIONS FOR CEREBRAL OEDEMA

Severe and overwhelming cerebral oedema can be accommodated within the intracranial vault by means of decompressive craniectomy. This allows accommodation of a median increase in intracranial volume of 75 cu. cm.

Decompressive Craniectomy for Focal Cerebral Oedema

This can be accomplished by either a hemispheric craniectomy commonly utilized in malignant middle cerebral artery strokes and posterior fossa decompressive craniectomy for cerebellar stroke with hydrocephalus and ICH.

Targeted localized craniectomy is also employed for cerebral oedema due to cerebral venous sinus thrombosis.

Multiple randomized control trials such as DECIMAL,[78] DESTINY I,[79] DESTINY II,[80] HAMLET,[81] and HeaDDFIRST[82] demonstrated that timely performance of decompressive hemicraniectomy in selected patients with 'malignant' ischaemic middle cerebral artery stroke can improve mortality and preserve functional outcome. Mortality related to surgical intervention is 20%, compared to 80% with medical management alone. The number needed to treat to prevent death is 4.

Lack of reliability in prediction of patients at high risk, lack of prompt neurosurgical referral, and historical provider, and institutional bias towards not performing decompressive craniectomy, along with a strong selection bias towards right hemispheric ischaemic stroke are barriers towards a standardized approach.

Decompressive Craniectomy in Traumatic Brain Injury

A recently published randomized control trial (Randomized Evaluation of Surgery with Craniectomy for Uncontrollable Elevation of Intracranial Pressure [RESCUEicp]) using decompressive craniectomy in patients with refractory ICH following TBI concluded that at six months while there was lower mortality in recipients of decompressive craniectomy, there were higher rates of vegetative state, lower severe disability, and higher upper severity compared to medical care.[83]

MEDICAL MANAGEMENT OF CEREBRAL OEDEMA

As cerebral oedema is a significant predictor of treatment outcome, it is important for timely and effective strategies to prevent life-threatening formation of cerebral hernia. General measures include avoidance of agitation, pain, fever and shivering, maintenance of euvolemia, euglycaemia and facilitation of venous outflow (head-of-bed elevation to 30–45 degrees). Maintenance of cerebral perfusion pressure is paramount to maintain cerebral blood flow and avoidance of hypoxia, hypercapnia, hyponatraemia, hyperventilation, and maintaining $PaCO_2$ at 25–30 mmHg.[84]

PRACTICAL PEARLS IN THE MANAGEMENT OF CEREBRAL OEDEMA

Since cerebral and resultant ICH can be potentially life-threatening, prompt recognition and assessment of patients at high risk is warranted. A concerted effort including agreement on sodium, PCO_2,[2] mean arterial pressure (MAP), and CPP targets and a streamlined approach to clinical management response to declining neurological examination in the setting of worsening ICH cannot be overemphasized.

Table 26.3 highlights the basic and advanced strategies that can be utilized in the management of patients with cerebral oedema.

CONCLUSIONS

Cerebral oedema is frequently encountered in the neurocritical care unit and is a significant cause of morbidity and death. Timely and effective treatment is required to prevent complications related to cerebral

Table 26.3 Management of cerebral oedema

Diagnostic and management strategies
BASIC
Surveillance
• Serial GCS or FOUR score measurements (every 1 hour)
• Pupillary reactivity, pupilometer trending (NPI and constriction velocity) every 1 hour
• Serial CT imaging to trend midline shift, cisternal effacement
Medical Management
• Head of bed elevation 30–45 degrees
• Isotonic fluids, avoid dextrose containing solutions
• Maintain CPP 60–80 mmHg
• Prevent and treat hypoxia (SpO_2 goal >90%)
• Prevent and treat hyponatraemia (sodium >135 mEq/L)
• Treat pain, agitation, and distress
• Normothermia protocol
• Steroids for vasogenic cerebral oedema associated with brain tumours
ADVANCED *In addition to the above measures*
Surveillance
• Frequent sodium checks (every 4–6 hours)
• Frequent serum osmolality checks (every 6 hours)
Medical Management
• Secure airway
• Hyperventilation to PCO_2 30–35 mmHg
• 2% or 3% saline/acetate infusion (target sodium 140–155 mEq/L)
• Mannitol 0.5–1 gm/kg
• External CSF drainage
• 23.4% saline bolus (30–50 ml)
• Propofol bolus + infusion (200 mcg/kg/min)
• CPP manipulation
• Barbiturate coma
• Hypothermia (32–34°C)
Surgical management
• Decompression
• Mass evacuation

Abbreviations: GCS: Glasgow Coma Scale; NPI: Neurological pupil index; CT: computed tomography; CPP: continuous partial pressure; SpO_2: peripheral capillary oxygen saturation; CSF: cerebrospinal fluid; PCO_2: partial pressure of carbon dioxide.

oedema. Thus, a multimodal and algorithmic approach is needed in the clinical management of cerebral oedema. The study of the pathophysiology of cerebral oedema is significantly important as this has led to several discoveries that directly impact its treatment. Apart from the number of standard therapies commonly used, understanding the basic physiology of cerebral oedema has led to the identification of novel therapies targeting specific channels. Several studies have also highlighted the importance of neurosurgical intervention in selected cases to improve mortality and preserve functional outcome. More investigative studies are necessary to further develop targeted therapies for cerebral oedema.

REFERENCES

1. Tang G, Yang GY. Aquaporin-4. A potential therapeutic target for cerebral edema. *Int J Mol Sci* 2016;17(10). pii: E1413.

2. Manz HJ. The pathology of cerebral edema. *Hum Pathol* 1974;5(3):291–313.

3. Nakayama S, Amiry-Moghaddam M, Ottersen OP, Bhardwaj A. Conivaptan, a selective arginine vasopressin V1a and V2 Receptor antagonist attenuates global cerebral edema following experimental cardiac arrest via perivascular pool of aquaporin-4. *Neurocrit Care* 2016;24(2):273–82.

4. Rash JE, Yasumura T, Hudson CS, Agre P, Nielsen S. Direct immunogold labeling of aquaporin-4 in square arrays of astrocyte and ependymocyte plasma membranes in rat brain and spinal cord. *Proc Natl Acad Sci USA* 1998;95(20):11981–6.

5. Rao KV, Reddy PV, Curtis KM, Norenberg MD. Aquaporin-4 expression in cultured astrocytes after fluid percussion injury. *J Neurotrauma* 2011;28(3):371–81.

6. Manley GT, Fujimura M, Ma T, et al. Aquaporin-4 deletion in mice reduces brain edema after acute water intoxication and ischemic stroke. *Nat Med* 2000;6(2):159–63.

7. Thrane AS, Rappold PM, Fujita T, et al. Critical role of aquaporin-4 (AQP4) in astrocytic Ca2+ signaling events elicited by cerebral edema. *Proc Natl Acad Sci USA* 2011;108(2):846–51.

8. Bushong EA, Martone ME, Jones YZ, Ellisman MH. Protoplasmic astrocytes in CA1 stratum radiatum occupy separate anatomical domains. *J Neurosci* 2002;22(1):183–92.

9. Stokum JA, Gerzanich V, Simard JM. Molecular pathophysiology of cerebral edema. *J Cereb Blood Flow Metab* 2016;36(3):513–38.

10. Skold MK, von Gertten C, Sandberg-Nordqvist AC, Mathiesen T, Holmin S. VEGF and VEGF receptor expression after experimental brain contusion in rat. *J Neurotrauma* 2005;22(3):353–67.

11. Lennmyr F, Ata KA, Funa K, Olsson Y, Terent A. Expression of vascular endothelial growth factor (VEGF) and its receptors (Flt-1 and Flk-1) following permanent and transient occlusion of the middle cerebral artery in the rat. *J Neuropathol Exp Neurol* 1998;57(9):874–82.

12. Simard JM, Kent TA, Chen M, Tarasov KV, Gerzanich V. Brain oedema in focal ischaemia: molecular pathophysiology and theoretical implications. *Lancet Neurol* 2007;6(3):258–68.

13. Maugeri R, Schiera G, Di Liegro CM, Fricano A, Iacopino DG, Di Liegro I. Aquaporins and brain tumors. *Int J Mol Sci* 2016;17(7):E1029.

14. Steiner E, Enzmann GU, Lin S, et al. Loss of astrocyte polarization upon transient focal brain ischemia as a possible mechanism to counteract early edema formation. *Glia* 2012;60(11):1646–59.

15. Liang D, Bhatta S, Gerzanich V, Simard JM. Cytotoxic edema: mechanisms of pathological cell swelling. *Neurosurg Focus* 2007;22(5):E2.

16. Klatzo I. Presidential address. Neuropathological aspects of brain edema. *J Neuropathol Exp Neurol* 1967;26(1):1–14.

17. Vorbrodt AW, Lossinsky AS, Wisniewski HM, et al. Ultrastructural observations on the transvascular route of protein removal in vasogenic brain edema. *Acta Neuropathol* 1985;66(4):265–73.

18. Liu Y, Tang GH, Sun YH, et al. The protective role of Tongxinluo on blood-brain barrier after ischemia-reperfusion brain injury. *J Ethnopharmacol* 2013;148(2):632–9.

19. Gawlitza M, Fiedler E, Schob S, Hoffmann KT, Surov A. Peritumoral brain edema in meningiomas depends on aquaporin-4 expression and not on tumor grade, tumor volume, cell count, or Ki-67 labeling index. *Mol Imaging Biol* 2017;19(2):298–304.

20. Mou K, Chen M, Mao Q, et al. AQP-4 in peritumoral edematous tissue is correlated with the degree of glioma and with expression of VEGF and HIF-alpha. *J Neurooncol* 2010;100(3):375–83.

21. Stummer W. Mechanisms of tumor-related brain edema. *Neurosurg Focus* 2007;22(5):E8.

22. Guo H, Zhou H, Lu J, Qu Y, Yu D, Tong Y. Vascular endothelial growth factor: an attractive target in the treatment of hypoxic/ischemic brain injury. *Neural Regen Res* 2016;11(1):174–9.

23. Donkin JJ, Vink R. Mechanisms of cerebral edema in traumatic brain injury: therapeutic developments. *Curr Opin Neurol* 2010;23(3):293–9.

24. Mocco J, Prickett CS, Komotar RJ, Connolly ES, Mayer SA. Potential mechanisms and clinical significance of global cerebral edema following aneurysmal subarachnoid hemorrhage. *Neurosurg Focus* 2007;22(5):E7.

25. Badaut J, Brunet JF, Grollimund L, et al. Aquaporin 1 and aquaporin 4 expression in human brain after subarachnoid hemorrhage and in peritumoral tissue. *Acta Neurochir Suppl* 2003;86:495–8.

26. Cao S, Zhu P, Yu X, et al. Hydrogen sulfide attenuates brain edema in early brain injury after subarachnoid hemorrhage in rats: Possible involvement of MMP-9 induced blood-brain barrier disruption and AQP4 expression. *Neurosci Lett* 2016;621:88–97.

27. Claassen J, Carhuapoma JR, Kreiter KT, Du EY, Connolly ES, Mayer SA. Global cerebral edema after subarachnoid hemorrhage: frequency, predictors, and impact on outcome. *Stroke* 2002;33(5):1225–32.

28. Kawamata T, Mori T, Sato S, Katayama Y. Tissue hyperosmolality and brain edema in cerebral contusion. *Neurosurg Focus* 2007;22(5):E5.

29. Rosenberg GA. Ischemic brain edema. Prog Cardiovasc Dis. 1999;42(3):209–16.

30. Jha SK. Cerebral edema and its management. *Med J Armed Forces India* 2003;59(4):326–31.

31. Barzo P, Marmarou A, Fatouros P, Hayasaki K, Corwin F. Contribution of vasogenic and cellular edema to traumatic brain swelling measured by diffusion-weighted imaging. *J Neurosurg* 1997;87(6):900–7.

32. Forbes KP, Pipe JG, Heiserman JE. Evidence for cytotoxic edema in the pathogenesis of cerebral venous infarction. *AJNR Am J Neuroradiol* 2001;22(3):450–5.

33. Lou M, Lieb K, Selim M. The relationship between hematoma iron content and perihematoma edema: an MRI study. *Cerebrovasc Dis* 2009;27(3):266–71.

34. Ziai WC, Toung TJ, Bhardwaj A. Hypertonic saline: first-line therapy for cerebral edema? *J Neurol Sci* 2007;261(1-2):157–66.

35. Bhardwaj A. Osmotherapy in neurocritical care. *Curr Neurol Neurosci Rep* 2007;7(6):513–21.

36. Kaufmann AM, Cardoso ER. Aggravation of vasogenic cerebral edema by multiple-dose mannitol. *J Neurosurg* 1992;77(4):584–9.

37. Cho J, Kim YH, Han HS, Park J. Accumulated mannitol and aggravated cerebral edema in a rat model of middle cerebral artery infarction. *J Korean Neurosurg Soc* 2007; 42(4):337–41.

38. Nout YS, Mihai G, Tovar CA, Schmalbrock P, Bresnahan JC, Beattie MS. Hypertonic saline attenuates cord swelling and edema in experimental spinal cord injury: a study utilizing magnetic resonance imaging. *Crit Care Med* 2009;37(7):2160–6.

39. White H, Cook D, Venkatesh B. The use of hypertonic saline for treating intracranial hypertension after traumatic brain injury. *Anesth Analg* 2006;102(6):1836–46.

40. Zeng HK, Wang QS, Deng YY, Jiang WQ, Fang M, Chen CB, Jiang X. A comparative study on the efficacy of 10% hypertonic saline and equal volume of 20% mannitol in the treatment of experimentally induced cerebral edema in adult rats. *BMC Neurosci* 2010 Dec 10;11:153.

41. Wakai A, Roberts I, Schierhout G. Mannitol for acute traumatic brain injury. *Cochrane Database Syst Rev* 2007(1):CD001049.

42. Koenig MA, Bryan M, Lewin JL, 3rd, Mirski MA, Geocadin RG, Stevens RD. Reversal of transtentorial herniation with hypertonic saline. *Neurology* 2008;70(13):1023–9.

43. Lo WD, Betz AL, Schielke GP, Hoff JT. Transport of sodium from blood to brain in ischemic brain edema. *Stroke* 1987;18(1):150–7.

44. Foroutan S, Brillault J, Forbush B, O'Donnell ME. Moderate-to-severe ischemic conditions increase activity and phosphorylation of the cerebral microvascular endothelial cell Na+-K+-Cl- cotransporter. *Am J Physiol Cell Physiol* 2005;289(6):C1492–501.

45. Chen H, Luo J, Kintner DB, Shull GE, Sun D. Na(+)-dependent chloride transporter (NKCC1)-null mice exhibit less gray and white matter damage after focal cerebral ischemia. *J Cereb Blood Flow Metab* 2005;25(1):54–66.

46. Simard JM, Kahle KT, Gerzanich V. Molecular mechanisms of microvascular failure in central nervous system injury–synergistic roles of NKCC1 and SUR1/TRPM4. *J Neurosurg* 2010;113(3):622–9.

47. Vohra PK, Hoeppner LH, Sagar G, et al. Dopamine inhibits pulmonary edema through the VEGF-VEGFR2 axis in a murine model of acute lung injury. *Am J Physiol Lung Cell Mol Physiol* 2012;302(2):L185–92.

48. Simard JM, Chen M, Tarasov KV, et al. Newly expressed SUR1-regulated NC (Ca-ATP) channel mediates cerebral edema after ischemic stroke. *Nat Med* 2006;12(4):433–40.

49. Zeng HK, Wang QS, Deng YY, et al. Hypertonic saline ameliorates cerebral edema through downregulation of aquaporin-4 expression in the astrocytes. *Neuroscience* 2010;166(3):878–85.

50. Nakayama S, Migliati E, Amiry-Moghaddam M, Ottersen OP, Bhardwaj A. Osmotherapy with hypertonic saline attenuates global cerebral edema following experimental cardiac arrest via perivascular pool of aquaporin-4. *Crit Care Med* 2016;44(8):e702–10.

51. Huang L, Cao W, Deng Y, Zhu G, Han Y, Zeng H. Hypertonic saline alleviates experimentally induced cerebral oedema through suppression of vascular endothelial growth factor and its receptor VEGFR2 expression in astrocytes. *BMC Neurosci* 2016;17(1):64.

52. Zeng HK, Wang QS, Deng YY, et al. A comparative study on the efficacy of 10% hypertonic saline and equal volume of 20% mannitol in the treatment of experimentally induced cerebral edema in adult rats. *BMC Neurosci* 2010;11:153.

53. Qureshi AI, Suarez JI, Bhardwaj A, Mirski M, Schnitzer MS, Hanley DF, et al. Use of hypertonic (3%) saline/acetate infusion in the treatment of cerebral edema: Effect on intracranial pressure and lateral displacement of the brain. *Crit Care Med* 1998;26(3):440–6.

54. Ryu JH, Walcott BP, Kahle KT, et al. Induced and sustained hypernatremia for the prevention and treatment of cerebral edema following brain injury. *Neurocrit Care* 2013;19(2):222–31.

55. Hirsch KG, Spock T, Koenig MA, Geocadin RG. Treatment of elevated intracranial pressure with hyperosmolar therapy in patients with renal failure. *Neurocrit Care* 2012;17(3):388–94.

56. Ryken TC, McDermott M, Robinson PD, et al. The role of steroids in the management of brain metastases: a systematic review and evidence-based clinical practice guideline. *J Neurooncol* 2010;96(1):103–14.

57. Wen PY, Schiff D, Kesari S, Drappatz J, Gigas DC, Doherty L. Medical management of patients with brain tumors. *J Neurooncol* 2006;80(3):313–32.

58. Papadopoulos MC, Saadoun S, Binder DK, Manley GT, Krishna S, Verkman AS. Molecular mechanisms of brain tumor edema. *Neuroscience* 2004;129(4):1011–20.

59. Hedley-Whyte ET, Hsu DW. Effect of dexamethasone on blood-brain barrier in the normal mouse. *Ann Neurol* 1986;19(4):373–7.

60. Heiss JD, Papavassiliou E, Merrill MJ, et al. Mechanism of dexamethasone suppression of brain tumor-associated vascular permeability in rats. Involvement of the glucocorticoid receptor and vascular permeability factor. *J Clin Invest* 1996;98(6):1400–8.

61. Barnes PJ. Molecular mechanisms and cellular effects of glucocorticosteroids. *Immunol Allergy Clin North Am* 2005;25(3):451–68.

62. Pitzalis C, Pipitone N, Perretti M. Regulation of leukocyte-endothelial interactions by glucocorticoids. *Ann N Y Acad Sci* 2002;966:108–18.

63. Blecharz KG, Drenckhahn D, Forster CY. Glucocorticoids increase VE-cadherin expression and cause cytoskeletal rearrangements in murine brain endothelial cEND cells. *J Cereb Blood Flow Metab* 2008;28(6):1139–49.

64. Miller JD, Leech P. Effects of mannitol and steroid therapy on intracranial volume-pressure relationships in patients. *J Neurosurg* 1975;42(3):274–81.

65. Gutin PH. Corticosteroid therapy in patients with cerebral tumors: benefits, mechanisms, problems, practicalities. *Semin Oncol* 1975;2(1):49–56.

66. Bell BA, Smith MA, Kean DM, et al. Brain water measured by magnetic resonance imaging. Correlation with direct estimation and changes after mannitol and dexamethasone. *Lancet* 1987;1(8524):66–9.

67. Pegorini S, Braida D, Verzoni C, et al. Capsaicin exhibits neuroprotective effects in a model of transient global cerebral ischemia in Mongolian gerbils. *Br J Pharmacol* 2005;144(5):727–35.

68. Pegorini S, Zani A, Braida D, Guerini-Rocco C, Sala M. Vanilloid VR1 receptor is involved in rimonabant-induced neuroprotection. *Br J Pharmacol* 2006;147(5):552–9.

69. Xu W, Mu X, Wang H, et al. Chloride co-transporter NKCC1 inhibitor bumetanide enhances neurogenesis and behavioral recovery in rats after experimental stroke. *Mol Neurobiol* 2017;54(4):2406–14.

70. Wang J, Feng L, Zhu Z, et al. Aquaporins as diagnostic and therapeutic targets in cancer: how far we are? *J Transl Med* 2015;13:96.

71. Jin H, Li W, Dong C, Ma L, Wu J, Zhao W. Effects of different doses of levetiracetam on aquaporin 4 expression in rats with brain edema following fluid percussion injury. *Med Sci Monit* 2016;22:678–86.

72. Soltani Z, Khaksari M, Shahrokhi N, et al. Effect of estrogen and/or progesterone administration on traumatic brain injury-caused brain edema: the changes of aquaporin-4 and interleukin-6. *J Physiol Biochem* 2016;72(1):33–44.

73. Shi SS, Zhang HB, Wang CH, et al. Propofol attenuates early brain injury after subarachnoid hemorrhage in rats. *J Mol Neurosci* 2015;57(4):538–45.

74. Wang BF, Cui ZW, Zhong ZH, et al. Curcumin attenuates brain edema in mice with intracerebral hemorrhage through inhibition of AQP4 and AQP9 expression. *Acta Pharmacol Sin* 2015;36(8):939–48.

75. Gerstner ER, Duda DG, di Tomaso E, et al. VEGF inhibitors in the treatment of cerebral edema in patients with brain cancer. *Nat Rev Clin Oncol* 2009;6(4):229–36.

76. Cohen MH, Shen YL, Keegan P, Pazdur R. FDA drug approval summary: bevacizumab (Avastin) as treatment of recurrent glioblastoma multiforme. *Oncologist* 2009;14(11):1131–8.

77. Sheth KN, Elm JJ, Molyneaux BJ, et al. Safety and efficacy of intravenous glyburide on brain swelling after large hemispheric infarction (GAMES-RP): a randomised, double-blind, placebo-controlled phase 2 trial. *Lancet Neurol* 2016.

78. Vahedi K, Vicaut E, Mateo J, et al. Sequential-design, multicenter, randomized, controlled trial of early decompressive craniectomy in malignant middle cerebral artery infarction (DECIMAL Trial). *Stroke* 2007;38(9):2506–17.

79. Juttler E, Schwab S, Schmiedek P, et al. Decompressive surgery for the treatment of malignant infarction of the middle cerebral artery (DESTINY): a randomized, controlled trial. *Stroke* 2007;38(9):2518–25.

80. Juttler E, Unterberg A, Woitzik J, et al. Hemicraniectomy in older patients with extensive middle-cerebral-artery stroke. *N Engl J Med* 2014;370(12):1091–100.

81. Hofmeijer J, Kappelle LJ, Algra A, et al. Surgical decompression for space-occupying cerebral infarction (the Hemicraniectomy After Middle Cerebral Artery infarction with Life-threatening Edema Trial [HAMLET]): a multicentre, open, randomised trial. *Lancet Neurol* 2009;8(4):326–33.

82. Frank JI, Schumm LP, Wroblewski K, et al. Hemicraniectomy and durotomy upon deterioration from infarction-related swelling trial: randomized pilot clinical trial. *Stroke* 2014;45(3):781–7.

83. Hutchinson PJ, Kolias AG, Timofeev IS, et al. Trial of decompressive craniectomy for traumatic intracranial hypertension. *N Engl J Med* 2016;375(12):1119–30.

84. Stevens RD, Huff JS, Duckworth J, Papangelou A, Weingart SD, Smith WS. Emergency neurological life support: intracranial hypertension and herniation. *Neurocrit Care* 2012;17(Suppl 1):S60–5.

27

Hydrocephalus

P. Sundararajan and A. Lele

ABSTRACT

Hydrocephalus is a condition that occurs due to excessive cerebrospinal fluid (CSF) accumulation leading to increased intracranial pressure (ICP) and other detrimental consequences. Hydrocephalus can be present since birth or acquired at a later stage. It is broadly classified as communicating or non-communicating hydrocephalus based on the underlying mechanism. The clinical presentation varies depending on the age at which it presents. Several imaging modalities are available to diagnose, identify, and monitor hydrocephalus. Treatment options are limited and based on the individual requirements of the case.

KEYWORDS

Hydrocephalus; raised intracranial pressure (ICP); communicating; non-communicating; cerebrospinal fluid (CSF).

INTRODUCTION

Hydrocephalus is the impairment in the formation, flow, or absorption of cerebrospinal fluid (CSF) leading to ventricular enlargement. It is often detected in infants, children, and adults by symptoms of increased intracranial pressure (ICP).[1,2] It is estimated that hydrocephalus affects 1.1 in 1000 infants,[3] and about 20%–30% patients with aneurysmal subarachnoid haemorrhage (aSAH) experience either early or late hydrocephalus.[4] It results due to several causes which may be congenital or acquired. Classification of hydrocephalus is based upon the underlying mechanisms. This chapter provides an understanding of the causes, presentation, diagnosis, and management of this condition.

BASIC ANATOMY AND PHYSIOLOGY OF CEREBROSPINAL FLUID

The choroid plexus produces almost 70% to 80% of the total CSF. The brain parenchyma, spinal cord, and ependymal lining of the ventricles produce the remaining amount. Cerebrospinal fluid production occurs by a combination of filtration across the endothelium and active transport of sodium by the choroidal epithelia.

Most of it is secreted in the lateral ventricles and leaves the ventricles through the foramen of Monro to enter the third ventricle. From there, the CSF flows into the fourth ventricle through the aqueduct of Sylvius. It leaves the fourth ventricle by the median foramen of Magendie and lateral foramina of Luschka and enters the subarachnoid space. Cerebrospinal fluid is essentially absorbed into the internal jugular system via cranial parasagittal arachnoid granulations.

The normal CSF production rate in an adult is 0.35 ml/min (20 ml/hr or 500 ml/24 hours). The capacity of normal lateral and third ventricles is approximately 20 ml, whereas the total CSF volume in an adult is 120–150 ml.[5] Approximately 330–380 ml of CSF enters the venous circulation daily.[6] Hence, in normal circumstances CSF is recycled over three times each day.

CAUSES OF HYDROCEPHALUS

Hydrocephalus can occur due to a congenital defect or can be acquired later in life. Congenital hydrocephalus is present at birth and occurs mostly due to a developmental defect leading to obstruction to the flow of CSF. The most common cause of congenital hydrocephalus is

Table 27.1 Common causes of hydrocephalus

Congenital	Acquired
• Aqueductal stenosis	• Subarachnoid haemorrhage[*]
• Atresia of foramen of Monro	• Intracerebral haemorrhage[**]
• Myelomeningocele	• Intraventricular haemorrhage[#]
• Genetic abnormalities	• Traumatic brain injury[##]
• Arnold Chiari malformations	• Post-surgical (after decompressive craniectomy)[$]
• Dandy Walker malformations	• Tumours
• Maternal infections	• Meningitis
• Vascular malformations	• Arachnoid cyst
	• Nutritional
	• Idiopathic

*Connolly ES, Jr., Rabinstein AA, Carhuapoma JR, et al. Guidelines for the management of aneurysmal subarachnoid hemorrhage: a guideline for healthcare professionals from the American Heart Association/American Stroke Association. *Stroke* 2012;43(6): 1711–37.

**Hemphill JC, 3rd, Greenberg SM, Anderson CS, et al. Guidelines for the management of spontaneous intracerebral hemorrhage: a guideline for healthcare professionals from the American Heart Association/American Stroke Association. *Stroke* 2015;46(7):2032–60.

#Hanley DF, Lane K, McBee N, et al. Thrombolytic removal of intraventricular haemorrhage in treatment of severe stroke: results of the randomised, multicentre, multiregion, placebo-controlled CLEAR III trial. *Lancet* 2017.

##Poca MA, Sahuquillo J, Mataro M, Benejam B, Arikan F, Baguena M. Ventricular enlargement after moderate or severe head injury: a frequent and neglected problem. *J Neurotrauma* 2005;22(11): 1303–10.

$Vadivelu S, Rekate HL, Esernio-Jenssen D, Mittler MA, Schneider SJ. Hydrocephalus associated with childhood nonaccidental head trauma. *Neurosurg Focus* 2016;41(5):E8.

aqueductal stenosis preventing the drainage of CSF between the third and fourth ventricles in the brain. The other causes of congenital hydrocephalus include myelomeningocele, Arnold-Chiari malformation, inherited genetic abnormalities, idiopathic vascular malformations or may be due to maternal infections such as cytomegalovirus, toxoplasmosis, rubella, varicella, and mumps.[7] Table 27.1 highlights the common causes of hydrocephalus.

Hydrocephalus may be acquired when a blockage to the ventricles in the brain occurs due to meningitis, intracranial haemorrhages, head trauma, arachnoid cysts, tumours, nutritional disorders (hypo- or hyper-vitaminosis A) and teratogenesis. In premature babies, intraventricular haemorrhage can occur leading to a block in the CSF flow and plug arachnoid villi leading to hydrocephalus.

TYPES OF HYDROCEPHALUS

Hydrocephalus is broadly classified as communicative or non-communicative based on the presence or absence of CSF flow. This is one of the earliest classifications formulated in 1913 by the neurosurgeon Dandy Walker.[8] He injected neutral phenolsulphonphthalein into the lateral ventricle. If the dye was recovered within 20 minutes from the spinal subarachnoid space, the hydrocephalus was termed 'communicating' indicating the presence of a patent communication between the ventricles and the subarachnoid space. If no dye was recovered, the hydrocephalus was termed 'non-communicating' or obstructive.

Communicative Hydrocephalus

Communicative or non-obstructive hydrocephalus occurs due to the impairment of CSF absorption at the arachnoid villi. The malabsorption of CSF leads to its accumulation and subsequent increase in the ICP. Subarachnoid or intraventricular haemorrhage, meningitis, congenital absence of arachnoid villi are the common causes of a non-obstructive hydrocephalus (Figure 27.1).

Non-Communicative Hydrocephalus

Non-communicative or obstructive hydrocephalus is caused by obstruction to the flow of CSF at any part of the ventricular system. The obstruction may be in the lateral ventricles, foramen of Monro, third ventricle, aqueduct of Sylvius, fourth ventricle or subarachnoid spaces (Figure 27.2).

NORMAL PRESSURE HYDROCEPHALUS

Normal pressure hydrocephalus occurs in older adults. It is characterized by the pathological enlargement of ventricles with normal opening pressures on lumbar puncture, and a triad of clinical symptoms that include dementia, gait ataxia, and urinary incontinence.[9] The cause is most commonly idiopathic. Treatment with ventriculoperitoneal shunting of CSF is effective with marked improvement of symptoms.

Negative Pressure Hydrocephalus

Negative pressure and low pressure hydrocephalus are rare clinical entities usually presenting post neurosurgery with clinical and imaging features of hydrocephalus but with negative CSF pressure.[10] Cerebrospinal fluid leaks have been suggested to produce very low subarachnoid pressures which lead to negative pressure hydrocephalus.[11]

The very low subarachnoid pressures in turn produce a transmantle pressure gradient that generates a state in which ventriculomegaly can persist with negative ICP.[12] Treatment involves correction of the CSF leak, neck wrapping to increase brain turgor and allowing the pressure in the ventricles to rise to the level of the opening pressure of the valve, and reestablishing the CSF route.[11]

CLINICAL PRESENTATION

The clinical presentation of hydrocephalus differs in neonates and infants compared to older children and adults. The other influencing factors are the progression and duration of the underlying condition, the location of obstruction and method of compensation for the increase in ICP due to the accumulation of CSF in the ventricles. At 2 years of age, closure of cranial sutures normally occurs. In infants, up to 2 years of age the increase in ICP is compensated by the expansion of the infant skull due to the presence of fibrous sutures leading to disproportionate head growth.

Other symptoms include general irritability, poor feeding, vomiting, and slow attainment of milestones. Clinical signs include bulging, firm fontanelle, wide separation of the cranial sutures, and prominence of scalp veins. Late clinical signs found are the MacEwen sign and the 'setting sun' appearance of the eyes. The MacEwen sign is also called the cracked pot sign due to the characteristic sound heard on percussion of the skull. The setting sun appearance of the eyes occurs due to the pressure on the mid-brain tectum by CSF in the suprapineal recess.[13]

In older children and adults, closure of the cranial sutures leads to raised ICP, headache, vomiting, and drowsiness on accumulation of CSF. When hydrocephalus has developed insidiously, cognitive impairment, poor concentration, and behavioural changes occur. Visual disturbances and papilloedema are more common in adults than in neonates and infants. The Cushing's reflex which includes the triad of bradycardia, hypertension, and irregularities in breathing pattern is seen during massive elevation of ICP and should be treated promptly.[13]

DIAGNOSTIC STUDIES IN PATIENTS WITH HYDROCEPHALUS

Clinical Diagnosis of Hydrocephalus

Over the years, many diagnostic studies have been used to identify the location, aetiology, and severity of hydrocephalus to manage and treat the condition.

Congenital hydrocephalus is generally diagnosed prenatally or at birth with ultrasound scans done in the antenatal period or after birth until the closure of the anterior fontanelle.[14,15] The first prenatal signs of hydrocephalus may be visible on ultrasound around 18–20 weeks of gestation, the width of one or both ventricles are measured at the level of the glomus of the choroid plexus. If the width of the ventricles measures greater than or equal to 10 mm it can be significant.[15,16] Later in gestation, around 24 weeks in severe cases of cerebral ventriculomegaly, the banana sign and lemon sign can be seen.[15,17] The banana sign occurs when the cerebellum loses its normal central convexity and curves anteriorly, obliterating the cisterna magna and compressing parallel to the occipital bone to resemble a banana.[18,19] The lemon sign can be visualized in a transverse foetal sonogram at the biparietal diameter. There is a loss of normal convex contour of the frontal bones which appears flattened or inwardly scalloped.[18,20]

One of the notable features of congenital hydrocephalus is the ventriculomegaly which prevents the fusion of cranial sutures leading to progressive enlargement of the head. Rapidly increasing head circumference in an infant measured with a measuring tape along the maximal obtainable circumference is diagnostic.[21–23]

The large size and shape of the skull, sutural separation, thinning of the cranial bones with a 'beaten silver' appearance can be noted in patients with obstructive hydrocephalus on plain X-rays.[13]

Ventriculography done with serial X-rays using air or dyes as contrast was used to assess the size of the ventricles and flow of CSF in earlier years. It is highly invasive and can lead to several serious complications. This method has been largely replaced by non-invasive computed tomography (CT) and magnetic resonance imaging (MRI) studies.[13,24]

Study of the entire ventricular system and assessment of the underlying aetiology of hydrocephalus can be evaluated with the help of either CT or MRI imaging. Features such as ventriculomegaly (Evans' index >0.3), enlargement of the temporal ventricular horns, enlargement of the third ventricle, thinning and elevation of the corpus callosum, and narrowed cortical sulci when present in a combination are highly suggestive of hydrocephalus.[5,13,25]

Computed tomography is used to assess ventricular size, and the size of the fourth ventricle can be used to diagnose communicating and obstructive hydrocephalus; larger in the former, smaller in the latter.[5,25]

Chiari malformations and cerebellar or periaqueductal tumours are best detected with an MRI.[5] Communicating hydrocephalus can be detected by aqueductal flow void phenomenon in which there is an absence of hypointense signal from the third ventricle into the fourth ventricle. The presence of periventricular white matter hyper-intensities in T2-weighted (T2W) or fluid-attenuated inversion recovery (FLAIR) images is indicative of interstitial oedema seen in acute hydrocephalus.[5,25]

Computed tomography can demonstrate gross dilatation of ventricles but MRI is the best imaging modality to provide functional and anatomic information to aid in discriminating the underlying aetiology.[26]

Intracranial Pressure Monitoring in Patients with Hydrocephalus

Increased resistance to CSF outflow causes increases in ICP, thus ICP monitoring can help to diagnose young patients with mild symptoms, older patients with possible low-grade hydrocephalus and provide accurate assessments of the shunt function.[5,27–30] Intracranial pressure values >18 mmHg/ml/minute help in the diagnosis of active hydrocephalus in the elderly.[5] Studies show that continuous ICP monitoring can help in detection of elevated basal ICP, B waves, or plateau waves which aid in assessing the requirement for surgical shunt placements, functioning of shunts and the need for shunt revisions.[5,29,31,32]

The presence of abnormal plateau waves or B waves in patients with shunt placements could signify shunt obstruction, infection or malfunction. If the opening pressure of the shunt is above the ICP pressure, drainage of CSF is insufficient leading to increased ICP and the above changes. On the other hand, the shunt opening pressure can be too low leading to excessive CSF drainage and intracranial hypotension which can lead to disabling symptoms.[29,31,33]

Volume-adding tests such as ventricular or lumbar infusion studies with continuous ICP monitoring can help in diagnosing cases where there is chronic ventricular dilation accompanied by ICP that is not greatly raised which may be due to obstruction of CSF absorption or shunt malfunction. Such lumbar infusion tests and tap tests can predict patients who may benefit from shunt surgery.[29,32,34]

MANAGEMENT STRATEGIES FOR PATIENTS WITH HYDROCEPHALUS

Forming a strategy for treatment of hydrocephalus mainly depends on the underlying aetiology. In some cases, removal of tumours or treatment of infections can help resolve the condition, but in cases of progressive hydrocephalus with increased ICP, medical treatment options are limited and surgical options are the mainstay.

Medical Management

Medical management is not effective for the long-term treatment of hydrocephalus and is used for temporary relief until surgical intervention can be planned. Acetazolamide can decrease the production of CSF by inhibiting carbonic anhydrase, an enzyme abundantly present in the choroid plexus which is necessary for the formation of CSF.[13,35] Acetazolamide used in conjunction with furosemide has also been shown to benefit patients.[28]

Surgical Management

Introduction to Surgical Management of Hydrocephalus

Surgical management of hydrocephalus is based on the following concepts:

1. Reduction of CSF formation
   - Choroid plexus resection
   - Choroid plexus cauterization
2. Decompression of ventricles
   - Lumbar puncture
   - Ventriculostomy
3. Bypassing the obstruction in the ventricular system
   - Ventricular shunts
   - Endoscopic third ventriculostomy

Choroid Plexus Resection/Choroid Plexus Cauterization

Choroid plexus resection is the definitive treatment of choice in patients with choroid plexus papillomas causing hydrocephalus. In patients with choroid plexus hyperplasia, endoscopic coagulation of the choroid plexus has shown to correct hydrocephalus without resorting to shunt placement.[36–39] In infants with myelomeningocele, primary treatment of hydrocephalus with combined endoscopic third ventriculostomy and choroid plexus cauterization provides long-lasting relief that does not need shunt placement. [40,41]

Lumbar Puncture

Serial lumbar punctures performed to reduce the volume of CSF is a short-term option for the treatment of hydrocephalus.[42] It is used to treat patients with acute hydrocephalus after subarachnoid haemorrhage and communicating hydrocephalus.[38,42] An external drain can be attached after lumbar puncture for continuous drainage of CSF but is not feasible for prolonged use as it can lead to complications such as meningitis, retained catheter, local infection, headaches, and nerve root irritation.[43]

Ventriculostomy

Ventriculostomy or external ventricular drain (EVD) is primarily placed to temporarily divert CSF from the brain in patients with progressive hydrocephalus at risk for elevated ICP. It is a commonly performed bedside neurosurgical procedure and can be performed in the intensive care unit or the operating room. An antimicrobial impregnated (preferred), multi-orifice catheter is placed in the frontal horn of the lateral ventricle using anatomical landmarks. An external ventricular drain allows CSF diversion in addition to ICP monitoring and a potential conduit for administration of thrombolytics. Animal studies assessing the use of fibrinolytic therapy to prevent and manage post haemorrhagic hydrocephalus occurring due to intraventricular haemorrhage have shown limited success.[44–48] Clot Lysis: Evaluating Accelerated Resolution of Intraventricular Haemorrhage Phase III (CLEAR-III), a randomized placebo-controlled trial of irrigation of alteplase vs saline in patients with intraventricular haemorrhage despite showing reduction in mortality failed to demonstrate improvement in functional outcome (mRS at 180 days) with survivors left in a severe disabled state.[49]

Ventricular Shunts

Ventricular shunt insertion remains the most popular modality for treatment of hydrocephalus in adults and children. The underlying principle lies in bypassing the site of obstruction to CSF flow by diverting the CSF from ventricular cavity to a site where it is readily absorbed.[43,50] Shunts are used in cases of progressive hydrocephalus with increased ICP as well as in normal pressure hydrocephalus. Patients with ICH who require emergency CSF diversion and have elevated ICP, and those with thalamic haemorrhage are at higher risk for permanent ventricular shunt placement.[51] Approximately 30% of patients with aneurysmal SAH require permanent shunt placement.[52,53] Predictors of shunt requirement include elevated daily CSF output (greater than 78 ml/day),[54] or greater than 1500 ml in the first week.[55]

The shunt assembly comprises a proximal catheter located in the cerebral ventricles and a distal catheter draining into a selected site of CSF absorption, connected by a valve and reservoir incorporated into the shunt system.[13] The most common drainage site is the peritoneum known as the ventriculoperitoneal (VP) shunt. The other drainage sites are the pleural space (ventriculopleural shunt) and the right atrium (ventriculoatrial shunt).[56–58] Lumboperitoneal shunts are of use in the treatment of communicating hydrocephalus[59] and may be beneficial as first-line therapy in patients with idiopathic normal pressure hydrocephalus.[60]

Almost 50% of VP shunts placed fail within the first 2 years after insertion.[61] The most common causes of shunt malfunction are shunt obstruction, infection, migration, and CSF ascites.[62–65]

Endoscopic Third Ventriculostomy

In endoscopic third ventriculostomy (ETV), a small perforation is made in the floor of the third ventricle between the mammillary bodies and infundibular recess in the midline, allowing movement of CSF out of the blocked ventricular system and into the basal cisterns.[65–68] It is considered as a treatment of choice in conditions causing obstructive hydrocephalus.[2] It is also used to treat patients with shunt failure when there is an underlying obstructive hydrocephalus.[69–71] More recently, studies are being conducted to expand the indications for ETV to treat communicating hydrocephalus such as normal pressure hydrocephalus (NPH).[72–74] Absolute contraindication for ETV is the presence of obstruction at the level of the arachnoid villi or the venous flow in the superior sagittal sinus.[2]

Infants have poorly developed absorptive surfaces in the subarachnoid spaces and have an open anterior fontanelle with a soft skull making them poor candidates for ETV, hence the effectiveness of ETV under the age of 1 year is variable.[2,75,76]

The incidence of permanent complications after ETV are less. The most common complications encountered are fever, bleeding, hemiparesis, gaze palsy, memory disorders, altered consciousness, diabetes insipidus, weight gain, and precocious puberty. Complication rates after ETV is between 2%–15%.[75] Over the last 20 years, there has been a shift in the treatment of many types of hydrocephalus away from VP shunting and toward ETV.[77–79] The overall summary of medical and surgical management is given in Table 27.2.

COMPLICATIONS OF HYDROCEPHALUS

Hydrocephalus in most cases is a lifelong problem and complications can arise because of the condition itself or from the treatment initiated. All patients with hydrocephalus must be educated regarding symptoms that may arise in case of shunt failure and the need for regular follow-ups.[5] The presence of hydrocephalus and intraventricular haemorrhage is a poor prognostic

Table 27.2 Summary of medical and surgical management options in patients with hydrocephalus

Medical management		
Treatment	**Indication**	**Rationale**
Acetazolamide/Furosemide	Excessive CSF production	Reduction in CSF production
Fibrinolytics	Posthemorrhagic Hydrocephalus	Prevent obstruction of cerebrospinal fluid pathways due to blood clots[#]
Surgical management		
Choroid plexus resection/ Choroid plexus cauterization	Choroid plexus papilloma, Choroid plexus hyperplasia	Decreases CSF production[##]
Lumbar puncture	Acute hydrocephalus, Communicating hydrocephalus	Reduces CSF volume, provides temporary relief
Ventriculostomy	For all types of hydrocephalus	Reduce CSF volume, allows ICP monitoring[*,**]
Ventricular shunts	Obstructive hydrocephalus, Normal pressure hydrocephalus	Diverting CSF from ventricles to alternate absorption sites
Endoscopic third ventriculostomy (ETV)	Obstructive hydrocephalus, Shunt failure	CSF drainage into basal cisterns[##]

Abbreviation: CSF: cerebrospinal fluid.

#Hanley DF, Lane K, McBee N, et al. Thrombolytic removal of intraventricular haemorrhage in treatment of severe stroke: results of the randomised, multicentre, multiregion, placebo-controlled CLEAR III trial. *Lancet* 2017.

##Dewan MC, Naftel RP. The global rise of endoscopic third ventriculostomy with choroid plexus cauterization in pediatric hydrocephalus. *Pediatr Neurosurg* 2016.

*Connolly ES, Jr., Rabinstein AA, Carhuapoma JR, et al. Guidelines for the management of aneurysmal subarachnoid hemorrhage: a guideline for healthcare professionals from the American Heart Association/American Stroke Association. *Stroke* 2012;43(6):1711–37.

**Hemphill JC, 3rd, Greenberg SM, Anderson CS, et al. Guidelines for the management of spontaneous intracerebral hemorrhage: a guideline for healthcare professionals from the American Heart Association/American Stroke Association. *Stroke* 2015;46(7):2032–60.

indicator in patients with intracerebral haemorrhage (ICH).[80]

Complications of shunt placement include shunt collapse, infection, occlusion which cause an increase in the ICP requiring shunt revision.[56,81,82] More complications are noted in infants and children with hydrocephalus as they age. They are more prone for visual impairment because of episodes of increased ICP or oculomotor disturbances.[83,84] Hydrocephalus patients have reduced motor function, a lower-than-average adult intelligence quotient (IQ) and are more prone for epilepsy.[85,86]

CONCLUSIONS

Hydrocephalus is a condition which is commonly encountered. If it is not diagnosed and treated, it can lead to fatal complications. Congenital hydrocephalus can affect the mental and social development of children and there are multiple challenges to be faced in their treatment such as shunt infections and requirement of multiple surgeries. Our understanding of hydrocephalus is still incomplete and there are several studies being conducted

to identify the genetic basis of hydrocephalus and improve management of this condition.

REFERENCES

1. Desai B, Hsu Y, Schneller B, Hobbs JG, Mehta AI, Linninger A. Hydrocephalus: the role of cerebral aquaporin-4 channels and computational modeling considerations of cerebrospinal fluid. *Neurosurg Focus* 2016;41(3):E8.

2. Rekate HL. A contemporary definition and classification of hydrocephalus. *Semin Pediatr Neurol* 2009;16(1):9–15.

3. Tully HM, Dobyns WB. Infantile hydrocephalus: a review of epidemiology, classification and causes. *Eur J Med Genet* 2014;57(8):359–68.

4. Germanwala AV, Huang J, Tamargo RJ. Hydrocephalus after aneurysmal subarachnoid hemorrhage. *Neurosurg Clin N Am* 2010;21(2):263–70.

5. Pople IK. Hydrocephalus and shunts: what the neurologist should know. *J Neurol Neurosurg Psychiatry* 2002;73(Suppl 1): i17–22.

6. Moore KL DA. *Clinically Oriented Anatomy.* 4th ed: Lippincott Williams and Wilkins; 1999.

7. Koo H, Chi JG. Congenital hydrocephalus—analysis of 49 cases. *J Korean Med Sci* 1991;6(4):287–98.

8. Dandy WE, Blackfan KD. An experimental and clinical study of internal hydrocephalus. *JAMA* 1913;61(25): 2216–7.

9. Adams RD, Fisher CM, Hakim S, Ojemann RG, Sweet WH. Symptomatic occult hydrocephalus with 'normal' cerebrospinal-fluid pressure.a treatable syndrome. *N Engl J Med* 1965;273:117–26.

10. Pandey S, Jin Y, Gao L, Zhou CC, Cui DM. Negative-pressure hydrocephalus: a case report on successful treatment under intracranial pressure monitoring with bilateral ventriculoperitoneal shunts. *World Neurosurg* 2017;99:812.e7–812.e12.

11. Filippidis AS, Kalani MY, Nakaji P, Rekate HL. Negative-pressure and low-pressure hydrocephalus: the role of cerebrospinal fluid leaks resulting from surgical approaches to the cranial base. *J Neurosurg* 2011;115(5): 1031–7.

12. Hunn BH, Mujic A, Sher I, Dubey AK, Peters-Willke J, Hunn AW. Successful treatment of negative pressure hydrocephalus using timely titrated external ventricular drainage: a case series. *Clin Neurol Neurosurg* 2014;116: 67–71.

13. Venkataramana NK. Hydrocephalus Indian scenario—A review. *J Pediatr Neurosci* 2011;6(Suppl 1):S11–22.

14. Van Landingham M, Nguyen TV, Roberts A, Parent AD, Zhang J. Risk factors of congenital hydrocephalus: a 10 year retrospective study. *J Neurol Neurosurg Psychiatry* 2009;80(2):213–7.

15. Garne E, Loane M, Addor MC, Boyd PA, Barisic I, Dolk H. Congenital hydrocephalus—prevalence, prenatal diagnosis and outcome of pregnancy in four European regions. *Eur J Paediatr Neurol* 2010;14(2):150–5.

16. Gaglioti P, Oberto M, Todros T. The significance of fetal ventriculomegaly: etiology, short- and long-term outcomes. *Prenat Diagn* 2009;29(4):381–8.

17. Van den Hof MC, Nicolaides KH, Campbell J, Campbell S. Evaluation of the lemon and banana signs in one hundred thirty fetuses with open spina bifida. *Am J Obstet Gynecol* 1990;162(2):322–7.

18. Atalar MH, Salk I, Egilmez H. Classical signs and appearances in pediatric neuroradiology: a pictorial review. *Pol J Radiol* 2014;79:479–89.

19. Nicolaides KH, Campbell S, Gabbe SG, Guidetti R. Ultrasound screening for spina bifida: cranial and cerebellar signs. *Lancet* 1986;2(8498):72–4.

20. Thomas M. The lemon sign. *Radiology* 2003;228(1): 206–7.

21. Korobkin R. The relationship between head circumference and the development of communicating hydrocephalus in infants following intraventricular hemmorrhage. *Pediatrics* 1975;56(1):74–7.

22. Park TS SR. Pediatric. In: HR W, editor. *Youmans Neurological Surgery*. 2nd ed: WB Saunders Company. pp. 1381–422.

23. Rengachary SS WR. *Neurosurgery*. McGraw Hill Book Company; 1985. pp. 2125–56.

24. Kellermann K, Bliesener JA, Kyambi JM. Positive ventriculography using water-soluble contrast media in infants with myelomeningocele and hydrocephalus. *Neuropadiatrie* 1978;9(1):49–58.

25. Kartal MG, Algin O. Evaluation of hydrocephalus and other cerebrospinal fluid disorders with MRI: An update. *Insights Imaging* 2014;5(4):531–41.

26. Dincer A, Ozek MM. Radiologic evaluation of pediatric hydrocephalus. *Childs Nerv Syst* 2011;27(10):1543–62.

27. Boon AJ, Tans JT, Delwel EJ, et al. Dutch normal-pressure hydrocephalus study: prediction of outcome after shunting by resistance to outflow of cerebrospinal fluid. *J Neurosurg* 1997;87(5):687–93.

28. Borgesen SE, Gjerris F. Relationships between intracranial pressure, ventricular size, and resistance to CSF outflow. *J Neurosurg* 1987;67(4):535–9.

29. Geocadin RG, Varelas PN, Rigamonti D, Williams MA. Continuous intracranial pressure monitoring via the shunt reservoir to assess suspected shunt malfunction in adults with hydrocephalus. *Neurosurg Focus* 2007;22(4):E10.

30. Tisell M, Edsbagge M, Stephensen H, Czosnyka M, Wikkelso C. Elastance correlates with outcome after endoscopic third ventriculostomy in adults with hydrocephalus caused by primary aqueductal stenosis. *Neurosurgery* 2002;50(1):70–77.

31. Puca A, Anile C, Maira G, Rossi G. Cerebrospinal fluid shunting for hydrocephalus in the adult: factors related to shunt revision. *Neurosurgery* 1991;29(6):822–6.

32. Sussman JD, Sarkies N, Pickard JD. Benign intracranial hypertension. Pseudotumour cerebri: idiopathic intracranial hypertension. *Adv Tech Stand Neurosurg* 1998;24:261–305.

33. Foltz EL, Blanks JP. Symptomatic low intracranial pressure in shunted hydrocephalus. *J Neurosurg* 1988;68(3):401–8.

34. Raneri F, Zella MA, Di Cristofori A, Zarrino B, Pluderi M, Spagnoli D. Supplementary tests in idiopathic normal pressure hydrocephalus: a single center experience with a combined lumbar infusion test and tap test. *World Neurosurg* 2017.

35. Whitelaw A, Kennedy CR, Brion LP. Diuretic therapy for newborn infants with posthemorrhagic ventricular dilatation. *Cochrane Database Syst Rev* 2001(2):CD002270.

36. Bohara M, Hirabaru M, Fujio S, et al. Choroid Plexus Tumors: Experience of 10 cases with special references to adult cases. *Neurol Med Chir (Tokyo)* 2015;55(12): 891–900.

37. Cannon DM, Mohindra P, Gondi V, Kruser TJ, Kozak KR. Choroid plexus tumor epidemiology and outcomes: implications for surgical and radiotherapeutic management. *J Neurooncol* 2015;121(1):151–7.

38. Heep A, Engelskirchen R, Holschneider A, Groneck P. Primary intervention for posthemorrhagic hydrocephalus

in very low birthweight infants by ventriculostomy. *Childs Nerv Syst* 2001;17(1–2):47–51.

39. Passariello A, Tufano M, Spennato P, et al. The role of chemotherapy and surgical removal in the treatment of Choroid Plexus carcinomas and atypical papillomas. *Childs Nerv Syst* 2015;31(7):1079–88.

40. Hallaert GG, Vanhauwaert DJ, Logghe K, et al. Endoscopic coagulation of choroid plexus hyperplasia. *J Neurosurg Pediatr* 2012;9(2):169–77.

41. Warf BC, Campbell JW. Combined endoscopic third ventriculostomy and choroid plexus cauterization as primary treatment of hydrocephalus for infants with myelomeningocele: long-term results of a prospective intent-to-treat study in 115 East African infants. *J Neurosurg Pediatr* 2008;2(5):310–6.

42. Stone SS, Warf BC. Combined endoscopic third ventriculostomy and choroid plexus cauterization as primary treatment for infant hydrocephalus: a prospective North American series. *J Neurosurg Pediatr* 2014;14(5):439–46.

43. Hasan D, Lindsay KW, Vermeulen M. Treatment of acute hydrocephalus after subarachnoid hemorrhage with serial lumbar puncture. *Stroke* 1991;22(2):190–4.

44. Brinker T, Seifert V, Dietz H. Subacute hydrocephalus after experimental subarachnoid hemorrhage: its prevention by intrathecal fibrinolysis with recombinant tissue plasminogen activator. *Neurosurgery* 1992;31(2):306–11; discussion 11–2.

45. Julow J. Prevention of subarachnoid fibrosis after subarachnoid haemorrhage with urokinase. Scanning electron microscopic study in the dog. *Acta Neurochir (Wien)* 1979;51(1–2):51–63.

46. Mayfrank L, Kissler J, Raoofi R, et al. Ventricular dilatation in experimental intraventricular hemorrhage in pigs. Characterization of cerebrospinal fluid dynamics and the effects of fibrinolytic treatment. *Stroke* 1997;28(1):141–8.

47. Pang D, Sclabassi RJ, Horton JA. Lysis of intraventricular blood clot with urokinase in a canine model: Part 3. Effects of intraventricular urokinase on clot lysis and posthemorrhagic hydrocephalus. *Neurosurgery* 1986;19(4):553–72.

48. Whitelaw A, Rivers RP, Creighton L, Gaffney P. Low dose intraventricular fibrinolytic treatment to prevent posthaemorrhagic hydrocephalus. *Arch Dis Child* 1992;67(1 Spec No):12–4.

49. Hanley DF, Lane K, McBee N, et al. Thrombolytic removal of intraventricular haemorrhage in treatment of severe stroke: results of the randomised, multicentre, multiregion, placebo-controlled CLEAR III trial. *Lancet* 2017.

50. Chotai S, Medel R, Herial NA, Medhkour A. External lumbar drain: A pragmatic test for prediction of shunt outcomes in idiopathic normal pressure hydrocephalus. *Surg Neurol Int* 2014;5:12.

51. Zacharia BE, Vaughan KA, Hickman ZL, et al. Predictors of long-term shunt-dependent hydrocephalus in patients with intracerebral hemorrhage requiring emergency cerebrospinal fluid diversion. *Neurosurg Focus* 2012;32(4):E5.

52. Zaidi HA, Montoure A, Elhadi A, et al. Long-term functional outcomes and predictors of shunt-dependent hydrocephalus after treatment of ruptured intracranial aneurysms in the BRAT trial: revisiting the clip vs coil debate. *Neurosurgery* 2015;76(5):608–13; discussion 13–4; quiz 14.

53. Mehta V, Holness RO, Connolly K, Walling S, Hall R. Acute hydrocephalus following aneurysmal subarachnoid hemorrhage. *Can J Neurol Sci* 1996;23(1):40–45.

54. Tso MK, Ibrahim GM, Macdonald RL. Predictors of shunt-dependent hydrocephalus following aneurysmal subarachnoid hemorrhage. *World Neurosurg* 2016;86: 226–32.

55. Erixon HO, Sorteberg A, Sorteberg W, Eide PK. Predictors of shunt dependency after aneurysmal subarachnoid hemorrhage: results of a single-center clinical trial. *Acta Neurochir (Wien)* 2014;156(11):2059–69.

56. Kandasamy J, Jenkinson MD, Mallucci CL. Contemporary management and recent advances in paediatric hydrocephalus. *BMJ* 2011;343:d4191.

57. Shprecher D, Schwalb J, Kurlan R. Normal pressure hydrocephalus: diagnosis and treatment. *Curr Neurol Neurosci Rep* 2008;8(5):371–6.

58. Chitale VR, Kasaliwal GT. Our experience of ventriculoatrial shunt using Upadhyaya valve in cases of hydrocephalus associated with tuberculous meningitis. *Prog Pediatr Surg* 1982;15:223–36.

59. Yadav YR, Parihar V, Sinha M. Lumbar peritoneal shunt. *Neurol India* 2010;58(2):179–84.

60. Kazui H, Miyajima M, Mori E, Ishikawa M, Investigators S. Lumboperitoneal shunt surgery for idiopathic normal pressure hydrocephalus (SINPHONI-2): an open-label randomised trial. *Lancet Neurol* 2015;14(6):585–94.

61. Browd SR, Ragel BT, Gottfried ON, Kestle JR. Failure of cerebrospinal fluid shunts: part I: Obstruction and mechanical failure. *Pediatr Neurol* 2006;34(2): 83–92.

62. Arriada N, Sotelo J. Review: treatment of hydrocephalus in adults. *Surg Neurol* 2002;58(6):377–84; discussion 84.

63. Kariyattil R, Steinbok P, Singhal A, Cochrane DD. Ascites and abdominal pseudocysts following ventriculoperitoneal shunt surgery: variations of the same theme. *J Neurosurg* 2007;106(5 Suppl):350–3.

64. Piatt JH, Jr., Carlson CV. A search for determinants of cerebrospinal fluid shunt survival: retrospective analysis of a 14-year institutional experience. *Pediatr Neurosurg* 1993;19(5):233–41; discussion 42.

65. Reddy GK, Bollam P, Shi R, Guthikonda B, Nanda A. Management of adult hydrocephalus with ventriculoperitoneal shunts: long-term single-institution experience. *Neurosurgery* 2011;69(4):774–80; discussion 80–1.

66. Sandberg DI. Endoscopic management of hydrocephalus in pediatric patients: a review of indications, techniques, and outcomes. *J Child Neurol* 2008;23(5):550–60.

67. Fritsch MJ, Kienke S, Ankermann T, Padoin M, Mehdorn HM. Endoscopic third ventriculostomy in infants. *J Neurosurg* 2005;103(Suppl 1):50–3.

68. Bilginer B, Oguz KK, Akalan N. Endoscopic third ventriculostomy for malfunction in previously shunted infants. *Childs Nerv Syst* 2009;25(6):683–8.

69. Boschert J, Hellwig D, Krauss JK. Endoscopic third ventriculostomy for shunt dysfunction in occlusive hydrocephalus: long-term follow up and review. *J Neurosurg* 2003;98(5):1032–9.

70. Chhun V, Sacko O, Boetto S, Roux FE. Third ventriculocisternostomy for shunt failure. *World Neurosurg* 2015;83(6):970–5.

71. Hader WJ, Walker RL, Myles ST, Hamilton M. Complications of endoscopic third ventriculostomy in previously shunted patients. *Neurosurgery* 2008;63(Suppl 1): ONS168–74; discussion ONS74–5.

72. Gangemi M, Mascari C, Maiuri F, Godano U, Donati P, Longatti PL. Long-term outcome of endoscopic third ventriculostomy in obstructive hydrocephalus. *Minim Invasive Neurosurg* 2007;50(5):265–9.

73. Gangemi M, Maiuri F, Naddeo M, et al. Endoscopic third ventriculostomy in idiopathic normal pressure hydrocephalus: an Italian multicenter study. *Neurosurgery* 2008;63(1):62–7; discussion 7–9.

74. Gangemi M, Maiuri F, Buonamassa S, Colella G, de Divitiis E. Endoscopic third ventriculostomy in idiopathic normal pressure hydrocephalus. *Neurosurgery* 2004;55(1):129–34; discussion 34.

75. Yadav YR, Parihar V, Pande S, Namdev H, Agarwal M. Endoscopic third ventriculostomy. *J Neurosci Rural Pract* 2012;3(2):163–73.

76. Yadav YR, Jaiswal S, Adam N, Basoor A, Jain G. Endoscopic third ventriculostomy in infants. *Neurol India* 2006;54(2):161–3.

77. Kamalo P. Exit ventriculoperitoneal shunt; enter endoscopic third ventriculostomy (ETV): contemporary views on hydrocephalus and their implications on management. *Malawi Med J* 2013;25(3):78–82.

78. Kandasamy J, Yousaf J, Mallucci C. Third ventriculostomy in normal pressure hydrocephalus. *World Neurosurg* 2013;79(Suppl 2):S22 e1–7.

79. Dewan MC, Naftel RP. The global rise of endoscopic third ventriculostomy with choroid plexus cauterization in pediatric hydrocephalus. *Pediatr Neurosurg* 2016.

80. Bhattathiri PS, Gregson B, Prasad KS, Mendelow AD, Investigators S. Intraventricular hemorrhage and hydrocephalus after spontaneous intracerebral hemorrhage: results from the STICH trial. *Acta Neurochir Suppl* 2006;96:65–8.

81. Bierbrauer KS, Storrs BB, McLone DG, Tomita T, Dauser R. A prospective, randomized study of shunt function and infections as a function of shunt placement. *Pediatr Neurosurg* 1990;16(6):287–91.

82. Choux M, Genitori L, Lang D, Lena G. Shunt implantation: reducing the incidence of shunt infection. *J Neurosurg* 1992;77(6):875–80.

83. Persson EK, Anderson S, Wiklund LM, Uvebrant P. Hydrocephalus in children born in 1999–2002: epidemiology, outcome and ophthalmological findings. *Childs Nerv Syst* 2007;23(10):1111–8.

84. Andersson S, Persson EK, Aring E, Lindquist B, Dutton GN, Hellstrom A. Vision in children with hydrocephalus. *Dev Med Child Neurol* 2006;48(10): 836–41.

85. Kokkonen J, Serlo W, Saukkonen AL, Juolasmaa A. Long-term prognosis for children with shunted hydrocephalus. *Childs Nerv Syst* 1994;10(6):384–7.

86. Kulkarni AV, Shams I. Quality of life in children with hydrocephalus: results from the hospital for sick children, Toronto. *J Neurosurg* 2007;107(5 Suppl): 358–64.

28

Vasospasm

J. F. Wang and S. Wahlster

ABSTRACT

Cerebral vasospasm can occur due to infectious and inflammatory aetiologies, medication drug effect and as part of the reversible cerebral vasoconstriction syndrome (RCVS)/posterior reversible encephalopathy syndrome (PRES) spectrum. Most commonly described in aneurysmal subarachnoid haemorrhage (aSAH), vasospasm and delayed cerebral ischaemia (DCI) are major prognostic determinants after aneurysm rupture. Radiographic appearance of blood on computed tomography (CT), clinical severity at presentation and smoking are major risk factors for DCI. Close neurological monitoring is essential—acute clinical changes, combined with increasing transcranial Doppler (TCD) velocities warrant further workup. Catheter angiogram is the best study to detect vasospasm. CT-angiography (CT-A), CT-perfusion (CT-P), quantitative electroencephalography (qEEG), microdialysis, and additional modalities can be helpful to monitor patients. Current preventative strategies include euvolemia, normotension, and oral nimodipine for 21 days. If vasospasm is detected, induced hypertension, angioplasty, or intra-arterial vasodilators can be attempted to improve outcomes. Further studies are needed to identify a better understanding of underlying mechanisms and treatment strategies.

KEYWORDS

Vasospasm; delayed cerebral ischaemia (DCI); aneurysmal subarachnoid haemorrhage (aSAH); nimodipine; transcranial Doppler (TCD); angiography; angiogram; intra-arterial vasodilators.

INTRODUCTION

Cerebral vasospasm refers to prolonged and potentially reversible narrowing of the intracranial vasculature. Multiple causes of vasospasm have been described, including infectious, inflammatory, and drug-related aetiologies. Vasospasm is most frequently described and currently known to be mainly relevant in the setting of aneurysmal subarachnoid haemorrhage (aSAH), which will be the major focus of this chapter.

AETIOLOGIES

In addition to vasospasm due to aSAH, an increasing number of conditions causing narrowing of the cerebral vasculature have been described. The presentation and clinical course can vary significantly, frequently depending on the underlying aetiology.

Vasospasm in the setting of an infectious process is most typically encountered with varicella zoster virus,[1] Treponema pallidum,[2] and Mycobacterium tuberculosis[3] as the underlying pathogen. Inflammatory causes include primary angiitis of the central nervous system (CNS),[4] sarcoidosis,[5] systemic lupus erythematosus, Behcet's syndrome, polyarteritis nodosa, and granulomatosis with polyangitis.[6] Cocaine use can increase the risk for a drug-induced vasculopathy and ischaemic stroke due to excessive sympathetic activity and subsequent vasoconstriction. There are also reports of cocaine and other sympathomimetic drugs associated with reversible cerebral vasoconstriction syndrome (RCVS) and posterior reversible encephalopathy syndrome (PRES).[7]

Reversible cerebral vasoconstriction syndrome and PRES are recently described disease entities, which are becoming more frequently diagnosed over the past decades because of their increased recognition by physicians as well as advances in neuroimaging. They share many clinical features and are thought to be a part of an overlapping disease spectrum. The pathophysiology is currently not completely understood, but dysfunctional autoregulation of the cerebral vasculature and blood–brain barrier (BBB) are thought to play a role. The clinical picture can mimic aSAH with sudden onset headaches and focal neurological deficits as common presenting symptoms. Reversible cerebral vasoconstriction syndrome can present with SAH in about 25% of cases. Identified risk factors include uncontrolled hypertension, pregnancy (+/- eclampsia), history of head trauma or migraines, consumption of street drugs as well as a number of inciting medications, including antidepressants (selective serotonin reuptake inhibitors[SSRIs]), immunosuppressive drugs (cyclosporine, tacrolimus, sirolimus), chemotherapeutic agents (cyclophosphamide, cisplatin, bevacizumab), and oral contraceptives.[7]

DEFINITION

Vasospasm after aSAH can refer to a clinical or radiographical phenomenon as well as a combination of both. The exact nomenclature varies across literature. Terms that are used, at times interchangeably, include vasospasm, delayed cerebral ischaemia (DCI), delayed ischaemic deficits, delayed ischaemic neurological deficit, secondary cerebral ischaemia, symptomatic vasospasm, and cerebral infarction.

In order to maintain a uniform nomenclature, we will use the terms vasospasm and DCI. We define vasospasm as vessel lumen visualized on angiography (with or without clinical symptoms), and will refer to DCI according to the following definition proposed by Vergowen et al. 'focal neurological impairment (such as hemiparesis, aphasia, apraxia, hemianopia, or neglect), or a decrease of at least 2 points on the Glasgow Coma Score (GCS) for at least 1 hour, not apparent immediately after aneurysm occlusion, which cannot be attributed to other causes by means of clinical assessment, CT or magnetic resonance imaging (MRI) scanning of the brain, and appropriate laboratory studies'.[1] The same group also defined cerebral infarction related to DCI as 'cerebral infarction on CT or MR scan of the brain within 6 weeks after SAH, or on the latest CT or MR scan made before death within 6 weeks, or proven at autopsy, not present on imaging between 24–48 hours after early aneurysm occlusion and not attributable to other causes such as surgical clipping or endovascular treatment or intraparenchymal haematoma'.[1]

PATHOPHYSIOLOGY

The exact process resulting in DCI is not completely understood. The presence of angiographic vasospasm is strongly associated with DCI and thought to be caused by the exposure of blood products to the abluminal side of the arterial vessels resulting in vasoconstriction and triggering a complex cascade. The key step in this process involves haemoglobin and other erythrocyte products inducing free oxygen radical reactions, inflammation, and endothelial injury, which ultimately lead to impaired production of nitric oxide (NO) and increased levels of endothelin-1 (E-1).[8] Nitric oxide is an endogenous vasodilator synthesized by various nitric oxide synthase (NOS) enzymes. Gene studies have identified specific single nucleotide polymorphism (Thr786Cys) in the gene encoding endothelial NOS predicting a higher susceptibility to vasospasm after aSAH.[9] Endothelin-1 is a vasoconstrictor produced by endothelial cells and its receptor antagonists have been shown to decrease vasospasm in a dose-dependent fashion.[10]

However, only about 50% of patients with vasospasm develop DCI. Loss of autoregulation, variations in collateral anastomotic blood flow as well as epigenetic and metabolic variations are thought to be additional relevant factors. Other processes hypothesized to contribute to the pathophysiology of DCI include microthrombi formation, microvascular constriction, inflammatory cascades, BBB disruption, delayed cell apoptosis, and cortical spreading ischaemia—it is believed that the co-presence of these mechanisms in combination with vasospasm ultimately triggers DCI.

CLINICAL RISK FACTORS

The best predictor of vasospasm and DCI is the radiographic appearance of initial CT scan.[11] Haemorrhage volume, location of aSAH, persistence of haemorrhage over time, and clot density are all associated with an increased risk of DCI.[12] A Fisher grade ≥3 on CT scan is predictive of DCI. This is mainly due to clot formation secondary to thick cisternal blood as well as the presence of intraventricular haemorrhage (IVH).[13] Risk for vasospasm is equally high for patients with IVH and thick cisternal blood, and even higher if both findings are present or bilateral IVH is seen.[14] The Modified Fisher Scale integrates the presence of IVH into the scoring system as a predictor of DCI.[15] Table 28.1 shows the scoring methodology for the Fisher Scale and Modified Fisher Scale. Figure 28.1 shows the odds ratio for developing vasospasm based on grading within the Modified Fisher Scale.

Table 28.1 Classification of modified and original Fisher Scale scores

SAH classification	IVH	Fisher grade	Modified Fisher grade
Diffuse Thick SAH	Present	3	4
	Absent	3	3
Localized Thick SAH	Present	3	4
	Absent	3	3
Diffuse Thin SAH	Present	4	2
	Absent	2	1
Localized Thin SAH	Present	4	2
	Absent	1	1
No SAH	Present	4	2
	Absent	1	0

Abbreviations: SAH: subarachnoid hemorrhage; IVH: intraventricular hemorrhage.
Reprinted with permission from: Frontera et al. Prediction of symptomatic vasospasm after subarachnoid haemorrhage: the modified fisher scale. *Neurosurgery* 2006;59(1):21–7[9].

Clinical severity based on other scoring systems such as the World Federation of Neurological Surgeons Scale (WFNSS), Hunt and Hess Scale (HHS), and GCS have also been shown to be predictors of DCI. A multivariate analysis demonstrated the WFNSS to be the strongest predictor of these three grading systems.[16] A study of 307 patients found that patients presenting with a WFNSS grade 1–3, no or thin aSAH on CT and age >68 had very low risk of DCI and might be candidates for less frequent monitoring.[17]

A meta-analysis of 52 studies reported strong evidence for a higher risk of DCI in smokers as well as moderate evidence for an increased risk in patients with hyperglycaemia, hydrocephalus, history of diabetes mellitus, and systemic inflammatory response syndrome (SIRS) at presentation.[18] There is limited evidence that female gender, Japanese descent, hypertension, younger patient age, cocaine use, a prior history of migraines or use of selective serotonin reuptake inhibitors (SSRIs) could be risk factors.

The location of the ruptured aneurysm has been implied as a risk factor with contrasting results between studies. Some series report higher incidence of vasospasm with anterior cerebral artery (ACA)[11,19] or middle cerebral artery (MCA) aneurysms (Figure 28.2),[20] while a number of studies indicate no relationship between location of aneurysm and incidence of vasospasm.[21,22] Ruptured posterior cerebral artery (PCA) aneurysms are less likely to result in DCI.[23] Of note, spontaneous perimesencephalic or prepontine aSAH, not associated with aneurysm rupture, typically tends to clear quickly with a low risk of vasospasm. A growing number of serum biomarkers, including interleukin-6 (IL-6), tumour necrosis factor (TNF), S100 calcium-binding protein B (S100b), von Willebrand factor (vWF), E-1, and vascular endothelial growth factor (VEGF) have shown an association with increased DCI risk. However, more studies are required to further validate these findings.

DIAGNOSIS

One of the most dreaded complications of aSAH, DCI is a major determinant of functional outcome[24] and can occur in up to 30% of patients.[24] Vasospasm and DCI after aSAH typically occur between day 3–12,[25] after the onset of symptoms. They reach a peak in incidence and severity between 7–10 days,[26] and resolve by 14–21 days. Close neurological monitoring during this time period is essential. Table 28.2 shows the sensitivity, specificity, positive predictive value, and negative predictive value of different testing modalities.

Table 28.2 Sensitivity and specificity of different diagnostic modalities for delayed cerebral ischaemia

	Sensitivity (95% CI)	Specificity (95% CI)	PPV (95% CI)	NPV (95% CI)
NCT	0.56 (0.37–0.73)	0.71 (0.45–0.88)	0.78 (0.55–0.91)	0.48 (0.28–0.68)
CTP	0.84 (0.65–0.93)	0.79 (0.52–0.92)	0.88 (0.69–0.96)	0.73 (0.48–0.89)
CTA Moderate to severe spasm	0.64 (0.45–0.80)	0.50 (0.27–0.73)	0.70 (0.49–0.84)	0.44 (0.23–0.67)
CTA Severe spasm	0.40 (0.23–0.59)	0.71 (0.45–0.88)	0.71 (0.45–0.88)	0.40 (0.23–0.45)

Reprinted with permission from: Dankbaar, et al. Diagnosing delayed cerebral ischemia with different CT modalities in patients with subarachnoid haemorrhage with clinical deterioration. *Stroke* 2009;40(11):3493–8.

Delayed cerebral ischaemia can present with worsening headache, meningismus, decreased level of consciousness, or focal deficits, which frequently localize to the parent vessel of the ruptured aneurysm and can include hemiparesis, aphasia, apraxia, and neglect. Symptoms typically manifest with a gradual onset and can be heralded by agitation or behavioural changes. Sudden elevations in blood pressure may suggest that the cerebral vasculature is attempting to compensate for decreases in cerebral blood flow (CBF).[27]

The clinical neurological examination is paramount to diagnosis, particularly in patients who are awake. When clinically suspected, additional diagnostic studies are indicated to ensure prompt detection and treatment of DCI. However, DCI is a diagnosis of exclusion. Differential diagnosis is broad, especially in medically complex patients with aSAH, and includes non-neurological (e.g., fever, infection, medication effect, hyponatraemia) as well as neurological causes (e.g., seizures, ischaemia related to the coiling/clipping procedure or neurogenic cardiac injury). These aetiologies need to be considered and quickly ruled out.

In conjunction with serial neurological examinations, transcranial Doppler (TCD) is a non-invasive test that is used to screen for the development of vasospasm.[28,29] Ultimately, catheter angiogram is the gold standard diagnostic test and also allows for interventional treatments. The index of suspicion for DCI needs to be weighed against the risk of subjecting the patient to this invasive procedure. Diagnostic modalities that can provide additional information include CT-angiography (CT-A) and CT-perfusion (CT-P).[30,31] Continuous electroencephalogram (cEEG, MRI, brain tissue oxygen monitoring, and near-infrared spectroscopy[32] are newer that can provide additional information. However, their clinical utility is limited and their use is not considered standard practice at this point.

Transcranial Doppler

As a non-invasive, cost-effective, easily acquired bedside examination, TCD is a part of routine monitoring for patients with aSAH. Vasospasm typically manifests on TCD as increased velocities due to changes in vessel width. Transcranial Dopplers are usually obtained as early as the first or second day after aSAH to obtain a baseline, prior to the typical onset of vasospasm, and then repeated daily over the next 14 days. Sudden changes in the trend, especially concomitant with changes in neurological examination, should raise concern for vasospasm and trigger further diagnostic workup such as CT-A or

catheter angiogram. Figure 28.3 shows CT-A and catheter angiogram examples of vasospasm.

Vasospasm on TCD is often defined as increased mean blood flow velocities >120 cm/s or peak flow velocities >200 cm/s in the MCAs, but numbers need to be interpreted in a clinical context. Lindegaard ratio of MCA/ICA velocities >3 can help differentiate between hyperaemia (ratio is <3) and vasospasm (ratio >3).[33,34]

Transcranial Dopplers are operator dependent and require an experienced user. Thick temporal bones may preclude insonation and therefore some patients will not have an 'adequate window.' False positives can be seen with augmented blood pressure, and false negatives can occur due to diminished blood flow of various aetiologies. Other factors that influence cerebral flow velocity include fever, volume status, and acute changes in haematocrit.

Angiography

Catheter angiogram remains the gold standard diagnostic test. However, it can be difficult to determine whether the study is indicated, especially in patients with poor neurological status in whom it can be difficult to detect significant changes. Several studies show good correlations between catheter angiogram and CT-A.[35–37] In general, CT-A tends to overestimate the degree of stenosis and therefore can be a sensitive screening test to determine whether the patient is an appropriate candidate for an endovascular study, especially when there is uncertainty about the clinical presence of vasospasm. At times, the study can be limited due to 'beam-hardening' artefacts from clips/coils. Computed tomography-perfusion is another diagnostic tool, related to CT-A, that assesses CBF in terms of mean transit time and can identify patients with cerebral hypoperfusion and risk for infarction.[30,31] The study can be limited in patients with poor cardiac output.

Electroencephalogram (EEG)

In addition to detecting seizure activity, EEG is sensitive to cerebral ischaemia and has been shown to correlate with CBF in carotid endarterectomy.[38] Patterns found during ischaemia include focal attenuation, loss of fast activity, loss of sleep spindles, and 'axial bursts.' There is increasing interest in cEEG monitoring in aSAH patients, offering a real-time and non-invasive approach to monitor broad regions of the brain. Quantitative EEG (qEEG) analyses findings on cEEG, such as frequency, amplitude, and rhythm are used to computationally generate numerical values and ratios that can be clinically useful in diagnosing DCI. Studies have found that specific patterns, such as changes in alpha–delta ratio and alpha variability can detect evolution of DCI before clinical deterioration is noted.[39] Currently, the value of cEEG in aSAH patients is still being investigated and concerned findings should always be correlated with the clinical picture. A major challenge will be to ensure timely review of large data files by neurophysiology experts. Some of the quantitative modalities may allow for more efficient screening and easier interpretation by providers with no specific EEG expertise.

PREVENTION

Haemodynamic augmentation therapy or 'Triple H' therapy (hypertension, hypervolaemia, and haemodilution) was previously considered the standard of care for vasospasm prophylaxis. Multiple systematic reviews have since found that there is no evidence to support the use of these therapies as prophylaxis has the possibility of cardiopulmonary and renal complications.[40,41] We later discuss the use of haemodynamic augmentation as a treatment after vasospasm. In recent practice, there has been a shift from 'Triple H' therapy to maintenance of euvolemia and normotension.

Hyponatraemia, frequently encountered in aSAH patients, may increase the risk for vasospasm and is associated with cerebral infarction in poor-grade patients.[42,43] Common aetiologies include syndrome of inappropriate antidiuretic hormone secretion (SIADH) and cerebral salt wasting. Importantly, hyponatraemia in the setting of aSAH should not be treated with fluid restriction but rather with 3% hypertonic saline, combined with fludrocortisone administration (0.3 mg/day) in refractory cases. Hyponatraemia encountered in aSAH tends to be a time-limited process, which frequently spontaneously resolves after 14–21 days.

Anaemia has been associated with a higher likelihood of vasospasm and poor outcome in aSAH patients. However, the liberal use of blood transfusions and higher haemoglobin thresholds have not been shown to improve outcomes and are associated with increased medical complications.

Despite extensive research and numerous trials, effective medical therapies for preventing vasospasm are limited. Nimodipine is an L-type calcium channel antagonist counteracting the influx of calcium into vascular smooth muscle. While nimodipine has not been shown to be effective in preventing angiographic vasospasm, multiple randomized controlled trials (RCTs) have shown that prophylactic oral nimodipine improves outcome and reduces DCI and mortality.[44,45] A Cochrane review

found that the relative risk of poor outcome defined by most trials as death or dependence assessed between one and six months, when oral nimodipine was compared to control was 0.67 (95% CI 0.55–0.81).[45] Nimodipine is dosed at 60 mg every 4 hours and typically given for 21 days. In some patients who experience hypotension or major blood pressure drops after receiving nimodipine, the dose can be adjusted to 30 mg every 2 hours. Trials assessing the effect of intrathecal nimodipine are currently underway.

Several clinical trials have evaluated the utility of statins, endothelin-1 antagonists, anti-inflammatory drugs, dantrolene, magnesium, and antiplatelets as prophylaxis for vasospasm and DCI. There have been inconsistent results across small clinical trials regarding statin therapy. A recent meta-analysis found that prophylactic statin therapy did not produce a statistically significant reduction in TCD vasospasm, DCI, poor neurological outcome, or death.[46] A larger phase III trial using prophylactic statin therapy is underway. Clazosentan is an E-1 receptor antagonist that has shown reduced incidence of angiographic vasospasm[10] but subsequent trials failed to show benefit on clinical outcomes.[47] Several meta-analyses have found that magnesium was associated with a reduced incidence of DCI, but found no benefit in clinical outcomes.[48,49] A Cochrane review evaluated seven clinical trials utilizing antiplatelets as prophylaxis and found that poor outcome and DCI occurred less frequently, but the results were not statistically significant and patients on antiplatelets may have a higher risk of bleeding.[50] Therefore, antiplatelet agents after aSAH are not recommended.

Other treatments that have been investigated as potential preventative strategies include prophylactic angioplasty, intrathecal thrombolytic therapy, and continuous lumbar drainage. A phase II multicentre RCT found a reduction in the need for therapeutic angioplasty after prophylactic transluminal balloon angioplasty, but did not demonstrate a statistically significant benefit in primary outcome (Glasgow Outcome Score) and procedure-related vessel perforation led to poor outcomes in some patients.[51] Intrathecal thrombolytics are postulated to increase the clearance of blood in the ventricles and basal cisterns. A meta-analysis of five RCTs found significant reduction in poor outcomes, angiographic vasospasm, DCI, and hydrocephalus. However, there were significant differences in thrombolytic drug selection and administration method between trials, problems with randomization, and lack of distinguishing placebo.[52] Additional studies are needed before implementation in standard practice. Lumbar drainage after aSAH is hypothesized to promote

CSF circulation in the ventricles through subarachnoid spaces, evacuating a large reservoir of bloody CSF from the spinal cisterns, and removing spasmogenic agents in the cerebrospinal fluid. A retrospective analysis demonstrated that patients who underwent lumbar drain versus extraventricular drain (EVD) for symptomatic hydrocephalus had better outcomes.[53] However, this study was not randomized and therefore selection of patients in this study is questionable. A recent RCT found no benefit of lumbar drains and a higher rate of complications.[54]

TREATMENT

After making the diagnosis of vasospasm and/or DCI, there are several treatment options aimed at increasing cerebral perfusion, including haemodynamic augmentation, balloon angioplasty, and intra-arterially administered vasodilators.

As discussed above, prophylaxis against DCI includes euvolemia and maintenance of cerebral perfusion. In the setting of DCI, haemodynamic augmentation with induced hypertension using vasoactive agents has been linked with improved neurological outcome in case series.[55,56] The most common agents used in current practice are phenylephrine and norepinephrine, with initial goal blood pressure as a predefined target or a percentage increase from baseline blood pressure. The use of ionotropic agents such as dobutamine or milrinone are reasonable in the appropriate clinical context and may be considered in patients with concomitant heart failure. It is generally accepted that reassessing neurological status after reaching the initial goal is needed to determine if the treatment was adequate or a higher blood pressure goal is warranted. Induced hypertension is also not unreasonable in the setting of DCI and nimodipine-related hypotension. It is important to monitor intravascular volume status and signs of cardiopulmonary or renal complications resulting from induced hypertension.

Endovascular treatment such as percutaneous transluminal angioplasty (PTA) and/or intra-arterial (IA) vasodilators can be useful in DCI. Percutaneous transluminal angioplasty, also known as transluminal balloon angioplasty, is one of the most common endovascular interventions. Angiogram is first performed to identify arterial narrowing that could be responsible for neurological deficits. If identified, successive gradual balloon dilations are performed and adjunctive IA vasodilator therapy may also be administered concurrently. Clinical outcomes following PTA are quite variable in literature and a recent review found that 62% of patients showed clinical improvement

and TCD velocities on average improved by 69%.[57] A single randomized controlled trial of early prophylactic angioplasty after aSAH without angiographic vasospasm suggested a lower risk of DCI, but the risk of procedural complications ultimately resulted in no difference in outcomes.[51] Therefore, endovascular treatments are generally reserved for DCI that is not responsive to medical treatment and before neurologic deficits become permanent. Percutaneous transluminal angioplasty is limited to proximal large vessels, as it has limited ability to reach distal (i.e., distal MCA) or sharply angled vessels (e.g., ACA). In those cases, intra-arterial vasodilator therapy alone may be the treatment of choice. Possible PTA-related complications include vessel rupture, arterial dissection, thromboembolism, reperfusion haemorrhage, branch occlusion, retroperitoneal haematoma, and groin haematoma at the catheter site.

Intra-arterial vasodilators are often used in conjunction with PTA or alone in cases of vasospasm not amenable to balloon angioplasty such as distal vessels or diffuse non-focal disease. After identifying a potential treatment target by digital subtraction angiography (DSA), infusion of a vasodilator is started with monitoring of blood pressure, intracranial pressure, and neurological status. A wide range of pharmacological agents are used with papaverine, nimodipine, and nicardipine being the most common. Intra-arterial verapamil and milrinone have also been described, but the use of these agents is still largely under investigation. There is insufficient literature to guide the timing of intervention, need for re-treatment, clinical triggers for intervention and duration of treatment.[58] Therefore, these parameters vary widely between institutions and provider preference.

CONCLUSIONS

Vasospasm and DCI are serious causes of morbidity and mortality in patients who survive aneurysm rupture. A high index of suspicion should be maintained during the first 14 days after index aSAH, the period in which vasospasm usually occurs. Serial neurological examinations and TCDs are the mainstay screening tools. While catheter angiogram is the gold standard diagnostic tool and also allows intra-arterial vasodilator treatment after diagnosis is established, there are many other diagnostic tools used in practice and currently under investigation. The care of patients with aSAH has advanced significantly in recent decades, but further research is needed to improve understanding of pathophysiology, prophylaxis, diagnostic tools, and treatment of vasospasm.

REFERENCES

1. Gilden D, Cohrs RJ, Mahalingam R, Nagel MA. Varicella zoster virus vasculopathies: diverse clinical manifestations, laboratory features, pathogenesis, and treatment. *Lancet Neurol* 2009;8(8):731–40.

2. Flint AC, Liberato BB, Anziska Y, Schantz-Dunn J, Wright CB. Meningovascular syphilis as a cause of basilar artery stenosis. *Neurology* 2005;64(2):391–2.

3. Garg RK. Tuberculosis of the central nervous system. *Postgrad Med J.* 1999;75(881):133–40.

4. Salvarani C, Brown RD Jr, Calamia KT. Primary central nervous system vasculitis: analysis of 101 patients. *Ann Neurol* 2007 Nov;62(5):442–51.

5. Hoitsma E, Faber CG, Drent M, Sharma OP. Neurosarcoidosis: a clinical dilemma. *Lancet Neurol* 2004 Jul;3(7):397–407.

6. Calabrese LH, Duna GF, Lie JT. Vasculitis in the central nervous system. *Arthritis Rheum* 1997 Jul;40(7):1189–201.

7. Singhal AB, Hajj-Ali RA, Topcuoglu MA, Fok J, Bena J, Yang D, Calabrese LH. Reversible cerebral vasoconstriction syndromes: analysis of 139 cases. *Arch Neurol* 2011;68(8):1005–12.

8. Pluta RM, Hansen-Schwartz J, Dreier J, Vajkoczy P, Macdonald RL, et al. Cerebral vasospasm following subarachnoid hemorrhage: time for a new world of thought. *Neurol Res* 2009;31(2):151–8.

9. Khurana VG, Sohni YR, Mangrum WI, McClelland RL, O'Kane DJ, Meyer FB, Meissner I. Endothelial nitric oxide synthase gene polymorphisms predict susceptibility to aneurysmal subarachnoid hemorrhage and cerebral vasospasm. *J Cereb Blood Flow Metab* 2004;24(3):291–7.

10. Macdonald RL, et al. Clazosentan to overcome neurological ischemia and infarction occurring after subarachnoid hemorrhage (CONSCIOUS-1): randomized, double-blind, placebo-controlled phase 2 dose-finding trial. *Stroke* 2008;39(11):3015–21.

11. Fisher CM, Kistler JP, Davis JM. Relation of cerebral vasospasm to subarachnoid hemorrhage visualized by computerized tomographic scanning. *Neurosurgery* 1980;6(1):1–9.

12. Reilly C, et al. Clot volume and clearance rate as independent predictors of vasospasm after aneurysmal subarachnoid hemorrhage. *J Neurosurg* 2004;101(2):255–61.

13. Rosen DS, Macdonald RL. Subarachnoid hemorrhage grading scales: a systematic review. *Neurocrit Care* 2005;2(2):110–8.

14. Claassen J, et al. Effect of cisternal and ventricular blood on risk of delayed cerebral ischemia after subarachnoid hemorrhage: the Fisher scale revisited. *Stroke* 2001;32(9):2012–20.

15. Frontera JA, et al. Prediction of symptomatic vasospasm after subarachnoid hemorrhage: the modified fisher scale. *Neurosurgery* 2006;59(1):21–7; discussion 21–7.

16. Chiang VL, Claus EB, Awad IA. Toward more rational prediction of outcome in patients with high-grade subarachnoid hemorrhage. *Neurosurgery* 2000;46(1):28–35; discussion 35–6.

17. Crobeddu E, et al. Predicting the lack of development of delayed cerebral ischemia after aneurysmal subarachnoid hemorrhage. *Stroke* 2012;43(3):697–701.

18. de Rooij NK, et al. Delayed cerebral ischemia after subarachnoid hemorrhage: a systematic review of clinical, laboratory, and radiological predictors. *Stroke* 2013;44(1):43–54.

19. Abla AA, Wilson DA, Williamson RW, Nakaji P, McDougall CG, et al. The relationship between ruptured aneurysm location, subarachnoid hemorrhage clot thickness, and incidence of radiographic or symptomatic vasospasm in patients enrolled in a prospective randomized controlled trial. *J Neurosurg* 2014;120(2):391–7.

20. Graf CJ, Nibbelink DW. Cooperative study of intracranial aneurysms and subarachnoid hemorrhage. Report on a randomized treatment study. 3. Intracranial surgery. *Stroke* 1974;5(4):557–601.

21. Niizuma H, et al. [Angiographical study on cerebral vasospasm following rupture of intracranial aneurysm (2nd report) (author's transl)]. *No Shinkei Geka* 1978;6(9):863–9.

22. Saito I, Sano K. Vasospasm following rupture of cerebral aneurysms. *Neurol Med Chir (Tokyo)* 1979;19(1):103–7.

23. McGirt MJ, et al. Leukocytosis as an independent risk factor for cerebral vasospasm following aneurysmal subarachnoid hemorrhage. *J Neurosurg* 2003;98(6):1222–6.

24. Vergouwen MD, Ilodigwe D, Macdonald RL. Cerebral infarction after subarachnoid hemorrhage contributes to poor outcome by vasospasm-dependent and -independent effects. *Stroke* 2011;42(4):924–9.

25. Weir B, Grace M, Hansen J, Rothberg C. Time course of vasospasm in man. *J Neurosurg* 1978 Feb;48(2):173–8.

26. Dorsch NW, King MT. A review of cerebral vasospasm in aneurysmal subarachnoid haemorrhage Part I: Incidence and effects. *J Clin Neurosci* 1994 Jan;1(1):19–26.

27. Connolly ES Jr, Rabinstein AA, Carhuapoma JR, et al. American Heart Association Stroke Council; Council on Cardiovascular Radiology and Intervention; Council on Cardiovascular Nursing; Council on Cardiovascular Surgery and Anesthesia; Council on Clinical Cardiology. Guidelines for the management of aneurysmal subarachnoid hemorrhage: a guideline for healthcare professionals from the American Heart Association/American Stroke Association. *Stroke* 2012 Jun;43(6):1711–37.

28. Seiler R, Grolimund P, Huber P. Transcranial Doppler sonography. An alternative to angiography in the evaluation of vasospasm after subarachnoid hemorrhage. *Acta Radiol Suppl* 1986;369:99–102.

29. Lindegaard KF, Nornes H, Bakke SJ, Sorteberg W, Nakstad P. Cerebral vasospasm after subarachnoid haemorrhage investigated by means of transcranial Doppler ultrasound. *Acta Neurochir Suppl (Wien)* 1988;42:81–4.

30. Mir DI, Gupta A, Dunning A, et al. CT perfusion for detection of delayed cerebral ischemia in aneurysmal subarachnoid hemorrhage: a systematic review and meta-analysis. *AJNR Am J Neuroradiol* 2014 May;35(5):866–71.

31. Dankbaar JW, de Rooij NK, Velthuis BK, Frijns CJ, Rinkel GJ, van der Schaaf IC. Diagnosing delayed cerebral ischemia with different CT modalities in patients with subarachnoid hemorrhage with clinical deterioration. *Stroke* 2009;40(11):3493–8.

32. Hänggi D. Participants in the International Multi-Disciplinary Consensus Conference on the Critical Care Management of Subarachnoid Hemorrhage. Monitoring and detection of vasospasm II: EEG and invasive monitoring. *Neurocrit Care* 2011 Sep;15(2):318–23.

33. Vora YY, Suarez-Almazor M, Steinke DE, Martin ML, Findlay JM. Role of transcranial Doppler monitoring in the diagnosis of cerebral vasospasm after subarachnoid haemorrhage. *Neurosurgery* 1999;44(6):1237–47; discussion 1247–8.

34. Gonzalez NR, Boscardin WJ, Glenn T, Vinuela F, Martin NA. Vasospasm probability index: a combination of transcranial doppler velocities, cerebral blood flow, and clinical risk factors to predict cerebral vasospasm after aneurysmal subarachnoid hemorrhage. *J Neurosurg* 2007 Dec;107(6):1101–12.

35. Yoon DY, Choi CS, Kim KH, Cho BM. Multidetector-row CT angiography of cerebral vasospasm after aneurysmal subarachnoid hemorrhage: comparison of volume-rendered images and digital subtraction angiography. *AJNR Am J Neuroradiol* 2006 Feb;27(2):370–7.

36. Anderson GB, Ashforth R, Steinke DE, Findlay JM. CT angiography for the detection of cerebral vasospasm in patients with acute subarachnoid hemorrhage. *AJNR Am J Neuroradiol* 2000 Jun–Jul;21(6):1011–5.

37. Chaudhary SR, Ko N, Dillon WP, et al. Prospective evaluation of multidetector-row CT angiography for the diagnosis of vasospasm following subarachnoid hemorrhage: a comparison with digital subtraction angiography. *Cerebrovasc Dis* 2008;25(1–2):144–50.

38. Sharbrough FW, Messick JM, Sundt TM. Correlation of continuous electroencephalograms with cerebral blood flow measurements during carotid endarterectomy. *Stroke* 1973;4(4):674–83.

39. Rots ML, et al. Continuous EEG monitoring for early detection of delayed cerebral ischemia in subarachnoid hemorrhage: a pilot study. *Neurocrit Care* 2016;24(2):207–16.

40. Treggiari MM, et al. Systematic review of the prevention of delayed ischemic neurological deficits with hypertension, hypervolemia, and hemodilution therapy following subarachnoid hemorrhage. *J Neurosurg* 2003;98(5):978–84.

41. Rinkel GJ, et al. Circulatory volume expansion therapy for aneurysmal subarachnoid haemorrhage. *Cochrane Database Syst Rev* 2004(4):CD000483.

42. McGirt MJ, et al. Correlation of serum brain natriuretic peptide with hyponatremia and delayed ischemic neurological deficits after subarachnoid hemorrhage. *Neurosurgery* 2004;54(6):1369–73; discussion 1373–4.

43. Zheng B, et al. A predictive value of hyponatremia for poor outcome and cerebral infarction in high-grade aneurysmal subarachnoid haemorrhage patients. *J Neurol Neurosurg Psychiatry* 2011;82(2):213–7.

44. Barker FG, Ogilvy CS. Efficacy of prophylactic nimodipine for delayed ischemic deficit after subarachnoid hemorrhage: a metaanalysis. *J Neurosurg* 1996;84(3):405–14.

45. Dorhout Mees SM, et al. Calcium antagonists for aneurysmal subarachnoid haemorrhage. *Cochrane Database Syst Rev* 2007(3):CD000277.

46. Vergouwen MD, et al. Effect of statin treatment on vasospasm, delayed cerebral ischemia, and functional outcome in patients with aneurysmal subarachnoid hemorrhage: a systematic review and meta-analysis update. *Stroke* 2010;41(1):e47–52.

47. Macdonald RL, et al. Clazosentan, an endothelin receptor antagonist, in patients with aneurysmal subarachnoid haemorrhage undergoing surgical clipping: a randomised, double-blind, placebo-controlled phase 3 trial (CONSCIOUS-2). *Lancet Neurol* 2011;10(7):618–25.

48. Reddy D, et al. Prophylactic magnesium sulfate for aneurysmal subarachnoid hemorrhage: a systematic review and meta-analysis. *Neurocrit Care* 2014;21(2):356–64.

49. Zhao XD, et al. A meta analysis of treating subarachnoid hemorrhage with magnesium sulfate. *J Clin Neurosci* 2009;16(11):1394–7.

50. Dorhout Mees SM, et al. Antiplatelet therapy for aneurysmal subarachnoid haemorrhage. *Cochrane Database Syst Rev* 2007(4):CD006184.

51. Zwienenberg-Lee M, Hartman J, Rudisill N, Madden LK, Smith K, et al. Effect of prophylactic transluminal balloon angioplasty on cerebral vasospasm and outcome in patients with Fisher grade III subarachnoid hemorrhage: results of a phase II multicenter, randomized, clinical trial. *Stroke* 2008;39(6):1759–65.

52. Kramer AH, Fletcher JJ. Locally-administered intrathecal thrombolytics following aneurysmal subarachnoid hemorrhage: a systematic review and meta-analysis. *Neurocrit Care* 2011;14(3):489–99.

53. Klimo P, et al. Marked reduction of cerebral vasospasm with lumbar drainage of cerebrospinal fluid after subarachnoid hemorrhage. *J Neurosurg* 2004;100(2):215–24.

54. Olson DM, et al. Continuous cerebral spinal fluid drainage associated with complications in patients admitted with subarachnoid hemorrhage. *J Neurosurg* 2013;119(4):974–80.

55. Kosnik EJ, Hunt WE. Postoperative hypertension in the management of patients with intracranial arterial aneurysms. *J Neurosurg* 1976;45(2):148–54.

56. Brown FD, Hanlon K, Mullan S. Treatment of aneurysmal hemiplegia with dopamine and mannitol. *J Neurosurg* 1978;49(4):525–9.

57. Hoh BL, Ogilvy CS. Endovascular treatment of cerebral vasospasm: transluminal balloon angioplasty, intra-arterial papaverine, and intra-arterial nicardipine. *Neurosurg Clin N Am* 2005;16(3):501–16, vi.

58. Diringer MN, Bleck TP, Claude Hemphill J 3rd, Menon D, Shutter L, et al. Critical care management of patients following aneurysmal subarachnoid hemorrhage: recommendations from the Neurocritical Care Society's Multidisciplinary Consensus Conference. *Neurocrit Care* 2011;15(2):211–40.

29

Pneumocephalus

A. Lele

ABSTRACT

The presence of intracranial air can be expected in all patients after craniotomies. However, the presence of large quantities of air causing neurological deficits can occur sometimes with disastrous side effects. Prompt radiological diagnosis and appropriate medical and/or surgical interventions can often reduce morbidity and mortality.

KEYWORDS

Pneumocephalus, tension, skull fracture, hyperoxia, lumbar drain.

INTRODUCTION

Pneumocephalus is essentially a radiographic diagnosis of accumulation of gas within the intracranial vault which poses a major clinical significance. Commonly seen on post-craniotomy neuroimaging studies, a large amount of pneumocephalus (tension) has been known to cause significant decline in neurological function, including cerebral herniation. This chapter presents readers with up to date information regarding the following aspects of pneumocephalus: Epidemiology, types of pneumocephalus, its clinical presentation, radiographic diagnosis, clinical management, and complications.

EPIDEMIOLOGY AND MECHANISM OF PNEUMOCEPHALUS

Epidemiology

The exact incidence of pneumocephalus is largely unknown, as clinically insignificant pneumocephalus is mostly unreported.

Data from a large case series on patients with head injuries suggest incidence of pneumocephalus to be about 9.7%.[1] The reported incidence of postoperative pneumocephalus is 42%.[2] In patients after pituitary tumour resection, pneumocephalus is a rare occurrence, and only reported in 2 out of 480 transphenoidal surgeries in one case series.[3]

Mechanisms of Pneumocephalus

There are two theories about the accumulation of air within the intracranial vault: (1) the inverted bottle theory and (2) the ball-value theory.[4]

The inverted bottle theory proposes the creation of supratentorial pneumocephalus in patients undergoing posterior fossa surgeries where air entry into the intracranial compartment is similar to air entry into an inverted soda-pop bottle which prompted Lunsford and colleagues to call it the 'inverted pop-bottle syndrome'.[5] On the other hand, in the ball-valve theory, positive pressure such as during sneezing, coughing, and Valsalva manoeuvres can force air through a cranial defect.[4]

TYPES OF PNEUMOCEPHALUS

The major types (and their causes) of pneumocephalus are highlighted in Table 29.1.

CLINICAL PRESENTATION

The clinical presentation can be varied, from asymptomatic incidental finding on brain computed tomography (CT) images to cerebral herniation.[6,7]

The common symptoms include headaches, nausea, vomiting, irritability, dizziness and seizures. A gurgling sensation in the head has also been reported.[8]

Table 29.1 Types and causes of pneumocephalus

Type	Common causes
Traumatic	• Traumatic brain injury, skull fracture • Cranio-facial trauma with fractures of air sinuses or skull base[*]
Post-surgical	• Transphenoidal pituitary surgery (TSS) • Post-craniotomy • Posterior fossa surgeries[**] • Surgeries performed in a sitting position[#] • VP shunt placement
Spontaneous (non-traumatic)	• Otogenic pneumocephalus[##] • Gas producing organisms such as Klebsiella and Bacteroides, *Escherichia coli*, Peptosptreptococcus, Fusobacterium species, and *Streptococcus pyogenes*[@] • Tumours (epidermoid, etc.)[@@]
Complications of positive pressure ventilation	• Use of BIPAP or CPAP in patients with obstructive sleep apnoea in a postoperative setting after nasal or pituitary procedures
Complications of neuraxial and cranial procedures	• Lumbar drain (complication of overdrainage)[$] • Epidural catheter placement (loss of resistance to air technique)[$$] • Intraventricular pneumocephalus complicating external ventricular drain placement/removal[>]
Complications of hyperbaric oxygen therapy	• Extradural collection of air[>>] • Tension pneumocephalus in a patient with CSF leak[>>>]

Abbreviations: BIPAP: bi-level positive airway pressure; CPAP: continuous positive airway pressure; CSF: cerebrospinal fluid.

Sources:

*(1) Filipowicz Z. [Spontaneous traumatic pneumocephalus in fractures of the anterior cranial fossa]. *Chir Narzadow Ruchu Ortop Pol* 1963;28: 569–73. (2) Ruberti R, Benedetti A. [Considerations on some complications of cranial fractures involving the pneumatic cranio-facial cavities]. *Chir Ital* 1964;16:431–44. (3) Hubner K. [Acute complications of skull base fractures]. *Z Arztl Fortbild (Jena)* 1968;62(6):326–8. (4) Turner JS, Jr. Pneumocephalus with facial fractures. *Laryngoscope* 1968;78(5):713–26. (5) Jefferson A, Reilly G. Fractures of the floor of the anterior cranial fossa. The selection of patients for dural repair. *Br J Surg* 1972;59(8):585–92. (6) Mifka P. [Roentgenologic differential diagnosis of skull fractures]. *Hefte Unfallheilkd* 1972;111:45–49. (7) Mikulickova H, Bukackova A, Beran J, Krivanek M. [Pneumocephalus as a rare complication of mid-facial fractures]. *Cesk Stomatol* 1972;72(4):285–8. (8) Gaillard J, Haguenauer JP, Gignoux B, Dumolard P. [Fractures of the frontal sinus: therapeutic procedure]. *Ann Otolaryngol Chir Cervicofac* 1973;90(12):741–4. (9) Cesteleyn L, Akuamo-Boateng E, Kovacs B, Claeys TH, Bremerich A, Smith RG. [Complications of orbito-frontobasal fractures]. *Acta Stomatol Belg* 1992;89(2):95–112. (10) Mercuri V, House RJ. Temporomandibular joint air in fractures of the skull base. *Australas Radiol* 1992;36(2):129–30.

**(1) Steudel WI, Hacker H. Prognosis, incidence and management of acute traumatic intracranial pneumocephalus. A retrospective analysis of 49 cases. *Acta Neurochir (Wien)* 1986;80(3–4):93–99. (2) Sloan T. The incidence, volume, absorption, and timing of supratentorial pneumocephalus during posterior fossa neurosurgery conducted in the sitting position. *J Neurosurg Anesthesiol* 2010;22(1):59–66. (3) Satyarthee GD, Mahapatra AK. Tension pneumocephalus following transsphenoid surgery for pituitary adenoma—report of two cases. *J Clin Neurosci* 2003;10(4):495–7. (4) Schirmer CM, Heilman CB, Bhardwaj A. Pneumocephalus: case illustrations and review. *Neurocrit Care* 2010;13(1):152–8. (5) Lunsford LD, Maroon JC, Sheptak PE, Albin MS. Subdural tension pneumocephalus. Report of two cases. *J Neurosurg* 1979;50(4):525–7. (6) Celikoglu E, Hazneci J, Ramazanoglu AF. Tension pneumocephalus causing brain herniation after endoscopic sinus surgery. *Asian J Neurosurg* 2016;11(3): 309–10. (7) Foo LL, Chaw SH, Chan L, Ganesan D, Karuppiah R. [Intractable intraoperative brain herniation secondary to tension pneumocephalus: a rare life-threatening complication during drainage of subdural empyema]. *Rev Bras Anestesiol* 2016. (8) Dabdoub CB, Salas G, Silveira Edo N, Dabdoub CF. Review of the management of pneumocephalus. *Surg Neurol Int* 2015;6:155. (9) Karavelioglu E, Eser O, Haktanir A. Pneumocephalus and pneumorrhachis after spinal surgery: case report and review of the literature. *Neurol Med Chir (Tokyo)* 2014;54(5):405–7. (10) Steudel WI, Hacker H. Acute intracranial pneumocephalus: prognosis and management—a retrospective analysis of 101 cases. *Neurosurg Rev* 1989;12(Suppl 1):125–36. (11) Heckmann JG, Ganslandt O. Images in clinical medicine. The Mount Fuji sign. *N Engl J Med* 2004;350(18):1881. (12) Michel SJ. The Mount Fuji sign. *Radiology* 2004;232(2):449–50. (13) Beiko J, McDonald P. Tension pneumocephalus–the Mount Fuji sign. *Can J Neurol Sci* 2005;32(4):538–9. (14) Mattick A, Goodwin P. Mount Fuji sign on CT following trauma. *J Trauma* 2005;59(1):254. (15) Vanhoenacker FM, Herz R, Vandervliet EJ, Parizel PM. The Mount Fuji sign in tension pneumocephalus. *JBR-BTR* 2008;91(4):175. (16) Agrawal A, Singh BR. Mount Fuji sign with concavo-convex appearance of epidural haematoma in a patient with tension pneumocephalus. *J Radiol Case Rep* 2009;3(1):10–12. (17) Yamashita S, Tsuchimochi W, Yonekawa T, Kyoraku I, Shiomi K, Nakazato M. The Mount Fuji sign on MRI. *Intern Med* 2009;48(17):1567–8. (18) Shaikh N, Masood I, Hanssens Y, Louon A, Hafiz A. Tension pneumocephalus as complication of burr-hole drainage of chronic subdural haematoma: A case report. *Surg Neurol Int* 2010;1. (19) Nimjee SM, Zomorodi AR, Adamson DC. Conquering mount fuji: resolution of tension pneumocephalus with a foley urinary catheter. *Case Rep Radiol* 2011:164316. (20) Perez Redondo M, Alcantara Carmona S, Carrascosa Granada A. [Mount Fuji sign: tension pneumoencephalus]. *Med Intensiva* 2011;35(3):199.

(Cont'd)

Table 29.1 (*Cont'd*)

#(1) Hulett WB, Laing JW. Tension pneumocephalus and the sitting position. *Anesthesiology* 1976;45(5):578. (2) Kitahata LM, Katz JD. Tension pneumocephalus after posterior-fossa craniotomy, a complication of the sitting position. *Anesthesiology* 1976;44(5):448–50. (3) MacGillivray RG. Pneumocephalus as a complication of posterior fossa surgery in the sitting position. *Anaesthesia* 1982;37(7):722–5. (4) Pandit UA, Mudge BJ, Keller TS, et al. Pneumocephalus after posterior fossa exploration in the sitting position. *Anaesthesia* 1982;37(10):996–1001. (5) Standefer M, Bay JW, Trusso R. The sitting position in neurosurgery: a retrospective analysis of 488 cases. *Neurosurgery* 1984;14(6):649–58.

##(1) Vallejo LA, Gil-Carcedo LM, Borras JM, De Campos JM. Spontaneous pneumocephalus of an otogenic origin. *Otolaryngol Head Neck Surg* 1999;121(5):662–5. (2) Mohammed el R, Profant M. Spontaneous otogenic pneumocephalus. *Acta Otolaryngol* 2011;131(6):670–4.

@Shehu BB, Ismail NJ, Hassan I. Management of pneumocephalus in a resource limited environment: review from sub-Saharan Africa. *Brain Inj* 2007;21(12):1217–23.

@@(1) Clark JB, Six EG. Epidermoid tumor presenting as tension pneumocephalus. Case report. *J Neurosurg* 1984;60(6):1312–4. (2) Kinsley S, Dougherty J. Tension pneumocephalus related to an epidermoid tumor of ethmoid sinus origin. *Ann Emerg Med* 1993;22(2):259–61. (3) Gupta N, Rath GP, Mahajan C, Dube SK, Sharma S. Tension pneumoventricle after excision of third ventricular tumor in sitting position. *J Anaesthesiol Clin Pharmacol* 2011;27(3):409–11.

$(1) Chan EK, Meiteles LZ. Otogenic tension pneumocephalus caused by therapeutic lumbar CSF drainage for post-traumatic hydrocephalus: a case report. *Ear Nose Throat J* 2007;86(7):391–3, 405. (2) Saito K, Inamasu J, Kuramae T, Nakatsukasa M, Kawamura F. Tension pneumocephalus as a complication of lumbar drainage for cerebral aneurysm surgery—case report. *Neurol Med Chir (Tokyo)* 2009;49(6):252–4. (3) Pepper JP, Lin EM, Sullivan SE, Marentette LJ. Perioperative lumbar drain placement: an independent predictor of tension pneumocephalus and intracranial complications following anterior skull base surgery. *Laryngoscope* 2011;121(3):468–73. (4) Eltorai IM, Montroy RE, Kaplan SL, Ho WH. Pneumocephalus secondary to cerebrospinal fluid leak associated with a lumbar pressure ulcer in a man with paraplegia. *J Spinal Cord Med* 2003;26(3):262–9.

$$(1) Vasdev GM, Chantigian RC. Pneumocephalus following the treatment of a postdural puncture headache with an epidural saline infusion. *J Clin Anesth* 1994;6(6):508–11. (2) Lin HY, Wu HS, Peng TH, et al. Pneumocephalus and respiratory depression after accidental dural puncture during epidural analgesia—a case report. *Acta Anaesthesiol Sin* 1997;35(2):119–23. (3) McMurtrie R, Jr., Jan R. Subarachnoid pneumocephalus: a rare complication of epidural catheter placement. *J Clin Anesth* 2002;14(7):539–42. (4) Kasai K, Osawa M. Pneumocephalus during continuous epidural block. *J Anesth* 2007;21(1):59–61. (5) Ferrante E, Rubino F, Porrinis L. Pneumocephalus: a rare complication of epidural catheter placement during epidural blood patch. *Headache* 2014;54(3):539–40.

>Prabhakar H, Ali Z, Rath GP, Bithal PK. Tension pneumocephalus following external ventricular drain insertion. *J Anesth* 2008;22(3):326–7.

>>Michel L, Khanh NM, Cedric B, Eric K, Alain B, Alain F. Air in 'extra-dural space' after hyperbaric oxygen therapy. *J Trauma* 2007;63(4):961.

>>>Lee CH, Chen WC, Wu CI, Hsia TC. Tension pneumocephalus: a rare complication after hyperbaric oxygen therapy. *Am J Emerg Med* 2009;27(2):257 e251–253.

Pneumocephalus must be considered as a differential diagnosis in patients with acute or gradual neurological decline. Often not a first differential on the list of many for such an emergency, its diagnosis and prompt treatment warrants immediate assessment, clinically and radiographically.

The possibility of pneumocephalus must also be entertained in the differential diagnosis of delayed emergence from anaesthesia after neurosurgical procedures.

RADIOGRAPHIC DIAGNOSIS

Pneumocephalus is a radiological diagnosis of documentation of air within the intracranial space. Air is hypodense at a Hounsfield coefficient of -1000 on CT scans[4] (Figures 29.1 and 29.2). The sensitivity of plain X-ray for air is 2 ml while that of CT scan is 0.55 ml.[9] Tension pneumocephalus can occur at wide ranges of intracranial air volume. Volume ranges described range from 25 ml to 65 ml.[8]

In a study by Stuedel et al., 508 cases of acute head injuries underwent CT scanning. Intracranial air was seen in 49 (9.7%) cases.[1] The location of air in this study was in the extradural, subdural, or subarachnoid space. In 82% of patients, the diagnosis was made within 6 hours of the injury.[10]

One of the well-known radiographic signs of pneumocephalus is the Mount Fuji sign or bubbling brain.[11–24] First described in the 1980s, it essentially represents tenting of the frontal lobes due to accumulation of air. It may represent 'tension' pneumocephalus, which if associated with neurological decline necessitates immediate decompression.

The presence of pneumocephalus on postoperative brain images is common after craniotomies. Otherwise, the presence of pneumocephalus on CT brain should raise the suspicion of disruption of sinuses and entrainment of air within the intracranial compartment with downstream effects such as susceptibility to CSF leak.

Anatomically, air accumulation may occur in any intracranial compartment, including subdural, extradural, intraventricular, subarachnoid, intraparenchymal and epidural spaces and may provide a clue towards the underlying pathology.

CLINICAL MANAGEMENT

Table 29.2 highlights the medical and surgical management of pneumocephalus.

Table 29.2 Management of pneumocephalus

Preventative ***Pneumocephalus/CSF leak precautions in high risk patients***
• Head of bed elevation to 30 degrees above zero • Avoid Valsalva manoeuvres (Avoid sneezing, blowing nose, use of incentive spirometry, sucking liquids with straws) • Avoid use of NIPPV (BIPAP or CPAP)
Conservative medical management
• *Normobaric hyperoxia therapy* • Use of 100% FIO_2 via endotracheal tube • High flow O_2 with face mask vs nasal cannula (not suitable after nasal or pituitary procedures)
Surgical management
• Immediate decompression of tension pneumocephalus

Abbreviations: CSF: cerebrospinal fluid; NIPPV: Non-invasive positive pressure ventilation; BIPAP: bi-level positive airway pressure; CPAP: continuous positive airway pressure; FIO_2: fraction of inspired oxygen.

Medical Management of Pneumocephalus

Pneumocephalus Precautions

These precautions are commonly employed in patients with or at risk for CSF leak since they can worsen pneumocephalus. These measures include:

• Avoidance of nasal O_2, of a face mask of any kind.
• Avoidance of mask ventilation, including bi-level positive airway pressure (BIPAP)[25] or continuous positive airway pressure (CPAP).[26–28]
• Avoid sucking with the use of straws.
• Avoid use of incentive spirometry.
• Avoid nasal blowing,[29,30] coughing, or sneezing.[31,32]

In a recent study by White-Druzo et al., a majority of patients with obstructive sleep apnoea after transphenoidal pituitary surgery with a postoperative anterior skull base defect returned to use the CPAP weeks after surgery and they noted only two cases of pneumocephalus, allaying any concerns of potential safety of the use of early CPAP.[27] The exact timing to resumption of CPAP largely depends upon the individual patient and their continued risk for pneumocephalus or CSF leak, as pneumocephalus has been documented to occur even after one month of surgery.[33]

Pneumocephalus after craniotomy (role of nitrous oxide)

The fact that nitrous oxide use is associated with pneumocephalus is well-documented.[34–36] Mechanistically, it makes sense that if nitrous oxide is used 'air trapping' and 'expansion of air pocket' makes it likely to exacerbate

pre-existing pneumocephalus. It is thus recommended to avoid nitrous oxide in patients at high risk of developing pneumocephalus, but the data against routine use of this agent is not truly conclusive.[36]

Pneumocephalus Management

Most pneumocephali will get absorbed without any clinical manifestations. Conservative management as highlighted in Table 29.2 results in reabsorption in 85% of cases in about 2–3 weeks.[9]

The use of hyperoxic therapy is common to all described management strategies. The commonly employed techniques include placement of high-flow O_2 via nasal cannula or given via a non-rebreather mask (NRBM). Absorption rates over 24 hours are better using NRBM (65%) than breathing room air (31%).[37]

Hyperbaric oxygen has been used to treat pneumocephalus.[38–40] The rationale being that air bubbles under greater than 1 atmospheric pressure will disintegrate faster than air bubbles at 1 atmospheric pressure. Faster reabsorption rates along with reduction in rate of meningitis and reduction in hospital stay was observed in one study.[39] Caution must be used while using this therapy as hyperbaric oxygen has resulted in pneumocephalus in high-risk patients.[41,42]

SURGICAL MANAGEMENT OF PNEUMOCEPHALUS

Controlled decompression has been achieved via placement of lumbar drainage for CSF. This technique allows for immediate decompression of tension pneumocephalus as well as provides a conduit for continuous CSF drainage to allow healing and sealing of dural tears.[43] Lumbar drain management can complicate pneumocephalus.[44–46] Tension pneumocephalus often requires immediate neurosurgical consultation with prompt decompression.

COMPLICATIONS

Pneumocephalus may be asymptomatic, present with focal neurological deficits, or manifest with signs and symptoms of intracranial hypertension. In a study by Stuedel et al. on 508 patients, injuries associated with a pneumatocoele or single intracranial air bubble, and those with frontobasal lesions had the best prognosis, while multiple air bubbles was a sign of poor prognosis.[1] The presence of pneumocephalus on brain CT was one of the factors associated with higher mortality after sniper headshot injuries.[47] Cerebral herniation can potentially complicate tension pneumocephalus.[6,7,48] Infectious complications are partly attributable to the presence of CSF leak which can then predispose patients to meningitis.[23,49]

CONCLUSIONS

Pneumocephalus, a common presence after a neurosurgical procedure on neuroimaging, and after craniofacial trauma is usually benign and a potentially treatable neurosurgical emergency. Prompt recognition and management is as crucial as it is to implement preventative measures for exacerbation and avoid evolution to potentially life-threatening tension pneumocephalus.

REFERENCES

1. Steudel WI, Hacker H. Prognosis, incidence and management of acute traumatic intracranial pneumocephalus. A retrospective analysis of 49 cases. *Acta Neurochir (Wien)* 1986;80(3–4):93–99.

2. Sloan T. The incidence, volume, absorption, and timing of supratentorial pneumocephalus during posterior fossa neurosurgery conducted in the sitting position. *J Neurosurg Anesthesiol* 2010;22(1):59–66.

3. Satyarthee GD, Mahapatra AK. Tension pneumocephalus following transsphenoid surgery for pituitary adenoma—report of two cases. *J Clin Neurosci* 2003;10(4):495–7.

4. Schirmer CM, Heilman CB, Bhardwaj A. Pneumocephalus: case illustrations and review. *Neurocrit Care* 2010;13(1): 152–8.

5. Lunsford LD, Maroon JC, Sheptak PE, Albin MS. Subdural tension pneumocephalus. Report of two cases. *J Neurosurg* 1979;50(4):525–7.

6. Celikoglu E, Hazneci J, Ramazanoglu AF. Tension pneumocephalus causing brain herniation after endoscopic sinus surgery. *Asian J Neurosurg* 2016;11(3):309–10.

7. Foo LL, Chaw SH, Chan L, Ganesan D, Karuppiah R. [Intractable intraoperative brain herniation secondary to tension pneumocephalus: a rare life-threatening complication during drainage of subdural empyema]. *Rev Bras Anestesiol* 2016.

8. Dabdoub CB, Salas G, Silveira Edo N, Dabdoub CF. Review of the management of pneumocephalus. *Surg Neurol Int* 2015;6:155.

9. Karavelioglu E, Eser O, Haktanir A. Pneumocephalus and pneumorrhachis after spinal surgery: case report and review of the literature. *Neurol Med Chir (Tokyo)* 2014;54(5):405–7.

10. Steudel WI, Hacker H. Acute intracranial pneumocephalus: prognosis and management—a retrospective analysis of 101 cases. *Neurosurg Rev* 1989;12(Suppl 1):125–36.

11. Heckmann JG, Ganslandt O. Images in clinical medicine. The Mount Fuji sign. *N Engl J Med* 2004;350(18): 1881.

12. Michel SJ. The Mount Fuji sign. *Radiology* 2004;232(2): 449–50.

13. Beiko J, McDonald P. Tension pneumocephalus–the Mount Fuji sign. *Can J Neurol Sci* 2005;32(4):538–9.

14. Mattick A, Goodwin P. Mount Fuji sign on CT following trauma. *J Trauma* 2005;59(1):254.

15. Vanhoenacker FM, Herz R, Vandervliet EJ, Parizel PM. The Mount Fuji sign in tension pneumocephalus. *JBR-BTR* 2008;91(4):175.

16. Agrawal A, Singh BR. Mount Fuji sign with concavo-convex appearance of epidural haematoma in a patient with tension pneumocephalus. *J Radiol Case Rep* 2009;3(1): 10–12.

17. Yamashita S, Tsuchimochi W, Yonekawa T, Kyoraku I, Shiomi K, Nakazato M. The Mount Fuji sign on MRI. *Intern Med* 2009;48(17):1567–8.

18. Shaikh N, Masood I, Hanssens Y, Louon A, Hafiz A. Tension pneumocephalus as complication of burr-hole drainage of chronic subdural hematoma: A case report. *Surg Neurol Int* 2010;1.

19. Nimjee SM, Zomorodi AR, Adamson DC. Conquering mount fuji: resolution of tension pneumocephalus with a foley urinary catheter. *Case Rep Radiol* 2011:164316.

20. Perez Redondo M, Alcantara Carmona S, Carrascosa Granada A. [Mount Fuji sign: tension pneumoencephalus]. *Med Intensiva* 2011;35(3):199.

21. Prakash B, Pranesh MB, Parimalam N, Harish Kumar R. Hyperostosis frontalis interna mimicking Mount Fuji sign. *J Assoc Physicians India* 2011;59:181–3.

22. Pruss H, Klingebiel R, Endres M. Tension pneumocephalus with diplegia and deterioration of consciousness. *Case Rep Neurol* 2011;3(1):48–49.

23. Himeno T, Takeshima S, Kubo S, Hara N, Takamatsu K, Kuriyama M. [Tension pneumocephalus complicated from bacterial meningitis—a report of case presenting 'Mount Fuji sign' in brain CT]. *Rinsho Shinkeigaku* 2013; 53(6):478–81.

24. Bartholomeus MG, de Leeuw FE. Neurological picture. 'Bubbling brain'. *J Neurol Neurosurg Psychiatry* 2008; 79(6):671.

25. Kopelovich JC, de la Garza GO, Greenlee JD, Graham SM, Udeh CI, O'Brien EK. Pneumocephalus with BiPAP use after transsphenoidal surgery. *J Clin Anesth* 2012;24(5):415–8.

26. Zlotnik D, Taylor G, Simmoneau A, Viot-Blanc V, Devys JM. [Two cases of pneumocephalus following noninvasive continuous positive airway ventilation after transsphenoidal neurosurgery]. *Ann Fr Anesth Reanim* 2014;33(4):275–8.

27. White-Dzuro GA, Maynard K, Zuckerman SL, et al. Risk of post-operative pneumocephalus in patients with obstructive sleep apnea undergoing transsphenoidal surgery. *J Clin Neurosci* 2016;29:25–28.

28. Young AE, Nevin M. Tension pneumocephalus following mask CPAP. *Intensive Care Med* 1994;20(1):83.

29. Fix A, Lang VJ. A complication of forceful nose-blowing. *Am J Med* 2007;120(4):328–9.

30. Lojo Rial C, Oldfield M. Extensive pneumocephalus after nose blowing: an unusual cause of severe headache. *Br J Hosp Med (Lond)* 2010;71(11):652–3.

31. Birkent H, Durmaz A, Hidir Y, Erdem U, Tosun F. Sneezing-related orbital emphysema and pneumocephalus treated with transnasal endoscopic surgery. *J Otolaryngol Head Neck Surg* 2008;37(6):E167–9.

32. Zhang YX, Liu LX, Qiu XZ. A case report of diffuse pneumocephalus induced by sneezing after brain trauma. *Chin J Traumatol* 2013;16(4):249–50.

33. Salem-Memou S, Vallee B, Jacquesson T, Jouanneau E, Berhouma M. Pathogenesis of delayed tension intraventricular pneumocephalus in shunted patient: possible role of nocturnal positive pressure ventilation. *World Neurosurg* 2016;85:365, e317–320.

34. Frost EA. Nitrous oxide and intraoperative tension pneumocephalus. *Anesthesiology* 1983;58(2):197.

35. Theilen HJ, Heller AR, Litz RJ. Nitrous oxide-induced tension pneumocephalus after thoracic spinal cord surgery: A case report. *J Neurosurg Anesthesiol* 2008;20(3): 211–212.

36. Pasternak JJ, Lanier WL. Is nitrous oxide use appropriate in neurosurgical and neurologically at-risk patients? *Curr Opin Anaesthesiol* 2010;23(5):544–50.

37. Gore PA, Maan H, Chang S, Pitt AM, Spetzler RF, Nakaji P. Normobaric oxygen therapy strategies in the treatment of postcraniotomy pneumocephalus. *J Neurosurg* 2008;108(5):926–9.

38. Isakov Iu V, Anan'ev GV, Aide Kh B, Korol'kov Iu I. [Use of hyperbaric oxygenation in various complications of craniocerebral injury in the acute period]. *Zh Vopr Neirokhir Im N N Burdenko* 1981(4):15–18.

39. Paiva WS, de Andrade AF, Figueiredo EG, Amorim RL, Prudente M, Teixeira MJ. Effects of hyperbaric oxygenation therapy on symptomatic pneumocephalus. *Ther Clin Risk Manag* 2014;10:769–73.

40. Shih CC, Tsai SH, Liao WI, Wang JC, Hsu CW. Successful treatment of epidural anesthesia-induced severe pneumocephalus by hyperbaric oxygen therapy. *Am J Emerg Med* 2015;33(8):1116 e1111–3.

41. Michel L, Khanh NM, Cedric B, Eric K, Alain B, Alain F. Air in 'extra-dural space' after hyperbaric oxygen therapy. *J Trauma* 2007;63(4):961.

42. Lee CH, Chen WC, Wu CI, Hsia TC. Tension pneumocephalus: a rare complication after hyperbaric oxygen therapy. *Am J Emerg Med* 2009;27(2):257 e251–253.

43. Arbit E, Shah J, Bedford R, Carlon G. Tension pneumocephalus: treatment with controlled decompression via a closed water-seal drainage system. Case report. *J Neurosurg* 1991;74(1):139–42.

44. Chan EK, Meiteles LZ. Otogenic tension pneumocephalus caused by therapeutic lumbar CSF drainage for post-traumatic hydrocephalus: a case report. *Ear Nose Throat J* 2007;86(7):391–3, 405.

45. Saito K, Inamasu J, Kuramae T, Nakatsukasa M, Kawamura F. Tension pneumocephalus as a complication of lumbar drainage for cerebral aneurysm surgery–case report. *Neurol Med Chir (Tokyo)* 2009;49(6):252–4.

46. Pepper JP, Lin EM, Sullivan SE, Marentette LJ. Perioperative lumbar drain placement: an independent predictor of tension pneumocephalus and intracranial complications following anterior skull base surgery. *Laryngoscope* 2011;121(3):468–73.

47. Can C, Bolatkale M, Sarihan A, Savran Y, Acara AC, Bulut M. The effect of brain tomography findings on mortality in sniper shot head injuries. *J R Army Med Corps* 2016.

48. Kilincoglu BF, Mukaddem AM, Lakadamyali H, Altinors N. [Posttraumatic tension pneumocephalus causing herniation]. *Ulus Travma Acil Cerrahi Derg* 2003;9(1):79–81.

49. Odani N, Kitazono H, Deshpande GA, Hiraoka E. Severe sepsis due to otogenic pneumococcal meningitis with pneumocephalus without meningeal symptoms. *Intern Med* 2015;54(13):1661–4.

30

Central Nervous System Infections

N. J. Johnson and D. F. Gaieski

ABSTRACT

Central nervous system (CNS) infections are neurologic emergencies requiring prompt diagnosis and treatment, and vigilant monitoring for complications. Morbidity and mortality are typically related to diffuse cerebral oedema or mass effect leading to intracranial hypertension, seizures, neurocognitive sequelae, and hearing loss. This chapter provides the reader with basic and advanced practical knowledge regarding the management of the critically ill patient with CNS infection.

KEYWORDS

Central nervous system (CNS) infection; meningitis; encephalitis; brain abscess; spinal abscess; epidural abscess; meningoencephalitis.

INTRODUCTION

Infections of the central nervous system (CNS) can be devastating, often requiring admission to the intensive care unit (ICU). Owing to the great potential for morbidity and death, intensivists must remain vigilant for numerous complications associated with these diseases. This chapter presents readers with up to date information regarding varied aspects of critical care for the patient with CNS infection including anatomy and terminology, epidemiology, pathophysiology, diagnosis, management, complications, and outcomes of bacterial meningitis, viral meningitis, and encephalitis; CNS abscess; and CNS infections in the immunocompromised patient.

ANATOMY AND TERMINOLOGY

Meningitis results from inflammation of the meninges and subarachnoid space. Inflammation of the brain parenchyma and spinal cord is termed encephalitis and myelitis, respectively. Meningitis is most commonly caused by infections due to viruses or bacteria, but may be caused by fungi, protozoa, or mycobacteria.[1,2] Many of the pathogens that cause viral meningitis also cause encephalitis. Central nervous system abscess includes pyogenic infection of the brain parenchyma, subdural space (often termed subdural empyema), and epidural space (both of the spine and cranium) and can occur simultaneous with meningoencephalitis.

BACTERIAL MENINGITIS

Epidemiology

There are approximately 500,000 cases of bacterial meningitis per year worldwide with 170,000 deaths and as many survivors with disability.[1,2] In the United States, the incidence of bacterial meningitis is three cases per 100,000 persons per year, but nearly 500 cases per 100,000 are diagnosed each year in the 'meningitis belt' of Africa (21 countries from Senegal to Ethiopia).[2]

Pathophysiology

Streptococcus pneumoniae and *Neisseria meningitidis* are the first and second most common causative organisms of community-acquired bacterial meningitis.[3] The widespread use of vaccination against *Haemophilus influenzae* type b has dramatically decreased the incidence of *H. influenzae* type b meningitis. Both *N. meningitidis* and *S. pneumoniae* are transmitted by aerosolized droplets of respiratory secretions and are transmitted via the bloodstream to the CNS resulting in a profound inflammatory response. This produces vasogenic oedema, as well as obstruction of CSF flow and resorption, leading to obstructive and communicating hydrocephalus and interstitial oedema. The combination of vasogenic and interstitial oedema leads to increased intracranial pressure (ICP) and altered level of consciousness.[1]

Predisposing and associated conditions put the individual at risk for meningitis due to other organisms. The most important antecedent illnesses for pneumococcal meningitis are pneumonia, acute otitis media, and acute sinusitis. The causative organisms of meningitis associated with otitis media, mastoiditis, or sinusitis are Streptococci spp., gram-negative anaerobes, *Staphylococcus aureus*, Haemophilus spp., and Enterobacteriaceae. *Listeria monocytogenes* is an important aetiologic organism for meningitis in older adults (>55 years old), those with chronic illness (diabetes, alcoholism), immunocompromised individuals, and pregnant women. Patients with congenital or acquired deficiency in the terminal common complement pathway (C3 and C5–C9), immunoglobulin deficiency, or asplenia are at risk for meningitis due to encapsulated organisms, specifically *N. meningitidis* and *S. pneumoniae*. Staphylococci, gram-negative bacilli, and anaerobes are the most common organisms causing meningitis in the postoperative neurosurgical patient.[4]

Diagnosis

Clinical Presentation

The vast majority of adults with community-acquired bacterial meningitis present with at least two of the following four symptoms: fever, headache, nuchal rigidity, or altered level of consciousness.[5–7] In a series of 493 episodes of bacterial meningitis in adults, fever was the most common finding and was present in 95% of patients at presentation, while another 4% became febrile during the next 24 hours.[8] Seizures are also a common presentation among adults with community-acquired bacterial meningitis.[9]

Nuchal rigidity or meningismus, which occurs when the neck resists passive flexion is the classic sign of meningeal irritation. In a recent review, nuchal rigidity had a pooled sensitivity of 70% for the diagnosis of meningitis and may be difficult to assess in patients with altered levels of consciousness.[10] Kernig and Brudzinski signs have also been classically described in bacterial meningitis. Recent studies suggest that Kernig sign and Brudzinski sign have poor sensitivity and specificity for the diagnosis of bacterial meningitis.[11]

Laboratory Evaluation

In order to diagnose meningitis, a lumbar puncture should be performed to sample the cerebrospinal fluid (CSF). A list of recommended CSF studies is shown in Table 30.1. Cerebrospinal fluid should routinely be sent for cell count, protein, glucose estimation, gram stain, and culture. It is often helpful to obtain an opening pressure when a CNS infection is suspected. Cerebrospinal fluid lactate has also been proposed as a marker for bacterial meningitis. The CSF abnormalities characteristic of bacterial meningitis are as follows: an opening pressure greater than 180 mm H_2O, an increased number of white blood cells (often 100–1000/µL or more) with a predominance of polymorphonuclear leukocytes, a decreased glucose concentration, and an elevated protein concentration.[12]

Imaging Studies

Cranial computed tomography (CT) prior to lumbar puncture is recommended in adult patients who meet any of the following criteria: (1) immunocompromised state due to human immunodeficiency virus (HIV) infection, immunosuppressive therapy, and/or bone marrow or solid-organ transplantation; (2) history of central nervous system disease (mass lesion, stroke, or focal infection); (3) new-onset seizure (within 1 week of presentation); (4) papilloedema; (5) abnormal level of consciousness; or (6) focal neurological deficit. The benefit of obtaining a CT scan prior to lumbar puncture must be weighed against the risk of delaying diagnosis and treatment, particularly antibiotics and corticosteroids in suspected bacterial

Table 30.1 Cerebrospinal fluid diagnostic studies for meningitis

Routine Studies
Cell count with differential
Glucose and protein
Lactic acid concentration
Gram stain and bacterial culture
Immunocompromised Host or Clinical Concern
India ink and fungal culture
Viral culture
Acid-fast smear and *Mycobacterium tuberculosis* culture
Cryptococcal antigen
Histoplasma antigen
Viral polymerase chain reaction (PCR) studies

meningitis.[13] In acute bacterial meningitis, cranial CT or magnetic resonance imaging (MRI) post-contrast administration may demonstrate diffuse meningeal enhancement.

Treatment

Patients with bacterial meningitis may present with altered mental status, seizures, cerebral herniation, and shock. Profound alterations in consciousness may necessitate endotracheal intubation. Patients with suspected meningococcal meningitis should be placed in respiratory isolation and precautions should be taken by healthcare providers performing invasive procedures, especially endotracheal intubation. Empiric antimicrobial and dexamethasone therapy should be started as rapidly as possible, with dexamethasone administered prior to or concomitant with administration of the first antibiotic. Antibiotics should not be delayed to obtain imaging studies or CSF samples via lumbar puncture.[5]

Empiric Antimicrobial Therapy

The choice of antibiotic for empiric therapy is based on the patient's age and any associated conditions that may have predisposed to CNS infection. Empiric therapy in children older than 1 month of age and adults should include a third- or fourth-generation cephalosporin (either ceftriaxone or cefepime) plus vancomycin.[14–18] Ampicillin should be added to the empiric regimen for coverage of *Listeria monocytogenes* in individuals over the age of 55 years and in individuals with impaired cell-mediated immunity due to a chronic illness, organ transplantation, pregnancy, AIDS, malignancy, or immunosuppressive therapy. Gentamicin is added to ampicillin in critically ill patients with *L. monocytogenes* meningitis. Empiric therapy in the postoperative neurosurgical patient should include a combination of vancomycin plus meropenem or ceftazidime. Meropenem has excellent activity against gram-negative bacilli, including *Pseudomonas aeruginosa*, but does not cover all anaerobic bacteria.[18]

Corticosteroid Therapy

A substantial body of experimental and clinical data demonstrates that dexamethasone therapy reduces meningeal inflammation leading to lower mortality, reduction in neurological sequelae, and a reduced frequency of sensorineural hearing loss.[19–27] In a meta-analysis of randomized controlled trials of adjuvant corticosteroids in the treatment of acute bacterial meningitis (18 studies involving 2,750 patients were included), the following was determined: (1) for children in high-income countries, there was a protective effect of corticosteroids on severe hearing loss overall and favourable point estimates for severe hearing loss in non-*Haemophilus* meningitis and for short-term neurological sequelae, and (2) in adults with acute bacterial meningitis, 36 of 308 (11.7%) who received corticosteroids died compared with 69 of 315 (21.9%) in the placebo group.[28] Practice guidelines for the management of bacterial meningitis recommend the use of dexamethasone (0.15 mg/kg every 6 hours for 2 to 4 days) in adults with suspected or proven pneumococcal meningitis.[29,30] The first dose should be administered 10 to 20 minutes before, or at least concomitant with, the first dose of antimicrobial agent.

Temperature Management

A recent randomized controlled trial (RCT) of induced moderate hypothermia, with hypothermia induced by rapid infusion of chilled saline and maintained at 32°C–34°C for 48 hours in 98 comatose adults with severe bacterial meningitis was stopped early for possible harm (20% absolute increase in mortality in the treatment arm).[31] There are no data to support maintenance of euthermia in patients with CNS infections, though this approach is reasonable and is a cornerstone of management in patients with severe brain injury.

Prophylaxis

Chemoprophylaxis for meningococcal meningitis is recommended for every person who has had close contact with the index patient. Rifampin is recommended in a dose of 600 mg every 12 hours for 2 days for adults. Rifampin should not be prescribed during pregnancy; ceftriaxone can be used instead.[1]

Complications

Numerous complications can be seen in bacterial meningitis, (Table 30.2) and a key role of the neurointensivist is to anticipate and address these complications.

Intracranial Hypertension

Elevated ICP is the most common cause of death in severe meningitis and has been associated with increased mortality and poor neurological outcome.[32,33] Inflammation due to CNS infection produces vasogenic oedema, as well as obstruction of CSF flow and resorption leading to obstructive and communicating hydrocephalus and interstitial oedema, all of which contribute to increased ICP and an altered level of consciousness.[1]

Table 30.2 Complications of bacterial meningitis

Seizures
Status epilepticus
Cerebral oedema
Intracranial hypertension and herniation
Septic shock
Multi-organ dysfunction
Healthcare-associated complications
    Nosocomial infection
    Venous thromboembolism
Persistent neurologic deficit
    Sensorineural hearing loss
    Cranial nerve palsy
    Hemiparesis or quadriparesis
    Aphasia

Intracranial pressure monitoring should be considered in patients with an altered level of consciousness. No strict guidelines exist, but some authors advocate for placement of an ICP monitor in all patients with a Glasgow Coma Scale (GCS) score ≤9 or with GCS = 10 plus an elevated CSF opening pressure >40 cm H_2O.[32,34]

Drainage of CSF should be considered in patients with elevated ICP.[34] In addition to reducing ICP, CSF removal may take out purulent material from the subarachnoid space and potentially relieve CSF outflow obstruction. In one series, CSF drainage was necessary in approximately half of the patients who required ICP monitoring.[32] Cerebrospinal fluid removal via external ventricular or lumbar drain has been associated with improved outcome.[34,35]

Elevated intracranial pressure should also be treated with standard supportive measures such as head elevation to 30 degrees, maintenance of normothermia, and eucapnia. Other therapies such as hyperosmotic agents, barbiturate infusion, vasopressor infusion to target supranormal mean arterial pressure, and decompressive craniectomy may be considered for refractory cases.[36,37] A treatment strategy targeting cerebral perfusion pressure (CPP) has been shown to be superior to an ICP-targeted approach in one paediatric study.[38]

Seizures

Approximately 20% of patients with meningitis develop seizures.[9,32] Cortical inflammation, cortical ischaemia, intraparenchymal haemorrhage, and cerebral oedema are thought to create epileptogenic foci. Clinical risk factors for seizures include severe systemic or CNS inflammation, a structural CNS lesion, pneumococcal meningitis, and other predisposing conditions such as a distant focus of infection or immunocompromised state.[9] Central nervous system infections, specifically meningitis and encephalitis, are risk factors for nonconvulsive seizures and status epilepticus. Clinicians should have a low threshold for electroencephalography (EEG) monitoring in this population.[5,39]

Status epilepticus should be treated with benzodiazepines (lorazepam 2–4 mg IV, repeat every 5–10 minutes), antiepileptic agents (phenytoin 20 mg/kg IV), and possibly endotracheal intubation followed by deep sedation with benzodiazepines, propofol, or barbiturates.[40] No evidence exists to support the routine use of antiepileptics for seizure prophylaxis.

Outcomes

Bacterial meningitis is a devastating disease associated with substantial mortality and morbidity. The major causative bacteria, *S. pneumoniae* and *N. meningitis*, are associated with case-fatality rates of 30% and 7%, respectively, in high-income countries.[41] In one series of patients with severe community-acquired bacterial meningitis admitted to the ICU, overall mortality was 11%.[42] Disease severity, determined by the APACHE II score was predictive of outcome. Neurological sequelae, including hearing loss, developmental disorders, and neuropsychological impairment occur in up to 50% of survivors of the disease.[1,7,41]

VIRAL MENINGITIS AND ENCEPHALITIS

Epidemiology and Pathophysiology

The reported annual incidences of viral meningitis is 219 per 100,000 in infants under 1 year, 27.8 per 100,000 in children under 14 years, and 7.6 per 100,000 people aged 16 and older.[43]

The enteroviruses are the most common cause of viral meningitis and encephalitis and account for at least 60% of cases.[19,20] Enteroviruses are often transmitted through the faecal-oral route and more rarely via respiratory droplets. Following enteroviruses, the next two most common causes of viral meningitis are the arboviruses and herpes viruses.[20] Arboviruses, particularly those that are mosquito borne, are typical in the summer and autumn months. Of the 150 arboviral species known to cause disease in humans, the La Crosse and West Nile viruses are the most common aetiologies of meningitis and encephalitis. The West Nile virus is now endemic throughout the contiguous United States, with over 161,000 human neuroinvasive disease cases, and 1549 deaths reported since 1999.[44]

The herpes virus family includes several viruses, many of which can cause viral meningitis and encephalitis. Herpes simplex viruses (HSV) account for the vast majority of cases. Herpes simplex virus-2 is the cause of genital herpes and frequently causes viral meningitis after primary infection. This occurs in about one-third of females and 10% of men with primary infection.[45] Varicella-zoster virus (VZV) is often transmitted via respiratory droplets. Herpes simplex virus and VZV are highly neurotropic and become latent within neuron cell bodies.[43]

Rabies is a lyssa virus infection resulting in acute encephalitis that is virtually always fatal. Although no high quality reporting mechanisms exist, estimates of global burden in 2010 ranged from 26,400 to 61,000 deaths.[46] Considerable geographical variation exists worldwide, with 95% of rabies cases in humans occurring in Africa and Asia. Dogs are the source of infection in more than 99% of cases in humans.[46]

Diagnosis

Clinical Presentation

The classic clinical presentation of viral meningitis is a febrile illness followed by nuchal rigidity and headache. Between 55% and 90% of patients with viral meningitis present with fever.[47–49] Other symptoms include photophobia, nausea, and vomiting.

Encephalitis, depending on its aetiology and the anatomic location of the brain it affects, may present more subtly with findings such as behavioural or personality changes, hallucinations, bizarre behaviour, neurologic deficits, or seizures.[50] Acute flaccid paralysis, myoclonus, and bulbar dysfunction have also been described in West Nile encephalitis.[44] Aphasia, or a disturbance of taste or smell, has been described in HSV encephalitis.[45] Aversion to water, refusal to swallow, and marked agitation are classic for rabies.[46]

Laboratory Evaluation

The classic CSF abnormalities in viral meningitis are listed in Table 30.3. The presence of red blood cells may indicate a haemorrhagic type of encephalitis, such as HSV. Cerebrospinal fluid polymerase chain reaction (PCRs) are available for the enteroviruses, HSV-2, and HIV, all of which are typically available in 24 to 48 hours. A CSF PCR is available for one of the arthropod-borne viruses, West Nile virus, but the PCR has poor sensitivity.[44] The diagnosis of rabies virus infection is made clinically and confirmed by viral antigens or ribonucleic acid (RNA) detected in saliva or hair follicles.[46]

Table 30.3 Classic cerebrospinal fluid characteristics in meningitis

Characteristic	Normal	Bacterial	Viral	Fungal
WBCs (cells/μL)	<5 (mononuclear)	>1,000	<1,000	<1,000
% PMNs	0	>80	<50	<50
Glucose (mg/dL)	>40	<40	>40	<40
Protein (mg/dL)	<50	>200	<200	>200
Gram stain	–	+	–	–

Abbreviations: CSF: cerebrospinal fluid; PMN: polymorphonuclear neutrophil; WBC: white blood cell.

Imaging Studies

Computed tomography and MRI are the imaging procedures that are most commonly performed. Electroencephalography has also been used in the past to aid in the diagnosis of viral meningitis and encephalitis. In HSV-1 encephalitis, at 48 hours after symptom onset, the majority of patients will have hyperintensity in the inferior and medial temporal lobe on fluid-attenuated inversion recovery (FLAIR) and diffusion-weighted imaging (DWI) MRI sequences.[50] There are no imaging findings specific for other types of viral meningitis but a number of findings in both West Nile disease and rabies have been described.[44,51]

Treatment

Treatment for most cases of viral meningitis and encephalitis is supportive. Acyclovir (10 mg/kg every 8 hours) is the recommended agent for HSV-1 and VZV meningitis and encephalitis. A number of therapies for West Nile have been investigated, but no study has documented efficacy.[44]

Prevention, pre-exposure vaccination, and post-exposure prophylaxis with a combination of rabies immune globulin and vaccination are the optimal strategies to prevent mortality from rabies. The 'Milwaukee protocol' is a controversial intensive care strategy that was developed for a patient who survived a bat bite despite not having received post-exposure prophylaxis and presenting with encephalitis.[52] Numerous patients have failed this experimental protocol.[46]

Complications

Complications of viral meningitis and encephalitis include hyponatraemia, most often due to inappropriate secretion of antidiuretic hormone, and seizures. Herpes simplex virus encephalitis is associated with an especially high prevalence of seizures. Patients with meningitis or encephalitis may also be at risk for hospital-acquired complications such as healthcare-associated pneumonia and venous thromboembolism due to prolonged immobility and impaired consciousness.[42]

Outcomes

Most cases of viral meningitis are self-limiting conditions with no neurological sequelae. In the case of HSV encephalitis, the likelihood and quality of survival are strongly related to the neurological condition of the patient at the treatment start time and his or her age. Younger patients who have more favourable neurologic examination outcomes are more likely to survive without deficits.[53]

Most patients with West Nile virus infection recover fully, though prolonged neurological sequelae have been described.[44] Approximately 10% of patients with neuroinvasive West Nile disease die, and advanced age is the most important risk factor for death. Rabies encephalitis is nearly always fatal in unimmunized patients.

CENTRAL NERVOUS SYSTEM ABSCESS

Epidemiology

Central nervous system abscess is rare, with a reported incidence of brain parenchymal abscess ranging from 0.4 to 0.9 cases per 100,000, though rates are higher in immunosuppressed patients.[54–57] The prevalence of spinal abscess is increasing. Approximately 20 years ago, spinal epidural abscess was diagnosed in approximately 1 of 20,000 hospital admissions.[58] The prevalence has doubled in the past two decades, owing to an aging population, increase in use of spinal instrumentation, and vascular access, and the spread of injection drug use.[59–63]

Pathophysiology

Central nervous system abscesses, which include intraparenchymal brain abscess, subdural empyema, and intracranial or spinal epidural abscess are typically associated with spread of contiguous or remote infections, injection drug use, surgery, trauma, or instrumentation.[54] In the case of brain abscess, bacteria enter through contiguous spread in about half of the cases and through haematogenous dissemination in about one-third of cases with unknown mechanisms accounting for the remaining cases.[54,64]

Pathogenic mechanisms of CNS abscess are dependent both on the aetiology and predisposing conditions.[54,58,64] Abscess formation occurring after surgery, instrumentation, or trauma, is most often caused by S. aureus, S. epidermidis, or gram-negative bacilli. CNS abscess due to contiguous spread from sinusitis, otitis, or odontogenic infection is frequently caused by Streptococcus and Staphylococcal species, though polymicrobial infections are possible. Haematogenous spread of bacteria is associated with underlying cardiac disease (e.g., endocarditis or congenital heart defects), pulmonary arteriovenous malformations, skin or soft tissue infections, injection drug use, or indwelling medical devices; Staphylococcus and Streptococcus species are often identified in these infections.[54,58,64]

Diagnosis

Clinical Presentation

The presentation of CNS abscess is variable. The most frequent clinical manifestation of brain parenchymal abscess is headache; fever and altered level of consciousness are frequently absent.[54] Up to 25% of patients present with seizures. Back pain (present in about 75% of patients), fever (50% of patients), and neurologic deficit (30% of patients) are the three most common symptoms in spinal epidural abscess.[65–66]

Central nervous system abscess may present with focal neurologic deficit or seizure. Patients may have clinical evidence of sinusitis, otitis media, facial or skull fracture, or remote infection (e.g., stigmata of endocarditis, skin or soft tissue infection).[54]

Laboratory Evaluation

In brain abscess, lumbar puncture is typically not helpful for diagnosis and should be performed with extreme caution.[54] Cerebrospinal fluid cultures reveal an aetiologic organism only 25% of the time. In three quarters of patients with spinal epidural abscess whose CSF is evaluated, high levels of protein and pleocytosis suggestive of parameningeal inflammation are found but are not specific for epidural infection.[59]

Imaging Studies

Cranial CT with contrast or MRI are the preferred imaging modalities in brain abscess. Classically, a ring-enhancing lesion with low T1 central intensity, high T2 central intensity without FLAIR attenuation, and a high DWI signal centrally is described on MRI. One prospective study involving 115 patients with 147 cystic brain lesions, which included 97 patients with brain abscess, showed that DWI had a sensitivity and specificity for the differentiation of brain abscesses from primary or metastatic cancers of 96% (positive predictive value, 98%; negative predictive value, 92%).[67] Both MRI with intravenous administration of gadolinium and myelography followed by CT of the spine are highly sensitive (>90%) in diagnosing spinal epidural abscess, but plain CT (with or without intravenous contrast) is not sufficiently sensitive to exclude the diagnosis.[58]

Treatment

The diagnosis of brain or spinal abscess should prompt immediate neurosurgical or spine surgical consultation, and empiric antimicrobials targeted at the most likely pathogens should be promptly given. Empirical antimicrobial regimens for CNS abscess should typically cover streptococci and staphylococci with ceftriaxone or cefepime, with consideration for coverage against methicillin-resistant *Staphylococcus aureus* with vancomycin and anaerobic bacteria with metronidazole.[23]

Complications and Outcomes

Currently, 70% of patients with brain abscess have a good outcome with no or minimal neurological sequelae, although data on functional and neuropsychological evaluation after brain abscess are lacking.[54] For spinal epidural abscess, the single most important predictor of the final neurological outcome is the patient's neurological status immediately before surgery.[58]

CENTRAL NERVOUS SYSTEM INFECTIONS IN THE IMMUNOCOMPROMISED PATIENT

A number of CNS infections may affect the immunocompromised host. HIV can present as acute meningitis at the time of seroconversion. Lymphocytic choriomeningitis virus transmitted by rodents is the causative agent in 15% of cases in which a virus is identified.[68] Human immunodeficiency virus infection is associated with meningitis due to *Cryptococcus neoformans* and brain abscess caused by *Toxoplasma gondii* or *Mycobacterium tuberculosis*.[54,64,69] Patients who have received solid organ transplants are at risk for nocardial and fungal brain abscesses. Fungi are responsible for up to 90% of cerebral abscesses among recipients of solid-organ transplants.[54,70,71] A variety of viruses, including measles, mumps, adenovirus, and other herpes viruses (such as human herpes virus 6) may cause meningitis in immunocompromised or unvaccinated individuals.[68]

Fungal meningitis typically presents more indolently, with symptoms of headache, fever, fatigue, and weight loss evolving over several days, typically in patients with underlying immunosuppression.[72] Lumbar puncture often shows markedly increased CSF opening pressure in patients with fungal meningitis. Tuberculous meningitis also has a protracted course and a vague nonspecific presentation consisting of fever, weight loss, night sweats, and malaise, often without headache and meningismus.[73]

Patients with suspected fungal meningitis should be treated with antifungals targeted at the most likely aetiologic agents. If there is a high index of suspicion for fungal meningitis such as prior history of the disease or systemic fungal infections, and the patient is declining rapidly, empiric Amphotericin B can be considered.[5] Preferred antimycobacterial regimens for tuberculous meningitis or CNS abscess include isoniazid, rifampin, pyrazinamide, and ethambutol. Initial antimicrobial regimens for other CNS infections are listed in Table 30.4.

Table 30.4 Therapy for selected uncommon central nervous system infections

Pathogens	Risk factors	Initial treatment
Herpes viruses (HSV, VZV)	Previous infection; immunosuppression	HSV meningitis: acyclovir 10 mg/kg IV; VZV meningitis: acyclovir 15 mg/kg IV
Rabies virus	Animal bite	Rabies vaccination, Rabies immune globulin, 'Milwaukee protocol'
West Nile virus	Mosquito exposure	None available
Borrelia burgdorferi (Lyme disease)	Tick bite	Lyme meningitis/encephalitis: ceftriaxone 2 g
Treponema pallidum (syphilis)	Sexual activity, syphilis infection	Penicillin G 3–4 million units IV
Nocardia *spp.*	HIV, immunosuppression	Trimethoprim-sulphamethoxazole 15 mg/kg/day IV
Toxoplasma gondii	HIV, immunosuppression	Pyrimethamine 200 mg + sulphadiazine 1 g + leucovorin

Cryptococcus neoformans	HIV, immunosuppression	Amphotericin B 1 mg/kg IV + flucytosine 25 mg/kg
Candida *spp.*	Immunosuppression, injection drug use	Amphotericin B 1 mg/kg IV
Aspergillus *spp.*	Immunosuppression	Amphotericin B 1 mg/kg IV

*Intraventricular vancomycin administration: children 10 mg/day, adults 20 mg/day.

CONCLUSIONS

Infections of the central nervous system are life-threatening neurological emergencies that require prompt diagnosis and treatment. Neurointensivists must be vigilant for serious complications, including cerebral oedema, intracranial hypertension, and seizures.

REFERENCES

1. van de Beek D, de Gans J, Tunkel AR, Wijdicks EFM. Community-acquired bacterial meningitis in adults. *N Engl J Med* 2006;354:44–53.

2. World Health Organization. Bacterial meningitis. Available at: http://www.who.int/csr/disease/meningococcal/en/ (accessed July 2, 2018).

3. Weisfelt M, de Gans J, van der Poll T, et al. Pneumococcal meningitis in adults: new approaches to management and prevention. *Lancet Neurol* 2006;5:332–42.

4. Tunkel AR, Scheld WM. Pathogenesis and pathophysiology of bacterial meningitis. *Clin Microbiol Rev* 1993;6:118–36.

5. Gaieski DF, Nathan BR, Weingart SD, Smith WS. Emergency neurologic life support: meningitis and encephalitis. *Neurocrit Care* 2012;17(Suppl 1):S66–72.

6. Thomas KE, Hasbun R, Jekel J, Quagliarello VJ. The diagnostic accuracy of Kernig's sign, Brudzinski's sign, and nuchal rigidity in adults with suspected meningitis. *Clin Infect Dis* 2002;35:46–52.

7. van de Beek D, de Gans J, Spanjaard L, et al. Clinical features and prognostic factors in adults with bacterial meningitis. *N Engl J Med* 2004;351:1849–59.

8. Durand ML, Calderwood SB, Weber DJ, et al. Acute bacterial meningitis in adults—a review of 493 episodes. *N Engl J Med* 1993;328:21–8.

9. Zoons E, Weisfelt M, de Gans J, et al. Seizures in adults with bacterial meningitis. *Neurology* 2008;70:2109–15.

10. Attia J, Hatala R, Cook DJ, Wong JG. The rational clinical examination. Does this adult patient have acute meningitis? *JAMA* 1999 Jul 14;282(2):175–81.

11. Ward MA, Greenwood TM, Kumar DR. Josef Brudzinski and Vladimir Mikhailovich Kernig: signs for diagnosing meningitis. *Clin Med Res* 2010;8:13–7.

12. Straus SE, Thorpe KE, Holroyd-Leduc J. How do I perform a lumbar puncture and analyze the results to diagnose bacterial meningitis? *JAMA* 2006;296(16):2012–22.

13. Tunkel AR, Hartman BJ, Kaplan BA, et al. Practice guidelines for the management of bacterial meningitis. *Clin Infect Dis* 2004;39:1267–84.

14. American Academy of Pediatrics, Committee on Infectious Diseases. Therapy for children with invasive pneumococcal infections. *Pediatrics* 1997;99:289–99.

15. Kaplan SL, Mason EO Jr. Management of infections due to antibiotic-resistant *Streptococus pneumoniae*. *Clin Microbiol Rev* 1998;11:628–44.

16. Ahmed A. A critical evaluation of vancomycin for treatment of bacterial meningitis. *Pediatr Infect Dis J* 1997;16:895–903.

17. Viladrich PF, Gudiol F, Linares J, et al. Evaluation of vancomycin for therapy of adult pneumococcal meningitis. *Antimicrob Agents Chemother* 1991;35:2467–72.

18. Roos KL, van de Beek D. Bacterial meningitis. In: Roos KR, Tunkel AR, eds. *Handbook of Clinical Neurology*. Edinburgh: Elsevier;2010. pp. 51–63.

19. Mustafa MM, Ramilo O, Olsen KD, et al. Tumor necrosis factor in mediating experimental *Haemophilus influenzae* type b meningitis. *J Clin Invest* 1989;84:1253–9.

20. Kern JA, Lamb RJ, Reed JC, et al. Dexamethasone inhibition of interleukin 1 beta production by human monocytes. *J Clin Invest* 1988;81:237–44.

21. Tauber MG, Khayam-Bashi H, Sande MA. Effects of ampicillin and corticosteroids on brain water content, cerebrospinal fluid pressure, and cerebrospinal fluid lactate levels in experimental pneumococcal meningitis. *J Infect Dis* 1985;151:528–34.

22. Lebel MH, Freij BJ, Syrogiannopoulos GA, et al. Dexamethasone therapy for bacterial meningitis; results of two double-blind, placebo-controlled trials. *N Engl J Med* 1988;319:964–71.

23. Odio CM, Faingezicht I, Paris M, et al. The beneficial effects of early dexamethasone administration in infants and children with bacterial meningitis. *N Engl J Med* 1991;324:1525–31.

24. Committee on Infectious Diseases, American Academy of Pediatrics. Dexamethasone therapy for bacterial meningitis in infants and children. *Pediatrics* 1990;86:130–3.

25. McIntyre PB, Berkey CS, King SM, et al. Dexamethasone as adjunctive therapy in bacterial meningitis: a meta-analysis of randomized clinical trials since 1988. *JAMA* 1997;278:925–31.

26. Girgis NI, Farid Z, Mikhail IA, et al. Dexamethasone treatment for bacterial meningitis in children and adults. *Pediatr Infect Dis J* 1989;8:848–51.

27. de Gans J, van de Beek D. The European dexamethasone in adulthood bacterial meningitis study investigators. Dexamethasone in adults with bacterial meningitis. *N Engl J Med* 2002;347:1549–56.

28. van de Beek D, de Gans J, McIntyre P, Prasad K. Corticosteroids for acute bacterial meningitis. *Cochrane Database Syst Rev* 2007;(1):CD004405.

29. Tunkel AR, Hartman BJ, Kaplan BA, et al. Practice guidelines for the management of bacterial meningitis. *Clin Infect Dis* 2004;39:1267–84.

30. Chaudhuri A, Martin PM, Kennedy PGE, et al. EFNS guideline on the management of community-acquired bacterial meningitis: report of an EFNS task force on acute bacterial meningitis in older children and adults. *Eur J Neurol* 2008;15:649–59.

31. Mourvillier B, Tubach F, van de Beek D, et al. Induced hypothermia in severe bacterial meningitis: a randomized clinical trial. *JAMA* 2013;310(20):2174–83.

32. Edberg M, Furebring M, Sjölin J, et al. Neurointensive care of patients with severe community-acquired meningitis. *Acta Anaesthesiol Scand* 2011 Jul;55(6):732–9.

33. Lindvall P, Ahlm C, Ericsson M, Gothefors L, Naredi S, Koskinen LO. Reducing intracranial pressure may increase survival among patients with bacterial meningitis. *Clin Infect Dis* 2004 Feb 1;38(3):384–90.

34. Glimåker M, Johansson B, Halldorsdottir H, et al. Neuro-intensive treatment targeting intracranial hypertension improves outcome in severe bacterial meningitis: an intervention-control study. *PLoS One* 2014;9(3):e91976.

35. Abulhasan YB, Al-Jehani H, Valiquette MA, et al. Lumbar drainage for the treatment of severe bacterial meningitis. *Neurocrit Care* 2013;19(2):199–205.

36. Cuthbertson BH, Dickson R, Mackenzie A. Intracranial pressure measurement, induced hypothermia and barbiturate coma in meningitis associated with intractable raised intracranial pressure. *Anaesthesia* 2004;59(9):908–11.

37. Perin A, Nascimben E, Longatti P. Decompressive craniectomy in a case of intractable intracranial hypertension due to pneumococcal meningitis. *Acta Neurochir (Wien)* 2008;150(8):837–42.

38. Kumar R, Singhi S, Singhi P, et al. Randomized controlled trial comparing cerebral perfusion pressure-targeted therapy versus intracranial pressure-targeted therapy for raised intracranial pressure due to acute CNS infections in children. *Crit Care Med* 2014 Aug;42(8):1775–87.

39. Laccheo I, Sonmezturk H, Bhatt AB, et al. Non-convulsive status epilepticus and non-convulsive seizures in neurological ICU patients. *Neurocrit Care* 2015;22(2):202–11.

40. Claassen J, Silbergleit R, Weingart SD, Smith WS. Emergency neurological life support: status epilepticus. *Neurocrit Care* 2012;17(Suppl 1):S73–8.

41. van de Beek D. Progress and challenges in bacterial meningitis. *Lancet* 2012;380(9854):1623–4.

42. Flores-Cordero JM, Amaya-Villar R, Rincón-Ferrari MD, et al. Acute community-acquired bacterial meningitis in adults admitted to the intensive care unit: clinical manifestations, management and prognostic factors. *Intensive Care Med* 2003;29(11):1967–73.

43. DeBiasi RL, Tyler KL. Viral meningitis and encephalitis. *Continuum (Minneap Minn)* 2006;12:58–94.

44. Petersen LR, Brault AC, Nasci RS. West Nile virus: review of the literature. *JAMA* 2013;310(3):308–15.

45. Corey L, Adams HG, Brown ZA, et al. Genital herpes simplex virus infections: clinical manifestations, course, and complications. *Ann Intern Med* 1983;98:958–72.

46. Crowcroft NS, Thampi N. The prevention and management of rabies. *BMJ* 2015;350:g7827.

47. Lee BE, Chawla R, Langley JM, et al. Paediatric investigators collaborative network on infections in Canada (PICNIC) study of aseptic meningitis. *BMC Infect Dis* 2006;6(68):1–8.

48. Singer J, Maur P, Riley J, et al. Management of central nervous system infections during an epidemic of enteroviral aseptic meningitis. *J Pediatr* 1980;96(3 Pt 2):559–63.

49. Wilfert C, Lehrman S, Katz S. Enteroviruses and meningitis. *Pediatr Infect Dis* 1983;2:333–41.

50. Whitley RJ, Soong SJ, Linneman C Jr, Liu C, Pazin G, Alford CA. Herpes simplex encephalitis. Clinical assessment. *JAMA* 1982;247:317–20.

51. Awasthi M, Parmar H, Patankar T, et al. Imaging findings in rabies encephalitis. *AJNR Am J Neuroradiol* 2001 Apr;22(4):677–80.

52. Willoughby RE Jr, Tieves KS, Hoffman GM, et al. Survival after treatment of rabies with induction of coma. *N Engl J Med* 2005;352:2508–14.

53. Whitley RJ, Soong SJ, Hirsch MS, et al. Herpes simplex encephalitis: vidarabine therapy and diagnostic problems. *N Engl J Med* 1981 Feb 5;304(6):313–8.

54. Brouwer MC, Tunkel AR, McKhann GM 2nd, van de Beek D. Brain abscess. *N Engl J Med* 2014 Jul 31;371(5):447–56.

55. Nicolosi A, Hauser WA, Musicco M, Kurland LT. Incidence and prognosis of brain abscess in a defined population: Olmsted County, Minnesota, 1935–1981. *Neuroepidemiology* 1991;10:122–31.

56. Helweg-Larsen J, Astradsson A, Richhall H, Erdal J, Laursen A, Brennum J. Pyogenic brain abscess, a 15 year survey. *BMC Infect Dis* 2012;12:332.

57. Selby R, Ramirez CB, Singh R, et al. Brain abscess in solid organ transplant recipients receiving cyclosporine-based immunosuppression. *Arch Surg* 1997;132:304–10.

58. Darouiche RO. Spinal epidural abscess. *N Engl J Med* 2006 Nov 9;355(19):2012–20.

59. Darouiche RO, Hamill RJ, Greenberg SB, Weathers SW, Musher DM. Bacterial spinal epidural abscess: review of 43 cases and literature survey. *Medicine (Baltimore)* 1992;71:369–85.

60. Pereira CE, Lynch JC. Spinal epidural abscess: an analysis of 24 cases. *Surg Neurol* 2005;63:(Suppl 1):S26–S29.

61. Akalan N, Ozgen T. Infection as a cause of spinal cord compression: a review of 36 spinal epidural abscess cases. *Acta Neurochir (Wien)* 2000;142:17–23.

62. Rigamonti D, Liem L, Sampath P, et al. Spinal epidural abscess: contemporary trends in etiology, evaluation, and management. *Surg Neurol* 1999;52:189–97.

63. Nussbaum ES, Rigamonti D, Standiford H, Numaguchi Y, Wolf AL, Robinson WL. Spinal epidural abscess: a report of 40 cases and review. *Surg Neurol* 1992;38:225–31.

64. Brouwer MC, Coutinho JM, van de Beek D. Clinical characteristics and outcome of brain abscess: systematic review and meta-analysis. *Neurology* 2014;82: 806–13.

65. Akalan N, Ozgen T. Infection as a cause of spinal cord compression: a review of 36 spinal epidural abscess cases. *Acta Neurochir* 2000;142:17–23.

66. Rigamonti D, Liem L, Sampath P, et al. Spinal epidural abscess: contemporary trends in etiology, evaluation, and management. *Surg Neurol* 1999;52:189–97.

67. Reddy JS, Mishra AM, Behari S, et al. The role of diffusion-weighted imaging in the differential diagnosis of intracranial cystic mass lesions: a report of 147 lesions. *Surg Neurol* 2006;66:246–50.

68. Rotbart HA. Viral meningitis. *Semin Neurol* 2000;20: 277–92.

69. Tan IL, Smith BR, von Geldern G, Mateen FJ, McArthur JC. HIV-associated opportunistic infections of the CNS. *Lancet Neurol* 2012;11:605–17.

70. Nelson CA, Zunt JR. Tuberculosis of the central nervous system in immunocompromised patients: HIV infection and solid organ transplant recipients. *Clin Infect Dis* 2011;53:915–26.

71. Baddley JW, Salzman D, Pappas PG. Fungal brain abscess in transplant recipients: epidemiologic, microbiologic, and clinical features. *Clin Transplant* 2002;16:419–24.

72. Salaki JS, Louria DB, Chmel H. Fungal and yeast infections of the central nervous system. A clinical review. *Medicine (Baltimore)* 1984; 63: pp. 108–32.

73. Alvarez S, McCabe WR. Extrapulmonary tuberculosis revisited: A review of experience at Boston City and other hospitals. *Medicine (Baltimore)* 1984;63:25–55.

31

Neuroprotective Strategies

K. T. Gobeske and S. Wahlster

ABSTRACT

Neuroprotective strategies that limit secondary damage following acute brain injury (ABI) have been identified in numerous experimental models. Despite promising results in animal studies, multiple human trials assessing therapeutic targets have failed. Increasing recognition of preclinical and clinical translational challenges, improvements in trial methodology, and formation of collaborative networks may result in opportunities for successful clinical trials going forward. Also, advanced monitoring techniques in clinical practice may lead to better understanding of human pathophysiology and the development of tailored treatment approaches for the individual patient.

KEYWORDS

Neuroprotection; neurologic injury; neurointensive care; pathologic mechanisms; cell signalling; inflammation.

INTRODUCTION

Acute brain injuries (ABIs) are amongst the greatest contributors to mortality, disability, and healthcare costs worldwide. Stroke alone is the second leading cause of death and third greatest source of Disability Adjusted Life Years.[1] In the USA, there are 52,000 deaths due to traumatic brain injury (TBI) each year,[2] and 5.3 million people live with TBI-related disabilities.[3] In Europe, TBI represents the leading cause of new permanent disability for people under the age of 40.[4] Intracranial haemorrhage (ICH) and hypoxic brain injury (HBI) following cardiopulmonary arrest (CA) are associated with significant mortality, morbidity, and disease burden.

The goal of neuroprotection is to improve outcomes by controlling secondary damage to the central nervous system (CNS). After the primary insult, a subsequent set of events is thought to significantly amplify the initial injury over the following hours and days. These secondary mechanisms tend to follow a finite set of pathways, even for varied causes of injury, and this allows therapeutic targets to be applied broadly across different conditions.[5] The longer time course over which secondary mechanisms progress also suggests a wider window for interventions.

MECHANISMS OF PATHOLOGY

Table 31.1 provides an overview of major secondary pathomechanisms. Many of these processes trigger a complex cascade of downstream effects, which can both be beneficial and detrimental. We outline some of the basic concepts—by no means exhaustive—and potential therapeutic interventions below.

Cell Migration and Paracrine Support

Cell viability in the brain is strongly dependent upon reciprocal signals from neighbouring cells and networks. Injury disrupts contact-dependent and activity-related trophic support, which prompts secondary inflammation and the uncovering of intrinsic cellular motifs suppressing growth and plasticity. Tonic inhibitors of neurite outgrowth, angiogenesis, migration, and axonal regeneration are increased. Mechanisms for axonal guidance also become perturbed. Identifying the receptors and signaling pathways responsible for these processes and their convergence with other inhibitory mechanisms will yield powerful tools to protect or restore neuronal connectivity after injury. New therapies that target the balance or synapse pruning vs formation, or

Table 31.1 Major mechanisms for secondary injury progression and neuroprotection

Cell Migration/Paracrine Support

- Chondroitin sulphate proteoglycan surface molecules → tonic inhibition of migration, proliferation
- Injury → ↑ CSPGs, glial scar components → PTP-σ receptor, ROCK pathway → ↓ axon outgrowth
- INF-γ, ROCK inhibitors, other CSPG ↓ → ↑ axon regrowth, progenitors
- Nogo, MAG, OMgp surface molecules → NgR1-Lingo1-p75 receptor complex → PTEN and RhoA pathways
- PTEN inhibits PI3K/AKT/mTOR → ↓ proliferation
- RhoA/ROCK/LIMK → ↓ outgrowth, migration, connectivity
- Semaphorins, ephrins, netrins, slits, CAMs → various receptors → repulsive>>attractant guidance cues
- Surface/secreted guidance molecules → inhibitory during injury:
- ↑ small GTPase activity → ↑ RhoA/ROCK/LIMK, ↓ Ras/Raf/MEK/ERK
- Cell damage → danger associated molecular patterns, other TLR activators → bind TLR2, TLR4
- Toll-like receptors → activate microglia/astrocytes → cytokine cascades → ↑inhibitory mechanisms
- Glial scar formation → cellular effects → ↓ neurite/cell migration, ↓ contact-dependent trophic support, ↑ CSPG activity[*]

Hypoxia Inducible Factor

- HIF: highly conserved dimeric transcription factor, master regulator of oxygen-dependent metabolism
- Acidosis, low O_2 tension, redox state enzyme/metal-ion → ↓ HIF breakdown → ↑ HIF activity
- Hypoxia → ↓ activity prolyl-4-hydroxylases, asparaginyl hydroxylases → ↑ HIF stability
- HIF → promoter response elements → transcription of VEGF, IGF, TGF, glucose transport proteins
- Treatments stabilizing HIF → ↓ damage from heme breakdown products, ↓ oxidative injury
- Balance of HIF1 vs HIF2 influences: survival, oedema, energy balance, regeneration, membrane stability[#]

Excitotoxicity/Calcium Signalling

- Cell injury, energy imbalance → membrane ion dysfunction → persistent depolarization
- Injury → rapid ↑ intracellular calcium → multiple calcium-related effectors and signalling pathways
- Phospholipase C → inflammatory pathways, IP3+DAG messengers, Ca^{++} channel opening, PKC activation
- Ca^{++} second messenger: motor protein function, apoptosis, fusion/binding proteins, vesicle release, etc.
- Neuronal/astrocyte electrical failure → pre/postsynaptic glutamate spillage → receptor activation
- AMPA/Kainate stimulation → K^+, Na^+, Ca^{++} flux → further loss of electrochemical gradient, energy failure
- NMDA overstimulation → Ca^{++} influx into multiple cell types → apoptosis, abnormal calcium signalling
- Calmodulin activation → activates many kinases and phosphatases, shapes activity of receptors/channels
- Calcium dysregulation has an essential role in excitotoxicity[@]

Neurotrophic/Growth Factors

- Following neurodevelopment → ↓ proliferative/regenerative capacity → support survival, adaptation
- BDNF, VEGF, IGF1, PDGF, CNTF, NGF, EGF, FGF, TGFb: similar neurotrophic roles via different receptors
- Tyrosine kinase and serine-threonine kinase receptors initiate neurotrophic factor downstream signalling
- Receptor subunit dimerization pattern → signalling cascade activation → downstream targets
- Growth factor and TGF-b family signalling may converge at the p38 MAPK signalling cascade
- Therapeutic target: essential downstream pathways, points of convergence; remove common inhibition

Energy Metabolism Imbalance

- Hypothermia, anaesthesia → ↓ metabolism → ↓ demand for oxygen, glucose, ATP, ↓ oxidative stress
- ↓ metabolic demand → ↓ vasodynamic flux → stabilized CSF dynamics → ↓ oedema
- ↓ metabolic demand → restore energy balance, ATP stores, electrochemical gradient → cell survival

(Cont'd)

Table 31.1 (*Cont'd*)

• Hypothermia → ↓ MMP9, ↓ aquaporin 4; ↑ endothelial tight junctions, ↑ astrocyte end foot coupling
• Hypothermia → altered expression AMPA GluR2 and NMDA NR2 subunits → ↓ excitotoxicity progression
• Hypothermia → ↓ BAX, ↑BCL-2, ↓FAS-FASL interaction → ↓ cytochrome-c release, caspase activation
• Hypothermia → ↑ BDNF/VEGF/GDNF/PDGF, ↑ angiogenesis, ↑ progenitor cells, ↑ neurite outgrowth
• Hypothermia → ↓ microglial activation, ↓ glial scar formation → detrimental and beneficial consequences
• Hypothermia anaesthesia → ↑ infections, ↑ medications, ↑ iatrogenic effects, ↑ coagulopathy[**]

Microglial Activation and Secondary Inflammation
• Microglia: CNS innate immune cells
• Injury → DAMPs → TLR2/TLR4 → cytokine cascades → microglial activation → M1/M2 phase subtypes
• Injury → monocyte influx → adopt microglial identity ≠ expansion from resident microglial progenitors
• M1 phase: induced INF-γ, TNF-α; express iNOS, CD32, CD16, CD86, CD11b; produce IL-1b, IL-6, GM-CSF
• M2 phase: induced IL4; express Arg1, CD206, TGM2, c-Myc, CCL22, EGR2, produce IL-10, CXCL12, TGF-b
• Early after injury → ↑ CCL2/CCR2 activity → ↑ monocyte infiltration, secondary inflammation
• Later after injury → ↑ CX3CL1/CX3CR1 → unspecified or M2 subtypes → mixed beneficial/detrimental
• Later after injury → ↑ CXCL12/CXCR4 → M2 subtypes, anti-inflammatory → ↑ neurotrophic factors
• M1/M2 polarity therapeutic target: minocycline, rosiglitazone, azithromycin, metformin, valproic acid[##]

Cortical Spreading Depression
• Injury → altered cortical electrophysiology → slow spreading waves depolarization, depressed activity
• Persistent depolarizations → ↑ electrochemical energy → ↑metabolism → neurovascular coupling
• Waves of oligemia/hyperaemia → regional hypoxia, hypoglycaemia, acidosis → neuron/astrocyte swelling
• Astrocyte swelling, dysfunction → ↓ buffering, K+ reuptake → energy failure, excitotoxicity[@@]

Cell-Based Strategies
• 3 strategies: supply exogenous cells, maximize endogenous potential, gene therapy/cell-based delivery
• durable, injury-site and cell-type specific, protective *and* restorative, innate mechanisms
• Neural Stem Cells: other progenitors cannot replace neurons/astrocytes/oligodendrocytes
• Induced Pluripotent Stem Cells: patient-specific, differentiation to neural lineage, risk forming tumours
• Marrow-lineage cells ≠ mesenchymal stem cells: cannot become NSCs, can supply trophic factors
• Endogenous NSCs: limited number, hippocampus/ventricles neurogenic niche, can be amplified/directed
• Cell vector engineering: manipulate for targeted migration and expression of desired factors
• Viral vector engineering: manipulate for gene delivery to specific place, cell-type, timing
• Vector properties: titre, infection rates, dividing/non-dividing cells, neural tropism, stable integration
• Vector types: adeno-associated, lentivirus, retrovirus, herpes virus, transposon/CRISPR/non-viral systems

Abbreviations: CSPGs: chondroitin sulphate proteoglycans; PTP-σ: protein tyrosine kinase sigma receptor; ROCK: rho associated kinase; INF-γ: interferon gamma; MAG: myelin associated glycoprotein; Nogo: neurite outgrowth inhibitor; OMgp: oligodendrocyte myelin glycoprotein; NgR1: Nogo-66 receptor 1; Lingo1: leucine rich repeat and immunoglobin-like domain-containing protein 1; PTEN: phosphatase and tensin homolog; PI3K: phosphoinositide 3-kinase; AKT: protein kinase B; mTOR: mammalian target of rapamycin; LIMK: LIM domain kinase, etc.

Notes:

*(1) Dyck SM, Karimi-Abdolrezaee S. Chondroitin sulfate proteoglycans: key modulators in the developing and pathologic central nervous system. *Exp Neurol* 2015;269:169–87. (2) Ohtake Y, Li S. Molecular mechanisms of scar-sourced axon growth inhibitors. *Brain Res* 2015;1619:22–35. (3) Forgione N, Fehlings MG. Rho-ROCK inhibition in the treatment of spinal cord injury. *World Neurosurgery* 2014;82(3–4):e535–539. (4) Roloff F, Scheiblich H, Dewitz C, Dempewolf S, Stern M, Bicker G. Enhanced neurite outgrowth of human model (NT2) neurons by small-molecule inhibitors of Rho/ROCK signaling. *PloS One* 2015;10(2):e0118536.

#Kumar H, Choi D-K. Hypoxia inducible factor pathway and physiological adaptation: a cell survival pathway? *Mediators Inflamm* 2015;2015:584758.

@(1) Lai TW, Zhang S, Wang YT. Excitotoxicity and stroke: identifying novel targets for neuroprotection. *Prog Neurobiol* 2014 Apr;115:157–88. (2) Brini M, Calì T, Ottolini D, Carafoli E. Neuronal calcium signaling: function and dysfunction. *Cell Mol Life Sci CMLS* 2014 Aug;71(15):2787–814.

(*Cont'd*)

Table 31.1 *(Cont'd)*

**(1) Liu L, Yenari MA. Therapeutic hypothermia: neuroprotective mechanisms. *Front Biosci J Virtual Libr* 2007 Jan 1;12:816–25. (2) Zhao H, Steinberg GK, Sapolsky RM. General versus specific actions of mild-moderate hypothermia in attenuating cerebral ischemic damage. *J Cereb Blood Flow Metab* 2007;27(12):1879–94. (3) Yenari MA, Han HS. Neuroprotective mechanisms of hypothermia in brain ischaemia. *Nat Rev Neurosci* 2012;13(4):267–78.

##(1) Chen Z, Trapp BD. Microglia and neuroprotection. *J Neurochem* 2016;136(Suppl 1):10–17. (2) Xia C-Y, Zhang S, Gao Y, Wang Z-Z, Chen N-H. Selective modulation of microglia polarization to M2 phenotype for stroke treatment. *Int Immunopharmacol* 2015;25(2):377–82.

@@(1) Wu D. Neuroprotection in experimental stroke with targeted neurotrophins. *NeuroRx J Am Soc Exp Neurother* 2005;2(1):120–8. (2) Hartings JA, Shuttleworth CW, Kirov SA, et al. The continuum of spreading depolarizations in acute cortical lesion development: Examining Leão's legacy. *J Cereb Blood Flow Metab* 2017;37(5):1571–94.

that selectively augment permissive signals while blocking inhibitory ones may have unheralded benefits.[6–9]

Excitotoxicity

Glutamate excitotoxicity is a major pathological mechanism in ABI and many other neurologic diseases. Injured cells cannot maintain membrane ion pumps and electrochemical balance. This causes persistent glutamate release followed by overstimulation of N-methyl-D-aspartic acid or N-methyl-D-aspartate (NMDA) and α-amino-3-hydroxy-5-methyl-4-isoxazolepropionic acid receptor (AMPA) receptors, leading to further fluxes of Ca^{++} and other ions. Cellular swelling, membrane damage, and apoptosis are direct consequences. Despite a well-established pathophysiology, numerous efforts using glutamate receptor antagonists have not yet been proven effective. A major challenge is to develop a drug that inhibits receptors specifically during excitotoxicity to avoid global side effects.[10,11]

Growth Factors

Neurotrophic factors are essential regulatory signaling molecules for CNS development and the maintenance of cell populations throughout life. They foster cell survival, proliferation, and synaptic plasticity at baseline while promoting recovery following injury.[12]

Significant overlaps in functions of different growth factors suggest a point of convergence in their downstream signalling cascades. Discovering mechanisms that inhibit the nascent cellular capacity for growth and regeneration may lead to interventions that can unblock the lost restorative potential of endogenous cell populations following injury. Numerous mechanisms supporting cell proliferation during development become inhibited around the same time, and the targeted removal of a common method for inhibition could have enormous therapeutic potential.

Temperature Regulation

Inducing hypothermia to reduce metabolic demand and preserve non-injured tissue is a well-established concept. Each degree decreased below normothermia provides a 5%–7% reduction in brain oxygen and glucose consumption.[13,14]

Other benefits of hypothermia include reducing oedema and intracranial pressure (ICP), inflammation, vascular permeability and blood–brain barrier (BBB) breakdown, cellular necrosis, and apoptosis.[15,16] Numerous studies in animal models have shown profound benefits, but human trials have had variable results (reviewed in detail in subsequent sections).

Microglial Activation and Secondary Inflammatory Consequences

The inflammatory response to CNS injury is governed by both innate immune cells (microglia) and cells migrating from peripheral populations across the damaged BBB. Products of injured cells trigger the production of cytokines that initiate other immune/inflammatory cell functions and shape the course of secondary/tertiary pathologic progression. Activated microglia can take on pro-inflammatory (M1) or anti-inflammatory (M2) roles depending upon local signals. Understanding and supporting anti-inflammatory components of cytokine signalling is an area of active study. New treatments promoting microglial M2 phase commitment may have a broad and powerful impact.[17,18]

Hormones

Numerous preclinical studies have suggested anti-apoptotic, anti-inflammatory, and antioxidant properties for female sex hormones. Oestrogen may promote cellular repair and proliferation of neural stem cells while progesterone may attenuate excitotoxicity, apoptotic pathways, and diffuse axonal injury (DAI) in experimental TBI models.[19] Thyrotropin-releasing hormone (TRH) may increase cerebral blood flow (CBF) while controlling inflammation and glutamate release. Erythropoietin (EPO) also may limit inflammation, excitotoxicity, and oedema. However, none of these agents has demonstrated significant clinical benefit.

Animal studies with glucocorticoids have shown beneficial and detrimental effects; human trials demonstrated detrimental effects in ICH, TBI, and possibly a marginal benefit in acute spinal cord injury (SCI).

Diketopiperazines are novel dipeptides similar to an active metabolite of TRH that can target numerous pathomechanisms and which have displayed a favourable safety profile and relevant therapeutic window of >8 hrs.[20] Yet their efficacy in larger human trials remains to be proven.

Hypoxia Inducible Factor

Hypoxia inducible factor (HIF) is an evolutionarily conserved transcription factor that is a master regulator of cellular responses to oxygen. Hypoxia inducible factor degradation by oxygen-sensitive enzymes becomes blocked in hypoxic conditions leading to increased production of HIF-induced genes. Thus acidosis, low oxygen tension, and haeme/metal-ion compounds induce HIF to increase angiogenesis, glucose supply and utilization, and neurotrophic factors supporting cell proliferation, migration, and survival. New treatments may target tissue- and time-specific HIF subunit expression. The interaction with nuclear factor kappa-light-chain-enhancer of activated B cells (NF-κB) also possess a potential therapeutic mechanism.[21–23]

Cortical Spreading Depression

Cortical spreading depression (CSD) was first observed in the cortex of rabbits following seizures, and has since been seen with migraine, stroke, subarachnoid haemorrhage (SAH) and TBI. Cortical spreading depression can be produced by applying high concentration KCl to the cortical surface and it can be recorded with electrodes measuring strong spreading depolarisations travelling 2–5 mm/min followed by hyperpolarization and depressed activity lasting 15–30 minutes. Experimental local hypoxia, hypoglycaemia, Na^+/K^+ pump failure, glutamate excitotoxicity, and trauma also can induce CSD. Altered neuronal excitability, metabolic activity, neural circuit responsiveness, and hypoxia-related signalling are associated with injury beyond the primary insult. Generation/recovery of spreading depolarization is a metabolically intense process causing a period of reactive hyperaemia followed by oligaemia. In normal tissue, these repeated waves of depolarization/repolarization coupled with hyperaemia/oligaemia typically do not outstrip demand-supply parameters. In the setting of a critical injury, decompensation of neurovascular coupling results in cortical spreading ischaemia (CSI) or terminal depolarisations. Mitochondrial energy failure and initiation of cellular programmes for apoptosis lead to expanding areas of cell death around the primary injury site, significantly augmenting the extent of injury.

New methods to probe CSD non-invasively in real-time using advanced electroencephalography (EEG), magnetoencephalography (MEG), and transcranial magnetic stimulation (TMS) will illuminate this previously hidden important process. Potential treatments targeting ion channels (e.g., antiepileptic drugs), histone deacetylase inhibitors (HDAC) inhibition, endothelin antagonism, and calcitonin gene-related peptide (CGRP) activity may help to control this central mechanism for injury progression.[24,25]

Cell-Based Therapy, Gene Therapy, and Cell Cycle Programming

Cell- and gene-based therapies hold great promise both to protect and restore CNS function. Patient-derived, engineered stem cells that will hone precisely to a defined place and time are more desirable than generic progenitor-type cells from general sources.

Cell-based therapies may involve exogenous replacement, endogenous facilitation or genetic manipulation of cells with restorative capacity. Presently, only neural-lineage exogenous cells can directly restore injury within the CNS. Non-neural lineage cells can be powerful vectors providing trophic support and can be engineered for increasingly potent and specific actions. The capabilities of extant neural stem/progenitor cells residing within limited neurogenic niches can be amplified and directed by manipulating key cell signalling pathways and genetic processes. The next-generation viral vectors for tailored gene delivery can directly and permanently alter cellular functions involved in recovery.[26,27]

TRANSLATIONAL CHALLENGES

Despite promising animal studies, numerous clinical trials assessing neuroprotective treatments have failed to show improved outcomes. Critical analysis of both preclinical and clinical studies will be important to improve the process of translation.[28]

Multiple methodological issues need to be reconciled to assure that preclinical studies have clinical relevance. While the mechanism of injury can be standardized in animal models, in contrast to the variability of human presentations, there is variable expression of pathology between animal strains, sex, and species.

Experimental models frequently do not accurately reflect human pathology. Likewise, there may be poor translation between animal models and human disease for issues of pharmacokinetics, pharmacodynamics, therapeutic window, and CNS drug penetration. The timing of treatment in animal studies also can occur much earlier and more consistent compared to clinical trials. Experimental animals often receive anaesthesia or other medications before the injury is applied. Many of these agents may affect neuronal function as well as metabolism of the tested drug.[29] Parameters for determining the sample size for an experiment also are different for animal studies, for instance the intention-to-treat concept is not a common practice.

The lack of strategies defining an appropriate sample size has led to many underpowered clinical trials in the past, which may have masked a significant therapeutic benefit. Improved statistical methodology and the formation of multi-centre consortiums yield promise for more accurate estimates and larger sample sizes in future studies. Appropriate patient selection and stratification of patients accounting for severity of injury and other potential confounders may also help detect relevant effects for subsets of populations. Establishing the clinically therapeutic window and targeted enrolment in that timeframe will lead to improved evaluation of intervention. Lastly, more nuanced outcome measures are needed to capture significant effects. Current measures of neurological function such as the modified Rankin Scale (mRS) or the Extended Glasgow Outcome Scale (GOS-E) can lead to oversimplification of outcomes and miss potentially relevant improvements in cognitive status or other domains. Overall, improved selection and methodology will be crucial for the success of future trials.

CLINICAL MODALITIES FOR NEUROPROTECTION

Despite the lack of clinical data supporting neuroprotective strategies, some major advances have been made in the treatment of ABI. Overall, ICU care in units with neurologic expertise has shown to improve patient outcomes. Improved knowledge of disease processes has led to better recognition of complications and prompt treatment. Also, negative trials have been informative in guiding clinical practice such as the abandonment of aggressive blood transfusion strategies after finding lack of improved outcomes while noticing increased medical complications.

We review some basic concepts that are currently applied in clinical practice to reduce further neurological damage following ABI and decrease mortality as well as disability.

Reperfusion and Autoregulation

The treatment of acute ischaemic stroke (AIS) has dramatically evolved over the past decades with the implementation of intravenous tissue plasminogen activator (IV-tPA) and endovascular mechanical thrombectomy (EMT). Multiple studies have demonstrated an association between recanalization and improved clinical outcomes in AIS.[30] The risks of haemorrhagic conversion and reperfusion injury needs to be carefully weighed in each patient before proceeding with IV-tPA or EMT. Endovascular treatment with intra-arterial vasodilators and/or balloon angioplasty is also a therapeutic option for patients with vasospasm and delayed cerebral ischaemia (DCI) after aneurysmal SAH, although clinical outcomes in trials have been variable. In both AIS and SAH, perfusion based neuroimaging can be used as a tool to identify potentially salvageable tissue which is at risk for ischaemia.

Cerebral autoregulation is the ability of the brain to maintain a constant CBF despite varying cerebral perfusion pressures (CPP). A common strategy, while not validated by successful clinical trials, is to target a CPP range at which autoregulation, and subsequently CBF, is best preserved. Cerebral blood flow can be estimated by various monitoring strategies (transcranial Doppler [TCD], ICP, or brain tissue oxygen monitoring, near infrared spectroscopy).[31,32]

Therapeutic Hypothermia

In addition to decreasing metabolic demand, mild to moderate therapeutic hypothermia (TH) is thought to have multiple potentially protective effects, including lowering elevated ICP, decreasing production of free radicals, mitochondrial dysfunction, and inflammatory responses as well as suppression of epileptic activity.

Therapeutic hypothermia after neurological injury has been studied extensively for a variety of neurological conditions. The greatest efficacy of mild TH is seen in the treatment of neonatal hypoxic-ischaemic encephalopathy.[33,34] Improved outcomes of TH were also demonstrated in HBI following cardiac arrest (CA) with a number needed to treat (NNT) of 6 to prevent one unfavourable outcome in select patient populations.[35,36] These findings resulted in the wide implementation of cooling after CA, but this practice was challenged by a recent larger study comparing TH to targeted temperature management (TTM). Patients maintained at 33°C vs 36°C after CA had equal neurological outcomes and mortality rates across all subgroups.[37] It is not clear if potential benefits in the

33°C group were offset by higher rates of confounding exposures and side effects. This trial also raised the question whether just preventing the detrimental effects of hyperthermia itself was neuroprotective, rather than the actions of hypothermia to reduce metabolic demand.

Clinical trials in TBI, stroke, SCI, and status epilepticus (SE) have shown mixed results. While some ICUs treat elevated ICPs after TBI with hypothermia, there is mixed data supporting this practice. Most studies of TH in TBI are limited by small numbers. While a recent larger trial showed unfavourable results when TBI patients had ICP treated with hypothermia,[38] a subsequent large meta-analysis suggests that cooling may be beneficial in adults with TBI, with equivocal results in children.[39,40]

Feasibility trials have demonstrated that TH is generally safe after stroke.[41–43] Some studies have suggested trends towards improved outcomes and slight improvement in haemorrhagic conversion rates and signs of reperfusion injury,[44–46] while others failed to demonstrate beneficial effects. A large international multicentre phase III trial of mild hypothermia after stroke is ongoing.[47]

Few small studies have assessed the effect of TH following ICH suggesting some benefits in peri-haemorrhage oedema and mortality.[48–50] Phase II trials are ongoing.

A recent trial of TH in SE did not show any significant neurological improvement, however, a decrease in the duration of seizures was observed.[51]

Clinical challenges encountered with cooling include haemodynamic instability, impairment of coagulation cascades, and extensive shivering (additional sedation and paralysis may be required). Various methods to induce hypothermia, including external devices (cooling blankets), internal probes (bladder, intravascular or intranasal approach) are widely available, and pharmacological methods are also being developed.

Intracranial Pressure Control

Various types of severe ABI result in increased ICP, mostly due to cytotoxic and/or vasogenic oedema or space-occupying lesions (various types of ICH, including epidural haemorrhage [EDH], subdural haemorrhage [SDH], intraparenchymal haemorrhage [IPH], SAH, and contusions), resulting in direct mass effect. Elevated ICP can significantly worsen primary injury in multiple ways: herniation and/or compression of vital brain structures leading to subsequent irreversible damage, and diminished perfusion due to limiting blood flow to adjacent areas leading to additional ischaemic insults.

The key steps to appropriate clinical management include recognizing conditions in which elevated ICP can pose a significant threat (large ischaemic middle cerebral artery [MCA] and cerebellar strokes, ICH with certain size/location), knowing concerned clinical signs as well as timeframe during which a patient is at risk for elevated ICP.

Details regarding pathophysiology and treatment options of increased ICP are outlined in Chapter 25 ('Intracranial Hypertension').[31,32]

Seizure Control

Seizures are frequently encountered in different types of ABI, such as ischaemic stroke, SAH, TBI, and ICH and are thought to worsen outcomes by increasing metabolic demand, ICP as well as CSD/risk of CSI, or excitotoxicity due to excessive brain activity. The exact location, type, and duration of the event are additional factors determining the need for aggressive treatment. Status epilepticus has been associated with increased mortality and poor outcomes, and prompt treatment is crucial to diminish further brain injury. Patients with SE are also at high risk for subsequent non-convulsive seizures and SE (up to 48% within 24 hrs). Continuous EEG should be strongly considered after a prolonged seizure, especially if the clinical examination remains concerning.

FUTURE DIRECTIONS

Further exploration of underlying pathomechanisms and their implementation from bench to bedside are paramount to identify effective neuroprotective strategies. Challenges of translational research are being recognized, as reviewed above, and need to be addressed for future trials. Another promising approach is the evaluation of multipotential drugs with a broader impact on the complex processes that occur after ABI. Non-pharmacological approaches, such as exercise, calorie restriction, and environmental enrichment have shown to activate endogenous neuroprotective factors and pathways, and research to develop drugs targeting these pathways is ongoing.

A major topic of ongoing investigation is the assessment of effects that various sedative/anaesthetic drugs may have on ICP, cerebral metabolism, and the pathophysiology of neuronal injury. As many ICU patients or ABI patients requiring surgery are heavily exposed to these agents, further knowledge about their potential beneficial or harmful effects in various patient populations may lead to changes in practice.

Continuously evolving advances in multimodal monitoring aims to gain further insight into human pathophysiology and identify patterns that warrant emergent intervention. Although yet to demonstrate improved outcomes, invasive monitoring techniques and their correlation with various parameters and trends (such as ICP, CBF, EEG, vital signs, etc.) may lead to treatment approaches accounting for the complexity of each individual patient. The development of significant serum biomarkers is also an active area of research. The formation of large consortia across the globe and collaborative acquisition of data in large cohorts will lead to increased opportunities for successful clinical trials.

CONCLUSIONS

There is an enormous need for better understanding and treatments of acute neurologic injuries. The complexity of the underlying pathophysiology and design of clinical trials has limited progress to date. Yet despite the manifold ways that an initial CNS injury may occur, there is increasing evidence that the mechanisms of secondary injury progression may be more limited. Since these typically are the largest overall contributors to pathology, new studies to clarify the pathways of secondary injury will have greater payoff for future therapies.

REFERENCES

1. Hankey GJ. The global and regional burden of stroke. *Lancet Glob Health* 2013 Nov;1(5):e239–240.
2. Coronado VG, McGuire LC, Sarmiento K, et al. Trends in traumatic brain injury in the U.S. and the public health response: 1995–2009. *J Safety Res* 2012 Sep;43(4):299–307.
3. Centers for Disease Control and Prevention (CDC). CDC grand rounds: reducing severe traumatic brain injury in the United States. *MMWR Morb Mortal Wkly Rep* 2013;62(27):549–52.
4. Peeters W, van den Brande R, Polinder S, et al. Epidemiology of traumatic brain injury in Europe. *Acta Neurochir (Wien)* 2015;157(10):1683–96.
5. Stocchetti N, Taccone FS, Citerio G, et al. Neuroprotection in acute brain injury: an up-to-date review. *Crit Care (Lond England)* 2015 Apr 21;19:186.
6. Dyck SM, Karimi-Abdolrezaee S. Chondroitin sulfate proteoglycans: Key modulators in the developing and pathologic central nervous system. *Exp Neurol* 2015 Jul;269:169–87.
7. Ohtake Y, Li S. Molecular mechanisms of scar-sourced axon growth inhibitors. *Brain Res* 2015;1619:22–35.
8. Forgione N, Fehlings MG. Rho-ROCK inhibition in the treatment of spinal cord injury. *World Neurosurgery* 2014 Oct;82(3–4):e535–539.
9. Roloff F, Scheiblich H, Dewitz C, Dempewolf S, Stern M, Bicker G. Enhanced neurite outgrowth of human model (NT2) neurons by small-molecule inhibitors of Rho/ROCK signaling. *PloS One* 2015;10(2):e0118536.
10. Lai TW, Zhang S, Wang YT. Excitotoxicity and stroke: identifying novel targets for neuroprotection. *Prog Neurobiol* 2014;115:157–88.
11. Brini M, Calì T, Ottolini D, Carafoli E. Neuronal calcium signaling: function and dysfunction. *Cell Mol Life Sci CMLS* 2014 Aug;71(15):2787–814.
12. Wu D. Neuroprotection in experimental stroke with targeted neurotrophins. *NeuroRx J Am Soc Exp Neurother.* 2005 Jan;2(1):120–28.
13. Erecinska M, Thoresen M, Silver IA. Effects of hypothermia on energy metabolism in mammalian central nervous system. *J Cereb Blood Flow Metab* 2003;23(5):513–30.
14. Liu L, Yenari MA. Therapeutic hypothermia: neuroprotective mechanisms. *Front Biosci J Virtual Libr;* 12:816–25.
15. Zhao H, Steinberg GK, Sapolsky RM. General versus specific actions of mild-moderate hypothermia in attenuating cerebral ischemic damage. *J Cereb Blood Flow Metab* 2007;27(12):1879–94.
16. Yenari MA, Han HS. Neuroprotective mechanisms of hypothermia in brain ischaemia. *Nat Rev Neurosci* 2012; 13(4):267–78.
17. Chen Z, Trapp BD. Microglia and neuroprotection. *J Neurochem* 2016 Jan;136(Suppl 1):10–17.
18. Xia C-Y, Zhang S, Gao Y, Wang Z-Z, Chen N-H. Selective modulation of microglia polarization to M2 phenotype for stroke treatment. *Int Immunopharmacol* 2015 Apr; 25(2):377–82.
19. Sayeed I, Stein DG. Progesterone as a neuroprotective factor in traumatic and ischemic brain injury. *Prog Brain Res* 2009;175:219–37.
20. Faden AI, Movsesyan VA, Knoblach SM, Ahmed F, Cernak I. Neuroprotective effects of novel small peptides in vitro and after brain injury. *Neuropharmacology* 2005 Sep;49(3):410–24.
21. Kumar H, Choi D-K. Hypoxia inducible factor pathway and physiological adaptation: a cell survival pathway? *Mediators Inflamm* 2015;2015:584758.
22. Sen T, Sen N. Treatment with an activator of hypoxia-inducible factor 1, DMOG provides neuroprotection after traumatic brain injury. *Neuropharmacology* 2016 Aug;107:79–88.
23. Smeyne M, Sladen P, Jiao Y, Dragatsis I, Smeyne RJ. HIF1α is necessary for exercise-induced neuroprotection while HIF2α is needed for dopaminergic neuron survival in the substantia nigra pars compacta. *Neuroscience* 2015; 295:23–38.
24. Kramer DR, Fujii T, Ohiorhenuan I, Liu CY. Cortical spreading depolarization: Pathophysiology, implications, and future directions. *J Clin Neurosci*, Official J Neurosurg Soc Australas. 2016 Feb;24:22–27.
25. Hartings JA, Shuttleworth CW, Kirov SA, et al. The continuum of spreading depolarizations in acute cortical lesion development: Examining Leão's legacy. *J Cereb Blood Flow Metab* 2017;37(5):1571–94.

26. Weston NM, Sun D. The potential of stem cells in treatment of traumatic brain injury. *Curr Neurol Neurosci Rep* 2018;18(1):1.

27. Snyder BR, Boulis NM, Federici T. Viral vector-mediated gene transfer for CNS disease. *Expert Opin Biol Ther* 2010 Mar;10(3):381–94.

28. Kabadi SV, Faden AI. Neuroprotective strategies for traumatic brain injury: improving clinical translation. *Int J Mol Sci* 2014;15(1):1216–36.

29. Statler KD, Alexander H, Vagni V, et al. Comparison of seven anesthetic agents on outcome after experimental traumatic brain injury in adult, male rats. *J Neurotrauma* 2006;23(1):97–108.

30. Goyal M, Menon BK, van Zwam WH, et al. Endovascular thrombectomy after large-vessel ischaemic stroke: a meta-analysis of individual patient data from five randomised trials. *Lancet (Lond Engl)* 2016;387(10029):1723–31.

31. Tasneem N, Samaniego EA, Pieper C, et al. Brain multimodality monitoring: a new tool in neurocritical care of comatose patients. *Crit Care Res Pract* 2017;2017: 6097265.

32. Frontera J, Ziai W, O'Phelan K, et al. Second neurocritical care research conference investigators. Regional brain monitoring in the neurocritical care unit. *Neurocrit Care* 2015 Jun;22(3):348–59.

33. Gluckman PD, Wyatt JS, Azzopardi D, et al. Selective head cooling with mild systemic hypothermia after neonatal encephalopathy: multicentre randomised trial. *Lancet (Lond Engl)* 2005;365(9460):663–70.

34. Shankaran S, Laptook AR, Ehrenkranz RA, et al. Whole-body hypothermia for neonates with hypoxic-ischemic encephalopathy. *N Engl J Med* 2005 Oct 13;353(15): 1574–84.

35. Bernard SA, Gray TW, Buist MD, et al. Treatment of comatose survivors of out-of-hospital cardiac arrest with induced hypothermia. *N Engl J Med* 2002 Feb 21; 346(8):557–63.

36. Hypothermia after Cardiac Arrest Study Group. Mild therapeutic hypothermia to improve the neurologic outcome after cardiac arrest. *N Engl J Med* 2002;346(8):549–56.

37. Nielsen N, Wetterslev J, Cronberg T, et al. Targeted temperature management at 33°C versus 36°C after cardiac arrest. *N Engl J Med* 2013;369(23):2197–206.

38. Andrews PJD, Sinclair HL, Rodriguez A, et al. Hypothermia for intracranial hypertension after traumatic brain injury. *N Engl J Med* 2015 Dec 17;373(25):2403–12.

39. Crompton EM, Lubomirova I, Cotlarciuc I, Han TS, Sharma SD, Sharma P. Meta-analysis of therapeutic hypothermia for traumatic brain injury in adult and pediatric patients. *Crit Care Med* 2017;45(4):575–83.

40. Adelson PD, Wisniewski SR, Beca J, et al. Comparison of hypothermia and normothermia after severe traumatic brain injury in children (Cool Kids): a phase 3, randomised controlled trial. *Lancet Neurol* 2013 Jun;12(6): 546–53.

41. De Georgia MA, Krieger DW, Abou-Chebl A, et al. Cooling for acute ischemic brain damage (COOL AID): a feasibility trial of endovascular cooling. *Neurology* 2004; 63(2):312–7.

42. Hemmen TM, Raman R, Guluma KZ, et al. Intravenous thrombolysis plus hypothermia for acute treatment of ischemic stroke (ICTuS-L): final results. *Stroke* 2010; 41(10):2265–70.

43. Lyden P, Hemmen T, Grotta J, et al. Results of the ICTuS 2 Trial (Intravascular cooling in the treatment of stroke 2). *Stroke* 2016 Dec;47(12):2888–95.

44. Horn CM, Sun C-HJ, Nogueira RG, et al. Endovascular Reperfusion and Cooling in Cerebral Acute Ischemia (ReCCLAIM I). *J Neurointerventional Surg* 2014 Mar; 6(2):91–95.

45. Piironen K, Tiainen M, Mustanoja S, et al. Mild hypothermia after intravenous thrombolysis in patients with acute stroke: a randomized controlled trial. *Stroke* 2014 Feb;45(2):486–91.

46. Su Y, Fan L, Zhang Y, et al. Improved neurological outcome with mild hypothermia in surviving patients with massive cerebral hemispheric infarction. *Stroke* 2016 Feb;47(2):457–63.

47. van der Worp HB, Macleod MR, Bath PMW, et al. EuroHYP-1: European multicenter, randomized, phase III clinical trial of therapeutic hypothermia plus best medical treatment vs. best medical treatment alone for acute ischemic stroke. *Int J Stroke*, Official J Int Stroke Soc. 2014 Jul;9(5):642–5.

48. Kollmar R, Juettler E, Huttner HB, et al. Cooling in intracerebral hemorrhage (CINCH) trial: protocol of a randomized German-Austrian clinical trial. *Int J Stroke* 2012 Feb;7(2):168–72.

49. Staykov D, Wagner I, Volbers B, Doerfler A, Schwab S, Kollmar R. Mild prolonged hypothermia for large intracerebral hemorrhage. *Neurocrit Care* 2013;18(2): 178–83.

50. Rincon F, Friedman DP, Bell R, Mayer SA, Bray PF. Targeted temperature management after intracerebral hemorrhage (TTM-ICH): methodology of a prospective randomized clinical trial. *Int J Stroke* 2014;9(5): 646–51.

51. Legriel S, Lemiale V, Schenck M, et al. Hypothermia for neuroprotection in convulsive status epilepticus. *N Engl J Med* 2016 22;375(25):2457–67.

Part VI

Metabolic Care

Editor: Michel Torbey

32

Glycaemic Control in Neurocritical Care

S. Hafeez, D. Greene-Chandos, and M. T. Torbey

ABSTRACT

The presence of stress hyperglycaemia has been associated with acute neurologic injury, its initial presence is either a marker of the severity of the disease and or a causative mechanism of secondary cerebral injury and a potential therapeutic target. The available evidence in different populations of neurocritically ill patients—traumatic brain injury (TBI), aneurysmal subarachnoid haemorrhage (aSAH), stroke, intracerebral haemorrhage (ICH), and status epilepticus (SE)—shows that the avoidance of severe hyperglycaemia: serum glucose >180 mg/dL and avoidance of hypoglycaemia <80 mg/dL are likely excellent clinical guidelines to follow to lessen neurologic morbidity and prevent worse outcomes.

KEYWORDS

Cerebral microdialysis; traumatic brain injury (TBI); aneurysmal subarachnoid haemorrhage (aSAH); acute ischaemic stroke; intracerebral haemorrhage (ICH); stress hyperglycaemia.

INTRODUCTION

Abnormal glucose levels are extraordinarily common in critically ill patients. The traditional thinking has been that abnormal glucose levels were related to bacterial consumption of glucose and hyperglycaemia as a marker of strong and protective adrenal response. However, since a seminal trial was published in 2001 by Van de Berghe[1] showing a significant decrease in mortality with very tight glycaemic control via continuous insulin therapy in surgical critical care patients; hyperglycaemia has become a therapeutic target for intense study.

The incidence of hyperglycaemia varies from 15%–50% in critically ill patients. It is often associated with nausea, abdominal pain, seizures, altered consciousness, and focal neurological deficits. Symptoms of hyperglycaemia are not easily identified in neurocritical care patients due to the confounding effect of cerebral injury and altered mental status.[1–4] Both glycaemic states cause a wide variety of biochemical, radiographical, and clinical changes that are associated with poor outcomes in diverse critically ill populations. In this chapter, we will focus on neurologically ill patients specifically-traumatic brain injury (TBI), aneurysmal subarachnoid haemorrhage (aSAH), acute ischaemic stroke (AIS), intracerebral haemorrhage (ICH), and status epilepticus (SE).[1] In neurocritically ill patients, we are starting to understand the optimal glucose control in different neurocritical care diseases. Prevention of severe hyperglycaemia is vital in keeping homoeostasis during the acute phase of neurologic injury and helps prevent further secondary neurologic injury and inflammation. What is being studied in more detail is what constitutes optimal glucose control in different disease states and at what time points should hyperglycaemia be allowed.[5,6]

GENERAL CRITICAL CARE GUIDELINES

Several large clinical trials have failed to definitively define the optimal glucose range in critically ill patients. Initial trials by van dan Berghe generated significant enthusiasm because they found an association between tight glucose control and decreased mortality. In critically ill septic patients with multi-organ failure, glucose levels maintained at 80–110 mg/dL decreased mortality from 8% to 4.6%.[1]

Several associations and societies—American Diabetes Association, American College of Physicians, American Association of Clinical Endocrinologists, and Society of Critical Care Medicine immediately adopted the findings and recommended tight glucose control targets ranging from <150 mg/dL or 110–140 mg/dL.[7–9]

However, since then, three large randomized controlled trials (RCTs) were conducted: (1) GLUCONTROL; (2) Volume Substitution and Insulin Therapy in Severe Sepsis (VISEP); and (3) Normoglycaemia in Intensive Care Evaluation–Survival Using Glucose Algorithm Regulation (NICE-SUGAR). However, these could not reproduce the results of the original trial. The results from these trials cast a shadow of confusion on the optimal glucose levels in critically ill patients. Soon thereafter, the Society of Critical Care Medicine updated their guidelines, which recommended avoidance of severe hyperglycaemia ≥180 mg/dL.[7] While most societies and clinicians have not come to a consensus on optimal glycaemic range, most agree that hypoglycaemia should be avoided.[10,11] Today, there are no large RCTs evaluating optimal glucose management in acute neurologically injured patients, however, good observational and cohort data will be examined below.

HYPERGLYCAEMIA IN NEUROCRITICAL CARE

Stress hyperglycaemia is associated with a wide range of primary brain injuries such as TBI, SAH, ICH, ischaemic stroke, and SE. This secondary hyperglycaemia is secondary to the cerebral and systemic inflammatory response triggered within hours of injury and lasting several days.[4,5] The cerebral injury results in increased cerebral metabolic demand and energy expenditure to maintain cellular ion gradients, causes local ischaemia, induces cerebral vasospasm, and increases capillary permeability. All of these ongoing cerebral processes propagates stress hyperglycaemia. Coupled with systemic inflammatory responses from other injuries—acute lung injury or acute respiratory distress syndrome (ARDS), microcirculatory shock, and hypertension; the constant inflammatory assault propagates the stress hyperglycaemic response.[12–15] Initially, clinicians and scientists hypothesized that this stress hyperglycaemic response is protective or at least provides the substrates necessary to fight the inflammatory response. However, scientists and clinicians have shown that stress hyperglycaemia is associated with a myriad of negative consequences: increased mortality, increased intensive care unit (ICU) length of stay, acute kidney injury, anaemia, polyneuropathy, and increased incidence of nosocomial infection.[14] It is unclear if stress

hyperglycaemia is a marker of initial severity of injury or a causative mechanism of secondary cerebral injury and a viable target for early therapy.

BACKGROUND PHYSIOLOGY AND MICRODIALYSIS STUDIES

During brain injury, both neurons and astrocytes have strong demands for energy and are exquisitely intolerant of low energy states and process excessive glucose.[12,13] In hyperglycaemia, the astrocytes and neurons become overloaded with glucose and cause free radical formation and oxidative injury. This activates N-methyl-D-aspartate (NMDA) receptors causing calcium excitotoxicity and release of intracellular calcium into the affected tissue. This results in increased local lactic acidosis and initiates apoptosis and microglial migration.[13] Local lactic acidosis and peri-ischaemic cortical depolarization become clinically relevant and can be identified via microdialysis, electrocorticography, and imaging studies. In animal models, there are two main glucose transporters in the brain that affect glucose regulation. The glucose transporter (GLUT) 1 found in the blood–brain barrier (BBB) mediates glucose uptake from extracellular fluid into astrocytes, oligodendroglia, and microglia. The GLUT3 transporter located on neurons allows for passive movement of neuronal glucose.[4] This is important because in severe TBI, the GLUT3 is upregulated and facilitates neuronal uptake of glucose while the GLUT1 is downregulated and results in less glucose to the supportive cell structures. This is likely a protective mechanism against hypoglycaemia.[15,16]

Another piece of the puzzle is related to mitochondrial changes during brain injury. Mitochondria are the powerhouses of the cell and provide aerobic energy to the neurons and surrounding cytoarchitecture. After a cerebral injury, the cerebral mitochondria become damaged and aerobic oxidative phosphorylation shuts down which in turn forces the neuron to begin anaerobic glycolysis and increases lactate production. Lactate is then metabolized to pyruvate to generate adenosine triphosphate (ATP). This results in an elevated lactate–pyruvate ratio (LPR). Elevated LPR, when measured in microdialysis studies in brain injured patients has shown to be associated with poor outcome and local cerebral ischaemia.[12,14,15] When the LPR becomes highly elevated in a hypoglycaemic state, the brain is said to undergo a cerebral metabolic energy crisis, which previous authors have defined as LPR >40 with a microdialysis glucose level of <0.7 mmol/L.[12,13] A simplistic answer to this problem would be to ensure normal serum glucose levels in brain injured patients, however, due to the several issues mentioned above – glucose receptor dysfunction, interruption of glucose shuttling, mitochondrial damage, peri-ischaemic cortical depolarization, and local ischaemia—normal glucose levels may not be enough to ensure cerebral hypoglycaemia is not occurring.[17–19]

TRAUMATIC BRAIN INJURY

Cerebral hyperglycaemia is associated with poor outcomes in severe TBI or trauma as best evidenced by the corticosteroid randomisation after significant head injury (CRASH trial) and the International Mission for Prognosis and Clinical Trial (IMPACT) database and several large single centre studies.[20–24] Severe TBI is associated with widespread inflammatory response and stress hyperglycaemia. The treatment of hyperglycaemia in severe TBI is controversial as intensive therapy can cause several hypoglycaemic episodes but excess hyperglycaemia is harmful. Five previous RCTs compared intensive vs conventional glycaemic targets and found no difference in mortality but found a difference in neurological recovery.[25] One study in particular showed an increased mortality risk for a single episode of serum glucose >200 mg/dL. A single centre RCT showed that intensive insulin therapy in severe TBI patients

demonstrated a mean decrease of 2.7 days in ICU length of stay but no difference in Glasgow Outcome Scale – Extended (GOS-E), mortality, or infection rate. It is important to note that no hypoglycaemic episodes were reported.[25] Intensive glucose control in several trials was associated with a lower risk of poor neurological outcome (58% vs 68%). Most of these studies allowed serum glucose in the control arm to be relatively high ≥200 mg/dL.[15] Cerebral microdialysis studies tell a paradoxical story of glucose control in TBI. Two studies show that during intensive insulin therapy, despite normal serum glucose (120–150 mg/dL), the brain is under significant metabolic distress from hypoglycaemia – increased lactate/pyruvate ratio and increased glutamate – without an improvement in mortality or neurological outcome.[12,13] Therefore, following serum glucose or cerebral glucose levels and what targets to aim for is still under investigation. The optimal approach to glycaemic control in TBI remains largely unknown.

Contusions and haematoma expansion in moderate and severe TBI is very common and the aetiology of their expansion is still under investigation. Animal models suggest that early hyperglycaemia in subjects with contusions from moderate TBI was associated with increased contusion area and neutrophil accumulation, suggesting that acute hyperglycaemia is present when cerebral inflammation is occurring (Table 32.1).[26]

Table 32.1 Intensive insulin therapy in traumatic brain injury

Study*	No. of patients	Intensive glucose control range	Conventional range	Hypoglycaemia definition	Nutrition initiation	Outcome
Coester	88	80–110 mg/dL	<180 mg/dL	<80 mg/dL	EN ASAP	• No mortality benefit
Yang	240	80–110 mg/dL	Target 180–200 mg/dL	<40 mg/dL	IV dextrose for 24 hr then EN or PN	• No mortality benefit • Lower infection rate • Improved neurologic outcome at 6 months
Bilotta	97	80–120 mg/dL	<220 mg/dL	<80 mg/dL	EN or PN ASAP	• No mortality benefit • No neurologic benefit outcome • Shorter ICU stay • More episodes of hypoglycaemia
Finfer	391	80–110 mg/dL	140–180 mg/dL	<40 mg/dL	EN ASAP	• No mortality benefit • No neurologic benefit outcome

* (1) Coester A, et al. Intensive insulin therapy in severe traumatic brain injury: a randomized trial. *J Trauma* 2010 Apr;68(4):904–11. (2) Yang M, et al. Intensive insulin therapy on infection rate, days in NICU, in-hospital mortality and neurological outcome in severe traumatic brain injury patients: a randomized controlled trial. *Int J Nurs Stud* 2009 Feb 20;46(6):753–8. (3) Bilotta F, et al. Intensive insulin therapy after severe traumatic brain injury: A randomized clinical trial. *Neurocrit Care* 2008;9(2):159–66. (4) Finfer S, et al. Intensive versus conventional glucose control in critically ill patients with traumatic brain injury: long-term follow-up of a subgroup of patients from the NICE–SUGAR study. *Intensive Care Med* 2015 Jun;41(6):1037–47.

ANEURYSMAL SUBARACHNOID HAEMORRHAGE

The main goal of therapy in aSAH patients is reducing further cerebral injury by treating the causes of cerebral vasospasm and minimizing delayed cerebral ischaemia (DCI). Maintenance of homoeostasis is key in the treatment of SAH—normothermia, normovolaemia, and normotension. Normoglycaemia is no different. However, there is a balance between increased cerebral glucose demand and hyperglycaemia-inducing inflammation.[27,28] In aSAH, admission hyperglycaemia and persistent hyperglycaemia is common and associated with development of symptomatic cerebral vasospasm, DCI, cerebral infarction, and worse outcomes compared to patients with normal blood glucose levels.[28] There are several theories and probable explanations as to why aSAH is associated with hyperglycaemia such as activation of the hypothalamic-pituitary-adrenal axis, catecholamine surges, increased cytokine production, insulin resistance, and activation of glycogenolysis and gluconeogenesis.[29]

Cerebral Vasospasm

One of the most common complications of aSAH is cerebral vasospasm. It occurs in approximately 30% of patients with aSAH. Currently only one proven therapy, oral nimodipine, is associated with improved outcomes of aSAH. Thus, there is a rush to find neuroprotective agents to treat DCI and demonstrate physiological targets that improve outcomes—one of those targets being hyperglycaemia. Hyperglycaemia has been linked to the presence or worsening of cerebral vasospasm. A retrospective study of 352 patients at a single centre demonstrated an association of mean admission and inpatient glucose values with development of symptomatic cerebral vasospasm. Multiple in vitro and in vivo studies have linked hyperglycemia with alterations in vascular tone to demonstrate an inhibition of vasodilation and increasing vasoconstriction.[30] Microdialysis studies conducted in patients across all grades of aSAH show blood glucose levels >140 mg/dL is independently associated with unfavourable outcome.[31] The Guidelines for the management of aSAH by the American Heart Association/American Stroke Association (AHA/ASA) addresses hyperglycaemia in two regards. First, for patients undergoing cerebral aneurysm surgery, the guidelines suggest that intraoperative hyperglycaemia with glucose concentrations above 129 mg/dL have been associated with alteration of cognition; and neurological deficits with glucose concentrations above 152 mg/dL. Hence hyperglycaemia should be avoided.

The second recommendation is strict avoidance of hypoglycaemia.[32,33] Otherwise, there is no current recommendation from the AHA/ASA guidelines as to what optimal serum glucose should be postoperatively, through the vasospasm period, and thereafter.[34]

ACUTE ISCHAEMIC STROKE

Ischaemic stroke is responsible for significant morbidity, disability, and healthcare expenditure in the US. The best treatments for stroke patients centres on secondary stroke prevention and reduction of morbidity and disability. Several areas of research are underway to reduce morbidity and mortality—early types of physical therapy, blood pressure control, agents to reduce cerebral oedema, and primary neuroprotective agents.[35,36] Another key therapeutic target has been stress hyperglycaemia. Accumulating evidence has suggested that hyperglycaemia is associated with poor outcomes. Post-stroke hyperglycaemia has also been associated with increased cerebral oedema, haemorrhagic transformation, lower likelihood of arterial recanalization, increased inflammation, and free radical production in the penumbral area, and deterioration of neurological state.[36–40] In acute ischaemic stroke, several different cellular processes occur simultaneously to cause brain injury: parenchymal and axonal hypoxic-ischaemic damage, microglia activation and migration, and cellular apoptosis. These processes are collectively responsible for primary injury from ischaemic stroke, however, these processes then activate a secondary inflammatory response that causes post-stroke hyperglycaemia.[41]

Therefore, the question again comes: is post-stroke hyperglycaemia a marker of severity of initial illness or a causal mechanism of secondary injury? In an attempt to address this conundrum, several prospective studies have been done: the UK glucose insulin stroke trial (GIST-UK),[39] the intensive vs subcutaneous insulin in patients with hyperacute stroke (INSULINFARCT)[38] trial, and the Glycaemia in Acute Stroke (GLIAS)37 trial. Initially, the aim of the GLIAS study was to establish a higher limit of serum glucose associated with poor outcome. The nearly 500 patient study concluded a serum glucose level of 155 mg/dL or greater was associated with poor outcome, independent of pre-existing diabetes mellitus.[38,39] Therefore, the next natural step in this area occurred with the GIST-UK trial, which was designed to use glucose/insulin/potassium infusion to maintain normoglycaemia. The RCT of 933 patients resulted in lower glucose levels in the experimental arm. However, 4-week mortality was not improved. The study also suffered from significant selection bias.[39] The INSULINFARCT study hypothesized intensive insulin therapy (IIT) compared to subcutaneous insulin therapy would improve outcome. One hundred and eighty patients with acute stroke were randomized to receive either therapy during the first 24 hours following acute ischaemic stroke. It was shown that IIT in the first 24 hours was associated with larger infarct growth and was not recommended. The largest trial being currently conducted is the Stroke Hyperglycaemia Insulin Network Effort (SHINE). The SHINE trial is aiming at studying 1,400 patients from approximately 60 enrolling sites that hypothesizes the treatment of hyperglycaemic acute ischaemic stroke patients with targeted glucose concentration (80 mg/dL–130 mg/dL) will be safe and result in improved 3-month outcome after stroke. The control group uses sliding scale insulin to keep glucose less than 180 mg/dL.[40] Collectively, these studies suggest that tight glucose control has not shown any improvement in outcome—likely from several episodes of hypoglycaemia—but prevention of severe hyperglycaemia is paramount.

Ischaemic Penumbra

The ischaemic penumbra is an area of brain in a low flow state that a stroke has not yet fully claimed; and if blood flow is restored to that area of parenchyma it can be saved. Although restoring blood flow is the most major factor, the penumbral area also requires sufficient energy supply. Hyperglycaemia has been associated with worsening the ischaemic penumbra.[36,41] During a stroke, glucose transporters decrease cellular uptake of available glucose to the infarcted tissue and upregulate it in the penumbral tissue to increase glucose uptake. These changes suggest the brain has an adaptive response to increase energy stores to the penumbral tissue and increased oxygen extraction.[42,43] However, in acute stroke patients with magnetic resonance imaging (MRI) scans showing perfusion-diffusion mismatch, higher blood glucose concentration correlated with less percentage of mismatch indicating poor collateral flow from long-standing hyperglycaemia or peri-ischaemic cortical depolarization from hyperglycaemia and further local ischaemia.[44]

Hyperglycaemia and Intravenous Tissue Plasminogen Activator

The link between hyperglycaemia and haemorrhagic transformation of an ischaemic stroke after tissue plasminogen activator (TPA) treatment is an intriguing association. In a retrospective evaluation of outcomes in a trial of TPA in 138 stroke patients, baseline serum glucose was the only independent predictor of haemorrhagic transformation. The overall rate of symptomatic bleeds was only 9%; however, in patients with serum glucose greater than 200 mg/dL, the rate was 25% (Table 32.2).[45–47]

INTRACEREBRAL HAEMORRHAGE

The AHA/ASA management of intracerebral haemorrhage guidelines does not give a specific recommendation on glucose range. They only mention hypoglycaemia should be avoided. The only class I recommendation is that glucose should be monitored and both hyperglycaemia and hypoglycaemia avoided.[48] These recommendations are largely based on retrospective cohort studies in which hyperglycaemia has been associated with poor outcome, increased mortality, and increased haematoma expansion in spontaneous intracerebral haemorrhage (sICH) patients.[49–52]

A similar and significant inflammatory response is caused by sICH, related to size of haemorrhage. Initial leukocytosis and systemic inflammatory response syndrome (SIRS) response in sICH is not associated with any type of infection but a marker of severity of illness and interestingly associated with presence of intraventricular haemorrhage.[49] Compared to TBI and SAH, the prognostic implication of hyperglycaemia and haematoma volume expansion is directly proportional to poor outcome and mortality in patients with sICH.[48–50] Therefore, in sICH, early intensive insulin therapy may be more warranted to prevent early oedema formation and haematoma expansion. Specifically related to sICH, there is an increased hospital length of stay (LOS) in patients who present with hyperglycaemia and have persistent hyperglycaemia throughout their stay. Significant fluctuations in glucose levels in patients with poorly controlled diabetes mellitus are likely an association with poor pre-morbid status.[50,51]

There are several upcoming clinical trials associated with glucose control and sICH. These studies should be sufficiently powered to answer the question of what is the optimal glucose levels patients with spontaneous ICH should be kept at to promote early neuron-astrocyte architecture repair and removal of necrotic cellular debris and prevent ischaemia to the peri-haematoma penumbra.

PERIOPERATIVE GLUCOSE CONTROL

In patients with pre-existing diabetes mellitus, uncontrolled hyperglycaemia is associated with suboptimal

Table 32.2 Intensive insulin therapy in acute ischaemic stroke

Study*	No. of patients	Conventional range or placebo	Intensive glucose range	Hypoglycaemia definition	Nutrition initiation	Outcome
Gray, GISTUK 2007	899	<306 mg/dL	72–126 mg/dL	<72 mg/dL	Not mentioned	• No change in mRS or GOS or death
Rosso, INSULIN INFARCT 2012	180	<126 mg/dL	90.9–126 mg/dL	<54 mg/dL	Not mentioned	• No change in infarct growth • Increased infarct growth in persistent occlusion
McCormick, GKI 2010	40	<306 mg/dL	72–126 mg/dL	<72 mg/dL	Not mentioned	• No change in infarct growth • Increased infarct growth in persistent occlusion
Bruno, THIS 2008	46	<200 mg/dL	<130 mg/dL	<60 mg/dL	Physician discretion, majority within 24 h	• Trend towards better outcome in tight control group
Johnston, GRASP 2009	74	<300 mg/dL	70–110 mg/dL 70–200 mg/dL	<55 mg/dL	EN or PO within 24 hours	• Trend towards better outcome in tight control group
Kreisel, 2009	40	<200 mg/dL	80–1100 mg/dL	<60 mg/dL	Physician discretion	• Intensive insulin control was well-tolerated
Staszewski, 2010	50	<180 mg/dL	81–126 mg/dL	<60 mg/dL	PO within 24 hours	• No improvement in outcome
Walters, 2006	25	N/A	90–144 mg/dL	N/A	Physician discretion	• Intensive insulin control was well-tolerated

*(1) Rosso, et al. Intensive versus subcutaneous insulin in patients with hyperacute stroke: results from the randomized INSULINFARCT trial. *Stroke* 2012 Sep;43(9)2343–9. (2) Gray, et al. Glucose-potassium-insulin infusions in the management of post-stroke hyperglycaemia: the UK Glucose Insulin in Stroke Trial (GIST-UK). *Lancet Neurol* 2007 May;6(5):397–406. (3) McCormick, et al. Randomized, controlled trial of insulin for acute poststroke hyperglycaemia. *Ann Neurol* 2010;67:570–8. (4) Bruno, et al. Treatment of Hyperglycemia in Ischemic Stroke (THIS): a randomized pilot trial. *Stroke* 2008;39:384–9. (5) Johnston, et al. Glucose regulation in Acute Stroke Patients (GRASP) trial: a randomized pilot trial. *Stroke* 2009;40:3804–9. (6) Kreisel SH, Berschin UM, Hammes HP, et al. Pragmatic management of hyperglycaemia in acute ischaemic stroke: safety and feasibility of intensive intravenous insulin treatment. *Cerebrovasc Dis* 2009;27:167–75. (7) Staszewski J, Brodacki B, Kotowicz J, Stepien A. Intravenous insulin therapy in the maintenance of strict glycaemic control in nondiabetic acute stroke patients with mild hyperglycaemia. *J Stroke Cerebrovasc Dis* 2010;20:150–54. (8) Walters MR, Weir CJ, Lees KR. A randomised, controlled pilot study to investigate the potential benefit of intervention with insulin in hyperglycaemic acute ischaemic stroke patients. *Cerebrovasc Dis* 2006;22:116–22.

outcomes in neurosurgery—increased craniotomy wound infections, peripheral nerve root lesions in spinal surgery, paralytic ileus, increased LOS, and hospital cost. There are also several downstream systemic effects that occur—increased nosocomial infections, acute kidney injury, cardiac arrhythmias, and longer length of mechanical ventilator support.[52,53] Intraoperatively, use of aggressive intraoperative strategies with insulin infusions in patients with high HbA1c levels and frequent finger stick glucose measurements are suggested to maintain euglycaemia.[54–56]

STATUS EPILEPTICUS

Severe hyperglycaemia and even moderate to severe hypoglycaemia can cause seizures in a non-brain injured patient. In patients with a brain injury, SE results in severe glutamate excitotoxicity and significant metabolic demand. Retrospective cohort studies have shown hyperglycaemia to be associated with more difficult seizure control and worse outcomes.[57]

CONCLUSIONS

The presence of stress hyperglycaemia has been associated with acute neurologic injury. It is either a marker of the severity of disease and or a causative mechanism of secondary cerebral injury and a potential therapeutic target. It is most likely that both points of view are simultaneously true. The avoidance of severe hyperglycaemia: serum glucose >180 mg/dL and avoidance of hypoglycaemia <80 mg/dL are likely excellent guidelines to follow. Further studies in neurocritical care patients will hopefully shed some light as to what optimal glucose levels should be to promote the best patient outcomes.

REFERENCES

1. van den Berghe G. Intensive insulin therapy in critically ill patients. *N Engl J Med* 2001;345:1359–67.
2. Egi M, Bellomo R, Stachowski E, et al. Blood glucose concentration and outcome of critical illness: the impact of diabetes. *Crit Care Med* 2008;36(8):2249–55.
3. Frankenfield DC, Omert LA, Badellino MM, et al. Correlation between measured energy expenditure and clinically obtained variables in trauma and sepsis patients. *J Parenter Enteral Nutr* 18 (1994;18):398–403.
4. Shi J, Dong B, Mao Y, et al. Review: Traumatic brain injury and hyperglycaemia, a potentially modifiable risk factor. *Oncotarget* Sept 2016.
5. Rostami E. Glucose and the injured brain-monitored in the neurointensive care unit. *Front Neurol* 2014;5:91.
6. Griesdale DE, de Souza RJ, van Dam RM, et al. Intensive insulin therapy and mortality among critically ill patients: a meta-analysis including NICE-SUGAR study data. *CMAJ* 2009.
7. Ichai C, Preiser JC, Société Française d'Anesthésie-Réanimation, et al. C International recommendations for glucose control in adult non diabetic critically ill patients. *Critical Care* 2010;14(5):R166.
8. Jacobi J, Bircher N, Krinsley J, et al. Guidelines for the use of an insulin infusion for the management of hyperglycaemia in critically ill patients. *Crit Care Med* 2012;40.
9. Qaseem A, Humphrey LL, Chou R, et al. Use of intensive insulin therapy for the management of glycaemic control in hospitalized patients: A clinical practice guideline from the American College of Physicians. *Ann Intern Med* 2011 Feb 15;154(4):260–7.
10. Vriesendorp TM, DeVries JH, van Santen S, et al. Evaluation of short-term consequences of hypoglycaemia in an intensive care unit. *Crit Care Med* 2006;34(11):2714–8.
11. Mechanick JI, Handelsman Y, Bloomgarden ZT. Hypoglycemia in the intensive care unit. *Curr Opin Clin Nutr Metab Care* 2007;10(2):193–6.
12. Vespa P, Boonyaputthikul R, McArthur DL, et al. Intensive insulin therapy reduces microdialysis glucose values without altering glucose utilization or improving the lactate/pyruvate ratio after traumatic brain injury. *Crit Care Med* 2006;34(3):850–6.
13. Oddo M, Schmidt JM, Carrera E, et al. Impact of tight glycaemic control on cerebral glucose metabolism after severe brain injury: A microdialysis study. *Crit Care Med* 2008 Dec;36(12):3233–8.
14. Hertz L, Peng L, Dienel GA. Energy metabolism in astrocytes: high rate of oxidative metabolism and spatiotemporal dependence on glycolysis/glycogenolysis. *J Cereb Blood Flow Metab* 2007;27:219–49.
15. Meierhans R, Béchir M, Ludwig S, et al. Brain metabolism is significantly impaired at blood glucose below 6 mm and brain glucose below 1 mm in patients with severe traumatic brain injury. *Critical Care* 2010,14:R13.
16. Kuo T, McQueen A, Chen TC, Wang JC. Regulation of glucose homeostasis by glucocorticoids. *Adv Exp Med Biol* 2015; 872:99–126.
17. Layon AJ, Gabrielli A, Friedman WA. Chapter 15. Endocrine Issues in Neurocritical Care. *Textbook of Neurointensive Care*. London: Springer–Verlag, 2013; pp. 293–313.
18. Griesdale DE, Tremblay MH, McEwen J, et al. Glucose control and mortality in patients with severe traumatic brain injury. *Neurocrit Care* 2009 Dec;11(3):311–6.
19. Kramer AH, Roberts DJ, Zygun DA. Optimal glycaemic control in neurocritical care patients: a systematic review and meta-analysis. *Crit Care* 2012 Oct 22;16(5):R203.
20. Lam J. Hyperglycemia and neurological outcome in patients with head injury. *J Neurosurg* 1991 Oct;75(4):545–51.
21. Rovlias, Kotsou. The influence of hyperglycaemia on neurological outcome in patients with severe head injury. *Neurosurgery* 2000 Feb;46(2):335–42; discussion 342–3.
22. van Beek JG, Mushkudiani NA, Steyerberg EW. Prognostic value of admission laboratory parameters in trauma brain injury: results from the IMPACT study. *J Neurotrauma* 2007 Feb;24(2):315–28.
23. Young B, Ott L, Dempsey R, et al. Relationship between admission hyperglycaemia and neurologic outcome of severely brain-injured patients. *Ann Surg* 1989 Oct; 210(4):466–73.
24. Roberts I, Yates D, Sandercock P, et al. CRASH trial collaborators. Effect of intravenous corticosteroids on death within 14 days in 10,008 adults with clinically significant head injury (MRC CRASH trial): randomised placebo-controlled trial. *Lancet* 2004;364:1321–28.
25. Bilotta F, Caramia R, Cernak I, et al. Intensive insulin therapy after severe traumatic brain injury: A randomized clinical trial. *Neurocrit Care* 2008;9(2):159–66.
26. Kinoshita K, Kraydieh S, Alonso O, et al. Effect of posttraumatic hyperglycaemia on contusion volume and neutrophil accumulation after moderate fluid-percussion brain injury in rats. *J Neurotrauma* 2002 Jun;19(6):681–92.
27. Schlenk F, Vajkoczy P, Sarrafzadeh A. Inpatient hyperglycaemia following aneurysmal subarachnoid

hemorrhage: relation to cerebral metabolism and outcome. *Neurocrit Care* 2009;11:56–63.

28. Kruyt ND, Biessels GJ, de Haan RJ, et al. Hyperglycemia and clinical outcome in aneurysmal subarachnoid haemorrhage: a meta-analysis. *Stroke* 2009;40(6): e424–30.

29. Kruyt ND. Hyperglycemia in aneurysmal subarachnoid hemorrhage: a potentially modifiable risk factor for poor outcome. *J Cereb Blood Flow Metab* (2010)30:1577–87.

30. Badjatia N, Topcuoglu MA, Buonanno FS, et al. Relationship between hyperglycaemia and symptomatic vasospasm after subarachnoid haemorrhage. *Crit Care Med* 2005 Jul;33(7):1603–9; quiz 1623.

31. Helbok R, Schmidt JM, Kurtz P, et al. Systemic glucose and brain energy metabolism after subarachnoid hemorrhage. *Neurocrit Care* 2010;12(3):317–23.

32. Connolly ES, Rabinstein AA, Carhuapoma JR, et al. Guidelines for the management of aneurysmal subarachnoid hemorrhage AHA/ASA. *Stroke* 2012;43:1711–37.

33. Pasternak JJ, McGregor DG, Schroeder DR, et al. IHAST Investigators. Hyperglycemia in patients undergoing cerebral aneurysm surgery: its association with long-term gross neurologic and neuropsychological function. *Mayo Clin Proc* 2008;83:406–17.

34. Fleming I and Busse R. Molecular mechanisms involved in the regulation of the endothelial nitric oxide synthase. *Am J Physiol Regul Integr Comp Physiol* 2003 Jan;284(1): R1–12.

35. Parsons MW, Barber PA, Desmond PM, et al. Acute hyperglycaemia adversely affects stroke outcome: a magnetic resonance imaging and spectroscopy study. *Ann Neurol* 2002 Jul;52:20–28.

36. Savopoulos C. Is management of hyperglycaemia in acute phase stroke still a dilemma? *J Endocrinol Invest* 2016 Nov 21.

37. Fuentes B, Castillo J, San José B, et al. The prognostic value of capillary glucose levels in acute stroke: the Glycemia in Acute Stroke (GLIAS) study. *Stroke* 2009 Feb;40(2):562–8.

38. Rosso C, Corvol JC, Pires C, et al. Intensive versus subcutaneous insulin in patients with hyperacute stroke: results from the randomized INSULINFARCT trial. *Stroke* 2012 Sep;43(9):2343–9.

39. Gray CS, Hildreth AJ, Sandercock PA, et al. Glucose-potassium-insulin infusions in the management of post-stroke hyperglycaemia: the UK Glucose Insulin in Stroke Trial (GIST-UK). *Lancet Neurol* 2007 May; 6(5):397–406.

40. Connor JT. Broglio KR, Durkalski V, et al. SHINE Trial: an adaptive trial design case study. *Trials* 2015 Mar 4; 16:72.

41. Kruyt ND, Biessels GJ, Devries JH, et al. Hyperglycemia in acute ischemic stroke: pathophysiology and clinical management. *Nat Rev Neurol* 2010 Mar;6(3):145–55.

42. Zhang J, Yang Y, Sun H, et al. Hemorrhagic transformation after cerebral infarction: current concepts and challenges. *Ann Transl Med* 2014 Aug;2(8):81.

43. Zhang WW, Zhang L, Hou WK, et al. Dynamic expression of glucose transporters 1 and 3 in the brain of diabetic rats with cerebral ischemia reperfusion. *Chin Med J (Engl)* 2009 Sep 5;122(17):1996–2001.

44. Bang OY, Saver JL, Lee KH, et al. Characteristics of patients with target magnetic resonance mismatch profile: data from two geographically and racially distinct populations. *Cerebrovascular Disease* 2010;29(1):87–94.

45. Els T, Klisch J, Orszagh M, et al. Hyperglycemia in patients with focal cerebral ischemia after intravenous thrombolysis: influence on clinical outcome and infarct size. *Cerebrovasc Dis* 2002;13(2):89–94.

46. Demchuk AM, Morgenstern LB, Krieger DW, et al. Serum glucose level and diabetes predict TPA-related intracerebral hemorrhage in acute ischemic stroke. *Stroke* 1999 Jan;30(1):34–39.

47. Sugiura Y. Predictors of symptomatic intracranial hemorrhage after endovascular therapy in acute ischemic stroke with large vessel occlusion. *J Stroke Cerebrovasc Dis* 2017 Apr;26(4):766–71.

48. Hemphill JC, et al. Guidelines for the management of spontaneous intracerebral hemorrhage. *Stroke* 2015;STR.0000000000000069.

49. Behrouz R, Hafeez S, Miller CM. Admission leukocytosis in intracerebral hemorrhage: Associated factors and prognostic implications. *Neurocrit Care* 2015 Dec;23(3): 370–3.

50. Zhao Y, Yang J, Zhao H, et al. The association between hyperglycaemia and the prognosis of acute spontaneous intracerebral hemorrhage. *Neurol Res* 2016 Dec 26:1–6.

51. Song EC, Chu K, Jeong SW, et al. Hyperglycemia exacerbates brain edema and perihematomal cell death after intracerebral haemorrhage. *Stroke* 2003 Sep;34(9):2215–20.

52. Liu J, Gao BB, Clermont AC, et al. Hyperglycemia induced cerebral hematoma expansion is mediated by plasma kalikrein. *Nat Med* 2011 Feb;17(2):206–10.

53. Godoy DA, Napoli MD, Biestro A, et al. Perioperative glucose control in neurosurgical patients. *Anesthesiology Research and Practice* 2012.

54. Dhinsa BS, Khan WS, Puri A, et al. Management of the patient with diabetes in the perioperative period. *Journal of Perioperative Practice* 2010;20(10):364–7.

55. Girard M, Schricker T. Perioperative glucose control: living in uncertain times-continuing professional development. *Canadian Journal of Anesthesia* 2011;58(3):312–29.

56. Godoy TA, Di Napoli M, Rabinstein AA. Treating hyperglycaemia in neurocritical patients: benefits and perils. *Neurocritical Care* 2010;13(3):425–38.

57. Mayer S, Claassen J, Lokin J, et al. Refractory status epilepticus frequency, risk factors, and impact on outcome. *Arch Neurol* 2002;59(2):205–10.

33

Arterial Blood Gas Analysis

T. Sabbouh, D. Greene-Chandos, and M. T. Torbey

ABSTRACT

Arterial blood gases (ABG) are an essential diagnostic tool for evaluating critically ill patients because they reflect the interaction between the pulmonary and the cardiovascular systems. By measuring pH (acidity), partial pressures of carbon dioxide ($PaCO_2$) and oxygen (PaO_2), ABG analysis provides an insight on the acid base, respiratory, and oxygenation status of the patient, respectively. Blood gases can be altered in response to metabolic and respiratory processes, which will be described in this chapter. If a compensatory response to a primary disorder is not sufficient, then a mixed disorder is present. Arterial blood gases should be analysed with consideration in cases of temperature changes.

KEYWORDS

Arterial blood gas (ABG); acid-base disorders; metabolic disorders; respiratory disorders; compensatory responses; mixed disorders.

INTRODUCTION

Arterial blood gas (ABG) is a test that measures the arterial pressure of oxygen (PaO_2), arterial pressure of carbon dioxide ($PaCO_2$), acidity (pH), bicarbonate (HCO_3), and base excess (BE). Such information is crucial when caring for critically ill patients as they monitor indices of oxygenation, ventilation, and acid-base balance. Compensatory responses to a primary disorder, mixed acid-base disorders, and temperature changes should be considered when analysing blood gases.

THE PARAMETERS OF ARTERIAL BLOOD GASES

The five key parameters measured in ABG are the following: pH, PaO_2, $PaCO_2$, HCO_3, and BE.[1] These parameters are summarized in Table 33.1.

Acidity, or pH

The pH is a reflection of the hydrogen concentration within the body and represents the body's ability to maintain a balance between acidic and alkaline substances.

The hydrogen concentration and therefore the pH are influenced by respiratory gases and many solutes such as sodium, potassium, chloride, and HCO_3.[2]

Table 33.1 Arterial blood gas parameters

ABG Parameters		
pH (range)	>7.45	Alkalaemia
	7.36–7.44	Normal
	<7.35	Acidaemia
PaO_2 (mmHg)	80–100	Normal
	<80	Hypoxia
$PaCO_2$ (mmHg)	>45	High
	35–45	Normal
	<35	Low
HCO_3 (mEq/L)	>26	High
	22–26	Normal
	<22	Low
BE (deficit/excess)	−2 to +2	Normal

Partial Pressures of Oxygen (PaO$_2$)

The PaO$_2$ is a measurement of the amount of O$_2$ in the arterial blood (dissolved in the plasma) which is usually less than 3% of the total oxygen in the blood (the rest is carried by haemoglobin).[3] PaO$_2$ is controlled by the amount of O$_2$ diffusing from the alveoli into the blood. Clinically, it offers crucial information about hypoxaemia and helps adjusting oxygen delivery to critically ill patients.[3]

Partial Pressures of Carbon Dioxide (PaCO$_2$)

The PaCO$_2$ is a measurement of the amount of CO$_2$ in the arterial blood and is referred to as the respiratory component as it is indicative of ventilation.[1]

Bicarbonate (HCO$_3$)

The HCO$_3$ is alkaline and vital in the pH buffering system to maintain a stable acid-base balance within the body. Around 70% of CO$_2$ is carried in the form of HCO$_3$ from the tissues to the lungs for excretion.[4]

Base Excess

Base excess is the amount of strong acid required to titrate blood to a pH of 7.40 when the patient's temperature is 37°C and PaCO$_2$ equal to 40 mmHg.[4] A base deficit (negative number) indicates the amount of strong base needed to be added to each litre of blood to achieve a pH of 7.40, whereas a BE (positive reading) indicates the amount of strong acid needed to be added to each litre of blood to return the pH to 7.40. Base excess suggests the amount of buffer that is readily present to reversibly bind hydrogen ions.[4]

Other Parameters

Also measured in the ABG analysis are other solutes within the blood such as sodium, potassium, glucose, lactate, as well as haemoglobin (Hb) and haematocrit. These parameters notify physicians about significant fluctuations that may necessitate further investigations.[2]

ACID-BASE BALANCE

Large amounts of acids are produced by adults daily which needs to be excreted, metabolized to neutral non-charged molecules, and/or buffered to avoid fatal acidaemia. The sources of these acids are divided into three categories:[5]

- Approximately 15,000 mmol of CO$_2$ is produced daily, which combines with water to produce carbonic acid (H$_2$CO$_3$) (equation 1). Carbon dioxide is eliminated from the body by the lungs.

- Several thousand mmol of organic acids from metabolic reactions (lactic acid and citric acid) are produced daily. These acids are neutralized into neutral products (such as glucose), CO$_2$, and water. Normally, their steady state concentration in the extracellular fluid is stable and low because the generation and utilization rates of these organic acids are equivalent.

- Approximately 50 to 100 mEq of nonvolatile acid is produced daily such as sulphuric acid, which is derived from the metabolism of sulphur-containing amino acids in the diet. These acids are excreted by the kidneys.

Renal excretion of acids is attained in two ways. The first way is the combination of hydrogen ions with urinary buffers resulting in titratable acids such as urate, creatinine, and phosphate (HPO$_4^{2-}$ + H$^+$ → H$_2$PO$_4^-$).[5] The second way is via ammonia to form ammonium (NH$_3$ + H$^+$ → NH$_4^+$). The major adaptive response to increase in acid quantities is an increase in ammonia production derived from the breakdown of glutamine.[5]

Assessment of the acid-base status is achieved by determining the components of bicarbonate-carbon dioxide buffer system in the blood:

$$Dissolved\ CO_2 + H_2O \Leftrightarrow H_2CO_3 \Leftrightarrow HCO_3 + H^+$$
(equation 1)

Using analytical electrodes, the pH and PaCO$_2$ are calculated. Using the Henderson–Hasselbalch equation, serum bicarbonate (HCO$_3$) is calculated as:[6]

$$pH = 6.10 + \log ([HCO_3] \div [0.03 \times PaCO_2]),$$
(equation 2)

where pH is equal to (–log [H$^+$]); 6.10 is the dissociation constant of this reaction; 0.03 is the solubility coefficient for CO$_2$ in the blood; and PaCO$_2$ is the partial pressure of carbon dioxide in the blood.

ACID-BASE DISORDERS

Acidaemia defines the state of low blood pH (pH <7.36) while acidosis is used to describe the processes leading to these states. Alkalaemia defines the state of high blood pH (pH > 7.45) while alkalosis is used to describe the process leading to these states.[6]

In situations where the body cannot maintain an acid-base balance, severe acidaemia or alkalaemia result in devastating consequences on many organ systems. These consequences are summarized in Table 33.2.

Table 33.2 Consequences of severe acid-base disturbances

Organ system	Acidaemia (pH <7.20)	Alkalaemia (pH >7.60)
Cardiovascular	↓ contractility, arteriolar vasodilation, ↓ mean arterial pressure and cardiac output, ↓ response to catecholamines, ↑ risk of arrhythmias	Arteriolar vasoconstriction, ↓ coronary blood flow, ↑ risk of arrhythmias
Respiratory	Hyperventilation, ↓ respiratory muscle strength	Hypoventilation
Metabolic	↑ potassium, insulin resistance	↓ potassium, calcium, magnesium, phosphorus
Neurological	Altered mental status	Altered mental status, seizures, tetany

Reference: Haber RJ. A practical approach to acid-base disorders. *Western Journal of Medicine* 1991;155(2):146.

Conferring to traditional concepts of acid-base physiology, the $[H^+]$ in the extracellular fluid is determined by the balance between $PaCO_2$ and HCO_3 in the fluid. The relationship is expressed as follows:[6]

$$[H^+] = 24 \times (PaCO_2/HCO_3) \qquad \text{(equation 3)}$$

The ratio of $PaCO_2/HCO_3$ categorizes the primary acid-base disorders and their compensatory responses and are shown in Table 33.3.[6]

Primary Acid-Base Disorders

According to equation 3, any alteration in either $PaCO_2$ or HCO_3 will lead to a change in the $[H^+]$ of extracellular fluid. A respiratory acid-base disorder results from alterations in $PaCO_2$ levels. An increase in $PaCO_2$ results in respiratory acidosis, whereas a decrease in $PaCO_2$ results in respiratory alkalosis. On the other hand, a metabolic acid-base disorder results from alterations in HCO_3. An increase in HCO_3 results in metabolic alkalosis, whereas a decrease in HCO_3 results in metabolic acidosis.[6]

Compensatory Responses

Depending on the type of primary acid-base disorder, a compensatory respiratory or renal response takes place in

Table 33.3 Primary acid-base disorders and compensatory responses

Primary disorder	Primary change	Compensatory response
Metabolic acidosis	↓ HCO_3	↓ $PaCO_2$
Metabolic alkalosis	↑ HCO_3	↑ $PaCO_2$
Respiratory acidosis	↑ $PaCO_2$	↑ HCO_3
Respiratory alkalosis	↓ $PaCO_2$	↓ HCO_3

Reference: Haber RJ. A practical approach to acid-base disorders. *Western Journal of Medicine* 1991;155(2):146.

an attempt to limit the change in pH.[6] The magnitude of compensatory responses will be described in the next section.

- When a metabolic acid-base disorder occurs, a compensatory respiratory response occurs in the same direction (i.e., an increase in HCO_3 is accompanied by an increase in $PaCO_2$; a decrease in HCO_3 is accompanied by a decrease in $PaCO_2$). The respiratory compensation is usually a rapid response that starts within 30 minutes and is complete within 12 to 24 hours.[6]

- When a respiratory acid-base disorder occurs, the compensatory metabolic response occurs in two phases. The first phase which occurs immediately is the result of whole body buffering mechanisms and leads to a small change in HCO_3. The second phase, the renal phase, which is a delayed response occurs if the respiratory disorder lasts for more than minutes to hours. The changes in HCO_3 occurs in the same direction as $PaCO_2$ in order to limit the changes in pH. The renal compensation which takes between three to five days is mediated by alteration in hydrogen ion secretion (i.e., increase in H^+ secretion in respiratory acidosis and decrease in H^+ secretion in respiratory alkalosis).[6]

Responses to Metabolic Acid-Base Disorders

In response to a metabolic acid-base disorder, the peripheral chemoreceptors located in the carotid body at the carotid bifurcation in the neck gets activated resulting in a change in minute ventilation.[6]

Metabolic Acidosis

The compensatory response to metabolic acidosis is a rapid increase in minute ventilation (tidal volume and respiratory rate) that leads to a subsequent decrease in $PaCO_2$.[5] For each reduction of 1 mEq/L in HCO_3,

$PaCO_2$ is expected to fall approximately 1.2 mmHg; thus giving the following equation:[7]

Expected $PaCO_2 = 40 - [1.2 \times (24 - \text{current HCO}_3)]$, (equation 4)

where 40 represents a normal $PaCO_2$ in mmHg, and 24 represents a normal HCO_3 in mEq/L.

For example, in a metabolic acidosis with a plasma HCO_3 of 12 mEq/L, the expected $PaCO_2$ is $40 - 1.2 \times (24 - 12) = 25.6$ mmHg. If the measured $PaCO_2$ is >25.6 mmHg, then there is secondary respiratory acidosis. If the measured $PaCO_2$ is <25.6 mmHg, then there is secondary respiratory alkalosis.

Several other predictive relationships have been suggested to conclude the appropriate respiratory compensation to metabolic acidosis. The results of these formulae are generally the same, and the reader may choose the equation he/she finds easiest to implement. These include:

$PaCO_2 = 1.5 \times HCO_3 + 8 \pm 2$ (Winter's equation) (equation 5)[5]

$PaCO_2 = HCO_3 + 15$ (equation 6)[8]

$PaCO_2$ should be identical to the decimal digits of arterial pH (e.g., 27 mmHg when arterial pH is 7.27)[8]

There is a limit to the maximum respiratory compensation that could be achieved. When severe metabolic acidosis is present (HCO_3 <6 mEq/L), the $PaCO_2$ cannot drop lower than 8–12 mmHg; this limitation is mostly as a result of respiratory muscle fatigue.[9]

The next step in assessing metabolic acidosis is the calculation of serum anion gap and determining the presence of a mixed acid-base disorder. This step is further described later in this chapter.

Metabolic Alkalosis

The compensatory response to metabolic alkalosis is a decrease in minute ventilation with a subsequent increase in $PaCO_2$.[10] However, this response is not as vigorous as the response to metabolic acidosis because the peripheral chemoreceptors are not very sensitive under normal conditions, so they are easier to stimulate than inhibit. The respiratory compensation to metabolic alkalosis increases $PaCO_2$ by 0.7 mmHg for every 1 mEq/L elevation of HCO_3. In severe metabolic alkalosis, $PaCO_2$ usually does not increase above 55 mmHg.[11,12] The equation given below explains the magnitude of response to metabolic alkalosis.[5]

$\Delta PaCO_2 = 0.7 \times \Delta HCO_3$ (equation 7)

Under normal conditions, $PaCO_2$ is 40 mmHg, and HCO_3 is 24 mEq/L; thus the following relationship is obtained:

Expected $PaCO_2 = 40 + [0.7 \times (\text{current HCO}_3 - 24)]$ (equation 8)

For example, in a metabolic alkalosis with a plasma HCO_3 of 42 mEq/L, the expected $PaCO_2$ is 52.6 mmHg. This is only a mild elevation in $PaCO_2$ demonstrating the relative weakness of the response to metabolic alkalosis. If the measured $PaCO_2$ <52.6 mmHg, then there is concomitant respiratory alkalosis; if the measured $PaCO_2$ is >52.6 mmHg, then there is concomitant respiratory acidosis.

The classification of metabolic alkalosis necessitates the determination of urinary chloride levels, the blood pressure, plasma renin activity, and plasma aldosterone levels. A summary of classification of metabolic alkalosis is provided in Table 33.4.

Responses to Respiratory Acid-Base Disorders

The compensatory response to alterations in $PaCO_2$ occurs in the proximal tubules of the kidneys where bicarbonate absorption is regulated to correct bicarbonate plasma levels. The renal response is slow and takes between three to five days to reach completion; therefore, the respiratory

Table 33.4 Approach to metabolic alkalosis

Urinary chloride	Saline responsiveness	Examples
<20	Saline-responsive	Gastrointestinal losses (vomiting, nasogastric intubation drainage, villous adenoma) Prior diuretics, volume depletion Laxatives, cystic fibrosis
>20	Saline-resistant	Hypertensive (primary hyperaldosteronism, secondary hyperaldosteronism, non-aldosterone) Hypotensive or normotensive (diuretics, exogenous alkali, Barter's, Gitelman's)

acid-base disorders are categorized into acute and chronic disorders.

Respiratory Acidosis

The compensatory response to acute respiratory acidosis results in an increase of serum HCO_3 by about 1 mEq/L for every 10 mmHg increase in $PaCO_2$.[10] Respiratory acidosis is considered chronic after the completion of three to five days. During chronic respiratory acidosis, the serum HCO_3 will rise by 3.5 to 4 mEq/L for every 10 mmHg increase in $PaCO_2$.[10] The relationships between $PaCO_2$ and HCO_3 are depicted in the following equations:

For acute respiratory acidosis:

$$\uparrow HCO_3 = 0.1 \times \Delta PaCO_2 \qquad \text{(equation 9)}^{[10,13]}$$

For chronic respiratory acidosis:

$$\uparrow HCO_3 = 0.4 \times \Delta PaCO_2 \qquad \text{(equation 10)}^{[14]}$$

Under normal conditions, $PaCO_2$ is 40 mmHg.

For example, in an acute increase in $PaCO_2$ to 60 mmHg, HCO_3 should increase by $0.1 \times (60 - 40) = 2$ mEq/L. Whereas, for a chronic increase in $PaCO_2$ to 60 mmHg, HCO_3 should increase by $0.4 \times 20 = 8$ mEq/L.

Respiratory Alkalosis

The compensatory response to acute respiratory alkalosis results in a decrease of serum HCO_3 by 2 mEq/L for every 10 mmHg decrease in $PaCO_2$. If the process persists for more than three to five days, the disorder is then considered chronic and serum HCO_3 would drop by 4–5 mEq/L for every 10 mmHg decrease in $PaCO_2$.[14] The relationships between $PaCO_2$ and HCO_3 are depicted in the following equations:

For acute respiratory alkalosis:

$$\downarrow HCO_3 = 0.2 \times \Delta PaCO_2 \qquad \text{(equation 11)}^{[15]}$$

For chronic respiratory alkalosis:

$$\downarrow HCO_3 = 0.5 \times \Delta PaCO_2 \qquad \text{(equation 12)}^{[11]}$$

Under normal conditions, $PaCO_2$ is 40 mmHg.

For example, in an acute decrease in $PaCO_2$ to 20 mmHg, the drop in HCO_3 should be $0.2 \times 20 = 4$ mEq/L. Whereas for a chronic decrease in $PaCO_2$ to 20 mmHg, the drop in HCO_3 should be $0.5 \times 20 = 10$ mEq/L.

The respiratory pathway controls CO_2 elimination and any disorder that affects any part of the pathway will result in either respiratory acidosis or alkalosis. The pathway includes the respiratory centres in the central nervous system, the peripheral nervous system, the respiratory muscles, chest wall and pleura, upper airways, and lungs. The most common causes of respiratory acidosis include airway obstruction, acute lung diseases, chronic lung diseases, opioids and sedatives, and weakening of the respiratory muscles.[16] On the other hand, the most common causes of respiratory alkalosis include hysteria, high altitude, early salicylate intoxication, and pulmonary embolism.[16]

A summary of primary acid-base disorders and their compensatory responses are summarized in Table 33.5.

Additionally, acid-base nomograms can be used readily to determine the nature and degree of compensatory response.

THE ANION GAP

In seriously ill patients, metabolic acidosis can be provoked by a combination of culprits thus requiring further workup to determine the most likely cause.

The anion gap (AG) is a rough approximation of the relative excess of unmeasured anions, and therefore is used to assess if metabolic acidosis is caused by the

Table 33.5 The predictive equations for assessing compensatory responses to primary acid-base disorders

Primary disorder	Compensatory response
Metabolic acidosis	Expected $PaCO_2 = 40 - [1.2 \times (24 - \text{current } HCO_3)]$ $PaCO_2 = 1.5 \times HCO_3 + 8 \pm 2$
Metabolic alkalosis	Expected $PaCO_2 = 40 + [0.7 \times (\text{current } HCO_3 - 24)]$
Acute respiratory acidosis	$\uparrow HCO_3 = 0.1 \times \Delta PaCO_2$
Chronic respiratory acidosis	$\uparrow HCO_3 = 0.4 \times \Delta PaCO_2$
Acute respiratory alkalosis	$\downarrow HCO_3 = 0.2 \times \Delta PaCO_2$
Chronic respiratory alkalosis	$\downarrow HCO_3 = 0.5 \times \Delta PaCO_2$

build-up of non-volatile acids (e.g., lactic acid) or primary loss of bicarbonate (e.g., diarrhoea) or diminished renal acid excretion.[10] Anion gap is defined as the difference between unmeasured cations (UC) and unmeasured anions (UA). The most important determinants of AG include sodium (Na), chloride (Cl), and HCO_3.[17]

To reach an electrochemical balance, the concentration of positively charged cations must be equivalent to the concentration of negatively charged anions. Thus, we can deduce the following relationship:[18]

$$Na + UC = (Cl + HCO_3) + UA$$

Reorganizing the terms of this relationship yields the following:

$$UA - UC = Na - (Cl + HCO_3)$$

The difference UA − UC is a measure of the relative excess of unmeasured anions, and is called the AG:[10]

$$AG = Na - (Cl + HCO_3) \qquad \text{(equation 13)}$$

The normal range of serum AG was previously between 7 and 13 mEq/L. However, over the past years, there has been an improvement in the analytical instruments used to measure Cl which resulted in an upward drift in the AG normal range. As a result, the normal value of serum AG is now averaging 6 mEq/L and ranging between 3 to 10 mEq/L. Moreover, it is really crucial to inquire in each laboratory about the baseline values as different laboratories may not be using the same analytical instruments.[10]

In normal patients, the main unmeasured anion responsible for serum AG is albumin, which under normal physiological pH, is negatively charged. Therefore, in cases of hypoalbuminaemia, the normal value of AG should be adjusted downwards. For every 1 g/dL (10 g/L) fall in serum albumin concentration, the serum AG decreases by 2.3 to 2.5 mEq/L. The following formula explains this relationship:[19]

$$\text{Corrected serum AG} = (\text{serum AG measured}) + (2.5 \times [4.5 - \text{observed serum albumin}]) \qquad \text{(equation 14)}$$

Moreover, marked hyperkalaemia, hypercalcaemia, and/or hypomagnesaemia may affect the analysis of AG as these cations are unmeasured. For instance, a serum potassium level of 6 will decrease the AG by 2 mEq/L.[10]

On a separate note, less common disorders have an impact on serum AG. For instance, the negatively charged protein immunoglobulin A (IgA) in IgA myeloma will elevate serum AG, while the positively charged protein immunoglobulin G in multiple myeloma will decrease serum AG.[10]

Metabolic acidosis with AG is classified as follows: high AG, normal AG, and mixed high and normal AG. Mixed disorders are tackled separately in this chapter. Table 33.6 gives a summary of the major causes of metabolic acidosis with AG.

High AG metabolic acidosis develops when the accumulating acid is any strong acid other than hydrogen chloride. The hydrogen ions are retained and will bond with bicarbonate reducing the latter's concentration,

Table 33.6 Classification of metabolic acidosis according to anion gap

Anion gap	Aetiologies	Examples
Increased AG (>12 mEq/L)	Lactic acidosis	Lactic acidosis type A from impaired tissue oxygenation Lactic acidosis type B from either increased generation or decreased clearance D-lactic acidosis from short bowel syndrome
	Renal failure	Uraemia
	Ingestions	Methanol, ethylene glycol, propylene glycol, iron tablets, salicylates
	Ketoacidosis	Diabetic, alcoholic, starvation
Normal AG (8–12 mEq/L)	Renal	Renal tubular acidosis Early renal failure
	Gastrointestinal	Diarrhoea, hyperalimentation
	Medications	Acetazolamide, spironolactone, sevelamer, cholestyramine
	Dilutional Addison disease	Rapid infusion of bicarbonate-free IV fluids

while the elevation in lactate levels (unmeasured anion) will raise the serum AG.[17]

Normal (hyperchloraemic) AG metabolic acidosis is usually produced by loss of HCO_3 or HCO_3 precursors. When HCO_3 is lost, Cl replaces it without any change in serum AG based on their equimolar relationship.[19] Moreover, fluids lost by the body (e.g., stools, urine, pancreatic secretions) contain elevated HCO_3 concentrations and reduced Cl concentration. In addition to that, the resultant hypovolaemia will favour retention of ingested or infused Cl (isotonic saline).[20,21]

MIXED DISORDERS

Mixed disorders are acid-base disturbances with more than one primary disorder at the same time. If compensation is less or greater than predicted, one should suspect a mixed disorder. Table 33.7 shows few examples of mixed acid-base disorders.

The Gap–Gap Ratio or Delta–Delta Ratio

In the case of high AG metabolic acidosis, it is possible to identify a concomitant metabolic acid-base disorder (a normal AG metabolic acidosis or metabolic alkalosis). This is achieved by performing Gap-Gap ratio (also known as delta-delta ratio), which is comparing the AG excess (difference between the measured and normal AG) to the HCO_3 deficit (the difference between the measured and normal HCO_3 in plasma).[22] By considering 12 mEq/L as a normal AG and 24 mEq/L as a normal HCO_3, the following relationship arises:[22]

$$AG\ excess/HCO_3\ deficit = (AG - 12)/(24 - HCO_3)$$
(equation 15)

Ratio <1

If the ratio of AG excess to HCO_3 deficit is less than 1, this indicates the presence of high AG metabolic acidosis and normal AG (hyperchloraemic) metabolic acidosis.[22]

A classic case is a patient with diabetic ketoacidosis (DKA) presenting with high AG metabolic acidosis. After

Table 33.7 Mixed acid-base disorders with compensations being greater of less than expected

Parameter	Condition
$PaCO_2$ too low	Concomitant primary respiratory alkalosis
$PaCO_2$ too high	Concomitant primary respiratory acidosis
HCO_3 too low	Concomitant primary metabolic acidosis
HCO_3 too high	Concomitant primary metabolic alkalosis

treating DKA with insulin and fluids, acidosis persists. This is because with aggressive isotonic saline, a normal AG (hyperchloraemic) metabolic acidosis will replace the high AG.[9,22] The serum bicarbonate remains low in this situation, but the gap–gap ratio falls below 1 as the acidosis switches from high AG to normal AG. Therefore, monitoring the serum HCO_3 alone will create a false impression that DKA is persisting, while the gap–gap ratio provides better insight on the acid-base status of the patient.[22,23]

Ratio = 1 or 2

If the ratio of AG excess to HCO_3 deficit is between 1 and 2, then the acid-base disorder is a pure metabolic acidosis.[24,25]

Ratio >2

If the ratio of AG excess to HCO_3 deficit is more than 2, this indicates the presence of high AG metabolic acidosis and concomitant metabolic alkalosis. This is a crucial consideration in the intensive care unit (ICU) setting in which nasogastric suction and diuretics are more commonly used.[25]

TEMPERATURE EFFECT ON BLOOD GAS ANALYSIS

Changes in the body temperature have a significant influence on the measurement of blood gases. The blood gas analysers constantly analyse blood samples at a temperature of 37°C, and therefore results are not correct if body temperature alters from 37°C.[22,26]

According to Henry's law, the partial pressure of a gas (oxygen and carbon dioxide) is proportional to its concentration at a given temperature and pressure. As temperature decreases, the solubility of oxygen and carbon dioxide in any fluid, including blood, increases causing the partial pressures of these gases to drop.[24,27–29]

For a normal body temperature, PO_2 equal to or greater than 60 mmHg (8 kPa) guarantees sufficient tissue oxygenation.[29] According to Bacher,[5,29] PO_2 should always be adjusted for current body temperature in hypothermic patients.

The pH varies with PCO_2 during variations in body temperature. Therefore, with hypothermia, as PCO_2 decreases, pH increases. The true PCO_2 and pH values can be calculated from the following formulae:

$$PCO_2(T) = pCO_2(37) \times 10^{[0.021 \times (T-37)]};$$
(equation 16)[30]

$$pH_T = pH_{37} - [0.0146 + 0.0065(pH_{37} - 7.4)](T\text{-}37),$$
(equation 17)[30]

where $pCO_2(T)$ represents patient's temperature-corrected PCO_2, $pCO_2(37°C)$ represents patient's PCO_2 at 37°C, T is the current body temperature (°C), pH_T represents true pH at current body temperature, and pH_{37} is pH at 37°C.

For example, the following ABG was obtained for a neurocritical care unit patient: pH = 7.508; pCO_2 = 30.6 mmHg; pO_2 = 61.6 mmHg; HCO_3 = 22 mEq/L; patient's temperature = 30°C. Without taking into consideration the body temperature, one would assume that this patient has alkalaemia secondary to decreased pCO_2. However, after adjusting pH and pCO_2 using equations 16 and 17, the corrected values become 7.405 and 43 mmHg respectively, which is equivalent to a normal ABG.[29]

Arterial Blood Gas Examples

Approach:

1. Determine whether there is acidaemia (pH <7.35) or alkalaemia (pH >7.45).
2. Determine the primary acid-base disorder.
3. Determine whether the compensation is sufficient or not. If the acid-base disorder is not fully compensated, then it is a mixed disorder.
4. Determine the AG in the case of metabolic acidosis.
5. Determine the presence of a mixed acid-base disorder in the case of high AG metabolic acidosis using the gap–gap (delta–delta) ratio.

Here we present four different examples of acid-base disorders. The normal AG is considered to be 12 mEq/L in all examples. The patient's temperature is considered to be 37°C in all examples.

Examples

Example 1:
Determine the acid-base disorder of the given ABG:
ABG: pH = 7.54; $PaCO_2$ = 56 mmHg; PaO_2 = 89 mmHg; HCO_3 = 47 mEq/L; BE = 23
Serum: Na = 133 mEq/L; Cl = 95 mEq/L; HCO_3 = 47 mEq/L

Example 2:
Determine the acid-base disorder of the given ABG:
ABG: pH = 7.16; $PaCO_2$ = 29 mmHg; PaO_2 = 57 mmHg; HCO_3 = 12 mEq/L; BE = −3
Serum: Na = 130 mEq/L; Cl = 90 mEq/L; HCO_3 = 12 mEq/L; albumin = 2.1 g/L.

Example 3:
Determine the acid-base disorder of the given ABG:
ABG: pH = 7.16; $PaCO_2$ = 20 mmHg; PaO_2 = 57 mmHg; HCO_3 = 14 mEq/L.

Serum: Na = 130 mEq/L; Cl = 105 mEq/L; HCO_3 = 14 mEq/L.

Example 4:
Determine the acid-base disorder of the given ABG:
ABG: pH = 6.90; $PaCO_2$ = 34 mmHg; PaO_2 = 60 mmHg; HCO_3 = 11 mEq/L.
Serum: Na = 140 mEq/L; Cl = 90 mEq/L; HCO_3 = 11 mEq/L.

Answers

Example 1:
- pH >7.45; therefore, there is alkalaemia.
- HCO_3 >26 mEq/L; therefore, there is metabolic alkalosis.
- Compensation: expected $PaCO_2$ = 40 + 0.7 × (47 − 24) = 56 mmHg. The expected $PaCO_2$ is equal to the one in the given ABG.
- This is not metabolic acidosis, so AG is not required.
- This is not high AG metabolic acidosis, so gap–gap ratio is not required.

Final diagnosis: Compensated metabolic alkalosis.

Example 2:
- pH <7.35; therefore, there is acidaemia.
- HCO_3 <22 mEq/L; therefore, there is metabolic acidosis.
  $PaCO_2$ <35 mmHg, is it a compensation or a respiratory disorder?
- Compensation: expected $PaCO_2$ = 40 − 1.2 × (24 − 12) = 25.6 mmHg. The given $PaCO_2$ (29 mmHg) is higher than the expected $PaCO_2$; therefore, there is respiratory acidosis.
- Metabolic acidosis is present; therefore, AG needs to be calculated:
  AG = 130 − (90 + 12) = 28 mEq/L.
  Albumin is low, therefore AG corrected = 28 + 2.5 (4.5 − 2.1) = 34 mEq/L.
  This implies that there is high AG metabolic acidosis.
- High AG metabolic acidosis is present; therefore, gap–gap ratio needs to be calculated:
  (34 − 12)/(24 − 12) = 1.833. The ratio falls between 1 and 2; therefore, there is no concomitant metabolic alkalosis or normal AG metabolic acidosis.

Final diagnosis: High AG metabolic acidosis and respiratory acidosis.

Example 3:
- pH <7.35; therefore, there is acidaemia.
- HCO_3 <22 mEq/L; therefore, there is metabolic acidosis.

$PaCO_2$ <35 mmHg, is it a compensation or a respiratory disorder?

- Compensation: expected $PaCO_2 = 40 - 1.2 \times (24 - 14)$ = 28 mmHg. The given $PaCO_2$ (20 mmHg) is lower than the expected $PaCO_2$; therefore, there is respiratory alkalosis.
- Metabolic acidosis is present; therefore, AG needs to be calculated:
AG = 130 − (105 + 14) = 11 mEq/L.
AG is normal. This implies that there is normal AG metabolic acidosis.
- Gap–gap ratio is not required in the case of normal AG metabolic acidosis.

Final diagnosis: Normal AG metabolic acidosis and respiratory acidosis.

Example 4:
- pH <7.35; therefore, there is acidaemia.
- HCO_3 <22 mEq/L; therefore, there is metabolic acidosis. $PaCO_2$ <35 mmHg, is it a compensation or a respiratory disorder?
- Compensation: expected $PaCO_2 = 40 - 1.2 \times (24 - 11)$ = 24.4 mmHg. The given $PaCO_2$ (34 mmHg) is higher than the expected $PaCO_2$; therefore, there is respiratory acidosis.
- Metabolic acidosis is present; therefore, AG needs to be calculated:
AG = 140 − (90 + 11) = 39 mEq/L.
This implies that there is high AG metabolic acidosis.
- High AG metabolic acidosis is present; therefore, gap–gap ratio needs to be calculated:
(39 − 12)/(24 − 11) = 2.07. The ratio is >2; therefore, there is concomitant metabolic alkalosis.

Final diagnosis: Respiratory acidosis, metabolic alkalosis, and high AG metabolic acidosis.

CONCLUSIONS

Measurement of ABG offers vital information in critically ill patients. Measurement of PaO_2 provides data on oxygenation, while measurement of pH, $PaCO_2$, and BE provide sufficient data to accurately assess simple and complex acid-base disturbances (metabolic and respiratory acidosis and alkalosis) as well as ventilation (respiratory acidosis and alkalosis). Patients' temperatures should always be considered when analysing blood gases.

REFERENCES

1. Adam S. *Critical Care Nursing: Science and Practice.* Oxford: Oxford University Press; 2017.
2. Siggaard-Andersen O. Acid-base balance. *Encyclopedia of Respiratory Medicine.* 2005:1–6.
3. Foxall F. *Arterial Blood Gas Analysis: An Easy Learning Guide.* United Kingdom: M&K Update Ltd; 2008.
4. Shapiro BA, Peruzzi WT, Kozelowski-Templin R. *Clinical Application of Blood Gases.* Maryland: Mosby; 1994.
5. Rose BD. *Clinical Physiology of Acid-base and Electrolyte Disorders.* McGraw-Hill; 1977.
6. Wagner PD. The physiological basis of pulmonary gas exchange: implications for clinical interpretation of arterial blood gases. *European Respiratory Journal* 2015;45(1):227–43.
7. Siggaard-Andersen O. *The Acid-base Status of the Blood.* Copenhagen: Munksgaard; 1974.
8. Adrogué HJ, Gennari FJ, Galla JH, Madias NE. Assessing acid–base disorders. *Kidney International* 2009;76(12):1239–47.
9. Marino PL. *Marino's the ICU Book.* Philadelphia: Lippincott Williams & Wilkins; 2013.
10. Adrogué HJ, Madias NE. Secondary responses to altered acid-base status: the rules of engagement. *J Am Soc Nephrol* 2010;21(6):920–3.
11. Wiederseiner J-M, Muser J, Lutz T, Hulter HN, Krapf R. Acute metabolic acidosis: characterization and diagnosis of the disorder and the plasma potassium response. *J Am Soc Nephrol* 2004;15(6):1589–96.
12. Pierce NF, Fedson DS, Brigham KL, Mitra RC, Sack RB, Mondal A. The ventilatory response to acute base deficit in humans: time course during development and correction of metabolic acidosis. *Annals of Internal Medicine* 1970;72(5):633–40.
13. Bushinsky DA, Coe FL, Katzenberg C, Szidon JP, Parks JH. Arterial PCO2 in chronic metabolic acidosis. *Kidney International* 1982;22(3):311–4.
14. Albert MS, Dell RB, Winters RW. Quantitative displacement of acid-base equilibrium in metabolic acidosis. *Annals of Internal Medicine* 1967;66(2):312–22.
15. Fulop M. A guide for predicting arterial CO2 tension in metabolic acidosis. *Am J Nephrol* 1997;17(5):421–4.
16. Javaheri S, Shore NS, Rose B, Kazemi H. Compensatory hypoventilation in metabolic alkalosis. *Chest Journal* 1982;81(3):296–301.
17. Arbus GS, Hebert LA, Levesque PR, Etsten BE, Schwartz WB. Characterization and clinical application of the significance band for acute respiratory alkalosis. *New England Journal of Medicine* 1969;280(3):117–23.
18. Martini T, Menzies D, Dial S. Re-evaluation of acid-base prediction rules in patients with chronic respiratory acidosis. *Canadian Respiratory Journal* 2003;10(6):311–5.
19. Krapf R, Beeler I, Hertner D, Hulter HN. Chronic respiratory alkalosis: the effect of sustained hyperventilation on renal regulation of acid–base equilibrium. *New England Journal of Medicine* 1991;324(20):1394–401.
20. Emmett M, Narins RG. Clinical use of the anion gap. *Medicine* 1977;56(1):38–54.

21. Narins RG, Emmett M. Simple and mixed acid-base disorders: a practical approach. *Medicine* 1980;59(3): 161–82.

22. Kraut JA, Madias NE. Serum anion gap: its uses and limitations in clinical medicine. *Clinical Journal of the American Society of Nephrology* 2007;2(1):162–74.

23. Garibotto G, Sofia A, Robaudo C, et al. Kidney protein dynamics and ammoniagenesis in humans with chronic metabolic acidosis. *Journal of the American Society of Nephrology* 2004;15(6):1606–15.

24. Gabow PA. Disorders associated with an altered anion gap. *Kidney International* 1985;27(2):472–83.

25. Feldman M, Soni N, Dickson B. Influence of hypoalbuminemia or hyperalbuminemia on the serum anion gap. *Journal of Laboratory and Clinical Medicine* 2005;146(6):317–20.

26. van Hoeven KH, Joseph RE, Gaughan WJ, et al. The anion gap and routine serum protein measurements in monoclonal gammopathies. *Clinical Journal of the American Society of Nephrology* 2011;6(12):2814–21.

27. Rackow E, Mecher C, Astiz M, Goldstein C, McKee D, Weil M. Unmeasured anion during severe sepsis with metabolic acidosis. *Circulatory Shock* 1990;30(2): 107–15.

28. Gabow PA, Kaehny WD, Fennessey PV, Goodman SI, Gross PA, Schrier RW. Diagnostic importance of an increased serum anion gap. *New England Journal of Medicine* 1980;303(15):854–8.

29. Kellum JA, Elbers PW. *Stewart's Textbook of Acid-base.* 2nd ed. Amsterdam: AcidBase.org; 2009.

30. Haber RJ. A practical approach to acid-base disorders. *Western Journal of Medicine* 1991;155(2):146.

34

Management of Fever in the Intensive Care Unit

A. Sawalha and M. Torbey

ABSTRACT

Fever is a common finding in intensive care unit (ICU) patients. It can originate from variable causes that range from infectious to non-infectious in nature. Furthermore, some of them are life-threatening, making careful assessment for such patients essential and lifesaving. Assessment will start with careful history taking, physical examination, and some investigations. After that the treatment decision will be taken based on the underlying diseases, as fever has been reported to have serious side effects in specific situations, including acute brain injury, while it has a beneficial role in patients with mild infections. Treatment measures range from antipyretic medications to cooling techniques. Induced normothermia can trigger a shivering response which must be controlled as it has side effects that might eliminate any beneficial role of fever treatment.

KEYWORDS

Fever; normothermia; central line associated blood stream infections (CLABSI); infection; antipyretics; shivering.

INTRODUCTION

In 2008, the American College of Critical Care Medicine and the Infectious Diseases Society of America published a guideline for the management of new onset fever in the intensive care unit (ICU). They defined 'fever' as a body temperature of 38.3°C (101°F) or higher.[1]

Fever is a common finding in ICU patients with an incidence of up to 70%.[2] New onset fever in ICU patients usually leads to an unnecessary number of diagnostic evaluations including laboratory tests and radiological assessments, which have a high financial burden on the health care system. Hence understanding the pathophysiology and the aetiology of fever is important to provide cost-effective clinical care. Both infectious and non-infectious causes are equally responsible for fever in ICU patients.[3,4] A careful evaluation for both causes is recommended.

In this chapter, we discuss the pathophysiology of fever in ICU patients, aetiology of fever, as well as the diagnostic approach and its management.

PATHOPHYSIOLOGY

Fever triggers a complex pathophysiological body response. It involves a release of cytokines that will alter the temperature set point in the hypothalamus. Fever induces the production of heat shock proteins (HSPs), which are essential for cellular survival during stress. Heat shock proteins are thought to have a role in decreasing the core temperature through decreasing the production of pro-inflammatory cytokines, which emphasizes the concept of temperature control in fever, compared to hyperthermia in terms of pathophysiology.[3] There are a huge number of pyrogens that stimulates the release of interleukin (IL)-6, IL-8, IL-1β and tumour necrosis factor (TNF), which induce synthesis of prostaglandin E2 (PGE2) within the preoptic nucleus of the anterior hypothalamus. When PGE2 acts on the hypothalamus, it initiates local cyclic adenosine monophosphate (cAMP) production,[3] that alters the hypothalamic thermostat leading to increase in sympathetic activity, shivering, and reduction in heat loss through the body.[4,5]

Another mechanism of fever production can be explained through damage to the central nervous system, which can induce hypothalamic dysfunction and disturb the regulation of the body temperature leading to fever.[3] This is well exemplified in stroke patients.[4] The presence of blood in cerebrospinal fluid (CSF), especially the intraventricular space can mechanically irritate the hypothalamic thermoregulatory centres resulting in fever.[6,7] This might explain why fever occurs in 70% of patients with subarachnoid haemorrhage.[8]

METHODS TO MEASURE THE BODY TEMPERATURE IN INTENSIVE CARE UNIT PATIENTS

The most commonly used sites for temperature management are the oral cavity, axilla, tympanic membrane, rectum, bladder, skin, central veins, and pulmonary artery.[4] Although multiple sites are available for temperature measurement, it is advisable to use the same site during the patient stay in the ICU.[4] Rectal temperature is 0.5°C higher than oral temperature, while axillary temperature is 0.1°C lower than oral temperature.[4,9] The temperature difference could be even wider in ICU patients. In ICU patients, oral temperature drops compared to tympanic or cutaneous temperature since patients may leave their mouth open due to intubation and ventilatory support.[10] Measuring oral, axillary or cutaneous temperature is not recommended in the ICU patient.[1,4]

Pulmonary artery catheter (PAC) has been the gold standard to measure core body temperature.[4] Since most patients do not require PAC and cannot be maintained for long periods of time, it is considered to be an impractical method for measuring core body temperature.[8] Other alternative methods can be used, which are accurate and practical at the same time. The most accurate way for assessment of core body temperature is through the oesophagus. The sensor should be in the lower 1/3rd of the oesophagus, close to the heart and aorta to increase its accuracy.[8] Another alternative is measuring temperature from the urinary bladder. The disadvantage of this technique is being highly dependent on urinary flow. It should not be used in oliguric/anuric patients and should be interpreted carefully in patients with increased urine production like diabetic patients.[8] Rectal temperature measurement is also a reliable tool, but it fails to detect rapid changes in core body temperature because the rectum has no thermoreceptors, and this lag time might be up to 1 hour.[8] Another limitation to the measurement of rectal

temperature is the risk it carries for posing bacteraemia in neutropenic patients.[11]

DIFFERENTIAL DIAGNOSES OF FEVER IN THE INTENSIVE CARE UNIT

The 2008 guidelines for management of new onset fever in the ICU stressed the great influence of non-infectious causes of fever in the ICU.[1] In fact, 50% of fever cases reported in the ICU were attributed to non-infectious causes.[3,4] A reflexive ordering of blood tests, urine tests, and early initiation of empiric antibiotics is not recommended. This approach adds unnecessary costs and risks to patient care.[4,12] Careful evaluation is the key to reach the optimum diagnosis and treatment.

The wide differential diagnosis of fever in the ICU makes the diagnosis challenging. The magnitude of fever might be helpful in this situation to narrow the differential diagnosis in some cases. Fevers between 38.3°C (101°F) and 38.8°C (101.8°F) carries both possibilities of being infectious or non-infectious, and thus it has a wide differential diagnosis. Fevers between 38.9°C (102°F) and 41°C (105.8°F) can be assumed to be infectious. Fevers ≥41.1°C (106°F) are usually non-infectious.[13] Examples of both infectious and non-infectious fevers are listed in Table 34.1, and selected causes will be discussed briefly in the next section.

Infectious Causes

Catheter-Associated Blood Infections

Central venous catheters (CVC) are very common in the ICU. The insertion site, insertion technique, and duration of the catheter play an important role in fever aetiology in ICU patients. In fact, central line associated

Table 34.1 Causes of fever in the ICU

Infectious causes	Non-infectious causes
Catheter-associated blood infection	Heat stroke
Ventilator-acquired pneumonia (VAP)	Postoperative fever
Surgical site infection (SSI)	Drug fever
Sinusitis	Acalculous cholecystitis
Clostridium difficile colitis	Neuroleptic malignant syndrome
Urinary tract infection	Serotonin syndrome
Endocarditis	Intracranial haemorrhage

blood stream infections (CLABSI) are considered to be one of the most common causes of fever in the ICU.[3] The use of full barrier precautions, shorter duration of catheter life, use of antibiotic impregnated catheters, avoidance of femoral venous access, and care by a central-line team are factors associated with a lower risk of CLABSI.[4,13]

The most common causative organisms are *Staphylococcus aureus*, coagulase-negative Staphylococcus, and Enterococcus. These gram-positive organisms have gained resistance for many beta-lactam antibiotics and even to vancomycin. They have the capability to form biofilms, thus removal of the CVC is an important part of the treatment of CLABSI.[4] Gram-negative organisms such as *Escherichia coli*, *Klebsiella pneumoniae*, and *P. aeruginosa* are also important causes of infection. Gram negative bacteria have an endotoxin in their wall, which might manifest with symptoms of sepsis.[3] As both bacteria and yeast colonize the skin, one should suspect Candida related blood infections, especially in patients who are receiving total parenteral nutrition or empiric broad-spectrum antibacterial agents through CVC.[4] Among Candida species, *Candida albicans* is the most frequently identified with the reason of blood stream infections.[3]

Surgical Site Infections

Surgical site infections (SSIs) should be highly suspected with any fever within 96 hours post-surgery.[1] The risk of postoperative SSI is about 2%–5%.[14] Clinical signs of SSI include purulence and erythema at the surgical site and in some cases wound dehiscence.[3]

Risk factors for SSI include anatomic location of the surgical site, degree of contamination, poor sterilization technique, and use of the prophylactic antibiotics. Previously mentioned risk factors emphasize the importance of proper skin preparation preoperatively and wound dressing,[15] as well as the use of appropriate prophylactic antibiotics[16] in decreasing the risk of SSIs.

Urinary Tract Infection

Urinary tract infection (UTI) is more frequent in patients with indwelling urinary catheter. It is more common in females than males and in patients who received antibiotics.[17] The routine evaluation of patients with suspected UTI is to get a mid-stream, clean catch urine sample, but this is not the case in ICU patients. Instead, we use the catheter to get the urine sample.[4] Sterilization of the rubber port of the catheter prior to collection of

the sample and analysing the sample within 1 hour of the sample collection is mandatory to avoid bacterial proliferation in the sample.[1]

Ventilator-Associated Pneumonia

Ventilator-associated pneumonia (VAP) is reported in 10%–25% of patients on ventilator during their stay in the ICU.[3,18] Its attributable mortality can be as high as 10%.[19] Although chest X-ray has low diagnostic yield in stable, non-intubated patients with suspicion of pneumonia, it is appropriate for use in critically ill patients, on ventilator, with a new onset of fever in the ICU.[20,21] There was no difference regarding the reduction of antibiotic use and improvement of clinical outcome when simple tracheal aspiration and culture was compared to more invasive procedures like bronchoalveolar lavage to definitively establish the diagnosis of VAP.[22] Risk factors for VAP identified include endotracheal intubation and altered levels of consciousness, delayed extubation, age >60 years, and an existing chronic lung disease.[3]

Sinusitis

The incidence of sinusitis is around 8% in ICU patients.[23] It is more common in patients who had the endotracheal, nasotracheal, or nasogastric tube, as these indwelling tubes cause mucosal damage and introduce bacteria, thus increasing the risk of infection.[4] Nasal insertion of the tubes was more associated with sinusitis development compared to oral placement.[24]

As many critically ill patients cannot communicate to express facial pain, studies to diagnose sinusitis are recommended. Computed tomography (CT) scan is the gold standard for the diagnosis.[4] As transportation of patients outside the ICU is difficult, ultrasound was introduced as an alternative to CT scan. Although ultrasound has lower sensitivity compared to a CT scan, its specificity is very high (95%), easy to learn, and it is a non-invasive and repeatable method of diagnosis.[4,25]

Clostridium Difficile Colitis

The frequent use of broad spectrum empiric antibiotics in the ICU puts many patients at risk of developing *Clostridium difficile* infection. Patients affected by *C. difficile* develop watery diarrhoea and leukocytosis. In those patients who received systemic antibiotics in the last 30 days, three individual stools specimens are required to confirm a positive toxin assay.[4]

Non-Infectious Causes

Postoperative Fever

Almost 30% of all surgical patients develop fever in the first 72 hours after surgery.[4,26] It is caused by secretion of endogenous pyrogens into the blood stream,[3] or by the lingering side effect of anaesthesia.[4] It is usually self-limited and does not need any therapeutic intervention.[2] Fever which develops after 96 hours of the operation is more likely to be infectious and needs further evaluation to exclude infection.[3] Other indicators for infection rather than benign postoperative fever could be elevated white blood cell (WBC) count and in patients who have had bowel resection or cancer surgery.[27]

Drug Fever

Drug fever is defined as a disorder characterized by fever coinciding with administration of a drug and resolving after discontinuation of the drug when no other aetiology for the fever is evident after a careful physical examination and laboratory investigation.[28] Its incidence is about 10% of all hospital admissions.[4] Most common medications that cause drug fever are antiepileptics, antibiotics, chemotherapeutics, diuretics, heparin, and antiarrhythmics.[3,4] Drug fever diagnosis is challenging since it can occur days after administration and subside days after stopping the offending medication.[3]

Acalculous Cholecystitis

The diagnosis of acalculous cholecystitis is difficult in sedated patients as they cannot report right upper quadrant pain and present only with fever. A high diagnostic suspicion is necessary because this condition has a high mortality rate if untreated.[29] Imaging techniques like ultrasonography or CT scan are diagnostic and demonstrate the classic radiological findings of cholecystitis, which are gallbladder distension, thickening of the gallbladder wall, presence of pericholecystic fluid, and intraluminal slugging.[4] The risk factors include trauma, surgery, positive-pressure ventilation, total parenteral nutrition, sedation, immunosuppression, transfusion of blood products, and hypotension.[3]

Thromboembolism

Immobility, vascular injury, and underlying malignancies are important risk factors for developing thromboembolism.[3] Fever in thromboembolic diseases is a questionable finding and looking for other causes of fever is advisable in those patients with thromboembolic disease and fever. In a prospective study where they measured the temperature of patients suspected to have deep vein thrombosis (DVT) during the duplex examination, only 4.6% of patients with DVT had fever >101°F.[30]

APPROACH TO THE FEBRILE PATIENT IN INTENSIVE CARE UNIT

History and Physical Examination

History and physical examination are the most important factors in the search for a fever aetiology. Obtaining direct history from patients in the ICU might be difficult because many of them will be sedated or intubated, but a careful review of the patient's past medical history will provide most of the risk factors that will narrow the list of differential diagnoses.

Physical examination must include devices attached to the patient, including intravascular catheters, endotracheal tube, nasogastric tube, and urinary bladder catheter. Skin examination might reveal warmth, erythema, or purulence at the site of intravascular catheters or at the surgical site. Abdominal examination might reveal localized tenderness in cholecystitis or diverticulitis, while generalized tenderness might suggest peritonitis. Examination must also include head and neck, lung and genitalia examination.

Treatment Decision

The decision whether to treat fever or not remains controversial. It is necessary to remember that fever is a symptom of an underlying disease. Several studies have reported altered mortality and morbidity rates with fever treatment for specific conditions. In patients with acute brain injury, fever may increase intracranial pressure (ICP) leading to worse outcomes.[31] Another study reported a decreased mortality in patients with infection when fever occurred in the first 24 hours of ICU admission, while fever ≥40°C in non-infectious situations was associated with increased mortality.[32] Fever treatment remains an individualized decision depending on the underlying disease. The impact of fever treatment in a few specific situations in the ICU will be discussed in brief.

Traumatic Brain Injury

Fever has been associated with poor neurological outcome and increased mortality.[31,33] Several treatment approaches targeting fever control in acute brain injury have been studied.

A bicentre, prospective, randomized trial compared conventional fever control (CFC) vs aggressive fever control (AFC) in the neurocritical care unit. Conventional fever control temperature goal was ≤37.9°C with standardized, stepwise fever management starting with acetaminophen 500 mg PO or by nasogastric tube. When the temperature remained above the threshold for another hour, fever management was escalated on an hourly basis with ibuprofen 500 mg PO followed by pethidine 100 mg intravenous (IV) and finally with a surface cooling blanket. On the other hand, AFC temperature goal was to maintain it at 36.5°C with an endovascular cooling device. Infectious complications were higher in the AFC group (94% vs 78%), but no difference in other major adverse effects including: sepsis, bacteraemia, and cerebral oedema. Although AFC significantly reduced the fever burden, it did not find a significant difference in neurologic outcome or overall rate of adverse events.[34]

Another approach to fever treatment was whether traumatic brain injury (TBI) patients should undergo hypothermia therapy or maintain normothermia. The idea behind prophylactic hypothermia treatment is to preserve body cells in the presence of high metabolic stress. Current evidence supports the prophylactic use of hypothermia treatment post cardiac arrest from acute coronary syndrome for neuroprotection and improves the neurological outcome.[35,36] This was not the case for patients with TBI. According to the 4th edition of the Brain Trauma Foundation guidelines for the management of severe TBI, prophylactic hypothermia was not recommended to improve the outcomes in patients with diffuse injury.

Cerebrovascular Accident

According to a multicentre, randomized, placebo-controlled clinical trial, paracetamol might have a beneficial effect on functional outcome in patients admitted with a body temperature of 37°C–39°C.[37]

Sepsis

A multicentre randomized controlled trial was done on 200 patients with sepsis to study the effect of external cooling on the outcome of patients with sepsis. The study found that the number of patients with 50% vasopressor dose decrease was significantly more common in the external cooling group. It also found that shock reversal during the ICU stay was significantly more common in patients who received external cooling as well as day-14 mortality was significantly lower in the cooling group.[38]

TREATMENT

The timing of fever treatment remains controversial. The commitment to treat fever does not justify starting antimicrobials prophylactically. Although some studies found the use of non-steroidal anti-inflammatory drugs (NSAIDs) or acetaminophen for fever control in septic patients to be associated with increased 28-day mortality,[39] other studies found a beneficial role of pyrexia treatment in those patients as mentioned earlier, especially when associated with early use of antibiotics in septic and immunocompromised patients.[40–42]

Decreasing the body temperature can be done pharmacologically or through cooling. Treating fever should not delay the essential workup for infectious causes.[3,8] Medications used frequently are paracetamol and ibuprofen.[4] The use of acetaminophen is preferred over the use of ibuprofen in patients with gastrointestinal bleeding, coagulopathy, or renal disease.[3,4] According to the Ohio State University Medical Center (OSUMC) targeted temperature management (TTM) protocol, the recommended dose of acetaminophen is 650 mg q4h and the maximum dose is 4000 mg per day. It should be scheduled for only 48 hours; and the patient should be reassessed every 48 hours. If scheduled acetaminophen is ordered, the liver function test should be done every 3 days. Ibuprofen can be used with caution in later stages where pyrexia is still not responding to both acetaminophen and external cooling.

Cooling Techniques

Four modes of heat transfer constitute the basis of interventions to promote heat loss: (1) evaporation (water sprays or sponge baths), (2) conduction (ice packs), (3) convection (fans), and (4) radiation (exposure of skin). Cooling can be achieved through external or internal cooling measures.[4] External cooling reduces body temperature by promoting heat loss without affecting the hypothalamic set point. In patients with temperature elevations caused by impaired thermoregulation, such as after a brain injury, antipyretic agents are usually ineffective, and temperature reduction may only be achieved by external cooling.[8] External cooling is the second step in TTM according to the OSUMC protocol, and it is done by applying external cooling blanket and ice packs to the groin, axilla, and neck regions.

Intravascular cooling can be done by cold saline infusion[4] or by using intravascular devices that allow cold saline to circulate inside it and exchange heat with blood without direct contact.[8] Internal cooling is the third therapeutic line when two doses of acetaminophen and application of external cooling measures failed to control the fever. In this stage, ibuprofen should also be administered. The recommended dose is 400 mg q4h, and maximum daily dose is 2400 mg. Internal cooling

Table 34.2 The Columbia anti-shivering protocol

Step	Medication	Dose	Mechanism
0 'general measures'	Acetaminophen	650–1000 mg every 4–6 hours	Decreases pyrogenic response in the brain
	Buspirone	30 mg every 8 hours	Has synergistic effect with opioids to lower the shivering threshold
	Skin counter-warming	43°C is the maximum temperature	Heat generated on skin will partially inhibit shivering response
	Magnesium Sulphate	0.5–1 mg/h IV, till blood level reaches 3–4 mg/dL	Cutaneous vasodilatation, thus increases skin temperature
1 'mild sedation'	Dexmedetomidine	0.2–1.5 mcg/kg/h	Has synergistic effect with opioids to lower the shivering threshold
	Opioid	Meperidine 50–100 mg IM or IV	Lowers the shivering threshold
2 'Moderate sedation'	Dexmedetomidine and Opioid	Doses as above	Lowers the shivering threshold
3 'Deep sedation'	Propofol	50–75 mcg/kg/min	Mildly reduces the vasoconstriction and shivering thresholds
4 'Neuromuscular blockade'	Vecuronium	0.1 mg/kg IV	A paralytic agent to prevent shivering. Reserved for hypothermic patients not able to achieve control with deep sedation

measures involves intermittent cold saline gastric lavage and saline infusion. An intravenous 4°C cold saline bolus of 500–1000 ml through large bore peripheral IV for refractory high-grade fever is recommended.

If both internal and external cooling measures failed with a temperature of >99.5°F (37.5°C) after 10 hours of initial therapies, a surface cooling device should be used. The overall fever treatment is described in the algorithm in Figure 34.1, according to the OSUMC TTM protocol.

SHIVERING CONTROL

One of the side effects related to normothermia maintenance is the induction of shivering. When the patient temperature drops below the shivering point, shivering will be induced to preserve the body temperature. In patients with acute brain injury, the thermoregulatory point is elevated. Hence any drop of temperature below the shivering point, even to normothermia, will induce shivering.[8] An observational study concluded that shivering during induced normothermia is associated with a significant decrease of brain tissue oxygenation (PbtO$_2$), and that decreases brain tissue oxygenation.[43] Shivering also led to change in the utilization of carbohydrates, lipids, and proteins in critically ill patients.[8] This is why uncontrolled shivering can eliminate many benefits of fever control, which makes combating and preventing shivering crucial when inducing and maintaining normothermia. In Table 34.2,

the stepwise shivering control is discussed according to The Columbia Anti-Shivering Protocol.[44] The goal of this stepwise protocol is to maintain the patient with no to minimal shivering. Both steps 3 and 4 require mechanical ventilation.

CONCLUSIONS

Fever is very common in the ICU. Although treatment of fever has shown benefit in critically ill neurological and neurosurgical patients, this is definitely not a reason to start prophylactic antibiotics. Fever workup should be initiated and antibiotics should only be started with either positive cultures or a high suspicion of infection aetiology. A protocol approach to treatment is the key for consistency in implementation and to enhance adoption of the fever management approach.

REFERENCES

1. O'Grady NP, Barie PS, Bartlett JG, et al. Guidelines for evaluation of new fever in critically ill adult patients: 2008 update from the American College of Critical Care Medicine and the Infectious Diseases Society of America. *Crit Care Med* 2008;36(4):1330–49.

2. Circiumaru B, Baldock G, Cohen J. A prospective study of fever in the intensive care unit. *Intensive Care Med* 1999; 25(7):668–73.

3. Pradhan A, Caplivski D. Fever in the ICU. In: *Critical Care*. Oropello JM, Pastores SM, Kvetan V, eds. 2016. New York: McGraw-Hill Education.

4. Yandle G, deBoisblanc BP. Persistent Fever. In: *Principles of Critical Care*. 4th ed, Hall JB, Schmidt GA, Kress JP, eds. 2015. New York: McGraw-Hill Education.

5. Rosenthal TC, Silverstein DA. Fever. What to do and what not to do. *Postgrad Med* 1988;83(8):75–84.

6. Frosini M, et al. Rectal temperature and prostaglandin E2 increase in cerebrospinal fluid of conscious rabbits after intracerebroventricular injection of hemoglobin. *Exp Brain Res* 1999;126(2):252–8.

7. Mayer S, et al. Clinical trial of an air-circulating cooling blanket for fever control in critically ill neurologic patients. *Neurology* 2001;56(3):292–8.

8. Badjatia N. Fever Management. CONTINUUM: Lifelong Learning in Neurology. *Critical Care Neurology* 2009;15(3): 83–99.

9. Sund-Levander M, Forsberg C, and Wahren LK. Normal oral, rectal, tympanic and axillary body temperature in adult men and women: a systematic literature review. *Scand J Caring Sci* 2002;16(2):122–8.

10. Neff J, et al. Effect of respiratory rate, respiratory depth, and open versus closed mouth breathing on sublingual temperature. *Res Nurs Health* 1989;12(3):195–202.

11. Dzarr AA, Kamal M, Baba AA. A comparison between infrared tympanic thermometry, oral and axilla with rectal thermometry in neutropenic adults. *European Journal of Oncology Nursing* 2009;13(4):250–4.

12. Krein SL, et al. Preventing device-associated infections in US hospitals: national surveys from 2005 to 2013. *BMJ Qual Saf* 2015;24(6):385–92.

13. Marik PE. Fever in the ICU. *Chest* 2000;117(3):855–69.

14. Anderson DJ, et al. Strategies to prevent surgical site infections in acute care hospitals. *Infect Control Hosp Epidemiol* 2008;29(Suppl 1):S51–61.

15. Fry DE. Surgical site infections and the surgical care improvement project (SCIP): evolution of national quality measures. *Surg Infect (Larchmt)* 2008;9(6):579–84.

16. Barie PS, Eachempati SR. Surgical site infections. *Surg Clin North Am* 2005;85(6):1115–35, viii-ix.

17. Bagshaw SM, Laupland KB. Epidemiology of intensive care unit-acquired urinary tract infections. *Curr Opin Infect Dis* 2006;19(1):67–71.

18. Chastre J, Fagon JY. Ventilator-associated pneumonia. *Am J Respir Crit Care Med* 2002;165(7):867–903.

19. Melsen WG, et al. Estimating the attributable mortality of ventilator-associated pneumonia from randomized prevention studies. *Crit Care Med* 2011;39(12):2736–42.

20. Strain DS, et al. Value of routine daily chest x-rays in the medical intensive care unit. *Crit Care Med* 1985;13(7):534–6.

21. Hejblum G, et al. Comparison of routine and on-demand prescription of chest radiographs in mechanically ventilated adults: a multicentre, cluster-randomised, two-period crossover study. *Lancet* 2009;374(9702):1687–93.

22. Canadian Critical Care Trials Group. A randomized trial of diagnostic techniques for ventilator-associated pneumonia. *N Engl J Med* 2006;355(25):2619–30.

23. George DL, et al. Nosocomial sinusitis in patients in the medical intensive care unit: a prospective epidemiological study. *Clin Infect Dis* 1998;27(3):463–70.

24. Rouby JJ, et al. Risk factors and clinical relevance of nosocomial maxillary sinusitis in the critically ill. *Am J Respir Crit Care Med* 1994;150(3):776–83.

25. Puhakka T, et al. Validity of ultrasonography in diagnosis of acute maxillary sinusitis. *Arch Otolaryngol Head Neck Surg* 2000;126(12):1482–6.

26. Garibaldi RA, et al. Evidence for the non-infectious etiology of early postoperative fever. *Infect Control* 1985;6(7):273–7.

27. de la Torre SH, Mandel L, Goff BA. Evaluation of postoperative fever: usefulness and cost-effectiveness of routine workup. *Am J Obstet Gynecol* 2003;188(6): 1642–7.

28. Mackowiak PA, LeMaistre CF. Drug fever: a critical appraisal of conventional concepts. An analysis of 51 episodes in two Dallas hospitals and 97 episodes reported in the English literature. *Ann Intern Med* 1987;106(5): 728–33.

29. Huffman JL, Schenker S. Acute acalculous cholecystitis: a review. *Clin Gastroenterol Hepatol* 2010;8(1):15–22.

30. Kazmers A, Groehn H, Meeker C. Do patients with acute deep vein thrombosis have fever? *Am Surg* 2000;66(6): 598–601.

31. Badjatia N. Hyperthermia and fever control in brain injury. *Crit Care Med* 2009;37(Suppl 7):S250–7.

32. Young PJ, et al. Early peak temperature and mortality in critically ill patients with or without infection. *Intensive Care Med* 2012.

33. Doyle JF, Schortgen F. Should we treat pyrexia? And how do we do it? *Critical Care* 2016;20(1):303.

34. Broessner G, et al. Prophylactic, endovascularly based, long-term normothermia in ICU patients with severe cerebrovascular disease: bicenter prospective, randomized trial. *Stroke* 2009;40.

35. Ibrahim K, et al. High rates of prasugrel and ticagrelor non-responder in patients treated with therapeutic hypothermia after cardiac arrest. *Resuscitation* 2014; 85(5):649–56.

36. Arrich J, et al. Hypothermia for neuroprotection in adults after cardiopulmonary resuscitation. *Cochrane Database Syst Rev* 2016;2:CD004128.

37. den Hertog HM, et al. The Paracetamol (Acetaminophen) In Stroke (PAIS) trial: a multicentre, randomised, placebo-controlled, phase III trial. *The Lancet Neurology* 2009;8(5):434–40.

38. Schortgen F, et al. Fever control using external cooling in septic shock: a randomized controlled trial. *Am J Respir Crit Care Med* 2012 May 15;185(10):1088–95.

39. Lee BH, et al. Association of body temperature and antipyretic treatments with mortality of critically ill patients with and without sepsis: multi-centered prospective observational study. *Crit Care* 2012;16(1):R33.

40. Gaieski DF, et al. Impact of time to antibiotics on survival in patients with severe sepsis or septic shock in whom early goal-directed therapy was initiated in the emergency department. *Crit Care Med* 2010;38(4):1045–53.

41. Kumar A, et al. Duration of hypotension before initiation of effective antimicrobial therapy is the critical determinant of survival in human septic shock. *Crit Care Med* 2006;34(6):1589–96.

42. Viscoli C, Varnier O, Machetti M. Infections in patients with febrile neutropenia: epidemiology, microbiology, and risk stratification. *Clin Infect Dis* 2005;40(Suppl 4): S240–5.

43. Oddo M, et al. Effect of shivering on brain tissue oxygenation during induced normothermia in patients with severe brain injury. *Neurocrit Care* 2010;12(1): 10–16.

44. Choi HA, Ko SB, Presciutti M, et al. Prevention of shivering during therapeutic temperature modulation: the Columbia anti-shivering protocol. *Neurocrit Care* 2011 Jun;14(3):389–94.

35

Therapeutic Hypothermia in Neurocritical Care

A. Hinduja and M. Torbey

ABSTRACT

Therapeutic hypothermia (TH), or targeted temperature management (TTM), the process of intentionally lowering the core body temperature, is potentially a powerful neuroprotective strategy available for treatment of acute brain injury. Although it has been used for several centuries to improve neurological outcomes in patients with acute brain injuries, its popularity has been renewed recently. Following acute brain injury, marked elevations in temperature are frequently observed triggering complex metabolic and neurochemical changes that potentiates secondary injury thus leading to poor neurological outcomes. Although TH has been applied in various neurological conditions, currently the highest level of evidence in improving neurological outcomes has been in comatose patients from ventricular fibrillation or pulseless ventricular tachycardia cardiac arrest. Several studies evaluating the optimal age group; depth, duration, and rate of achievement of TH specific to various neurological disorders are required to validate its therapeutic benefit.

KEYWORDS

Therapeutic hypothermia (TH); targeted temperature management; cooling; neurocritical care; brain injury; fever.

INTRODUCTION

Therapeutic hypothermia (TH) is induced reduction in the core body temperature owing to its neuroprotective benefits as a treatment protocol in acute brain injury. Its use in medicine dates to about 5000 years ago, but has gained significant interest in the last century. Historically, TH was used to provide anaesthesia during amputations, prevent replication of malignant cells, and reduce complications during cardiac surgery.[1,2] Despite several animal studies, case reports, series and uncontrolled studies reporting possible benefits of improved neurological outcome from induced hypothermia after cardiac arrest and traumatic brain injury (TBI); the use of TH in clinical practice remains highly limited due to side effects, lack of consensus on the ideal duration and goal-targeted temperature, and major limitations in the infrastructure.

The term TH has been replaced by a more specific term 'targeted temperature management' (TTM) to represent a specific temperature target besides providing specific information on various phases of hypothermia (induction, maintenance, and rewarming phase). Therapeutic hypothermia has been historically classified into mild (34.5°C–36.5°C), moderate (32°C–34.5°C), marked (28°C–32°C) and profound (<28°C) hypothermia. Over time there has been an evolution in several cooling methods but are broadly divided into two categories: external and internal cooling methods. Various techniques employed in the induction of TH using external cooling methods include use of cooling blankets, ice packs, alcohol baths, cold water immersion, cold saline gastric lavage, and local cooling using helmet devices. Despite its non-invasive nature, these carry several disadvantages, such as high nursing requirements, intense vasoconstriction leading to shivering, slow onset to achieve the desired temperature, and erratic temperature maintenance. Alternatively, the internal cooling method provides less variation in the targeted temperature but requires the placement of an invasive central venous catheter to achieve TH.

MECHANISM OF NEUROPROTECTION

Following acute brain injury, marked elevations in temperature are frequently observed. Fever can trigger complex metabolic and neurochemical changes that potentiates secondary injury. Proposed mechanisms of hyperthermia include diffuse mechanisms like sympathetic tone, inflammation, direct damage to the thermoregulatory centres in the hypothalamus and pons, and presence of blood in the ventricles. Elevations in temperature lead to release of neurotransmitters, increase in intracellular glutamate concentrations, potentiate the sensitivity of neurons to excitotoxic injury, and increase neuronal intracellular acidosis and inhibition of protein kinases responsible for synaptic transmission and cytoskeletal function.[3] Fever following acute brain injury has been associated with poor outcome in various neurological conditions. TH offers neuroprotection by several mechanisms which include: reduction of cerebral metabolic rate leading to reduction in cellular oxygen and glucose requirements; reduced mitochondrial dysfunction thus leading to improvement in energy homoeostasis; reduction and prevention of apoptosis; reduction of excitotoxic, oxidative, and inflammatory effect by targeting ischaemic-reperfusion; attenuation of reperfusion injury; minimizing cortical depolarization' depression of immune response and potentially harmful pro-inflammatory reactions; reduced permeability of blood–brain barrier (BBB) and vessel wall resulting in reduction of oedema; and reduced permeability of cellular membranes resulting in improvement of cellular homoeostasis thus reducing the release of excitatory neurotransmitters following injury.[3]

Potential indications for the use of therapeutic hypothermia are highlighted in the subsequent section.

POST CARDIAC ARREST

The documented use of TH for cardiac arrest dates back to more than 200 years ago. The 'Russian Method of Resuscitation' consisted of covering a patient with snow hoping for return of spontaneous circulation (ROSC) was initially described in 1803.[2] Therapeutic hypothermia has regained its recognition in the last decade as a neuroprotective strategy in victims of cardiac arrest after two randomized, prospective clinical trials demonstrated its benefits in the post resuscitative phase.

In a multicentre, randomized, controlled European trial, patients resuscitated within 60 minutes of ventricular fibrillation (VF) cardiac arrest were randomly assigned to undergo TH with a target temperature of 32°C to 34°C for 24 hours followed by passive rewarming over 8 hours or standard treatment with normothermia with the primary end point being blinded assessment of neurological outcome at 6 months and secondary outcome being mortality at 6 months and rate of complications at 7 days.[4] Patients enrolled in the TH group achieved their target temperature within 8 hours (IQR, 4–16). Marked improvement in neurological outcome (55% versus 39%, p = 0.009, risk ratio 1.40, 95% CI, 1.08–1.81) and reduction in mortality (p = 0.02) was observed in the TH group compared to normothermia. No significant differences in rate of complications were observed between both cohorts (p = 0.70). Simultaneously another randomized, controlled trial in Australia, enrolled patients with 2 hours of ROSC following VF cardiac arrest to TH with a target temperature of 33°C for 12 hours or normothermia.[5] A significant improvement in neurological outcome was observed following TH (p = 0.046), which demonstrated further significance after adjustment of baseline differences in age and time from collapse to ROSC (p = 0.011, odds ratio 5.25, 95% CI, 1.47–18.76).

Impact of Degree, Time to Initiation and Setting of Therapeutic Hypothermia on Outcomes

The TTM, a large multicentre, international trial randomly assigned 950 patients within 240 minutes of out-of-hospital cardiac arrest (OHCA) irrespective of the initial rhythm to either 33°C or 36°C.[6] The target temperature was achieved within 4 hours and maintained for 24 hours followed by rewarming for 8 hours. No significant difference in all-cause mortality at 6 months was observed between both groups (p = 0.51). No significant differences in secondary outcomes at 180 days in terms of mortality or poor neurological function using the Cerebral Performance Category scale (CPC)(p = 0.78) and modified Rankin scale (mRS)(p = 0.87) was observed. A subsequent substudy of the TTM demonstrated increased mortality from prolonged time to ROSC with a hazard ratio of 1.02 per minute (95% CI 1.01–1.02) but lack of association with the level of TTM (p = 0.85).[7] Additionally, prolonged time to ROSC was associated with reduced odds of survival with a favourable neurological outcome using both CPC and mRS with no significant interaction at the level of TTM.

While animal studies have demonstrated improved outcomes from early initiation of TH and increased rate of cooling, human studies have reported mixed results. The Italian Cooling Experience (ICE) Study Group conducted a multicenter observational clinical study that compared the outcomes of patients that underwent TH into early-initiation group (TH started <2 hours since cardiac arrest) and late-initiation group (TH started >2 hours since cardiac arrest).[8] Despite lack of significant differences in neurological outcomes between both groups at discharge and at 6 months, higher mortality was observed in the early-initiation TH group compared to the late-initiation group. While some studies have demonstrated conflicting findings, others failed to demonstrate superiority in neurological outcome from early initiation in the hospital, prehospital setting, or during cardiopulmonary resuscitation, thus suggesting that factors besides timing of induction of TH and time to reach target temperature play a major impact in determining the final neurological outcome.[9–13] Some of the key reasons for conflicting results of various studies and meta-analysis include variability in the targeted temperature, study methodology, time to induction, method of cooling, time to ROSC, and quality of cardiopulmonary resuscitation.

Although TH is widely used to provide neuroprotection to comatose patients resuscitated from cardiac arrest from shockable rhythms, its use has been expanded to those that sustained a cardiac arrest from nonshockable rhythms. Although several observational studies have demonstrated a favourable neurological outcome and survival from the use of TH in post-cardiac-arrest patients with initial nonshockable rhythm, others have demonstrated conflicting studies.[14–16] Thus its use in nonshockable rhythm needs large multicenter trials to clarify its benefit in other rhythms.

Upcoming Trials that May Provide Further Clarifications in Therapeutic Hypothermia

1. The time-differentiated TTM after OHCA trial, a multicentre, randomized, parallel-group, assessor-blinded clinical trial (TTH48 trial) has been designed to compare the duration of TTM at 33°C ± 1°C for either 24 or 48 hours following presumed cardiac arrest.[17]

2. The HYPERION trial, a multicentre, randomized, controlled, assessor-blinded, superiority trial has been designed to provide us the answer if TH is beneficial in comatose patients resuscitated after nonshockable cardiac arrest.[18] It plans to enrol 584 successfully resuscitated nonshockable cardiac arrest patients to either TH between 32.5°C and 33.5°C or normothermia between 36.5°C and 37.5°C for 24 hours with blinded assessment of primary outcome at 90 days using the CPC scale.

ISCHAEMIC STROKE

Ischaemic stroke is the leading cause of death and disability worldwide. Hyperthermia among ischaemic stroke patients has been associated with worsening stroke severity, infarct size, mortality, and poor outcomes.[19] Therapeutic hypothermia using various modalities and temperature ranges has been used in ischaemic strokes to provide neuroprotection and for management of cerebral oedema. Therapeutic hypothermia is the most potent neuroprotectant in animal models of acute ischaemic stroke because of its multiple physiological targets. While data on the appropriate depth of TH among humans with ischaemic stroke is lacking, animals with ischaemic stroke subjected to various temperature targets have demonstrated reduction in infarct size, cerebral oedema, and improved functional outcomes at 34°C.[20]

Therapeutic Hypothermia for Neuroprotection in Ischaemic Strokes

The Copenhagen Stroke Study, a safety case-control study in ischaemic strokes demonstrated the feasibility of surface cooling in 17 awake patients with ischaemic stroke within 12 hours of symptom onset to a targeted temperature of 35°C for 6 hours and compared them to 56 controls.[21] No significant differences in mortality (p = 0.50) and outcome at 6 months (p = 0.21) from the use of TH were observed.

The COOL AID (Cooling for Acute Ischaemic Brain Damage), an open pilot safety and feasibility study subjected 10 stroke patients within 6 hours of symptom onset to surface cooling with a target temperature of 32°C for 12–72 hours.[22] Although it demonstrated safety from use of TH, all patients were intubated, sedated, and paralyzed to prevent shivering and a longer time to achieve the targeted temperature. To overcome this time lag, the COOL AID trial, a pilot feasibility trial randomized 18 ischaemic stroke patients within 12 hours of symptom onset to TH with a targeted temperature of 33°C using endovascular cooling device and compared them to 22 controls.[23] Therapeutic hypothermia was achieved in 13 of 18 patients within a mean time of 77 min (SD 44). It demonstrated feasibility in achieving the targeted temperature faster than previous trials with the additional advantage of managing these patients without intubation and sedation. No significant differences in the diffusion-weighted imaging (DWI) lesion growth and clinical outcome was observed.

To broaden the scope of TH, The Intravascular Cooling in the Treatment of Stroke (ICTuS) study, an uncontrolled, multicentre feasibility study was performed on 18 awake ischaemic stroke patients presenting within 12 hours of symptom onset. The patients were subjected to TH with a targeted temperature of 33°C for a period of 12–24 hours.[24] It demonstrated that the endovascular cooling catheter was well tolerated in these patients and also patients who received proactive management of shivering using intravenous meperidine and oral buspirone achieved the lowest targeted temperature (33.7 ± 0.7°C vs 35.6 ± 1.0°C). Besides this study demonstrated lack of increase in the incidence or severity of adverse effects from extension of TH to 24 hours from the 12-hour timeframe.

Another pilot neuroprotective study combined intravenous caffeinol for 2 hours within 4 hours from stroke onset and mild TH (surface or endovascular to achieve a targeted temperature of 33°C–35°C) within 5 hours from stroke onset for 24 hours among 18 ischaemic stroke patients that received intravenous thrombolysis.[25] No significant adverse effects from combined use of tissue plasminogen activator, TH, and caffeinol was observed.

The Intravenous Thrombolysis Plus Hypothermia for Acute Treatment of Ischemic Stroke (ICTuS-L) study, a randomized controlled trial was designed to assess the safety and feasibility of coupling TH using the endovascular cooling catheter with intravenous alteplase in acute ischaemic strokes presenting within 6 hours of symptom onset.[26] Patients who presented within 3 hours of symptom onset received intravenous thrombolysis and were randomised to a targeted temperature of 33°C for 24 hours followed by gradual rewarming for 12 hours or normothermia. Those who presented within 3–6 hours of symptom onset were randomized to intravenous thrombolysis or no thrombolysis and TH or no TH resulting in four combinations. In total, 59 patients were enrolled, of which 58 patients were included in the intention-to-treat analysis (28 in the TH group and 30 to normothermia). Although the incidence of pneumonia was significantly higher in the TH group (p = 0.001), no significant differences in mortality or 3-month functional outcomes were observed, thus demonstrating preliminary safety and feasibility among ischaemic stroke patients.

Ongoing Trials

The Intravascular Cooling in the Treatment of Stroke (ICTuS) 2/3 Trial, a prospective, randomized, single-blinded,

multicentre phase 2–3 study has been designed to achieve faster cooling by the addition of 4°C saline infusions to the ICTuS protocol with scrupulous pneumonia surveillance and requirement of catheter placement within 2 hours of completion of thrombolysis.[27] The target temperature of 33°C will be achieved within 6 hours of symptom onset and maintained for 24 hours with gradual rewarming for 12 hours. For the management of shivering, meperidine, buspirone and skin warming will be used with additional meperidine boluses for breakthrough shivering. If shivering could not be controlled without respiratory compromise, the target temperature will be increased in 0.5°C increments until shivering is stopped (permissive hypothermia). All patients will have their head of bed elevated, nasogastric tube inserted to drain the gastric contents and reduce the aspiration risk, besides aggressive surveillance for pneumonia using the Centres for Disease Control and Prevention (CDC) definition for prompt initiation of antibiotics in suspected cases. The phase 2 results demonstrated no significant reduction in mortality, 3-month functional outcome, and adverse events. Pneumonia occurred in 19% of TH compared to 10% in normothermic patients (95% CI) 1.99 (0.63–6.98).

The EuroHYP-1, an international, multicentre, phase 3, randomized, open-label clinical trial with blinded outcome assessment is designed to determine the benefit of TH (using surface or endovascular devices) in acute ischaemic stroke.[28] It plans to enrol 1500 awake patients with acute ischaemic stroke within 90 minutes of initiation of thrombolysis or 90 minutes of admission among alteplase-ineligible patients to a targeted temperature of 34°C–35°C within 6 hours of symptom onset and maintained for 24 hours. Shivering will be controlled using pethidine and buspirone. The primary outcome is mRS at 3 months with secondary outcomes being measures of death, dependency, infarct size, growth, swelling, and haemorrhagic transformation on brain imaging.

Massive Hemispherical Infarction

Moderate TH was induced in 50 patients with complete middle cerebral artery (MCA) strokes within 22 ± 9 hours of symptom onset and maintained for 24–72 hours with passive warming over 17 hours (11–24 hours) to determine its efficacy in reduction of raised intracranial pressure (ICP).[29] Intracranial pressure monitoring device was inserted at 21 hours (6–32 hours) and monitored for 3–7 days. Elevated ICP was treated with intermittent boluses of hypertonic saline, mannitol, and glycerine. Elevated

ICP was significantly reduced in the TH group (p<0.05). Four (8%) patients died within 3 days while still under TH (2 from cardiac failure, 1 from coagulopathy, 1 from raised ICP) while 15 additional patients (30%) died after 3 days, during or after the rewarming phase from rebound increase in ICP and fatal herniation. A shorter rewarming phase (<16 hours) was associated with pronounced rise of ICP (p>0.05).

Another study compared the outcomes of 36 ischaemic stroke patients with at least two-thirds of the MCA territory between those treated with moderate TH (33°C for 71 ± 21 hours) or hemicraniectomy.[30] Despite lack of differences in their baseline characteristics, mortality was significantly higher in those treated with TH compared to the standard hemicraniectomy (47% vs 12%, p = 0.02), majority of these related to raised ICP, thus concluding that hemicraniectomy is superior in massive MCA strokes. A recent study evaluated the impact of TH in elderly patients (>60 years) with more than two-thirds of MCA stroke that were ineligible for hemicraniectomy.[31] Therapeutic hypothermia with a targeted temperature of 33°C was initiated at 30.3 ± 23.0 hours and maintained for 76.7 ± 57.1 hours in 11 patients with a mortality of 18% (2 patients), thus this might serve as an alternative strategy in the elderly with massive strokes who are ineligible for hemicraniectomy.

INTRACEREBRAL HAEMORRHAGE

Spontaneous intracerebral haemorrhage (sICH) is associated with greater mortality than ischaemic stroke. Fever is an independent predictor of early neurological deterioration, suggesting that fever might cause secondary cerebral injury. The duration of fever among patients with ICH is independently associated with poor outcome in a dose-related response. In animal models, TH has demonstrated a reduction in disruption of blood-brain barrier and reduced cerebral oedema.

In humans, a pilot study compared 12 patients with supratentorial ICH >25 ml to a targeted temperature of 35°C for 10 days with 25 controls.[32] Since the natural course of evolution of oedema is characterized by a marked increase in the first week and maximum over the second week, a prolonged duration of TH of 10 days was selected in this study. No significant differences between absolute haematoma size in the TH group and controls were observed (58 ± 29 ml versus 57 ± 31 ml, p = 0.98). A significant increase in the size of peri-haematoma oedema was observed in the controls compared to the TH group at day 14 compared to baseline (day 1, 40 ± 28 ml to day 14, 88 ± 47 ml vs day 1, 53 ± 43 ml to day 14,

57 ± 45 ml, p = 0.035). Besides, progressive improvement in functional outcomes was observed in the TH group at 3 months and 12 months. Similarly, a promising trend towards improved outcomes was observed after ongoing enrolment of 25 patients to TH, thus supportive of promising results from its use.[33] A meta-analysis of preclinical studies demonstrated significant reduction in oedema (p<0.0001), BBB leakage (p<0.0001) and improved behavioural outcomes (p<0.0001) from the use of TH compared to normothermia, thus a potentially effective therapy in acute ICH that warrants future research.[34]

Ongoing Trial

Cooling in intracerebral haemorrhage (CINCH) trial, a prospective, multicentre, and interventional, randomized, parallel, two-arm (1:1) phase 2 trial with blinded end-point adjudication has been proposed to determine the impact of TH on the survival and reduction in ICH volume compared to conventional treatment.[35] The primary outcome measure of this study is the total lesion volume on computed tomography (CT) (ICH plus perihaematoma oedema) on day 8 ± 0.5 and day 11 ± 0.5 and mortality after 30 days. The secondary end points that will be evaluated include in-hospital mortality, and mortality and functional outcome at 90 and 180 days.

SUBARACHNOID HAEMORRHAGE

The use of TH in subarachnoid haemorrhage (SAH) dates back to 1954 when it was used as a neuroprotectant to minimize the effect of anoxia during surgical repair of the aneurysm.[36] The 'Intraoperative Hypothermia for Aneurysm Surgery Trial' evaluated the impact of TH during acute aneurysmal SAH clipping procedures. This multicentre trial randomly assigned 1001 patients with good grade SAH (World Federation of Neurological Surgeons score of I, II, or III) to intraoperative TH with a target temperature of 33°C or normothermia. The study demonstrated no significant differences in mortality, discharge destination, and Glasgow outcome scores at 3 months (p = 0.32). However, postoperative bacteraemia was common in the TH arm compared to controls (p = 0.05). This negative result might be attributed to the selection of those with lack of profound brain injury given the inclusion of those with good clinical condition.

Since fever is commonly observed following acute brain injury, aggressive management of fever and maintenance of normothermia amongst patients with SAH was associated with reduction in rates of poor outcome at 12 months (p = 0.004). In an exploratory matched controlled study of poor grade SAH (Hunt and Hess Scale [HHS] >3 and World Federation of Neurological Societies Scale >3), 12 patients subjected to mild TH (35°C) <48 hours after ICTuS for a prolonged duration (7 ± 1 days) were compared with 24 matched controls. Therapeutic hypothermia neither influenced the occurrence nor the duration of angiographic vasospasm, but reduced the degree of macrovascular spasm and the peak spastic velocities (p<0.05). A marked reduction in the frequency of delayed cerebral ischaemia was observed in the TH group (87.5% versus 50%) with a relative risk reduction of 43% and preventive risk ratio of 0.33 (95% CI, 0.14–0.77, p = 0.036) with a trend towards favourable functional outcome (66.7% versus 33.3%, p = 0.06), thus this might be a promising neuroprotective therapy that warrants larger studies.

A pilot study among patients with aneurysmal SAH demonstrated no significant difference in survival or functional outcome from the use of TH with or without decompressive hemicraniectomy (DHC) when compared to DHC alone for the management of global cerebral oedema and refractory ICP, thus it may be less promising for refractory ICP in these patients.[37]

TRAUMATIC BRAIN INJURY

The mortality and morbidity from TBI continues to remain a major problem. The positive effect of TH in closed head injury was first demonstrated by Rosomoff in the 1950s. When compared to normothermia, hypothermic mongrel dogs subjected to targeted temperature of 25°C had a five-fold increase in survival time with reduction in brain volume and cerebrospinal fluid pressure. Cooling induces a reduction in brain metabolism by 5% per 1°C reduction in core temperature leading to vasoconstriction and reduction in brain volume, thus decreasing ICP. Based on these mechanisms several clinical studies have been undertaken to determine its benefit in patients with TBI. Therapeutic hypothermia for TBI has two broad aims: first to control raised ICP and second, to provide neuroprotection. Several case control studies and smaller studies demonstrated a reduction in ICP, improvement of cerebral perfusion pressure and a trend in improved outcomes from use of TH, thus providing the basis of several trials in both adult and paediatric populations with TBI.

The National Acute Brain Injury: Hypothermia (NABIS:H) study, a prospective, multicentre, randomized trial compared the benefits of TH with a target temperature of 33°C initiated by surface cooling within 6 hours after injury for 48 hours followed by gradual rewarming with normothermic patients.[38] No significant difference in clinical outcome at 6 months was observed between both cohorts. Despite major differences in the time taken to achieve the targeted temperature, no significant relation between time to reach the target temperature and outcome was observed. In a subgroup analysis, patients >45 years of age had worse outcomes compared to those ≤45 years or younger (p = 0.001). Among patients ≤45 years who were hypothermic on admission, 52% assigned to TH had poor outcomes compared to 76% in the normothermia group (p = 0.02) suggesting that patients who are hypothermic on admission should not be rewarmed. Due to a weak evidence of improved outcomes in patients who were hypothermic on admission subject to TH compared to those in the normothermia group (p = 0.09), and to address the criticisms, the NABIS: H II study was attempted.[39] It was a randomized, multicentre trial that randomized patients with severe TBI who were 16–45 years of age within 2.5 hours of injury to TH of 33°C for 48 hours or normothermia. It was terminated early for futility given the lack of difference in clinical outcome at 6 months. A subgroup analysis of a small subset of patients that underwent surgical evacuation of intracerebral haematoma demonstrated improved outcome from TH (p = 0.02). A similar multicentre randomized controlled trial conducted in Japan showed lack of beneficial effects from use of TH for 48 hours among severe TBI patients with low ICP.[40] The Cool Kids trial demonstrated lack of improvement from use of TH in the paediatric population, thus justifying the fact that short-term hypothermia for 48 hours might not beneficial in patients with TBI.

The use of TH in management of raised ICP was evaluated in the Eurotherm3235 trial.[41] Traumatic brain injury patients with persistently elevated ICP that failed stage 1 treatments (mechanical ventilation and sedation) were randomly assigned to TH versus standard of care (osmotherapy) as stage 2 treatments. Upon failure to control ICP, stage 3 treatments (barbiturates, decompressive craniectomy) were used. Therapeutic hypothermia with a target temperature of 32°C–35°C was maintained for at least 48 hours following which treatment was continued if necessary to control raised ICP or rewarming. This trial was suspended early due to worse clinical outcome at 6 months in the TH group (p = 0.04). Despite these results, there were fewer occurrences of failure in controlling ICP in the TH group compared to controls. The other pitfall of this trial is the fact that hypothermia was maximal at day 3 following which patients were rewarmed or upgraded to stage 3 therapies. Similarly, the Brain-Hypothermia Study Group (B-HYPO) randomized severe TBI patients (GCS 4–8) to either prolonged TH (32°C–34°C) for ≥72 hours followed by gradual rewarming or fever control.[42] No significant differences in poor outcome were observed between both groups. Since cerebral oedema peaks between 3–5 days, rather than targeting the benefits of medium-term TH on neuroprotection, studies have evaluated the effects of TH for >3 days among severe TBI patients. In severe TBI patients (Glasgow Coma Scale [GCS] ≤8), TH of 33°C–35°C from 3–14 days demonstrated marked reduction in ICP and mortality with increased rate of favourable outcome.[43] The same group demonstrated improved outcome from long-term TH (average of 5 days) compared to short-term TH amongst TBI with mass effect and midline shift >1 cm. Currently, two ongoing clinical trials—POLAR-RCT an Australian trial to determine if early prophylactic TH between 3–7 days at 33°C and the LTH-1 Chinese study to determine if cooling to 34°C–35°C between 5 and 14 days leads and outcomes at 6 months are undergoing which may provide future clarifications.

MENINGITIS

Despite aggressive care, the mortality and morbidity among patients with bacterial meningitis is high.[44,45] Animal studies and case reports demonstrated beneficial results with moderate TH in those affected with meningitis.[46,47] To confirm this an open label, multicentre clinical trial was conducted among comatose adults (GCS of ≤8 for <12 hours) with community-acquired bacterial meningitis which randomized patients to TH (32°C–34°C) for 48 hours followed by passive rewarming versus control.[48] The primary outcome was Glasgow Outcome Scale (GOS) scores at 3 months with a score of 5 as favourable outcome and a score of 1–4 as unfavourable outcome. The trial was prematurely terminated at the request of the data safety monitoring board (DSMB) after enrolment of 98 patients because of higher mortality observed in the hypothermia group compared to controls (51% vs 31%, relative risk [RR], 1.99; 95% CI, 1.05–3.77; p = 0.04) but after adjustment of the age, GCS score, and sepsis, no significant association between TH and mortality was observed (hazard ratio [HR], 1.76; 95% CI, 0.89–3.45; p = 0.10). No significant difference in unfavourable outcome between both groups was observed (p = 0.10). These results were similar in the subset of patients with pneumococcal meningitis. The major pitfalls include a higher prevalence of septic shock in the TH group compared to control (37% vs 20%), greater percentage

of death from systemic reasons in the TH group (44% vs 38%), higher percentage of death in those with septic shock (HR 2.54; 95% CI, 1.31–4.94) despite lack of significant differences in overall mortality between both groups. Although no significant difference in primary outcome was observed, a larger proportion of patients had a fairly good outcome (GOS 4 = 20% vs 12% and GOS 3 = 14% vs 31%), thus indicative of marginal benefit.

A subsequent historic control study compared patients with community acquired bacterial meningitis with GCS ≤9, respiratory failure and breath holding index ≤0.835 (using transcranial Doppler [TCD]) or optic nerve sheath diameter (ONSD) ≥6 mm demonstrated by marked reduction of hospital mortality (OR = 0.059; 95% CI 0.017–0.211) and adverse neurological outcome (OR = 0.209; 95% CI 0.082–0.534) in the TH group.[49] The downside to this study was breath-holding index is in indirect evaluation of raised ICP and thus improved outcomes might be possible from control of ICP rather than the neuroprotection from TH.[50] Thus with two major conflicting studies, future trials are required to determine the accuracy.

HEPATIC ENCEPHALOPATHY

Acute liver failure (ALF) is a rare catastrophic condition that carries a high mortality despite aggressive supportive intensive care management and in severe cases requires liver transplant for survival. Cerebral oedema progressing to raised intracranial hypertension and herniation remains one of the leading causes of death in ALF. Hyperammonaemia increases the cerebral metabolism of ammonia resulting in overproduction of intracellular glutamine, an osmotic active agent that leads to astrocyte swelling. The cerebral blood flow is increased by various factors that lead to oxidative stress and release of inflammatory cytokines. Besides alterations in glutamate reuptake mechanisms further escalates this process leading to progressive brain swelling. The use of TH in ALF had been proposed due to its ability to protect against cerebral oedema by various mechanisms: normalization of cerebral blood flow, decreased cerebral metabolic rate, decreased cytokine production, decreased conversion of glutamate to glutamine. Therapeutic hypothermia has demonstrated benefit in controlling ICP in anecdotal reports of patients with ALF and in animal studies.

To determine the benefit of TH in ALF, a multicentre retrospective cohort analysis of ALF patients in the US Acute Liver Failure Study Group with Grade III and IV hepatic analysis was performed.[51] Therapeutic hypothermia was used in 97 patients (8%) and 1135 patients (92%) were not cooled. A higher percentage of patients with TH had ICP monitoring (39.2% vs 22% controls, p<0.001). No significant difference in 21-day overall survival and transplant-free survival was observed between both cohorts. For acetaminophen induced liver failure TH improved survival in patients <25 years old (OR = 2.735, 95% CI = 1.001–7.467) but worsened for patients ≥64 years (OR = 0.167, 95% CI = 0.028–0.999). Therapeutic hypothermia had no impact on outcome in patients with non-acetaminophen liver failure. Besides no significant differences in mortality from neurological complications was observed between both cohorts (p = 0.75).

To evaluate the efficacy of TH in ALF, a pragmatic multicentre randomized controlled trial (RCT) of TTM in ALF was performed.[52] Patients with ALF, high-grade encephalopathy, and ICP monitoring were randomized to TTM of 34°C or 36°C (control) for a period of 72 hours. No significant difference in sustained elevation of ICP was observed from the use of TH (p = 0.56). No significant difference in adverse events or overall mortality was observed from the use of TH, thus providing confirmation that prophylactic use of TH did not prevent the development or limit cerebral oedema in patients with ALF. Thus it may be reserved as a short-term rescue therapy in patients with refractory ICP. It is currently unclear what the temperature target, duration, and rate of rewarming should be in patients with ALF. Future studies in patients with ALF are needed to determine the subset of patients it might provide benefit.

SPINAL CORD INJURY

Spinal cord injury (SCI) is a catastrophic neurological condition that leads to devastating consequences. Although advances in medicine have reduced the morbidity and mortality, it still continues to remain a major burden to the individual and the health care system. Following the initial trauma, axonal disruption, and vascular and metabolic changes occur leading to secondary injury from inflammation, adverse immune reactions, apoptosis-induced cell death, necrosis, and further nerve and axonal damage leading to demyelination.[53] There is increased production of free radicals, endogenous opioids, and release of excitatory neurotransmitters. Cell death around the epicentre further promotes Wallerian degeneration and demyelination. There is limited regenerative capacity and thus a significantly reduced likelihood of long-term recovery. Currently, no proven treatments offer protection against the consequences of SCI, thus the great need to discover cytoprotective treatments.

Although TH was used for several neurological conditions, its use in SCI came into the spotlight when Kevin Everett, who played for the national football league sustained a severe, incomplete cervical spinal cord injury but made significant recovery from the use of TH and early decompressive surgery. Levi reported the feasibility and safety of TH initiated in a case study of 14 patients with SCI for 48 hours with a target temperature of 33°C followed by gradually controlled rewarming. Subsequent studies that compared cases with controls demonstrated improvement in outcomes in 35.5%–42.8% of patients from the use of systemic TH (using the American Spinal Injury Association and International Medical Society of Paraplegia Impairment Scale–AIS).[54,55] In another prospective series of 20 SCI patients subjected to local TH (localized deep spinal cord cooling) with a dural temperature of 6°C within 8 hours of injury in addition to surgical decompression and steroids, 80% of patients with complete cord injury made some recovery in motor or sensory function. The mean improvement in neurological level of injury in all patients was 1.05.[56] The Miami Project to Cure Paralysis and the Department of Neurological Surgery at the University of Miami, Miller School of Medicine is currently recruiting for a randomized clinical trial, which may provide more definitive evidence of whether modest TH is safe and efficacious in acute SCI.

STATUS EPILEPTICUS

Therapeutic hypothermia has demonstrated antiepileptic and neuroprotective properties in animal models and case series in human beings with seizures.[57,58] Based on these promising results, the HYPERNATUS (Hypothermia for Neuroprotection in Convulsive Status Epilepticus), a large multicentre trial randomized 270 critically ill patients with convulsive status epilepticus to TH with standard care or standard care alone.[59] Although the rates of progression to electroencephalography-confirmed status epilepticus on the first day was lower from the use of TH (11% vs 22%; OR, 0.40; 95% CI, 0.20–0.79; p = 0.009), no significant difference in the functional outcome using the GOS score of 5 from the use of TH was observed (OR, 1.22; 95% CI, 0.75–1.99; p = 0.43). Although no major significant differences between the subgroup analyses were observed, a trend towards improvement in functional outcome in those ≤65 years from TH was observed. Besides no significant differences in other secondary outcomes – refractory status epilepticus, super refractory status epilepticus, length of ICU stay, length of hospital stay, and in-hospital mortality were observed.

The major criticism to this study is the use of GOS as a primary outcome in a disease entity of heterogeneous aetiology. The outcomes of patients with seizures is highly variable and dependent on the aetiology, thus despite the fact of lack of impact in outcome, it might be used as a temporary measure to control further neuronal injury from ongoing seizures.

CONCLUSIONS

The use of TH has emerged as a major breakthrough in the treatment of neurological injuries. While several challenges in its safe and effective application, patient comfort, management of shivering, and complications has been overcome in the recent decade many questions still remain unanswered. Currently, the highest level of evidence in the use of TH is amongst comatose patients with ROSC after VF/pVT (pulseless ventricular tachycardia cardiac arrest). Several studies evaluating the optimal age group, depth, duration, and rate of achievement of TH specific to various disease conditions are required in order to broaden its clinical use.

REFERENCES

1. Alzaga AG, Cerdan M, Varon J. Therapeutic hypothermia. *Resuscitation* 2006;70(3):369–80.

2. Varon J, Acosta P. Therapeutic hypothermia: past, present, and future. *Chest* 2008;133(5):1267–74.

3. Polderman KH. Induced hypothermia and fever control for prevention and treatment of neurological injuries. *Lancet* 2008;371(9628):1955–69.

4. Hypothermia after cardiac arrest study G. Mild therapeutic hypothermia to improve the neurologic outcome after cardiac arrest. *N Engl J Med* 2002;346(8):549–56.

5. Bernard SA, Gray TW, Buist MD, et al. Treatment of comatose survivors of out-of-hospital cardiac arrest with induced hypothermia. *N Engl J Med* 2002;346(8):557–63.

6. Nielsen N, Wetterslev J, Cronberg T, et al. Targeted temperature management at 33 degrees C versus 36 degrees C after cardiac arrest. *N Engl J Med* 2013;369(23):2197–206.

7. Kjaergaard J, Nielsen N, Winther-Jensen M, et al. Impact of time to return of spontaneous circulation on neuroprotective effect of targeted temperature management at 33 or 36 degrees in comatose survivors of out-of hospital cardiac arrest. *Resuscitation* 2015;96:310–6.

8. Italian Cooling Experience Study G. Early-versus late-initiation of therapeutic hypothermia after cardiac arrest: preliminary observations from the experience of 17 Italian intensive care units. *Resuscitation* 2012;83(7):823–8.

9. Sendelbach S, Hearst MO, Johnson PJ, Unger BT, Mooney MR. Effects of variation in temperature management on cerebral performance category scores in patients who received therapeutic hypothermia post cardiac arrest. *Resuscitation* 2012;83(7):829–34.

10. Kim F, Nichol G, Maynard C, et al. Effect of prehospital induction of mild hypothermia on survival and neurological status among adults with cardiac arrest: a randomized clinical trial. *JAMA* 2014;311(1):45–52.

11. Perman SM, Ellenberg JH, Grossestreuer AV, et al. Shorter time to target temperature is associated with poor neurologic outcome in post-arrest patients treated with targeted temperature management. *Resuscitation* 2015;88:114–9.

12. Uribarri A, Bueno H, Perez-Castellanos A, et al. Impact of time to cooling initiation and time to target temperature in patients treated with hypothermia after cardiac arrest. *Eur Heart J Acute Cardiovasc Care* 2015;4(4):365–72.

13. Bernard SA, Smith K, Finn J, et al. Induction of therapeutic hypothermia during out-of-hospital cardiac arrest using a rapid infusion of cold saline: The RINSE Trial (Rapid Infusion of Cold Normal Saline). *Circulation* 2016;134(11):797–805.

14. Perman SM, Grossestreuer AV, Wiebe DJ, Carr BG, Abella BS, Gaieski DF. The utility of therapeutic hypothermia for post-cardiac arrest syndrome patients with an initial nonshockable rhythm. *Circulation* 2015;132(22):2146–51.

15. Sung G, Bosson N, Kaji AH, et al. Therapeutic hypothermia after resuscitation from a non-shockable rhythm improves outcomes in a regionalized system of cardiac arrest care. *Neurocrit Care* 2016;24(1):90–96.

16. Dumas F, Grimaldi D, Zuber B, et al. Is hypothermia after cardiac arrest effective in both shockable and nonshockable patients?: insights from a large registry. *Circulation* 2011;123(8):877–86.

17. Kirkegaard H, Rasmussen BS, de Haas I, et al. Time-differentiated target temperature management after out-of-hospital cardiac arrest: a multicentre, randomised, parallel-group, assessor-blinded clinical trial (the TTH48 trial): study protocol for a randomised controlled trial. *Trials* 2016;17(1):228.

18. Lascarrou JB, Meziani F, Le Gouge A, et al. Therapeutic hypothermia after nonshockable cardiac arrest: the HYPERION multicenter, randomized, controlled, assessor-blinded, superiority trial. *Scand J Trauma Resusc Emerg Med* 2015;23:26.

19. Reith J, Jorgensen HS, Pedersen PM, et al. Body temperature in acute stroke: relation to stroke severity, infarct size, mortality, and outcome. *Lancet* 1996;347(8999):422–5.

20. Kollmar R, Blank T, Han JL, Georgiadis D, Schwab S. Different degrees of hypothermia after experimental stroke: short- and long-term outcome. *Stroke* 2007;38(5):1585–9.

21. Kammersgaard LP, Rasmussen BH, Jorgensen HS, Reith J, Weber U, Olsen TS. Feasibility and safety of inducing modest hypothermia in awake patients with acute stroke through surface cooling: A case-control study: the Copenhagen Stroke Study. *Stroke* 2000;31(9):2251–6.

22. Krieger DW, De Georgia MA, Abou-Chebl A, et al. Cooling for acute ischemic brain damage (cool aid): an open pilot study of induced hypothermia in acute ischemic stroke. *Stroke* 2001;32(8):1847–54.

23. De Georgia MA, Krieger DW, Abou-Chebl A, et al. Cooling for Acute Ischemic Brain Damage (COOL AID): a feasibility trial of endovascular cooling. *Neurology* 2004;63(2):312–7.

24. Lyden PD, Allgren RL, Ng K, et al. Intravascular Cooling in the Treatment of Stroke (ICTuS): early clinical experience. *J Stroke Cerebrovasc Dis* 2005;14(3):107–14.

25. Martin-Schild S, Hallevi H, Shaltoni H, et al. Combined neuroprotective modalities coupled with thrombolysis in acute ischemic stroke: a pilot study of caffeinol and mild hypothermia. *J Stroke Cerebrovasc Dis* 2009; 18(2):86–96.

26. Hemmen TM, Raman R, Guluma KZ, et al. Intravenous thrombolysis plus hypothermia for acute treatment of ischemic stroke (ICTuS-L): final results. *Stroke* 2010;41(10):2265–70.

27. Lyden PD, Hemmen TM, Grotta J, Rapp K, Raman R. Endovascular therapeutic hypothermia for acute ischemic stroke: ICTuS 2/3 protocol. *Int J Stroke* 2014;9(1):117–25.

28. van der Worp HB, Macleod MR, Bath PM, et al. EuroHYP-1: European multicenter, randomized, phase III clinical trial of therapeutic hypothermia plus best medical treatment vs. best medical treatment alone for acute ischemic stroke. *Int J Stroke* 2014;9(5):642–5.

29. Schwab S, Georgiadis D, Berrouschot J, Schellinger PD, Graffagnino C, Mayer SA. Feasibility and safety of moderate hypothermia after massive hemispheric infarction. *Stroke* 2001;32(9):2033–5.

30. Georgiadis D, Schwarz S, Aschoff A, Schwab S. Hemicraniectomy and moderate hypothermia in patients with severe ischemic stroke. *Stroke* 2002;33(6):1584–8.

31. Jeong HY, Chang JY, Yum KS, et al. Extended use of hypothermia in elderly patients with malignant cerebral edema as an alternative to hemicraniectomy. *J Stroke* 2016;18(3):337–43.

32. Kollmar R, Staykov D, Dorfler A, Schellinger PD, Schwab S, Bardutzky J. Hypothermia reduces perihemorrhagic edema after intracerebral hemorrhage. *Stroke* 2010;41(8):1684–9.

33. Staykov D, Wagner I, Volbers B, Doerfler A, Schwab S, Kollmar R. Mild prolonged hypothermia for large intracerebral hemorrhage. *Neurocrit Care* 2013;18(2):178–83.

34. Melmed KR, Lyden PD. Meta-Analysis of pre-clinical trials of therapeutic hypothermia for intracerebral hemorrhage. *Ther Hypothermia Temp Manag* 2016.

35. Kollmar R, Juettler E, Huttner HB, et al. Cooling in intracerebral hemorrhage (CINCH) trial: protocol of a randomized German-Austrian clinical trial. *Int J Stroke* 2012;7(2):168–72.

36. Botterell EH, Lougheed WM, Scott JW, Vandewater SL. Hypothermia, and interruption of carotid, or carotid and vertebral circulation, in the surgical management of intracranial aneurysms. *J Neurosurg* 1956;13(1):1–42.

37. Karnatovskaia LV, Lee AS, Festic E, Kramer CL, Freeman WD. Effect of prolonged therapeutic hypothermia on intracranial pressure, organ function, and hospital outcomes among patients with aneurysmal subarachnoid hemorrhage. *Neurocrit Care* 2014;21(3):451–61.

38. Clifton GL, Miller ER, Choi SC, et al. Lack of effect of induction of hypothermia after acute brain injury. *N Engl J Med* 2001;344(8):556–63.

39. Clifton GL, Valadka A, Zygun D, et al. Very early hypothermia induction in patients with severe brain injury (the National Acute Brain Injury Study: Hypothermia II): a randomised trial. *Lancet Neurol* 2011;10(2):131–9.

40. Shiozaki T, Hayakata T, Taneda M, et al. A multicenter prospective randomized controlled trial of the efficacy of mild hypothermia for severely head injured patients with low intracranial pressure. Mild Hypothermia Study Group in Japan. *J Neurosurg* 2001;94(1):50–54.

41. Andrews PJ, Sinclair HL, Rodriguez A, et al. Hypothermia for intracranial hypertension after traumatic brain injury. *N Engl J Med* 2015;373(25):2403–12.

42. Maekawa T, Yamashita S, Nagao S, Hayashi N, Ohashi Y. Brain-Hypothermia Study G. Prolonged mild therapeutic hypothermia versus fever control with tight hemodynamic monitoring and slow rewarming in patients with severe traumatic brain injury: a randomized controlled trial. *J Neurotrauma* 2015;32(7):422–9.

43. Jiang J, Yu M, Zhu C. Effect of long-term mild hypothermia therapy in patients with severe traumatic brain injury: 1-year follow-up review of 87 cases. *J Neurosurg* 2000;93(4):546–9.

44. van de Beek D, de Gans J, Spanjaard L, Weisfelt M, Reitsma JB, Vermeulen M. Clinical features and prognostic factors in adults with bacterial meningitis. *N Engl J Med* 2004;351(18):1849–59.

45. van de Beek D, de Gans J, Tunkel AR, Wijdicks EF. Community-acquired bacterial meningitis in adults. *N Engl J Med* 2006;354(1):44–53.

46. Irazuzta JE, Pretzlaff R, Rowin M, Milam K, Zemlan FP, Zingarelli B. Hypothermia as an adjunctive treatment for severe bacterial meningitis. *Brain Res* 2000;881(1):88–97.

47. Lepur D, Kutlesa M, Barsic B. Induced hypothermia in adult community-acquired bacterial meningitis—more than just a possibility? *J Infect* 2011;62(2):172–7.

48. Mourvillier B, Tubach F, van de Beek D, et al. Induced hypothermia in severe bacterial meningitis: a randomized clinical trial. *JAMA* 2013;310(20):2174–83.

49. Kutlesa M, Lepur D, Barsic B. Therapeutic hypothermia for adult community-acquired bacterial meningitis-historical control study. *Clin Neurol Neurosurg* 2014;123:181–6.

50. Engrand N, Welschbillig S, Taylor G. Comment on: Therapeutic hypothermia for severe adult community-acquired

bacterial meningitis. *Clin Neurol Neurosurg* 2016;145: 102–3.

51. Karvellas CJ, Todd Stravitz R, Battenhouse H, Lee WM, Schilsky ML. Group USALFS. Therapeutic hypothermia in acute liver failure: a multicenter retrospective cohort analysis. *Liver Transpl* 2015;21(1):4–12.

52. Bernal W, Murphy N, Brown S, et al. A multicentre randomized controlled trial of moderate hypothermia to prevent intracranial hypertension in acute liver failure. *J Hepatol* 2016;65(2):273–9.

53. Maybhate A, Hu C, Bazley FA, et al. Potential long-term benefits of acute hypothermia after spinal cord injury: assessments with somatosensory-evoked potentials. *Crit Care Med* 2012;40(2):573–9.

54. Levi AD, Casella G, Green BA, et al. Clinical outcomes using modest intravascular hypothermia after acute cervical spinal cord injury. *Neurosurgery* 2010;66(4):670–7.

55. Dididze M, Green BA, Dietrich WD, Vanni S, Wang MY, Levi AD. Systemic hypothermia in acute cervical spinal cord injury: a case-controlled study. *Spinal Cord* 2013;51(5):395–400.

56. Hansebout RR, Hansebout CR. Local cooling for traumatic spinal cord injury: Outcomes in 20 patients and review of the literature. *J Neurosurg Spine* 2014;20(5):550–61.

57. Niquet J, Gezalian M, Baldwin R, Wasterlain CG. Neuroprotective effects of deep hypothermia in refractory status epilepticus. *Ann Clin Transl Neurol* 2015;2(12):1105–15.

58. Corry JJ, Dhar R, Murphy T, Diringer MN. Hypothermia for refractory status epilepticus. *Neurocrit Care* 2008; 9(2):189–97.

59. Legriel S, Lemiale V, Schenck M, et al. Hypothermia for neuroprotection in convulsive status epilepticus. *N Engl J Med* 2016;375(25):2457–67.

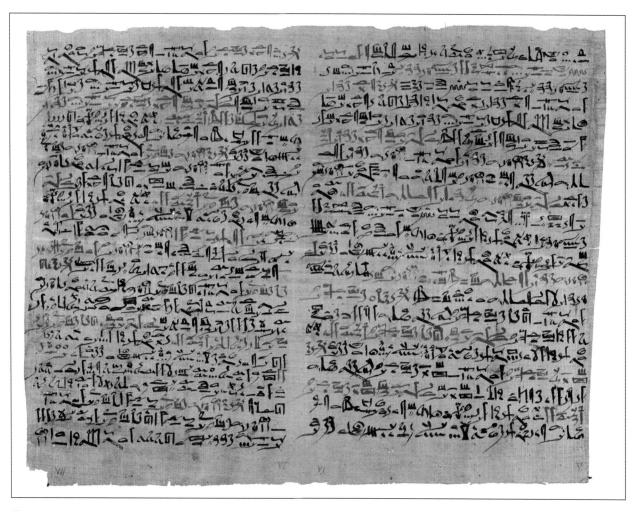

Figure 1.1 Edwin Smith Papyrus is the oldest surviving surgical document.

Source: Jeff Dahl. Edwin Smith Papyrus v2.jpg. Available at: https://commons.wikimedia.org/wiki/File:Edwin_Smith_Papyrus_v2.jpg.

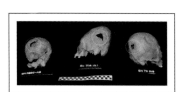

Figure 1.2 Three trepanned skulls from the Copacabana Peninsula in the Titicaca Basin, dating from 800 BC to AD 1000.
Reprinted with permission from: Juengst SL, Chávez SJ. Three trepanned skulls from the Copacabana Peninsula in the Titicaca Basin, Bolivia (800 BC-AD 1000). *Int J Paleopathol* 2015;9:20–27.

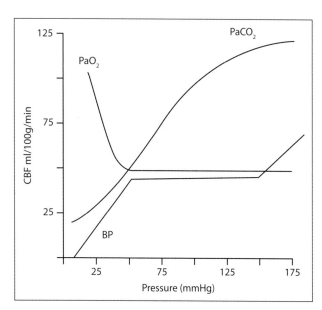

Figure 2.1 Cerebrovascular autoregulation and effect of $PaCO_2$ and PaO_2 on cerebral blood flow (CBF).

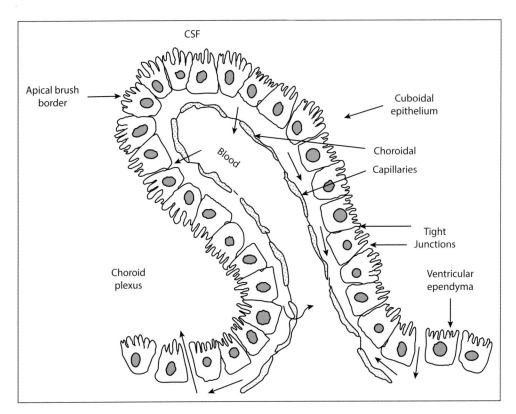

Figure 3.1 Structure of the choroid plexus.

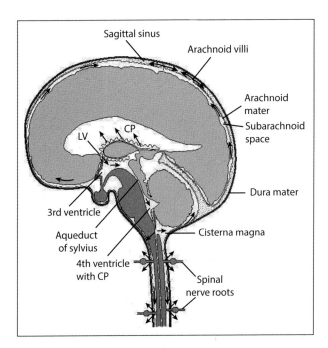

Figure 3.2 Circulation of the cerebrospinal fluid (CSF).

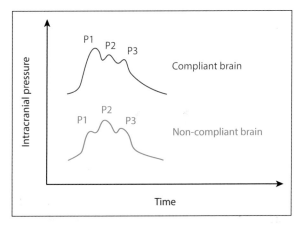

Figure 3.3 Cerebrospinal fluid waveforms when the intracranial compliance is normal (top waveform) and when intracranial compliance is reduced (bottom waveform).

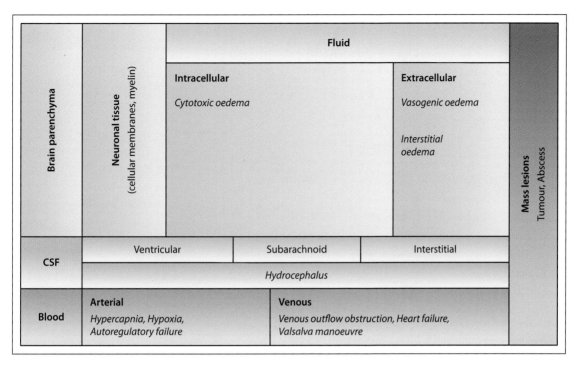

Figure 4.1 Components of intracranial volume. This graphical representation shows the intracranial contents in their approximate relative proportions, and gives examples (in italics) of states which may increase the volume of each component.

Source: Author's own creation.

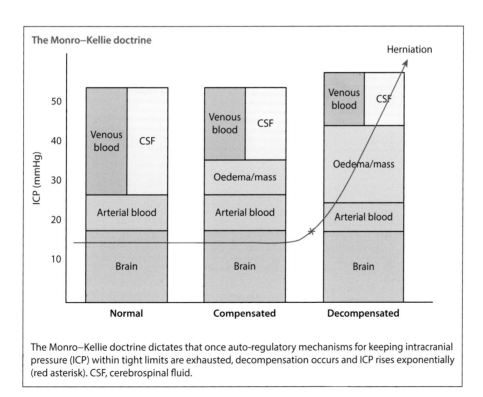

Figure 4.2 Intracranial compensation for expanding mass. This schematic diagram demonstrates how displacement of CSF is the first compensatory mechanism for an increase in intracranial mass, followed by reduction in venous volume.

Reproduced with permission from: Wykes V, Vindlacheruvu R. Intracranial pressure, cerebral blood flow and brain oedema. *Surgery (Oxford)*. 2015;33(8): pp. 355–62.

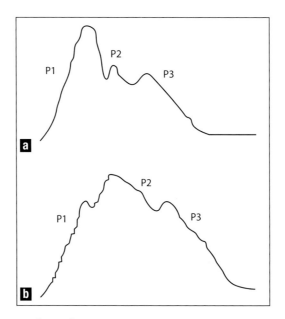

Figure 4.3 The four phases of intracranial compliance curve.
Reproduced with permission from: Ross N, MDa, Eynon CA, MDb. *Current Anaesthesia & Critical Care*. (2005) 16, 255–261.

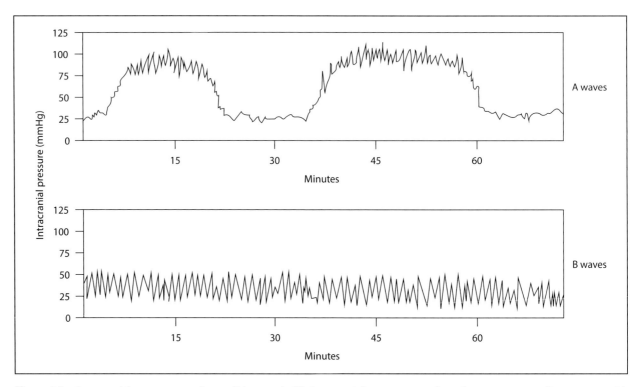

Figure 4.4 Intracranial pressure waveforms: (A) normal; (B) intracranial pressure waveform from a non-compliant system with P2 exceeding P1.
Source: Ross N, Eynon GA. Intracranial pressure monitoring. *Trends in Anaesthesia and Critical Care*. 2005;16(4):255–61.

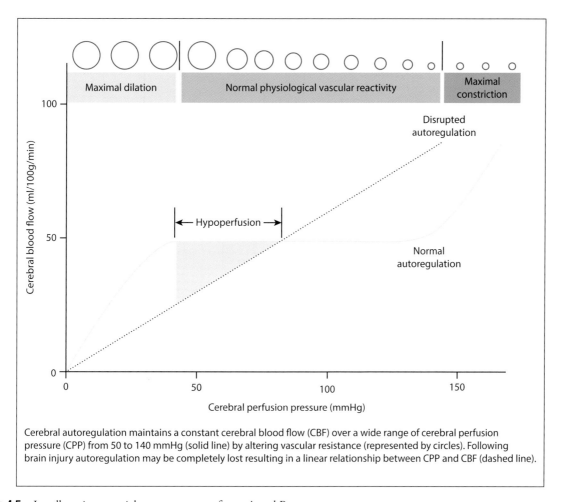

Cerebral autoregulation maintains a constant cerebral blood flow (CBF) over a wide range of cerebral perfusion pressure (CPP) from 50 to 140 mmHg (solid line) by altering vascular resistance (represented by circles). Following brain injury autoregulation may be completely lost resulting in a linear relationship between CPP and CBF (dashed line).

Figure 4.5 Lundberg intracranial pressure waves of type A and B.

Source: Ross N, Eynon GA. Intracranial pressure monitoring. *Trends in Anaesthesia and Critical Care*. 2005;16(4):255–61.

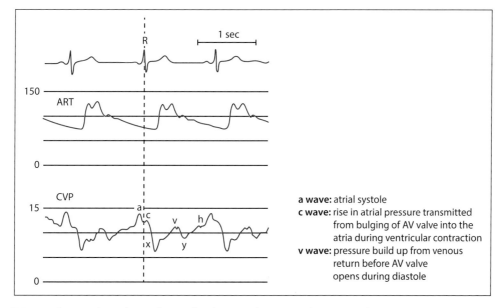

a wave: atrial systole
c wave: rise in atrial pressure transmitted from bulging of AV valve into the atria during ventricular contraction
v wave: pressure build up from venous return before AV valve opens during diastole

Figure 6.1 CVP waveform and its relationship to the electrocardiogram and ABP waveforms.

Reprinted with permission from: Pittman JA, Ping JS, Mark JB. *Int Anesthesiol Clin* 2004;42:13–30, Lippincott Williams & Wilkins.

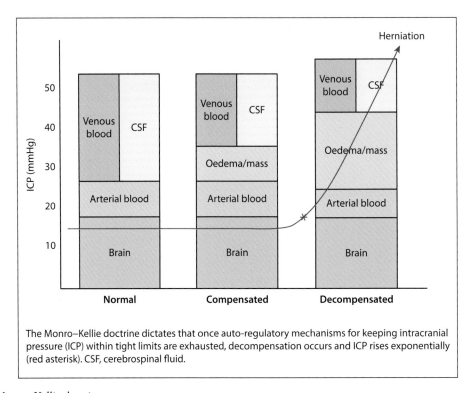

The Monro–Kellie doctrine dictates that once auto-regulatory mechanisms for keeping intracranial pressure (ICP) within tight limits are exhausted, decompensation occurs and ICP rises exponentially (red asterisk). CSF, cerebrospinal fluid.

Figure 8.1 The Monro–Kellie doctrine.

Reproduced with permission from: Ross N, MDa, Eynon CA, MDb. *Current Anaesthesia & Critical Care.* (2005) 16, 255–261.

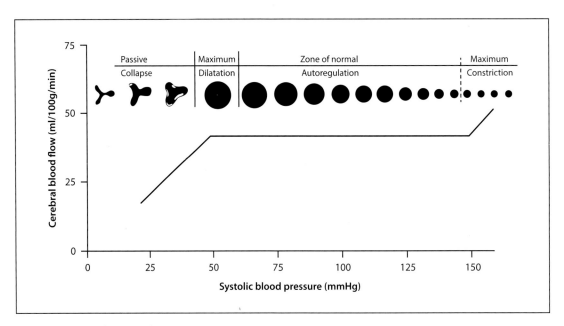

Figure 8.2 Cerebral vessel autoregulation curve.

Reproduced with permission from: Ross N, MDa, Eynon CA, MDb. Current Anaesthesia & Critical Care. (2005) 16, 255–261.

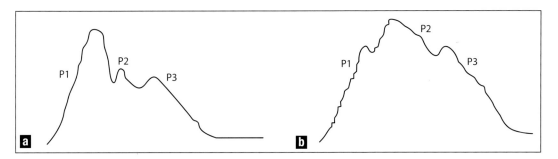

Figure 8.3 Components of ICP waveform and changes with increasing ICP.

Reprinted with permission from: Ross N, Eynon CA. Intracranial pressure monitoring. *Current Anaesthesia & Critical Care* (2005);16:255–61.

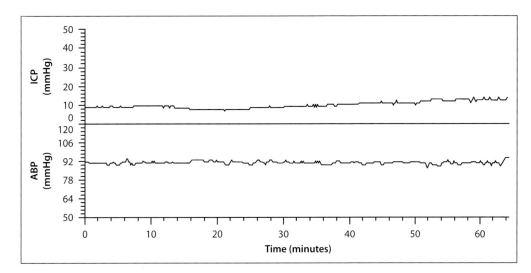

Figure 8.4 Low and stable ICP.

Reprinted with permission from: Ross N, Eynon CA. Intracranial pressure monitoring. *Current Anaesthesia & Critical Care* (2005);16:255–61.

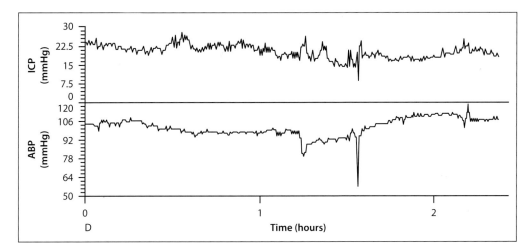

Figure 8.5 High and stable ICP.

Reprinted with permission from: Czosnyka M, Pickard JD. Monitoring and interpretation of intracranial pressure. *Journal of Neurology, Neurosurgery & Psychiatry* 2004;75:813–21, BMJ Publishing group.

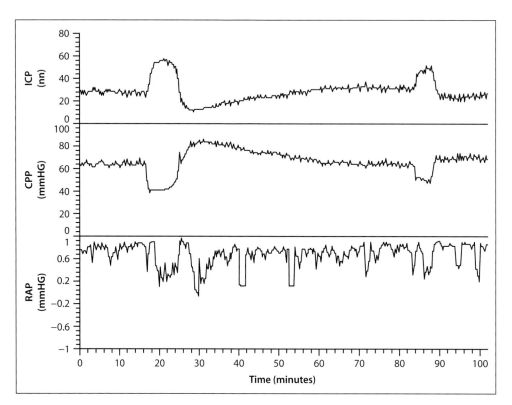

Figure 8.6   Lundberg A waves.

Reprinted with permission from: Czosnyka M, Pickard JD. Monitoring and interpretation of intracranial pressure. *Journal of Neurology, Neurosurgery & Psychiatry* 2004;75:813–21, BMJ Publishing group.

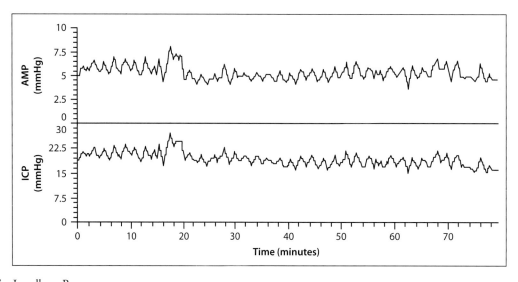

Figure 8.7   Lundberg B waves.

Reprinted with permission from: Czosnyka M, Pickard JD. Monitoring and interpretation of intracranial pressure. *Journal of Neurology, Neurosurgery & Psychiatry* 2004;75:813–21, BMJ Publishing group.

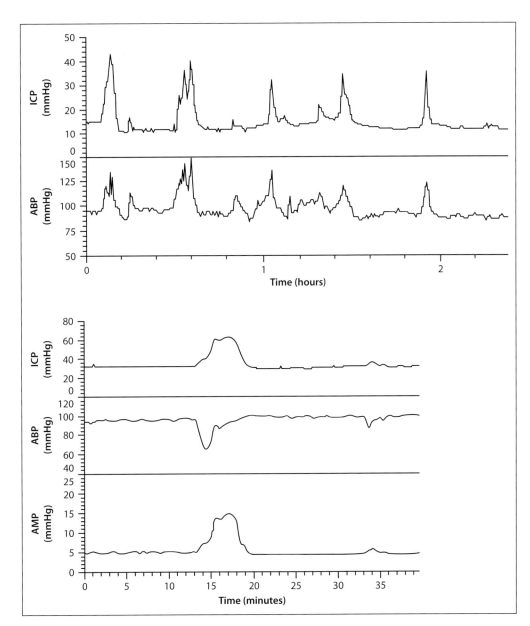

Figure 8.8   ICP changes related to arterial pressure changes and hyperemia.

Reprinted with permission from: Czosnyka M, Pickard JD. Monitoring and interpretation of intracranial pressure. *Journal of Neurology, Neurosurgery & Psychiatry* 2004;75:813–21, BMJ Publishing group.

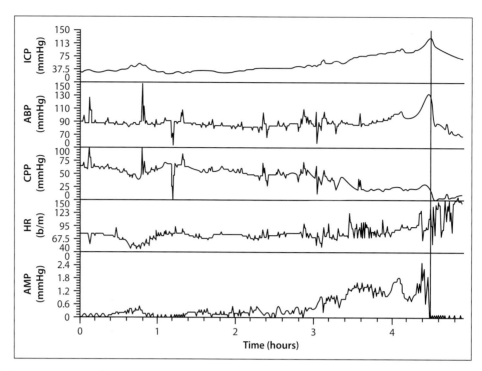

Figure 8.9 Refractory intracranial hypertension.

Reprinted with permission from: Czosnyka M, Pickard JD. Monitoring and interpretation of intracranial pressure. *Journal of Neurology, Neurosurgery & Psychiatry* 2004;75:813–21, BMJ Publishing group.

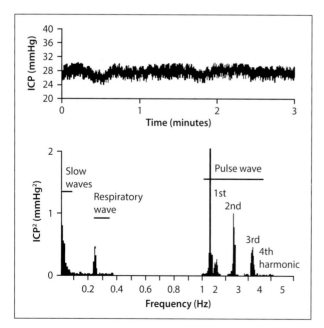

Figure 8.10 ICP waveform analysis.

Reprinted with permission from: Czosnyka M, Pickard JD. Monitoring and interpretation of intracranial pressure. *Journal of Neurology, Neurosurgery & Psychiatry* 2004;75:813–21, BMJ Publishing group.

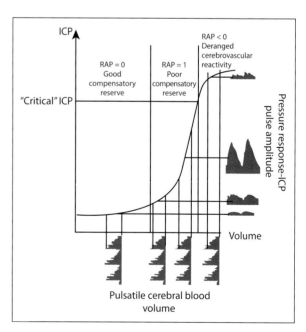

Figure 8.11 RAP and pressure–volume curve.

Reprinted with permission from: Czosnyka M, Pickard JD. Monitoring and interpretation of intracranial pressure. *Journal of Neurology, Neurosurgery & Psychiatry* 2004;75:813–21, BMJ Publishing group.

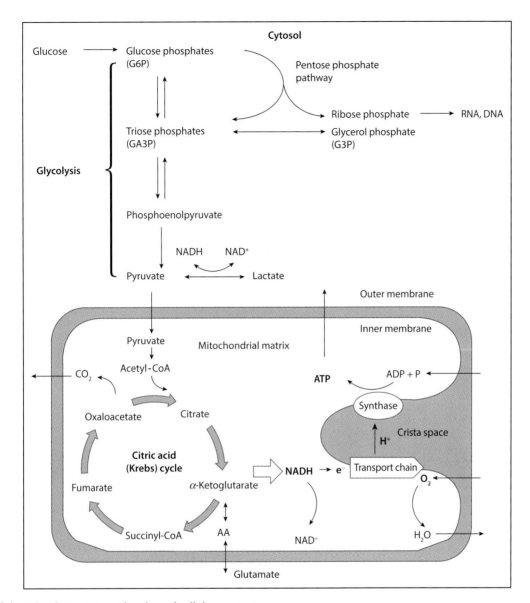

Figure 10.1 Glycolysis, citric acid cycle, and cellular respiration.
Reprinted with permission from: Buitrago Blanco MM, Prashant GN, Vespa PM. Cerebral metabolism and the role of glucose control in acute traumatic brain injury. *Neurosurg Clin N Am* 2016;27:453–63, Elsevier.

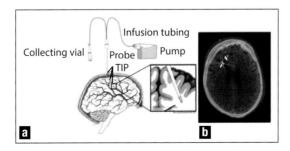

Figure 10.2 Cerebral microdialysis system.
Reprinted with permission from: Buitrago Blanco MM, Prashant GN, Vespa PM. Cerebral metabolism and the role of glucose control in acute traumatic brain injury. *Neurosurg Clin N Am* 2016;27:453–63, Elsevier.

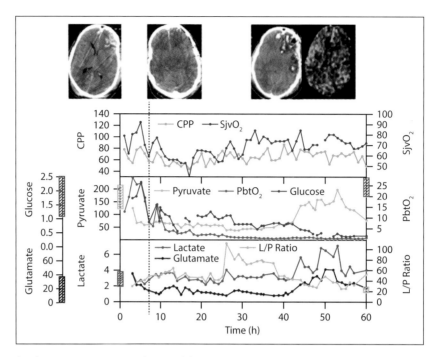

Figure 10.3 Regional ischaemia in a patient with severe TBI.

Reprinted with permission from: Lazaridis C, Robertson CS. The role of multimodal invasive monitoring in acute traumatic brain injury. *Neurosurg Clin N Am* 2016;27(4):509–17, Table 1, Elsevier.

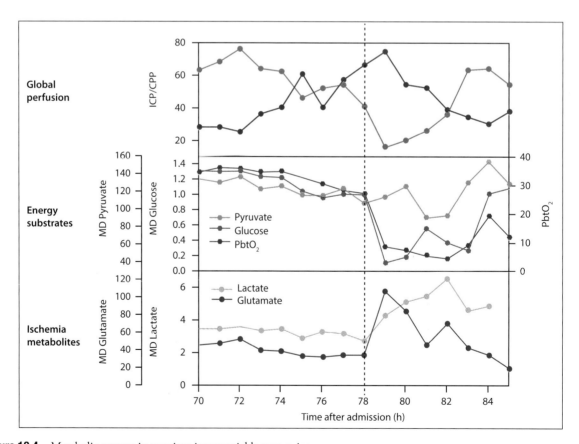

Figure 10.4 Metabolic pattern in transient intracranial hypertension.

Reprinted with permission from: Lazaridis C, Robertson CS. The role of multimodal invasive monitoring in acute traumatic brain injury. *Neurosurg Clin N Am* 2016;27(4):509–17, Table 1, Elsevier.

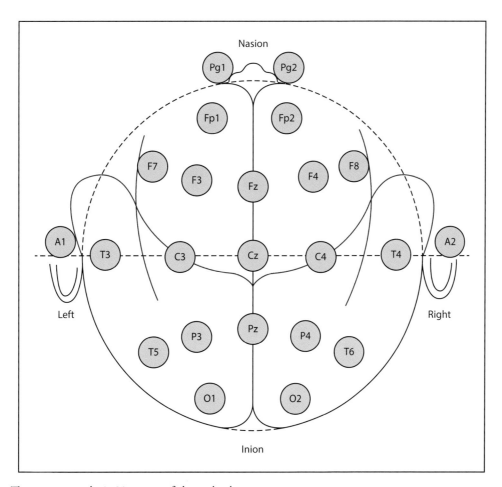

Figure 11.1 The international 10–20 system of electrode placement.

Reprinted with permission from: Michael J. Aminoff. *Aminoff's Electrodiagnosis in Clinical Neurology*. 6th ed. Electroencephalography: General Principles and Clinical Applications, Pages 37–84. Copyright 2012, Elsevier.

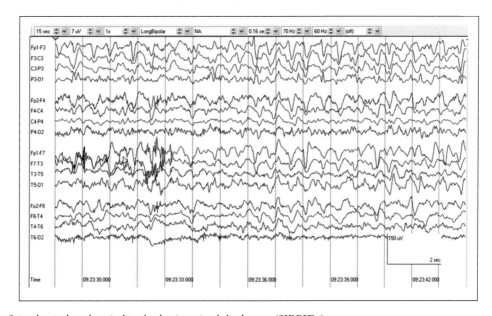

Figure 11.2 Stimulus-induced periodic, rhythmic or ictal discharges (SIRPIDs).

Reprinted with permission from: Wittman JJ, Jr., Hirsch LJ. Continuous electroencephalogram monitoring in the critically ill. *Neurocrit Care* 2005;2:330–41, Springer.

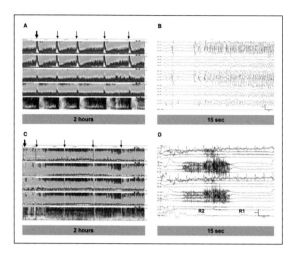

Figure 11.3 Compressed spectral array for seizure detection.

Reprinted with permission from: Williamson CA, Wahlster S, Shafi MM, Westover MB. Sensitivity of compressed spectral arrays for detecting seizures in acutely ill adults. *Neurocrit Care* 2014;20:32–9, Springer.

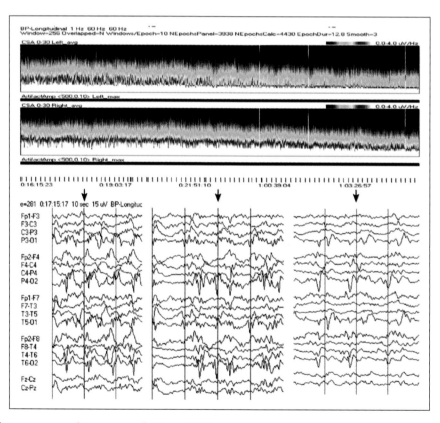

Figure 11.4 Resolving non-convulsive status epilepticus – CSA.

Reprinted with permission from: Wittman JJ, Jr., Hirsch LJ. Continuous electroencephalogram monitoring in the critically ill. *Neurocrit Care* 2005;2:330–41, Springer.

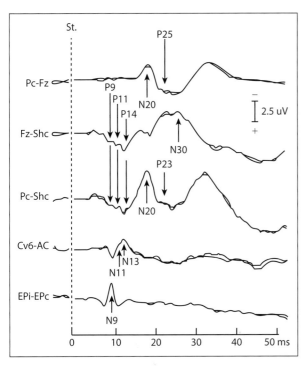

Figure 11.5 Somatosensory evoked potential.

Modified and reprinted with permission from: Cruccu G, Aminoff MJ, Curio G, et al. Recommendations for the clinical use of somatosensory-evoked potentials. *Neurophysiol* 2008;119:1705–19, Elsevier.

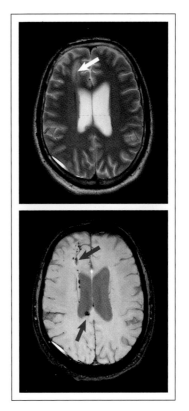

Figure 12.1 Diffuse axonal injury.
Courtesy: Parthiban Balasundaram.

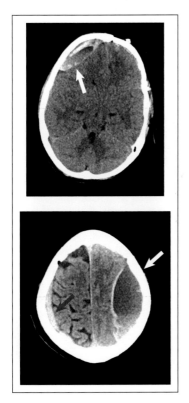

Figure 12.2 Extra-dural haemorrhage.
Courtesy: Parthiban Balasundaram.

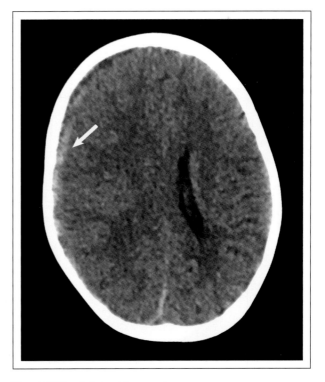

Figure 12.3 Subdural haemorrhage.
Courtesy: Parthiban Balasundaram.

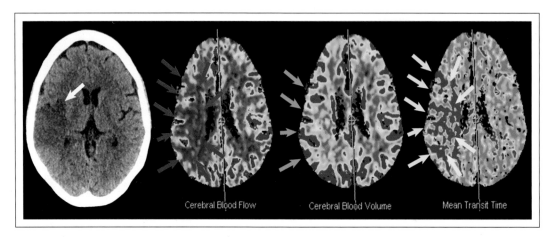

Figure 12.4 Acute stroke.
Courtesy: Parthiban Balasundaram.

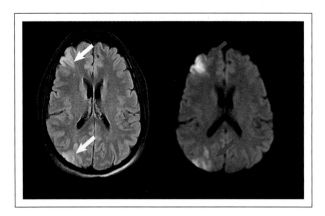

Figure 12.5 Border zone infarcts.
Courtesy: Parthiban Balasundaram.

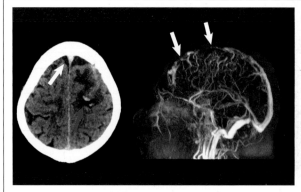

Figure 12.6 Cortical venous thrombosis (CVT).
Courtesy: Parthiban Balasundaram.

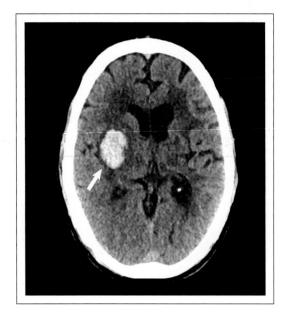

Figure 12.7 Intracerebral haemorrhage.
Courtesy: Parthiban Balasundaram.

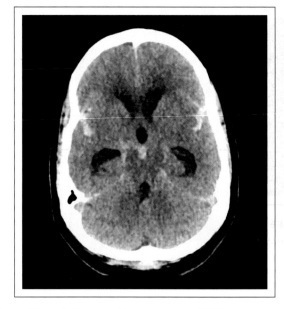

Figure 12.8 Subarachnoid haemorrhage (SAH).
Courtesy: Parthiban Balasundaram.

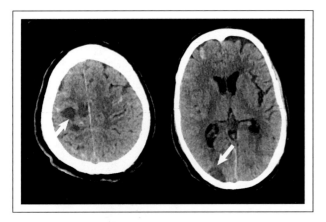

Figure 12.9 Vasospasm.
Courtesy: Parthiban Balasundaram.

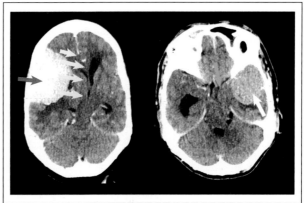

Figure 12.10 Herniations.
Courtesy: Parthiban Balasundaram.

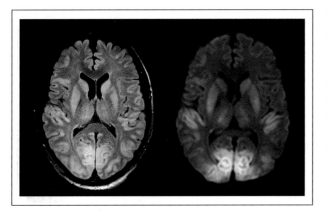

Figure 12.11 Hypoxic injury.
Courtesy: Parthiban Balasundaram.

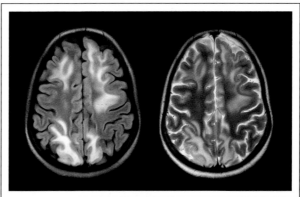

Figure 12.12 PRES.
Courtesy: Parthiban Balasundaram.

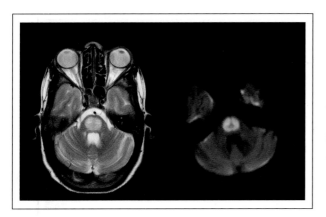

Figure 12.13 Osmotic demyelination.
Courtesy: Parthiban Balasundaram.

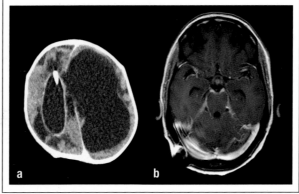

Figure 12.14a and b Ventriculitis/Meningitis.
Courtesy: Parthiban Balasundaram.

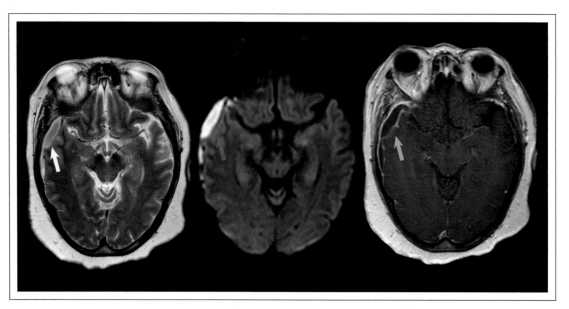

Figure 12.15 Subdural empyema.
Courtesy: Parthiban Balasundaram.

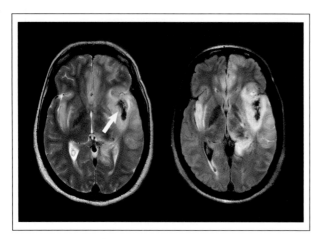

Figure 12.16 Herpes encephalitis.
Courtesy: Parthiban Balasundaram.

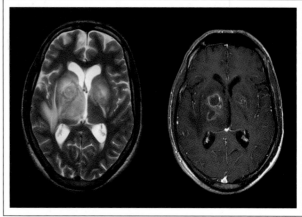

Figure 12.17 Toxoplasmosis.
Courtesy: Parthiban Balasundaram.

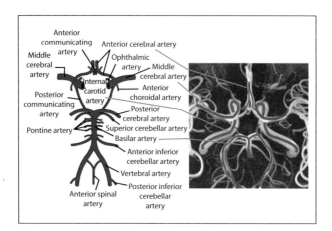

Figure 13.1a Cerebral arteries and their main branches.

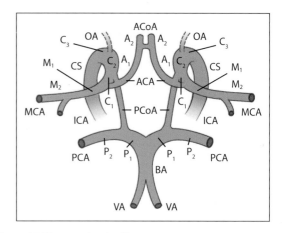

Figure 13.1b Circle of willis.

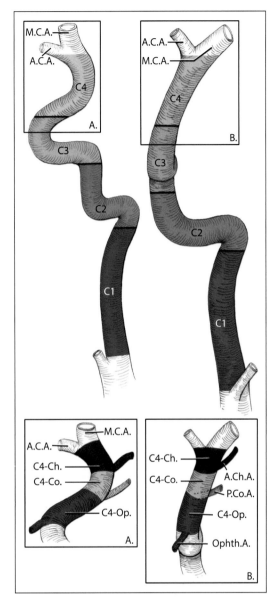

Figure 13.2 Internal carotid artery segments.

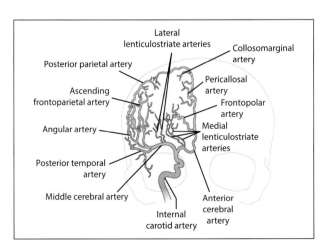

Figure 13.3a Sagittal view.

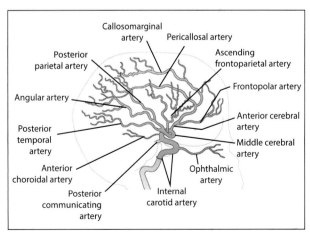

Figure 13.3b Coronal view.

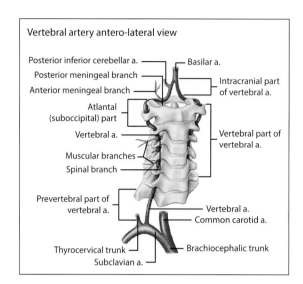

Figure 13.4 The vertebral artery (VA) after originating from the subclavian artery enters the cervical canal at the level of the sixth cervical vertebra and progresses up to the foramen magnum intracranial part where it gives off the posterior inferior cerebellar artery (terminal branch) before merging with the contralateral VA into the basilar artery (BA).

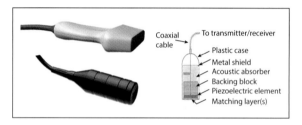

Figure 13.5 Pizoelectric probes used for TCCD (top) and for TCD (bottom).

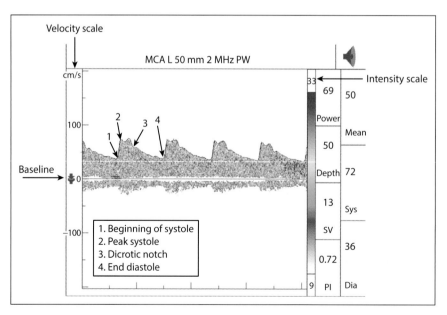

Figure 13.6 'Fast Fourier transform' (FFT), also known as spectral analysis, is used to produce a two-dimensional image on the screen. The curve is further elaborated to gain several important diagnostic parameters: peak systolic velocity, telediastolic velocity, mean velocity, Gosling's 'pulsatility index (PI)' and Pourcelot's 'resistance index (RI)'.

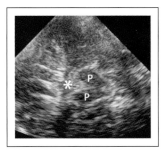

Figure 13.7 On grayscale images, the hypoechoic heart-shaped cerebral peduncles (P) and echogenic star-shaped basilar cistern (*) are the reference landmarks for the circle of Willis.

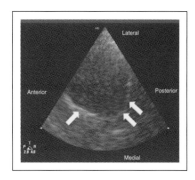

Figure 13.8 Correct probe/grayscale images orientation. Contralateral skull bone in displayed as the hyperechoic line on the medial side.

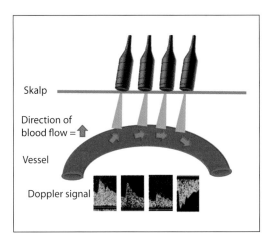

Figure 13.9 Changes in Doppler signal flow velocity according to FFT detected as blood flow direction variations towards and away from the insonation probe occur.

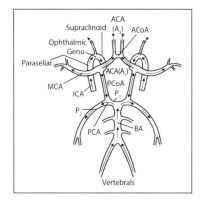

Figure 13.10 Blood flow direction in the vessels of the circle of Willis.

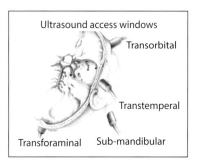

Figure 13.12 Correct position of TCD/TCCD probe according to the acoustic window selected for vessels intonation.

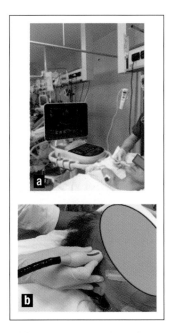

Figure 13.11a and b Transtemporal window TCCD.

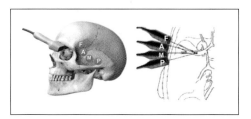

Figure 13.13 Position of the TCCD and TCD probes respectively in the ophthalmic and the temporal region in order to insonate the anterior and posterior parts of the circle of Willis.

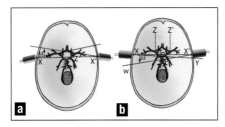

Figure 13.14 Position of the probe in the temporal region to insonate the anterior and posterior parts of the circle of Willis. A, Line X–X′ indicates a frontal plane that runs through the regular placement of the probe on either side and, simultaneously, perpendicular to the sagittal midline of the skull. Z′ indicates the site of the intracranial internal carotid artery bifurcation. The X′-Z′ distance is 63 ± 5 mm. The angle μ is the angle with which the probe is aimed more anteriorly toward the middle cerebral artery and anterior cerebral artery segments. This angle was found to be 6 ± 1.1 degrees. B, The angle ω indicates the angle with which the beam is directed more posteriorly to insonate the top (T) of the basilar artery (BA) and the P1 segments (P′) on both sides. This angle was found to be 4.6 ± 1.2 degrees. The BA bifurcation could be insonated at depths of 78 ± 5 mm, corresponding to the distance X–T or X′-T, respectively. Y indicates the fictional point at which the pathway of the beam then transits the contralateral skull—that is, approximately 2 to 3 cm behind the external acoustic meatus. The P2 segments (P) can also be insonated if the beam is directed even more posteriorly and slightly caudally (line X′-P). W lies approximately 5 cm behind the contralateral external acoustic meatus.

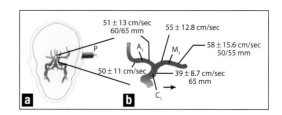

Figure 13.15 Position of the probe in the temporal region to insonate the anterior and posterior parts of the circle of Willis. A, Line X–X′ indicates a frontal plane that runs through the regular placement of the probe on either side and, simultaneously, perpendicular to the sagittal midline of the skull. Z′ indicates the site of the intracranial internal carotid artery bifurcation. The X′-Z′ distance is 63 ± 5 mm. The angle μ is the angle with which the probe is aimed more anteriorly toward the middle cerebral artery and anterior cerebral artery segments. This angle was found to be 6 ± 1.1 degrees. B, The angle ω indicates the angle with which the beam is directed more posteriorly to insonate the top (T) of the basilar artery (BA) and the P1 segments (P′) on both sides. This angle was found to be 4.6 ± 1.2 degrees. The BA bifurcation could be insonated at depths of 78 ± 5 mm, corresponding to the distance X–T or X′-T, respectively. Y indicates the fictional point at which the pathway of the beam then transits the contralateral skull—that is, approximately 2 to 3 cm behind the external acoustic meatus. The P2 segments (P) can also be insonated if the beam is directed even more posteriorly and slightly caudally (line X′-P). W lies approximately 5 cm behind the contralateral external acoustic meatus.

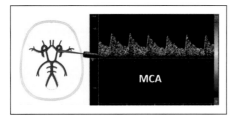

Figure 13.16 Transtemporal window allows the examination of the terminal portion of the internal carotid artery, its bifurcation into the middle and the anterior cerebral arteries, and the posterior cerebral artery.

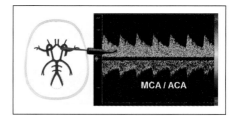

Figure 13.17 Transtemporal window allows the examination of the terminal portion of the internal carotid artery, its bifurcation into the middle and the anterior cerebral arteries, and the posterior cerebral artery.

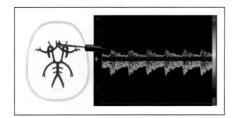

Figure 13.18 Transtemporal window allows the examination of the terminal portion of the internal carotid artery, its bifurcation into the middle and the anterior cerebral arteries, and the posterior cerebral artery.

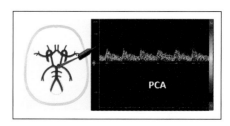

Figure 13.19 Transtemporal window allows the examination of the terminal portion of the internal carotid artery, its bifurcation into the middle and the anterior cerebral arteries, and the posterior cerebral artery.

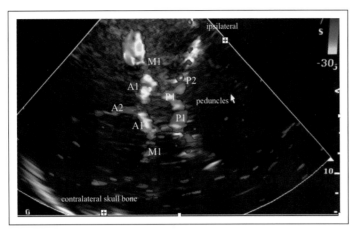

Figure 13.20 Illustration of a typical transtemporal transcranial colour-coded duplex sonography (TCCD) examination. For initial spatial orientation, the examination is started with a large-scale, B-mode cranial view, which is usually achieved at a depth of 14 to 17 cm. Visualization of the hyperechoic contralateral skull proves the presence of adequate transcranial ultrasound penetration. If the hypoechoic, heart-shaped midbrain (peduncles) and the hyperechoic sphenoid bone can be visualized, then the correct insonation plane has been achieved. For the colour-mode examination, the insonation depth is reduced to 8 to 10 cm; the precommunicating (P1) and postcommunicating (P2) segments of the posterior cerebral artery (PCA) can be visualized as they follow the edge of the midbrain. More anteriorly, the sphenoidal (M1) and the insular (M2) parts of the middle cerebral artery (MCA), and the precommunicating (A1) part of the anterior cerebral artery (ACA) can be depicted. In rare cases, and with excellent bone insonation conditions (as illustrated), the entire circle of Willis can be displayed. The distal part of the internal carotid artery (ICA) is also assessable with the probe tilted downward.

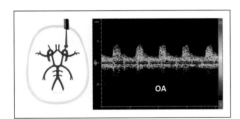

Figure 13.21 Ophthalmic artery intonation through the transorbital window: flow is directed towards the probe.

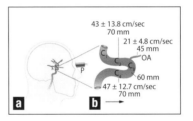

Figure 13.22a and b Transorbital approach to the insonation of the intracranial segments of the ICA.

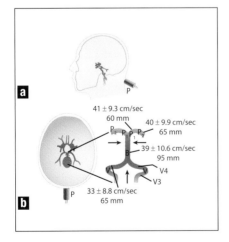

Figure 13.23a and b Probe orientation and typical insonation depths and flow velocities for VAs and BA through the transforaminal window.

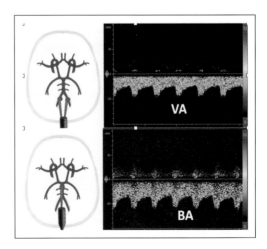

Figure 13.24 Colour Doppler flowmetry for VA (upper) and BA (lower).

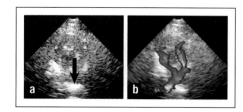

Figure 13.25a and b Illustration of a typical suboccipital (or transforaminal) transcranial colour-coded duplex sonography (TCCD) examination. A, For initial spatial orientation, the examination is started with a large-scale, B-mode cranial view, which is usually achieved at a depth of 11 to 13 cm. Visualization of the hypoechoic foramen magnum (asterisks) and the hyperechoic clivus (arrow) proves the adequacy of transcranial ultrasound penetration. B, For the colour-mode examination, the insonation depth is usually reduced to 8 to 11 cm, visualizing segments (V4) of both vertebral arteries (VAs) as they follow the edges of the foramen magnum. The Y-shaped conjunction of the VAs with the basilar artery (BA) is usually located close to the clivus. Note, however, that the origin of the BA is highly variable and all three arteries are not always visible within the same insonation plane.

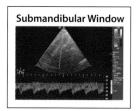

Figure 13.26 Illustrates intonation of ICA by means of a TCCD machine through the submandibular window. Doppler velocity signal is away from the probe.

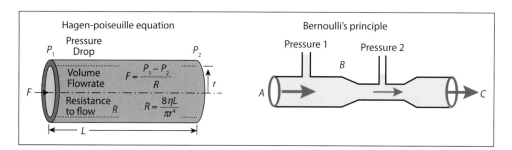

Figure 13.27 The Hagen-Poiseuille equation (left) defines the flow through a tube and how this flow is affected by the attributes of the tube; the length and radius, and the attributes of the fluid; the viscosity. Note that resistance to flow is inversely proportional to the fourth power of the radius. On the right, the pictured explain Bernoulli Principle which states that "For a non-compressible, non-viscous fluid undergoing laminar flow, the sum of the pressure, kinetic and potential energies per unit volume remains a constant at all points along the line of flow". Mathematically represented by P + 1/2*p v2 + pgh = constant, where:

> P = Pressure
> g = Acceleration due to gravity (m/s2)
> h = Height of the tube
> p = Density of liquid
> v = Velocity of fluid

This is a perfect system so all the energy is conserved as either pressure energy, potential (or stored) energy, and the energy existing as flow. We assume no loss of energy through heat caused by friction within the fluid or caused by drag on the tube's walls. This means that if we alter the energy of one portion of the system, it has an effect on the rest of the system. So if the kinetic energy rises, the potential energy and pressure must fall. When we apply the Bernoulli principle in our practice we can ignore the portion due to gravity to make life a little simpler. Consider our tube with a narrowing, as there are no leaks, the volume of fluid at point A is the same at point C. Consequently, the narrowing at point B means that the fluid has to speed up in order to fulfill this continuity. Bernoulli equation can be then so simplified:

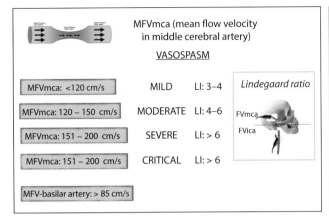

Figure 13.28 Summary of flow velocities ranges and LI ratio for detection of cerebral vasospasm.

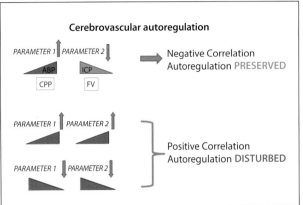

Figure 13.29 Cerebrovascular autoregulation mechanisms.

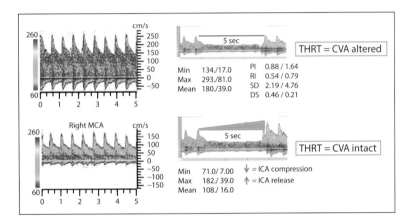

Figure 13.30 Transient Hyperaemic Response Test: when cerebrovascular autoregulation (CVA) is altered (upper graph) after carotid compression and release no velocity modification in the ipsilateral MCA is observed because the arteriolar bed is not able to vasodilate in order to compensate the drop in cerebral perfusion pressure. On the contrary, when CVA is preserved (lower graph), after carotid compression and release, a transient increase in peak flow velocity for two heart cycles and a ensuing return to basal values are observed as a consequence of arteriolar bed adaptations.

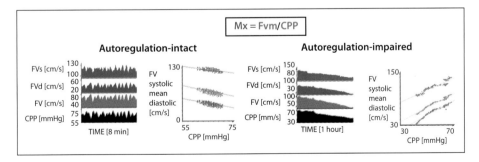

Figure 13.31 Mean flow velocity index (Mx) is calculated as the moving correlation coefficient between mean flow velocity (Fvm) and CPP. The graphs show that when CVA is intact between the two variables a negative or null correlation exists whereas when CVA is impaired Fvm and CPP fluctuate in the same direction (positive correlation).

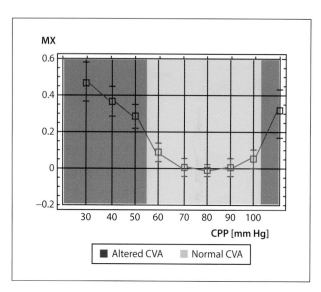

Figure 13.32 Mx plotted against CPP. The graph shows that a null Mx is observed for a range of CPP values in which CVA is physiologically ensured.

Courtesy: Czosnyka M.

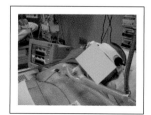

Figure 13.33 TCD bedside continuous monitoring.

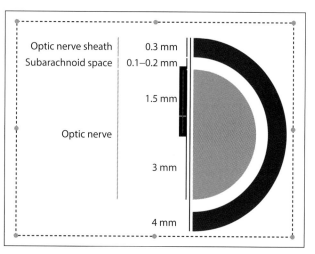

Figure 13.34 Schematic representation of the optic nerve and its sheath cross-sections.

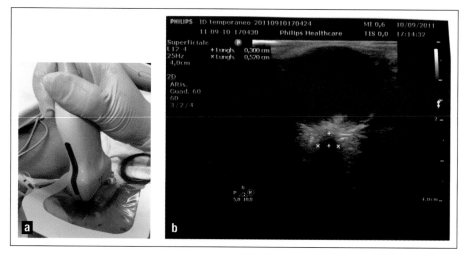

Figure 13.35a and b ONSD intonation technique: a linear ultrasound 7.5–10.5 MHz probe is gently placed over the upper temporal eyelid, after applying ultrasound conducting gel, and power is reduced to prevent retinal damage (left image). ONSD is visualised posteriorly to the eyeball as a hypoechoic structure extending from the retina posteriorly. The optic nerve sheath is subtly more echogenic and surrounds the nerve. Measurements are taken 3 mm behind the retina in two different axes (right image).

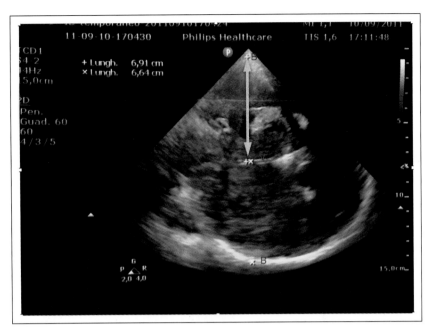

Figure 13.36 Midline shift (MLS) measurement by using ultrasound: Ipsilateral and contralateral bone table and (B) the third ventricle, identified as a double hyperechogenic image over the midbrain (V). The distance between the external bone table and the centre of the third ventricle is then measured bilaterally (yellow arrow).

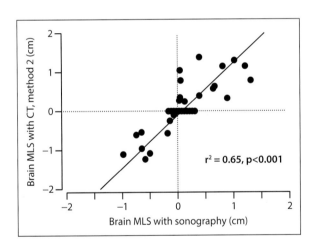

Figure 13.37 Correlation between sonography and CT method for MLS assessment. CT, computed tomography; MLS, midline shift.

Courtesy: Motuel et al. Assessment of brain midline shift using sonography in neurosurgical ICU patients *Critical Care*. (2014) 18:676.

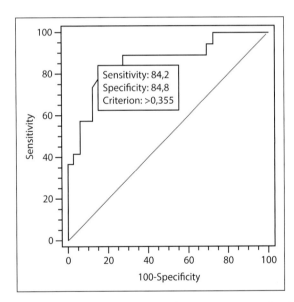

Figure 13.38 Receiver operating characteristic curve for the detection of a CT MLS >0.5 cm with TCS. CT, computed tomography; MLS, midline shift; TCS, transcranial sonography.

Courtesy: Motuel et al. Assessment of brain midline shift using sonography in neurosurgical ICU patients. *Critical Care*. (2014) 18:676.

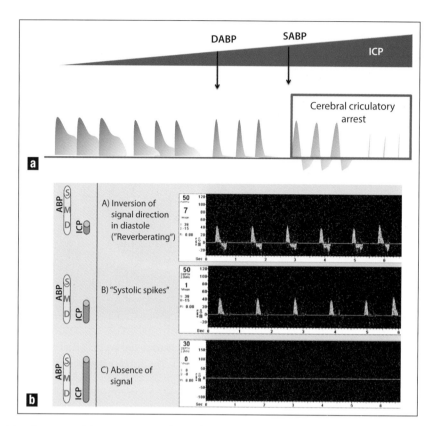

Figure 13.39a and b Intracranial hypertension and circulatory arrest. Transcranial Doppler changes in middle cerebral artery (MCA) mean flow with progressive increase in intracranial pressure (ICP). a. The initial stage has a typical pattern of systolic peaks with progressive reduction in diastolic velocities. b. The three patterns that correspond to intracranial circulatory arrest are shown: biphasic oscillating flow, systolic spike flow, and zero flow. Notes: D- diastolic arterial pressure; S- systolic arterial pressure.

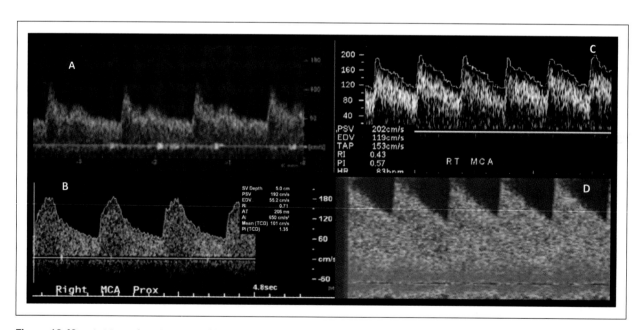

Figure 13.40 *A.* Normal MCA; *B.* Mild MCA stenosis: mild stenosis was defined as systolic peak velocity 140 to 209 cm/s; *C.* Moderate MCA stenosis: moderate stenosis was defined as a systolic peak velocity from 210 to 280 cm/s; *D.* Severe MCA stenosis: severe stenosis was defined as a systolic peak velocity above 280 cm/s.

Reprinted with permission from: Jaroslaw Krejza, Rong Chen, Grzegorz Romanowicz, et al. Sickle cell disease and transcranial Doppler imaging. *Stroke* 2011;42:81–86.

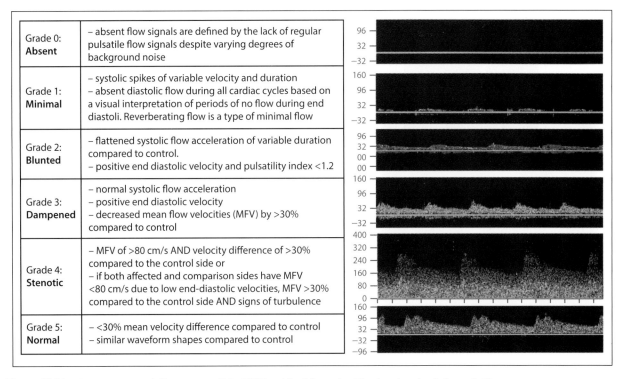

Grade 0: **Absent**	– absent flow signals are defined by the lack of regular pulsatile flow signals despite varying degrees of background noise
Grade 1: **Minimal**	– systolic spikes of variable velocity and duration – absent diastolic flow during all cardiac cycles based on a visual interpretation of periods of no flow during end diastoli. Reverberating flow is a type of minimal flow
Grade 2: **Blunted**	– flattened systolic flow acceleration of variable duration compared to control. – positive end diastolic velocity and pulsatility index <1.2
Grade 3: **Dampened**	– normal systolic flow acceleration – positive end diastolic velocity – decreased mean flow velocities (MFV) by >30% compared to control
Grade 4: **Stenotic**	– MFV of >80 cm/s AND velocity difference of >30% compared to the control side or – if both affected and comparison sides have MFV <80 cm/s due to low end-diastolic velocities, MFV >30% compared to the control side AND signs of turbulence
Grade 5: **Normal**	– <30% mean velocity difference compared to control – similar waveform shapes compared to control

Figure 13.41   Description and illustration of the TIBI residual flow classification (grades 0 through 5).

Source: Demchuk AM, Burgin WS, Christou I, et al. Thrombolysis in brain ischemia (TIBI) transcranial Doppler flow grades predict clinical severity, early recovery, and mortality in patients treated with intravenous tissue plasminogen activator. *Stroke* 2001 Jan;32(1):89–93.

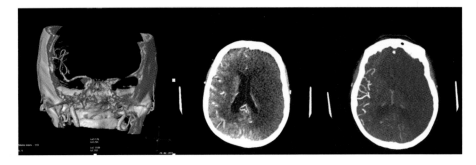

Figure 13.42   Left MCA occlusion on CT angiography.

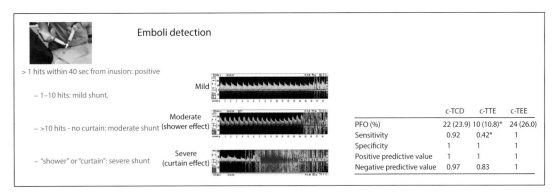

Emboli detection

> 1 hits within 40 sec from inusion: positive

– 1–10 hits: mild shunt,   Mild

– >10 hits - no curtain: moderate shunt   Moderate (shower effect)

– "shower" or "curtain": severe shunt   Severe (curtain effect)

	c-TCD	c-TTE	c-TEE
PFO (%)	22 (23.9)	10 (10.8)*	24 (26.0)
Sensitivity	0.92	0.42*	1
Specificity	1	1	1
Positive predictive value	1	1	1
Negative predictive value	0.97	0.83	1

Figure 13.43   Microemboli detection with TCD after injection of normal saline mixed with air. Cut off for positivity of the test and appearance of the detected disturbances on the Doppler signal. It is also displayed accuracy of TCD in diagnosis PFO when compared with TEE.

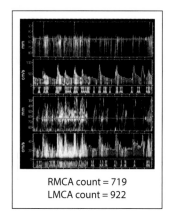

Figure 13.44 Hyperintensity thromboembolic signal (HITS).

RMCA count = 719
LMCA count = 922

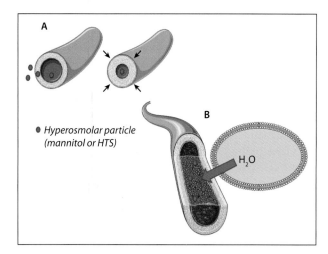

A

B

• Hyperosmolar particle
(mannitol or HTS)

H_2O

Figure 15.1 Osmotherapy MOA.

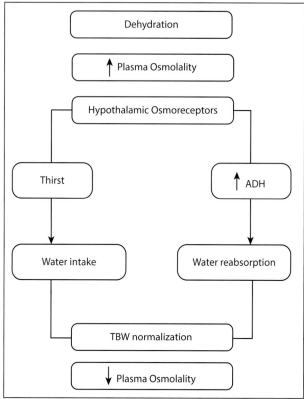

Dehydration

↑ Plasma Osmolality

Hypothalamic Osmoreceptors

Thirst

↑ ADH

Water intake

Water reabsorption

TBW normalization

↓ Plasma Osmolality

Figure 23.1 Water homoeostasis.

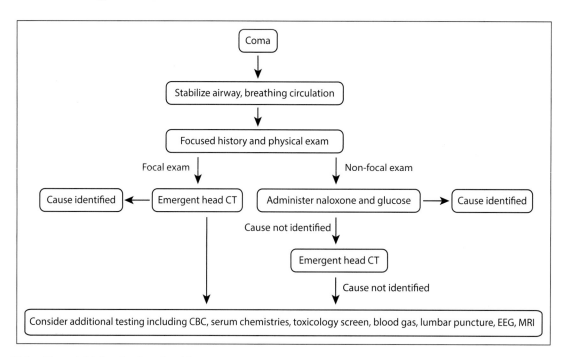

Coma

Stabilize airway, breathing circulation

Focused history and physical exam

Focal exam

Non-focal exam

Cause identified ← Emergent head CT

Administer naloxone and glucose → Cause identified

Cause not identified

Emergent head CT

Cause not identified

Consider additional testing including CBC, serum chemistries, toxicology screen, blood gas, lumbar puncture, EEG, MRI

Figure 24.1 Coma initial evaluation algorithm.

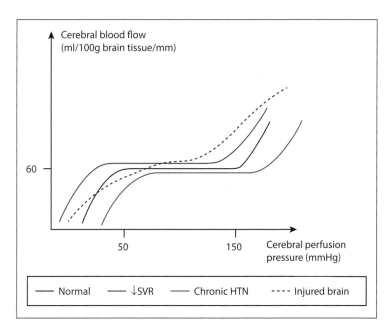

Figure 25.1 Cerebral autoregulation.

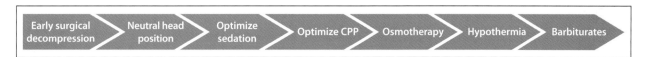

Figure 25.2 Algorithm for IH management.

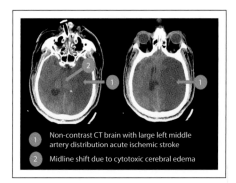

Figure 26.1 CT brain with large middle artery stroke with cerebral oedema.

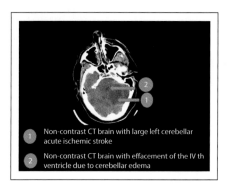

Figure 26.2 CT brain with cerebellar stroke with cerebral oedema.

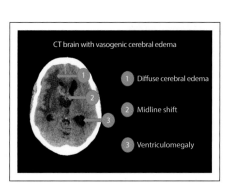

Figure 26.3 CT brain with cerebral oedema associated with brain tumour.

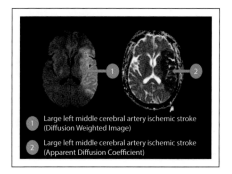

Figure 26.4 MRI demonstrating cytotoxic cerebral oedema.

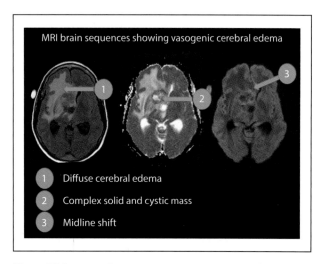

Figure 26.5 MRI demonstrating vasogenic cerebral oedema.

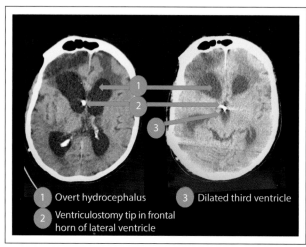

Figure 27.1 Obstructive hydrocephalus in patient with intracerebral haemorrhage with intraventricular extension.

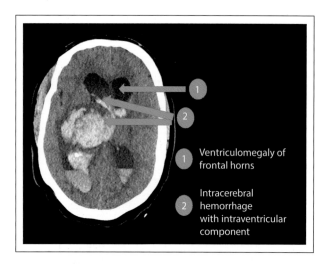

Figure 27.2 Communicative hydrocephalus with external CSF diversion.

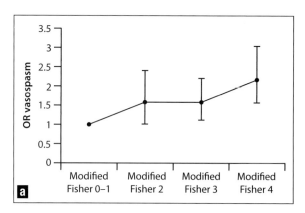

Figure 28.1 Odds ratios for risk of symptomatic vasospasm in the original and modified Fisher CT rating scales. The risk of vasospasm progressively increases for each modified Fisher grade (A). OR, odds ratio. Vertical bars represent 95% confidence intervals.

Reprinted with permission from: Frontera et al. Prediction of symptomatic vasospasm after subarachnoid haemorrhage: the modified fisher scale. *Neurosurgery.* 2006;59(1):21–7.

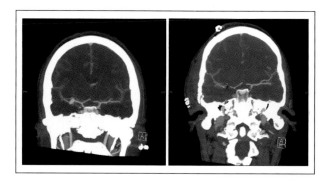

Figure 28.2 Left: CT-A demonstrating right middle cerebral artery aneurysm on admission. Right: CT-A now shows vasospasm seven days after aneurysm treatment.

Courtesy: Mike Levitt, MD, University of Washington.

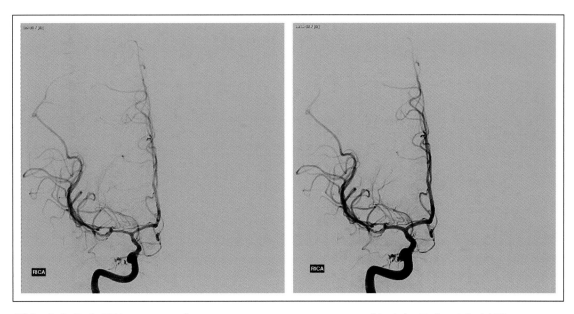

Figure 28.3 Left: Right ICA angiogram demonstrates severe vasospasm on post-bleed day 7 after right MCA aneurysm rupture and coiling. Right: Right ICA angiogram obtained after angioplasty and intra-arterial nicardipine.
Courtesy: Mike Levitt, MD, University of Washington.

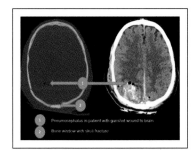

Figure 29.1 Traumatic pneumocephalus in patient with gunshot wound to head.

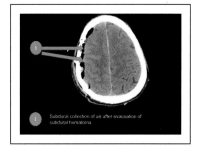

Figure 29.2 Subdural collection of air after evacuation of subdural haematoma.

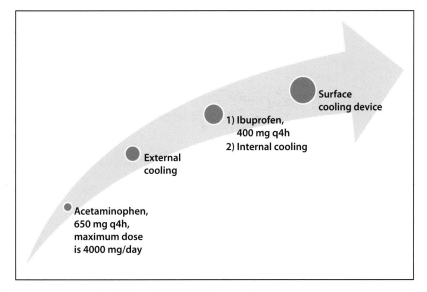

Figure 34.1 Ohio State University Medical Center (OSUMC) targeted temperature management protocol.

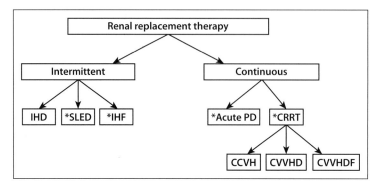

Figure 39.1 Modalities of renal replacement therapy.

*Useful in haemodynamically unstable patients.

Abbreviations: HD: Haemodialysis; SLED: slow extended dialysis; CRRT: continuous renal replacement therapy; CVVH: continuous venovenous haemofiltration; CVVHD: continuous venovenous haemodialysis; CVVHDF: continuous venovenous haemodiafiltration.

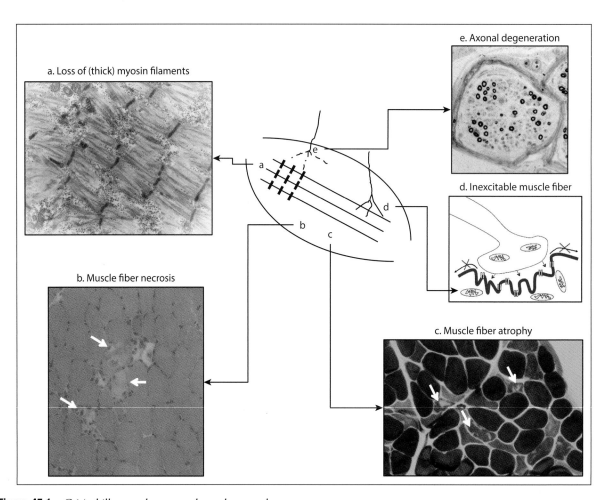

Figure 45.1 Critical illness polyneuropathy and myopathy.

Reproduced with permission from: Latronico N, et al. 'Critical illness myopathy', *Current Opinion in Rheumatology* 2012;24(6):616–22. Copyright © 2012 Wolters Kluwer Health.

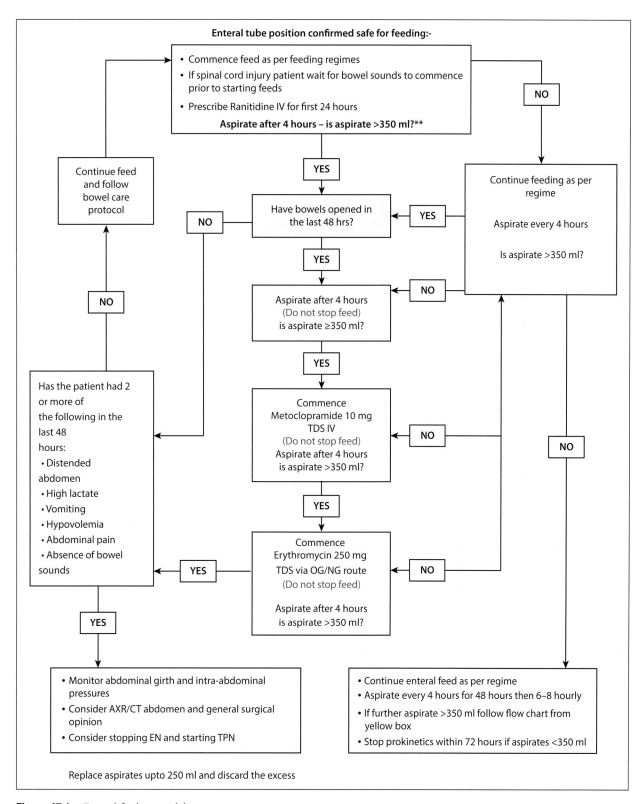

Figure 47.1 Enteral feeding guideline.

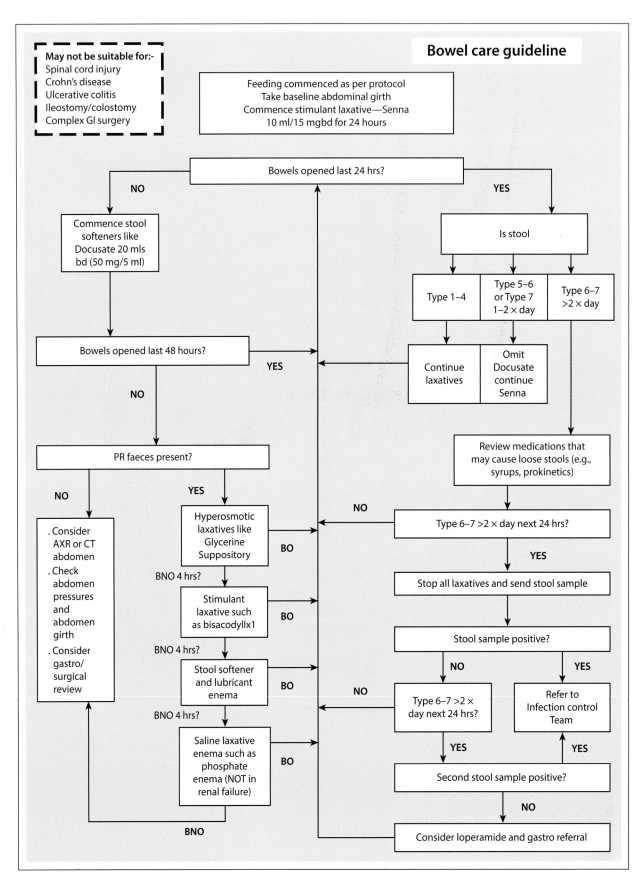

Figure 47.2 Bowel care guideline.

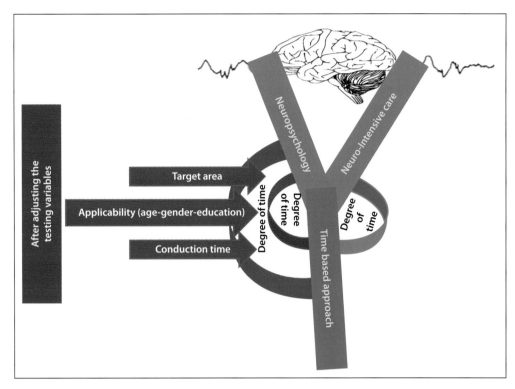

Figure 50.1 Cognitive test and functional outcomes scales.

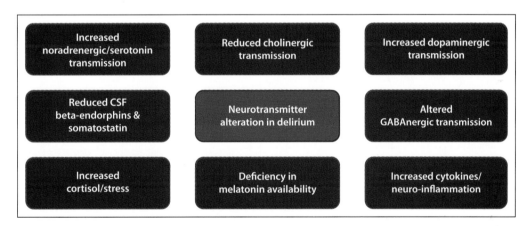

Figure 51.1 Neurochemical alteration in patients with delirium.

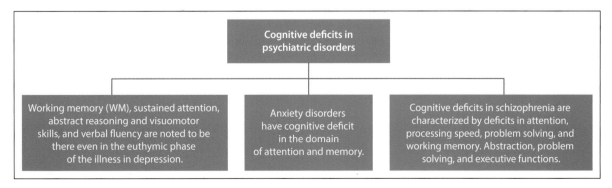

Figure 52.1 Cognitive deficits in psychiatric disorders.

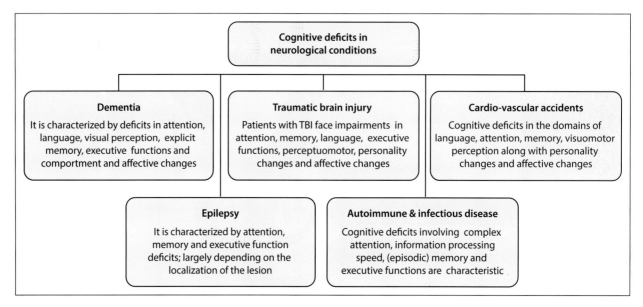

Figure 52.2 Cognitive defi cits in neurological conditions.

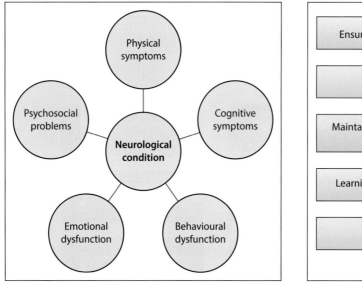

Figure 52.3 Problems faced by survivors of neurological conditions.

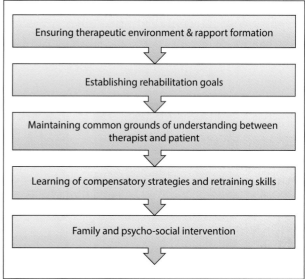

Figure 52.4 Principles of NR in neurointensive care.

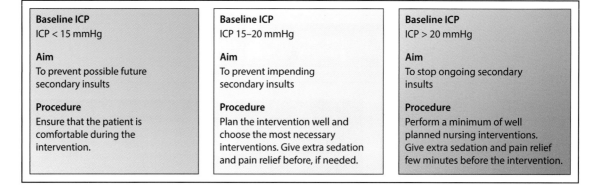

Figure 57.1 Decision-making tool for nursing interventions in a NICU.

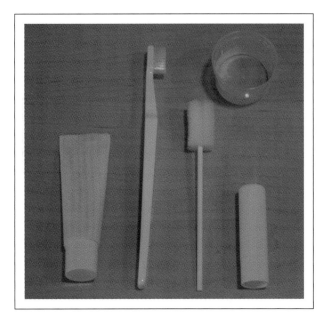

Figure 57.2 Oral care devices, no foaming toothpaste, toothbrush, oral swab, lip balsam and chlorhexidine 0.1–0.2% mouthwash.

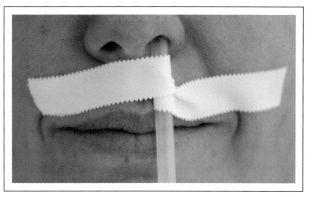

Figure 57.3 Fixation of a nasogastric tube in a way that reduces the risk for pressure ulcer inside the nose.

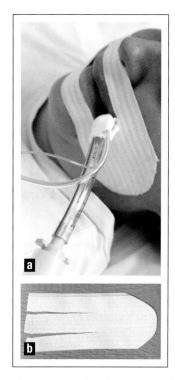

Figure 57.5 Tube fixation with adhesive tape (Figure 5a) and outline how to cut the adhesive tape (Figure 5b).

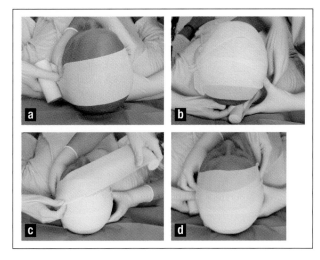

Figure 57.4 Outline how to apply a head bandage. (1) Put a sterile non-adhesive dressing over the surgery wounds and over tubes and catheters (e.g. ICP measuring devices). (2) Use a sterile elastic bandage and make the first laps from the right ear to the left ear and then back and forth to cover the top of the head (Figure 57.4a). (3) Make laps around the head to secure the first passes of bandage. The bandage should be placed low down on the neck, over the ears and down to the eyebrows (Figure 57.4b and c). (4) Fix the bandage with some tape (Figure 57.4d).

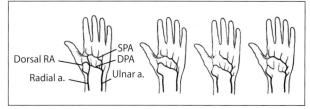

Figure 59.1 Variation in anatomy.
Reprinted with permission from: Ruengsakulrach P, Eizenberg N, Fahrer C, Fahrer M, Buxton BF. Surgical implications of variations in hand collateral circulation: Anatomy revisited. *The Journal of Thoracic and Cardiovascular Surgery.* 122(4):682–6.

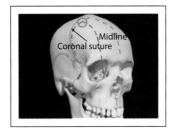

Figure 61.1 Kocher's point: mid-pupillary line (2–4 cm or two fingerbreadths lateral to the midline) and 2–3 cm anterior to the coronal suture (fingerbreadth in front of coronal suture, mid-pupillary line).

Reproduced with permission from: Intracranial pressure monitoring. *European Journal of Anaesthesiology (EJA)* 2008;25:192–5.

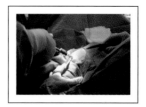

Figure 61.2 Drilling procedure to create burr hole. Intracranial pressure monitoring. *European Journal of Anaesthesiology (EJA)* 2008;25:192–5.

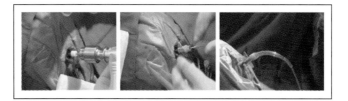

Figure 61.3 Insertion of transducer tipped catheter in the brain parenchyma.

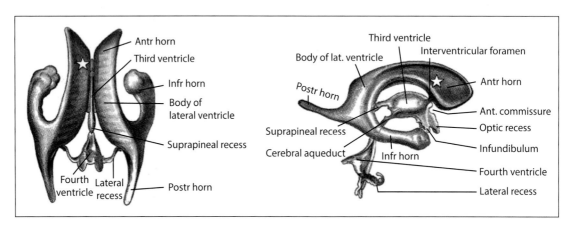

Figure 62.1 Lateral and anterior view of the cerebral ventricular system. Distal catheter target is marked with white stars.
Reproduced with permission from: Daube JR. *Handbook of Clinical Neurophysiology*. Elsevier

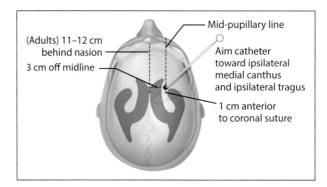

Figure 62.2 Kocher's point is located 1–2 cm anterior to the coronal suture in the mid-pupillary line.
Reproduced with permission from: Ganti L. *External ventricular drain placement*. Springer Nature.

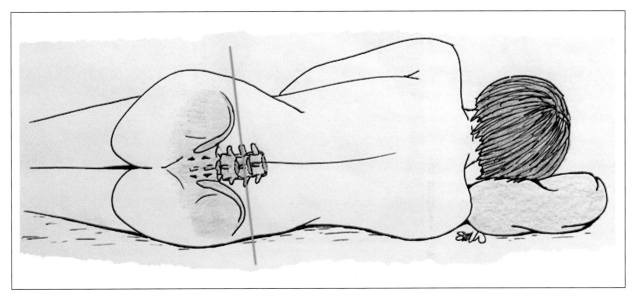

Figure 63.1 The intersection of the intercristal line and midline is a common landmark for the L3–4 interspace. This may vary depending on body habitus.

Courtesy: Sheena M. Weaver.

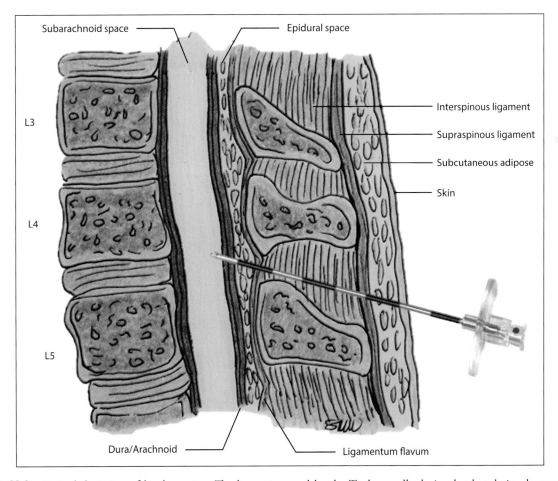

Figure 63.2 Sagittal depiction of lumbar spine. The layers traversed by the Touhy needle during lumbar drain placement are labelled.

Courtesy: Sheena M. Weaver.

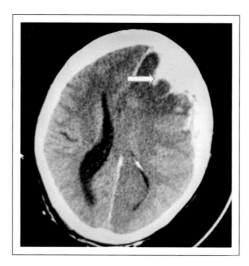

Figure 64.1 Chronic subdural haematoma.

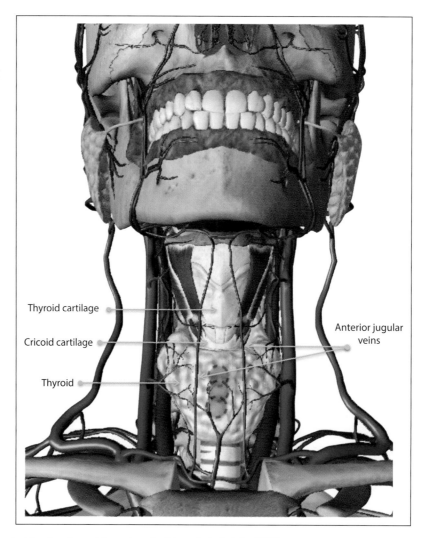

Thyroid cartilage

Cricoid cartilage

Thyroid

Anterior jugular veins

Figure 65.1 Anatomical landmarks and insertion site (dotted circles) for PDT.

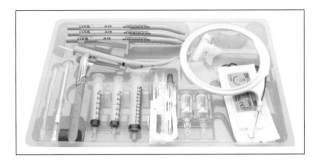

Figure 65.2 Blue Rhino™ kit.

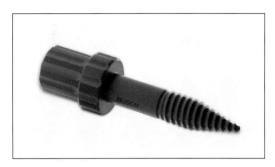

Figure 65.3 PercuTwist screw.

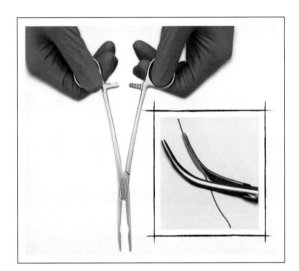

Figure 65.4 Criggs' guide wire dilating forceps.

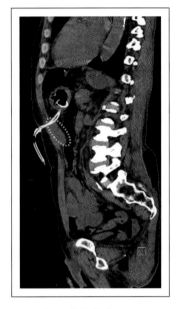

Figure 66.1 Uncomplicated PEG placement in a scaphoid virgin abdomen resulting in full-thickness penetration of small bowel (outlined by double-dashed oblique oval), Left parasagittal view.

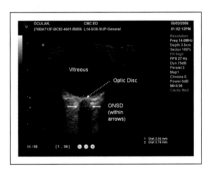

Figure 67.1 Ultrasound image showing the hyper echoic optic nerve sheath (arrows point to the outer margins of the ONS) and optic disc.

Reprinted with permission from: Tayal VS, Neulander M, Norton HJ, Foster T, Saunders T, Blaivas M. Emergency department sonographic measurement of optic nerve sheath diameter to detect findings of increased intracranial pressure in adult head injury patients. *Ann Emerg Med.* 2007;49(4):508–14.

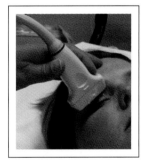

Figure 67.2 Positioning of the ultrasound probe during the measurement of ONSD. (Please note: this image does not show the presence of the sterile transparent dressing prior to the application of the ultrasound gel.)

Reprinted with permission from: Tayal VS, Neulander M, Norton HJ, Foster T, Saunders T, Blaivas M. Emergency department sonographic measurement of optic nerve sheath diameter to detect findings of increased intracranial pressure in adult head injury patients. *Ann Emerg Med.* 2007;49(4):508–14.

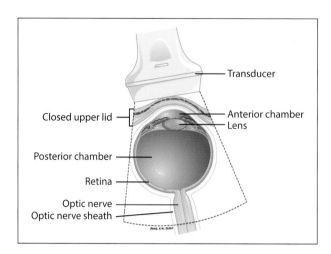

Figure 67.3 Diagram showing the optic nerve sheath anatomy with respect to the ultrasound probe position.
Reprinted with permission from: Tayal VS, Neulander M, Norton HJ, Foster T, Saunders T, Blaivas M. Emergency department sonographic measurement of optic nerve sheath diameter to detect findings of increased intracranial pressure in adult head injury patients. *Ann Emerg Med.* 2007;49(4):508–14.

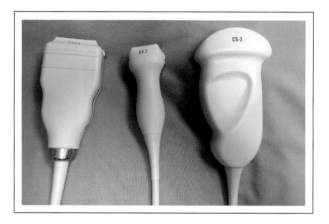

Figure 68.1 Three commonly used probes for point-of-care ultrasound in critically ill patients. From left to right, these are the high-frequency linear probe, the low frequency phased array probe and the low frequency curved array probe.

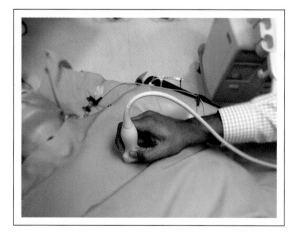

Figure 68.2 Ultrasound probe positioning for acquiring the parasternal long axis view of the heart. The marker is pointed towards the patient's right shoulder.

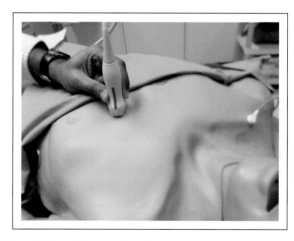

Figure 68.3 Ultrasound probe positioning for acquiring the parasternal short axis view of the heart. The marker is pointed towards the patient's left shoulder.

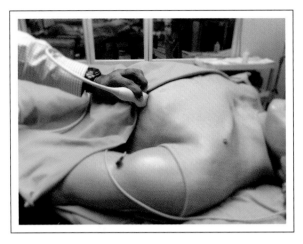

Figure 68.4 Ultrasound probe positioning for acquiring the apical four-chamber view of the heart. The marker is pointed towards the patient's left side.

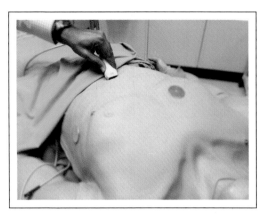

Figure 68.5 Ultrasound probe positioning for acquiring the subcostal four-chamber view of the heart. The marker is pointed towards the patient's left side. Notice that the probe is held from above, to allow for a flatter imaging angle.

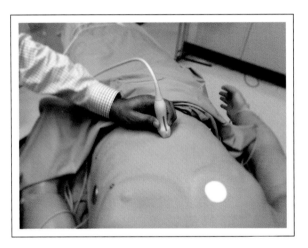

Figure 68.6 Ultrasound probe positioning for acquiring the subcostal view of the inferior vena cava. The marker is pointed towards the patient's head.

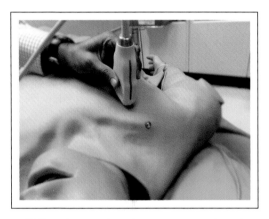

Figure 68.7 Ultrasound probe positioning for ultrasound evaluation of the lung. The probe is positioned in a cephalad-caudad direction, to allow for imaging of two ribs and the intercostal space in between. The examination should be repeated across multiple intercostal spaces bilaterally, including on the anterior and the lateral, and if possible, posterior chest walls.

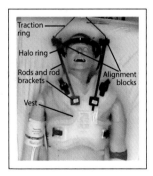

Figure 69.1 Halo Brace System. Halo system following application. Traction ring is optional component. Alignment blocks allow for adjusting alignment by loosening rods and adjusting flexion/extension of head as well as antero-posterior position as necessary.
Courtesy: Sheena M. Weaver.

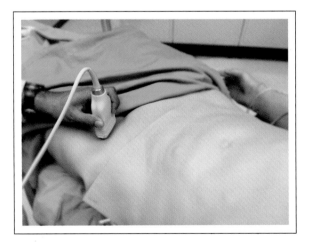

Figure 68.8 Ultrasound probe positioning for ultrasound evaluation of the common femoral vein.

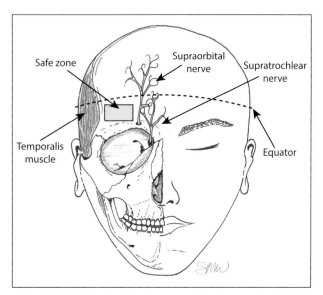

Figure 69.2 Anatomy of the safe zone.
Courtesy: Sheena M. Weaver.

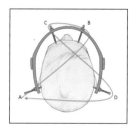

Figure 69.3 Crossed pin tightening pattern.
Courtesy: Sheena M. Weaver.

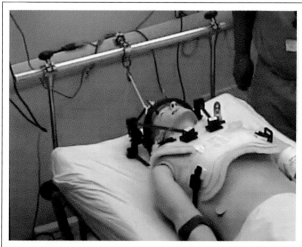

Figure 69.4 Halo with traction apparatus. Halo brace with traction setup. Leave rods in place, non-tightened such that the halo ring and cervical spine can reduce prior to rod placement. Tighten rods following reduction or achievement of desired alignment.
Courtesy: Sheena M. Weaver.

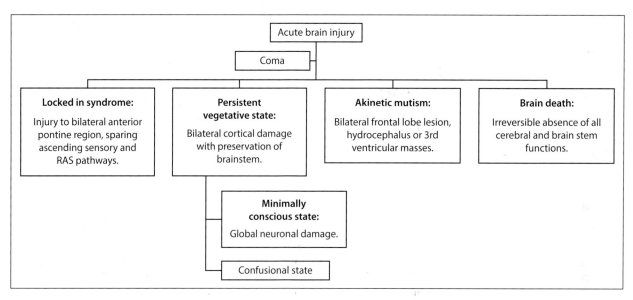

Figure 72.1 Clinical syndromes.

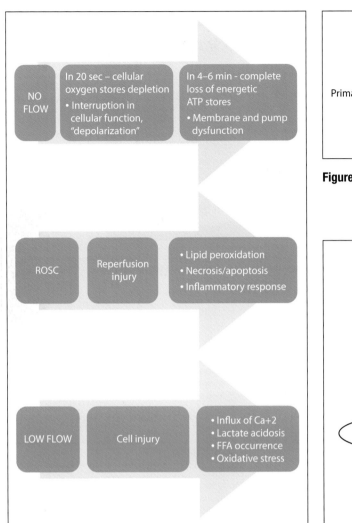

Figure 72.2 Neuropathology of HIE.

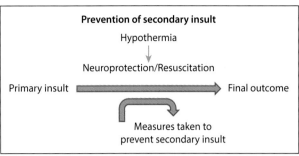

Figure 72.3 To prevent secondary insult.

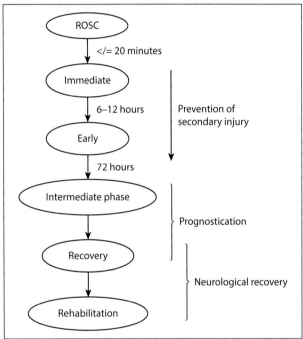

Figure 72.4 Phases of post-cardiac arrest syndrome.

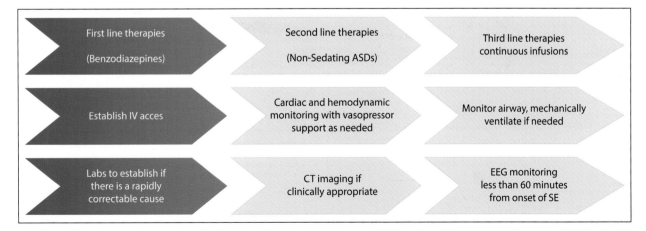

Figure 73.1 Diagram depicting the basic parallel components of care for a patient in SE.

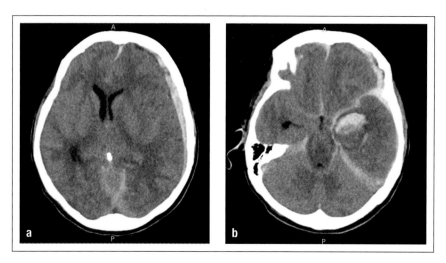

Figure 73.2 a-b Two axial CT images of the brain showing subarachnoid haemorrhage, a left temporal haemorrhage and a left subdural haematoma.

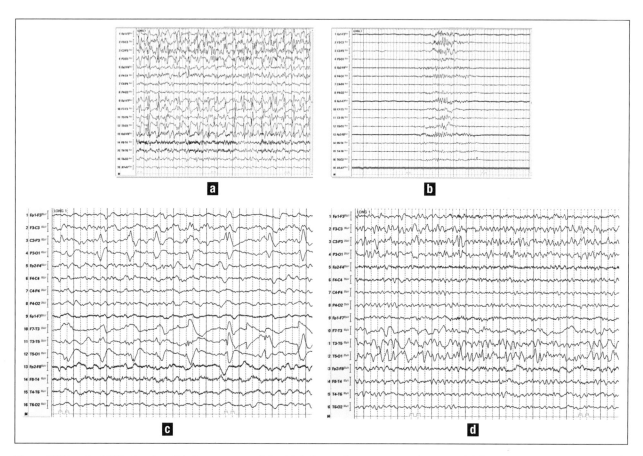

Figure 73.3 a-d EEG showing (A) the presence of focal left hemispheric status epilepticus, (B) burst-suppression pattern with about one burst every 10 seconds achieved while the patient was on IV midazolam, (C) an example of left-sided periodic discharges that became less frequent, and (D) final appearance of a near normal background pattern.

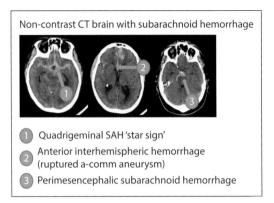

1. Quadrigeminal SAH 'star sign'
2. Anterior interhemispheric hemorrhage (ruptured a-comm aneurysm)
3. Perimesencephalic subarachnoid hemorrhage

Figure 74.1 Non-contrast CT scan demonstrating a SAH.

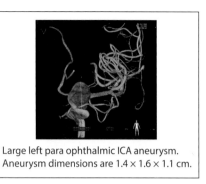

Large left para ophthalmic ICA aneurysm. Aneurysm dimensions are 1.4 × 1.6 × 1.1 cm.

Figure 74.2 3-reconstruction image from a digital subtraction cerebral angiogram demonstrating large left paraophthalmic aneurysm.

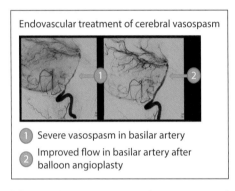

1. Severe vasospasm in basilar artery
2. Improved flow in basilar artery after balloon angioplasty

Figure 74.3 Cerebral angiogram with vasospasm in the basilar artery.

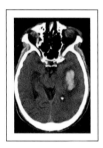

Figure 75.1 Left hemispheric intracerebral haemorrhage.

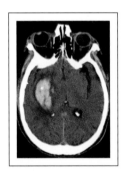

Figure 75.2 Cerebral angio CT scan showing the 'spot sign' within a right hemispheric intracerebral haemorrhage.

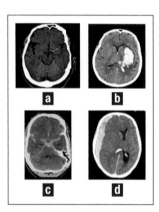

Figure 76.1 Aetiology of acute stroke in the middle cerebral artery territory.

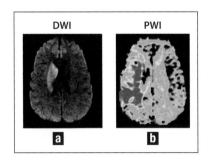

Figure 76.2 Acute stroke.
Courtesy: Parthiban Balasundaram.

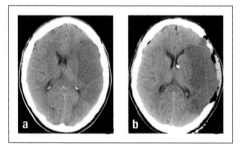

Figure 76.3 Malignant MCA infarction.
Courtesy: Parthiban Balasundaram.

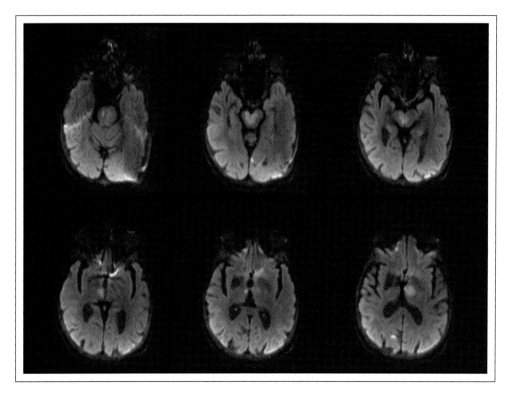

Figure 77.1 An MRI brain demonstrating restricted diffusion affecting thalami and large parts of the midbrain and pons.
Courtesy: Dr Xuemei Cai from Tufts University, Boston, USA.

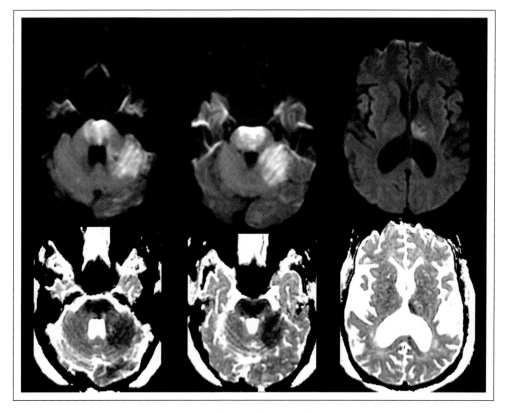

Figure 77.2 An MRI brain demonstrating restricted diffusion affecting thalami and large parts of the midbrain and pons.
Courtesy: Dr Xuemei Cai from Tufts University, Boston, USA.

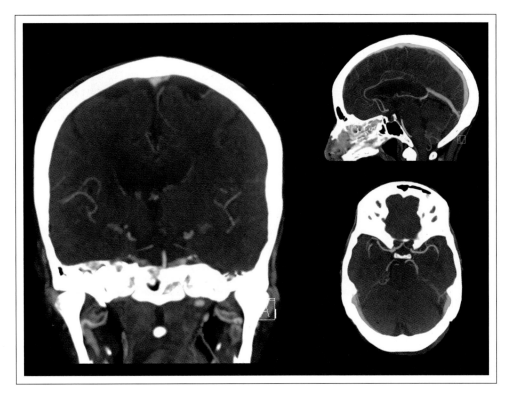

Figure 77.3 An emergent CT/CT-A of head and neck revealing a fully occlusive thrombus at the 'top of the basilar artery'.
Courtesy: Dr Xuemei Cai from Tufts University, Boston, USA.

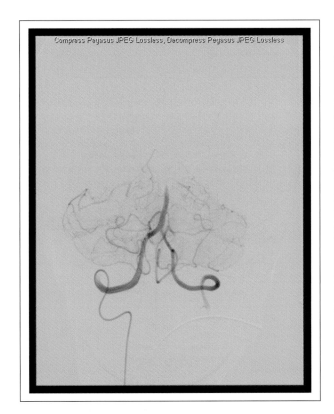

Figure 77.4 A CT-A revealing successful recanalization achieved within 4 hours from symptom onset.
Courtesy: Dr Xuemei Cai from Tufts University, Boston, USA.

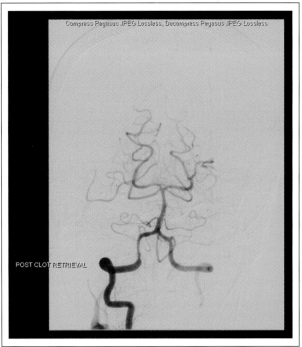

Figure 77.5 A CT-A revealing successful recanalization achieved within 4 hours from symptom onset.
Courtesy: Dr Xuemei Cai from Tufts University, Boston, USA.

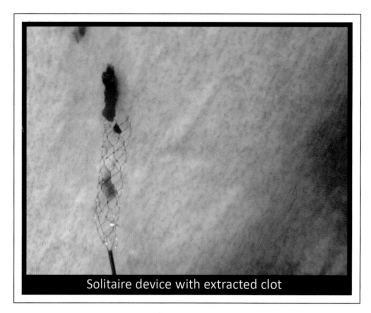

Figure 77.6 Endovascular treatment for clot retrieval, solitaire device with extracted clot.
Courtesy: Dr Xuemei Cai from Tufts University, Boston, USA.

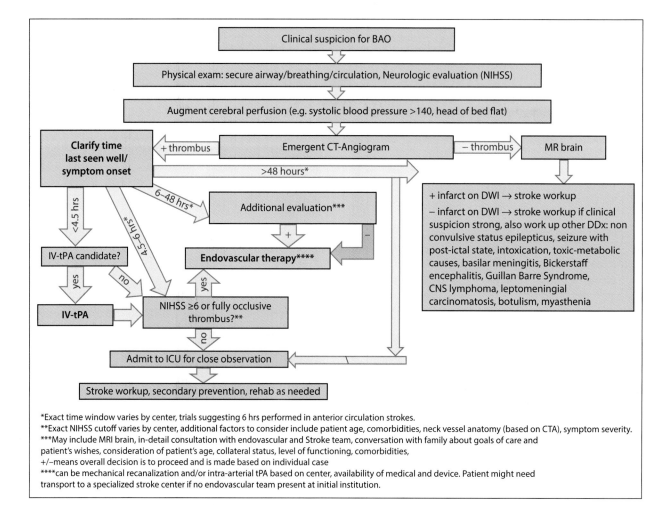

Figure 77.7 Suggested algorithm for approach in a patient with BAO.
Courtesy: Sarah Wahlster.

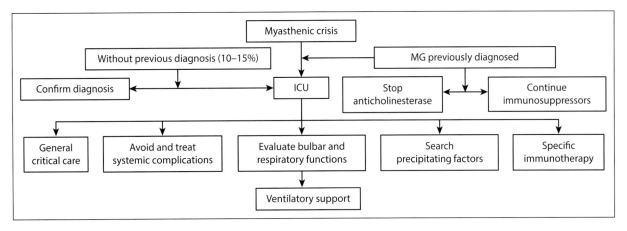

Figure 78.1 Algorithm for myasthenic crisis management.

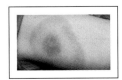

Figure 79.1 Distinctive rash of Lyme disease.

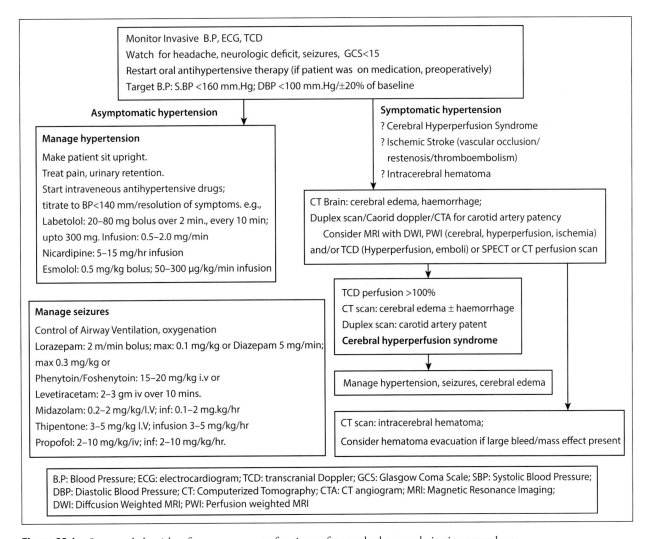

Figure 80.1 Suggested algorithm for management of patients after cerebral revascularization procedures.

Monitor Invasive BP, ECG, Heart Rate, Oxygen Saturation, TCD, Volume status, Urine output; ICP, CPP in high risk patients

Watch for headache, vomiting, seizures, neurologic deficit, GCS<15

Perform Check angiography (to confirm complete resection of AVM)

Maintain euvolemia

Start prophylactic antiepileptic therapy (e.g. phenytoin: loading dose-15–20 mg/kg, IV, over 30 minutes, followed by 100 mg IV, every 8 hours titrated to plasma level, for 7 days; or, Levetiracetam: loading dose- 1000 mg IV/orally; followed by 500 mg IV/orally, BID × 7 days) or restart therapy if patient already on antiepileptic medication

Start Antihypertensive therapy (if preoperatively on therapy and/or to maintain target

Maintain SBP slightly lower than baseline values, preferably between 90–110 mm.Hg/MAP- 70 mm.Hg.)

Features of intracranial hypertension

CT scan (haemorrhage, cerebral edema, cerebral hyperemia)

TCD: vasomotor paralysis

Cerebral angiography (AVM remnant; vasospasm, stagnation in feeder/draining vessels; delayed circulation)

MRI brain with DWI if CT scan is negative and cerebral infarction is suspected.

Cerebral Hyperperfusion Syndrome

Medical management: Control of hypertension, seizures, cerebral edema.

Surgical management: Emergent surgical evacuation of a large intracranial hematoma; Decompressive craniectomy.

Withdrawal of intensive measures guided by clinical signs of neurological recovery, BP, ICP, CPP, TCD monitoring.

BP: Blood Pressure; ECG: electrocardiogram; TCD: Transcranial Doppler Ultrasound; ICP: Intracranial pressure; CPP: Cerebral Perfusion Pressure; GCS: Glasgow Coma Scale; AVM: arteriovenous malformation; SBP: systolic blood pressure; MAP: mean arterial pressure; CT scan: Computerized Tomography; MRI: Magnetic Resonance Imaging; DWI: Diffusion weighted Imaging

Figure 80.2 Neurointensive care management of patients who have undergone obliteration of cerebral arteriovenous malformations.

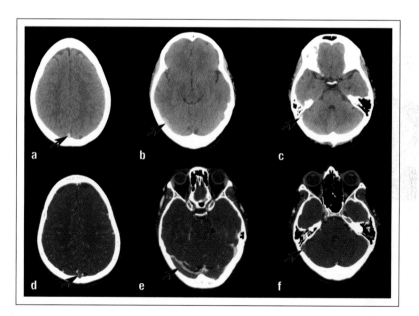

Figure 81.1 CT (A-C) and CTV (D-F) performed at the time of admission demonstrated thrombus (arrows) in the posterior superior sagittal sinus (A and D) extending through to the right transverse sinus (B and E) into the right sigmoid sinus (C and F) and proximal right internal jugular vein.

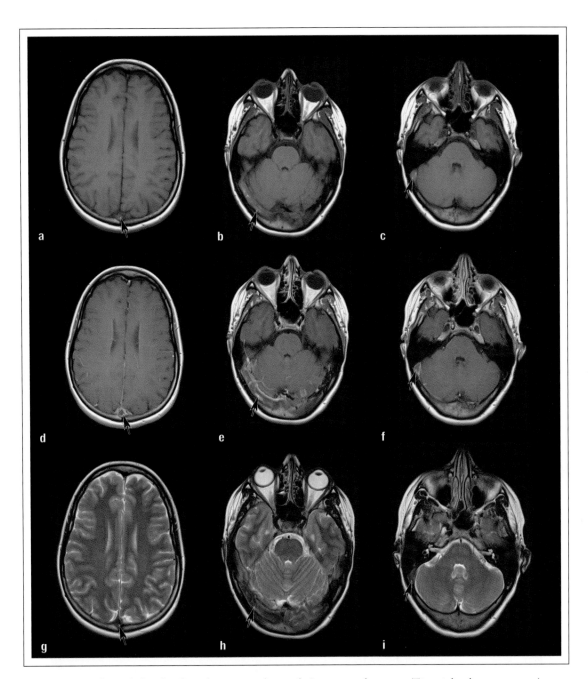

Figure 81.2 MRI performed shortly after admission to hospital. Sequences shown are T1-weighted pre-contrast (top row, a-c), T1-weighted post-contrast (middle row, d-f), and T2-weighted (bottom row, g-i). No mass lesions or other focal parenchymal lesions were identified. The images again show the extensive thrombus (arrows) in the posterior superior sagittal sinus (a, d and g), right transverse sinus (b, e and h) and right sigmoid sinus (c, f and i).

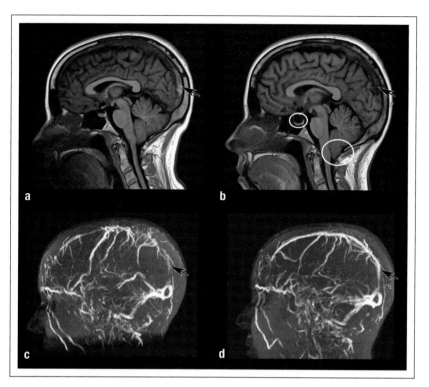

Figure 81.3 Sagittal T1-weighted MRI (top row) and MR venography time-of-flight (bottom row) performed shortly after admission to hospital (a and c) and 18 months later (b and d). The thrombus (seen as a hyperintensity on the T1-weighted MRI) in the posterior superior sagittal sinus (arrows, a and c) has significantly reduced in the interval between the two scans. Cerebellar tonsil descent (larger white ellipse), a partially empty sella (smaller white ellipse) and ectatic optic nerve sheaths on the scan performed at 18 months suggest the development of intracranial hypertension. On the MRV time-of-flight sequences, there is evidence of recanalization of the posterior superior sagittal sinus (arrows).

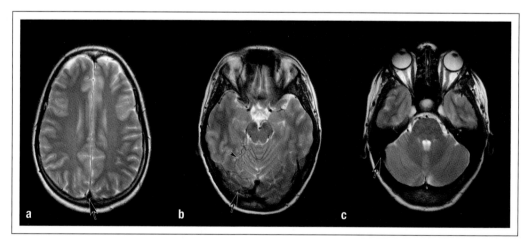

Figure 81.4 MR imaging performed 18 months following diagnosis. T2-weighted imaging (a and b) demonstrating recanalization (large arrows) of the posterior aspect of the SSS (a), right transverse sinus (b) and sigmoid sinus (c). In addition, prominent vessels (small arrow, b) overlying the right tentorium are visible and represent expanded collaterals relating to chronic thrombosis.

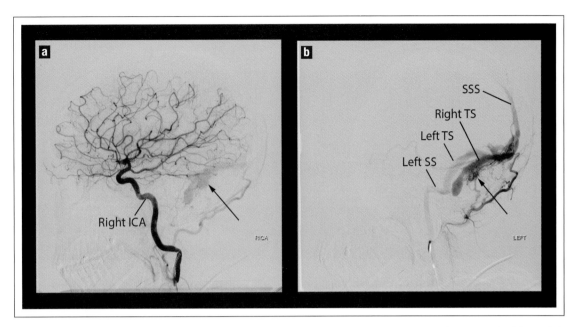

Figure 81.5 Digital subtraction angiography performed 18 months after the initial diagnosis of CVT. Early filling of the right transverse sinus due to a tentorial dural arteriovenous fistula (arrow) is demonstrated (a), along with occlusion of the right sigmoid sinus (b), which is consequently not visible (normally seen as a continuation of the right transverse sinus). Abbreviations: ICA, internal carotid artery; SS, sigmoid sinus; SSS, superior sagittal sinus; TS, transverse sinus.

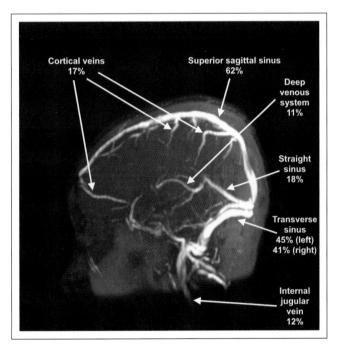

Figure 81.6 Labelled MRV head imaging showing the commonest sites for CVT within the cerebral venous system. Figures based on data from the ISCVT cohort. Percentages summate to more than 100% due to some patients having thrombus in multiple locations.

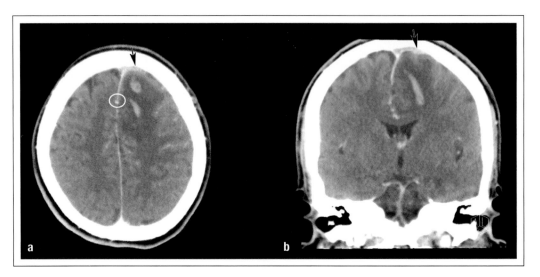

Figure 81.7 Post-contrast axial (a) and coronal (b) cranial CT imaging of a 44-year-old female with CVT. There is a large area of hypodensity in the left superior frontal lobe with parenchymal haemorrhage as well as frontal convexity subarachnoid blood (arrow). In addition, the anterior superior sagittal sinus and adjacent cortical veins appeared hyperdense (white ellipse), in keeping with CVT.

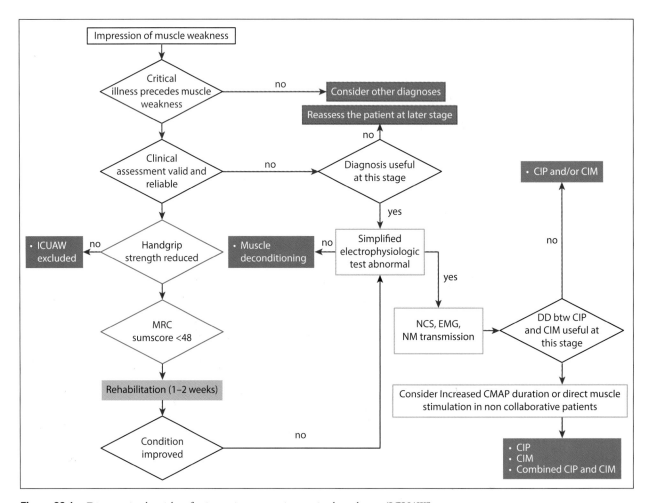

Figure 83.1 Diagnostic algorithm for intensive care unit-acquired weakness (ICUAW).

Reprinted with permission from: Latronico N, Gosselink R. A guided approach to diagnose severe muscle weakness in the intensive care unit. *Rev Bras TerIntensiva.* 2015;27(3):199–201, with permission from the Editor.

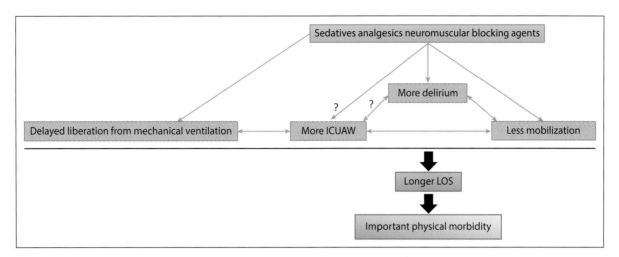

Figure 83.2 Relationship between ICU-acquired weakness (ICUAW), delirium and mobilization.
Reprinted with permission from: Latronico N, Herridge M, Hopkins RO, et al. The ICM research agenda on intensive care unit acquired weakness. *Intensive Care Med.* 2017. In press. With permission from the Editor. Springer.

Part VII

Respiratory Care

Editor: Edward Manno

Respiratory Care for Neurological Patients

E. M. Manno

ABSTRACT

Airway management and respiratory care for neurological patients require special skills and knowledge of the disease processes that lead to respiratory support. Loss of consciousness leads to loss of airway control and airway management depends upon the nature and location of the injury. Abnormal breathing patterns provide neurological localization and diagnostic information. Specific modes of ventilation can be tailored to specific neurological diseases. This chapter reviews these acute processes and the application of respiratory principles to acute neurological disease.

KEYWORDS

Airway management; acute neurological disease; abnormal respiratory patterns; respiratory care; airway management in neurological disease.

INTRODUCTION

A significant number of patients with neurological injury will require endotracheal intubation and mechanical ventilation. Patients with neurological injury who require mechanical ventilation have increased morbidity and mortality. Neurological injury requiring mechanical ventilation may occur secondary to a depressed level of consciousness or due to direct or indirect injury to the structures involving the processes of respiration and airway control. The neurological patient presents a unique set of challenges both for airway and respiratory management. Extubation of the neurological patient has similar challenges.

In this chapter we review the basics of airway management and mechanical ventilation with focus on specific neurological diseases and complications that affect these processes.

AIRWAY MANAGEMENT

Airway management of the neurological patient has specific challenges which may be based on the nature of the injury. Indications for intubation of the neurological patient are listed in Table 36.1. In general reasons for intubation

Table 36.1 Indications for intubation of the neurological patient

Immediate	Apnoea
	Airway obstruction
	Inability to tolerate bag mask ventilation
Urgent	GCS score <9
	Prevention of aspiration
	Oedema of larynx
	High cervical spine injury
Controlled	Hyperventilation for rapid intracranial pressure (ICP) control
	Lower cervical spine injury
	Pulmonary contusion
	Flail chest
	Congestive heart failure
	Aspiration
	Therapeutic or diagnostic procedures in the uncooperative patient
	High metabolic demand from work of breathing

Adapted from: Souter MJ, Manno EM. Ventilatory management and extubation criteria of the neurological/neurosurgical patient. *The Neurohospitalist* 2013;1:39–45.

in the neurological patient are based on aetiologies of loss of airway control. Patients with a depressed level of consciousness, oftentimes defined as a Glasgow Coma Scale score (GCS) of less than 8, traditionally have required endotracheal intubation. The rationale for this is that with a depressed level of consciousness, pharyngeal tone is lost and the patient is at high risk for aspiration. The National Trauma Databank reported an increase in aspiration pneumonia and worse outcomes in head trauma patients that were not immediately intubated.[1] Subsequent studies have supported this concept.[2,3]

Loss of pharyngeal tone produces a set of circumstances which can compromise airway patency. A depressed level of consciousness will lead to loss of control of the tongue which can occlude the pharynx when the patient is placed supine. This coupled with the effect of a hypotonic pharyngeal wall will result in a range of obstruction from sonorous breathing to complete occlusion of the airway. Nasal flaring and intercostal in-drawing of the thorax are objective findings that can be found under these conditions. Treatment is with manoeuvres that relieve the obstruction. This can include a jaw thrust which is performed by placing the fingers under the posterior aspect of the jaw and pulling forward. A tight fitting cervical collar can provide temporary benefit by lifting the jaw forward. Patient's however most likely will require some more permanent means of maintaining airway patency including endotracheal intubation or placement of the tracheostomy. In some circumstances a nasal or pharyngeal airway can be successful in relieving partial obstructions. Care must be taken in the placement of these devices to avoid damage to the soft tissues and teeth.[4]

Airway management of the patient with head and neck trauma require special considerations. Endotracheal intubation may occur in the case of severe head trauma for control of intracranial hypertension (IH). Under these circumstances hyperventilation leads to vasoconstriction of the small arteries and arterioles resulting in decreased cerebral blood flow (CBF), decreased cerebral blood volume (CBV) with subsequent lowering of overall CBV and intracranial pressure (ICP).

A significant proportion of trauma patients will have an unstable spine. Around 5%–10% of patients with moderate or severe head injury will have an unstable cervical spine and half of those will have sustained cord injury.[5] Endotracheal intubation in these patients require meticulous management of the airway. Direct laryngoscopy can be performed quickly but requires an additional individual to provide in-line manual stabilization of the head and neck. Similarly direct laryngoscopy in the setting of the cervical collar can impair the view of the larynx. Even with manual stimulation direct laryngoscopy can cause up to 3–5 mm of C5–C6 subluxation. Video laryngoscopy reduces but does not eliminate cervical subluxation. While video laryngoscopy can provide good views of the glottis, the tracheal tube cannot always be guided through the cords. Thus, the preferred method for endotracheal intubation in patients with possible cervical neck injury is fibreoptic intubation. This however requires an experienced operator and may delay intubation until the appropriate equipment is available.[4,5]

Specific medications may be required to optimize endotracheal intubation in the neurological patient. In general endotracheal intubation should occur quickly and efficiently using the least amount of sedation required to complete the procedure. Care should be taken to avoid sedative hypotension and the possibility of decreased cerebral perfusion during the procedure. Close monitoring of blood pressure and judicious use of short-acting vasopressors may be needed during intubation. Specific medications and their dosages for endotracheal intubation are listed in Table 36.2. Opiates are used to decrease the cough reflex and blunt the induced hypertensive response of laryngeal manipulation. They are sympatholytic and often result in a reduction in blood pressure. Propofol similarly can be used for induction but oftentimes can precipitate hypotension. Ketamine has less cardiovascular side effects but has been associated with increased ICP. The significance of this increase in ICP is unclear since documentation of decreased cerebral perfusion with the use of ketamine is lacking.[6] Benzodiazepines may help with muscle rigidity encountered in certain neurological conditions.

Etomidate has several advantages for use in endotracheal intubation of the neurological patient. It has minimal cardiovascular effects and does not increase ICP. It also has little effect on respiration and may allow the patient to breathe with supplemental oxygen rather than bag mask ventilation prior to endotracheal intubation. Etomidate has been associated with adrenal insufficiency and should only be used once during a hospitalization.

Paralytics are valuable in facilitating endotracheal intubation but will impair neurological assessment of the patient. In patients where frequent neurological assessments are critical, paralytics should be avoided if endotracheal intubation can be safely performed without their use. Succinylcholine is a short-acting depolarizing paralytic commonly used in endotracheal intubation. It is avoided in the immobilized patient, patients with

Table 36.2 Induction agents commonly used in intubation of the neurological patient

Drug	Dosing	Comments/Concerns
Sedatives		
Propofol	2.2.5 mg/kg	Short duration of action
Etomidate	0.3 mg/kg	Adrenal suppression, occasional fasciculations
Midazolam	0.3–0.35 mg/kg	Less hypotension, useful in muscle rigidity
Ketamine	0.5–1.5 mg/kg	Sympathomimetic, associated with hallucinations
Opiates		
Morphine	100–200 mcg/kg	Histamine release, hypotension, nausea
Fentanyl	2–5 mcg/kg	Muscle rigidity in high doses
Alfentanil	20–50 mcg/kg	Muscle rigidity in high doses
Paralytics		
Succinylcholine	1–1.5 mg/kg	Short acting, hyperkalaemia in states of immobilization or muscle damage
Rocuronium	0.6 mg/kg	Slower onset variable pharmacokinetics
Vecuronium	0.08–0.1 mg/kg	Hepatic metabolism
Cisatracurium	0.15–0.2 mg/kg	Eliminated by plasma esterases, safe in hepatic and renal failure

Adapted from: Souter MJ, Manno EM. Ventilatory management and extubation criteria of the neurological/neurosurgical patient. *The Neurohospitalist* 2013;1:39–45.

muscle injury, or the patient with recurrent seizures due to concerns of developing life-threatening hyperkalaemia.[4] The non-depolarizing paralytic agents do not have these concerns but will impair neurological assessment for a variable amount of time. In general, the shortest acting agents are preferred unless paralysis is being used to supplement the treatment of IH.

ABNORMAL BREATHING PATTERNS

Breathing is a coordinated effort involving multiple supratentorial and brainstem areas. A variety of respiratory patterns can develop in various metabolic and neurological injuries. Many can have diagnostic and localizing value. Recognition of these patterns can aid in the diagnosis and treatment of specific disorders.

The 'neurology of respiration' is complex and has been the subject of many historical manuscripts and texts.[7] An in-depth description of this process has been reviewed in a recent textbook and is beyond the scope of this chapter.[8] A basic understanding of the neuroanatomy involved and the respiratory patterns that develop with a variety of neurological injuries however is extremely valuable.

Respiration maintains normal oxygenation and acid-base balance. It is regulated by a group of neurons located in the pons and lower medulla. The generation of the respiratory rhythm probably originates from a group of neurons in the ventral lateral medulla that are labelled the ventral respiratory group (VRG). These neurons rhythmically fire through mechanisms that are ill-defined but are modulated by chemoreceptor inputs from the carotid bodies, mechanical receptors from the limbs, and neuronal input from the pons.[8,9] Pontine neurons labelled as the pneumotaxic centre influence the VRG through a polysynaptic connection that modulates the rhythm of the discharges originating from the VRG. This pneumotaxic centre receives inputs from the stretch receptors in the lung which are stimulated during inspiration.[10] The pneumotaxic centre and the VRG receive inputs from the forebrain and cerebellum. Forebrain input allows for behavioural control over respiration and cerebellar input influences the precision and regularity of respiration.[7]

Abnormalities in respiratory breathing patterns approximate but do not precisely correlate with the forebrain or brainstem areas that are affected. The classic description of these abnormal respiratory patterns is defined in Plum and Posner's text.[7] Post-hyperventilation apnoea and Cheyne–Stokes respiration are typically found in patients with bilateral forebrain damage or impairment. They are common to disease processes that directly or indirectly affect the bilateral hemispheres of the cerebral cortex. This respiratory pattern can be found in head trauma, bilateral cerebral infarctions, hypertensive encephalopathies, uraemia, metabolic and hepatic encephalopathies, general sedation or anaesthesia, or congestive heart failure (possibly due to hypoperfusion).[7,8]

Central neurogenic hyperventilation defined as sustained and deep hyperpnoea is a commonly encountered respiratory pattern in the intensive care unit (ICU). It is most often seen in pulmonary processes that stimulate the peripheral receptors in the lung. It is encountered in pneumonia, congestive heart failure and pleural-based pulmonary diseases. Similarly meningitis, hepatic coma, or subarachnoid blood can stimulate the respiratory centres directly. Certain medications such as salicylates have a similar effect. Central neurogenic hyperventilation secondary to primary neurological injury is exceedingly rare. Direct hypothalamic stimulation from tumours or haemorrhages can reproduce this respiratory pattern. Destructive lesions of the brainstem tegmentum in strokes has been reported to result in sustained hyperventilation.[7]

Ataxic breathing or irregular disordered respiration represents a functional disruption of the primary respiratory neuronal population.[7] Slowly expanding lesions in the posterior fossa which disrupt cerebellar input to these neurons will also lead to this respiratory pattern. More rapid expansion of cerebellar lesions leads to apnoea.

Apneustic or agonal respirations can be a terminal respiratory pattern. Direct respiratory cramps at the end of respiration is encountered with medullary infarcts, tumours, or haemorrhages. It is commonly seen with basilar artery occlusions.

Respiratory patterns can also be affected by spinal cord injury and breathing patterns may reflect the level of injury. The most common cervical injury in spinal cord trauma occurs at the level of C5–C6.[11] Patients with injury to the spinal cord at that level can have a variable level of preserved phrenic nerve and subsequent diaphragmatic function. Patients however will lose intercostal and abdominal muscle use. The resultant respiratory pattern is one without abdominal paradox. Under these circumstances the chest will involute in with inspiration. Patients will breathe best when placed supine with this level of injury. Contrary to this level of injury, higher cervical injuries result in loss of phrenic nerve function. This is an unstable respiratory situation where patients can only use their scalene and accessory muscles for inspiration. Patients will need immediate endotracheal intubation.[12]

MODES OF MECHANICAL VENTILATION

The 'traditional' modes of mechanical ventilation have employed the use of a set volume of lung inflation combined with a set rate of ventilation to deliver a required minute volume of ventilation. In assist-control ventilation each 'triggered' ventilator effort of the patient results in a delivered set volume of inflation. Thus, the minute volume is determined by the respiratory rate of the patient.[13] As each respiration has a set delivered volume of inflation, this mode of ventilation is consider a means of full ventilator support designed to decrease the overall work of breathing.

Intermittent mandatory volume ventilation delivers a set volume of inflation at a set respiratory rate. Thus, the patient over a minute has a mandated minute ventilation delivered by the ventilator. The patient can breathe over the set rate but these breaths will not initiate the set volume of inflation. Since the inherent patients' respiratory rate may not be aligned with the ventilator set rate, a 'synchronized' form of intermittent mandatory ventilation was developed to deliver an inflation volume only at the onset of inspiration.

Volume ventilation has fallen into relative disfavour secondary to concerns of ventilator-induced lung injury from over-distention of lung alveoli.[14]

Pressure control ventilation initiates insufflation until a preset lung pressure is attained. Over-distention injury can be avoided but lung volumes are variable and blood gases need to be followed closely to ensure adequate oxygenation and acid-base balance. A potential disadvantage of this ventilator mode is oftentimes sedation and paralysis are required to maintain treatment. This is required in order to achieve the needed inspiratory time to expiratory time ratio required to make this mode of ventilation effective for gas exchange. This may limit its usefulness in the neurological patient that requires close neurological monitoring.

Pressure support ventilation is a mode of ventilation where the patient breathes spontaneously. In this mode each breath is augmented by a set pressure. For neurological patients without an acute pulmonary process, this may be a mode of choice since it is well-tolerated and may not require significant sedation. It also allows evaluation of the patient's respiratory pattern. Most ventilators however will not allow the patient to display a Cheyne–Stokes respiratory pattern if the apnoea period is prolonged. Under these circumstances, the ventilator will default to an intermittent mandatory volume mode of ventilation.

Newer ventilator modes of mechanical ventilation have been developed in an attempt to remedy some of the potential limitations of traditional modes of ventilation. Dual control modes are modes of ventilation that allow variations in pressure augmentation to provide a set tidal or minute volume. Pressure augmentation can occur within each breath to ensure a specific tidal volume or between breaths to ensure a set minute volume.[15]

Airway pressure release ventilation or bi-level ventilation is a ventilator mode where a high and low pressure is set and ventilation occurs when pressure is released from the higher set pressure. This mode has gained some popularity since it has some degree of inherent positive pressure associated at all times thus maximizing oxygenation while being comfortable for respiration. Proportional assist ventilation and proportional pressure support are mechanical modes of ventilation where the ventilator generates pressure in proportion to the patients' effort.[15]

Neurally adjusted ventilator-assisted modes of ventilation utilizes an electrical oesophageal probe to measure diaphragmatic contractility to titrate ventilatory flow rates.[16] These modes of ventilation have been reported to improve ventilator synchrony. The utility of these modes of ventilation in patients with neurological injury has not been studied.

ACUTE RESPIRATORY DISTRESS SYNDROME

Acute respiratory distress syndrome (ARDS) is a term used to describe an acute inflammatory condition of the alveolar-capillary membrane that leads to increased alveolar permeability and subsequent interstitial oedema.[17] The syndrome varies from congestive heart failure since the condition occurs in the absence of high pulmonary wedge pressures. The aetiology of this condition is unclear but is believed to be initiated through a systemic activation of neutrophils which adhere to the vascular endothelium of the pulmonary capillaries.[18] Predisposing factors to the development of this syndrome involve any process that activates a systemic inflammatory response. In the neurological patient this can be isolated or can be due to multisystem trauma, sepsis, aspiration, transfusion syndromes, or subarachnoid haemorrhage. Diagnostic criteria include acute onset, the presence of a predisposing condition, bilateral infiltrates on chest X-ray, pressure of arterial oxygen (PaO_2)/Fraction of inspired oxygen (FiO_2) <200 mmHg, and a pulmonary artery occlusion pressure <18 mmHg.[19] More recently an update of this definition stratified the severity of ARDS based on the PaO_2/FiO_2 ratio.[20]

Mortality of this condition remains high with reported mortalities of >40% in moderate and severe cases.[21–23]

No specific treatment outside of the use of lower tidal volumes has been proven useful in this process. The technique of using low tidal ventilation (4–8 ml/kg) is designed to prevent further volume-induced trauma to an already compromised pulmonary endothelium.[14,24] Interventions that may provide some survival benefits include the uses of higher levels of positive end expiratory pressure (PEEP), use of neuromuscular blockade, and decreases in driving pressures.[25,26] The use of steroids has been controversial and remains unproven. Similarly, prone positioning has shown improvements in oxygenation and appears promising but definitive improvements in mortality have been lacking.[27] More recently the use of extracorporeal life support has been utilized for this condition and awaits the results of an ongoing randomized trial.[28]

VENTILATOR-ASSOCIATED PNEUMONIA

Ventilator-associated pneumonia (VAP) is a complication of prolonged endotracheal intubation. The associated mortality remains high up to 40%.[29,30] Ventilator-associated pneumonia has gained considerable attention because of significantly greater hospital length of stay and increased associated hospital costs. The increased prevalence of multidrug resistant organisms has made the diagnosis and treatment increasingly important.[31] Early diagnosis is important since delays in treatment lead to increased mortality however, inappropriate initial antimicrobial therapy has similarly been associated with excess mortality in patients with VAP.[32,33]

Risk factors for VAP include the duration of hospitalization, recent antibiotic exposure, and duration of endotracheal intubation. Patients at risk for developing antibiotic-resistant bacteria include patients from a long-term acute care facility, those with recent hospitalizations, immunosuppressed patients, patients on haemodialysis, and patients receiving gastric acid suppression.[30,34] Early onset VAP defined within the first 4–5 days of mechanical ventilation was initially thought to be caused by more antibiotic susceptible organisms. More recent evidence however suggested that this may not actually occur.[35]

The diagnosis for VAP is difficult since many non-infectious conditions can mimic VAP. More stringent diagnostic criteria increase specificity but lack the sensitivity needed to make an early diagnosis. Most clinicians use the finding of a new or progressive radiographic infiltrate and at least one clinical feature of pneumonia including fever, leukocytosis, worsening oxygenation, or an increase in pulmonary tracheal secretions.[36] The lack of diagnostic certainty has led to the categorization of ventilator associated events versus the terminology of VAP.

Traditional methods of obtaining respiratory cultures have significant limitations. Contamination and colonization is common. Bronchial samples obtained with traditional bronchoscopy or through minimally invasive techniques are better suited for culturing than traditional tracheal aspirations. Newer microbial techniques are gaining increasing applicability including nucleic acid amplification tests and proteonomic technologies. Multiplex automated digital microscopic evaluation of bacterial volatile organic compounds is currently being evaluated.[30]

Timely and appropriate administration of antibiotics is crucial towards treating VAP. Delaying therapy even by a few hours is associated with increased mortality.[33] Beta-lactam and carbapenem antibiotics remain the mainstay of treatment, however, appropriate dosing must be given to ensure optimal antimicrobial exposure. Early and appropriate therapy may obviate the need for extensive courses of treatment. Newer data supports antimicrobial treatment for 7–8 days.[37] The exception being difficult to treat *Pseudomonas aeruginosa* infection and other non-fermenters as they can experience higher rates of recurrence with shorter treatment regimens.[38]

NEUROGENIC PULMONARY OEDEMA

Neurogenic pulmonary oedema is a condition of acute pulmonary oedema that occurs in the setting of massive sympathetic discharge. It has been reported in animal studies with acute increases in intracranial pressure and is found in disease processes with similar increases in intracranial pressure.[39] These include changes in intracranial pressure secondary to head trauma, subarachnoid haemorrhage, intracerebral haemorrhage, or any acute intracranial process that raises intracranial pressure.

The proposed mechanisms include sympathetically mediated endothelial damage. This occurs secondary to activation of the contractile myofibril elements of the endothelium leading to endothelial leakage of proteinaceous fluid into the pulmonary interstitium. This is exacerbated by pulmonary veno-constriction leading to an abrupt but transient increase in pulmonary pressures.[40]

The diagnosis is typically not difficult in the setting of an acute neurological catastrophe. Pulmonary fluid is typically exudative secondary to endothelial damage. This however can be complicated by myocardial stunning which often occurs with pulmonary endothelial damage.[41]

Treatment includes diuresis and evaluation of cardiac functioning. In the event of cardiac stunning vasopressors improving cardiac index are preferred to avoid hypotension and worsening pulmonary oedema. Fortunately, this diagnosis is self-limited and can improve rapidly.

PULMONARY EMBOLI

Pulmonary emboli are common in both neurological and neurosurgical populations. Estimates of deep venous thrombosis range from 30%–40% in postoperative neurosurgical patients.[42] Immobilization and paralysis in many patients with neurological injury predispose this population to embolic complications. Anticoagulation remains the mainstay of treatment; however, recent neurosurgery or head trauma may preclude the use of anticoagulation. In these situations vena cava filters are preferred. External pneumatic compression devices should be used in all patients when possible. The current recommendation for prophylactic mini dose heparin or other heparinoids is increasingly advocated within a shorter time period of neurological insult.[43]

PULMONARY COMPLICATIONS IN NEUROLOGICAL DISEASE

Mechanical ventilation is required for a number of acute neurological conditions. Complicated neurosurgical procedures may require extended periods of mechanical ventilation. Similarly, spinal cord trauma and head injury may require prolonged periods of immobilization and ventilation. Mechanical ventilation however in acute neurological processes portend a worse outcome than those not requiring mechanical ventilation. Mortality rates as high as 75% have been reported for ischaemic strokes and intracerebral haemorrhages that require mechanical ventilation.[44]

Pulmonary complication rates have been reported at 10% for ischaemic strokes and close to a third of patients with intracerebral haemorrhage. The most common complication for intracerebral haemorrhages have been reported to be pneumonia, either aspiration- or ventilator-associated and pulmonary oedema. Interestingly, the rates of pulmonary emboli and development of ARDS are not as pervasive in these disease processes. Pulmonary complications are more common in patients with lower GCS and portend a longer length of stay and worse outcomes in these populations.[45]

WEANING AND EXTUBATION OF NEUROLOGICAL PATIENTS

Many neurological patients in an intensive care setting remain intubated for primarily maintenance of airway patency or for a depressed level of consciousness. Traditionally, neurological patients have remained intubated until they reach some ill-defined level of consciousness. However, one prospective study of brain injured patients found that delaying extubation based solely on a patients' level of consciousness led to an increase in pulmonary complications, increased length of stay, and worse outcomes.[46] A prospective randomized pilot trial of early extubation has been performed.[47] A funded trial examining early versus late extubation in this patient population has recently been done.

Early evidence suggests that if airway control of secretions can be maintained, early extubation may be preferable.

CONCLUSIONS

The management of airway disorders is complex in neurologically ill patients. For proper respiratory care, special skills and knowledge of the disease process are imperative. Certain respiratory signs and symptoms are suggestive of underlying neurological condition and are diagnostic in nature. Therefore, it is of utmost importance to thoroughly understand respiratory principles and its application in acute neurological conditions.

REFERENCES

1. Marshall LF, Becker DP, Bowers SA, et al. The national traumatic coma databank. Part 1: Design, purpose, goals and results. *J Neurosurg* 1983;59:276–84.

2. Holly LT, Kelly DF, Counelis GJ, Blinman T, McArthur DL, Cryer HG. Cervical spine trauma associated with moderate and severe head injury: Incidents, risk factors, and injury characteristics. *J Neurosurg* 2002;96:285–91.

3. Holland MC, Mackersie RC, Morabito D, et al. The development of acute lung injury is associated with worse neurological outcome in patients with severe brain injury. *J Trauma* 2003;55:106–111.

4. Souter MJ, Manno EM. Ventilatory management and extubation criteria of the neurological/neurosurgical patient. *The Neurohospitalist* 2013;1:39–45.

5. Wetsch WA, Carlistcheck M, Spelten O, et al. Success rates and endotracheal tube insertion times of experienced emergency physicians using 5 video laryngoscopes: A randomized trial in a simulated trapped car accident victim. *Eur J Anaesthesiol* 2011;28:849–58.

6. Himmelseher S, Durieux ME. Revising a dogma: ketamine for patients with neurological injury? *Anesth Analg* 2005; 101:524–34.

7. Plum F, Posner JB. The pathologic physiology of signs and symptoms of coma. In: Plum F, Posner JB, editors. *The Diagnosis of Stupor and Coma*. 3rd ed. Philadelphia: F. A. Davis Co, 1982; pp. 1–73.

8. Bolton CF, Chen R, Wijdicks EFM, Zifko UA. Anatomy and physiology of the nervous system control of respiration. In: *Neurology of Breathing*. Philadelphia: Butterworth/Heinemann, 2004; pp. 19–35.

9. Richter DW, Ballanyi K, Ramirez JM. Respiratory rhythm generation. In: Miller AD, Bianchi AL, Bishop BP, eds. *Neural Control of the Respiratory Muscles*. New York: CRC Press, 1997; pp. 119–30.

10. St. John WM. Neurogenesis of patterns of automatic ventilator activity. *Prog Neurobiol* 1998;56:97–117.

11. Chen-Gadol AA, Pichelman MA, Manno EM. Management of head trauma and spinal cord injury in adults. In: *Neurological Therapeutics: Principles and Practice*. UK, London: Noseworthy JH Martin Dunitz, 2003;1221–37.

12. Luce JM, Tyler ML, Pierson DJ. *Intensive Respiratory Care*. Philadelphia: Saunders, 1984; pp. 67–69.

13. Marino PL. Modes of Assisted Ventilation. In: Marino PL ed. *The ICU Book*, 3rd ed. Philadelphia: Lippincott Williams and Wilkins, 2007: pp. 473–89.

14. The Acute Respiratory Distress Syndrome Network. Ventilation with lower tidal volumes as compared with traditional tidal volumes for acute lung injury and the acute respiratory distress syndrome. *N Engl J Med* 2000; 342:1301–8.

15. Samtanilla JI, Daniel B, Mei-Ean Y. Mechanical Ventilation. *Emerg Med Clin N Am* 2008;26:849–62.

16. Sinderby C, Beck J. Proportional assist ventilation and neutrally adjusted ventilator assist-better approaches to ventilator synchrony? *Clin Chest Med* 2008;29:329–42.

17. Villar J. What is the acute respiratory distress syndrome? *Respir Care* 2011;56:1539–45.

18. Abraham E. Neutrophils and acute lung injury. *Crit Care Med* 2003;31 (suppl):S195–S199.

19. Bernard GR, Artigas A, Brigham KL, et al. The American-European Consensus Conference on ARDS. *Am J Respir Crit Care Med* 1994;149:818–24.

20. Ranieri VM, Rubenfeld GD, Thompson BT, et al. Acute respiratory distress syndrome: the Berlin definition. *JAMA* 2012;307:2526–33.

21. Villar J, Blanco J, Kacmarek RM. Current incidence and outcome of the acute respiratory distress syndrome. *Curr Opin Crit Care* 2016;22:1–6.

22. Caser EB, Zandonade E, Pereira E, at el. Impact of distinct definitions of acute lung injury on its incidence and outcome in Brazilian ICUs: a prospective evaluation of 7133 patients. *Crit Care Med* 2014;42:574–82.

23. Phua J, Badia JR, Adhikari NKJ, et al. Has mortality from acute respiratory distress syndrome decreased over time? *Am J Respir Crit Care Med* 2014;42:574–82.

24. Dreyfuss D, Saumon G. Ventilator induced lung injury. *Am J Respir Crit Care Med* 1998;157:294–323.

25. Briel M, Meade M, Mercat A, et al. Higher vs lower positive end expiratory pressure in patients with acute lung injury and acute respiratory distress syndrome: systemic review and meta-analysis. *JAMA* 2010;303:865–73.

26. Papazian L, Forel JM, Gacouin A, et al. Neuromuscular blockers in early acute respiratory distress syndrome. *N Engl J Med* 2010;363:1107–116.

27. Guerin C, Reignier J, Richard JC, et al. Prone positioning in severe acute respiratory syndrome. *N Engl J Med* 2013; 368:2159–68.

28. Leligdowicz A, Fan E. Extracorporeal life support for severe acute respiratory distress syndrome. *Curr Opin Crit Care* 2015;21:13–19.

29. Bekaert M, Tinsit J-F, Vansteelsndt S, et al. Attributable mortality of ventilator associated pneumonia: A reappraisal using causal analysis. *Am J Respir Crit Care* 2011;184: 1133–9.

30. Guillamet CV, Kollef MH. Update on ventilator associated pneumonia. *Curr Opin Crit Care* 2015;21:430–8.

31. Magiorakos A-P, Srinivasan A, Carey RB, et al. Multidrug-resistant extensively drug-resistant Hennepin drug resistant bacteria: An international expert proposal for interim standard definitions for acquired resistance. *Clin Microbiol Infect*, Office of Publ Eur Soc Clin Microbiol Infect Dis. 2012;18:268–81.

32. Kumar A, Roberts D, Wood KE, et al. Duration of hypotension before initiation of effective antimicrobial therapy is to critical determinate of survival and human septic shock. *Crit Care Med* 2006;34:1589–96.

33. Ferrer R, Martin-Loeches I, Phillips G, et al. Empiric antibiotic treatment reduces mortality and severe sepsis and septic shock from the first hour: Results from a guideline based performance improvement program. *Crit Care Med* 2014;42:1749–55.

34. Koulenti D, Lisboa T, Brun-Buisson C, et al. Spectrum of practice in the diagnosis of nosocomial pneumonia in patients requiring mechanical ventilation and European intensive care units. *Crit Care Med* 2009;37:2360–8.

35. Restrepo MI, Peterson J, Fernandez JF, et al. Comparison of the bacterial etiology of early onset and late onset ventilator associated pneumonia and subjects enrolled into large clinical studies. *Respir Care* 2013;58: 1220–5.

36. American Thoracic Society, Infectious Diseases Society of America. Guidelines for the management of adults with hospital-acquired ventilator associated and healthcare associated pneumonia. *Am J Respir Crit Care Med* 2005; 171:388–416.

37. Dimopoulos G, Poulakou G, Pneumatikos IA, et al. Short versus long duration antibiotic regimens for ventilator associated pneumonia: Systematic review and meta-analysis. *Chest* 2013;144:1759–67.

38. Chastre J, Wolff M, Fagon J-Y, et al. Comparison of 8 versus 15 days of antibiotic therapy for ventilator associated pneumonia and adults: Randomized trial. *JAMA* 2003;90:2588–98.

39. Shivalkar B, Van Loon J, Wieland W, et al. Variable effects of explosive or gradual increase of intracranial pressure on myocardial structure and function. *Circulation* 1993;87:230–9.

40. Malik AB. Mechanisms of neurogenic pulmonary edema. *Circulation Research* 1985;57:1–18.

41. Gajic O, Manno EM. Neurogenic pulmonary edema: another multiple hit model of acute lung injury. *Crit Care Med* 2007;35:1979–80.

42. Swann KW, Black PM. Deep venous thrombosis and pulmonary emboli in neurosurgical patients: a review. *J Neurosurg* 1984;61:1055–62.

43. Hemphill JC, Greenberg SM, Anderson CS, et al. Guidelines for the management of spontaneous intracerebral hemorrhage. *Stroke* 2015;46:2032–60.

44. Gujjar AR, Deibert E, Manno EM, et al. Mechanical ventilation for ischemic stroke and intracerebral hemorrhage: indications, timing, and outcome. *Neurology* 1998;51:447–51.

45. Maramattom BV, Weigand S, Reinalda M, et al. Pulmonary complications after intracerebral hemorrhage. *Neurocritical Care* 2006;5:115–19.

46. Coplin WM, Pierson DJ, Cooley KD, et al. Implications of extubation delay in brain injured patients meeting standard weaning criteria. *Am J Respir Crit Care Med* 2000;161:1530–6.

47. Manno EM, Rabinstein AA, Wijdicks EFM, et al. A prospective trial of elective extubation in brain injured patients meeting extubation criteria for ventilatory support: a feasibility study. *Crit Care* 2008;12:R138.

Part VIII

Cardiovascular Care

Editor: Manee Raksakietisak

37

Cardiovascular Care for Neurological Patients

M. Raksakietisak

ABSTRACT

The cardiovascular care includes early detection and prompt management of cardiovascular problems to diminish serious consequences. There are three different cardiovascular problems commonly associated with neurological conditions discussed in the subsequent section, including but not limiting to hypertension, hypotension, and arrhythmias. Apart from this, cardiac arrest also manifests with numerous neurological disorders. The hypertensive response to high intracranial pressure (ICP) is the modulating factor. Subarachnoid haemorrhage (SAH), traumatic brain injury (TBI), and stroke need tight control of blood pressure (BP). The neurogenic stunned myocardium (NSM), spinal shock, sepsis, and others can cause hypotension. While treating the causes, supportive care like fluid therapy, inotropes, and/or vasopressors should be given immediately to provide adequate cerebral perfusion pressure (CPP).

Neurogenic stunned myocardium, neuromuscular diseases, spinal injury, epilepsy, and strokes are associated with arrhythmias. The treatment is the shared responsibility of critical care physicians and cardiologists.

Brain herniation and non-neurological problems can contribute to cardiac arrest. The reversible causes need to be identified and treated for successful resuscitation.

The post-cardiac-arrest care includes treatment of the precipitating causes and supportive care. The target temperature management (32°C–36°C) is recommended at least for 24 hours.

KEYWORDS

Hypertension; cardiovascular care; haemodynamics; hypotension; neurogenic stunned myocardium (NSM); arrhythmias; cardiac arrest; post-cardiac-arrest care; targeted temperature management (TTM).

INTRODUCTION

Brain injury from either trauma, surgery, or diseases can result in several systemic organ dysfunctions. Among different organ dysfunctions, the cardiovascular system is commonly affected and ensuing consequences such as unstable haemodynamics (hypertension or hypotension), dysrhythmia or arrhythmias (benign or significant), stunned myocardium, or even cardiac arrest are frequently encountered by intensivists. These cardiovascular abnormalities undoubtedly relate to poor outcome. Early detection and prompt management is crucial to diminish these complications.

HYPERTENSION

Hypertension is one of the most common conditions seen in the general population and also in neurointensive care patients and leads to myocardial infarction, left ventricular failure, haemorrhagic stroke or intracerebral haemorrhage (ICH), renal failure, and death if it is not detected early and treated appropriately.[1–3]

Causes of Hypertension

There are several causes of hypertension in neurointensive care patients. They are neurological and non-neurological causes. Among a constellation of causes, the common neurological causes are postoperative pain, delirium, increased intracranial pressure (ICP), and paroxysmal sympathetic hyperactivity (PSH).

Some can be easily treated and there is no need for antihypertensive drugs. After excluding other causes, essential hypertension should be treated with antihypertensive drug(s) (Table 37.1).[1–3]

Symptoms and Signs

Most patients admitted to the neurointensive care usually are asymptomatic but patients may develop headache, visual disturbance, restlessness, or even chest pain suggestive of hypertension. In the intensive care unit (ICU), hourly or continuous intra-arterial blood pressure (BP) monitoring (invasive BP monitoring) is routinely performed in order to detect BP alterations.[1–3]

Management

As far as management is concerned, the treatable causes should be corrected. The increased ICP is associated with vomiting, visual disturbance, dilated pupil, restlessness, and so on. Emergency imaging may be

required to diagnose the cause(s) of increased ICP. The hypertensive response to high ICP or Cushing reflex (hypertension and bradycardia) is the modulating factor unlike the cathecholamine release stimulated by the central nervous system (tachycardia and hypertension).[1–3]

The important but conflicting issues are the level of blood pressure that requires treatment and the level to which blood pressure should be lowered and there are no absolute conclusions. In neurocritical care, one situation differs from the other. For example, hypertension caused by raised ICP differs from hypertension from subarachnoid haemorrhage (SAH) or post-craniotomy. There are several neurological conditions that need special care during meticulous management of hypertension.

Subarachnoid Haemorrhage

Blood pressure management in SAH is challenging and differs from time to time, e.g., before or after treatment of cerebral aneurysm or after cerebral vasospasm. Before definite treatment either with a surgical clip or radiological coiling of the aneurysm, the systolic blood pressure (SBP) should be kept below 140 mmHg for fear of aneurysmal rupture. After treatment, BP should be kept higher for

Table 37.1 Organs, causes and treatment of hypertension in critically ill patients

Organ	Causes	Treatment
CVS	Discontinuation of antihypertensive drugs Essential (primary) hypertension Administration of vasopressor drugs	Resume medication Antihypertensive drugs Stop vasopressor drugs
CNS	Pain (most common after surgery) Delirium Paroxysmal sympathetic hyperactivity (PSH) Increased intracranial pressure (ICP) Withdrawal symptoms	Analgesic drug Sedatives Antihypertensive drugs (β blocker) Lowering ICP Sedatives
Renal	Bladder distention Fluid overload Renal failure	Bladder catheterization Diuretic drug Antihypertensive drugs
Respiratory	Hypoxaemia/hypercarbia	Oxygen therapy/mechanical ventilation
Endocrine/Metabolic	Hypoglycaemia Intoxication Steroid administration Cushing syndrome	Check blood glucose Check for substance abuse Antihypertensive drugs Antihypertensive drugs
Drug-induced hypertension	Erythropoietin, NSAIDs, phenethylamines, steroids, tyrosine kinase inhibitors, hormonal contraceptives, etc.	Consider using the alternative drugs Antihypertensive drugs

Sources: (1) Salgado DR, Silva E, Vincent JL. Control of hypertension in the critically ill: a pathophysiological approach. *Ann Intensive Care* 2013;3(1):17. (2) Zaidi G, Chichra A, Weitzen M, Narasimhan M. Blood pressure control in neurological ICU patients: What is too high and what is too low? *Open Crit Care Med J* 2013;6(Suppl 1:M3):46–55. (3) Jurca SJ, Elliott WJ. Common substances that may contribute to resistant hypertension, and recommendations for limiting their clinical effects. *Curr Hypertens Rep* 2016 Oct;18(10):73.

prevention of cerebral vasospasm but not too high to cause cardiac or other complications. If vasospasm occurs, normally BP augmentation is suggested.[4]

The American Heart Association (AHA)/American Society of Anesthesiologists (ASA) guidelines[5] for the management of aneurysmal SAH recommend that between the time of symptom and aneurysm obliteration, BP should be controlled with a titratable antihypertensive agent to balance the risk of stroke, hypertension-related bleeding, and maintenance of cerebral perfusion pressure (CPP). The European Stroke Organization[6] suggests that until clipping or coiling of the aneurysm, SBP should not exceed 180 mmHg and if the blood pressure is lowered, mean arterial pressure (MAP) should be kept at least above 90 mmHg.

Despite lack of randomized controlled trials, induced hypertension to prevent and treat vasospasm is still being used by clinicians. Caution is generally recommended as it may increase the risk for hypertensive encephalopathy and haemorrhagic transformation of ischaemia.

Traumatic Brain Injury

According to the Brain Trauma Foundation Traumatic Brain Injury Guidelines 2016,[7] the target CPP in a traumatic brain injury (TBI) patient is 60–70 mmHg and the minimum optimal CPP threshold being unclear may depend upon the autoregulatory status of the patient (level IIB). Maintaining SBP at >100 mmHg for patients 50 to 69 years old, or at >110 mmHg or above for patients 15 to 49, or >70 years old may be considered to decrease mortality and improve outcomes (level III). During CPP management by increasing MAP, there is a risk of hyperaemia if pressure autoregulation is lost.[7]

Paroxysmal sympathetic hyperactivity (PSH) is an autonomic dysfunction characterized by paroxysmal increase in sympathetic and motor activity. It occurs after severe acquired brain injury. The clinical features are tachycardia, hypertension, tachypnoea, hyperthermia, diaphoresis, and increased motor activity. The PSH is associated with poor outcome and a beta blocker is used to control BP with some success but the drug dose needs to be carefully titrated to avoid unwanted hypotension.[8]

Stroke

Intracerebral haemorrhage: Although it is less common than ischaemic stroke, ICH is more life threatening and less treatable. From the INTERACT 2 (Intensive Blood Pressure Reduction in Acute Cerebral Hemorrhage Trial) clinical trial,[9] 2,839 spontaneous ICH participants were randomly assigned to target SBP 110–139 mmHg or

140–179 mmHg to attest the effectiveness of intensive and standard BP reduction protocols. It was shown that intensive BP lowering was safe, resulted in more favourable functional outcomes and better overall quality of life. This landmark trial makes big changes in BP management in international guidelines. In 2014, the European Stroke Organization recommended that in acute ICH (onset <6 hr), the intensive BP reduction (SBP <140 mmHg in <1 hr) is safe and may be superior to the previously higher target of SBP <180 mmHg.[10] Later in 2015, the AHA/ASA updated their guidelines for the management of spontaneous ICH. Acute lowering of SBP for patients with BP between 150 and 220 mmHg to 140 mmHg is safe considering that there is no contraindication to acute BP treatment.[11]

A recent trial, ATACH 2 (Antihypertensive Treatment of Acute Cerebral Hemorrhage), included 1,000 patients with the same target SBP as INTERACT 2 but the result showed no benefit. In the ATACH 2 trial, participants were included more early within 4.5 hours of onset of stroke and all of them had initial BP in the higher range (>180 mmHg).[12]

Acute ischaemic stroke and transient ischaemic attack: From the ASA guidelines for strokes in 2013, a patient who otherwise is eligible for acute reperfusion therapy except that BP is >185/110 mmHg: Antihypertensive drug(s) (labetalol or nicardipine) can be used. Management of BP during and after recombinant tissue plasminogen activator (rt-PA) or other acute reperfusion therapy is to maintain BP at or below 180/105 mmHg. In patients who are not treated with rt-PA, it is advised to lower the BP cautiously only if it is greater than 220/120 mmHg.[13]

Antihypertensive Drugs

Antihypertensive drugs are classified according to their structures and functions. In acute hypertensive crisis in neurocritical care, vasodilators are not the best option because they can increase cerebral blood volume (CBV) and ICP. In a patient with intracranial hypertension (IH), reducing MAP can reduce CPP, so ICP should be lowered before starting antihypertensive drugs. Beta-adrenergic blocking agents are a good option and the most commonly used is labetalol. The MAP should not be reduced more than 20% in the first hour. If acute reduction of cardiac output is a great concern, the dihydropyridine calcium channel blocker, e.g., nicardipine has little negative effect on heart rate and contractility. The combination of more than one antihypertensive drug can be used and finally if others fail, use sodium nitroprusside.

Table 37.2 The commonly used antihypertensive drugs in neurocritical care

Drugs	Dose	Onset	Half-life	Metabolism
Labetalol	10–20 mg over 1–2 min, may repeat one time	5–10 min	6 hr	Hepatic conjugation
Esmolol	Bolus: 500 µg/kg (over 1 min) Infusion: 50–300 µg/kg/min	1–2 min	9 min	Plasma esterase
Nicardipine	Bolus: not recommended 5 mg/h IV, titrate up by 2.5 mg/hr every 5–15 minutes, maximum 15 mg/hr	5–10 min	2–4 hr	Hepatic CYP3A4
Nimodipine (oral)	60 mg every four hours	1 hr	1–2 hr	Hepatic
Clavedipine	Bolus: not recommended Infusion: 1–2 mg/hr Max 32 mg/hr	1–2 min	1–15 min	Plasma and tissue esterases
Nitroprusside	Bolus: not recommended Infusion: 0.25–4 µg/kg/min Max 10 µg/kg/min	1–2 min	<10 min	Erythrocytes Hepatic methylation Cyanide toxicity

Sources: (1) Zaidi G, Chichra A, Weitzen M, Narasimhan M. Blood pressure control in neurological ICU patients: What is too high and what is too low? *Open Crit Care Med J* 2013;6(Suppl 1:M3):46–55. (2) Jauch EC, Saver JL, Adams HP Jr, Bruno A, Connors JJ, Demaerschalk BM, et al. Guidelines for the early management of patients with acute ischemic stroke: a guideline for healthcare professionals from the American Heart Association/American Stroke Association. *Stroke* 2013;44(3):870–947. (3) Kiser TH. Cerebral vasospasm in critically ill patients with aneurysmal subarachnoid hemorrhage: Does the evidence support the ever-growing list of potential pharmacotherapy interventions? *Hosp Pharm* 2014;49(10):923–41.

In SAH, oral nimodipine is widely used for reducing severity of neurological deficits in patients with cerebral vasospasm, although there is no evidence of changes in cerebral angiography. Intravenous nicardipine is another alternative for cerebral vasospasm (Table 37.2).[2,13,14]

HYPOTENSION

Hypotension should be quickly assessed as either real or artefact of the measurement. Prompt diagnosis and treatment are important because prolonged hypotension results in poor perfusion and organ damage.[15]

Causes of Hypotension

There are several causes of hypotension, e.g., hypovolaemia (absolute or relative), decreased myocardial contraction, arrhythmias, or decreased systemic vascular resistance (Table 37.3).

Although hypotension is caused by several factors, the initial management includes fluid and/or vasopressor or inotrope to increase the BP. Afterwards, the cause needs to be identified and treated correctly. Some causes have similar symptoms and signs, therefore it is sometimes difficult to identify like anaphylaxis from antibiotics.[16] A single dose of etomidate given during emergency intubation can suppress the adrenal gland for more

Table 37.3 Causes of hypotension

Decreased preload	Hypovolaemia Inadequate fluid replacement Ongoing blood loss (in multiple trauma) Diuresis (hyperglycaemia, mannitol) Relative hypovolaemia Sepsis (due to vasodilatation, leakage) Positive-pressure ventilation (decreased venous return) Pulmonary embolism Pneumothorax Cardiac tamponade
Decreased contractility	Neurogenic stunned myocardium Myocardial ischaemia and infarction Congestive heart failure Sepsis Drugs (antihypertensive, antidysrhythmics) Hypothyroidism
Arrhythmias	Sinus bradycardia 2 or 3 degrees AV block Atrial fibrillation (AF) with block Sinus tachycardia Supraventricular tachycardia (SVT) Atrial fibrillation (AF) with rapid ventricular response Ventricular tachycardia, ventricular fibrillation

Decreased systemic vascular resistance	Sepsis
	Anaphylaxis
	Transfusion reaction
	Adrenal insufficiency
	Sympathetic block from spinal shock

Source: Kumar A, Unligil U, Parrillo JE. Circulatory shock. In: Parrillo JE, Dellinger RP, editors. *Critical Care Medicine*. China: Elsevier Saunders; 2014: pp. 299–324.

than 24 hours and might cause relative adrenal insufficiency.[17]

There are several neurological conditions that need special care for hypotension: (1) Sepsis; (2) Head injury; (3) Neurogenic stunned myocardium (NSM) or Neurogenic stress cardiomyopathy; and (4) Spinal shock from spinal cord injury (SCI). We discuss each of these in the next few paragraphs and devote a separate section to NSM.

Sepsis

In neurocritical care, many patients are unconscious or given sedatives. These patients are vulnerable to infections, e.g., respiratory tract infection, especially ventilator-associated pneumonia, urinary tract infection (UTI), catheter-line infection, etc. In order to avoid infection, prevention using proper hand hygiene, oropharyngeal decontamination, and other methodologies are very important. Routine screening for severe sepsis is useful for the early implementation of therapy in potentially infected seriously ill patients.

Sepsis guidelines: We address a part of sepsis guideline 2012[18] in this chapter, with respect to fluid therapy and vasopressor/inotropic drug management.

- **Fluid therapy in severe sepsis**: Crystalloid is recommended as the initial fluid for resuscitation. Hydroxyethyl starches should not be used in view of their potential harm. Albumin can be co-administered in fluid resuscitation when patients require substantial amounts of crystalloids. However, there is still no recommendation as to the type of crystalloid to use.

  In hypoperfusion with suspicion of hypovolaemia, a minimum of 30 ml/kg of crystalloids need to be achieved. More rapid administration and greater amounts of fluid may be needed in some patients. Fluid challenge is continued as long as there is haemodynamic improvement in dynamic (e.g., pulse pressure variation) or static (e.g., central venous pressure) cardiovascular parameters.

  Red blood cell transfusion occurs only when haemoglobin concentration decreases to <7.0 g/dL to target a haemoglobin concentration of 7.0–9.0 g/dL in adults.

Fluid composition can cause unwanted side effects such as altering the pH balance. The metabolism of organic anions such as lactate and acetate leads to the production of bicarbonate and can cause metabolic alkalosis. The use of Ringer's lactate affects the inability to use lactate as a marker of hypoperfusion. It should not be used in septic patients with lactic acidosis and hepatic dysfunction and disruption of lactate clearance. Ringer's acetate is an alternative balanced crystalloid that may be used in patients with diabetic lactic acidosis and those with impaired hepatic metabolism. Normal saline (NS) is a non-balanced crystalloid that can result in hyperchloraemic non-anion gap metabolic acidosis. Another concern about normal saline is its potential risk for acute kidney injury.[19] However, in neurointensive care patients, serum sodium is an important factor for maintaining fluid balance between intravascular and interstitial brain water. These factors, along with many others, must be considered when selecting a fluid for volume resuscitation.

In 2015, Raghunathan et al.[20] published the retrospective cohort study of 60,734 ICU patients comparing balanced and non-balanced crystalloids in a human population being treated for sepsis. They assessed the use of NS, NS with balanced crystalloids, NS with colloids, and a combination of all three together. Administering a combination of NS and balanced crystalloids together resulted in a mortality of 17.69%, which was significantly lower than the mortality rate of patients treated with NS only (20.19%) or NS with colloids (24.16%) or NS with balanced crystalloids and colloids (19.23%). The administration of balanced crystalloids was consistently associated with lower mortality, whether colloids were used (relative risk, 0.84; 95% CI, 0.76–0.92) or not (relative risk, 0.79; 95% CI, 0.70–0.89).

- **Vasopressor therapy**: To achieve a target MAP of 65 mmHg, norepinephrine is recommended as the first choice of vasopressor. Adding epinephrine or vasopressin (0.03 unit/min) or dopamine is sometimes needed to maintain adequate BP. Dopamine can be used as the first line vasopressor for patients with low risk of tachyarrhythmias and absolute or relative bradycardia.
- **Inotropic drugs**: A dobutamine infusion of up to 20 µg/kg/min will be administered or added to the vasopressor (if in use) in the presence of myocardial dysfunction or ongoing hypoperfusion despite adequate volume resuscitation.

Head injury

Severe cases of TBI require neurocritical care. The aim is to stabilize haemodynamics and systemic oxygenation to prevent further brain injury. Arterial hypotension is a major risk. Hypotension reduces CPP and increases ICP due to cerebral vasodilation. The common causes of hypotension in TBI are hypovolaemia, systemic inflammatory response, drugs (mannitol), and others. Traumatic brain injury may shift the autoregulation curve to the right and/or lose the autoregulation. So even a small change of MAP can cause brain ischaemia or hyperaemia. It also disrupts the blood–brain barrier (BBB) and causes brain oedema. The brain oedema after TBI can be cytotoxic or vasogenic. Traumatic brain injury can cause sympathetic stimulation, so BP is maintained despite hypovolaemia. Mannitol has been liberally used in many TBI patients and worsens the patient's volume status. To prevent severe hypotension, the routine use of mannitol and intravascular dehydration should be avoided. From the Brain Trauma Foundation Traumatic Brain Injury Guidelines 2016, the target CPP in a TBI patient is 60–70 mmHg. Maintaining SBP at >100–110 mmHg may decrease mortality and improve outcomes.[21]

Spinal Shock From Spinal Cord Injury

Spinal shock accompanies SCI during the acute phase. A sudden disruption of the centre of the sympathetic system in the spinal cord leads to spinal shock. The severity of the spinal shock depends on the level of cord injury. Spinal shock usually lasts days to weeks with an average of 4–12 weeks. Neurogenic shock consists of bradycardia, severe arterial hypotension and hypothermia. SBP <90 mmHg in the supine position, which is not the result of hypovolaemia due to haemorrhage or dehydration is characteristic of neurogenic shock. The lack of compensatory vasoconstriction, secondary to disruption in sympathetic activity contributes to low blood pressure, especially in postural changes (orthostatic hypotension).

Treatment: Treatment implies correction of bradycardia and hypotension. As a first step, give intravenous fluids and use chronotropic and/or inotropic medications. The vasopressors like norepinephrine, dobutamine, and dopamine can be used. The spinal cord perfusion pressure must be maintained. Prolonged or severe hypotension results in spinal cord ischaemia. An MAP of at least 85 mmHg is necessary to maintain spinal cord perfusion and help prevent secondary ischaemia.[22,23]

NEUROGENIC STUNNED MYOCARDIUM (NSM)

Neurogenic stunned myocardium or neurogenic stress cardiomyopathy is characterized by electrocardiography (ECG) changes, increased cardiac biomarker, reversible left ventricular dysfunction (cardiomyopathy) but no defect in coronary perfusion. It results from excessive release of cathecholamines at the cardiac nerve terminal. It is related to subarachnoid haemorrhoid or other neurologic aetiologies.

Neurogenic stunned myocardium can cause minimal clinical effects, but sometimes it is very severe and leads to cardiogenic shock and neurogenic pulmonary oedema.

Diagnosis

Electrocardiography changes can be of any kind. The ST segment changes (T wave inversion and U wave) and QT prolongation are the most common and sometimes look like acute coronary syndrome. Arrhythmias can be benign or malignant but severe arrhythmias are quite uncommon. The most common arrhythmias are sinus arrhythmias and atrial fibrillation.

The elevation of cardiac biomarkers (troponins, especially troponin I) is found in 20%–37% of patients and reaches its peak in 24–72 hours. Clinical severity has been shown to relate to troponin levels. Brain natriuretic peptide (BNP) is also elevated and correlates well with troponin, wall motion abnormalities, low left ventricular ejection fraction (LVEF) and pulmonary oedema.

Many echocardiographic wall motion abnormalities (apical or non-apical or global hypokinesia) can occur. Left ventricular apical ballooning similar to stress cardiomyopathy (Takotsubo disease) and severe global hypokinesis has been documented. Myocardial wall motion abnormalities are outside of the normal coronary vascular distribution and can vary from segmental changes to global hypokinesis. The majority of wall motion abnormalities are in the basal and middle parts with apical sparing. It is likely that the changes correspond to localization of cardiac sympathetic nerve terminals.

The new technique 'speckle strain' echocardiography can reliably detect NSM, although estimating LVEF is still the standard method. This technique has been developed as an alternative to quantify global and segmental myocardial function. The Doppler and 2D imaging identify an acoustic thumb print in the reflected ultrasound called 'speckle'. This permits specific segments to be tracked and the amount of deformation of each segment can be quantified.

The use of coronary angiography to diagnose NSM is still considered an invasive procedure and has some limitations. Computed tomography (CT) coronary angiography is non-invasive with 80% accuracy and so is not always suitable but remains promising. Magnetic resonance imaging (MRI) is also an alternative for diagnosis.

It is important to differentiate NSM from acute coronary syndrome but it is not always easy. For a definite diagnosis, the coronary angiography is needed, but it is rarely used due to its invasiveness. Factors favouring NSM are wide ranges of ECG changes, modest increase in cardiac biomarkers, and inconsistency between ECG changes and echocardiography.

Treatment

All the NSM patients need to be closely monitored for haemodynamic changes. Some patients develop cardiogenic shock and pulmonary oedema. The cardiogenic shock is treated with inotrope to optimize cardiac output and maintain CPP. In severe cases, an intra-aortic balloon pump may be required. Severe arrhythmias or sudden cardiac arrest is a rare event. Arrhythmias should be treated according to types and haemodynamic consequences. Drugs that prolong the QTc interval such as antidepressants should be avoided.[24,25]

Although cardiomyopathy is reversible, patients with NSM exhibit poor outcome and high mortality.

ARRHYTHMIAS

There are several neuroanatomic sites that influence heart rhythm and rate, myocardial function, and vascular tone. These locations include the insular cortex, amygdala, paraventricular, hypothalamus, and various sites in the brainstem and spinal cord.[21] In the neurointensive care setting, arrhythmias are very common with various causes. For example, NSM is not only associated with ST segment changes but also cardiac arrhythmias.[21,22] Atrial fibrillation is a leading cause of ischaemic stroke. Many neuromuscular diseases are associated with cardiac dysfunction and arrhythmias.[21] Acute spinal injury can cause sinus bradycardia and atrio-ventricular block (AV block).[19,20]

Most of the arrhythmias or dysrhythmias generally do not require treatment, e.g., atrial premature contractions and unifocal ventricular premature contractions. However, some arrhythmias e.g., atrial fibrillation needs lifelong treatment. The management of arrhythmias is the shared responsibility of critical care intensivists and cardiologists. The arrhythmias may arise from intrinsic cardiac pathology or from secondary causes, e.g., myocardial infarction, some metabolic or perfusion problems, and specific causes need to be identified. The common secondary causes of arrhythmias are presented in Box 37.1.

Box 37.1 The secondary causes of arrhythmias

Increased/decreased sympathetic/parasympathetic activity

Electrolyte imbalance especially hypokalaemia or hyperkalaemia, hypomagnesaemia

Hypoxaemia/hypercapnia

Metabolic acidosis or alkalosis

Myocardial ischaemia/infarction

Increased intracranial pressure

Neurogenic stunned myocardium

Drug toxicity: digoxin, amiodarone, opioids

Malignant hyperthermia/hyperthyroidism or hypothyroidism

Source: Trohman R, Attaya S. Cardiac arrhythmias. In: Parrillo JE, Dellinger RP, eds. *Critical Care Medicine*. China: Elsevier Saunders; 2014. pp. 515–47.

Management

In this chapter we cover only acute care of common arrhythmias.

Sinus tachycardia: It is a normal response to physiological, pharmacological, or pathological changes. The tachycardia resolves after these conditions become normal or near normal. The causes are shown in Table 37.4.[26]

Table 37.4 Causes of sinus tachycardia

System	Examples
Cardiovascular	Hypovolaemia Heart failure Anaemia Pulmonary embolism Sepsis
Neurogenic	Pain Agitation, anxiety, fear Sympathetic stimulation
Metabolic	Sepsis Hyperthyroid Fever, shivering Carcinoma Acidosis
Respiratory	Hypoxaemia/hypercarbia
Pharmacologic	Sympathomimetic drugs, e.g., dopamine, epinephrine Vagolytic drugs, e.g., atropine Vasodilators, e.g., nitrates Bronchodilators, e.g., terbutaline, salbutamol

Source: Trohman R, Attaya S. Cardiac arrhythmias. In: Parrillo JE, Dellinger RP, eds. *Critical Care Medicine*. China: Elsevier Saunders; 2014. pp. 515–47.

Table 37.5 Causes of sinus bradycardia

System	Examples
Cardiovascular	SA node dysfunction Myocardial infarction (inferior wall)
Neurogenic	Increased intracranial pressure Spinal shock Vagal stimulation Autonomic instability (carotid hypersensitivity)
Metabolic	Hypothyroid Hypothermia Gram negative sepsis
Respiratory	Hypoxaemia/hypercarbia (late sign)
Pharmacologic	Opioids, e.g., fentanyl, sufentanil CVS drugs: β blocker, calcium channel blocker, digoxin, amiodarone Sedative: dexmedetomidine Anticholinesterase reversal: pyridostigmine

Source: Trohman R, Attaya S. Cardiac arrhythmias. In: Parrillo JE, Dellinger RP, eds. *Critical Care Medicine*. China: Elsevier Saunders; 2014. pp. 515–47.

Sinus bradycardia: Sinus bradycardia is usually benign and requires no treatment. It is common in young and fit adults but it can be a sign of some pathological conditions (Table 37.5). The heart rate can be increased with atropine, dopamine, or epinephrine. Temporary or permanent pacing is used in some persistent bradycardia with symptoms.[26]

Atrial fibrillation/flutter: Ischaemic strokes can result from cardiac embolism. Atrial fibrillation/flutter (AF) is mostly preventable and oral anticoagulants (old and new) can be used effectively to prevent atrial thrombus. The risk should be assessed by using a simple risk score such as CHA$_2$DS$_2$-VASc, and an oral anticoagulant should be prescribed for all who are at risk.[27] The treatment of AF includes anticoagulants, rate control, and rhythm control. We discuss these treatments in greater detail in the next few paragraphs.

Anticoagulants

In patients with non-valvular AF, the risk of ischaemic stroke should be assessed by using simple risk scores such as the CHA$_2$DS$_2$-VASc score, and an oral anticoagulant should be prescribed for those who are at risk regardless of the presence of permanent, persistent or paroxysmal AF. For decades, targeting an international normalized ratio (INR) of 2.0–3.0 with the vitamin K antagonist,

warfarin, has been the standard of care. Nevertheless, in real life, one-third of eligible patients with AF receive no anticoagulants, and over half of the patients on warfarin achieve suboptimum INR levels. Bleeding risk assessment should also be part of the clinical decision-making process. In most cases, an elevated bleeding risk score should not be used as a reason to withhold anticoagulation but rather reversible risk factors should be identified and potentially corrected. New oral anticoagulants, e.g., dabigatran, apixaban, rivaroxaban, and edoxaban[28] are as effective as or superior to vitamin K antagonists for the prevention of stroke and systemic embolism with a significant reduction in haemorrhagic stroke, a faster onset and offset and without need for anticoagulant monitoring. In AF patients with rheumatic mitral stenosis or a mechanical heart valve prosthesis or patients on dialysis, vitamin K antagonists remain the only anticoagulant option.

Immediate reversal of the anticoagulant effect is indicated in life-threatening bleeding such as intracerebral haemorrhage. These decisions are best made by a multidisciplinary team involving a haematologist, cardiologist, surgeon, and the intensivist. For vitamin K antagonists, fresh frozen plasma, vitamin K, and prothrombin complex concentrates are recommended. For new non-vitamin-K anticoagulants, administration of prothrombin complex concentrates should be considered. At the time of this writing, dabigatran is the only new oral anticoagulant that has a specific antidote available. Idarucizumab is a clinically available humanized antibody fragment that binds dabigatran and rapidly and dose-dependently reverses its effects.[29]

Rate Control

During AF, the atria cannot eject blood properly resulting in reduced stroke volume and cardiac output by 20%–30%. The fast ventricular rate or rapid ventricular response (RVR) further reduces ventricular filling time and stroke volume.

Rate control is the treatment for nearly all patients with AF, even when a rhythm control strategy is attempted. Rate control is the approach of choice for patients with new onset or acute AF or with acute recurrences. Rate control can be a first choice treatment for patients who do not require sinus rhythm (e.g., elderly patients with no or minor symptoms). Rate control is the only option when rhythm control fails or the risks of restoring sinus rhythm outweigh the benefits.

Before beginning a rate control treatment, AF with RVR (like sinus tachycardia) could indicate specific disorders needing further management such as volume resuscitation.

Table 37.6 Rate controlling intravenous drugs in atrial fibrillation

Drugs	Intravenous administration	Caution
β blockers		
Metoprolol tartrate	2.5–5.0 mg bolus over 2 min up to four doses	Asthma
Esmolol	500 μg/kg intravenous bolus over 1 min, followed by 50–300 μg/kg per min	Acute heart failure
Non-dihydropyridine calcium antagonists		
Verapamil	2.5–10 mg bolus over 2 min	Heart failure with reduced ejection fraction
Diltiazem	0.25 mg/kg bolus over 2 min, then 5–15 mg/hr*	
Digitalis glycosides		
Digoxin	0.5 mg bolus (0.75–1.5 mg over 24 hours in divided doses)**	Wolff–Parkinson–White syndrome
Other		
Amiodarone	300 mg over 30–60 min followed by 900–1200 mg over 24 hr (preferably via central venous catheter)	Prolonged QT syndrome

*adapt doses in hepatic and renal impairment.
**adapt doses in renal impairment.
Sources: (1) Trohman R, Attaya S. Cardiac arrhythmias. In: *Critical Care Medicine*. Parrillo JE, Dellinger RP, eds. China: Elsevier Saunders; 2014. pp. 515–47. (2) Van Gelder IC, Rienstra M, Crijns HJ, Olshansky B. Rate control in atrial fibrillation. *Lancet* 2016;388:818–28. doi:10.1016/S0140-6736(16)31258–2.

The drugs widely used to reduce the ventricular rate during AF are β blockers, non-dihydropyridine calcium-channel antagonists, cardiac glycosides (digoxin), and amiodarone. The choice of rate controlling drugs, alone or in combination, depends on symptoms, comorbidities, and potential side-effects (Table 37.6).

Rhythm Control

Many AF patients have substantial symptoms despite ventricular rate control and require restoration of sinus rhythm to improve their cardiac output and quality of life. The restoration and maintenance of sinus rhythm are referred to as rhythm control. Rhythm control could be achieved by electrical or pharmacological cardioversion or catheter ablation.

Postoperative AF is very common post cardiac surgery but less frequent during neurocritical care. Although many AFs terminate spontaneously within hours or days, some can persist for longer. Here we focus on acute care and emergency management.

Electrical Cardioversion

In haemodynamically compromised patients with new onset AF, synchronized electrical cardioversion is indicated. In the more elective setting, cardioversion carries a risk of stroke in patients who are not anticoagulated. Thus, patients who have been in AF longer than 48 hours should start anticoagulant therapy at least three weeks before cardioversion. When early cardioversion is preferred, a transoesophageal echocardiogram should be performed to exclude left atrial thrombi before attempting cardioversion. After giving mild to moderate sedation, cardioversion using biphasic defibrillators with 100 J or more and antero-posterior electrode placement are recommended.[26,31]

Pharmacological Cardioversion

Unlike direct current cardioversion, pharmacological cardioversion with an antiarrhythmic drug obviates the need for conscious sedation. However, the success rate for pharmacological cardioversion is lower.[31] Various drugs can be used as shown in Table 37.7.

The patients undergoing pharmacological cardioversion require continuous clinical and ECG monitoring during drug administration and afterwards because of the risk of proarrhythmic events such as ventricular arrhythmia, sinus node arrest, or atrioventricular block. Amiodarone can be used for rate and rhythm control and it is also effective for other tachyarrhythmias.[26,31]

New ventricular arrhythmias need an assessment in electrolytes, acid-base status, and oxygenation/ventilation.

Table 37.7 Antiarrhythmic drugs used to restore sinus rhythm in patients with atrial fibrillation

Drugs	Intravenous administration	Caution
Class Ic		
Flecainide	2 mg/kg over 10 min	Abnormal ventricular function
Propafenone	2 mg/kg over 10–20 min	Severe obstructive lung disease
Class III		
Amiodarone	300 mg over 30–60 min followed by 900–1200 mg over 24 hr	Prolonged PR, QRS, and QT intervals, lung fibrosis, hepatic impairment; thyroid dysfunction
Sotalol	80–160 mg twice daily	Asthma, renal impairment, left ventricular dysfunction, QTc>450 ms, sinus bradycardia; <50 bpm, second or third degree AV block
Multichannel blocker		
Vernakalant	3 mg/kg dose over 10 min and A second infusion of 2 mg/kg (if AF persists after 10 min)	Proarrhythmia

Sources: (1) Trohman R, Attaya S. Cardiac arrhythmias. In: *Critical Care Medicine*. Parrillo JE, Dellinger RP, eds. China: Elsevier Saunders; 2014. pp. 515–47. (2) Piccini JP, Fauchier L. Rhythm control in atrial fibrillation. *Lancet* 2016;388:829–40. doi:10.1016/S0140-6736(16)31277–6.

The 12-lead ECG is used for differentiating monomorphic from polymorphic ventricular tachycardia (VT) and also ST segment analysis. A symptomatic patient with non-sustained ventricular arrhythmias and premature ventricular contractions (PVCs) without structural heart disease needs no treatment. Sustained VT with haemodynamic instability should be treated with cardioversion/defibrillation (100–200 J), while stable tachycardia can be treated with amiodarone or beta-blockers. Lidocaine remains another option although it is not a first line treatment. The recurrence of arrhythmias is still high, so the implantable cardioverter defibrillator (ICD) should be considered, especially in patients with poor left ventricular function.[26]

CARDIAC ARREST

Although neurogenic cardiovascular problems are common and related to poor prognosis, sudden cardiac arrest or death is a rare event. The mechanism is unclear but may relate to QTc prolongation from some drugs such as antipsychotics or antiarrhythmics.

Some patients with neuromuscular disorder were reported having sudden cardiac arrest. They present with a positive family history for sudden cardiac arrest palpitations, arterial hypertension, ECG abnormalities (bundle branch block, bifascicular block, QT-prolongation, increased QT variability, early repolarization, T-wave alternans, and VT). The neuromuscular disorders in which sudden cardiac death was frequently reported include myotonic

dystrophy type 1, mitochondrial disorders, laminopathy, desminopathy, Danon disease, and amyotrophic lateral sclerosis.[32]

Seizure-related cardiac arrhythmias are frequently reported and have been implicated as a potential mechanism of Sudden Unexpected Death in Epilepsy (SUDEP). During seizure, asystole, bradycardia, and AV conduction block happen, but most are self-limiting. Postictal arrhythmias are mostly found following convulsive seizures and often associated with near SUDEP. The postictal arrhythmias include asystole, AV block, and the less prevalent AF and VF.[33]

In the ICU, all patients have continuous monitoring and some already have been intubated with controlled ventilation. If cardiac arrest occurs, with prompt resuscitation and readily available drugs and equipment, the survival rate should be high. From the Bergum D et al. study,[34] the causes of arrests could be neurological problems (sudden increase in ICP, sudden intracranial haemorrhage, and brain herniation) or non-neurological problems such as respiratory problems (hypoxaemia), cardiovascular problems (myocardial infarction, severe arrhythmias) and during cardiac arrest, most ECG rhythms are non-shockable (systole/pulseless electrical activity or PEA). So the causes (5H and 5T), need to be identified and treated and that may make resuscitation more successful.[35] But unfortunately, not all causes could be known. Patient records and pre-arrest clinical symptoms are good information and most frequently used in these circumstances.[32]

Sustained ICH and acute brain herniation are catastrophic neurological events that require immediate recognition and treatment to prevent irreversible injury and death. The cardinal signs of transtentorial (uncal) herniation are an acute loss of consciousness associated with ipsilateral pupillary dilation and contralateral hemiparesis. The standard care of raised ICP should be implemented in all cases. Surgery is considered for patients who have failed medical management. Decompressive surgical interventions include (1) placement of an external ventricular drain (ventriculostomy), (2) evacuation of extra-axial lesion (e.g., epidural haematoma), (3) resection of intracerebral lesion, (4) removal of brain parenchyma, and (5) decompressive craniectomies.[33,36,37]

POST-CARDIAC-ARREST CARE

Only few cardiac arrests are treated in the ICU. Some patients are resuscitated rapidly and have a very brief period of cardiac arrest and are too well to benefit from intensive care. Some patients are too sick to benefit from being taken care in the ICU or some have no return of spontaneous circulation. Post-cardiac-arrest care is addressed as the fifth link in the chain of survival. The post-cardiac-arrest care includes treatment of the precipitating cause of cardiac arrest combined with the assessment and mitigation of ischaemia-reperfusion injury to multiple organ systems.

Post-Cardiac-Arrest Syndrome

Post-cardiac-arrest syndrome is described as a combination of pathophysiological changes after cardiac arrest which include ischaemic/reperfusion response, post-cardiac arrest myocardial dysfunction and anoxic-ischaemic brain injury.

Post-cardiac-arrest brain injury: After cardiac arrest, the pathophysiological changes related to the brain include impaired cerebral autoregulation, cerebral oedema, and neuronal degeneration. The clinical manifestations are coma (GCS <8), seizure, myoclonus cognitive dysfunction, impaired temperature control, vegetative state, and brain death.

Post-cardiac-arrest myocardial dysfunction: Post-cardiac-arrest myocardial dysfunction is caused by myocardial stunning after the ischaemic process despite the return of normal coronary perfusion. Patients manifest with hypotension, arrhythmias, or cardiovascular instability. It is reversible and has good recovery. It is necessary to differentiate this from acute coronary syndrome which is a major leading cause of cardiac arrest and may need

immediate treatment like coronary intervention and recanalization.

Systemic ischaemic/reperfusion response: Ischaemic/reperfusion response triggers immunological, cardiovascular, and coagulation pathways and leads to multi-organ failure. Many cytokines and endotoxins are released and affect the patient's outcome. The systemic inflammatory response impairs vasoregulation, causes volume depletion, and hypotension. It also impairs tissue oxygen delivery and utilization and increases susceptibility to infection. The stress response also stimulates the adrenal gland and causes hyperglycaemia. Furthermore, low level of cortisol is related to poor outcome.

Persistent precipitating pathologies: The pathophysiology of post-cardiac-arrest syndrome is more complicated by the precipitating pathology that causes the cardiac arrest itself. Diagnosis and management of persistent precipitating pathologies such as acute coronary syndrome (ACS), pulmonary diseases, haemorrhage, sepsis, and others are mandatory.[38]

Management

Airway and Breathing

Patients who experience a very brief period of cardiac arrest and have immediate response to resuscitation may not require intubation. However, most of the patients who have persistent precipitating cause(s) of cardiac arrests definitely need intubation and controlled ventilation.

Maintaining the pressure of arterial carbon dioxide ($PaCO_2$) within a normal physiological range (end-tidal CO_2 30–40 mmHg or $PaCO_2$ 35–45 mmHg). A higher $PaCO_2$ may be permissible in patients with acute lung injury or high airway pressures. Mild hypocapnia might be useful as a temporary measure to treat cerebral oedema, but hyperventilation might cause cerebral vasoconstriction. In a hypothermic patient, the $PaCO_2$ might be higher than the actual value.[39]

In order to avoid hypoxia, the highest oxygen concentration should be used until the arterial oxyhaemoglobin saturation (SpO_2) or the partial pressure of arterial oxygen (PaO_2) can be measured. The fraction of inspired oxygen (FiO_2) can be decreased if the SpO_2 is 94% or greater.[39]

Haemodynamic Management

Post-cardiac-arrest patients often have unstable haemodynamics, which can occur for multiple reasons that include the underlying aetiology of the arrest as well as the ischaemia-reperfusion injury or myocardial dysfunction from the arrest. Avoiding and immediately correcting hypotension (SBP less than 90 mmHg, MAP less than 65 mmHg) during post-resuscitation care may be reasonable. The optimal BP would be different for various patients.

Targeted Temperature Management

The targeted temperature management (TTM) (32°C–36°C) is recommended for comatose adult patients with return of spontaneous circulation (ROSC) after cardiac arrest (out of or in hospital cardiac arrest, and shockable or non-shockable) and 24 hours was selected as the minimum recommended time. The committee recommends against routine use of prehospital cooling with rapid infusion of large volumes of cold intravenous fluid immediately after ROSC. Hyperthermia or fever is associated with poor outcome. It may be reasonable to actively prevent fever in comatose patients after TTM. Therapeutic hypothermia is associated with several complications such as increased systemic vascular resistance, decreased cardiac output, cold diuresis, hypovolaemia, arrhythmias, impaired coagulation, and reduced immunological response.[40]

Other Aspects of Neurological Care

An electroencephalogram (EEG) for the diagnosis of seizure should be promptly performed and interpreted, and then should be monitored frequently or continuously in comatose patients. The anticonvulsant regimens for the treatment of status epilepticus may be considered after cardiac arrest.

Glycaemic control in critically ill patients is controversial and efforts to tightly control glucose at low levels have been associated with increased frequency of hypoglycaemic episodes that may be detrimental. The benefit of any specific target range of glucose management is uncertain in adults with ROSC after cardiac arrest.[39]

Extracorporeal Life Support

In case of refractory cardiac arrest (>10–30 min) without ROSC and with unknown causes of cardiac arrest, extracorporeal life support can support organ perfusion while waiting for the investigations. Veno-arterial extracorporeal membrane oxygenation (VA-ECMO) can be used for this purpose and it is implemented into the new AHA Cardiopulmonary Resuscitation (CPR) Guidelines 2015.[35] It is called extracorporeal cardiopulmonary resuscitation (ECPR). Due to the complexity and expertise requirement, the ECPR programme should be started in experienced and high-volume extracorporeal membrane

oxygenation (ECMO) centres. For cardiac arrest due to accidental hypothermia (drowning) or intoxication, ECPR should be considered even with cardiac arrest lasting longer than 60 minutes. Better outcome is obtained when ECPR is combined with mechanical CPR, therapeutic hypothermia, and percutaneous coronary intervention.[41]

PREDICTION

The earliest time for prognostication using clinical examination in patients treated with TTM where sedation or paralysis could be a confounder may be 72 hours after return to normothermia or 72 hours after cardiac arrest in patients who are not treated with TTM. There are several tests used to predict outcome.[39] These are:

- Pupillary reflex: In comatose patients who are treated or not treated with TTM, the absence of pupillary reflex to light at 72 hours or more after cardiac arrest or after TTM may predict poor neurological outcome.
- Motor movement: Due to high false positive rate, the findings of either absent motor movements or extensor posturing or the presence of simple myoclonus (distinguished from status myoclonus which has continuous, repetitive myoclonic jerks lasting more than 30 minutes) *should not* be used alone for predicting a poor neurological outcome.

    In combination with other diagnostic tests at 72 or more hours after cardiac arrest, the presence of status myoclonus during the first 72 to 120 hours after cardiac arrest may predict poor neurological outcomes.

- Electroencephalogram: In comatose patients who are treated with TTM, the persistent absence of EEG reactivity to external stimuli at 72 hours after cardiac arrest and persistent burst suppression on EEG after rewarming may predict a poor outcome.

    Intractable and persistent (more than 72 hours) status epilepticus in the absence of EEG reactivity to external stimuli may predict poor outcome.

- Evoked potentials: Bilateral absence of the N20 somatosensory evoked potentials (SSEP) wave 24 to 72 hours after cardiac arrest or after rewarming is a predictor of poor outcome.
- Imaging tests: The marked reduction of the grey white ratio on brain CT obtained within 2 hours after cardiac arrest may predict a poor outcome. The extensive restriction of diffusion on brain MRI at 2–6 days after cardiac arrest in combination with other established predictors may predict a poor neurological outcome.
- Blood test: Neuron-specific enolase (NSE) and S-100B are the two most commonly examined blood

markers. Studies of NSE and S-100B reported that initial S-100B levels were higher in patients with poor outcome compared to patients with good outcome, and that NSE levels would increase over 72 hours in patients with poor outcome relative to patients with good outcome. However, studies did not identify specific blood levels of these proteins. In conclusion, the blood levels of NSE and S-100B should not be used alone to predict a poor neurologic outcome.[39]

CONCLUSIONS

The cardiovascular care for neurosurgical patients is very important. The patients could experience hypotension, hypertension, arrhythmias, or even cardiac arrest. The neurointensivists need to know the pathophysiology and management for these conditions. The cardiologists also play an important role for further cardiac investigations and treatment.

REFERENCES

1. Salgado DR, Silva E, Vincent JL. Control of hypertension in the critically ill: a pathophysiological approach. *Ann Intensive Care* 2013;3(1):17.

2. Zaidi G, Chichra A, Weitzen M, Narasimhan M. Blood pressure control in neurological ICU patients: What is too high and what is too low? *Open Crit Care Med J* 2013;6(Suppl 1:M3):46–55.

3. Jurca SJ, Elliott WJ. Common substances that may contribute to resistant hypertension, and recommendations for limiting their clinical effects. 2016 Oct;18(10):73.

4. Carcel C, Sato S, Anderson CS. Blood pressure management in intracranial hemorrhage: Current challenges and opportunities. *Curr Treat Options Cardiovasc Med* 2016; 18(4):22. doi:10.1007/s11936-016-0444-z.

5. Connolly ES Jr, Rabinstein AA, Carhuapoma JR, Derdeyn CP, Dion J, Higashida RT, et al. Guidelines for the management of aneurysmal subarachnoid hemorrhage: a guideline for healthcare professionals from the American Heart Association/American Stroke Association. *Stroke* 2012;43(6):1711–37.

6. Steiner T, Juvela S, Unterberg A, Jung C, Forsting M, Rinkel G. European Stroke Organization. European Stroke Organization guidelines for the management of intracranial aneurysms and subarachnoid haemorrhage. *Cerebrovasc Dis* 2013;35(2):93–112.

7. Carney N, Totten AM, O'Reilly C, et al. Guidelines for the management of severe traumatic brain injury. 4th ed. *Neurosurgery* 2017 Jan 1;80(1):6–15.

8. Lump D, Moyer M. Paroxysmal sympathetic hyperactivity after severe brain injury. *Curr Neurol Neurosci Rep* 2014;14(11):494. doi:10.1007/s11910-014-0494-0.

9. Anderson CS, Heeley E, Huang Y, et al. Rapid blood-pressure lowering in patients with acute intracerebral hemorrhage. *N Engl J Med* 2013;368(25):2355–65.

10. Steiner T, Al-Shahi Salman R, Beer R, et al. European Stroke Organisation (ESO) guidelines for the management of spontaneous intracerebral hemorrhage. *Int J Stroke* 2014;9(7):840–55. doi:10.1111/ijs.12309.

11. Hemphill JC 3rd, Greenberg SM, Anderson CS, et al. Guidelines for the management of spontaneous intracerebral hemorrhage: a guideline for healthcare professionals from the American Heart Association/American Stroke Association. *Stroke* 2015;46:2032–60.

12. Qureshi AI, Palesch YY, Barsan WG, et al. Intensive blood-pressure lowering in patients with acute cerebral hemorrhage. *N Engl J Med* 2016;375(11):1033–43.

13. Jauch EC, Saver JL, Adams HP Jr, Bruno A, Connors JJ, Demaerschalk BM, et al. Guidelines for the early management of patients with acute ischemic stroke: a guideline for healthcare professionals from the American Heart Association/American Stroke Association. *Stroke* 2013;44(3):870–947.

14. Kiser TH. Cerebral vasospasm in critically ill patients with aneurysmal subarachnoid hemorrhage: Does the evidence support the ever-growing list of potential pharmacotherapy interventions? *Hosp Pharm* 2014;49(10):923–41.

15. Kumar A, Unligil U, Parrillo JE. Circulatory shock. In: Parrillo JE, Dellinger RP, eds. *Critical Care Medicine.* China: Elsevier Saunders; 2014: pp. 299–324.

16. Lohsiriwat V, Sriyoscharti S, Raksakietisak M, Leelarasamee A. Three-day unrecognized cefazolin anaphylaxis in a case undergoing coronary bypass graft surgery. *J Med Assoc Thai* 2012;95(6):825–9.

17. Raksakietisak M, Ngamlamiad C, Duangrat T, Soontarinka S, Raksamani K. The changes in cortisol levels during cardiac surgery: A randomized double-blinded study between two induction agents etomidate and thiopentone. *J Med Assoc Thai* 2015;98(8):775–81.

18. Dellinger RP, Levy MM, Rhodes A, et al. Surviving Sepsis Campaign Guidelines Committee including the Pediatric Subgroup. Surviving sepsis campaign: international guidelines for management of severe sepsis and septic shock: 2012. *Crit Care Med* 2013;41(2):580–637.

19. Avila AA, Kinberg EC, Sherwin NK, Taylor RD. The use of fluids in sepsis. *Cureus* 2016;8(3):e528. doi:10.7759/cureus.528

20. Raghunathan K, Bonavia A, Nathanson BH, et al.: Association between initial fluid choice and subsequent in-hospital mortality during the resuscitation of adults with septic shock. *Anesthesiology* 2015;123(6):1385–93.

21. Kinoshita K. Traumatic brain injury: pathophysiology for neurocritical care. *J Intensive Care* 2016;4:29.doi:10.1186/s40560-016-0138-3.

22. Grigorean VT, Sandu AM, Popescu M, et al. Cardiac dysfunctions following spinal cord injury. *J Med Life* 2009;2(2):133–45.

23. Popa C, Popa F, Grigorean VT, et al. Vascular dysfunctions following spinal cord injury. *J Med Life* 2010;3(3): 275–85.

24. Raad B. Cardiac manifestations of neurologic disorders. 1. Neurologic complications of systemic disease. *Continuum (Minneap Minn)* 2011;17:13–26.

25. Kerro A, Woods T, Chang JJ. Neurogenic stunned myocardium in subarachnoid hemorrhage. *J Crit Care* 2016;38:27–34.

26. Trohman R, Attaya S. Cardiac arrhythmias. In: Parrillo JE, Dellinger RP, eds. *Critical Care Medicine*. China: Elsevier Saunders; 2014. pp. 515–47.

27. Friberg L, Rosenqvist M, Lindgren A, Terént A, Norrving B, Asplund K. High prevalence of atrial fibrillation among patients with ischemic stroke. *Stroke* 2014;45(9):2599–605. doi:10.1161/STROKEAHA.114.006070.

28. Freedman B, Potpara TS, Lip GY. Stroke prevention in atrial fibrillation. *Lancet* 2016;388:806–17. doi:10.1016/S0140-6736(16)31257-0.

29. Kirchhof P, Benussi S, Kotecha D, et al. 2016 ESC Guidelines for the management of atrial fibrillation developed in collaboration with EACTS. *Eur Heart J* 2016;37(38):2893–962.

30. Van Gelder IC, Rienstra M, Crijns HJ, Olshansky B. Rate control in atrial fibrillation. *Lancet* 2016;388:818–28. doi:10.1016/S0140-6736(16)31258-2.

31. Piccini JP, Fauchier L. Rhythm control in atrial fibrillation. *Lancet* 2016;388:829–40. doi:10.1016/S0140-6736(16) 31277-6.

32. Finsterer J, Stöllberger C, Maeztu C. Sudden cardiac death in neuromuscular disorders. *Int J Cardiol* 2016;203: 508–15. doi:10.1016/j.ijcard.2015.10.176.

33. van der Lende M, Surges R, Sander JW, Thijs RD. Cardiac arrhythmias during or after epileptic seizures. *J Neurol Neurosurg Psychiatry* 2016;87:69–74. doi:10.1136/jnnp-2015-310559.

34. Bergum D, Nordseth T, Mjølstad OC, Skogvoll E, Haugen BO. Causes of in-hospital cardiac arrest—incidences

and rate of recognition. *Resuscitation* 2015;87:63–8. doi:10.1016/j.resuscitation.2014.11.007.

35. Link MS, Berkow LC, Kudenchuk PJ, et al. Part 7: Adult Advanced Cardiovascular Life Support 2015 American Heart Association Guidelines Update for Cardiopulmonary Resuscitation and Emergency Cardiovascular Care. *Circulation* 2015;132(suppl 2):S444–S464.

36. Bergum D, Haugen BO, Nordseth T, Mjølstad OC, Skogvoll E. Recognizing the causes of in-hospital cardiac arrest—A survival benefit. *Resuscitation* 2015;97:91–96. doi:10.1016/j.

37. Stevens RD, Shoykhet M, Cadena R. Emergency neurological life support: Intracranial hypertension and herniation. *Neurocrit Care* 2015;23:S76–S82.

38. Nolan JP, Neumar RW, Adrie C, et al. Post-cardiac arrest syndrome: Epidemiology, pathophysiology, treatment, and prognostication: A scientific statement from the International Liaison Committee on Resuscitation; the American Heart Association Emergency Cardiovascular Care Committee; the Council on Cardiovascular Surgery and Anesthesia; the Council on Cardiopulmonary, Perioperative, and Critical Care; the Council on Clinical Cardiology; the Council on Stroke. *Resuscitation* 2008;79(3):350–79.

39. Chair CWC; Donnino MW; Fink EL; Geocadin RG. Part 8: Post–Cardiac Arrest Care 2015 American Heart Association Guidelines Update for Cardiopulmonary Resuscitation and Emergency Cardiovascular Care. *Circulation* 2015;132(suppl 1):S465–S482.

40. Michael W. Donnino. Temperature Management After Cardiac Arrest. An Advisory Statement by the Advanced Life Support Task Force of the International Liaison Committee on Resuscitation and the American Heart Association Emergency Cardiovascular Care Committee and the Council on Cardiopulmonary, Critical Care, Perioperative and Resuscitation. *Circulation* 2015;132: 2448–56.

41. Patroniti N. Post-cardiac arrest extracorporeal life support. *Best Pract Res Clin Anaesthesiol* 2015;29(4):497–508.

Part IX

Renal Care

Editor: Mohan Gurjar

38

Acute Kidney Injury

M. Gurjar and D. S. Bhadauria

ABSTRACT

Renal dysfunction, often encountered in critically ill patients has an impact on patient outcome. Updation with recent definitions, its limitations, role of newer biomarkers, and brain-kidney crosstalk is essential. Managing neurological critically ill patients with acute kidney injury (AKI) poses multiple challenges; including fluid and electrolyte management, presence of coagulopathy, use of hyperosmolar medication, radiographic contrast, dose adjustment of various drugs and nutrition. Also, there is a need of follow-up after AKI, as AKI and chronic kidney disease (CKD) are now recognized as related entities and probably represents a continuum of the disease process.

KEYWORDS

Renal dysfunction; critical care; acute kidney injury (AKI); neurological patient; biomarkers.

INTRODUCTION

Renal dysfunction is not uncommon in critically ill patients, including neurological patients. In the last 10–15 years our understanding about acute deterioration of renal function is much better with ever evolving clarity on its definition, pathophysiology as well as short- and long-term renal and patient outcome. There is scarcity of literature on acute kidney injury (AKI) specific for neurological patients.

DEFINITIONS, LIMITATIONS, AND NOVEL BIOMARKERS

Definitions

In 2004, the second international consensus conference of the acute dialysis quality initiative group proposed a classification scheme for acute renal failure (ARF), called 'RIFLE': **R**isk of renal dysfunction, **I**njury to the kidney, **F**ailure of kidney function, **L**oss of kidney function, and **E**nd-stage kidney disease (Table 38.1).[1] This classification is based on changes in glomerular filtration rate (GFR), serum creatinine (SCr) and/or urine output. In the RIFLE classification, first three—Risk, Injury, and Failure—are three levels of renal dysfunction, wherein the worst changes in SCr or urine output is used; and loss of kidney function and end-stage kidney disease are two clinical outcomes defined by the duration of loss of kidney function.

The concept of AKI defined in the RIFLE criteria was introduced to encompass the entire spectrum of ARF syndrome. In earlier literature, ARF was defined by more than 30 different definitions. The introduction of AKI terminology was the benchmark in recent literature, which had replaced the term ARF.

In further improving the definition and increasing sensitivity to identify more individuals at risk of AKI, a larger, multidisciplinary international group (AKI Network [AKIN]) proposed few modifications to the original RIFLE criteria known as AKIN criteria (2007).[2] In the AKIN criteria, 'Risk', 'Injury' and 'Failure' are replaced by Stage 1, Stage 2, and Stage 3, respectively (Table 38.2). Additionally in this criteria, Stage 1 (Risk) also includes an increase in SCr of at least 0.3 mg/dL within 48 hours; and for Stage 3 (Failure), the patient who received renal replacement therapy (RRT) regardless of SCr or urine output.

However, in a comparison of the RIFLE and AKIN criteria for diagnosis and classification of AKI among 120,123 intensive care unit (ICU) patients, the AKIN

Table 38.1 The RIFLE criteria for acute kidney injury (AKI)

Severity of renal dysfunction		Glomerular filtration rate (GFR) criteria	Urine output (UO) criteria
Increasing Severity	Risk	↑ SCr × 1.5 OR ↓ GFR >25%	UO <0.5 ml/kg/hr × 6 hr
	Injury	↑ SCr × 2 OR ↓ GFR >50%	UO <0.5 ml/kg/hr × 12 hr
	Failure	↑ SCr × 3 or ↓ GFR >75% or SCr >4mg/dL	UO <0.3 ml/kg/hr × 24 hr OR Anuria × 12 hr
	Loss	Persistent failure (complete loss) of kidney function >4 weeks	
	End-stage	End-stage kidney disease >3 months	

Note: For describing 'Failure', if classification defined by serum creatinine (SCr), use RIFLE-F$_C$; while RIFLE-F$_O$ should be used for classification achieved by urine output criteria.

Table 38.2 Acute kidney injury network (AKIN) criteria to classify AKI

Severity of renal dysfunction		Serum creatinine (SCr) criteria	Urine output (UO) criteria
Increasing Severity	Stage 1	↑ SCr × 1.5 OR ↑ ≥0.3 mg/dL in SCr	UO <0.5 ml/kg/hr × 6 hr
	Stage 2	↑ SCr × 2	UO <0.5 ml/kg/hr × 12 hr
	Stage 3	↑ SCr × 3 OR ↑ ≥0.5 mg/dL if baseline SCr > 4 mg/dL OR	UO <0.3 ml/kg/hr × 24 hr or Anuria × 12 hr or
		Patient who receive RRT (irrespective of the stage as per SCr or UO at the time of RRT)	

criteria did not improve sensitivity, robustness, and predictive ability of the definition and classification of AKI in the first 24 hours after admission to the ICU (AKIN Stage I and II, 18.1% and 10.1% vs RIFLE category 'R' and 'I' 16.2% and 13.6%).[3]

Currently, as per the Kidney Disease Improving Global Outcomes (KDIGO) clinical practice guideline for AKI published in March 2012, AKI is defined as any of the following:[4]

i. Increase in SCr by ≥0.3 mg/dL (≥26.5 µmol/L) within 48 hours; or
ii. Increase in SCr to ≥1.5 times the baseline, which is known or presumed to have occurred within the prior 7 days; or
iii. Urine volume <0.5 ml/kg/hr for 6 hours.

Limitations

The KDIGO also stressed the need of a single definition for practice and research; although in real time diagnosing AKI may not be possible with one of the definitions. Also, clinician may not know baseline SCr of the patient when presented with raised levels, which may lead to difficulty in distinguishing AKI from chronic kidney disease (CKD). Table 38.3 highlights a few case scenarios regarding the clinical application of the present definition.

It is not only limitation with the definition but also considering SCr in the definition as it is well-known that SCr is affected by some factors: non-modifiable (age, gender, and race) and modifiable (diet, muscle mass, exercise, some drugs, and volume status). Also, SCr level is a late reflection of deteriorating kidney function; as its

Table 38.3   Clinical application of definitions in the diagnosis of AKI

| Case | Serum creatinine (SCr) (mg/dL) | | | | | AKI diagnosis | |
	Baseline	Day 1	Day 2	Day 3	Day 7	Criteria 1 (≥0.3 mg/dL rise ≤48 hr)	Criteria 2 (50% rise from baseline)
a	0.5	0.6	0.7	0.8	0.7	No	Yes
b	1.0	1.1	1.2	1.3	1.6	No	Yes
c	0.9	0.9	1.1	1.2	1.3	Yes	No
d	Not known	2.2	1.9	1.2	1.1	No	Yes
e	Not known	1.5	1.6	1.8	1.7	Yes	Not known
f	Not known	2.5	2.4	2.3	2.0	No	Not known

level is insensitive to small changes in GFR and requires a decrease in GFR by >50% for an increase in SCr level, which occurs over 48–72 hours.[4,5]

Novel Biomarkers

In order to overcome the limitations of creatinine, in recent years, some biomarkers for AKI have been identified. Commonly studied biomarkers for AKI are: Neutrophil Gelatinase-Associated Lipocalin (NGAL), Kidney Injury Molecule (KIM-1), Cystatin C, and Interleukin-18.[6,7] Levels of NGAL rise as early as two hours after insult on the kidney. The diagnostic accuracy of these biomarkers for early diagnosis of AKI has been evaluated in some cohort of patients like post-cardiac surgery, post-renal transplant, patients having sepsis, cirrhosis, etc. Recent meta-analysis has shown that NGAL levels (both plasma and urine) had good diagnostic accuracy for early diagnosis of AKI after radiographic contrast exposure as well as among septic patients.[8,9] In some studies, it has also been shown that these biomarkers have a potential role in predicting the need of renal replacement therapy and mortality.[9]

EPIDEMIOLOGY, RISK FACTORS, AND OUTCOMES

The incidence of AKI from 9,449 trauma ICU patients is reported up to 18%.[10] Old age, female gender, presence of co-morbid illness and greater illness severity were at high risk for developing AKI. In these patients, each RIFLE category was independently associated with higher hospital mortality.[10]

In two different cohorts of neurological patients, 136 patients with severe traumatic brain injury (TBI) and 787 patients with aneurysmal subarachnoid haemorrhage (SAH), the incidence of AKI was found almost similar (23%).[11,12] In both studies, presence of AKI was associated with higher mortality.

Among stroke patients, 528 ischaemic and 829 intracerebral haemorrhage (ICH), incidence of AKI was 14% and 21%, respectively.[13] Acute kidney injury was associated with increased hospital mortality from ischaemic stroke (odds ratio [OR] 3.08; 95% confidence interval [CI] 1.49–6.35) but ICH was not (OR 0.82; 95% CI 0.50–1.35), even after adjusting for age, gender, race, and presence of other risk factors. Though, in the subset analysis of ICH patients who stayed >2 days, AKI was found to be associated with higher in-hospital mortality (OR 2.11; 95% CI 1.18–3.77).

In another study of 311 patients after resuscitation from out-of-hospital cardiac arrest, renal dysfunction was present in more than one-third patients (37%).[14] In this study, the presence of AKI requiring RRT was not found an independent predictor of survival.

In general, ICU patients admitted with sepsis, concomitant AKI is common during the first 24 hours of admission. Of 120,123 patients admitted in different ICUs from Australia, 33,375 had sepsis (27.8%); and among septic patients, 14,039 (42.1%) had concomitant AKI (septic AKI).[15] In comparison to non-septic AKI, septic AKI was associated with greater severity of AKI as per the RIFLE category, and also associated with longer duration of stay as well as higher mortality in the ICU across all strata of RIFLE categories.

Other than sepsis, common causes of AKI in critically ill patients admitted with normal renal functions include drugs (like aminoglycosides, amphotericin B, vancomycin, mannitol, etc.) and radiographic contrast exposure. Mannitol has been found to be an independent risk factor of AKI after cerebral trauma. Incidence of contrast-induced AKI (CI-AKI) in ICU patients has been reported in up to one-third of the patients.[16]

On the other side, there are infections (malaria, leptospirosis, bacterial endocarditis, meningococcal sepsis) and diseases (hypertension, various vasculitic syndrome, haemolytic uremic syndrome, acute and chronic liver failure), which lead to both renal dysfunction as well as brain injury.[17] The patho-mechanism of renal dysfunction depends upon the underlying cause of AKI, which includes acute tubular necrosis, tubular apoptosis, hypovolaemia, hypotension, malignant hypertension, or vasculitis.

BRAIN–KIDNEY CROSSTALK

Like typical examples of interaction between two organs, hepato-renal syndrome and cardio-renal syndrome, there are enough evidences available through animal studies that injury of either brain or kidney can lead to changes in other organ functions called brain–kidney crosstalk. This brain–kidney crosstalk is beyond the presence of common risk factors for both organ dysfunction like age and other co-existing co-morbidities. Also, this crosstalk is independent of new risk exposure during the management of either brain or renal pathological conditions, for example mannitol use in cerebral trauma leads to AKI; and use of steroid in vasculitis-associated AKI leads to steroid-induced psychosis.

Due to brain–kidney crosstalk, in the presence of AKI, neurological manifestations may include headache, visual disturbance, tremor, myoclonus, seizures, stupor or coma. Mechanisms associated with cerebral dysfunction secondary to AKI include:[18]

- *Impaired blood–brain barrier integrity:* Due to increased cytokine effects (increased production and decreased renal clearance) there is complement cascade activation, increased humoral immune response and increased production of reactive oxygen species; uraemic toxin retention; and hyperosmolar state (via increase in vascular endothelial growth factor).
- *Neurotransmitter derangement:* Decrease in cerebral catecholamines (norepinephrine, epinephrine, and dopamine) and increase in plasma catecholamines.
- *Acid-base disturbance (metabolic acidosis):* Intracellular acidosis causes alteration in neurotransmitter balance with excess ammonia cycling between neurons and astrocytes; and increased influx of sodium and calcium into the cell leading to cellular injury and cell death. Acidosis milieu also leads to arteriolar vasodilatation and ultimately cerebral oedema.
- *Organic osmolyte and brain water disturbance:* Increase in plasma urea leads to increase in astrocyte and neuronal urea concentration and intracellular osmolality, which is initially compensated by efflux of sodium, potassium, calcium, and other organic anions. Once this mechanism is exhausted, especially in the

presence of intracellular acidosis, these cells swell up. There are contradictory results from animal models for brain water content in the presence of AKI.
- *Alteration of drug pharmacokinetics:* Drugs that are excreted renally may result in toxicity (including central nervous system [CNS]) due to drug accumulation if dosages are not adjusted accordingly. Down-regulation of cell membrane transporters, namely organic anion transporters (OATs) and adenosine triphosphate (ATP)-dependent P-glycoprotein transporters play a major role in decreasing drug clearance in the presence of AKI.
- *Inflammatory cascade:* There are three waves of inflammatory cascade: (1) within minutes of renal ischaemia, surge of uric acid; (2) exocytosis of Weibel–Palade bodies releasing pro-inflammatory mediators (endothelin-1, large multimers of von Willebrand factor, interleukin-8, and angiopoietin-2); and (3) release of high mobility group box 1 protein and deoxyribonucleic acid (DNA) binding protein which leads to intense inflammatory response within hours of AKI.

Although AKI results in a generalized systemic inflammatory cascade, there are some specific inflammatory reactions in the brain like increase in keratinocyte-derived chemoattractant and granulocyte colony-stimulating factor and glial fibrillary acidic protein. Interestingly, increase of glial fibrillary acidic protein in the brain has been found only after AKI and not after acute liver injury in animal models.

On the other side, acute brain injury could lead to renal dysfunction which may manifest as hyponatraemia, reduced renal glomerular perfusion, or even AKI.[18] These are explained as follows.

- *Hyponatraemia:* This electrolyte imbalance is commonly present in patients with acute SAH and post pituitary surgery. Though the mechanism behind hyponatraemia may be different, the patient may be having either syndrome of inappropriate antidiuretic hormone secretion (SIADH) or cerebral salt (sodium) wasting (CSW). Syndrome of inappropriate antidiuretic hormone secretion and CSW have many similarities; it is very difficult to differentiate the cause of hyponatremia, particularly in patients with neurological diseases. But still, it is also essential to differentiate between SIADH and CSW as their management differs in many ways. Characteristically, in both conditions urine sodium concentration may be higher or normal; but patients with SIADH are euvolaemic or hypervolaemic, and patients with CSW are typically hypovolaemic. It is difficult to differentiate solely on the basis of volume status of patients but measuring fractional excretion and serum urate, plasma rennin and aldosterone levels may be useful in distinguishing between SIADH and CSW.

- *Reduced renal glomerular perfusion:* Acute brain injury leads to increased visceral sympathetic nervous system activation that may cause reduced renal glomerular perfusion.
- *Acute kidney injury:* Through increased sympathetic nervous system activation, the presence of intravascular haemolysis due to sustained hypertension and red cell thrombi in the glomeruli may lead to AKI after brain injury.

Interestingly, it has been found that donor brain death influences acute vascular rejection after kidney transplant in a recipient.[19] After brain death in a donor, the kidney is affected by haemodynamic changes, neurohormonal activation, and inflammatory response which results in reduced allograft survival.[20,21]

GENERAL AND SPECIFIC MANAGEMENT ISSUES IN NEUROINTENSIVE CARE

The presence of renal dysfunction in critically ill neurological patients (stroke, seizure, and TBI) poses multiple challenges to clinicians. Fluid and electrolyte management, presence of coagulopathy, use of hyperosmolar medication, radiographic contrast, and dose adjustment of various drugs in the presence of AKI are some of them. Most of the suggestions and recommendations mentioned below are from KDIGO guidelines for AKI.[4]

- *Fluid for resuscitation:* Use of isotonic crystalloids is preferred over colloids (albumin or starches) as the initial management for expansion of intravascular volume in patients without shock at risk for AKI or with AKI. Consider vasopressors in conjunction with fluids in patients with vasomotor shock with or at risk for AKI. There should be protocol-based management of haemodynamic and oxygenation parameters to prevent development or worsening of AKI in high-risk patients in the perioperative setting or in patients with septic shock. In anuric or oliguric patients, not only volume of fluid but also composition of fluid is important, especially sodium, potassium, and chloride content.
- *Hyperosmolar therapy:* In the management of patients with elevated ICP secondary to ischaemic or haemorrhagic stroke, hypoxic ischaemic injury, or due to metabolic cause like acute liver failure, use

of mannitol as hyperosmolar therapy is one of the important interventions. In the presence of AKI, use of mannitol is not advised. Also, the safety of hypertonic saline which is being used more frequently nowadays to control raised ICP is not clear in patients having AKI.

- *Diuretics:* Diuretics should not be used to prevent AKI or enhance kidney function recovery. Also, a diuretic is not suited for treatment of AKI, except in the management of volume overload. One should not use low-dose dopamine or fenoldopam or atrial natriuretic peptide (ANP) to prevent or treat AKI.
- *Other nephrotoxic drugs:* Intravenous aminoglycosides should be avoided if necessary, then give once daily dose and monitor for drug levels. If amphotericin B is required, then use lipid formulations of amphotericin B rather than conventional formulations.
- *N-acetylcysteine (NAC):* There should be no routine use of NAC for prevention of AKI in critically ill patients with hypotension or postsurgical AKI.
- *Contrast-induced AKI (CI-AKI):* For prevention of CI-AKI, use either iso-osmolar or low-osmolar iodinated contrast media with the lowest possible dose, rather than high-osmolar contrast media. Also, use intravenous isotonic sodium chloride along with NAC or isotonic sodium bicarbonate solution. If feasible, for the given clinical condition, give 3 ml/kg of normal saline over 1 hour before contrast exposure, then give 1 ml/kg for the next 4–6 hours. For example, in a 60 kg patient, give 200 ml of normal saline over 1 hour pre-contrast, then give the remaining 300 ml volume at 50–60 ml/hour. For prevention of CI-AKI do not use theophylline or fenoldopam. Also, do not use prophylactic intermittent haemodialysis (IHD) or hemofiltration (HF) for contrast-media removal.
- *Renal replacement therapy:* To start RRT, consider the broader clinical context, not single blood urea nitrogen (BUN) and/or creatinine thresholds alone. Consider for continuous renal replacement therapy (CRRT) rather than standard intermittent RRT for haemodynamically unstable patients. Use of CRRT is also preferred over intermittent RRT for AKI patients with acute brain injury or other causes of increased ICP or generalized brain oedema; as intermittent RRT increases ICP and decreases cerebral perfusion pressure (CPP). Intermittent RRT has also been found with higher mortality in a neurosurgical cohort of patients when compared with continuous dialysis, but choice is dependent on other factors also. (See Chapter 39, 'Renal Replacement Therapy'.) The dose of RRT to be delivered should be prescribed before starting each session of RRT.

- *Dialysis catheter:* While initiating RRT, use an uncuffed non-tunnelled dialysis catheter rather than a tunnelled catheter under ultrasound guidance and obtain a chest X-ray if the site is in a vein in the neck region. The choice of catheter site should be right jugular vein > femoral vein > left jugular vein > subclavian vein with preference for the dominant side. Do not use topical antibiotics over the skin insertion site or antibiotic locks for prevention of catheter-related infections of non-tunnelled dialysis.

- *Anticoagulants during dialysis:* If there is no contraindication for anticoagulation, then use either unfractionated or low-molecular weight heparin during intermittent RRT; and use preferably regional citrate anticoagulation instead of either unfractionated or low-molecular-weight heparin during CRRT. In patients with increased risk of bleeding, use regional citrate anticoagulation and do not use regional heparinization during CRRT. In patients with heparin-induced thrombocytopenia (HIT), heparin must be stopped and direct thrombin inhibitors such as argatroban used during RRT.

- *Dialysate buffer:* Use bicarbonate rather than lactate as a buffer in dialysate and replacement fluid for RRT in patients with AKI and circulatory shock or liver failure.

- *Nutrition:* In a critically ill patient, provide nutrition preferentially via the enteral route in patients with AKI. Achieve a total energy intake of 20–30 kcal/kg/d in patients with any stage of AKI. Avoid restriction of protein intake with the aim of preventing or delaying initiation of RRT. Administer 0.8–1.0 g/kg/d of protein in non-catabolic AKI patients without the need for dialysis; 1.0–1.5 g/kg/d in patients with AKI on RRT; and up to a maximum of 1.7 g/kg/d in patients on CRRT and in hypercatabolic patients. Insulin therapy could be considered to target plasma glucose below 180 mg/dL.

RECOVERY FOLLOW-UP

There is a need for follow-up after AKI, as AKI and chronic kidney disease (CKD) are now recognized as related entities and probably represent a continuum of the disease process. In a 2017 consensus statement by Acute Disease Quality Initiative (ADQI), the term acute kidney disease (AKD) has been proposed to define the course of disease after AKI.[22] Definitions:

- *Rapid reversal of AKI:* Complete reversal of AKI by KDIGO criteria within 48 hours of AKI onset.

- *Acute kidney disease (AKD):* Acute or subacute damage and/or loss of kidney function for a duration between 7 and 90 days after exposure to an AKI initiating

event. Outcome of AKD includes recovery, recurrence of AKI, progression of AKD and/or death. Stages 1, 2, and 3 of AKD are defined the same as for AKIN criteria. Stage 0 AKD is where reduced SCr is still higher than baseline but 1.5 times below Stage 0C AKD: SCr level <1.5 times baseline but not back to baseline level. Stage 0B AKD: continued evidence of ongoing injury/repair and/or indicators of loss of renal glomerular or tubular reserve. Stage 0A AKD: when there is absence of criteria for 0B and 0C AKD.

- *Chronic kidney disease (CKD):* Acute kidney disease that persists beyond 90 days is considered to be chronic kidney disease. These patients still have chances of renal recovery. Stage 0C CKD, where SCr does not come back to baseline, but within 1.5 times the baseline level. Stage 0B CKD, where SCr level returned to baseline, but still shows evidence of ongoing damage/injury (like elevated biomarkers) or loss of renal reserve. Stage 0A CKD, where there is no structural or damage markers for AKD present.

CONCLUSIONS

As per the KDIGO clinical practice guidelines, increase in SCr by as small as ≥0.3 mg/dL (≥26.5 μmol/l) within 48 hours is considered as AKI. It has been found that injury of either brain or kidney can lead to changes in other organ functions called brain–kidney crosstalk. Presence of AKI in critically ill neurological patients poses multiple challenges to clinicians, including fluid and electrolyte management, presence of coagulopathy, use of hyperosmolar medication, radiographic contrast, and dose adjustment of various drugs. Severity of AKI is independently associated with higher hospital mortality. Survivors need follow-up after discharge, as AKI and CKD are now recognized as related entities and probably represents a continuum of the disease process.

REFERENCES

1. Bellomo R, Ronco C, Kellum JA, Mehta RL, Palevsky P. Acute Dialysis Quality Initiative workgroup. Acute renal failure - definition, outcome measures, animal models, fluid therapy and information technology needs: the Second International Consensus Conference of the Acute Dialysis Quality Initiative (ADQI) Group. *Crit Care* 2004;8(4): R204–12.

2. Mehta RL, Kellum JA, Shah SV, et al. Acute Kidney Injury Network. Acute Kidney Injury Network: report of an initiative to improve outcomes in acute kidney injury. *Crit Care* 2007;11(2):R31.

3. Bagshaw SM, George C, Bellomo R. ANZICS Database Management Committee. A comparison of the RIFLE

and AKIN criteria for acute kidney injury in critically ill patients. *Nephrol Dial Transplant* 2008;23(5):1569–74.

4. Kidney Disease: Improving Global Outcomes (KDIGO) Acute Kidney Injury Work Group. KDIGO clinical practice guideline for acute kidney injury. *Kidney Int Suppl* 2012;2(1):1–138.

5. Slocum JL, Heung M, Pennathur S. Marking renal injury: can we move beyond serum creatinine? *Transl Res* 2012;159(4):277–89.

6. Schiffl H, Lang SM. Update on biomarkers of acute kidney injury: moving closer to clinical impact? *Mol Diagn Ther* 2012;16(4):199–207.

7. Fuhrman DY, Kellum JA. Biomarkers for Diagnosis, Prognosis and Intervention in Acute Kidney Injury. *Contrib Nephrol* 2016;187:47–54.

8. Tong J, Li H, Zhang H, et al. Neutrophil gelatinase-associated lipocalin in the prediction of contrast-induced nephropathy: a systemic review and meta-analysis. *J Cardiovasc Pharmacol* 2015;66(3):239–45.

9. Zhang A, Cai Y, Wang PF, et al. Diagnosis and prognosis of neutrophil gelatinase-associated lipocalin for acute kidney injury with sepsis: a systematic review and meta-analysis. *Crit Care* 2016;20:41.

10. Bagshaw SM, George C, Gibney RT, Bellomo R. A multi-center evaluation of early acute kidney injury in critically ill trauma patients. *Ren Fail* 2008;30(6):581–9.

11. Li N, Zhao WG, Zhang WF. Acute kidney injury in patients with severe traumatic brain injury: implementation of the acute kidney injury network stage system. *Neurocrit Care* 2011;14(3):377–81.

12. Zacharia BE, Ducruet AF, Hickman ZL, et al. Renal dysfunction as an independent predictor of outcome after aneurysmal subarachnoid hemorrhage: a single-center cohort study. *Stroke* 2009;40(7):2375–81.

13. Khatri M, Himmelfarb J, Adams D, Becker K, Longstreth WT, Tirschwell DL. Acute kidney injury is associated with increased hospital mortality after stroke. *J Stroke Cerebrovasc Dis* 2014;23(1):25–30.

14. Yanta J, Guyette FX, Doshi AA, Callaway CW, Rittenberger JC. Post cardiac arrest service. Renal dysfunction is common following resuscitation from out-of-hospital cardiac arrest. *Resuscitation* 2013;84(10):1371–4.

15. Bagshaw SM, George C, Bellomo R. ANZICS Database Management Committee. Early acute kidney injury and sepsis: a multicentre evaluation. *Crit Care* 2008;12(2):R47.

16. McCullough PA, Choi JP, Feghali GA, et al. Contrast-Induced Acute Kidney Injury. *J Am Coll Cardiol* 2016; 68(13):1465–73.

17. Davenport A. Renal replacement therapy in the patient with acute brain injury. *Am J Kidney Dis* 2001;37(3):457–66.

18. Nongnuch A, Panorchan K, Davenport A. Brain-kidney crosstalk. *Crit Care* 2014;18(3):225.

19. Sánchez-Fructuoso AI, Prats D, Marques M, et al. Does donor brain death influence acute vascular rejection in the kidney transplant? *Transplantation* 2004;78(1):142–6.

20. Morariu AM, Schuurs TA, Leuvenink HG, van Oeveren W, Rakhorst G, Ploeg RJ. Early events in kidney donation: progression of endothelial activation, oxidative stress and tubular injury after brain death. *Am J Transplant* 2008; 8(5):933–41.

21. Morrissey PE, Monaco AP. Donation after circulatory death: current practices, ongoing challenges, and potential improvements. *Transplantation* 2014;97(3):258–64.

22. Chawla LS, Bellomo R, Bihorac A, et al. Acute Disease Quality Initiative Workgroup 16. Acute kidney disease and renal recovery: consensus report of the Acute Disease Quality Initiative (ADQI) 16 Workgroup. *Nat Rev Nephrol* 2017;13(4):241–57.

39

Renal Replacement Therapy

D. S. Bhadauria and M. Gurjar

ABSTRACT

Neurointensive care patients may develop renal dysfunction, severe enough to require renal replacement therapy (RRT) either because of multiple traumatic injuries or brain injury secondary to systemic illness that also leads to kidney injury. Extracorporeal therapy in these patients is challenging as it may exacerbate preexisting brain injury by influencing haemodynamic and osmolar alterations. The type of renal replacement therapy in this subgroup of patients is an area of great debate because of the pros and cons associated with each type of extracorporeal therapy. Conventional intermittent haemodialysis is potentially known to increase intracranial pressure by increase in brain water content and worsening of preexisting haemorrhage because of anticoagulation of the extracorporeal circuit. While taking care of these patients, physicians should be aware of the physiological aspects of intracranial pressure (ICP) and cerebral blood flow (CBF), and how extracorporeal therapy influences these patients.

KEYWORDS

Neurologic patients; renal dysfunction; renal replacement therapy (RRT); haemodialysis; extracorporeal therapy; neurointensive care.

INTRODUCTION

Neurointensive care includes a wide spectrum of conditions related to neurology and patient populations, including patients with primary neurological disease as well as those with neurological complications arising out of medical or surgical illness. These patients at onset may have either normal renal function or preexisting renal dysfunction. These patients may require renal replacement therapy (RRT) due to severe worsening of renal function, which could be because of multiple traumatic injuries or brain injury secondary to systemic illness that also leads to kidney injury. They are also at risk of acute kidney injury (AKI) due to exposure to radiocontrast agents, sepsis, nephrotoxic drugs to treat sepsis and nonsteroidal anti-inflammatory drugs.

Acute kidney injury could be prevented by maintenance of hydration, an important clinical goal for preventing AKI, particularly due to contrast-induced nephropathy. Other measures are avoidance of multiple contrast exposure by selecting other imaging techniques wherever possible, and avoidance of nephrotoxic drugs if possible.[1] Prevention and general management of AKI is discussed in the previous chapter in detail.

Extracorporeal therapy in the neurointensive care patient is challenging as it may exacerbate preexisting brain injury by influencing haemodynamic and osmolar alterations. Conventional intermittent haemodialysis (intermittent HD, or IHD) is potentially known to increase intracranial pressure (ICP) by increase in brain water content, even in patients undergoing regular and stable maintenance HD.[2] Anticoagulation in the extracorporeal circuit could potentiate further haemorrhage. So the type of RRT in this subgroup of patients is an area of great debate among nephrologists and intensivists because of the pros and cons associated with each type of extracorporeal therapy. The physicians taking care of critically ill neurological patients require special training and knowledge about the physiological aspects of ICP, cerebral blood flow (CBF), and how extracorporeal therapy influences these patients.

This chapter reviews the role of RRT, its type, and its impact on neurointensive care patients with AKI.

PHYSIOLOGICAL CHANGES IN THE BRAIN DURING RENAL REPLACEMENT THERAPY

Intracranial compliance is an important consideration that complicates neurointensive care of patients. The cranium has a fixed volume inside, and the pressure–volume relationship is in a state of equilibrium and this is known as Monro–Kellie doctrine. This is a relationship between ICP; volume of brain tissue, blood, cerebrospinal fluid (CSF), and cerebral perfusion pressure (CPP). A change in volume of constituents of the cranium is compensated by reverse alteration in the volume of another mean increase in ICP and must cause a decline in CPP.[3]

Renal replacement therapy is beneficial for improving encephalopathy due to retention of azotaemic products causing uraemia by removing them and reducing toxic drug levels. However, it may cause paradoxical increase in ICP due to cerebral oedema or adversely affect this subgroup of patients by a different mechanism.

Rapid Removal of Urea

A rise in ICP could be because of dialysis disequilibrium syndrome in patients of IHD. However uremic patients also develop an increase in brain water content on treatment with IHD which leads to rise in ICP significantly in patients with cerebral oedema.[4,5] This phenomenon is akin to dialysis disequilibrium syndrome[6] seen soon after initiation of HD with a low sodium dialysate in severely uremic patients. Previously, this was thought to be due to rapid removal of urea from the plasma with little and slower losses from the CSF and brain creating an osmotic gradient and entry of water passing into the brain.[7] But later evaluation proved that the removal of urea from CSF is slower than that from plasma but urea removal was similar from the brain to that from plasma. In order to adapt for change in intracellular osmolality and prevent oedema, brain cell metabolism starts producing small molecular weight osmoles such as peptides, phosphate moieties, and other solutes known as idiogenic osmoles.[8]

INTRADIALYTIC HYPOTENSION

The ICP rises within the first hour of HD due to fall in blood pressure resulting in hypoperfusion of the brain and rebound rise in ICP. Avoidance of intradialytic hypotension is of utmost importance during IHD to minimize iatrogenic episodes of cerebral ischaemia.[3]

Supraphysiological Bicarbonate Concentration in Dialysate

Brain damage may be exacerbated in patients when undergoing IHD using high performance membrane dialyzers and dialysates having supraphysiological levels of bicarbonate. Higher dialysate bicarbonate concentrations ≥38 mmol/L may be detrimental as cerebrospinal pH is a little lower than that of blood under normal conditions and brain intracellular pH is still lower. This rapid increase in blood pH during dialysis sets up disturbances in equilibrium; as bicarbonate is being a charged molecule used to cross the cell membranes of cells slowly. So bicarbonate is used to get more chances of reacting with hydrogen ions in plasma water, which leads to the formation of carbon dioxide. This carbon dioxide then transverses the hydrophobic cell membranes rapidly and once again dissociates to generate hydrogen ions inside cells. This leads to paradoxical intracellular acidosis and generation of idiogenic osmoles intracellularly, hence increasing intracellular osmolality and increasing water entry into the cells. These paradoxical changes in cerebral acidity level (pH) affect the respiratory centre adversely, especially spontaneously breathing patients and increasing the risk and frequency of apnoeic episodes in this subgroup of patients.[6]

INDICATION OF RENAL REPLACEMENT THERAPY

The important issues in neurointensive care patients with AKI are timing, indications, and type of RRT. The emergency indications of RRT are refractory volume overload or pulmonary oedema, refractory metabolic acidosis, and refractory hyperkalaemia (K^+ >6.5 mEq/L), while planned indications could be oliguria for more than 24 hours, anuria for more than 12 hours, creatinine levels of more than 10.0 mg/dL and urea levels of more than 200 mg/dL.[9] The early initiation of RRT in critically ill patients is an issue of debate. It is still unclear whether early initiation without an emergency indication would provide any benefit to critically ill patients with AKI compared with late initiations of RRT. Two new randomized trials have evaluated this issue and found dramatically opposite outcomes.[10,11] Till further data are being made available, it is wise not to initiate RRT in critically ill patients without obvious clinical indications.

MODALITIES OF RENAL REPLACEMENT THERAPY

There are several modalities of RRT (Figure 39.1 and Table 39.1) in the armamentarium for the management of patients with AKI including IHD, 'hybrid' therapies

Table 39.1 Characteristic values in various forms of dialysis

Type of therapy	Transport mechanism	Urea clearance ml/min	UF lit/day
1. Intermittent haemodialysis	Diffusion + Convection	22–400	4–6
2. Slow extended dialysis	Diffusion + Convection	150–200	6–8
3. Continuous arteriovenous haemofilteration	Convection	7–10	0–12
4. Continuous venovenous haemofilteration	Convection	15–17	0–12
5. Continuous arteriovenous haemodiafiltration	Convection + Diffusion	16–39	4–12
6. Continuous venovenous haemodialysis	Convection + Diffusion	16–39	4–12
7. Peritoneal dialysis	Diffusion + Convection	12–17	1–3

Abbreviation: UF: Ultrafiltration.

such as sustained low-efficiency dialysis (SLED) and also known as extended duration dialysis (EDD) and continuous renal replacement therapy (CRRT), and peritoneal dialysis (PD).

Intermittent Haemodialysis

IHD is the principal mode of RRT in patients with AKI since a long time ago. The duration of single treatment session is 3 to 5 hours in various interval basis depending upon electrolyte disturbances, metabolic demands, metabolic acidosis, and volume status ranging from a schedule of twice weekly to alternate day or daily.[9]

The risk of intradialytic hypotension and cardiovascular instability during IHD can be decreased by cooling the dialysate to 35°C, and by increasing the dialysate sodium around 10 mEq/L above serum sodium[12] (Table 39.2). Measures like slowing down the IHD session with slower blood and dialysate flows, high dialysate sodium and cooling of dialysate may be as beneficial and prove equally effective as CRRT in prophylaxis against cerebral oedema. However, combinations of measures like prolonged intermittent RRT coupled with higher blood flow, warmed and low sodium dialysate may increase the risk of cerebral oedema.[13,14]

Continuous Renal Replacement Therapy

Continuous renal replacement therapy was developed to support patients who develop hypotension during conventional IHD, hence the primary indication of CRRT is haemodynamic instability. The CRRT includes a group of treatment modalities which are pump-driven and venovenous.[15] These modalities of venovenous CRRT differs from each other based on their principle solute removal: solute transport in continuous venovenous haemofiltration (CVVH) occurs by convection; solute transport in continuous venovenous haemodialysis (CVVHD) occurs by diffusion; solute transport in continuous venovenous haemodiafiltration (CVVHDF) occurs by convection and diffusion.[16] As such CRRTs are to be preferred in neurointensive care patients to slow down the rate of change in serum urea and bicarbonate to decrease the risk of brain oedema.[17,18]

Intracranial stability is better in CRRT than IHD because of much less changes in osmolality and urea and

Table 39.2 Precautions to be taken during haemodialysis in neurointensive care patients

Neurointensive condition	Target to be achieved	Clinical strategies
Cerebral oedema	Prevent hypotension	1. Minimum ultrafiltration rate 2. Blood volume monitoring 3. Long dialysis sessions 4. Cool dialysate temperature
	Keep serum urea <15 mmol/L	1. Daily dialysis sessions
	Keep serum sodium >145 mmol/L	1. High dialysate sodium
	Reduction of fall in plasma osmolality	1. Slower blood pump speed 2. Smaller surface area dialyzer 3. Bolus of hypertonic saline
Intracranial haemorrhage	Avoidance of anticoagulation during haemodialysis	1. Anticoagulation-free HD session or regional anticoagulation

bicarbonate levels.[19] This greater intracranial stability is also contributed by greater cardiovascular stability provided by CRRT and could be because of the important factor of thermal losses observed in this modality.[20]

Hybrid Therapies

The hybrid modalities are modified RRT provided by conventional haemodialysis machines for extended time duration with lower blood and dialysate flow rates.[21] A host of terms have been used for these therapies, including SLED, EDD, and sustained low-efficiency daily diafiltration (SLEDD-f). Solute clearance is enhanced by extending the duration of dialysis treatment while haemodynamic tolerability is provided by slower ultrafiltration. The amount of metabolic control and haemodynamic stability achieved with these hybrid therapies is comparable to that seen with CRRT.[22] However, there is paucity of data upon the use of this modality and its influence in neurointensive care patients.

Peritoneal Dialysis

Peritoneal dialysis (PD) is a continuous form of RRT and associated with slower solute clearances and more haemodynamic stability than IHD. As it is less efficient as a dialysis modality to provide adequate solute clearance, it may be less useful in hypercatabolic patients. It can also lead to worsening of brain oedema in neurointensive care patients because all the commercially available dialysate fluids are hyponatraemic and have high glucose content, with risk of exacerbating hyperglycaemia. Hypertonic glucose dialysate instillation and drainage can cause a decrease in right atrial filling, with subsequent reduction in cardiac output and decline in cerebral perfusion.[18,23]

In acute PD, pulmonary functions are compromised because of the instillation of large volumes into the peritoneal cavity. This results in a net reduction in PaO_2 because of increase in alveolar-arterial oxygen gradient and basal atelectasis.[24] In addition to this, cardiovascular instability may result because of sudden alteration in intraperitoneal volume due to draining out of fluid and resultant changes in cardiac filling pressures and systemic vascular resistance.[3] Tidal dialysis is the preferred mode of PD to minimize changes in plasma volume and stabilize cardiovascular and hence intracranial stability.[3]

SPECIFIC MANAGEMENT ISSUE RELATED TO ANTICOAGULATION DURING RENAL REPLACEMENT THERAPY

Systemic anticoagulation in neurointensive care is risky, particularly in patients with acute brain injury as they may develop intracerebral haemorrhage. Anticoagulant-free dialysis is possible for a short session of IHD but not for CRRT. For CRRT anticoagulation-free dialysis is cumbersome, yet possible by diluting the blood before entry into the dialyzer.[23] Regional anticoagulants, rather systemic anticoagulation should be used for the extracorporeal circuit, if required.[24] The most effective regional anticoagulants are citrate and prostacyclin.[25] Prostacyclin should be used cautiously as being a potent vasodilator it may cause a rise in ICP by the reduction of cerebral perfusion pressure.[26]

Regional Citrate Anticoagulation

This consists of continuous infusion of trisodium citrate solution (102 mmol/L) which is isoosmolar, into the arterial side of the dialyzer.[27] This leads to a fall in the free plasma calcium concentration because of binding of calcium to citrate, hence preventing the propagation of anticoagulation cascade. The dialyzer removes the citrate-calcium complex. The activated clotting time is kept above 200 seconds by adjusting the citrate infusion rate. The infusion of 5% calcium chloride into the venous return line at a rate of 0.5 ml/min is used to reverse this regional anticoagulation. Frequent plasma monitoring is important to prevent hypocalcaemia or hypercalcemia.[27]

COMPLICATIONS FROM HAEMODIALYSIS

Complications from HD include hypotension; nausea; vomiting; dialysis disequilibrium syndrome; muscle cramps; cardiac events such as arrhythmias, ischaemia; and sudden cardiac death; dialyzer reaction; hypoglycaemia; haemolysis; blood leak into the dialyzer; clotting of dialyzer circuit; and air embolism.

CONCLUSIONS

Continuous renal replacement therapy by virtue of providing cardiovascular and intracranial stability is the modality of choice in neurointensive care patients. Need of anticoagulation is a drawback of CRRT as systemic anticoagulants may provoke intracerebral haemorrhage. If anticoagulation is required, then regional anticoagulation is the choice. Peritoneal dialysis does not need anticoagulation but suboptimal solute clearances and cardiovascular followed by intracranial instability because of sudden changes in intraperitoneal volume are drawbacks. Intermittent HD may result in cerebral oedema and rise in ICP. Preventive measures like priming the circuit, change in electrolyte composition and temperature of the dialysate, and reduction in treatment time may provide cardiovascular and hence intracranial stability.

REFERENCES

1. Arkom Nongnuch, Kwanpeemai Panorchan, Andrew Davenport. *Critical Care* 2014;18(225):2–11.

2. Floerchinger B, Oberhuber R, Tullius SG. Effects of brain death on organ quality and transplant outcome. *Transplant Rev (Orlando)* 2012;26:54–59.

3. Davenport A. Renal replacement therapy in the patient with acute brain injury. *Am J Kidney Dis* 2001;37:457–66.

4. Khatri M, Himmelfarb J, Adams D, Becker K, Longstreth WT, Tirschwell DL. Acute kidney injury is associated with increased hospital mortality after stroke. *J Stroke Cerebrovasc Dis* 2014;23:25–30.

5. Silk DBA, Trewby PN, Chase RA, et al. Treatment of fulminant hepatic failure by polyacrylonitrile membrane hemodialysis. *Lancet* 1977;2:1–3.

6. Rosen SM, O'Connor K, Shaldon S. Hemodialysis disequilibrium syndrome. *BMJ* 1964;2:672–5.

7. Kennedy AC, Linton AL, Luke RG, Renfrew S, Dinwoodie A. The pathogenesis and prevention of cerebral dysfunction during dialysis. *Lancet* 1964;1:790–3.

8. Arieff AI. Dialysis disequilibrium syndrome: Current concepts on pathogenesis and prevention. *Kidney Int* 1994; 45:629–35.

9. Fry AC, Farrington K. Management of acute renal failure. *Postgraduate Medical Journal* 2006;82(964):106–116. doi:10.1136/pgmj.2005.038588.

10. Gaudry S, Hajage D, Schortgen F, et al. Initiation strategies for renal-replacement therapy in the intensive care unit. *N Engl J Med* 2016;375(2):122.

11. Zarbock A, Kellum JA, Schmidt C, et al. Effect of early vs delayed initiation of renal replacement therapy on mortality in critically ill patients with acute kidney injury: The ELAIN randomized clinical trial. *JAMA* 2016;315(20):2190.

12. Vinsonneau C, Camus C, Combes A, et al. Hemodiafe Study Group: Continuous venovenous haemodiafiltration versus intermittent haemodialysis for acute renal failure in patients with multiple organ dysfunction syndrome: a multicentre randomised trial. *Lancet* 2006;68:379–85.

13. Wu VC, Huang TM, Shiao CC, et al. NSARF Group: The hemodynamic effects during sustained low-efficiency dialysis versus continuous veno-venous hemofiltration for uremic patients with brain hemorrhage: a crossover study. *J Neurosurg* 2013;119:1288–95.

14. Davenport A. Changing the hemodialysis prescription for hemodialysis patients with subdural and intracranial hemorrhage. *Hemodial Int* 2013;17:S22–S27.

15. Wendon J, Smithies M, Sheppard M, et al. Continuous high volume venous-venous haemofiltration in acute renal failure. *Intensive Care Med* 1989;15:358–63.

16. Ronco C, Bellomo R. Basic mechanisms and definitions for continuous renal replacement therapies. *Int J Artif Organs* 1996;19:95–99.

17. Davenport A. Renal replacement therapy in the patient with acute brain injury. *Am J Kidney Dis* 2001;37:457–66.

18. Davenport A, Will EJ, Davison AM. Continuous vs. intermittent forms of haemofiltration and/or dialysis in the management of acute renal failure in patients with defective cerebral autoregulation at risk of cerebral oedema. *Contrib Nephrol* 1991;93:225–33.

19. Davenport A, Will EJ, Losowsky MS, Swindells S. Continuous arteriovenous hemofiltration in patients with hepatic encephalopathy and renal failure. *BMJ* 1987;295:1028–34.

20. Yagi N, LeBlanc M, Sakai K, Wright EJ, Paganini EP. Cooling effect of continuous renal replacement therapies in critically ill patients. *Am J Kidney Dis* 1999;32:1023–30.

21. Tolwani AJ, Wheeler TS, Wille KM. Sustained low-efficiency dialysis. *Contrib Nephrol* 2007;156:320–4.

22. Kielstein JT, Kretschmer U, Ernst T, et al. Efficacy and cardiovascular tolerability of extended dialysis in critically ill patients: a randomized controlled study. *Am J Kidney Dis* 2004;43:342–9.

23. Sherlock M, O'Sullivan E, Agha A, et al. The incidence and pathophysiology of hyponatraemia after subarachnoid haemorrhage. *Clin Endocrinol (Oxf)* 2006;64:250–4.

24. DeBroe M, Lins RL, DeBacker WA. Pulmonary aspects of dialysis patients. In: Jacobs C, Kjellstrand CM, Koch KM, Winchester JF eds. *Replacement of Renal Function by Dialysis*. 4th ed. MA: Boston, Kluwer, 1996; pp. 1034–48.

25. Davenport A. The coagulation system in the critically ill patient with acute renal failure and the effect of an extracorporeal circuit. *Am J Kidney Dis* 1996;30(suppl 4): S20–S27.

26. Ward DM. The approach to anticoagulation in patients treated with extracorporeal therapy in the ICU. *Adv Ren Replace Ther* 1997;4:160–73.

27. Davenport A. Anticoagulation in patients with acute renal failure treated with continuous renal replacement therapies. *Home Hemodialysis Int* 1998;2:41–60.

Part X

Haematological Care

Editor: Altan Sahin

Part II

40

Anaemia

A. A. Yilbas

ABSTRACT

Anaemia, which is one of the most common clinical conditions in critical care patients, is usually associated with worse outcomes like organ hypoperfusion, multiorgan failure, and death. The acutely injured brain is more vulnerable to further neuronal damage caused by impaired oxygen delivery and in addition, the patients in critical care units have increased oxygen demand due to mechanical ventilation, sepsis, fever, and infections. Due to these reasons, the target haemoglobin (Hb) level for transfusion is usually accepted as 8–9 g/dL in neurointensive care. However, all patients should be evaluated individually according to their physiological status in order to balance the risks of transfusion and decreased oxygen content. Physiological indicators of ischaemia such as brain tissue oxygen tension (PbtO$_2$), cerebral microdialysis, and jugular venous oxygen saturation (SjvO$_2$) are recommended as supportive transfusion triggers instead of just the Hb level. This chapter discusses the reasons, physiological effects, and management of anaemia in specialized conditions of neurointensive care.

KEYWORDS

Anaemia; haemoglobin (Hb); oxygen delivery; transfusion; neurointensive care.

INTRODUCTION

Anaemia is one the most common clinical conditions in critical care patients including approximately two-thirds at the time of intensive care unit (ICU) admission.[1] The World Health Organization (WHO) defines anaemia as haemoglobin (Hb) and haematocrit concentrations less than 12 g/dL and 36% in women and 13 g/dL and 39% in men.[2]

The normal human brain is selectively protected against anaemia due to the cerebral autoregulation process. Studies on healthy volunteers have demonstrated that normal cerebral function can be preserved until Hb levels decrease to about 5–7 g/dL.[3] In critical care patients who have an increased oxygen demand due to mechanical ventilation, sepsis, fever, and infections anaemia is usually associated with worse outcomes like organ hypoperfusion, multiorgan failure, and death. Besides the risks of anaemia, transfusion has its own adverse effects such as transfusion-related acute lung injury, increased nosocomial infections, longer hospital stay, and being an important predictor

of mortality.[4] Due to these reasons, the usual current practice is a restrictive red blood cell transfusion strategy even up to Hb ≈7 g/dL in critical care patients without serious cardiac disease. However, the acutely injured brain is more vulnerable to further neuronal damage caused by impaired oxygen delivery. Actually the optimal Hb level to avoid secondary cerebral insults in neurocritical patients with diseases like traumatic brain injury (TBI), stroke, or subarachnoid haemorrhage (SAH) is still not known. All patients should be evaluated individually according to their physiological status in order to balance the risks of transfusion and decreased oxygen content, but the common clinical practice in neurocritical care patients is to have a target Hb level approximately at 8–9 g/dL.[1,5]

PHYSIOLOGICAL EFFECTS OF ANAEMIA

Cardiovascular Response

Heart rate and contractility increase as a response to the stimulation of the sympathetic nervous system due to decrease in aortic and chemotactic perception of Hb. The decreased viscosity of blood also causes an increase in venous return and stroke volume. Thus, the normal cardiovascular system responds to isovolaemic anaemia with increased cardiac output (CO), stroke volume, and blood pressure. Besides this, the blood flow is redistributed in favour of cerebral and coronary circulations instead of splanchnic circulation as a protective mechanism.[1,6]

Tissues are protected from falling oxygen delivery by this compensatory increase in CO. However, this mechanism may not work appropriately in neurointensive care patients. A fact to keep in mind is that many of the neurointensive care patients have concomitant cardiac diseases in routine clinical practice. Even in the absence of a pre-existing cardiac disease; left ventricular systolic dysfunction, increase in creatine kinase, regional wall motion abnormalities, and electrocardiographic changes have been reported after acute aneurysmal SAH. All these factors may prevent an appropriate increase in CO in response to anaemia.[7]

Normally, CO is regulated to have systemic oxygen delivery (DO_2) about five times the systemic oxygen consumption (VO_2). In a simple way, estimated VO_2 corresponds to 3 cm^3/kg and DO_2 is oxygen content times the cardiac output, which is approximately 7.5 cm^3/kg/min. When compensatory changes to increase DO_2 in response to anaemia fail and DO_2–VO_2 ratio becomes <2:1, the result is anaerobic metabolism and lactic acidosis. In chronic anaemia patients, compensation by increased CO is usually enough to maintain DO_2–VO_2 ratio of >2:1. For an adult critical care patient, the estimated 3:1 DO_2–VO_2 would be approximately at a haemoglobin 10 g/dL and haematocrit 30%. However, in critical care patients resting VO_2 is usually higher than normal due to systemic inflammatory response and compensation to anaemia may require even greater CO increases in such cases. For example, in sepsis VO_2 increases up to 6 cm^3/kg. It could be challenging to cope with the increased workload on the heart, especially in situations of increased tissue demand like infections, surgical stress, and fever. The result may easily be extreme hypoxia or acute cardiac failure.[1,7,8]

Cerebral Oxygen Delivery and Cerebrovascular Response

Cerebral blood flow (CBF) and Hb are the major factors that affect cerebral oxygen delivery (cDO_2). The cDO_2 can be expressed by the following formula:

$$cDO_2 \text{ (mlO}_2\text{/min)} = [\text{CBF (L/min)} \times \text{Hb (g/dL)} \times \text{oxygen saturation (SaO}_2\text{) (\%)} \times 1.39 \text{ (mlO}_2\text{/gHb)}] + (0.003 \times \text{pressure of arterial oxygen [PaO}_2\text{])}$$

Cerebral perfusion pressure (CPP) can be defined as the difference between mean arterial pressure and cerebral venous pressure. Cerebral blood flow (CBF) is not just directly proportional to mean arterial pressure (MAP) due to cerebral autoregulation mechanisms which cause vasoconstriction of cerebral arterioles in response to raised CPP and vasodilation in response to decreased CPP. This means, the brain can maintain constant CBF through wide ranges of CPP and MAP. Similarly, reduction in blood oxygen content and decreased blood viscosity in anaemia causes cerebral vasodilation and increase in CBF to preserve oxygen delivery.[7,9] This vasodilation occurs due to the increased sympathetic activation of presynaptic β_2 adrenergic receptors and nitric oxide (NO) synthesis from the perivascular cerebral neurons. Nitric oxide is a vasodilating mediator that has been proven to regulate the increase in CBF in conditions like anaemia, hypoxia, hypercarbia, and acidosis.[10,11] Hypoxia inducible factor (HIF)-1α is also another regulator of oxygen homoeostasis which increases in the cerebral cortex because of anaemia. Increased NO stabilizes HIF-1α by limiting its degradation and so many neuroprotective mechanisms including glycolysis, angiogenesis, and stem cell proliferation are activated. Vascular endothelial growth factor (VEGF), erythropoietin (EPO), and inducible nitric oxide synthase (iNOS) are among the other biochemical mediators that take part in potential protective mechanisms of the cerebral cortex due to anaemia. However, most of these mediators have also experimentally demonstrated harmful effects via excitotoxicity, increased reactive oxygen species, apoptosis, inflammation or increased vascular permeability of the blood–brain barrier.[9]

There are many other physiological changes that may influence CBF. For example; when cerebral metabolic rate of oxygen ($CMRO_2$) is decreased due to factors like hypothermia or sedation, this will cause a reduction in CBF. Cerebral blood flow is also influenced by partial pressures of carbon dioxide ($PaCO_2$) and oxygen (PaO_2). The effect of PaO_2 is not usually prominent until PaO_2 levels fall to 60 mmHg.[1]

Mechanisms of adaptation can eventually fail to overcome reduced oxygen delivery as anaemia worsens or oxygen consumption increases. Cerebral vasodilation and increase in CBF may also worsen cerebral oedema and cause increased intracranial pressure (ICP) in neurocritical care patients. Red blood cell (RBC) transfusion and supplemental oxygen treatments are among the methods to improve cerebral DO_2.[12] Studies have shown that increased fraction of inspired oxygen (FiO_2) combined with controlled ICP improve outcome following TBI and acute SAH.[12,13] The optimal timing of RBC transfusion to improve cerebral DO_2 and avoid unnecessary adverse effects of transfusion is still not clear, but the literature supports that RBC transfusion increases DO_2 in neurocritical care patients whose Hb was less than 9 g/dL.[14]

POTENTIAL CAUSES OF ANAEMIA IN NEUROINTENSIVE CARE PATIENTS

Anaemia is simply the result of two possible pathophysiological conditions: decreased RBC production or increased RBC destruction and/or loss. In addition to the classical causes, there are some special processes which lead to an increased incidence of anaemia in critical care patients.

Impaired Erythropoietin Expression

Normally EPO levels increase as a response to decreased Hb. However, EPO levels are found to be inappropriately low in critical care patients. Release of proinflammatory cytokines (mainly interleukin [IL]-1β and tumour necrosis factor [TNF]-α) and decreased renal function are the main underlying mechanisms of blunting EPO response to anaemia.[15]

Impaired Iron Metabolism

Proinflammatory cytokines like IL-1β, IL-6, TNF-α and decreased EPO cause alterations in many steps of iron metabolism. Upregulation of some iron regulatory proteins also leads to impaired duodenal iron absorption and iron release from macrophages. The net result is decreased serum iron levels and limited availability of iron for erythropoiesis.[15,16]

Nutritional Deficiencies

A recent study has shown that the incidence of iron, B_{12}, and folic acid deficiencies in ICU patients were 9%, 2%, and 2%, respectively.[17] Nutritional deficiencies contribute to a small fraction of anaemia in the ICU but they are among the most easily treatable reasons.

Shortened Life Span of RBC

In inflammatory states like sepsis and trauma, some functional and structural changes mimic natural aging and result in a shortened life span of erythrocytes. These changes include decreased RBC deformability, induced apoptosis, decreased Hb content, increased oxidative lipids, and changes in intracellular calcium concentrations. The underlying mechanism is thought to be through proinflammatory cytokines and reactive oxygen species.[16]

Iatrogenic Loss

Diagnostic phlebotomy accounts for up to 30% of required blood transfusions in the ICU. Iatrogenic haemolysis due to transfusion reactions, rapidly infused hypotonic solutions or secondary to prosthetic heart valves, intra-aortic balloon pumps, etc. can also be important. Bleeding secondary to stress gastritis, especially in mechanically ventilated patients, patients with acute renal failure, or patients taking anticoagulative medicine can be another reason of iatrogenic blood loss.[5,16]

Drugs

In contrast to their proliferative effect on normal erythropoiesis at physiological levels, prolonged vasopressor infusions (norepinephrine and epinephrine), especially at high concentrations can inhibit haematopoietic precursor maturation. Calcium channel blockers, angiotensin receptor blockers, angiotensin converting enzyme inhibitors, and theophylline can also suppress erythropoietic response to anaemia.[18–20]

ANAEMIA IN SPECIAL CONDITIONS IN NEUROINTENSIVE CARE

Traumatic Brain Injury

Traumatic brain injury patients are vulnerable to secondary ischaemic injury and have higher critical CBF threshold. Anaemia is seen in varying degrees in 10%–69% of severe TBI and can cause secondary insults due to reduced cDO_2.[16]

Lower Hb values at hospital admission and also development of anaemia (Hb <9 g/dL) during ICU stay have been associated with worse outcome and increased mortality.[12,16,21] However, some other studies did not find any difference in important significant outcomes like mortality, organ failure, and length of ICU stay among patients who were treated with restrictive or liberal transfusion strategies.[22,23] Targeting a higher transfusion threshold of haemoglobin (10 g/dL) after severe TBI also increased the risk of progressive haemorrhagic injury. This is mostly related to the less deformable erythrocytes impairing cerebral microcirculation, especially in the older transfused blood.[24]

Reduction in brain tissue oxygen tension (PbtO$_2$) and jugular venous oxygen saturation (SjvO$_2$) are accepted as important predictors of worse outcome in TBI patients. However, the Hb level that causes brain tissue hypoxia (PbtO$_2$ <20 mmHg) is not exactly clear and varies according to each patient's physiological status. An Hb level of <9 g/dL is associated with lower mean PbtO$_2$ values. The <9 g/dL Hb, together with monitored PbtO$_2$ values <20 mmHg, is found more acceptable to predict worse outcomes than anaemia alone.[1,25] Measurement of PbtO$_2$ is also recommended by the Brain Trauma Foundation (BTF) to monitor oxygen delivery. Transfusion usually increases PbtO$_2$ but in some cases, especially when transfused blood is aged, even a reduction in PbtO$_2$ can be seen. Improvement in PbtO$_2$ is transient and does not always reflect an improvement in cerebral metabolism.[1,16,25]

Subarachnoid Haemorrhage

Angiographic vasospasm can occur during the first two weeks of aneursymal rupture and complicates about two-thirds of SAH cases. Magnetic resonance imaging (MRI) of SAH patients who survived showed that 50%–70% have cerebral infarction, which was not present at the beginning. Although the evidence of its efficacy is controversial, the classical 'triple-H' triad of treatment of SAH consists of haemodilution, hypervolaemia, and hypertension to improve CBF to overcome vasospasm, but the increase in CBF is not always directly proportional to changes in PbtO$_2$ and CMRO$_2$.[1] So, it is especially important for this patient group to prevent secondary insults due to decreased oxygen delivery because of the high risk of delayed ischaemia.[26]

Anaemia is present in nearly half of SAH patients. Anaemia usually develops on third or fourth day following the aneurysm rupture. The possible causes are haemodilution, rebleeding, surgical blood loss, and drug effects. Anaemia and RBC transfusion are both associated with poor clinical outcome and mortality.[1,16,21] Lower admission Hb levels are associated with increased risk of cerebral infarction regardless of SAH severity.[27] Although some studies have shown that RBC transfusions could help avoid vasospasm-induced cerebral ischaemia, some others suggest RBC transfusion as an independent risk factor for symptomatic vasospasm and delayed cerebral ischaemia.[1,22] The mechanism of vasospasm is thought to be related to local NO depletion and inflammation.[22] Also some other studies found an association between

RBC transfusion and increased risk of thrombotic events in SAH patients.[28]

It is not clear whether anaemia is a cause or a marker of poor outcome in case of SAH. The threshold for transfusion varies in different institutions, according to patient characteristics, clinical experience, and the possibilities of advanced neurological monitoring. A North American Survey about SAH including 282 clinicians showed that the preference was more restrictive RBC transfusion (mean Hb 7.85 g/dL) in low-grade SAH and more liberal transfusion strategy (mean Hb 8.58 g/dL) in patients with delayed cerebral ischaemia. The overall mean Hb concentration that the clinicians decided to transfuse in a high-grade patient (World Federation of Neurological Surgeons – WFNS Grade 4) was 8.19 g/dL. Also a majority of clinicians in the same survey were more likely to transfuse a patient with PbtO$_2$ <15 mmHg.[26]

Acute Ischaemic Stroke

In patients with acute ischaemic stroke (AIS), the oxygenation of penumbra is very critical because of the impaired CBF. Increased haematocrit and therefore increased blood viscosity is often observed in AIS patients. Elevated haematocrit can lead to impaired microvascular circulation in the penumbra and local thrombosis. Several studies have found a relationship between increased haematocrit and worse outcomes like greater infarct size, early mortality, and major disability after AIS.[12,22,29] The optimal haematocrit levels observed to be related with the best outcomes are 42%–45%.[16] Although animal studies have shown that mild anaemia (haematocrit 30%–36% and Hb 10–12 g/dL) could be better for cerebral oxygen delivery and neuroprotection, the improving effects of early haemodilution therapy has not been exactly proven in human beings.[1,22] The association between haematocrit levels and poor outcome after stroke is described as a 'U' shape. High haematocrit levels impair microcirculation, on the other hand low haematocrit levels decrease oxygen transport.[12,16,30] Severe acute haemodilution during cardiopulmonary bypass may even increase the risk of perioperative stroke.[31,32]

A previous history of RBC transfusion is also associated with increased risk of AIS. A Japanese study with a follow-up period of healthy subjects for 10 years found that RBC transfusion was a risk factor for AIS development.[33]

In the current guidelines of American Heart Association (AHA) Stroke Council, routine RBC transfusion or haemodilution does not have a role in the management of AIS.[34] The transfusion threshold for anaemic patients again is not clear for TBI and SAH. Recent studies suggest haemodilution with high doses of albumin may be effective in reducing infarct size and increasing the efficacy of thrombolytic therapy.[1,12]

Intracerebral Haemorrhage

Most patients with intracerebral haemorrhage (ICH) have hypoperfusion areas in the perihaematomal tissues. As oxygen extraction fraction in this perihaematomal area is not increased, the underlying mechanism is thought to be reduced cerebral metabolism instead of true ischaemia. So a major secondary insult is not expected due to mild anaemia.[1] However, both anaemia on admission and nadir Hb levels during hospital stay have been found to be associated with increased haemorrhage volumes and poor functional outcome. The larger bleeding volumes related to anaemia even in the case of normal platelet count might be associated with the impairment of platelet–platelet and platelet–endothelial interactions in these patients. The unfavourable effect of anaemia on outcomes were found especially more prominent in minor volume ICH patients.[35,36] The effect of RBC transfusion on outcome of patients with ICH is also contradictory.[21]

Elective Cranial Surgery

The data in literature regarding the effects of anaemia and RBC transfusion strategies (restrictive or liberal) on patients undergoing elective cranial surgery are very limited. The study by Seicean et al.[37] included 668 patients undergoing surgery for intracranial aneurysm, 59.9% of whom were treated for unruptured aneurysms. The study found that both preoperative anaemia and RBC transfusion were risk factors for perioperative complications and increased length of hospital stay. Another study including 6,576 elective neurosurgical patients found that perioperative anaemia was associated with prolonged hospital stay, but not mortality or complications. The difference was irrespective of severity of anaemia. However, one important limitation of this study was that anaemic patients were more likely to have concomitant co-morbidities and higher American Society of Anesthesiologists (ASA) status.[38]

OPTIMAL TRANSFUSION TRIGGER

Anaemia and RBC transfusion seem to be independent risk factors associated with poor outcome and mortality in neurocritical care patients. However, the studies in neurocritical care patients could not address a specific Hb level as the threshold for RBC transfusion. Current

Table 40.1 Signs of ischaemia accepted as transfusion triggers in neurocritical care patients

Haemoglobin	7–9 g/dL (especially together with other triggers)
$PbtO_2$	<15–20 mmHg
NIRS	<30% or more than 20% decrease from baseline
$SjvO_2$	<50% (for at least 10 min)
LPR	>35–40

evidence supports an individual based transfusion strategy instead of RBC transfusion based on a constant level of Hb which could be more useful for balancing the risks of transfusion and decreased oxygen content. Thus; in addition to the Hb levels, clinicians are in search for more physiological transfusion indicators using signals coming from the brain such as brain tissue oxygen tension or near infrared spectroscopy[22] (Table 40.1).

Brain Tissue Oxygen Tension

Brain tissue oxygen tension probes give the opportunity of continuous monitoring of the balance between regional oxygen supply and cellular oxygen consumption. Thus, it can help determine optimal targets for transfusion according to the physiological status of each patient.

The oxygen-sensitive $PbtO_2$ catheter with approximately 0.5 mm diameter can be placed into the brain parenchyma usually at bedside in the neurointensive care. Correct placement should be confirmed with a computerized tomography (CT) scan. Licox system (Gesellschaft für medizinische Sondentechnik, Kiel, Germany), Paratrend catheter (Diametrics Medical, High Wycombe, UK) and the Neurotrend catheter (modified from Paratrend catheter, Codman, Raynam, MA) are the main commercial types of $PbtO_2$ monitors. Multiparameter catheters which can measure $PbtO_2$, intracranial pressure (ICP), and brain temperature together are now also available. Although it is an invasive monitoring method, the complications like infection or device associated contusion are reported rarely.[39,40]

If the catheter is placed in an undamaged brain part, the measurement reflects global cerebral oxygenation. However, it can be positioned in the penumbra of a lesion to allow close monitoring of the brain part especially at risk. For example, in SAH, $PbtO_2$ probe could be placed in the brain region where maximal vasospasm is expected. According to animal studies and the studies in humans undergoing awake neurosurgery, $PbtO_2$ values between 25–30 mmHg appear to be normal. $PbtO_2$ <15 or 20 mmHg was accepted as a threshold for ischaemia in different studies. Especially in patients with TBI, not just the number, but also the duration and intensity of episodes of low $PbtO_2$ have been associated with poor outcome.[39–41]

Near-Infrared Spectroscopy

Near-infrared spectroscopy (NIRS) is a non-invasive, real-time method to indirectly measure regional cerebral oxygen saturation (rSO_2) with bilateral scalp frontal probes.[41,42] The measurement technique depends on the absorption of near-infrared light by oxygenated haemoglobin (HbO_2) and deoxygenated haemoglobin (HbD). In principle, tissue haemoglobin content (HbT) can be calculated as $HbT = HbO_2 + HbD$ and rSO_2 is the ratio of HbO_2 to HbT. As the cerebral vasculature consists of 15%–25% arterial and 75%–85% venous blood, rSO_2 value is towards the venous component and should be approximately 66%. Kurth et al.[43] investigated NIRS in piglets to determine hypoxic ischaemic threshold values. In this study, the mean baseline rSO_2 of piglets was 68%. Cerebral lactate concentrations increased when rSO_2 values was about 44%, minor and major electroencephalogram changes were seen when rSO_2 values were 42% and 37%, respectively. Clinical studies suggest that a decrease of more than 20% of baseline rSO_2 value should be considered as important. An rSO_2 of <30% indicates a serious problem in oxygen delivery.[44] However, the reference ranges for ischaemic thresholds, especially in neurointensive care patients are not clearly identified.[45,46]

Near-infrared spectroscopy directed strategies are suggested to improve postoperative neurological outcome in several types of major surgeries including on-pump cardiac surgeries.[47] The benefit of NIRS in detecting cerebral oxygenation changes due to RBC transfusion during cardiac surgery has been shown.[22] Low rSO_2 values indicate increased oxygen extraction fraction due to decreased CBF. Although the data is still contradictory, many studies have found good correlation between rSO_2 and invasive cerebral monitoring like $PbtO_2$ and $SjvO_2$.[46] Near-infrared spectroscopy correlated with blood loss in experimental models of haemorrhage and it is suggested to be considered for detecting regional haemoglobin desaturation during blood loss despite the potential limitations. Development in technology and further research probably may lead to usage of NIRS-based models as an alternative transfusion trigger in future.[48]

Jugular Venous Oxygen Saturation

This technique provides the measurement of global cerebral oxygenation through a jugular catheter which is inserted under fluoroscopy until the tip lies in the jugular bulb of the dominant side. The jugular bulb drains venous blood from cerebral hemispheres, cerebellum, and brainstem, and the contribution of extracranial circulation is smaller than 6.6% if the catheter tip is in the right position. Normal $SjvO_2$ values are between 55%–75%. The threshold for ischaemia is accepted as $SjvO_2$ <50% for at least 10 minutes. Low $SjvO_2$ values indicate tissue hypoxia due to several reasons like anaemia, vasospasm, excessive hyperventilation, and increased cerebral demand (fever, seizures, etc.). $SjvO_2$ values higher than 75% not just simply reflect hyperaemia but also a possibly decreased metabolic demand in the traumatized brain tissue.[41,42]

Episodes of $SjvO_2$ <50% or >75% were found associated with worse outcomes in TBI and SAH patients.[42] In one study including trauma patients, Hb levels were found less than 8 g/dL in patients with $SjvO_2$ <65%.[49] In another study, blood transfusion increased $SjvO_2$ only in patients whose values were <70%.[50]

There are some important limitations of $SjvO_2$ monitoring. First of all, regional changes, especially in the penumbra lesions can remain undiagnosed because of overshadowing from hyperaemic areas. The sensitivity is low. If the tip of the catheter is placed too distally, falsely high values could be gained due to the mixture from extracerebral venous blood. Although complications are rare and catheter placement is relatively simple; thrombosis, increased ICP, venous air embolism, pneumothorax, and infection can be seen. Artefacts due to catheter movements are common.[41,42] According to current knowledge, $SjvO_2$ monitoring alone does not seem enough to detect secondary insults and determine a threshold for transfusion. However, it can add complementary information as part of multimodal monitoring in neurointensive care.

Cerebral Microdialysis

Cerebral microdialysis, which is simply the analysis of extracellular fluid within the cerebral parenchyma allows bedside metabolic monitoring of glucose, lactate, pyruvate, glutamate, and urea levels via a sterile microdialysis catheter. Glucose, lactate, and pyruvate are among the primary markers of cerebral energy metabolism.[41] In case of ischaemia, extracellular glucose levels decrease due to increased consumption while there is a rise in lactate levels. The occurrence of these metabolic changes is usually seen at $PbtO_2$ levels <20 mmHg.[51] A large study including 223 patients showed that microdialysis markers were strongly related to long-term outcome.[52]

Increased lactate reflects a shift to anaerobic metabolism and so lactate to pyruvate ratio (LPR), especially gives information about tissue oxygenation. An LPR of >25 is considered as abnormal while LPR >40 is considered related with cell energy dysfunction.[41] In the North American survey,[26] LPR of 35–40 was the threshold considered critical for transfusion by most of the clinicians.

MANAGING ANAEMIA IN NEUROINTENSIVE CARE PATIENTS

Preventing Unnecessary Blood Loss

The impact of iatrogenic blood losses on anaemia and RBC transfusion in critical care patients is actually far more than estimated. Diagnostic phlebotomy is the cause of approximately 40–70 ml blood loss per day, which exceeds the normal healthy replacement rate. This condition, named as 'anaemia of chronic investigation' leads nearly up to 30% of blood transfusions in the ICU. As modern laboratory devices allow accurate analysis with less blood samples, it becomes easier to modify this factor. Using small volume or paediatric collection tubes, point of care testing, non-invasive Hb monitoring, grouping different laboratory tests to the same time and recycling the discarded volumes from indwelling arterial lines are among the strategies to prevent unnecessary loss. Although point of care devices and non-invasive Hb monitors reduce hospital costs and blood loss, the problems with suboptimal accuracy should be kept in mind.[15,16]

Red Blood Cell Transfusion

Red blood cell transfusion causes an increase in oxygen content and blood viscosity. However, some biochemical changes including loss of membrane phospholipids, oxidative protein damage, and reductions of adenosine triphosphate (ATP) occur in stored blood. The 2, 3–diphosphoglycerate levels decrease and even become nearly undetectable after one week of storage. Duration of blood storage is among the leading factors associated with adverse effects. In a study among cardiac surgery patients; mortality, sepsis, renal failure, and the need for mechanical ventilation were all higher in patients who received RBC transfusion >14 days compared to patients who received RBC transfusion <14 days.[1] Using fresh blood might increase the effect while reducing the risks of transfusion. Experimental animal studies showed that the increase in $PbtO_2$ was more in the fresh blood given group compared to stored blood, but the same effect could not be shown in human studies. Neurocognitive tests did not differ between patients transfused with RBC stored <5 hours and >14 days.[1]

Both anaemia and RBC transfusion are related to worse outcomes in neurointensive care. The Hb threshold to initiate transfusion still remains uncertain. Red blood cell transfusion is discussed in more detail in Chapter 42.

Human Recombinant Erythropoietin and Erythropoietin Stimulating Analogues

Erythropoietin synthesized by the kidneys is essential for the bone marrow to produce RBCs. In critical care patients, EPO gene expression is suppressed by pro-inflammatory cytokines like IL-1 and TNF-α. The responsiveness to EPO is also diminished.[53] A randomized controlled study including 1,302 critical care patients with anaemia showed that patients receiving recombinant human EPO needed less amount of transfusion and also had a better Hb increase from baseline.[4] However, studies were unable to find an improvement in mortality or significant outcome.[53]

Erythropoietin has also experimentally shown cell-protective and anti-apoptotic properties. It was thought to have benefits in neuroprotection, but studies in stroke or TBI patients did not show significant advantage. An ischaemic stroke trial of EPO even resulted in higher death rate in comparison with placebo. This result was probably due to patients requiring thrombolytic therapy.[54] The risk of thromboembolic events should be considered, especially in high risk groups like patients with cancer.[4]

Erythropoietin and EPO-stimulating analogues are not legally approved or could be recommended with certain evidence for ICU patients. In anaemic chronic renal disease patients and cancer patients, the recommended EPO doses respectively vary between 2000–8000 IU and 30,000–40,000 IU per week. The increase in the number of reticulocytes will be seen 3 or 4 days after the administration of EPO.[54]

Iron Supplementation

The combination of iron supplementation and EPO can improve erythropoiesis and increase Hb levels. Also, treatment failure with darbepoetin alpha, an EPO stimulating analogue, was shown to be decreased with supplemental iron. The recommended route of supplementation is intravenous rather than oral because intestinal absorption of iron is inhibited by hepcidin.

Vitamin B12 and folic acid supplementation may also be considered as an additional therapy to erythropoiesis stimulating agents to improve RBC production.[4,15]

Haemoglobin-Based Blood Substitutes

These artificial oxygen carriers seem to have a theoretical advantage for improving oxygen delivery. They were especially designed for patients suffering from acute massive haemorrhage because of a short half-life. However, they were associated with severe nephrotoxicity, impaired perfusion, perioperative stroke, increased myocardial infarction, and mortality in several studies. Currently, Hb-based blood substitutes are not approved in many countries and they have no role in routine practice.[1,15]

CONCLUSIONS

Anaemia is usually associated with worse outcomes like organ hypoperfusion, multi-organ failure, and death in critical care patients who have an increased oxygen demand due to mechanical ventilation, sepsis, fever, and infections. Both anaemia and RBC transfusions are associated with worse outcomes in neurocritical care patients.

A transfusion threshold of 7 g/dL Hb is usually accepted as safe in critical care patients without serious cardiac disease. However, the Hb level could be targeted approximately at 8–9 g/dL in neurocritical care patients as an acutely injured brain is more vulnerable to further neuronal damage caused by impaired oxygen delivery. Besides the Hb level, physiological indicators of ischaemia such as $PbtO_2$, cerebral microdialysis, and $SjvO_2$ can be recommended as supportive transfusion triggers.

REFERENCES

1. Kramer AH, Zygun DA. Anemia and red blood cell transfusion in neurocritical care. *Crit Care* 2009;13(3):R89.

2. International Nutritional Anemia Consultative Group (INACG), World Health Organization (WHO), United Nations Childrens Fund (UNICEF). Stoltzfus RJ, Dreyfuss ML, eds. Guidelines for the use of iron supplements to prevent and treat iron deficiency anemia. 1998. Available from: http://who.int/nutrition/publications/micronutrients/guidelines_for_Iron_supplementation.pdf.

3. Weiskopf RB, Kramer JH, Neumann M, et al. Acute severe isovolemic anemia impairs cognitive function memory in humans. *Anesthesiology* 2000;92:1646–52.

4. Morgan CA, Byul Sarah S, Forest CP. Transfusion-free treatment strategies for acute anemia in critical care. *JAAPA* 2016 Aug;29(8):38–44.

5. Moreb JS. Hematologic and coagulation implications of neurologic disease. In: Layon AJ, Gabrielli A, Friedman WA, eds. *Textbook of Neurointensive Care.* London: Springer-Verlag, 2013;322–7.

6. Hebert PC, Van der Linden P, Biro G, Hu LQ. Physiologic aspects of anemia. *Crit Care Clin* 2004;20(2):187–212.

7. Spinelli E, Bartlett RH. Anemia and transfusion in critical care: Physiology and management. *Journal of Intensive Care Medicine* 2016;31(5):295–306.

8. Kothaveale A, Banki NM, Kopelnik A, et al. Predictors of left ventricular regional wall motion abnormalities after subarachnoid hemorrhage. *Neurocrit Care* 2006,4: 199–205.

9. Hare GM, Tsui AK, McLaren AT, Ragoonanan TE, Yu J, Mazer CD. Anemia and cerebral outcomes: many questions, fewer answers. *Anesth Analg* 2008;107(4): 1356–70.

10. Joshi S, Young WL, Duong DH, et al. Intracarotid infusion of the nitric oxide synthase inhibitor, l-NMMA, modestly decreases cerebral blood flow in human subjects. *Anesthesiology* 2000;93:699–707.

11. Niwa M, Inao S, Takayasu M, et al. Time course of expression of three nitric oxide synthase isoforms after transient middle cerebral artery occlusion in rats. *Neurol Med Chir* 2001;41:63–72.

12. LeRoux P. Haemoglobin management in acute brain injury. *Curr Opin Crit Care* 2013;19(2):83–91.

13. Nangunoori R, Maloney-Wilensky E, Stiefel MDM, et al. Brain tissue oxygen based therapy and outcome after severe traumatic brain injury: a systematic literature review. *Neurocrit Care* 2012;17:131–8.

14. Dhar R, Scalfani MT, Zazulia AR, et al. Comparison of induced hypertension, fluid bolus, and blood transfusion to augment cerebral oxygen delivery after subarachnoid hemorrhage. *J Neurosurg* 2012;116:648–856.

15. Hayden SJ, Albert TJ, Watkins TR, Swenson ER. Anemia in critical illness: insights into etiology, consequences, and management. *Am J Respir Crit Care Med* 2012 May 15;185(10):1049–57.

16. Naidech AM, Kumar MA. Participants in the International Multidisciplinary Consensus Conference on Multimodality Monitoring. Monitoring of hematological and hemostatic parameters in neurocritical care patients. *Neurocrit Care* 2014 Dec;21(Suppl 2):S168–76.

17. McCully SP, Fabricant LJ, Kunio NR, et al. The International Normalized Ratio overestimates coagulopathy in stable trauma and surgical patients. *J Trauma Acute Care Surg* 2013; 75(6): 947–53.

18. Fonseca RB, Mohr AM, Wang L, Sifri ZC, Rameshwar P, Livingston DH. The impact of a hypercatecholamine state on erythropoiesis following severe injury and the role of IL-6. *J Trauma* 2005;59:884–9.

19. Linde T, Sandhagen B, Hagg A, Morlin C, Danielson BG. Decreased blood viscosity and serum levels of erythropoietin after anti-hypertensive treatment with

amlodipine or metoprolol: results of a cross-over study. *J Hum Hypertens* 1996;10:199–205.

20. Vlahakos DV, Marathias KP, Madias NE. The role of the renin–angiotensin system in the regulation of erythropoiesis. *Am J Kidney Dis* 2010;56:558–65.

21. Gruenbaum SE, Ruskin KJ. Red blood cell transfusion in neurosurgical patients. *Curr Opin Anaesthesiol* 2014 Oct; 27(5):470–3.

22. Leal-Noval SR, Múñoz-Gómez M, Murillo-Cabezas F. Optimal hemoglobin concentration in patients with subarachnoid hemorrhage, acute ischemic stroke and traumatic brain injury. *Curr Opin Crit Care* 2008 Apr; 14(2):156–62.

23. Boutin A, Chassé M, Shemilt M, et al. Red blood cell transfusion in patients with traumatic brain injury: A systematic review and meta-analysis. *Transfus Med Rev* 2016 Jan;30(1):15–24.

24. Vedantam A, Yamal JM, Rubin ML, Robertson CS, Gopinath SP. Progressive hemorrhagic injury after severe traumatic brain injury: effect of hemoglobin transfusion thresholds. *J Neurosurg* 2016 Nov;125(5):1229–34.

25. Oddo M, Levine JM, Kumar M, et al. Anemia and brain oxygen after severe traumatic brain injury. *Intensive Care Med.* 2012 Sep;38(9):1497–504.

26. Kramer AH, Diringer MN, Suarez JI, Naidech AM, Macdonald LR, LeRoux PD. Red blood cell transfusion in patients with subarachnoid hemorrhage: a multidisciplinary North American survey. *Crit Care* 2011;15(1):R30.

27. Kramer AH, Zygun DA, Bleck TP, Dumont AS, Kassell NF, Nathan B. Relationship between hemoglobin concentrations and outcomes across subgroups of patients with aneurysmal sub-arachnoid hemorrhage. *Neurocrit Care* 2009;10(2):157–65.

28. Kumar MA, Boland TA, Baiou M, et al. Red blood cell transfusion increases the risk of thrombotic events in patients with subarachnoid hemorrhage. *Neurocrit Care* 2014;20:84–90.

29. Allport LE, Parson MW, Butcher KS, et al. Elevated hematocrit is associated with reduced reperfusion and tissue survival in acute stroke. *Neurology* 2005; 65: 1382–7.

30. Tanne D, Molshatzki N, Merzeliak O, Tsabari R, Toashi M, Schwammenthal Y. Anemia status, hemoglobin concentration and outcome after acute stroke: a cohort study. *BMC Neurol* 2010;10:22.

31. Habib RH, Zacharias A, Schwann TA, et al. Adverse effects of low hematocrit during cardiopulmonary bypass in the adult: should current practice be changed? *J Thorac Cardiovasc Surg* 2003;125:1438–50.

32. Karkouti K, Djaiani G, Borger MA, et al. Low hematocrit during cardiopulmonary bypass is associated with increased risk of perioperative stroke in cardiac surgery. *Ann Thorac Surg* 2005; 80:1381–7.

33. Yamada S, Koizumi A, Iso H, et al. History of blood transfusion before 1990 is a risk factor for stroke and cardiovascular diseases: the Japan Collaborative Cohort Study (JACC study). *Cerebrovasc Dis* 2005;20:164–71.

34. Powers WJ, Derdeyn CP, Biller J, et al. American Heart Association Stroke Council. 2015 American Heart Association/American Stroke Association Focused Update of the 2013 Guidelines for the early management of patients with acute ischemic Stroke Regarding Endovascular Treatment: A Guideline for Healthcare Professionals From the American Heart Association/American Stroke Association. *Stroke* 2015 Oct;46(10):3020–35.

35. Kuramatsu JB, Gerner ST, Lücking H, et al. Anemia is an independent prognostic factor in intracerebral hemorrhage: an observational cohort study. *Crit Care* 2013 Jul 23;17(4):R148.

36. Kumar MA, Rost NS, Snider RW, et al. Anemia and hematoma volume in acute intracerebral hemorrhage. *Crit Care Med* 2009 Apr;37(4):1442–7.

37. Seicean A, Alan N, Seicean S, Neuhauser D, Selman WR, Bambakidis NC. Risks associated with preoperative anemia and perioperative blood transfusion in open surgery for intracranial aneurysms. *J Neurosurg* 2015 Jul;123(1): 91–100.

38. Alan N, Seicean A, Seicean S, Neuhauser D, Weil RJ. Impact of preoperative anemia on outcomes in patients undergoing elective cranial surgery. *J Neurosurg* 2014 Mar;120(3):764–72.

39. Huschak G, Hoell T, Hohaus C, Kern C, Minkus Y, Meisel HJ. Clinical evaluation of a new multiparameter neuromonitoring device: measurement of brain tissue oxygen, brain temperature, and intracranial pressure. *J Neurosurg Anesthesiol* 2009 Apr;21(2):155–60.

40. Mulvey JM, Dorsch NW, Mudaliar Y, Lang EW. Multimodality monitoring in severe traumatic brain injury: the role of brain tissue oxygenation monitoring. *Neurocrit Care* 2004;1(3):391–402.

41. LeRoux P. Invasive neurological and multimodality monitoring in the neuro ICU. In: Layon AJ, Gabrielli A, Friedman WA, eds. *Textbook of Neurointensive Care*. London: Springer-Verlag, 2013;127–40.

42. Haitsma IK, Maas AI. Advanced monitoring in the intensive care unit: brain tissue oxygen tension. *Curr Opin Crit Care* 2002 Apr;8(2):115–20.

43. Kurth CD, Levy WJ, McCann J. Near-infrared spectroscopy cerebral oxygen saturation thresholds for hypoxia-ischemia in piglets. *J Cereb Blood Flow Metab* 2002;22:335–41.

44. Andropoulos DB, Stayer SA, Diaz LK, Ramamoorthy C. Neurological monitoring for congenital heart surgery. *Anesth Analg* 2004;99:1365–75.

45. Menke J, Möller G. Cerebral near-infrared spectroscopy correlates to vital parameters during cardiopulmonary bypass surgery in children. *Pediatr Cardiol* 2014 Jan; 35(1):155–63.

46. Weigl W, Milej D, Janusek D, et al. Application of optical methods in the monitoring of traumatic brain injury: A review. *J Cereb Blood Flow Metab* 2016 Nov;36(11):1825–43.

47. Moerman A, De Hert S. Cerebral oximetry: the standard monitor of the future? *Curr Opin Anaesthesiol* 2015 Dec;28(6):703–9.

48. Torella F, Haynes SL, McCollum CN. Cerebral and peripheral near-infrared spectroscopy: an alternative transfusion trigger? *Vox Sang* 2002 Oct;83(3):254–7.

49. Scalea TM, Hartnett RW, Duncan AO, et al. Central venous oxygen saturation: a useful clinical tool in trauma patients. *Journal of Trauma* 1990;30:1539–43.

50. Adamczyk S, Robin E, Barreau O, et al. Contribution of central venous oxygen saturation in postoperative blood transfusion decision. *Annales Françaises d'Anesthesie et de Reanimation* 2009;28:522–30.

51. Bellapart J, Boots R, Fraser J. Physiopathology of anemia and transfusion thresholds in isolated head injury. *J Trauma Acute Care Surg* 2012 Oct;73(4):997–1005.

52. Timofeev I, Carpenter KL, Nortje J, et al. Cerebral extracellular chemistry and outcome following traumatic brain injury: a microdialysis study of 223 patients. *Brain* 2011;134(Pt 2):484–94.

53. Coleman T, Brines M. Science review: recombinant human erythropoietin in critical illness: a role beyond anemia? *Crit Care* 2004 Oct;8(5):337–41.

54. Jelkmann I, Jelkmann W. Impact of erythropoietin on intensive care unit patients. *Transfus Med Hemother* 2013 Oct;40(5):310–8.

41

Coagulopathy

B. Akca

ABSTRACT

Haemostatic abnormalities related to primary brain tumours also contribute to coagulopathy in neurointensive care. Traumatic brain injury (TBI) is often associated with coagulopathy and coagulopathy in turn is associated with prolonged stay in the neurointensive care unit. It has been shown that one-third of the patients with TBI show mild-severe coagulopathy upon admission to the hospital. The presence of coagulopathy has been linked to progression of ischaemic and haemorrhagic lesions and early identification of coagulopathy is important in the management of delayed brain injury. Antiplatelet agents (aspirin, clopidogrel, prasugrel, ticagrelor), vitamin K antagonists (warfarin), direct thrombin inhibitors (dabigatran), and factor Xa antagonists (rivaroxaban, apixaban, edoxaban) are mainly used for antithrombotic purpose. These drugs are known to predispose to the development of both acute and chronic subdural haematomas. Also patients on antithrombotic agents are thought to be at higher likelihood of presenting with larger haematomas or more severe neurological outcomes.

KEYWORDS

Neurointensive care; coagulopathy; anticoagulants; antiplatelets; haemostasis.

INTRODUCTION

Patients admitted to neurointensive care units and those requiring urgent surgical interventions due to primary brain tumours, traumatic brain injury (TBI) or intracranial haemorrhage (ICH) might also be using anticoagulant agents due to thromboembolic disorders. Anticoagulant therapy increases the risk of major bleeding complications in neurosurgical patients and so the clinical management of patients on anticoagulant therapy is really challenging.

Clinicians, especially neurointensivists and neuroanaesthetists, are expected to be up to the indications, contraindications, mechanism of action, and side effects of these drugs to manage these patients overall.

PRIMARY BRAIN TUMOURS

Haemostatic abnormalities related to primary brain tumours also contribute to the coagulopathic situation. Brain tumours mostly cause hypercoagulability and as a result of this consumptive period of coagulation, resultant hypocoagulability. In patients with intracranial tumours, many haemostatic abnormalities are reported. Common haemostatic abnormalities are prolonged thrombin time, abnormal levels of fibrinogen, and increased fibrin degradation products. From the mechanistic point of view, hyperfibrinolysis is the mechanism responsible for abnormalities in patients with primary brain tumours.[1] Apart from this, release of plasminogen activator factors from tumour cells or tissue factors from injured brain parenchyma during tumour removal is thought to be another main pathology of disseminated intravascular coagulation (DIC). Considering these findings together 'chronic' DIC with/without fibrinolysis appears to be the most common abnormalities in patients with intracranial tumours.[2]

TRAUMATIC BRAIN INJURY

Traumatic brain injury is often associated with coagulopathy,[3] and coagulopathy is associated with a prolonged stay in the neurointensive care unit (NICU).[4]

A study has elicited that one-third of the patients with TBI show mild to severe coagulopathy upon admission to the hospital.[5] In another study, it was found that this number is doubled on the first day of trauma.[6] The presence of coagulopathy has been linked to progression of ischaemic and haemorrhagic lesions,[7] and early identification of coagulopathy is critical in the management of delayed brain injury.[8] Early monitoring of coagulation with thromboelastometry (ROTEM) and thromboelastography (TEG) (to assess viscoelasticity of blood) may also contribute to early diagnosis of coagulopathy.[6] Risk factors for the development of coagulopathy are:[9]

- Severity of head trauma
- Glasgow Coma Scale (GCS) score ≤8
- Hypotension ≤90 mmHg
- Fluid administration ≥2000 ml before hospital admission; this parameter may independently be associated with coagulopathy in patients with TBI
- Age ≥75 years

Lustenberger and colleagues defined TBI associated coagulopathy as low platelet count and/or prolonged activated partial thromboplastin time (aPTT) and/or international normalized ratio (INR) occurring after admission to hospital (23 ±2 hours). In this study, it was shown that as the time interval to the onset of coagulopathy decreases, the magnitude of final injury increases.[4] The mortality rate of patients developing coagulopathy within the first day of TBI was 55% whereas mortality rate of patients developing coagulopathy later than the first day was 23%.[4] Therefore, coagulopathy is presumed to be a powerful predictor of outcome and prognosis in patients with TBI.

Alterations in coagulation parameters could easily be monitored against bleeding, but hypercoagulability is harder to define since there is no specific routine laboratory test.[7] By using thromboelastometry, blood could be assessed for both hypocoagulable and hypercoagulable states (global haemostatic function) in one single test since it takes into consideration the humoral, cellular, and fibrinolysis systems.[7]

In current practice, we cannot explain the exact mechanisms of TBI-associated coagulopathy, but there are some strong hypothetical assumptions. In healthy people, fibrinolytic mechanisms and coagulation cascade are balanced to prevent ischaemia (thrombosis) and bleeding. An imbalance between them leads to consumption coagulopathy.[6,9,10] Tissue factor (thromboplastin) (TF) is the main factor that initiates the extrinsic cascade of coagulation. Tissue factor

is highly expressed in the central nervous system.[11] Therefore, excessive release of cerebral TF into the circulation due to head trauma is assumed to be the main mechanism in TBI-associated coagulopathy. Tissue factor activates the extrinsic pathway of the cascade and as a result of this hyperactivation consumptive coagulopathy due to depletion of coagulation factors occurs. A second hypothesis suggests that a 'maladaptive' protein C response results in a depletion of protein C.[3] Another mechanism is that patients with TBI are found to be vulnerable to develop hyperfibrinolysis, which is associated with high mortality.[12] The principal effector of fibrinolysis is plasmin and tissue plasminogen activator (tPA) is the product of cleavage. Elevated tPA and increased fibrinogen degradation products (D-Dimer) could be seen in patients with TBI as a result of DIC.[13]

Carrick and colleagues concluded that patients with moderate to severe TBI are at risk for coagulopathy in several days (>72 hours[4]) after trauma, so laboratory parameters should be monitored.[13] The greatest risk factor for progression of haemorrhage is 'coagulopathy' on the first day of trauma.[7]

Laboratory Parameters

These are:

- *Prothrombin Time (PT)*: Sensitive to the depletion of coagulation factors (fVII, fV, fX, fII)
- *Partial Thromboplastin Time (PTT)*: Sensitive to the depletion of the factors in the intrinsic pathway (fXI, fIX, fVIII)
- *Thrombin Time (TT)*: Sensitive to the dysfunction of fibrinogen
- *Platelet Count (PC)*: This parameter could not give information about the function of platelets. Platelet function analyser (PFA-100) and platelet function assay (VerifyNow®) could be used for this purpose.
- *D-Dimer*: Sensitive to active fibrinolysis/DIC.[13]

Treatment

According to our knowledge, a guideline for the treatment of coagulopathy in patients with TBI does not exist. Therefore, adequate control of haemorrhage and its progression should be the aim of treatment. In most trauma centres, abnormal standard laboratory parameters (PT, PTT, TT, PC) are not corrected. These centres are advocating that correcting laboratory parameters does not alter the outcome of patients[14] and INR values <1.7 or aPTT <1.5 × normal are considered to indicate an adequate amount of clotting factors.[15]

Fresh Frozen Plasma

Prophylactic administration of fresh frozen plasma (FFP) was associated with an increase in delayed haematoma and mortality apart from benefit.[16] Fresh frozen plasma should only be used when real evidence for coagulopathy occurs.

Platelets

Platelet concentrates are recommended for patients with active bleeding.[5]

Antifibrinolytic Medication (Tranexamic Acid)

The CRASH-2 trial compared the effect of tranexamic acid with placebo in trauma patients, and tranexamic acid was found to be effective (use of tranexamic acid reduced mortality significantly in general trauma but not in TBI) when administered in the first 3 hours of trauma.[17]

Recombinant Factor VIIa

Recombinant factor VIIa (rFVIIa) was found to correct INR quickly and more economically in patients with TBI, allowing neurosurgical intervention more rapidly.[18,19] These findings should be replicated in prospective randomized controlled clinical trials for use in patients with TBI due to increased risk of thrombosis associated with the use of rFVIIa.

COAGULOPATHY IN PATIENTS ON ANTICOAGULANTS

As the population ages, the prevalence of nonvalvular atrial fibrillation, venous thromboembolism, prosthetic heart valves, transient ischaemic attack, and stroke increases and so the number of patients on antithrombotic (either antiplatelet or anticoagulant) therapy also increases.

Antiplatelet agents (aspirin, clopidogrel, prasugrel, ticagrelor), vitamin K antagonists (warfarin), direct thrombin inhibitors (dabigatran), factor Xa antagonists (rivaroxaban, apixaban, edoxaban) are mainly used for antithrombotic purpose. These drugs are known to predispose to the development of both acute and chronic subdural haematomas.[20] Also, patients on antithrombotic agents are thought to be at higher likelihood of presenting with larger haematomas or more severe neurological outcomes.[20] The cases in literature are limited, but there is strong evidence for increased expansion of intracranial haematomas with vitamin K antagonists.[21,22] Patients who develop an intracranial

haematoma while on anticoagulants are at an increased risk of mortality.

When compared with patients receiving warfarin, the incidence of life-threatening bleeding especially ICH is lower in patients on direct oral anticoagulants (DOACs), also known in literature as target-specific anticoagulants (dabigatran, rivaroxaban, apixaban, edoxaban).[23–26] Intracranial haemorrhage rates were statistically lower with dabigatran when either dosage was administered (110–150 mg twice a day).[27]

The management of patients admitted to neurointensive care units with ICH involves the reversal of the antithrombotic agent properly in possible situations and proceed with either surgical intervention or close surveillance. Therefore, clinicians are expected to know the pharmacokinetics and pharmacodynamics of these agents, laboratory monitorization of anticoagulation, drug interactions, and specific strategies for reversal.

ANTIPLATELET AGENTS

Acetylsalicylic Acid

Acetylsalicylic acid (ASA) inhibits cyclooxygenase (COX)-1 at small doses or both COX-1 and COX-2 at higher doses.[28] Inhibition of COX-1 blocks the formation of prostaglandin H2 and thromboxane A2 cannot be synthesized. Thromboxane. A2 activates platelets and stimulates their aggregation, therefore, platelet activation is impaired.[29] The effect of ASA on platelets is irreversible. After the discontinuation of aspirin intake, platelet function could be expected to increase by 10%–15% every day as a result of new platelet formation.[29]

P2Y$_{12}$ Receptor Antagonists

P2Y$_{12}$ receptors are adenosine diphosphate (ADP) receptors expressed on the surface of platelets, which can be blocked chemically and the overall effect of ADP on platelets is reduced.

- **Clopidogrel:** It is a prodrug, 85% of which is hydrolysed to an inactive metabolite. The active metabolite of the drug binds to P2Y$_{12}$ receptors irreversibly. The CYP450 dependency makes clopidogrel susceptible to drug interactions.
- **Prasugrel:** It is also a prodrug which is converted by CYP450 enzymes to its active metabolite. The active metabolite of the drug binds to P2Y$_{12}$ receptors irreversibly.
- **Ticagrelor:** It is a cyclopentyl-triazolo-pyrimidine, and binds reversibly to a different site on the P2Y$_{12}$ receptor.[29]

Glycoprotein IIb/IIIa Inhibitors

Glycoprotein (Gp) IIb/IIIa receptors are the most numerous proteins on the surface of platelets. Glycoprotein IIb/IIIa inhibitors block the adhesion of fibrinogen to the activated platelet, preventing the building of inter-platelet bridges.[29] These drugs are mostly used in neurovascular interventions through an intravenous route. Abciximab, eptifibatide, and tirofiban are the agents of this class.

Management of Bleeding

A similar incidence of intracerebral haematoma in patients on antiplatelet agents was reported to range from 0.2%–0.4%.[30] Mainly, the reversal strategy for antiplatelet drugs is transfusion of exogenous platelets since these drugs except for ticagrelor bind irreversibly to their targets.

Current guidelines recommend administering platelets only to patients who require neurosurgical intervention.[20] There is a paucity of literature on the use of platelet transfusions in TBI patients on antiplatelet drugs. A single retrospective study found no difference in mortality among 166 TBI patients receiving platelets compared with a matched group of 162 patients who did not receive platelet transfusion.[31,32]

Desmopressin may be an attractive agent for patients on antiplatelet drugs since its administration resulted in transfusion of fewer units of red cells, less blood loss, and a lower risk of reoperation due to bleeding in cardiac surgery.[33]

VITAMIN K ANTAGONISTS

Warfarin

Warfarin use increases a patient's risk for spontaneous ICH. The incidence of spontaneous haemorrhage is 7–10 times higher among patients taking warfarin compared to those not on anticoagulation.[34]

The coagulation factors II, VII, IX, and X require carboxylation in the liver. Vitamin K is essential for this process. Warfarin inhibits vitamin K epoxide reductase and blocks the formation of reduced vitamin K. The half-life of warfarin is 36–42 hours and it is metabolized by the liver. The effect of warfarin rapidly changes due to drug interactions and polymorphisms of the cytochrome P450 system.[35] Therefore, the degree of pharmacological coagulopathy should be closely monitored using INR. For most of the patients moderate anticoagulation is sufficient (INR: 2.0–3.0), but for patients with prosthetic mechanical heart valves, a higher INR value (2.5–3.5) is recommended.[34]

The most severe and potentially mortal complication in patients on warfarin is ICH.[36] Patients on anticoagulants suffering from ICH require timely and complete reversal of anticoagulation. Acute interventions minimizing ICH and haematoma size are critical for better outcomes in neurointensive care units.[37]

Management of Bleeding

Warfarin inhibits vitamin-K-dependent factors (fII, fVII, fIX, FX), so these factors should be repleted. There are different alternatives for repletion:

- *Vitamin K*: Administration of vitamin K is assumed effective in reversing warfarin effects. Intravenous administration is the preferred route. In guidelines (*American College of Chest Physicians Evidence-Based Clinical Practice Guidelines, 8th Edition, Guidelines on oral anticoagulation: third edition, Warfarin reversal: consensus guidelines on behalf of the Australasian Society of Thrombosis and Haemostasis*), dosages of 5–10 mg of vitamin K given by slow intravenous infusion is recommended for urgent reversal of warfarin.[38–40]

- *Fresh Frozen Plasma*: Fresh frozen plasma is a blood product available worldwide that contains vitamin-K-dependent factors which are depleted by warfarin. Fresh frozen plasma is deficient in factor IX. In urgent reversal, FFP administration could be used to replace these factors (15–20 ml/kg). This conventional technique is rather slow and ineffective since FFP is not a concentrated drug which means volume overload and before administering FFP, it should be thawed resulting in treatment delay. Also, every transfusion is a risk for infection transmission and transfusion-related acute lung injury (TRALI).[37]

- *Prothrombin Complex Concentrate*: Prothrombin complex concentrate (PCC) is a human plasma-derived concentrate that contains all the vitamin K-dependent coagulation factors in concentrated form.[41] Prothrombin complex concentrate is the fastest, most effective method of warfarin reversal in use. Target INR could be achieved within 15 minutes in 90% of patients (25–50 U/kg).[42] The adverse effect of PCC is mainly the risk of arterial/venous thrombosis (5%).

- *Recombinant Factor VIIa*: Recombinant factor VIIa is cloned from human clotting factor VII. Recombinant factor VIIa is an effective agent for radiographic stabilization of ICH and reversal of INR, but there is no evidence that usage of rfVIIa improves outcome of patients with ICH.[43] Recombinant factor VIIa is given through an intravenous route and its onset of action is almost 'immediate'. Due to thrombotic complications[44] and cost-effectivity, rfVIIa would not be the agent of 'first' choice.[20]

NOVEL ORAL ANTICOAGULANTS

Factor Xa and thrombin are the targets of this group of agents for anticoagulant treatment. Routine monitoring of anticoagulant effect is not required. Patients receiving novel anticoagulants had a reduced risk of stroke, systemic embolism, and mortality, and a smaller risk of fatal bleeding compared to patients on warfarin.[45] Also, anticoagulant effect of these drugs is much shorter than warfarin (Table 41.1).

Clinicians are still facing fatal bleeding in patients on novel anticoagulants needing urgent reversal. In those cases, timing of the last medication allows a clinician to estimate the time required for the drugs to be eliminated from circulation since pharmacokinetics of these agents are well-known.

Oral Direct Thrombin Inhibitors

Oral direct thrombin inhibitors, dabigatran etexilate is the prodrug form of dabigatran, a synthetic molecule which is an orally administered direct thrombin inhibitor.[27] Thrombin catalyses the final step in the cascade converting fibrinogen to fibrin.[46] Plasma levels peak in 1–3 hours. It is excreted by the kidneys (80%) and has a half-life of 12–14 hours.[47]

Ketoconazole, amiodarone, verapamil, and quinidine may increase plasma concentration of dabigatran since these drugs are P-glycoprotein inhibitors.[29]

Dabigatran prolongs aPTT and TT. As the commercial reagent in laboratories change, aPTT values vary and does not accurately reflect the quantity of dabigatran in circulation. Thrombin time is the most accurate test for detecting dabigatran even in very small quantities. If the TT is normal, then clinically relevant drug level is excluded. Ecarin clotting time (ECT) and dilute TT test could also be used for this purpose but these tests are not widely available. Prothrombin time has a low sensitivity for measuring the effects of dabigatran.[46]

A patient's renal function is an important consideration for elimination of dabigatran since this drug is excreted by the kidneys mostly.

Idarucizumab, a specific reversal agent—a monoclonal antibody fragment for dabigatran—binds selectively and reverses the anticoagulant effect of dabigatran within minutes.[48] Idarucizumab is administered as two 2.5 grams (a total of 5 grams) intravenous injections given over 15 minutes.

Oral activated charcoal could be useful for reducing dabigatran absorption following recent ingestion (within 2–3 hours).[46,49]

Haemodialysis could be considered for removal of dabigatran in cases of renal dysfunction since dabigatran has low plasma protein binding and small molecular size.[46,50]

Oral Factor Xa Inhibitors

Rivaroxaban, apixaban, and edoxaban are frequently used oral factor Xa inhibitors. The laboratory assessment of these drugs could be achieved by chromogenic assay for anti-factor Xa activity.[51] An agent-*andexanet alfa (Portola Pharmaceuticals, San Francisco, CA)* is expected to receive Food and Drug Administration (FDA) approval soon for urgent reversal of factor Xa inhibitors.[51] *Ciraparantag* is currently being studied in healthy volunteers as a reversal agent for all oral anticoagulants after taking promising results in animal studies. The mechanism of action of ciraparantag is binding anticoagulants with noncovalent hydrogen bonds.[50] Due to pharmacokinetic properties, haemodialysisis is not indicated to reverse these agents.

Rivaroxaban

Rivaroxaban selectively inhibits factor Xa in a reversible way. Plasma levels peak in 1–3 hours. Rivaroxaban is

Table 41.1 Characteristics of anticoagulant drugs

	Dabigatran	**Rivaroxaban**	**Apixaban**	**Edoxaban**
Mechanism of Action	Direct Thrombin Inhibitor	F Xa inhibitor	F Xa inhibitor	F Xa inhibitor
Half-life	12–14 hr	7–10 hr	8–15 hr	10–14 hr
Peak plasma concentration	1–3 hr	1–3 hr	2.5–4 hr	1–2 hr
Elimination	80% renal	50%/50% renal/hepatic	25% renal	50% renal
Drug interactions	P-glycoprotein inhibitors	P-glycoprotein inhibitors	CYP3Y4, P-glycoprotein inhibitors	P-glycoprotein inhibitors

excreted by the kidneys and liver and has a half-life of 7–10 hours. Co-treatment with CYP3A4 inhibitors should be avoided because it may lead to altered plasma concentrations.[29,52] In addition to factor Xa activity, PT/INR within normal ranges excludes significant levels of rivaroxaban.[51]

Apixaban

Apixaban inhibits both free and prothrombinase complex-bound factor Xa selectively. Plasma levels peak in 2.5–4 hours. Apixaban has a half-life of 8–15 hours. P-glycoprotein inhibitors may increase absorption. P-glycoprotein inducers (carbamazepine, phenobarbital, phenytoin, etc.) may cause a decreased concentration of apixaban.[28,52] For detecting the presence of apixaban, PT has limited sensitivity.[53]

Edoxaban

Edoxaban is a direct inhibitor of factor Xa. Plasma levels peak in 1–2 hours. Edoxaban has a half-life of 10–14 hours. The co-administration of P-glycoprotein inhibitors should be avoided. Patients with renal dysfunction and low body weight need dose adjustment.[29,54]

As a summary, if aPTT/PT/antifactor Xa tests are within normal range we can assume that the effect of novel oral anticoagulants is over.

CONCLUSION

The major concern in neurointensive care patients is that the intracranial area is a closed compartment. The tolerance threshold of enlargement of brain tissue due to bleeding is too narrow as long as the intracranial pressure correlates closely with morbidity and mortality of the patients. Therefore, coagulopathy in neurointensive care units is highly important concerning patients' neurological outcome. Clinicians should be well prepared in certain clinical situations leading to coagulopathy.

REFERENCES

1. Goh KY, et al. Haemostatic changes during surgery for primary brain tumours. *J Neurol Neurosurg Psychiatry* 1997;63(3):334–8.
2. Prasad KS, et al. Haemostatic derangement in patients with intracranial tumours. Br *J Neurosurg* 1994;8(6):695–702.
3. Maegele M. Coagulopathy after traumatic brain injury: incidence, pathogenesis, and treatment options. *Transfusion* 2013;53(Suppl 1):28S–37S.
4. Lustenberger T, et al. Time course of coagulopathy in isolated severe traumatic brain injury. *Injury* 2010;41(9):924–8.
5. Harhangi BS, et al. Coagulation disorders after traumatic brain injury. *Acta Neurochir (Wien)* 2008;150(2):165–75; discussion 175.
6. Greuters S, et al. Acute and delayed mild coagulopathy are related to outcome in patients with isolated traumatic brain injury. *Crit Care* 2011;15(1):R2.
7. Laroche M, et al. Coagulopathy after traumatic brain injury. *Neurosurgery* 2012;70(6):1334–45.
8. Stein SC, et al. Delayed brain injury after head trauma: significance of coagulopathy. *Neurosurgery* 1992;30(2):160–5.
9. Cohen MJ, et al. Early coagulopathy after traumatic brain injury: the role of hypoperfusion and the protein C pathway. *J Trauma* 2007;63(6):1254–61; discussion 1261–2.
10. Brohi K, et al. Acute coagulopathy of trauma: hypoperfusion induces systemic anticoagulation and hyperfibrinolysis. *J Trauma* 2008;64(5):1211–7; discussion 1217.
11. Eddleston M, et al. Astrocytes are the primary source of tissue factor in the murine central nervous system. A role for astrocytes in cerebral hemostasis. *J Clin Invest* 1993;92(1):349–58.
12. Schochl H, et al. Hyperfibrinolysis after major trauma: differential diagnosis of lysis patterns and prognostic value of thrombelastometry. *J Trauma* 2009;67(1):125–31.
13. Carrick MM, et al. Subsequent development of thrombocytopenia and coagulopathy in moderate and severe head injury: support for serial laboratory examination. *J Trauma* 2005;58(4):725–9; discussion 729–30.
14. Dzik WH. The James Blundell Award Lecture 2006: transfusion and the treatment of haemorrhage: past, present and future. *Transfus Med* 2007;17(5):367–74.
15. Allard CB, et al. Abnormal coagulation tests are associated with progression of traumatic intracranial hemorrhage. *J Trauma* 2009;67(5):959–67.
16. Etemadrezaie H, et al. The effect of fresh frozen plasma in severe closed head injury. *Clin Neurol Neurosurg* 2007;109(2):166–71.
17. CRASH-2 trial collaborators. Shakur H, Roberts I, Bautista R, et al. Effects of tranexamic acid on death, vascular occlusive events, and blood transfusion in trauma patients with significant haemorrhage (CRASH-2): a randomised, placebo-controlled trial. *Lancet* 2010;376(9734):23–32.
18. Bartal C, et al. Coagulopathic patients with traumatic intracranial bleeding: defining the role of recombinant factor VIIa. *J Trauma* 2007;63(4):725–32.
19. Stein DM, et al. Recombinant factor VIIa: decreasing time to intervention in coagulopathic patients with severe traumatic brain injury. *J Trauma* 2008;64(3):620–7; discussion 627–8.
20. Guha D, Macdonald RL. Perioperative management of anticoagulation. *Neurosurg Clin N Am* 2017;28(2):287–95.

21. Purrucker JC, et al. Early clinical and radiological course, management, and outcome of intracerebral hemorrhage related to new oral anticoagulants. *JAMA Neurol* 2016;73(2):169–77.

22. Huynh TJ, et al. Validation of the 9-point and 24-point hematoma expansion prediction scores and derivation of the PREDICT A/B scores. *Stroke* 2015;46(11):3105–10.

23. Levy JH. Discontinuation and management of direct-acting anticoagulants for emergency procedures. *Am J Emerg Med* 2016;34(11S):14–18.

24. Granger CB, et al. Apixaban versus warfarin in patients with atrial fibrillation. *N Engl J Med* 2011;365(11):981–92.

25. Patel MR, et al. Rivaroxaban versus warfarin in nonvalvular atrial fibrillation. *N Engl J Med* 2011;365(10):883–91.

26. Connolly SJ, et al. Dabigatran versus warfarin in patients with atrial fibrillation. *N Engl J Med* 2009;361(12):1139–51.

27. Pollack CV Jr., Bernstein R, Dubiel R, et al. Healthcare resource utilization in patients receiving idarucizumab for reversal of dabigatran anticoagulation due to major bleeding, urgent surgery, or procedural interventions: interim results from the RE-VERSE AD study. *J Med Econ* 2017;1–8.

28. Mega JL, Simon T. Pharmacology of antithrombotic drugs: an assessment of oral antiplatelet and anticoagulant treatments. *Lancet* 2015;386(9990):281–91.

29. Koenig-Oberhuber V, Filipovic M. New antiplatelet drugs and new oral anticoagulants. *Br J Anaesth* 2016;117(Suppl 2):ii74–ii84.

30. Campbell PG, et al. Emergency reversal of clopidogrel in the setting of spontaneous intracerebral hemorrhage. *World Neurosurg* 2011;76(1–2):100–4; discussion 59–60.

31. Downey DM, et al. Does platelet administration affect mortality in elderly head-injured patients taking antiplatelet medications? *Am Surg* 2009;75(11):1100–3.

32. Bachelani AM, et al. Assessment of platelet transfusion for reversal of aspirin after traumatic brain injury. *Surgery* 2011;150(4):836–43.

33. Desborough MJ, et al. Desmopressin for treatment of platelet dysfunction and reversal of antiplatelet agents: a systematic review and meta-analysis of randomized controlled trials. *J Thromb Haemost* 2017;15(2):263–72.

34. Steiner T, Rosand J, Diringer M. Intracerebral hemorrhage associated with oral anticoagulant therapy: current practices and unresolved questions. *Stroke* 2006;37(1):256–62.

35. Aiyagari V, Testai FD. Correction of coagulopathy in warfarin associated cerebral hemorrhage. *Curr Opin Crit Care* 2009;15(2):87–92.

36. Imberti D, et al. Emergency reversal of anticoagulation with a three-factor prothrombin complex concentrate in patients with intracranial haemorrhage. *Blood Transfus* 2011;9(2):148–55.

37. Bechtel BF, et al. Treatments for reversing warfarin anticoagulation in patients with acute intracranial hemorrhage: a structured literature review. *Int J Emerg Med* 2011;4(1):40.

38. Ansell J, et al. Pharmacology and management of the vitamin K antagonists: American College of Chest Physicians Evidence-Based Clinical Practice Guidelines. 8th Ed. *Chest* 2008;133(Suppl 6):160S–198S.

39. Guidelines on oral anticoagulation. 3rd ed. *Br J Haematol* 1998;101(2):374–87.

40. Baker RI, et al. Warfarin reversal: consensus guidelines on behalf of the Australasian Society of Thrombosis and Haemostasis. *Med J Aust* 2004;181(9):492–7.

41. Appelboam R, Thomas EO. Warfarin and intracranial haemorrhage. *Blood Rev* 2009;23(1):1–9.

42. Thachil J, Gatt A, Martlew V. Management of surgical patients receiving anticoagulation and antiplatelet agents. *Br J Surg* 2008;95(12):1437–48.

43. Mayer SA, et al. Efficacy and safety of recombinant activated factor VII for acute intracerebral hemorrhage. *N Engl J Med* 2008;358(20):2127–37.

44. Levi M, et al. Safety of recombinant activated factor VII in randomized clinical trials. *N Engl J Med* 2010;363(19):1791–800.

45. Miller CS, et al. Meta-analysis of efficacy and safety of new oral anticoagulants (dabigatran, rivaroxaban, apixaban) versus warfarin in patients with atrial fibrillation. *Am J Cardiol* 2012;110(3):453–60.

46. Siegal DM, Crowther MA. Acute management of bleeding in patients on novel oral anticoagulants. *Eur Heart J* 2013;34(7):489–498b.

47. Stangier J, et al. The pharmacokinetics, pharmacodynamics and tolerability of dabigatran etexilate, a new oral direct thrombin inhibitor in healthy male subjects. *Br J Clin Pharmacol* 2007;64(3):292–303.

48. Pollack CV Jr., et al. Idarucizumab for dabigatran reversal. *N Engl J Med* 2015;373(6):511–20.

49. vanRyn J, et al. Dabigatran etexilate—a novel, reversible, oral direct thrombin inhibitor: interpretation of coagulation assays and reversal of anticoagulant activity. *Thromb Haemost* 2010;103(6):1116–27.

50. Shih AW, Crowther MA. Reversal of direct oral anticoagulants: a practical approach. Am Soc Hematol Educ Program. *Hematology* 2016(1):612–9.

51. Weinberger J, Cipolle M. Optimal reversal of novel anticoagulants in trauma. *Crit Care Clin* 2017;33(1):135–52.

52. Dempfle CE. Direct oral anticoagulants—pharmacology, drug interactions, and side effects. *Semin Hematol* 2014;51(2):89–97.

53. Wong PC, et al. Apixaban, an oral, direct and highly selective factor Xa inhibitor: in vitro, antithrombotic and antihemostatic studies. *J Thromb Haemost* 2008;6(5):820–9.

54. Lip GY, Agnelli G. Edoxaban: a focused review of its clinical pharmacology. *Eur Heart J* 2014;35(28):1844–55.

42

Blood Transfusion

O. Arun

ABSTRACT

Blood transfusion (BT) is a common practice for critically ill patients. A majority of patients admitted to the intensive care unit often receive red blood cell (RBC) concentrates as a consequence of anaemia; platelets and plasma components are often given for various indications sometimes outside consensus guidelines. Although BT can be a life-saving therapy in some circumstances, many studies have pointed out increased morbidity and mortality due to serious complications and adverse reactions such as transfusion-related acute lung injury (TRALI), anaphylaxis, transfusion-associated circulatory overload (TACO), transfusion-associated bacterial sepsis, and transfusion-associated graft-versus-host disease (TA-GVHD). The appropriate use of blood products is essential due to the existence of potential risks as well as potential benefits for each patient. Indications and complications of various types of blood products with the major features and many aspects of BT in neurointensive care unit (NICU) patients are discussed in this chapter.

KEYWORDS

Blood transfusion (BT); blood products; transfusion practice; transfusion risks; critically ill.

INTRODUCTION

Blood is a suspension of red blood cells (RBCs) (also erythrocytes), white cells (leukocytes), and platelets in plasma. It is a vital fluid that has basically three functions in the human body: transportation, protection, and regulation. Erythrocytes constitute a major part of the cells in the blood and occupy ≈45% of total blood volume. They comprise iron-containing protein molecules haemoglobin (Hb), which is responsible for carrying almost all of the oxygen (O_2) in the blood. Deterioration in O_2 transportation is not only one of the potential restrictive factors for tissue oxygenation but also may worsen secondary brain injury in neurosurgical patients. The brain requires approximately 3.3 ml of O_2 per 100 g of brain tissue per minute thus adequate oxygen transportation is of crucial performance for blood, particularly for brain function.[1]

Anaemia is a common co-morbidity among intensive care unit (ICU) patients. While 60%–66% of patients are anaemic at admission, the incidence of anaemia is increased during their stay and detected in 97% of the patients at the end of the first week in ICU. The incidence of anaemia among neurocritical care patients is also high and quite variable according to their neurological pathology. Patients with traumatic brain injury (TBI), subarachnoid haemorrhage (SAH), acute ischaemic stroke, and intracranial haemorrhage (ICH) commonly develop anaemia and require blood transfusion (BT) in the Neurosurgical ICU. Although transfusion of blood and blood products is common in the neurointensive care unit (NICU) parallel with the rate of anaemia, the type of neurological injury influences the aims of transfusion and creates diversities among clinicians' transfusion strategies.[2]

A majority of BT is performed by packed red blood cell (PRBC) (also known as red cell concentrate or packed cells) transfusion. The basic goal of PRBC transfusion is to improve O_2 delivery (DO_2) to the tissues. Due to the inability of directly measuring DO_2 in the clinical practice, Hb is routinely measured as an indicator of transfusion requirement. Although restrictive blood transfusion strategy (Hb transfusion trigger of 7–8 g/dL^{-1}) is supported by recent studies when compared with liberal transfusion strategy (Hb transfusion trigger of 9–10 g/dL^{-1}), there has been a controversy regarding the optimal Hb level triggering blood transfusion in NICU patients.[3]

The appropriate use of blood products is essential due to the existence of potential risks as well as potential benefits for each patient. Indications and complications of various types of blood products with the major features and many aspects of BT in NICU patients are discussed in this chapter.

GENERAL FEATURES OF TRANSFUSION PRACTICE

Terminology of Blood Components

Until the late 1970s most of the transfusions were made by 'whole blood' without any processing to separate the components.[4] Today, major indications of whole blood transfusion are red cell replacement in acute blood loss with hypovolaemia, exchange transfusion, and unavailability of RBCs. Whole blood is rarely kept in hospital blood banks because of the more rigorous collection process, shorter shelf life, and greater risk of reaction due to the components of blood. Instead, to separate the whole blood into components is more convenient, cost-effective, and salutary and blood components are used substantially instead of whole blood in most of the developed and developing countries.[5]

The term 'blood product' is a general nomenclature and defines any therapeutic substance prepared from human blood. Another term 'blood component' refers to a blood product made from fresh whole blood and includes packed RBC (PRBC), fresh frozen plasma (FFP), platelets, cryoprecipitate, and granulocyte components. While the first three components mentioned above are obtained by centrifuging whole blood, cryoprecipitate is made from fresh plasma by putting the plasma through a freeze/thaw cycle and granulocyte concentrates are collected by haemapheresis. Another term 'plasma derivatives' defines plasma proteins prepared from large pools of human plasma under pharmaceutical manufacturing conditions, e.g., coagulation factors, immunoglobulin, and albumin.[5]

Apheresis is another way to obtain platelets, plasma, and red cells from whole blood. Basically, it is a medical technology in which the blood is taken from the donor and passed through an apparatus that separates one particular constituent and returns the remainder to the circulation. Centrifugation and filtration are the two main mechanisms of apheresis that depend on cellular blood components' different specific gravity and size, respectively. The components that can be collected with apheresis are double unit red cell collection (red cells), single donor platelet (SDP), harvesting platelets, leucapheresis (harvesting granulocytes, peripheral blood haematopoietic stem cell), plasmapheresis is (collecting normal plasma) and therapeutic plasma exchange (for exchanging with normal plasma after collecting and discarding the patient's plasma).[6]

Blood Components

A single whole blood donation contains 450–500 ml of blood with a minimum haematocrit (Hct) of 38%. Shelf life of whole blood is 21–35 days depending on the anticoagulant-preservative solution.[7] The donor's blood is drawn into a plastic pack containing 63 ml of an anticoagulant-preservative solution, usually citrate phosphate dextrose (CPD) (21-day storage time), CPD-adenine (CPDA) (35-day storage time), or new generation additive solutions (e.g., ADSOL) (42-day storage time). The citrate binds calcium and acts as an anticoagulant, and the glucose and adenine support red cell metabolism during storage. The preservative solution ADSOL contains adenine, dextrose, sorbitol, sodium chloride, and mannitol while SAGM is a saline solution containing added adenine, glucose, and mannitol. Almost all whole blood donations are processed to separate red cells, platelets, plasma, and granulocytes.[5] These components of blood are discussed in detail in the next few paragraphs.

Red Blood Cells

Red blood cell concentrate is a blood component obtained by removing a part of the plasma (and a variable number of platelets) from whole blood by centrifugation, without further manipulation or addition of additive solutions. It contains all the RBCs initially present, most of the leucocytes ($2.5–3 \times 10^9$) and a variable number of platelets. The Hct is between 65%–75% and the minimum Hb content is 45 g. The volume of RBC concentrate is 280 ± 50 ml.[8]

Red blood cell concentrate devoid of the buffy coat (the leucocyte-platelet layer) is another product that is obtained after separating plasma and buffy coat from RBCs by centrifugation. The white cell content must be below 1.2×10^9 and the mean platelet count $<20 \times 10^9$ per unit.

As in whole blood, preservative solutions can be added to RBCs to improve their shelf life. The volume of additive solution is between 80 and 110 ml. The product results in an Hct of 50%–70% (depends on the quantity of the additive solution, the method of centrifugation, and the amount of residual plasma) and a volume of 300–400 ml.[9]

Transfusion of RBCs should be based on the patient's clinical condition. The major rationale is to improve oxygen delivery to tissues. Indications for RBC transfusion include acute sickle cell crisis (for stroke prevention) or acute blood loss of greater than 1,500 ml or 30% of blood volume. Patients with symptomatic anaemia should be transfused if they cannot function without treating the anaemia.[10] It is expected from one unit of packed RBCs to increase the Hb level by 1 g/dL^{-1} (10 g/L^{-1}) and Hct by 3%.

Frozen (Cryopreserved) Red Blood Cells

Although the facility of storing RBCs in anticoagulant and additive systems gives life-saving consequences, during this process RBCs progressively deteriorate and with the prolonged storage time adverse clinical outcomes such as postoperative infections, prolonged length of hospital stay, multiple organ failure, and increased mortality can occur.[11] Cryopreservation is a process of storing at ultra-low temperatures with the aim of preventing the progressive cellular deterioration that has been linked to adverse clinical outcome. Ultra-low temperatures cease the biological activity of RBCs, which enables them to be preserved for prolonged periods of time. Glycerol, a cryoprotective additive, is used to prevent freezing damage by limiting ice crystal formation while minimizing solute effects and cellular dehydration during freezing.[12]

There are two freezing methods according to the glycerol concentration. With the low-glycerol method (LGM) RBCs are frozen rapidly with a final concentration of approximately 20% glycerol and stored at temperatures below −140°C while with the high-glycerol method (HGM) RBCs are frozen slowly with a final concentration of approximately 40% glycerol and stored at temperatures between −60°C and −80°C. With one of these techniques and correct storage conditions frozen RBCs can be kept available for at least 10 years.[12]

Frozen RBC units must be thawed rapidly to prevent recrystallization and a deglycerolization washing procedure is performed to reduce glycerol content. Incomplete deglycerolization may induce renal failure due to high concentrations of free Hb.[13] In the HGM frozen group RBCs require more extensive washing because of higher glycerol concentration and this may cause cellular loss particularly in older RBCs.[14] Although the post-thaw storage time is limited to 24 hours due to the potential risk of bacterial contamination, HGM frozen RBCs can be stored up to seven days in SAGM solution and up to 21 days in additive solution-3 (AS-3) after thawing.[15]

Frozen RBCs are primarily used when the RBC availability is limited or unpredictable. Apart from military oriented usage, one of the main scopes of frozen RBCs is the patient with complex immune-haematological profile in the absence of compatible donors.[16]

Effects of Storage on Red Blood Cells and Rejuvenation

Red blood cell storage lesion refers to the alterations in RBC quality and cellular functionality during ex vivo preservation in blood banks. These alterations can be classified into three categories: biochemical, biomechanical, and immunologic. Major biochemical changes during RBC storage are 2,3-diphosphoglycerate (DPG) and adenosine triphosphate (ATP) depletion, fall in S-nitrosothiol (SNO) bioactivity that mediate oxygen-sensitive vasodilator effect of RBCs, accumulation of oxidized lipid and protein species, and loss of chemokine scavenging capacity.[17] The biomechanical changes include alterations in corpuscle shape, deformability, osmotic fragility, and intracellular viscosity that are all important determinants of RBCs' haemodynamic function and survival in the circulation.[18] These morphological changes are attributed to various biochemical alterations in stored RBCs such as decrease in the level of ATP and 2,3-DPG, loss of membrane phospholipid with associated vesiculation, protein rearrangement, and lipid oxidation.[19] Improved renal allograft survival after allogeneic blood transfusion and some post-transfusional adverse effects such as nosocomial infections, transfusion-related acute lung injury (TRALI), and multi-organ failure points out some immune-modulatory effects of stored RBCs on recipients that were later referred as transfusion-related immunomodulation (TRIM).[20]

Rejuvenation is a process of restoring depleted metabolites particularly 2,3-DPG and ATP to improve the function and post-transfusion survival of stored red cells. The rejuvenating solution (Rejuvesol®) contains pyruvate, inosine, phosphate, and adenine. The solution is intended only for the extracorporeal rejuvenation of RBC and not for whole blood because the additional plasma may reduce the effectiveness of the rejuvenation process.[21]

Plasma Components

Plasma is the remaining portion after removing of cellular elements (i.e., RBCs and white blood cells

[WBCs]) and platelets by centrifugation of whole blood. Several different plasma preparations are available, including fresh frozen plasma (FFP), thawed plasma (TP), liquid plasma (LP), cryoprecipitate, and factor concentrates.

Fresh frozen plasma is obtained from whole blood by apheresis (also known as platelet pheresis) and is frozen at −18°C or colder. The size of the unit of plasma differs according to the obtaining technique. A unit of apheresis collection contains approximately 500 ml while single donor collection contains approximately 250 ml. Fresh frozen plasma contains functional amounts of coagulation factors V and VIII. Once it has been thawed, the plasma must be transfused within 24 hours, otherwise the concentrations of factor V and factor VIII begin to decline. Fresh frozen plasma needs to be blood type (ABO)-compatible, but does not require cross-matching or Rhesus (Rh) blood typing.

Thawed plasma is the FFP not transfused within 24 hours after being thawed. It can be transfused within 5 days after being thawed if stored at 1–6°C. Although some centres routinely use extended-TP internationally, there are no clinical studies evaluating its efficacy compared with FFP. Factor VIII (FVIII) is the worst affected factor in TP and its activity is mainly lost during the first 24 hours following thawing. Potential concerns with respect to the use of TP include the theoretical risk of bacterial contamination and increased levels of DEHP (di (2-ethylhexyl)phthalate) exposure.[22]

Cryoprecipitate is prepared by controlled thawing of FFP and collecting the precipitate that contains high molecular weight proteins, including FVIII, von Willebrand factor (vWf) and fibrinogen. The cryoprecipitate prepared from a single donor unit contains 80–300 units of FVIII and vWf, and 300–600 mg of fibrinogen in a volume of 20–50 ml. It is used in cases of hypofibrinogenaemia, which most often occurs in the setting of massive haemorrhage or consumptive coagulopathy. The usual dose in adults is typically two five-donor pools (equivalent to 10 single donor units) containing 3–6 g fibrinogen in a volume of 200–500 ml. Each unit will raise the fibrinogen level by 5–10 mg/dL^{-1} (0.15–0.29 μmol/L^{-1}).[23]

Liquid plasma is prepared by removing the cellular part from previously stored whole blood. Both LP and TP can be stored for extended periods (>24 hr) to reduce wastage and to improve rapid availability of plasma in massive transfusion protocols. It has limited use due to lack of FV and FVIII.[22]

The common indications of plasma transfusion in critically ill patients is inadequate haemostasis. Some examples of clinical situations for transfusion of plasma are as follows:

- Massive transfusion with coagulation deficiencies,
- Active bleeding with patients on Coumadin or who need to undergo an invasive procedure before vitamin K could reverse the anticoagulant effect,
- Transfusion or plasma exchange in patients with thrombotic thrombocytopenic purpura (TTP),
- Management of selected coagulation factor deficiencies when coagulation concentrates are unavailable,
- Management of rare specific plasma protein deficiencies

Although plasma components are widely used for the indications mentioned above, the benefit of plasma administration has been found limited and has not been supported with scientific evidence. The response to a plasma transfusion is directly proportional to the difference between the patient's levels of coagulation factors and that of the infused plasma. Plasma products are prone to be more efficient in patients with severe factor deficiencies than in patients with a mildly prolonged international normalized ratio (INR).[24,25]

Platelet Components

In order to prepare platelet concentrate, the platelets are separated from the buffy coat, pooled, and filtered to remove white cells. Another way is to collect is by platelet pheresis. Two techniques give similar results with respect to functionality of platelets but the procedure of platelet pheresis has an advantage of exposing the recipient to fewer donors than centrifugation. Storage at 22°C with agitation gives the best result for platelet function. As this temperature favours bacterial growth, culture of the platelet concentrates before clinical use is important to avoid donor infections.[26]

Platelet transfusion is indicated in patients with thrombocytopenia and/or platelets' functional defects. Clinical indications may be therapeutic or prophylactic:[27]

- Patients with a platelet count <10 × 10^3 platelets/microlitre to prevent spontaneous haemorrhage
- Patients with a platelet count <50 × 10^3 platelets/microlitre who are actively bleeding, are scheduled to undergo an invasive procedure, or have a qualitative intrinsic platelet disorder
- Patients with a platelet count <100 × 10^3 platelets/microlitre who have a central nervous system injury, multisystem trauma, are undergoing neurosurgery, or require an intrathecal catheter for anaesthesia
- Patients with a normal platelet count who have active bleeding and a reason for platelet dysfunction, such as a congenital platelet disorder, chronic antiplatelet therapy, or uraemia.

Heparin-induced thrombocytopenia (HIT), TTP, haemolytic-uraemic syndromes (HUS), disseminated intravascular coagulation (DIC), and immune thrombocytopenia (ITP) are special considerations where platelet transfusion is less effective and/or associated with deleterious effects. Thus, these conditions are considered as relative contraindications in platelet transfusion.[9]

An adult dose unit generally contains $2.5–3 \times 10^{11}$ platelets. In clinical practice it is usually intended with the dose as the number of whole blood donations (typically 4–6) that are pooled to provide the dosage. A single platelet pheresis procedure can provide an adult dose unit from a single donor. While the centrifugation of whole blood platelets from 4–5 donations constitutes one adult therapeutic dose, the apheresis procedure from 1 donor collection provides 1–3 adult therapeutic doses. Normally 4–6 single donor units should raise the platelet count by $20–40 \times 10^3$ platelets/microlitre. Increments will be less if there is splenomegaly, DIC, or septicaemia.[9]

Granulocyte Transfusion

Granulocyte transfusions can be used as supportive therapy in patients with life-threatening neutropenia and/or neutrophil dysfunction. Granulocytes can be prepared either by apheresis or from whole blood. The buffy coat contains a high concentration of white cells and platelets and can be used as a source to get the granulocyte-containing component. In the apheresis technique, donor premedication with steroids and granulocyte colony stimulating factor (G-CSF) facilitate higher granulocyte cell count in the collection than deriving from whole blood.[28] Despite the potential availability of this component, clinical trials have not so far established the effectiveness of granulocyte transfusion.

RED CELL IMMUNOLOGY AND COMPATIBILITY TESTING

The ABO System

The ABO blood group system was the first discovered and is still the most important system among 29 human blood group systems approved by the International Society of Blood Transfusion. This system contains four groups that are determined by the presence of A and B antigens on the surface of the RBCs, and of anti-A or anti-B antibodies (also called isohaemagglutinins) in the plasma (Table 42.1). Type A RBCs have the A antigen on their surface, those of type B have antigen B, type AB RBCs carry both antigens, while type O cells carry

Table 42.1 ABO blood groups

Blood group	ABO antigens on RBCs	ABO antibodies in plasma	Frequency (%)
Group O	None	Anti-A and Anti-B	45
Group A	A	Anti-B	40
Group B	B	Anti-A	10
Group AB	A and B	None	5

neither antigen. Antibodies against A or B antigens are produced in the healthy body starting from the first year of life by sensitization to environmental substances, such as food, bacteria, and viruses. Antibodies in the A- and B-type individuals are usually IgM-type but O-type individuals can also produce IgG-type antibodies. They attack and rapidly destroy red cells when encountered with the corresponding antigen resulting in a potentially lethal transfusion reaction. For example, anti-A antibodies attack the RBCs of Group A or AB and Anti-B antibodies attack the RBCs of Group B or AB.[29]

Subtypes of ABO blood groups are called subgroup or variant. About 20 subgroups of blood type A appears to have the most variation in subgroups, of which A1 and A2 are the most common (over 99%). A1 makes up about 80% of all A-type blood. Some individuals produce antibodies against other variants and discrepancies can be seen in rare cases when typing the blood.

Rhesus System

The Rh blood system was originally defined by a stimulated reaction between a rabbit antibody and RBCs of Rhesus monkeys. The system is defined by the presence or absence of Rh antigen representing the two blood types, Rh positive and Rh negative. In fact, it is far more complex than the ABO system and currently comprises 54 antigens. The D antigen was the first Rh antigen to be described and remains the most clinically important one due to its higher immunogenic capacity.[30]

In a Caucasian population, the RhD negative blood type is representing approximately 15% of the population. Unlike the ABO system, antibodies to RhD, mainly of the IgG class, do not exist in humans and occur only in RhD-negative individuals following a transfusion or pregnancy. Therefore, it is a routine practice for all blood transfusions to be compatible within the ABO system and for the D antigen of the Rh system. However, unlike the A and B antigens, the Rh antigens are present only on RBCs. Therefore, unlike for blood transfusion, they do not normally play a role in organ transplantation, and

Rh typing of organ donors and recipients is not a significant consideration.[31]

Compatibility Testing

Compatibility testing refers to the set of procedures for searching for antibodies in a patient's serum that may react with the donor's RBCs, in order to prevent any adverse reaction and to ensure maximum survival time for RBCs after the transfusion. Compatibility testing involves:

- Checking the patient's previous history of transfusion
- Checking the patient's ABO and RhD groups
- Performing antibody screening which can be done by several methods also known as serological techniques. Most of these methods involve searching for agglutination and/or haemolysis as the indicator of antigen-antibody interaction in the patients' plasma or serum
- Performing a cross-match which is testing the patient's serum against the donor red cells (also referred as major cross-match). In some centres, testing of the patient's red cells with donor serum (also referred as minor cross-match) is omitted because the donor's serum is checked during the grouping. Even if the patient's and donor's ABO and RhD groups are known, it is advised to perform a cross-match as the final serological test of compatibility to prevent any mistake regarding ABO grouping of the patient or donor[32]

The majority of laboratories now use automated testing with advanced information technology systems and electronic issues (computerized cross-match) for documentation and reporting of the results. Table 42.2 shows the compatibility information for RBCs and plasma between patient and donor blood groups.

Table 42.2 RBC compatibility table

Recipient	Donor							
	O–	O+	A–	A+	B–	B+	AB–	AB+
O–	✓	×	×	×	×	×	×	×
O+	✓	✓	×	×	×	×	×	×
A–	✓	×	✓	×	×	×	×	×
A+	✓	✓	✓	✓	×	×	×	×
B–	✓	×	×	×	✓	×	×	×
B+	✓	✓	×	×	✓	✓	×	×
AB–	✓	×	✓	×	✓	×	✓	×
AB+	✓	✓	✓	✓	✓	✓	✓	✓

Source: Inaba S, Nibu K, Takano H, et al. Potassium-adsorption filter for RBC transfusion: a phase III clinical trial. *Transfusion* 2000; 40:1469–74.

Table 42.3 ABO requirements for blood components

Whole Blood	Must be identical to that of the recipient
RBCs	Must be compatible with the recipient's plasma
Granulocytes Pheresis	Must be compatible with the recipient's plasma
Fresh Frozen Plasma	Must be compatible with the recipient's RBCs
Platelets Pheresis	All ABO groups are acceptable; components compatible with the recipient's RBCs are preferred
Cryoprecipitate	All ABO groups are acceptable

Whenever possible, patients should receive ABO-identical blood; however, it may be necessary to make alternative selections. Requirements for components and acceptable alternative choices are summarized in Table 42.3.

Washing Blood Products

Washing of blood products refers to the removing of plasma/supernatant in RBC/platelet products before transfusion. The basic aim is to prevent and/or eliminate possible complications associated with infusion of proteins present in a small amount of residual plasma in blood products. Washing can be performed with different techniques including a manual open-system technique, an automated cell washer, or an auto-transfusion device.[33] Washed units are depleted of 99% plasma proteins and 85% WBCs but they contain 10%–20% fewer RBCs than the original units. The shelf life of washed products is 24 hours in RBCs and 4 hours in platelets after washing. Some possible detrimental effects of washing are cellular loss, susceptibility to haemolysis, and functional deterioration of platelets.

Indications for washing are:

- Patients with IgA deficiency
- Prevention of allergic reactions not sensitive to antihistamine drugs
- Post-transfusion febrile reactions present even when leucodepleted RBCs are used[8]

Leucodepletion of Blood Products

During allogeneic blood transfusion, a large number of leucocytes pass to the recipient circulation recognized as foreign cells by the immune system that may lead to several adverse reactions such as febrile reactions. In order to avoid such reactions leukodepleted blood transfusion is required. The removal of WBCs (or leukocytes) from the blood products is termed as leucodepletion in Europe and leucoreduction in the US. Blood is considered leucodepleted if the total leucocyte content per unit of blood is $<5 \times 10^6$ and the red cell product should have retained at least 85% of the original red cells.[34] Methods of leucocyte removal from blood include filtering, red cell washing, centrifugation, and buffy coat removal, freezing and deglycerolization of red cells, and apheresis.[35] By using current generation (3rd and 4th) leucodepleted filters, the WBC count has reduced to greater than 99.9%.

The indications for leucodepleted products are:[6]

- Recommended indications
  - Prevention of febrile non-haemolytic transfusion reactions (FNHTRs) caused by the presence of antibodies to WBCs
    o Patients with recurrent FNHTR
    o Patients who need prolonged transfusion support
  - Reduction of the incidence of Cytomegalovirus (CMV) infections in
    o CMV-negative patients with congenital or acquired immunodeficiency
    o CMV-negative recipients of a bone marrow transplantation from a CMV-negative donor
    o Pregnant women, independently of their CMV serological status, given the possible immune-modulatory effect of the transfusion (re-activation of CMV)
  - Reduction of the risk of rejection in candidates for haematopoietic stem cell transplantation
  - Prevention of refractoriness to platelet transfusion
  - Intrauterine transfusions and transfusions to premature babies, neonates, and paediatric patients up to 1 year old
- Possible indications
  - Candidates for renal transplantation: The use of leucodepleted red cells prevents human leucocyte antigen (HLA) alloimmunisation and avoids the risk of transmission of CMV
  - Immunomodulation: There is insufficient evidence to recommend routine use of leucodepleted RBCs in surgical patients with the aim of preventing postoperative infections or recurrent neoplasms

Irradiation of Blood Components

Irradiation is the process by which an object is exposed to radiation. The main purpose of irradiating cellular blood components with either γ-rays or X-rays is the prevention of transfusion-associated graft versus host disease (TA-GVHD) in immune-deficient patients, foetuses, and very premature newborns.[36] The basic mechanism of irradiating is forming deoxyribonucleic acid (DNA) crosslinks that prevent lymphocyte replication without significantly damaging RBCs, platelets or granulocyte function.

With the exception of FFP, all kinds of blood/blood components have been reported to cause TA-GVHD and they should be considered for irradiation in patients with a risk of TA-GVHD.

Shelf lives of irradiated RBC products are shortened to 28 days after irradiation while there is no change in the shelf life of products of platelets and granulocytes.

Indications for Blood Irradiation

For patients with the following conditions, irradiation of blood should be performed before transfusion:[37,38]

- Cardiovascular surgery
- Surgical operations for cancers
- Congenital immune deficiencies
- Haematopoietic transplantation
- Foetuses and low-birth-weight infants
- Neonates requiring exchange transfusion
- Immune-compromised recipients of organ transplantation
- Aged recipients (>65 years old)
- Massive blood loss or severe trauma

Transfusion of irradiated blood should be considered for patients with the following conditions:

- Malignant lymphomas
- Leukaemia and other haematological malignancies
- Solid tumours undergoing treatment with high-dose chemotherapy or irradiation therapy

Irradiated products are not indicated for patients with human immunodeficiency virus (HIV) or acquired immunodeficiency syndrome (AIDS) due to the blockade of both host and donor lymphocytic response by the HIV infection. The dosage of irradiation should be between 15–50 Gy. There are some consequences of irradiation that include oncogenic potential, mutations of viruses in the blood, disturbances of the cellular functions of RBCs and platelets, and elevation of blood potassium levels.[39] As a result of these several drawbacks, alternative methods for preventing TA-GVHD including X-ray irradiation and pathogen inactivation protocols are still being search.

TRANSFUSION-TRANSMITTED INFECTIONS AND PATHOGEN INACTIVATION

Although the risk of transfusion-transmitted infections (TTIs) today is lower than ever, the possibility of

Table 42.4 Estimated rate of viral infection transmission

HIV-1,2	1:2,300,000
Hepatitis B	1:280,000–1:352,000
Hepatitis C	1:1,800,000
Hepatitis D	Risk unknown: presumed to be rare
Hepatitis A and E	Risk unknown: presumed to be rare
HTLV-I, II	1:2,993,000
Cytomegalovirus	Common
West Nile Virus	Uncommon, risk varies by season and location
Epstein–Barr Virus	Rare, limited to case reports

transmitting infectious organisms via blood products is still a major concern in BT practice. One of the important security steps against transfusion-transmitted infectious diseases is testing all donated blood for infectious agents and blood group antibodies before transfusion.

Viral infection transmissions can still occur even at acceptable rates due to the limited success of donor screening and laboratory testing (Table 42.4).[40] The donor samples can be checked for the reactivity of hepatitis B virus (HBV) surface antigen (HBsAg) and antibodies to HBV core antigen (anti-HBc), HIV-1 and HIV-2, human T-cell lymphotropic virus (HTLV) types I and II, and hepatitis C virus (HCV). Introduction of nucleic acid testing (NAT), rather than measuring pathogen-specific humoral immune responses in the donor has greatly helped to reduce the risk of TTIs.[41] It is a highly sensitive and specific molecular technique for viral nucleic acids that detects viral ribonucleic acid (RNA) or DNA earlier than the other screening methods. Nucleic acid testing has also significantly increased the sensitivity to detect infected blood components earlier in the 'window period' than antibody or antigen assays. The American Red Cross implemented the automated triplex NAT for HIV, HCV, and HBV. Cytomegalovirus and human herpes virus-8 (HHV-8) are transfusion-transmissible pathogens that can cause significant complications in immune-compromised recipients. The West Nile Virus; Parvovirus B19; and hepatitis A, E, and G viruses are some of the other viral agents that have been shown to be transmissible via blood transfusion.[42,43] The contents of tested agents can be variable and additional tests performed according to the epidemiology of infections in the population.

As a consequence of the increasing awareness and clinical relevance of bacterial contamination of blood components with effective screening tests, bacterial contamination has substantially declined. Autologous RBC units are

considered to be safe for bacterial infections and sepsis associated with transfusion of a bacterially contaminated RBC unit is a very rare event. On the contrary, bacterially contaminated platelets are the most common transfusion-transmitted disease source in transfusion practice.[44] Fresh frozen plasma and cryoprecipitate are very rarely significantly contaminated with bacteria because of storage under −18°C. Bacterial TTIs can be divided based on the origin of microorganisms; originate from the environment, skin of the transfused subject, or those that are likely derived from a donor bacteraemia. Bacterial contaminations most commonly occur during blood collection or handling of blood products, thus isolated bacteria usually belong to skin and/or gastrointestinal flora. General measures to reduce the risk of bacterial contamination include the search for donor eligibility, optimal blood product processing, handling and storage, skin preparation with improved donor arm disinfection, and removal of the first 30–40 ml of whole blood from the collection.

Several parasites that have been implicated in transfusion-associated transmission are Plasmodium spp. (can cause malaria by one of four species called *P. falciparum, P. vivax, P. malariae*, and *P. ovale*), *Trypanosoma cruzi* (aetiologic agent of Chagas disease), *Babesia microti* (aetiologic agent of babesiosis), and *Leishmania donovani*. Individuals from endemic areas of these parasites may be chronic carriers of the parasite and are potentially at risk of transmitting the parasite via transfusion of their blood.[45]

The unavailability of previous history of possible infectious agents, development of effective laboratory tests for each agent, and widespread application of these tests to all collected blood are major problems hindering the 100% success rate against infections. Search for more effective ways of sterilizing blood after collection brought out pathogen inactivation technology. 'Pathogen inactivation' refers to decreasing the amount of an infectious pathogen, either by physical removal (e.g., nanofiltration) or by inactivation technology. There are several methods for pathogen inactivation:

- Methods that damage lipids
  - Solvent/detergent treatment
- Methods that damage nucleic acids
  - Amotosalen and ultraviolet A (UV-A) light (Intercept™)
  - Riboflavin and UV light (Mirasol®)
  - Methylene blue and visible light
  - UV light alone

All of these technologies are available in Europe and in the USA, except methylene blue treatment and riboflavin plus UV light are not licenced in the USA. Pathogen inactivation technologies have several potential limitations regarding efficacy, possible toxicity, possible reduction in component quality, and cost.[45]

MONITORING OF TRANSFUSION

The patient should be observed before, during, and after the transfusion for the early detection of any adverse events or reactions. Adverse reactions can occur with all blood components and plasma derivatives. Before starting the transfusion, patient's general condition, baseline heart rate, blood pressure, temperature, and respiratory rate must be recorded. During the transfusion, these vital parameters must be checked and recorded as soon as the transfusion is started and 15 minutes after starting the transfusion. The first 15 minutes of the transfusion course is particularly important because severe transfusion reactions most commonly present during this period. Patient monitoring must be maintained at least every hour during transfusion. If an adverse event or reaction is suspected, the transfusion must be stopped immediately until the patient can be clinically evaluated and the vital signs including urinary output must be rechecked. Signs and symptoms of severe adverse reactions such as fever, flushing, urticaria, hypotension, anxiety/restlessness, and respiratory distress often begin in the first 15 minutes of the transfusion. If the patient has mild allergic reaction without signs of haemodynamic instability, laryngeal oedema, and tongue or lip swelling, the transfusion can be restarted after an effective antihistamine therapy. Monitoring and documentation of vital signs and general condition of the patient shall be repeated four hours after a successful and uneventful blood transfusion course. Inpatients should be observed for late reactions over the next 24 hours after the transfusion is completed.[46]

COMPLICATIONS OF TRANSFUSION

A transfusion reaction can be defined as any unfavourable transfusion-related event occurring in a patient during or after transfusion of blood components. The prevalence of these adverse reactions is highly parallel with the frequency of transfusion practice (Table 42.5).[47] In addition, these adverse events may present with a wide variety of signs and symptoms that require understanding and distinguishing from a coincidental complication of illness being treated (Table 42.6). Serious reactions and complications of blood transfusion are rare but can be life-threatening (Table 42.7). A major reason for most of these

Table 42.5 Prevalence of transfusion reactions

Type of transfusion reaction	Prevalence (per 100,000 units transfused)
Allergic transfusion reaction	112.2
Anaphylactic transfusion reaction	8
Acute haemolytic transfusion reaction	2.5–7.9
Delayed haemolytic transfusion reaction	40
Delayed serological transfusion reaction	48.9–75.7
FNHTR	1000–3000
HHTR	Unknown
Hypotensive transfusion reaction	1.8–9.0
Massive transfusion associated reactions (citrate, potassium, cold toxicity)	Unknown
Post-transfusion purpura	Unknown
Septic transfusion reaction	0.03–3.3 (product dependant)
TACO	10.9
TA-GVHD	Extremely rare (near 0%) with irradiation or pathogen reduction methods
Transfusion-associated necrotising enterocolitis	Unknown
TRALI	0.4–1.0 with mitigation (varies by component and post-implementation of risk mitigation strategy)

complications is transfusion of mismatched blood products and among these complications most common cause of morbidity and mortality is TRALI.[48]

Allergic and Anaphylactic Transfusion Reactions

Allergic reaction is defined as an immediate hypersensitivity response initiated by immunological mechanisms. Mild allergic reactions have only cutaneous manifestations such as localized or generalized urticaria, erythema, and pruritus, and usually resolve after administration of antihistamines. Anaphylaxis is a severe and life-threatening allergic reaction that is rapid in onset and affecting multiple organ systems evidenced by itchy rash, throat or tongue swelling, shortness of breath, nausea and vomiting, diarrhoea, cramping abdominal or pelvic

Table 42.6 Signs and symptoms of transfusion reactions

Cutaneous	Inflammatory	Cardiovascular	Respiratory	Gastrointestinal	Pain
Pruritis	Fever	Tachycardia	Tachypnea	Nausea	Headache
Urticaria	Chills	Bradycardia	Dyspnea	Vomiting	Chest
Erythema	Rigors	Hypotension	Wheezing	Diarrhoea	Substernal
Flushing		Hypertension	Rales		Abdominal
Pallor		Arrhythmia	Hoarseness		Back
Purpura		Shock	Stridor		Infusion site
Petechiae		Jugular venous distension	Pulmonary oedema, chest tightness		Proximal extremity
Cyanosis					
Jaundice					

Table 42.7 Complications of blood transfusion

Early
- Haemolytic reactions
  - Acute
  - Delayed
- Non-haemolytic febrile reactions
- Allergic reactions to proteins, IgA
- TRALI
- Reactions secondary to bacterial contamination
- Circulatory overload
- Air embolism
- Thrombophlebitis
- Hyperkalaemia
- Citrate toxicity
- Hypothermia
- Clotting abnormalities (after massive transfusion)

Late
- Transmission of infection
  - Viral (hepatitis A, B, C, HIV, CMV)
  - Bacterial (Treponeum pallidum, Salmonella)
  - Parasites (malaria, toxoplasma)
- Graft-versus-host disease
- Iron overload (after chronic transfusions)
- Immune sensitization (RhD antigen)

Reprinted with permission from: Melanie JM, Matthew JAW. Complications of blood transfusion. *Contin Educ Anaesth Crit Care Pain* 2006;6:225–9.

pain, light-headedness, tachycardia, and hypotension.[49] The term 'anaphylactoid' is used to point out the reactions that have clinical similarities to anaphylaxis under different mechanisms.

Allergic transfusion reactions occur during or within four hours of transfusion with a blood component. Although these reactions seem to occur most frequently with platelet transfusions and plasma, the incidence is variable depending on patient characteristics, product manufacturing, storage time, reporting rates, reaction definitions, and monitoring standards and it was shown that incidences of allergic reactions with platelets and RBCs were similar.[50]

Allergic hypersensitivity reactions are attributed to exposure to proteins or other allergenic soluble substances in the donor plasma that bind to preformed IgE or non-IgE antibodies on mast cells and basophils, resulting in the secretion of histamine. Another source of histamine is thought to be leucocytes in stored cellular blood components. Thus, the allergic transfusion reactions are more common with increasing storage time of blood components. Anaphylactic and anaphylactoid reactions are sometimes associated with class, subclass, and allotype-specific antibodies against IgA, particularly in IgA-deficient patients.[51]

If only cutaneous symptoms are present, the transfusion may be temporarily interrupted and H_1-blocking antihistamine (adults, 25–50 mg diphenhydramine intravenous or per oral) can be given to the patient. An H_2 blocker, such as cimetidine (adults, 300 mg intravenously) or ranitidine (adults, 50 mg intravenously), may be added to the H_1 blocker to induce resolution of the reaction. If symptoms resolve and no further symptoms occur, the transfusion may be resumed with the same unit of blood product and can be completed at a lower speed under direct observation of the patient. During the observation if symptoms recur and/or additional symptoms present, the transfusion must be stopped.

In severe allergic/anaphylactic reactions, transfusion must be stopped immediately. Epinephrine should be given (1:1000 IM, with 5–10 min intervals if required) if hypotension does not resolve after adequate crystalloid or colloid replacement intravenously and/or in the setting of life-threatening symptoms such as widespread urticarial reaction, facial or laryngeal oedema. Epinephrine may be given intravenously if the patient is unconscious or in shock. H_1 and H_2 blockers (except sedating antihistamines such as promethazine), bronchodilators, and glucocorticoids for intravenous administration as second-line drugs should be considered in addition to the epinephrine. Oxygen therapy should be administered as required with endotracheal intubation if there is significant upper airway obstruction.[52]

Routine premedication with antihistamines is not indicated in recipients who have no previous history of allergic transfusion reaction. Although close monitoring and observation of the patient is strongly recommended, there is no evidence to support routine prophylaxis with antihistamines or glucocorticoids in patients with previous mild allergic transfusion reactions. In patients with moderate to severe allergic transfusion reactions, reducing the plasma content of the unit by centrifugation or washing, or use of platelets stored in additive solutions in addition to premedication with antihistamines is recommended to reduce the incidence or decrease the severity of any future reaction. Patients who have had a prior life-threatening anaphylactic reaction can undergo testing for IgA deficiency to rule out a relative deficiency of IgA. Although there is no supporting evidence, IgA deficient patients shall receive blood components that lack IgA, either by washing or preparation of components from IgA-deficient blood donors.[53,54]

Haemolytic Transfusion Reactions

Haemolytic transfusion reactions (HTR) are classified as acute or delayed based on whether they occur within or after 24 hours of the transfusion, respectively. There is another distinction according to the localisation of haemolysis: intravascular or extravascular. Intravascular haemolysis is characterized by haemoglobinemia and haemoglobinuria while extravascular haemolysis is the lack of these signs and characterized by shortened survival of infused red cells.[55]

Acute Haemolytic Transfusion Reactions

Acute HTR may either be immune or non-immune. Immune-mediated acute HTRs are caused by transfusion of RBCs that are incompatible with the patient's anti-A, anti-B, or other RBC antibodies. The interaction of antibody with antigen on the RBC membrane can initiate complement activation and a systemic inflammatory response.

The most common reasons of these reactions originate from misidentification of blood sample, improper labelling of blood products, or infusion of properly labelled blood product to the wrong patient. The clinical

manifestations of these reactions such as chills and fever, pain (IV line back, chest), hypertension/hypotension, dyspnoea, gross haematuria and haemoglobinuria, DIC, acute renal failure, shock, and death are caused by intravascular or extravascular haemolysis occurring from antigen-antibody interaction. Fever with or without chills are the most common and might be the early symptom and is generally defined as 1°C increase in body temperature. If there is appearance of these symptoms and/or any change in vital signs or general condition of the patient, transfusion must be stopped and the recipient's ID and labels of blood component must be checked. While notifying the hospital blood bank urgently, supportive management shall be started. Hydration, alkalinisation of urine, and diuresis can be beneficial in the prevention of renal impairment. Corticosteroid therapy may be considered. In severe reactions, patients usually require ICU treatment with cardiovascular, renal, and respiratory supportive treatment. Patients shall be investigated for clinically significant bleeding that may be a sign of DIC.

Non-immune acute HTR can occur due to haemolysis of RBCs by physical disruptive factors such as co-administration of RBCs with an incompatible crystalloid solution (e.g., 5% dextrose solution), incorrect storage of blood, overheating in a blood warmer, and use of malfunctioning or non-validated administration systems.

Some haematologic abnormalities, particularly autoimmune haemolytic anaemia, can have presentations similar to HTR. If both immune and non-immune causes have been eliminated, an intrinsic RBC defect, such as glucose-6-phosphatase dehydrogenase deficiency as the potential cause of coincidental haemolysis should be considered. Furthermore, sickle cell anaemia, chronic liver disease, and active bleeding interfere with the diagnosis of HTRs.[56]

Delayed Haemolytic Transfusion Reactions

In this kind of HTRs, recipients have previously been immunised to a blood group antigen, usually by transfusion or pregnancy. After the exposure, antibody titre subsequently decreases to levels undetectable by routine tests. Re-exposure with RBCs expressing the relevant antigen produces a secondary immune response 24 hours to 28 days (usually in the first week) after the transfusion and results in intravascular haemolysis of transfused antigen-positive red cells.

Delayed HTRs are often asymptomatic but can be accompanied by either a fall or failure of haemoglobin increment, jaundice due to a rise in indirect bilirubin from destruction of RBCs, rarely splenomegaly, haemoglobinaemia, and haemoglobinuria. Fever, chest/abdominal or back pain, dyspnoea, chills, and hypertension are other possible clinical features. Most patients do not require treatment other than additional transfusions to maintain the desired haemoglobin. The therapeutic approach is similar with the acute form.[57]

Hyperhaemolytic Transfusion Reactions

Hyperhaemolytic transfusion reaction (HHTR) is a potentially life-threatening reaction characterized by accelerated intravascular haemolysis with a fall in Hb level below pre-transfusion level, markedly elevated lactate dehydrogenase (LDH), indirect hyperbilirubinemia, and haemoglobinuria.[58] Excessive drop in Hb levels indicate the haemolysis of both endogenous and transfused RBCs. Reticulocyte count typically drops during haemolysis while a dramatic increase can be detected during the recovery period. HHTR typically occurs in patients with haemoglobinopathies, particularly sickle-cell disease but also can be seen in those without underlying haemotologic disease. Acute and delayed forms are two distinct forms of HHTR. The acute form usually occurs less than seven days after transfusion and direct anti-globulin test (DAT) may be negative and serologic tests may fail to show RBC alloantibodies. In the delayed form DAT is positive and RBC alloantibodies are identified in the post-transfusion sample.[59] Thus, particularly in the acute phase, the diagnosis of HHTR requires a high index of suspicion.

Further transfusions can exacerbate haemolysis and avoidance is recommended in mild reactions. However, rapid haemolysis may cause severe anaemia and blood transfusion might be needed. In this situation, intravenous immunoglobulin (IVIG) and corticosteroids (e.g., methylprednisolone) are recommended.[59] In severe reactions additional IVIG, rituximab, and plasma exchange are also recommended.

Febrile Non-Haemolytic Transfusion Reactions

Febrile non-haemolytic transfusion reaction (FNHTR) defines as increase in body temperature ≥1°C during or within four hours following transfusion unrelated with haemolysis or other causes of fever such as infection, sepsis, etc. The incidence is 1–3% per unit transfused but can be higher in multi-transfused recipients. In mild reactions, usually fever is ≥38°C and the temperature rise is 1–1.5°C from pre-transfusion baseline without any chills, rigors, and respiratory distress and

haemodynamic instability. In severe cases, fever is >39°C and the temperature rise is ≥2.0°C from pre-transfusion baseline with chills and rigors. In all cases hypo/hypertension, tachycardia, headache, and flushing can be observed.[47]

In the presence of fever, the transfusion should be stopped immediately and the patient assessed closely for signs of infection or haemolysis. Exclusion of other important transfusion-related aetiologies is important in the diagnosis of FNHTRs. A possibility of septic transfusion reaction should be considered particularly after a platelet transfusion.[60] In the lack of any febrile illness and haemolytic reaction, the diagnosis of an FNHTR can be made. Checking for the history of previous transfusion reactions is also beneficial. Previous pregnancies and multiple transfusions should be established for alloimmunization potential that may increase the frequency of FNHTRs. Some clinicians prefer to continue the transfusion during the investigation phase if the patient has no symptoms and signs of haemolysis or an infection.[47]

Acetaminophen is the first choice of antipyretic agent in the treatment of febrile transfusion reactions. Although premedication with antipyretics before transfusion is not effective for the prevention of febrile reactions, prophylactic use of acetaminophen can be considered for patients with a history of FNHTR. Aspirin and non-steroidal anti-inflammatory drugs are contraindicated in patients receiving platelets due to the effects of these agents on platelet functions. Meperidine is an effective agent in the treatment of rigors. Most of the febrile reactions do not involve histamine release, thus antihistamines are not indicated. Steroids shall be considered with their anti-inflammatory effects when antipyretics are not effective or in patients with severe FNHTR. Slowing the speed of transfusion of blood component can be beneficial to prevent or decrease the severity of FNHTR. Pre- or post-storage of leucocyte reduction of blood components can successfully prevent febrile reactions in alloimmunized individuals.[52]

Hypotensive Transfusion Reactions

Acute hypotensive transfusion reactions (AHTRs) are characterized by early and abrupt onset of hypotension within 15 minutes of the start of transfusion and expected to resolve quickly (within 10 minutes) once transfusion is stopped.[61] Acute hypotension can be a component of various transfusion reactions, including bacterial contamination of blood products, acute haemolysis, TRALI, allergic reactions, and anaphylaxis. Acute hypotensive transfusion reaction is now considered as a distinct manifestation of transfusion reactions, thus it is important to observe the clinical features accompanying the drop in systolic and diastolic pressure to identify isolated AHTR.

Although the exact mechanism of AHTRs is probably multifactorial, activation of coagulation cascade and generation of bradykinin, a vasoactive nanopeptide is thought to be the principle mechanism for AHTR. Other possible mechanisms include the charge of filters used in leukoreduction and the contact of blood products with the tubes and surfaces of other devices.[62] Hypotensive reactions occur more commonly in chronic hypertensive patients taking angiotensin converting enzyme (ACE) inhibitor therapy.[63]

When a hypotensive reaction occurs during transfusion, the transfusion must be stopped immediately. There is no need for a specific treatment other than supportive therapy as the blood pressure is expected to rise gradually once the transfusion is stopped. Vasoactive drugs are not indicated ordinarily. The same blood product should not be restarted as the symptoms may reoccur. If AHTR occurs in a patient taking ACE inhibitor, switching this medication with another antihypertensive medication is recommended. The usage of bedside leukoreduction filters should be avoided.[64]

Massive Transfusion-Associated Reactions

Although the most common situation leading to massive transfusion is cardiac surgery, trauma is also one of the most frequent causes of massive BT, particularly in the ICU. There are various definitions of massive BT for adults in literature:[65]

- Replacement of one entire blood volume within 24 hours
- Transfusion of >10 units of PRBCs in 24 hours
- Transfusion of >20 units of PRBCs in 24 hours
- Transfusion of >4 units of PRBCs in 1 hour when ongoing need is predictable
- Replacement of 50% of total blood volume within 3 hours.

Massive transfusion reactions are multifactorial and related to both rate and large volume of the transfused blood and also seriousness of the underlying injury or illness that requires massive transfusion. Most of the reactions that possibly accompany BT can be more frequent and severe with massive transfusion. Among these complications metabolic and haemostatic abnormalities deserve particular attention.[47]

Citrate Toxicity

Citrate is used for anticoagulation of stored blood (3 g per unit of RBC) by chelating calcium. In a healthy adult, the liver metabolizes 3 g of citrate in 5 minutes.[66] Normally patients with normal liver function will tolerate the citrate load of blood components in the usual transfusion manner. However, infusion rates greater than 5 minutes per unit of RBC and liver or renal failure, and parathyroid dysfunction may drive citrate elevation, particularly with the transfusion of plasma or plasma-containing blood components.[67]

The primary deleterious effect of citrate toxicity is the drop of ionized calcium levels. Citrate anti-coagulates blood by binding to divalent cations such as calcium, magnesium, and zinc but symptoms of hypocalcaemia such as tingling, paraesthesia, tetanic symptoms, including muscle cramps, fasciculations, spasms, and changes in cardiac function, including alterations of cardiac depolarization (prolonged QT interval) and blunting of left ventricular response are predominant to symptoms of hypomagnesaemia. These clinical manifestations of hypocalcaemia are more likely to occur in patients who are in shock or are hypothermic. Citrate is rapidly metabolized to bicarbonate in mitochondria-rich tissue, such as liver, skeletal muscle, and kidney and metabolic alkalosis is reported as another well-known complication of massive blood transfusion.[68]

Mild citrate toxicity can be managed and/or prevented by slowing the rate of transfusion. When this is impossible and/or ineffective or signs and symptoms of hypocalcaemia occur, administration of supplemental calcium, usually calcium gluconate or calcium citrate is indicated. Measurement of a patient's ionized calcium level is beneficial to determine the need for calcium supplementation. Calcium should not be added into the blood component directly to avoid clot formation in the bag.[69]

Hyperkalaemia/Hypokalaemia

During storage of RBCs, potassium concentration of the unit supernatant increases due to the inhibition of Na^+/K^+-ATPase activity in RBC membranes. Potassium concentrations in PRBCs can range from 7–77 mEq/L^{-1} depending on the age of stored blood. Hyperkalaemia resulting from massive transfusion of older RBC units can cause significant cardiac complications and possibly cardiac arrest in some patients, particularly in children and adolescents with hypovolaemia.[70] Longer storage age and irradiation of the RBC product, rate and volume of RBC transfusion, age and weight of the patient, and presence of co-morbidities (hyperglycaemia, hypocalcaemia, hypothermia, acidosis, and renal insufficiency) are additional risk factors for transfusion-associated hyperkalaemic cardiac arrest. Electrocardiography (ECG) changes due to hyperkalaemia include peaked T waves, prolongation of the PR interval, and ventricular arrhythmia. For the prevention of hyperkalaemia, the rate of infusion should be limited to 0.5 ml/kg^{-1}/min^{-1}, particularly in patients with low blood volume such as neonates and infants.[71] Using fresh units of blood products, washing or plasma-reduced RBCs, and irradiated RBCs 12 hours before irradiation might be favourable. Using of inline potassium filters are also reported to be beneficial.[72] Insulin, glucose, calcium gluconate, and furosemide can be used in the treatment of hyperkalaemia.[47]

Hypokalaemia can be generated due to re-accumulation of potassium ions into potassium-depleted red cells and movement of potassium shift with protons in alkaloid blood after citrate metabolism to bicarbonate. The effect of hypokalaemia is decreased with the use of new generation RBC additive solutions such as Adsol. Therefore the complications of hypokalaemia are more likely when large numbers of plasma units rather than RBC units are transfused.[52]

Hypothermia (Cold Toxicity)

Hypothermia is defined as the body core temperature below 35°C (95°F) and generally classified as mild (32–35°C), moderate (28–32°C) and severe (<28°C).[73] Hypothermia has long been known as an important factor for mortality, early coagulopathy (because of platelet dysfunction), and multiple organ failure after traumatic haemorrhage.[74] Although rapid infusion of large quantities of cold (1–10°C) blood or RBC units has a tendency to induce cardiac arrhythmias and cardiac arrest, particularly in severe hypothermia, even small amounts of cold blood can be cardiotoxic if directly transfused into central venous lines. Another complication of hypothermia is impaired citrate and delayed drug metabolism.[52,75]

For routine transfusion at a standard rate and volume, blood products are suggested to be infused without warming if the patient is already warmed. However, even if the patient is warmed, it should be better to avoid transfusion of cold products through central venous lines. In case of an indication of warming blood products, inline blood warming devices or an approved external warming device that has a temperature monitor and a warning system detecting malfunction and haemolysis should be used. Uncontrolled overheating of RBCs particularly above 42°C can cause haemolysis and fatalities of red cells that can induce DIC and shock.[76,77]

Coagulopathy

Occurrence of coagulopathy during massive transfusion remains an important clinical problem. Coagulopathy during or after massive transfusion is secondary to a number of factors that can vary depending on the cause of haemorrhage:

- Hypothermia can participate in coagulopathy by causing reversible platelet dysfunction and enhancing fibrinolysis.[78]
- As RBCs have been shown to enhance thrombin generation and activated platelet responsiveness, the haematocrit level and/or haemoglobin concentration is an important factor for haemostatic function. Although optimal haematocrit or haemoglobin concentration for appropriate haemostasis is unknown, haematocrit as high as 35% is thought to be required.[79]
- Haemodilution is often thought to be the most important haemostatic abnormality associated with massive transfusion. Coagulopathy is attributed to dilution of platelets and clotting factors that occurs as the lost blood is initially replaced with crystalloid/colloid solutions and PRBCs. This relationship is thought not to be so simple and exact and affected by several factors including the dynamics of blood loss, the difficulties in estimating true blood loss, the inter-individual variations in clotting factor levels, and the functionality of organ systems involved in haemostasis, i.e., the liver, spleen, and bone marrow.[80] Thus, haemodilution *per se* is thought not to be the single factor for coagulopathy.
- The increased acid load from massive transfusion of RBC units may also contribute to coagulopathy. With increasing storage time, the acidity (pH) of RBC units gradually decrease due to production of lactic acid. Usually, the transfusion of an aged RBC unit with a low pH is not expected to cause acid-base disturbance due to high buffering capacity of plasma in the circulation. However, massive transfusion of PRBCs can further increase acid load and deteriorate coagulopathy, particularly in patients who are already acidotic.[81]
- Large volumes of FFP that have excess amounts of citrate anticoagulant may develop hypocalcaemia. Ionized calcium is an essential element in the coagulation pathways and binding of citrate to calcium may induce hypocalcaemia and contribute to coagulopathy.[80]
- Although specific component therapy provides both logistic and economic benefits, massive transfusion of modern RBC components that lack platelets and coagulation factors may lead to coagulopathy at an earlier stage than whole blood.[80]

Various studies subjected to the inspection of laboratory parameters and responses to various haemostatic components in patients developing bleeding diathesis suggested that platelet deficits were more important than coagulation factor deficiencies. Low fibrinogen and platelet levels have been shown as better predictors of haemostatic failure than prothrombin time (PT) and partial thromboplastin time (PTT). Instead of prophylactic replacement of haemostatic components, replacement of platelets and coagulation factors in the massively transfused patients by using platelets counts, the PT, aPTT, and fibrinogen levels would be preferable. Recently, it has been suggested that point-of-care haemostasis assays such as thromboelastography (TEG) and rotational thromboelastometry (ROTEM) might be better at assessing coagulopathy in patients requiring massive transfusion.[82]

TRANSFUSION-ASSOCIATED CIRCULATORY OVERLOAD

Transfusion-associated circulatory overload (TACO) is a severe acute complication of transfusion in which pulmonary oedema develops primarily due to excessive quantity of transfused blood components or an excessive rate of transfusion. True incidence of TACO is unknown due to the lack of specific clinical parameters and/or laboratory tests but its estimated frequency is about 1%–8% of patients who are transfused.[83] The frequency appears to be higher in hospitalized patients, especially those in the ICU. It can be often serious that 20% of patients require intensified care and attributed mortality can be as high as 28%–39%.[84]

As the pathogenesis of TACO is similar to the causes of acute congestive heart failure, it is also described as cardiogenic dyspnoea due to volume overload. Increase in hydrostatic pressure due to an increase in central venous pressure and pulmonary blood volume can cause fluid extravasation into the alveolar space. Inflammatory processes are also thought to be involved in the pathogenesis. Risk factors for the generation of TACO include extremes of age (<3 years, >60 years), pre-existing cardiac (left ventricular dysfunction) and renal disease, pre-existing fluid overload, female gender, small stature, low body weight, recent vasopressor treatment and hypoalbuminaemia. Positive fluid balance, larger amount of plasma transfused, and faster blood product infusion rate were also found to be associated with an increased likelihood of TACO in critically ill patients.[85] Although the average amount of RBC transfusion triggering TACO is 2 units, transfusion of a single unit can be sufficient to induce the reaction.[86]

The clinical manifestations of TACO include respiratory distress (dyspnoea, orthopnoea), headache, seizures, cyanosis, tachycardia, hypertension, a wide pulse pressure, jugular venous distension, increased pulmonary wedge pressure, and lower extremity oedema. Rales and/or wheezing and S3 heart sound can be identified on lung and cardiac examination, respectively.[87] Although there are some guidelines published by the International Society for Blood Transfusion, the British Committee for Standards in Haematology of the British Society for Haematology, and the U.S. Biovigilance Network, the evaluation and diagnosis of TACO can be problematic due to the lack of uniformly accepted set of diagnostic criteria.[88] There is no universally accepted definition of TACO but new onset or acute exacerbation ≥3 of the following are required for diagnosis:[89]

- Respiratory distress
- Raised brain natriuretic peptide (BNP or NT-pro-BNP)
- Increased central venous pressure
- Left heart failure
- Positive fluid balance
- Pulmonary oedema

The differential diagnosis of TACO includes TRALI, septic transfusion reactions, and acute haemolytic transfusion reactions. Patients with TRALI present with respiratory distress due to acute onset of pulmonary oedema and have some clinical features that can create challenges in distinguishing it from TACO. However, TRALI is characterized by hypotension and low-grade fever without cardiomegaly, occurring most typically within one to two hours of transfusion. Pulmonary capillary wedge pressure (PCWP) is normal or low. Comparison of the clinical and laboratory features of TRALI and TACO are presented in Table 42.8.[90]

Assessment of patients regarding intravascular volume and fluid balance, and determination of cardiac, renal, and respiratory functions before transfusion is important for the prevention of TACO. For patients at high risk, an appropriate rate of transfusion (<2–4 ml/kg^{-1}/h^{-1}) and monitoring fluid balance during and after transfusion are recommended. In patients with impaired cardiovascular reserve and large transfusion requirement, administration of a diuretic therapy immediately before transfusion should be considered. If signs and symptoms suggest TACO, transfusion should be stopped immediately. Supplemental oxygen and diuretic therapy should be instituted as needed. Sitting or reverse Trendelenburg positions are favourable if possible.[91]

Table 42.8 Comparison of clinical and laboratory features of TACO and TRALI

Feature	TRALI	TACO
Body temperature	Fever can be present	Unchanged
Blood pressure	Hypotension	Hypertension
Respiratory symptoms	Acute dyspnoea	
Neck veins	Unchanged	Can be distended
Auscultation	Rales	Rales, S3 may be present
Chest radiograph	Diffuse, bilateral infiltrates	
Ejection fraction	Normal, decreased	Decreased
PA occlusion pressure	≤18 mmHg	>18 mmHg
Pulmonary oedema fluid	Exudate	Transudate
Fluid balance	Positive, even, negative	Positive
Response to diuretic	Minimal	Significant
White count	Transient leucopenia	Unchanged
BNP	<200 pg/ml	>1200 pg/ml
Leucocyte antibodies	Donor leucocyte antibodies present, Cross-match incompatibility between donor and recipient	Donor leucocyte antibodies may or may not be present, positive results can suggest TRALI even with true TACO cases

Reprinted with permission from: Skeate RC, Eastlund T. Distinguishing between transfusion-related acute lung injury and transfusion associated circulatory overload. *Curr Opin Hematol* 2007 Nov;14(6):682–7.

TRANSFUSION-RELATED ACUTE LUNG INJURY

Acute non-cardiogenic pulmonary oedema occurring immediately after transfusion of donor plasma that contains leukoagglutinin is termed as TRALI. Although it is conferred to occur more common with platelets, FFP, and whole blood, transfusion of any blood component that includes plasma can cause TRALI. Furthermore, TRALI-related deaths are more common with RBC transfusions in developed countries. The incidence is estimated to be 1 in 5,000 units transfused but reports of TRALI are increasing parallel with the growing attention to the syndrome.[92] Like TACO, TRALI is more common among critically ill patients and the incidence is estimated to reach 5%–8%.[93]

The definition of TRALI is clinical and it can be considered in patients developing new signs and symptoms of acute lung injury (ALI)/acute respiratory distress syndrome (ARDS) during or within six hours after transfusion with the lack of ALI/ARDS risk factors other than transfusion such as septic shock, Mendelson's syndrome, near drowning, DIC, pulmonary contusion, and pneumonia.[94] TRALI can also occur in patients having other risk factors for ALI and diagnosis can be challenging in such patients.

TRALI can occur in all age groups and equally in both sexes. Specific risk factors related to both recipient and blood component transfused have been reported. Liver transplantation surgery, chronic alcohol abuse, shock, higher peak airway pressure during mechanical ventilation support, current smoking, higher interleukin (IL)-8 levels, and positive fluid balance are identified risk factors for TRALI.[95] Critically ill patients appear to have the highest risk. Emergency cardiac surgery, haematologic malignancy, massive transfusion, and higher Acute Physiology and Chronic Health Evaluation II (APACHE II) scores are additional risk factors for patients under intensive care therapy. Plasma or whole blood from female donors, transfusion of increased volume of highly reactive anti-human leucocyte antigen (HLA) Class II antibody and anti-human neutrophil antigen (HNA) antibody are additional risk factors for TRALI associated with blood components.[95]

The main mechanism leading to ALI involves sequestration of activated neutrophils within the pulmonary capillaries. Although the exact mechanism of how a transfusion is associated with neutrophil activation has not been fully understood, two hypotheses have been suggested: antigen–antibody hypothesis (immune mechanism) and the two-event hypothesis (non-immune mechanism). According to the antigen–antibody hypothesis, antibodies to HLA Class II and I and HNA may bind to recipient neutrophils and trigger the activation. It has been known that female donors have a much higher prevalence of anti-HLA antibodies than do male donors due to exposure to foetal alloantigen during pregnancy.[96] But interestingly, the presence of leucocyte antibodies in donors has been observed to be common while the occurrence of TRALI is uncommon. Antibodies directed against the HNA 3a antigen have also been found to be associated with several TRALI cases.[97]

The generally accepted theory for TRALI pathogenesis is two-event hypothesis.[98] The first event is related to the underlying clinical condition of the patient, e.g., sepsis, which alters the reactivity of the endothelium leading to sequestration and priming of neutrophils in the lung (priming refers to shifting neutrophils to a high responsive state). The second event is activation of primed neutrophils by transfusion of a stored blood product. As a result of neutrophil activation, cytokines, reactive oxygen species, oxidases, and proteases are released and damage the pulmonary capillary endothelium that causes inflammatory pulmonary oedema.[98]

Recently, two different models have been introduced related to the 'two-event theory'. The 'threshold model' represents the combination of multiple causal factors reaching a certain cumulative pathogenic threshold that results in TRALI. In the 'sufficient-cause model' individual contributing factors have been pointed out as a combination in a sufficient way to cause TRALI. Although these two models have some limitations, they are thought to be better equipped than the two-event model to describe the multi-causal nature of TRALI.[99]

The clinical presentation of TRALI includes dyspnoea, tachypnoea, hypoxaemia, cyanosis, tachycardia, fever, hypothermia, and hypotension or hypertension. In previously intubated patients, elevated peak and plateau airway pressures and pink frothy airway secretions coming from the endotracheal tube can be seen. Although the clinical presentation of TRALI can delay as long as six hours, the symptoms usually can be seen at any time even within minutes after the initiation of transfusion.

TRALI is a clinical diagnosis and should be considered when a patient develops hypoxaemic respiratory insufficiency during or shortly after transfusion of any blood product. The diagnostic criteria for TRALI contains the following issues:[100]

- The presence of new ARDS occurring during or within six hours after blood product administration
- Hypoxaemia documented with peripheral pulse oximetry (SpO_2) ≤90% on room air or the pressure of arterial oxygen (PaO_2)/fraction of inspired oxygen (FIO_2) ratio is <300 mmHg
- Abnormal chest radiograph that demonstrate bilateral pulmonary infiltrates

The differential diagnosis of TRALI includes other clinical conditions that can manifest with respiratory distress following transfusion such as TACO, septic and haemolytic transfusion reactions, and anaphylaxis.[101]

When TRALI is suspected, the transfusion should be stopped immediately and the case should be reported to the blood bank for quarantine of other units from the same donation to investigate the presence of HLA and possibly HNA antibodies. The recipient's vital signs should be evaluated particularly for hypoxia and hypotension. Management of TRALI is mainly supportive and a majority of the patients need oxygen supplementation. Although non-invasive respiratory support with continuous positive airway pressure (CPAP) or bi-level positive airway pressure (BiPAP) may be sufficient in less severe cases, invasive mechanical ventilation is often required. During mechanical ventilation support, restrictive tidal volume strategy might be appropriate in patients with TRALI like other forms of ALI such as ARDS. Hypovolemic and hypotensive patients may need haemodynamic support with vasopressors. TRALI is the leading cause of transfusion-related mortality and the mortality rates have been reported as high as 41%–67%, particularly for patients requiring ICU admission and ventilator support. Although patients who recover from TRALI do not appear to have additional risk for recurrent episodes following future transfusions, a preventive transfusion strategy with avoiding plasma containing blood products would be appropriate.[92,101]

TRANSFUSION-ASSOCIATED GRAFT-VERSUS-HOST DISEASE

Transfusion-associated graft-versus-host disease is a rare but lethal complication developed after infusion of viable allogeneic donor lymphocytes that proliferate and attack the recipient's own tissues resulting in dysfunction of the skin, liver, gastrointestinal tract, and bone marrow. Although TA-GVHD has some similar clinical manifestations with hematopoietic cell transplantation associated GVHD, it is quite different with being unresponsive to immune-suppressive therapy and high mortality rates around 80%–90%. Bone marrow aplasia arising from immune attack mediated by the transfused lymphocytes is the main reason for lethality. In transplantation-associated GVHD, engrafted lymphoid cells in the bone marrow are of donor origin and exempted from any immune reaction.[102]

The incidence of TA-GVHD in immune-competent recipients is not known, but in immune-compromised patients it is estimated to be 0.1%–1.0%. Routine irradiation of cellular blood components as a preventive strategy in developed countries such as Japan has resulted in the decline in incidence. The incidence may be affected from genetic variability within a population, as well as the incidence of consanguineous marriage in immune-competent recipients.[103]

TA-GVHD does not occur after most transfusions because the donor lymphocytes are destroyed by the recipient's immune system. Immunodeficiency and a specific type of partial HLA matching between the donor and recipient are the two main pathophysiological factors that may inhibit this protective mechanism. Severely immune-deficient patients such as recipients of haemopoietic stem cell transplantation or patients with congenital immunodeficiency affecting T cells or Hodgkin's and non-Hodgkin's lymphoma and acute and chronic leukaemia; those in need of neonatal exchange transfusions; and patients taking high-dose chemotherapy (e.g., purine analogue drugs, alemtuzumab, or anti-thymocyte globulin for aplastic anaemia) or radiotherapy because of solid tumours are at increased risk for the disease.[104] Besides these two main factors, there are some minor factors that may be relevant as a risk factor such as the age of the component (the number of viable lymphocytes diminishes with storage) and lymphocyte dose (although leucodepletion does not prevent TA-GVHD). TA-GVHD has been reported after the administration of most blood products such as non-irradiated whole blood, PRBCs, platelets, granulocytes, and fresh, non-frozen plasma. Frozen, deglycerolized red cells, FFP, and cryoprecipitate are exceptions. Minimal necessary dose required to produce disease in a susceptible host has been reported to be approximately 10^7 lymphocytes kg^{-1}.[105] The lymphocyte content of the blood components per unit is generally below the amount that is required for producing TA-GVHD.

The clinical presentation of TA-GVHD includes fever, skin rash, and desquamation, abdominal pain, vomiting, diarrhoea, hepatitis, cough, and pancytopenia, and typically occurs 1–6 weeks after transfusion. Erythematous maculopapular rash is observed usually on the trunk, and then spreads into the extremities, including the palms and soles and may progress into generalized erythroderma and toxic epidermal necrosis. Liver is not affected in all patients but there is usually mild to moderate elevation of bilirubin and liver enzymes. Pancytopenia, abnormal liver function tests, and electrolyte abnormalities are the main laboratory findings associated with TA-GVHD. The main responsible factor for mortality, which is uncontrolled infections, frequently occurs within three weeks after the onset of TA-GVHD related to pancytopenia and liver failure.[106]

Diagnosis of TA-GVHD can be challenging. Non-specific clinical features of TA-GVHD can be attributed to the underlying illness and have limited diagnostic value. A skin biopsy from the affected area can support the diagnosis with non-specific features including lymphocytic infiltration, basal layer vacuolization, and satellite dyskeratosis. Documentation of donor-derived cells, chromosomes or DNA in the blood or affected tissues of the recipient (chimerism) is more valuable for the diagnosis and can be obtained by several methods including amplified fragment-length polymorphism analysis, short tandem repeat analysis, variable number tandem repeat analysis, and human microsatellite markers or cytogenetic analysis.[107] In the differential diagnosis of TA-GVHD, a variety of medical problems and systemic illnesses such as viral and bacterial infections, drug reactions, liver failure, underlying malignancy, and haemophagocytic syndromes should be considered.

There is no effective treatment for TA-GVHD at present and overall mortality is greater than 90%. Corticosteroids, azathioprine, anti-thymocyte globulin, methotrexate, and cyclosporine have been used without considerable success despite some limited case reports resulting in complete recovery.[108] Thus, identifying patients at risk for TA-GVHD and implementing preventive strategies are of primary importance. Irradiating cellular blood components with gamma rays or X-rays is considered to be the standard preventive strategy. Pathogen reduction technology to disrupt the residual lymphocytes' ability to proliferate is not sufficient alone for at risk patients regarding TA-GVHD.

TRANSFUSION-RELATED IMMUNOMODULATION

Transfusion-related immunomodulation (TRIM) refers to the down-regulation of the recipient's cellular immune response after allogeneic BT. TRIM has been associated with alterations in immune function including decreased helper T-cell count, decreased helper/suppressor T-lymphocyte ratio, decreased lymphocyte response to mitogens, decreased natural killer cell function, defective antigen presentation, decreased monocyte/macrophage phagocytic function, and reduction in cell-mediated immunity.[109] Although there are some beneficial effects such as enhanced survival of renal allografts and reduced recurrence rate of Crohn's disease, the possible detrimental clinical consequences of TRIM are recurrence of resected malignancies, postoperative bacterial infections, activation of opportunistic infections, transfusion-related multiple organ dysfunction syndrome, and increased short-term (up to 3 months) mortality.[110] Allogeneic mononuclear cells or their soluble products have been thought to mediate these effects. Using autologous blood or pre-storage leucofiltered blood can mitigate the adverse effects of TRIM.

PHYSIOLOGICAL PARAMETERS OF TISSUE OXYGENATION

Arterial blood flow and its oxygen content (CaO$_2$) are the main determinants of the amount of oxygen delivered

Table 42.9 Factors that influence cerebral blood flow

- Arterial blood pressure
- Intracranial pressure
- Venous outflow
- Blood viscosity
- $PaCO_2$
- PaO_2
- Collateral flow
- Vasoreactivity
- Status of cerebral autoregulation

Source: Zauner A, Muizelaar JP. Chapter 5. Brain metabolism and cerebral blood flow. In: Reilly P, Bullock R eds. *Head Injury*. London: Chapman & Hall, 1997.

to the brain. Thus oxygen delivery to the brain can be expressed by the following equation:

$$DO_2 \, (ml \, O_2/min) = CBF \, (L/min) \times CaO_2$$

Cerebral blood flow (CBF) is influenced and regulated by a number of factors (Table 42.9). The net driving force for the flow is defined as the cerebral perfusion pressure (CPP), which is the difference between mean arterial (blood) pressure (MAP) and the cerebral venous pressure (CVP). Due to the close relationship between CVP and intracranial pressure (ICP), the latter is widely used instead of CVP.

$$CPP = MAP - ICP \, (CVP)$$

Hagen-Poiseuille equation can be used to describe the parameters affecting the flow through the cerebral vasculature:

$$Flow = (\pi \, r^4 \Delta) / 8 \, \eta L$$
(r = radius, P = pressure, L = length, and η = viscosity)

This equation gives the relation between discharge, dynamic viscosity of the fluid, diameter of the pipe, and the pressure gradient (which is negative) along the direction of flow for a steady uniform laminar flow through circular pipes. When this equation is applied to a fluid, changing the radius of the pipe creates a dramatic effect on flow.[111]

Cerebral autoregulation is a function of cerebral vascular response to changes in CPP and in a normal brain changes in CPP between 50–130 mmHg produce only minimal changes in CBF due to effective cerebral vasodilatation and/or vasoconstriction (the 'r' in the above equation). Autoregulation can be impaired in neurocritical care patients following ischaemia, trauma or subarachnoid haemorrhage and normal autoregulation range altered such that CBF is directly dependent on CPP and a satisfactory MAP in a normal individual cannot be sufficient to maintain adequate CBF. Briefly, loss of cerebral autoregulation makes the brain more vulnerable to both hypoperfusion and hyperperfusion.[111]

The oxygen content of arterial blood can be expressed by the following equation:

$$CaO_2 = (Hb \times SaO_2 \times k_1) + (k_2 \times PaO_2)$$

where Hb = Haemoglobin (g/L^{-1}), SaO_2 = Arterial Hb oxygen saturation (%), PaO_2 = Arterial oxygen partial pressure (in mmHg); k_1 is defined further.

Oxygen is carried in arterial blood in two forms: Combined with Hb and dissolved in plasma. In a healthy individual, more than 98% of oxygen is bound to Hb. Although the O_2 binding capacity of each gram of Hb molecule is 1.39 ml in theory (k_1 above, termed Hüfner's constant), due to the presence of abnormal forms of Hb, such as carboxyhaemoglobin and methaemoglobin in variable amounts, this capacity reduces to 1.31 ml/g^{-1}. The amount of dissolved O_2 in plasma is <2% when breathing air and determined by the solubility coefficient of O_2 (k_2 above 0.003) and PaO_2. Under normal atmospheric pressure, dissolved part of oxygen in blood is insignificant even at high flow of inspired O_2 (FiO_2). Thus Hb is one of the key factors regarding transportation of oxygen in blood.[112]

EFFICACY OF RBC TRANSFUSION

The primary goal of RBC transfusion is to improve tissue DO_2 and increase tissue oxygen concentration and consumption. It was shown that a majority of RBC transfusions in the ICU have been administered for low Hb levels and not for haemorrhage.[113] The basic assumption in RBC transfusion is that increasing low Hb levels with RBC transfusion will restore the tissue hypoxia caused by low Hb concentration.

In neurocritical care patients, several factors including hypoxaemia, hypovolaemia, raised ICP, vasospasm, failure of cerebral autoregulation, and disruption of flow-metabolism coupling may contribute to impair cerebral DO_2.[114] Oxygen uptake (VO_2) remains independent of DO_2 over a wide range of values due to the adaptation of oxygen extraction ratio ($O_2ER = VO_2/DO_2$) to the changes in DO_2, but this compensatory mechanism has limits and when cardiac output is acutely reduced by acute blood withdrawal, anaemia, or hypoxaemia, oxygen extraction ratio (O_2ER) increases (SvO_2 decreases) and VO_2 remains quite stable, until DO_2 falls below a critically low threshold (DO_{2crit}, the point at which the maximum O_2ER is reached), when VO_2 starts to fall. Under DO_{2crit} level, VO_2 becomes DO_2 dependant and brain tissue with a high O_2ER is particularly vulnerable to ischaemia and secondary brain injury.[115] Thus with a RBC transfusion, improving DO_2 without a concomitant improvement in VO_2 would be an important limiting factor to restore adequate tissue oxygenation and to prevent cerebral ischaemia in the management of critically ill neurological patients.

The degree of anaemia at the initiation of transfusion is the main factor affecting the extent of DO_2 enhanced by RBC transfusion. Increased blood viscosity due to the augmentation of haematocrit may decrease cardiac output so that DO_2 may not adequately increase following RBC transfusion. In critically ill patients, underlying cardiac and/or pulmonary functional deteriorations can impair tissue oxygenation and the severity of tissue oxygenation impairment at the initiation of transfusion may affect the extent of VO_2 enhanced by RBC transfusion. A review of 18 clinical studies investigating the effects of RBC transfusions on DO_2/VO_2 relationship in critically ill patients showed that despite an increase in haematocrit and CaO_2 by RBC transfusions, an increase in DO_2 and VO_2 was observed only in 14 and 5 studies, respectively.[116] The lack of increase in VO_2 after RBC transfusion can be in part due to dysfunction of stored RBC because of storage lesions such as decrease in 2,3-DPG, ATP depletion and release of pro-inflammatory substances that result in a left shift of the oxyhaemoglobin dissociation curve, and increase in erythrocyte deformability.

Tissue oxygen delivery also depends on RBC flow regulation in the microcirculation. The microcirculation is usually defined as a part of the vascular tree comprising blood vessels smaller than 100 µm, including arterioles, capillaries, and venules. Apart from oxygen transportation, RBCs also seem to maintain the perfusion of microcirculation and restore functional capillary density.[117,118] According to recent findings, the RBC can also use Hb as an oxygen sensor that can modulate blood flow by releasing nitric oxide (NO) and/or ATP that are important regulatory mechanisms for maintaining adequate tissue oxygen concentration.[119,120]

Monitoring DO_2 for the purpose of measuring the effectiveness of BT is complex and cannot be routinely applicable. Continuous monitoring of mixed venous oxygen saturation (SvO_2) via pulmonary artery catheterization can be used to evaluate the oxygen supply/demand balance but technical limitations such as insertion and placement difficulties and potential complications related with the catheter itself have emerged as the search for a more practical parameter. Central venous oxygen saturation ($ScvO_2$) measuring via a regular central venous catheterization coupled with a fibre optic lumen was recently proposed as a parameter for evaluating O_2 demand/supply adequacy.[121] Although it is accepted as a validated monitoring parameter for VO_2/DO_2 balance and suggested as a suitable prognostic factor in critically ill patients, there are various theoretical and technical limitations particularly coming from the different measurement sites of $ScvO_2$ (joining point of coronary sinus in the right auricle) and SvO_2 (pulmonary artery). Thus, further studies that give additional data regarding the determinants of $ScvO_2$ and the relationship between $ScvO_2$ and the physiology of circulation seem to be essential to ensure a reliable interpretation in different clinical situations.[122]

CONCLUSIONS

In this chapter prominent features of blood components, procedure of transfusion, and possible pitfalls, and adverse reactions are presented. Although BT is an important clinical practice with life-saving therapeutic potentials of blood products, errors in transfusion procedure and adverse reactions can induce morbidities and mortality and limit this favourable potential. Therefore, prompt recognition and correct diagnosis of adverse reactions with effective treatment will ensure safety of the transfusion practice.

REFERENCES

1. Allen S. *Critical Care Medicine: Perioperative Management.* 2nd ed. Philadelphia: Lippincott Williams & Wilkins: 2002.

2. Hayden SJ, Albert TJ, Watkins TR, Swenson ER. Anemia in critical illness: insights into etiology, consequences, and management. *Am J Respir Crit Care Med.* 2012 May 15;185(10):1049–57.

3. Hebert PC, Wells G, Blajchman MA, et al. A multicenter, randomized, controlled clinical trial of transfusion requirements in critical care. Transfusion requirements in critical care investigators, Canadian Critical Care Trials Group. *New England Journal of Medicine* 1999;340(6):409–17.

4. Giangrande PLF. The history of blood transfusion. *British Journal of Haematology* 2000;110:758–67.

5. McClelland DBL. *Handbook of Transfusion Medicine.* 4th ed. London: TSO (The Stationery Office). 2007.

6. Basu D, Kulkarni R. Overview of blood components and their preparation. *Indian J Anaesth* 2014 Sep-Oct;58(5):529–37.

7. Circular of Information. American Association of Blood Banks, America's Blood Centers and the American Red Cross. 2007.

8. Liumbruno G, Bennardello F, Lattanzio A, Piccoli P, Rossetti G. Recommendations for the transfusion of red blood cells. *Blood Transfus* 2009 Jan;7(1):49–64.

9. World Health Organization. Blood Transfusion Safety Team. *The Clinical Use of Blood: Handbook.* 2001 Geneva.

10. Klein HG, Spahn DR, Carson JL. Red blood cell transfusion in clinical practice. *Lancet* 2007;370(9585):415–26.

11. Vamvakas EC. Meta-analysis of clinical studies of the purported deleterious effects of "old" (versus "fresh") red blood cells: are we at equipoise? *Transfusion* 2010;50:600–10.

12. Scott KL, Lecak J, Acker JP. Biopreservation of red blood cells: past, present, and future. *Transfus Med Rev* 2005;19:127–42.

13. Henkelman S, Noorman F, Badloe JF, Lagerberg JW. Utilization and quality of cryopreserved red blood cells in transfusion medicine. *Vox Sang* 2015 Feb;108(2):103–12.

14. Pallotta V, D'Amici GM, D'Alessandro A, et al. Red blood cell processing for cryopreservation: from fresh blood to deglycerolization. *Blood Cells Mol Dis* 2012;48:226–32.

15. Bohonek M, Petras M, Turek I, et al. Quality evaluation of frozen apheresis red blood cell storage with 21-day postthaw storage in additive solution 3 and saline-adenine-glucose-mannitol: Biochemical and chromium-51 recovery measures. *Transfusion* 2010;50:1007–13.

16. García-Roa M, Del Carmen Vicente-Ayuso M, Bobes AM, et al. Red blood cell storage time and transfusion: current practice, concerns and future perspectives. *Blood Transfus* 2017 May;15(3):222–31.

17. Bennett-Guerrero E, Veldman TH, Doctor A, et al. Evolution of adverse changes in stored RBCs. *Proc Natl Acad Sci* 2007;104:17063–68.

18. Almac E, Ince C. The impact of storage on red cell function in blood transfusion. *Best Pract Res Clin Anaesthesiol* 2007;21:195–208.

19. Hess JR, Greenwalt TG. Storage of red blood cells: new approaches. *Transfus Med Rev* 2002;16:283–95.

20. Blajchman MA. Immunomodulatory effects of allogeneic blood transfusions: Clinical manifestations and mechanisms. *Vox Sang* 1998;74:315–9.

21. Hess JR, Solheim BG. Red blood cell metabolism, preservation, and oxygen delivery. In: Simon TL, McCullough J, Snyder EL, Solheim BG, Trauss GS, eds. *Rossi's Principles of Transfusion Medicine.* West Sussex: John Wiley & Sons, Ltd., Chichester, 2016. doi:10.1002/9781119013020.ch9.

22. Cardigan R, Green L. Thawed and liquid plasma–what do we know? *Vox Sang* 2015;109(1):1–10.

23. Callum JL, Karkouti K, Lin Y. Cryoprecipitate: the current state of knowledge. *Transfus Med Rev* 2009;23(3):177–88.

24. Liumbruno G, Bennardello F, Lattanzio A, Piccoli P, Rossetti G. Italian Society of Transfusion Medicine and Immunohaematology (SIMTI) Work Group. Recommendations for the transfusion of plasma and platelets. *Blood Transfus* 2009 Apr;7(2):132–50.

25. Abdel-Wahab OI, Healy B, Dzik WH. Effect of fresh-frozen plasma transfusion on prothrombin time and bleeding in patients with mild coagulation abnormalities. *Transfusion* 2006;46:1279.

26. Schrezenmeier H, Seifried E. Buffy-coat-derived pooled platelet concentrates and apheresis platelet concentrates: which product type should be preferred? *Vox Sang* 2010 Jul 1;99(1):1–15.

27. Slichter SJ. Evidence-based platelet transfusion guidelines. *Hematology* Am Soc Hematol Educ Program. 2007:172–8.

28. Atallah E, Schiffer CA. Granulocyte transfusion. *Curr Opin Hematol* 2006 Jan;13(1):45–9.

29. Hosoi E. Biological and clinical aspects of ABO blood group system. *J Med Invest* 2008 Aug;55(3–4):174–82.

30. Poole J. Blood Group Incompatibility. In: eLS. Chichester: John Wiley & Sons Ltd. Jan 2003. http://www.els.net [doi:10.1038/npg.els.0002096].

31. Cooling L. Carbohydrate blood groups. In: Simon TL, McCullough J, Snyder EL, Solheim BG, Trauss GS, eds. *Rossi's Principles of Transfusion Medicine.* Chichester, West Sussex: John Wiley & Sons, Ltd., Jan 2003. doi:10.1002/9781119013020.ch13.

32. *Safe Blood and Blood Products.* Module 3: Blood group serology. Geneva: World Health Organization; 2009.

33. Keir AK, Wilkinson D, Andersen C, Stark MJ. Washed versus unwashed red blood cells for transfusion for the prevention of morbidity and mortality in preterm infants. *Cochrane Database Syst Rev* 2016 Jan 20;(1):CD011484.

34. Tayler VV. Technical Manual. 13th ed. Maryland, USA: AABB. 1999;175–6.

35. Kumar H, Gupta PK, Mishra DK, Sarkar RS, Jaiprakash M. Leucodepletion and Blood Products. *MJAFI* 2006;62(2):174–7.

36. Mintz PD, Wehrli G. Irradiation eradication and pathogen reduction. Ceasing cesium irradiation of blood products. *Bone Marrow Transplant* 2009;44(4):205–11.

37. Asai T, Inaba S, Ohto H, et al. Guidelines for irradiation of blood and blood components to prevent post transfusion graft-vs.-host disease in Japan. *Transfus Med* 2000 Dec;10(4):315–20.

38. Rühl H, Bein G, Sachs UJH. Transfusion-associated graft-versus-host disease. *Transfus Med Rev* 2009;23(1):62–71.

39. Asai T, Inaba S, Ohto H, et al. Guidelines for irradiation of blood and blood components to prevent post-transfusion graft-vs.-host disease in Japan. *Transfus Med* 2000 Dec;10(4):315–20.

40. Fiebig E, Busch M. Infectious disease screening. 16th ed; Bethesda: American Association of Blood Banks, 2008; pp. 241–82.

41. Snyder EL, Dodd RY. Reducing the risk of blood transfusion. *Hematology* Am Soc Hematol Educ Program. 2001:433–42.

42. Circular of Information for the Use of Human Blood and Blood Components; 2009. Available from: http://www.aabb.org/Documents/About_Blood/Circulars_of_Information/coi0809r.pdf.

43. Cannon MJ, Operskalski EA, Mosley JW, Radford K, Dollard SC. Lack of evidence for human herpes virus-8 transmission via blood transfusion in a historical US cohort. *J Infect Dis* 2009;199(11):1592–8.

44. Blajchman MA, Beckers EAM, Dickmeiss E, Lin L, Moore G, Muylle L. Bacterial detection of platelets: current problems and possible resolutions. *Transfus Med Rev* 2005;19(4):259–72.

45. Lindholm PF, Annen K, Ramsey G. Approaches to minimize infection risk in blood banking and transfusion practice. *Infect Disord Drug Targets* 2011 Feb;11(1):45–56.

46. World Health Organization. The clinical use of blood: handbook. 2002;56–8.

47. Delaney M, Wendel S, Bercovitz RS, et al. Biomedical Excellence for Safer Transfusion (BEST) Collaborative. Transfusion reactions: prevention, diagnosis, and treatment. *Lancet* 2016;388(10061):2825–36.

48. Maxwell MJ, Wilson MJA. Complications of blood transfusion. *Contin Educ Anaesth Crit Care Pain* 2006;6(6):225–9.

49. Simons FE, Ardusso LR, Bilò MB, et al. and the World Allergy Organization. World Allergy Organization anaphylaxis guidelines: summary. *J Allergy Clin Immunol* 2011;127:587, e1–22.

50. Kleinman S, Chan P, Robillard P. Risks associated with transfusion of cellular blood components in Canada. *Transfus Med Rev* 2003;17:120–62.

51. Miller RD. Transfusion therapy. In: Miller RD. ed. *Anaesthesia*. Philadelphia, PA: Churchill Livingstone, 2000; 1613–44.

52. Fadeyi EA, Pomper GJ. Febrile, allergic, and nonimmune transfusion reactions. In: Simon TL, McCullough J, Snyder EL, Solheim BG, Trauss GS, eds. *Rossi's Principles of Transfusion Medicine*. Chichester, West Sussex: John Wiley & Sons, Ltd., 2016. doi: 10.1002/9781119013020.ch58.

53. Tinegate H, Birchall J, Gray A, et al. and the BCSH Blood Transfusion Task Force. Guideline on the investigation and management of acute transfusion reactions. Prepared by the BCSH Blood Transfusion Task Force. *Br J Haematol* 2012;159:143–53.

54. Sandler SG, Eder AF, Goldman M, Winters JL. The entity of immunoglobulin A-related anaphylactic transfusion reactions is not evidence based. *Transfusion* 2015;55:199–204.

55. Davenport RD, Bluth MH. Hemolytic transfusion reactions. In: Simon TL, McCullough J, Snyder EL, Solheim BG, Trauss GS, eds. *Rossi's Principles of Transfusion Medicine*. Chichester, West Sussex: John Wiley & Sons, Ltd., 2016. doi: 10.1002/9781119013020.ch57.

56. Sahu S, Hemlata, Verma A. Adverse events related to blood transfusion. *Indian J Anaesth* 2014;58(5):543–51.

57. Strobel E. Hemolytic Transfusion Reactions. *Transfus Med Hemother* 2008;35(5):346–53.

58. Win N. Hyperhemolysis syndrome in sickle cell disease. *Expert Rev Hematol* 2009;2:111–115.

59. Win N, Sinha S, Lee E, Mills W. Treatment with intravenous immunoglobulin and steroids may correct severe anemia in hyperhemolytic transfusion reactions: case report and literature review. *Transfus Med Rev* 2010 Jan;24(1):64–67.

60. Jacobs MR, Smith D, Heaton WA, Zantek ND, Good CE, and the PGD Study Group. Detection of bacterial contamination in prestorage culture-negative apheresis platelets on day of issue with the Pan Genera Detection test. *Transfusion* 2011;51:2573–82.

61. Popovsky MA. *Transfusion Reactions*. Bethesda, MD: AABB Press; 2001:222.

62. Arnold DM, Molinaro G, Warkentin TE, et al. Hypotensive transfusion reactions can occur with blood products that are leukoreduced before storage. *Transfusion* 2004;44:1361–66.

63. Sweeney JD, Dupuis M, Mega AP. Hypotensive reactions to red cells filtered at the bedside, but not to those filtered before storage, in patients taking ACE inhibitors. *Transfusion* 1998;38:410–11.

64. Kalra A, Palaniswamy C, Patel R, Kalra A, Selvaraj DR. Acute hypotensive transfusion reaction with concomitant use of angiotensin-converting enzyme inhibitors: a case report and review of the literature. *Am J Ther* 2012 Mar;19(2):e90–4.

65. Chidester SJ, Williams N, Wang W, Groner JI. A pediatric massive transfusion protocol. *J Trauma Acute Care Surg* 2012;73:1273–7.

66. Kramer L, Bauer E, Joukhadar C, et al. Citrate pharmacokinetics and metabolism in cirrhotic and noncirrhotic critically ill patients. *Crit Care Med* 2003;31:2450–5.

67. Kai Li, Yuan Xu. Citrate metabolism in blood transfusions and its relationship due to metabolic alkalosis and respiratory acidosis. *Int J Clin Exp Med* 2015;8(4):6578–84.

68. Dzik WH, Kirkley SA. Citrate toxicity during massive blood transfusion. *Transfus Med Rev* 1988;2:76–94.

69. Meikle A, Milne B. Management of prolonged QT interval during a massive transfusion: calcium, magnesium or both? *Can J Anaesth* 2000;47:792–5.

70. Lee AC, Reduque LL, Luban NL, Ness PM, Anton B, Heitmiller ES. Transfusion-associated hyperkalemic cardiac arrest in pediatric patients receiving massive transfusion. *Transfusion* 2014;54:244–54.

71. Strauss RG. RBC storage and avoiding hyperkalemia from transfusions to neonates & infants. *Transfusion* 2010;50:1862–5.

72. Inaba S, Nibu K, Takano H, et al. Potassium-adsorption filter for RBC transfusion: a phase III clinical trial. *Transfusion* 2000;40:1469–74.

73. Marx J. *Rosen's Emergency Medicine: Concepts and Clinical Practice*. Mosby/Elsevier. 2006. 2239.

74. Reynolds BR, Forsythe RM, Harbrecht BG, et al. Inflammation and host response to injury investigators. Hypothermia in massive transfusion: have we been paying enough attention to it? *J Trauma Acute Care Surg* 2012 Aug;73(2):486–91.

75. Smith HM, Farrow SJ, Ackerman JD, Stubbs JR, Sprung J. Cardiac arrests associated with hyperkalemia during red blood cell transfusion: a case series. *Anesth Analg* 2008 Apr;106(4):1062–9.

76. Hirsch J, Menzebach A, Welters ID, Dietrich GV, Katz N, Hempelmann G. Indicators of erythrocyte damage after microwave warming of packed red blood cells. *Clin Chem* 2003;49:792–9.

77. Poder TG, Nonkani WG, Tsakeu Leponkouo É. Blood warming and hemolysis: A systematic review with meta-analysis. *Transfus Med Rev* 2015 Jul;29(3):172–80.

78. Hardy JF, de Moerloose P, Samama CM. The coagulopathy of massive transfusion. *Vox Sang* 2005 Oct;89(3):123–7.

79. Blajchman MA, Bordin JO, Bardossy L, Heddle NM. The contribution of the haematocrit to thrombocytopenic bleeding in experimental animals. *Br J Haematol* 1994;86:347–50.

80. Spahn DR, Rossaint R. Coagulopathy and blood component transfusion in trauma. *Br J Anaesth* 2005;95(2):130–9.

81. Ferrara A, MacArthur JD, Wright HK, Modlin IM, McMillen MA. Hypothermia and acidosis worsen coagulopathy in the patient requiring massive transfusion. *Am J Surg* 1990;160:515–8.

82. Davenport R, Khan S. Management of major trauma haemorrhage: treatment priorities and controversies. *Br J Haematol* 2011;155:537–48.

83. Lieberman L, Maskens C, Cserti-Gazdewich C, et al. A retrospective review of patient factors, transfusion practices, and outcomes in patients with transfusion-associated circulatory overload. *Transfus Med Rev* 2013;27:206–12.

84. Parmar N, Pendergrast J, Lieberman L, Lin Y, Callum J, Cserti-Gazdewich C. The association of fever with transfusion-associated circulatory overload. *Vox Sang* 2017 Jan;112(1):70–78.

85. Menis M, Anderson SA, Forshee RA, et al. Transfusion-associated circulatory overload (TACO) and potential risk factors among the inpatient US elderly as recorded in Medicare administrative databases during 2011. *Vox Sang* 2014;106:144.

86. Lavoie J. Blood transfusion risks and alternative strategies in pediatric patients. *Paediatr Aneasth* 2011;21:14–24.

87. Popovsky MA. Transfusion-associated circulatory overload: the plot thickens. *Transfusion* 2009 Jan;49(1):2–4.

88. Popovsky MA. Breathlessness and blood: a combustible combination. *Vox Sang* 2002;83(Suppl 1):147–50.

89. CDC. NHSN Biovigilance component, hemovigilance module surveillance protocol v2.1.3. Atlanta: Centers for Disease Control and Prevention, 2014.

90. Skeate RC, Eastlund T. Distinguishing between transfusion related acute lung injury and transfusion associated circulatory overload. *Curr Opin Hematol* 2007;14(6):682–7.

91. Andrzejewski C, McGirr. Nursing hemotherapy bedside biovigilance in the recognition and management of suspected transfusion reactions. In: Popovsky M ed. *Transfusion Reactions*. Bethesda, MD: AABB Press, 2012: pp. 551–7.

92. Toy P, Lowell C. TRALI–definition, mechanisms, incidence and clinical relevance. *Best Pract Res Clin Anaesthesiol* 2007 Jun;21(2):183–93.

93. Vlaar AP, Binnekade JM, Prins D, et al. Risk factors and outcome of transfusion-related acute lung injury in the critically ill: a nested case-control study. *Crit Care Med* 2010;38:771.

94. Toy P, Popovsky MA, Abraham E, et al. Transfusion-related acute lung injury: Definition and review. *Crit Care Med* 2005;33:721–6.

95. Toy P, Gajic O, Bacchetti P, et al. Transfusion-related acute lung injury: incidence and risk factors. *Blood* 2012;119:1757.

96. Triulzi DJ, Kakaiya R, Schreiber G. Donor risk factors for white blood cell antibodies associated with transfusion-associated acute lung injury: REDS-II leukocyte antibody prevalence study (LAPS). *Transfusion* 2007;47:563.

97. Davoren A, Curtis BR, Shulman IA, et al. TRALI due to granulocyte-agglutinating human neutrophil antigen-3a (5b) alloantibodies in donor plasma: A report of 2 fatalities. *Transfusion* 2003;43:641.

98. Silliman CC. The two-event model of transfusion-related acute lung injury. *Crit Care Med* 2006;34:S124.

99. Middelburg RA, van der Bom JG. Transfusion-related acute lung injury not a two-hit, but a multicausal model. *Transfusion* 2015 May;55(5):953–60.

100. Kleinman S, Caulfield T, Chan P, et al. Toward an understanding of transfusion-related acute lung injury: statement of a consensus panel. *Transfusion* 2004;44:1774.

101. Vlaar AP, Juffermans NP. Transfusion-related acute lung injury: a clinical review. *Lancet* 2013;382:984–94.

102. Gehrie EA, Snyder EL, Ryder AB. Transfusion-associated graft-versus-host disease. In: Simon TL, McCullough J, Snyder EL, Solheim BG, Trauss GS, eds. *Rossi's Principles of Transfusion Medicine*. Chichester, West Sussex: John Wiley & Sons Ltd., 2016. doi: 10.1002/9781119013020.ch60.

103. Aoun E, Shamseddine A, Chehal A, et al. Transfusion-associated GVHD: 10 years' experience at the American University of Beirut-Medical Center. *Transfusion* 2003;43:1672.

104. Schroeder ML. Transfusion-associated graft-versus-host disease. *Br J Haematol* 2002;117:275.

105. von Fliedner V, Higby DJ, Kim U. Graft-versus-host reaction following blood product transfusion. *Am J Med* 1982;72:951.

106. US Centers for Disease Control and Prevention. The National Healthcare Safety Network (NHSN) Manual: Biovigilance Component v2.1.3. Atlanta, GA: Division of Healthcare Quality Promotion, National Center for Emerging Zoonotic Infectious Diseases. [2016 January 5]. Available from: http://www.cdc.gov/nhsn/pdfs/biovigilance/bv-hvprotocol-current.pdf.

107. Rühl H, Bein G, Sachs UJ. Transfusion-associated graft-versus-host disease. *Transfus Med Rev* 2009 Jan;23(1): 62–71.

108. Hutchinson K, Kopko PM, Muto KN, et al. Early diagnosis and successful treatment of a patient with transfusion-associated GVHD with autologous peripheral blood progenitor cell transplantation. *Transfusion* 2002;42:1567–72.

109. Blajchman MA. Transfusion immunomodulation or TRIM: What does it mean clinically? *Hematology* 2005;10(Suppl 1):208–14.

110. Vamvakas EC, Blajchman MA. Transfusion-related immunomodulation (TRIM): An update. *Blood Reviews* 2007;21:327–48.

111. Kramer AH, Zygun DA. Anemia and red blood cell transfusion in neurocritical care. *Crit Care* 2009;13(3):R89.

112. McLellan SA, Walsh TS. Oxygen delivery and haemoglobin. *Continuing Education in Anaesthesia Critical Care & Pain* 2004;4(4):123–6.

113. Corwin HL, Gettinger A, Pearl RG, et al. The CRIT Study: Anemia and blood transfusion in the critically ill – current clinical practice in the United States. *Crit Care Med* 2004;32:39–52.

114. Mendelow AD. Pathophysiology of delayed ischaemic dysfunction after subarachnoid haemorrhage: experimental and clinical data. *Acta Neurochirurgica* Supplementum 1988;45:7–10.

115. Jamnicki M, Kocian R, van der Linden P, Zaugg M, Spahn DR. Acute normovolemichemodilution: physiology, limitations, and clinical use. *J Cardiothorac Vasc Anesth* 2003;17(6):747–54.

116. Hebert PC, McDonald BJ, Tinmouth A. Clinical consequences of anemia and red cell transfusion in the critically ill. *Crit Care Clin* 2004 Apr;20(2): 225–35.

117. Cabrales P, Intaglietta M, Tsai AG. Transfusion restores blood viscosity and reinstates microvascular conditions from hemorrhagic shock independent of oxygen carrying capacity. *Resuscitation* 2007;75: 124–34.

118. Sakr Y, Chierego M, Piagnerelli M, et al. Microvascular response to red blood cell transfusion in patients with severe sepsis. *Crit Care Med* 2007;35:1639–44.

119. Wallis JP. Nitric oxide and blood: a review. *Transfus Med* 2005;15:1–11.

120. Ellsworth ML. The red blood cell as an oxygen sensor: what is the evidence? *Acta Physiol Scand* 2000;168: 551–9.

121. Surve RM, Muthuchellappan R, Rao GS, Philip M. The effect of blood transfusion on central venous oxygen saturation in critically ill patients admitted to a neurointensive care unit. *Transfus Med* 2016 Oct;26(5):343–8.

122. RBC compatibility table. American National Red Cross. December 2006. Retrieved 2008-07-15.

43

Deep Venous Thrombosis

F. Uzumcugil

ABSTRACT

Venous thromboembolism (VTE) and its complications constitute one of the main causes of cardiovascular death. Neurological pathologies have high risk for the development of VTE due to long-term immobility and increased embolus formation caused by pathological changes in the endothelium. Despite the high risk for VTE in patients with neurological pathologies, there is considerable reluctance in using thromboprophylaxis for those patients. Thromboprophylaxis can be provided by mechanical and pharmacological methods. The reluctance is mainly for pharmacological prophylaxis, which may lead to major bleeding leading to detrimental effects. It is important to determine the patients at high risk for VTE to start thromboprophylaxis. In addition, it is important to determine patients at risk for major bleeding to decide for pharmacological prophylaxis. The pathologies such as brain tumours, stroke, trauma, spinal cord injuries (SCIs), surgical interventions, and intracranial haemorrhage (ICH) are also important to determine the method for thromboprophylaxis. All have individualized concerns and should be considered *a priori*.

KEYWORDS

Thromboprophylaxis; neurointensive care; neurosurgery; neurology.

INTRODUCTION

The estimated worldwide incidence of venous thromboembolism (VTE) has been reported to be 1–2 cases/1000 in a year, but a rate of 4/1000 in a year has also been reported.[1] In all patients, the complications of VTE is the third most common cause of cardiovascular death following myocardial infarction and ischaemic stroke.[2] In adult intensive care unit (ICU) patients, the prevalence of clinically evident deep vein thrombosis (DVT) or pulmonary embolism (PE) is reported to be 20/1000 patients with a frequency of at least 14.5/1000 patients despite pharmacological thromboprophylaxis.[3,4] The ICU patients diagnosed to have neurological pathologies have high risk of death from VTE due to secondary venous stasis caused by paralysis and increased risk of embolus formation caused by endothelial activation, especially in patients with brain neoplasms and rheumatologic or inflammatory diseases affecting either central or peripheral nervous system.[5–8] Ischaemic

or haemorrhagic stroke also increases the risk of clot formation due to secondary effects on the endothelium.[9] Although the risk for VTE in neurological patients is high, there are major concerns regarding both the neurological pathology and the patient leading to the reluctance in using thromboprophylaxis in those patients. This chapter on thromboprophylaxis in patients with neurological pathologies is based on recommendations of the National Institute for Health and Care Excellence (NICE) guidelines which have been updated in 2015; and Neurocritical Care Society recommendations. The neuropathologies are briefly discussed separately in terms of those recommendations.[10]

According to the NICE recommendations, all patients should be assessed on admission in terms of increased risk of VTE. The risk factors for thromboembolism are generally suggested to be active cancer or cancer treatment, age over 60 years, critical care admission, dehydration, thrombophilia, body mass index over 30 kg/m², one or more co-morbidities (e.g., heart disease; metabolic, endocrine, respiratory pathologies; acute infectious diseases; inflammatory conditions), the evidence of VTE history of the patient personally or a first-degree relative, the use of hormone replacement therapy, the use of oestrogen-containing contraceptives, and phlebitis of varicose veins. The *medical* patients who (1) had or are expected to have reduced mobility for three or more days, (2) are expected to have gradually decreasing mobility compared to their normal status, or (3) have one or more of the risk factors of thromboembolism are accepted to have increased risk. On the other hand, *surgical* patients with one or more of; (1) surgery lasting more than 90 min (including total anaesthetic and surgical time) or if the surgery involves the pelvis or lower extremities, (2) acute surgery for inflammatory or intra-abdominal problem, (3) anticipated significant reduced mobility, and (4) one or more risk factors for VTE are accepted to have increased risk.[10]

Prior to offering pharmacological prophylaxis, all patients should be assessed for risk of bleeding; and the patients with risk of bleeding should not be offered pharmacological prophylaxis unless VTE risk outweighs bleeding risk. The NICE recommendations suggest active bleeding, acquired bleeding disorders (e.g., acute liver failure), the ongoing use of anticoagulants which increase the risk of bleeding (e.g., warfarin with INR >2), expected spinal or epidural anaesthesia or lumbar puncture within the next 12 hours; or previous spinal or epidural anaesthesia or lumbar puncture within 4 hours, acute stroke, platelets $<75 \times 10^9/L$, blood pressure $\geq230/120$ mmHg; uncontrolled hypertension, and inherited bleeding disorder without treatment (e.g., haemophilia, von Willebrand disease) as risk factors for bleeding.[10]

Within 24 hours of admission and whenever the clinical situation changes, the risks both for VTE and bleeding should be reassessed to ensure that the methods for prophylaxis are used properly and to identify the adverse events related to prophylaxis itself.[10]

METHODS FOR THROMBOPROPHYLAXIS

Prophylaxis for VTE can be provided by both mechanical and pharmacological methods.[11–13] Mechanical prophylaxis consists of compression stockings (CS) and intermittent pneumatic compression (IPC) devices, whereas, pharmacological prophylaxis includes unfractionated heparin (UFH), low-molecular-weight heparin (LMWH) (e.g., enoxaparin sodium, tinzaparin sodium, or dalteparin sodium) or fondaparinux sodium.[14]

Intermittent pneumatic compression devices in combination with or without CS are used as the standard of care at most institutions for thromboprophylaxis in patients undergoing neurosurgery. The efficacy of IPC is optimal when they are used continuously.[5] Intermittent pneumatic compression was reported to reduce the incidence of proximal DVT in patients undergoing craniotomy.[15] In a meta-analysis, it was reported that there was a non-significant trend towards IPC over CS; whereas, IPC was also reported to provide benefit in preventing PE compared to placebo.[16]

Due to the risk of intracranial haemorrhage (ICH), pharmacologic prophylaxis is not employed frequently in many neurosurgical units. Low molecular weight heparin was previously shown to be of clear benefit over CS.[15] In a study, the rate of DVT development was reduced from 32% in patients receiving prophylaxis by only CS, to 17% in patients receiving prophylaxis by CS combined with LMWH 40 mg/day.[17] In a similar study, comparing nadroparin with CS in 485 patients of which 400 underwent surgery for central nervous system (CNS) tumours, the rate of DVT development was reduced from 26% to 19% and the rate of DVT with PE development was reduced from 12% to 7%.[13] In studies comparing LMWH with IPC in patients undergoing neurosurgery, a regimen of enoxaparin was employed; in a study by Dickinson et al.[18] it was reported to be of no benefit, while increasing the risk of bleeding, whereas, in a study by Kurtoglu et al.,[19] it was also reported to be of no benefit, but without increasing the risk of bleeding.[18,19]

The randomized data reveals that LMWH is of clear benefit compared to CS for thromboprophylaxis. Raslan et al.[5] suggested that LMWH might be more effective than UFH due to the evidence that LMWH was shown to be superior to CS; and UFH was to be superior to placebo. However, when LMWH and UFH are compared, both these methods were found to be equivalent.[5,20,21]

The reluctance from using pharmacological prophylaxis depends most commonly on the potential for increasing the risk of bleeding. However, studies comparing LMWH with mechanical prophylaxis reported no significant increase in either ICH, minor or major bleeding. Similarly, UFH was also reported to cause no significant increase in ICH or other bleeding events compared to non-pharmacological techniques. In a study by Dickinson et al.,[18] heparin prophylaxis which was initiated preoperatively resulted in increased risk of ICH, whereas in the Collen et al. study, early initiation of pharmacological prophylaxis was not suggested to cause a trend towards rise in the risk of ICH.[16]

The evidence reveals that pharmacological prophylaxis neither proves to be better than mechanical prophylaxis nor causes increased risk for ICH or any other major bleeding events. The ACCP guidelines recommend sequential compression devices (SCD) for patients undergoing neurosurgery. LMWH or UFH, remaining to be the alternatives, are suggested to be used in high-risk patients.[22]

BRAIN TUMOURS

Patients with cancer are more vulnerable to development of VTE in the postoperative period. Venous thromboembolism including both PE and DVT was reported to have a 2- to 7-fold increased risk in cancer patients leading to higher mortality and morbidity.[14] The risk of VTE is higher in brain neoplasms due to the nature of management including high-dose corticosteroid treatment, pharmacologically induced dehydration and major surgery, as well as, pathological neovascularization, damage to vascular endothelium during surgery and the release of brain thromboplastin leading to a hypercoagulable state and immobility in the postoperative period.[5,14,23] Patients undergoing surgery for glioma or meningioma were reported to have a risk of VTE within a range of 3–31%, with a risk for PE of 5% associated with a mortality rate as high as 50%.[14] Prophylaxis for VTE in cancer patients was shown to decrease the risk of 1-year mortality.[24]

In a review reporting the risk of VTE to be increased during the course of malignant glioma, possible risk factors for the development of VTE were defined as 'the presence of lower extremity paresis, the histologically diagnosed glioblastoma multiforme (GBM), age over 60 years, large tumour size, chemotherapeutic agent use, and duration of surgery over 4 hours'.[25] In a large retrospective analysis, the cumulative incidence of symptomatic VTE in patients with malignant glioma was reported to be 7.5%, 55% of which were diagnosed within 61 days of major surgery, with a rate of 16.1 events per 100 persons/year during the first 6 months. In this analysis, the risk factors for VTE were defined as old age, histopathology demonstrating GBM, three or more chronic co-morbidities, and a neurosurgical procedure within 61 days. Moreover, the development of VTE was reported to cause increased risk of death within 2 years.[26] The American College of Chest Physicians guidelines recommends the addition of LMWH for neuro-oncological patients because of this high-risk for VTE.[14,22]

The VTE prophylaxis is more frequently used for benign cerebral tumours than primary brain tumours,

which are more prone to development of VTE, as well as, major bleeding in the postoperative period, which is the major factor that hinders the use of prophylaxis for VTE after neurosurgery.[14] Haemorrhage within the tumour itself is a major concern, as well as, ICH. The NICE guidelines recommend the use of mechanical devices for VTE prophylaxis, while pharmacological prophylaxis is recommended for patients who are defined to be at 'low-risk' for major bleeding, although neurosurgery is not easy to define the degree of risk for bleeding.[27] Intracranial haemorrhage rates were investigated previously in patients undergoing neurological surgery and receiving pharmacological prophylaxis for VTE, and were reported to be similar in patients with meningioma (6.0%), metastases (4.4%), glioblastoma (6.2%), and astrocytoma (5.4%).[28,29] Despite this data, the preference of prophylaxis proved no difference between benign and malignant pathologies.[14] The use of prophylaxis for VTE in patients undergoing surgery for cerebral neoplasms were previously investigated; and 39.2% was reported to receive mechanical prophylaxis alone, 13% to receive pharmacological prophylaxis alone and 18.1% to receive a combination of both.[14] One-third of the patients were reported not to receive any kind of prophylaxis, whereas, as per a survey, 76% of neurosurgery patients were reported to use mechanical thromboprophylaxis following surgery for brain tumours.[30]

In a study by Turpie et al.,[31] CS alone, CS in combination with IPC, and no prophylaxis were compared and a reduction in frequency of DVT from 20% in patients without prophylaxis to 9% in both treatment arms was reported. In a similar study addressing 70 patients, of which 39 were operated due to brain neoplasms, IPC, and IPC in combination with CS were found to have similar rates of DVT.[32] In contrast to those studies, Wautrecht et al.[33] found that IPC in combination with CS was superior to CS alone in brain tumour surgery. The results of these studies suggest that mechanical prophylaxis is superior to no prophylaxis and IPC in combination with CS may be superior to CS alone.[5]

In a study by Constantini et al.,[34] UFH 5000 SC (subcutaneous) 12 hr was initiated 2 hours prior to surgery and compared to placebo in terms of safety; and it was reported that there was no increase in intraoperative blood loss or any difficulty in providing haemostasis, however, significant ICH developed in one patient in the heparin group and in two patients in the placebo group. Multimodal prophylaxis comprised either enoxaparin 40 mg/day or UFH 5000 SC 12 hr in combination with IPC, CS, and screening for thromboembolism by using low extremity venous ultrasonography, was reported to have comparable low rates of VTE after surgery for brain tumours.[2]

In a meta-analysis, including data from 827 patients, 80% of which were to have brain tumours, the timing of initiation of prophylaxis was addressed. Out of 827 patients, 110 patients received prophylaxis prior to surgery and the remaining received prophylaxis within 24 hours after surgery. Treatment strategies consisted of different regimens including enoxaparin 40 mg/day with IPC, nadroparin 7500 anti-Xa U/day, enoxaparin 20 mg/day, and UFH 5000 SC 8 hr compared to control regimens of either IPC or placebo. The rate of VTE development reduced to 16% in LMWH or UFH-treated patients from 29% of control groups; whereas, the rate of bleeding was 2.3% in the heparin group and 1.4% in the control group.[35,36]

In high-grade gliomas, the rate of VTE was reported to be 5% in patients receiving thromboprophylaxis with graded compression stockings (GCS) in combination with either 40 mg enoxaparin, 2500 IU dalteparin or 5000 IU dalteparin without any haemorrhagic complications. Dalteparin 5000 IU was also shown to prevent VTE without causing any bleeding complications during its use for a median period of 6.3 months in a study including 63 patients of newly diagnosed GBM.[37] In a study comparing enoxaparin started within 48 h after surgery with no prophylaxis, no difference was reported in terms of ICH (12.5 vs 12.9%, respectively).[5] However, in a similar study by Dickinson et al., enoxaparin was reported to increase the risk of ICH when initiated preoperatively in patients with brain tumours. This trial also concluded that many neurosurgeons were reluctant to use pharmacological prophylaxis in those patients.[18]

The Neurocritical Care Society recommends[1] LMWH or UFH upon hospitalization in brain tumour patients, if the risk of major bleeding and signs of haemorrhagic conversion are ruled out (strong recommendation, moderate-quality evidence).

STROKE

An IPC device initiated within 0–3 days after stroke was reported to provide a reduction of 3.6% (95% confidence interval (CI); 1.4–5.8%) in the risk of VTE.[38] LMWH was reported to be superior over UFH for the prevention of DVT in patients with acute ischaemic stroke (AIS); revealing a reduction of 43% in the risk of VTE compared with UFH (relative risk (RR) 0.57, 95% CI; 0.44–0.76, p = 0.0001).[39]

The Neurocritical Care Society recommends[1] pharmacological prophylaxis as soon as it is feasible in patients with AIS (strong recommendation and high-quality evidence). If the patient with AIS has restricted mobility, prophylactic dose LMWH is recommended over prophylactic dose UFH in combination with IPC (strong recommendation and high-quality evidence). The use of UFH, LMWH and/or IPC in the immediate postsurgical or endovascular period in patients undergoing hemicraniotomy or endovascular interventions, is suggested, except when patients receive recombinant tissue plasminogen activator (rtPA). Prophylaxis should be delayed for 24 hours in case of rtPA use (weak recommendation and low-quality evidence). The use of CS in AIS cannot be recommended due to insufficient evidence, despite no evidence of harm.

The NICE guidelines also do not offer anti-embolism stockings, foot impulse or neuromuscular electrical stimulation devices for stroke. NICE recommends considering to offer prophylactic dose of LMWH (or UFH for patients with renal impairment or renal failure) to continue until the acute event is stabilized; if the diagnosis for haemorrhagic stroke is excluded and the risk of bleeding into another site or a haemorrhagic transformation is ruled out and if the patient has one or more of; (1) major restriction of mobility, (2) VTE history, (3) dehydration, and (4) comorbidities such as malignant pathologies.[10]

INTRACRANIAL HAEMORRHAGE

The risk of VTE in ICH is considerably high, that the prevalence of symptomatic DVT has been estimated to be 1%–2% in retrospective observational studies. However, in prospective observational studies employing venous ultrasonography for screening the incidence of DVT, it was reported to be 20%–40%.[40,41] The risk of VTE in ICH is estimated to be 2–4 times as high as AIS.

In patients with acute ICH, the use of either UFH or LMWH for thromboprophylaxis proved to reduce the risk of PE significantly (RR 0.37, 95% CI; 0.17–0.80, p = 0.01) compared to no prophylaxis; without any significant difference in the development of DVT, expansion in haematoma or mortality.[42] Pharmacological prophylaxis for VTE in ICH was reported to reduce the risk of symptomatic DVT (RR 0.31, 95% CI; 0.21–0.42) and pulmonary embolism (RR 0.7, 95% CI; 0.47–1.03) without any effect on haematoma expansion (RR 0.24, 95% CI; 0.05–1.13) or mortality (RR 1.05, 95% CI; 0.46–2.36).[43]

The Neurocritical Care Society recommends[1] IPC and/or CS in patients with ICH on admission over no prophylaxis (strong recommendation, high-quality evidence). If haematoma is stabilized and there is no ongoing coagulopathy, prophylactic doses of subcutaneous UFH or LMWH is suggested to be started within 48 hours of admission (weak recommendation, low-quality evidence). Patients on pharmacological prophylaxis are also suggested to continue the use of mechanical prophylaxis by IPC (weak recommendation, low-quality evidence).

ANEURYSMAL SUBARACHNOID HAEMORRHAGE

The thromboprophylaxis in aneurysmal subarachnoid haemorrhage (aSAH) is not a frequently addressed issue in studies. Most commonly the recommendations are based on observations in patients with AIS. The patients with aSAH have an increased risk of VTE leading to an incidence of DVT and PE as high as 1.5%–24% and 1.2%–2%, respectively. VTE is associated with an increased risk of pulmonary/cardiac complications, infectious complications, such as pneumonia and sepsis, and vasospasm.[44]

Early mobilization, the use of IPC devices or combination of IPC with anticoagulants were suggested to be effective for thromboprophylaxis in aSAH.

Unfractionated heparin at doses of 5000 IU SC either BID or TID was reported to be effective, however, the use of UFH BID was suggested to be safer than TID in terms of increased risk of bleeding.[16] LMWH has been shown to increase bleeding compared to mechanical thromboprophylaxis techniques. LMWH is expected to prevent 8–36 VTE events per 1000 patients, whilst leading to 4–22 bleeding events per 1000 patients. Hence, LMWH was suggested to be more harmful causing SAH, rather than preventing thromboembolism. In aSAH, screening by lower extremity Doppler ultrasonography may be a safe technique, however, it may not be cost-effective.[45]

The Neurocritical Care Society recommends[1] that in patients with aSAH, UFH is recommended for prophylaxis except in patients with unsecured ruptured aneurysm scheduled for surgical intervention (strong recommendation, low-quality evidence). IPC use is recommended to be started on admission (strong recommendation, moderate-quality evidence). In patients whose aneurysm is secured by surgery or coiling, UFH is recommended for thromboprophylaxis at least 24 hours after the intervention (strong recommendation, moderate-quality evidence).

TRAUMATIC BRAIN INJURY

In trauma patients who survived the first 24 hours, PE is the third leading cause of death. Reduction in mobility, activation of procoagulants, and prolonged ventilation are the leading factors contributing to the development of VTE in trauma patients making traumatic brain injury (TBI) an independent risk factor for thromboembolism.[1]

There is no standard for initiation of thromboprophylaxis by either UFH, LMWH, or IPC in patients with TBI. In a study by Nathan's et al., more than four days of delay in initiation of pharmacological thromboprophylaxis caused patients to have a three-fold increase in DVT and patients with head injury were reported to receive prophylaxis delayed for more than four days twice as likely.[46] Moreover, in a retrospective review the trauma patients with head injury were reported to have 3–4 times more risk for the development of DVT compared to the ones without head injury (RR 2.67, 95% CI; 1.69–4.20).[47]

LMWH for thromboprophylaxis is recommended for multi-trauma patients without head injury, however, there is no sufficient data to recommend the use of LMWH in patients with traumatic ICH.[12]

The Neurocritical Care Society recommends[1] IPC to be initiated within 24 hours of admission or within 24 hours after the craniotomy is completed (weak recommendation, low-quality evidence). LMWH or UFH is recommended to be initiated within 24–48 hours of the presentation of patients with TBI or ICH or after 24 hours of craniotomy (weak recommendation, low-quality evidence). Mechanical devices such as IPC is recommended to be used in TBI (weak recommendation, low-quality evidence).

SPINAL CORD INJURY

The prevalence of DVT in paralytic spinal cord injury (SCI) was reported to be as high as 18%–100% within the first 12 weeks and PE was reported to be 4.6%–14%. The risk was reported to be at its highest within the first 2 weeks and decreased after the first 3 months. Although the rates decreased further after 6 months, DVT remains to be a risk even several months after injury.[48,49] The incidence of DVT was reduced from 26% to 2% with thromboprophylaxis comprised of LMWH combined with early mobilization (within 72 hours) compared to LMWH combined with late mobilization (in 8–28 days, mean 12 days). IPC devices are not sufficient alone to prevent the development of DVT, hence if pharmacological prophylaxis is contraindicated for the patient, screening for DVT is recommended to be considered as well as placement of IVC filter in the established presence of DVT.[50–52]

The Neurocritical Care Society recommends[1] UFH or LMWH in combination with mechanical prophylaxis preferably IPCs over no prophylaxis and over mechanical prophylaxis alone. Prophylaxis is recommended to be started as early as possible within 72 hours of injury (strong recommendation, high-quality evidence). LMWH or adjusted dose UFH is recommended as soon as the bleeding is controlled (strong recommendation, moderate-quality evidence). IPC in combination with either LMWH or UFH is recommended within 24 hours after elective craniotomy (strong recommendation, moderate-quality evidence).

SPINAL SURGERY

As per the Neurocritical Care Society,[1] ambulatory spinal surgery with unique positioning of prone or kneeling has been reported to be associated with zero risk of VTE, hence, IPC devices are recommended to be considered for use alone only in those patients (weak recommendation, low-quality evidence). Ambulation in combination with mechanical prophylaxis alone or with LMWH is recommended for patients undergoing standard spinal surgery, whereas combined therapy (GCS or IPC + LMWH + ambulation) is recommended for patients with increased risk of thromboembolism (strong recommendation, moderate-quality evidence).

THE PLACEMENT OF EXTERNAL VENTRICULAR DRAINS

External ventricular drains (EVD) are indicated for acute hydrocephalus caused by SAH, intraventricular or intraparenchymal haemorrhage, infection, brain tumours or shunt failure, as well as severe TBI.[53,54] However, the benefits can be offset by haemorrhagic or infectious complications. The Neurocritical Care Society developed recommendations for EVD management. In the context of this chapter, EVD placement in patients with high-risk for VTE are briefly discussed.

The Neurocritical Care Society recommends mechanical prophylaxis in case of contraindication for anticoagulants for patients scheduled for EVD placement, recognizing the adverse outcomes of ICH, especially the progression in already existing haemorrhages. The society accepts the priority of avoidance of ICH over avoidance of relatively small risk of PE in the absence of pharmacological prophylaxis.[53]

Heparin is only recommended for high-risk patients for VTE, provided that the contraindications for anticoagulants are resolved.[52] Subcutaneous UFH may be superior in prevention of VTE against the risk of haemorrhage compared to LMWH, but there is no sufficient data to make any recommendation. However,

LMWH may be considered for high-risk patients for VTE.[15,53] There is no sufficient data to make any suggestion on the timing of pharmacological prophylaxis for patients undergoing placement of EVD, whereas, the initiation of pharmacological prophylaxis is recommended to be initiated within 1–4 days after ICH or traumatic haemorrhage is secured and stabilized.[55,56] As it is well recognized that ICH complications from EVD decreases over time, thromboprophylaxis may be used in the days following EVD placement; probably within 72 hours (at the latest) provided that any existing haemorrhage is stabilized.[53]

The Neurocritical Care Society recommends[53] thromboprophylaxis during immobilization (strong recommendation, low-quality evidence). The recommendations are against routine use of inferior vena cava (IVC) filters for primary thromboprophylaxis (strong recommendation, low-quality evidence). Mechanical prophylaxis (SCD or IPC) is recommended in case of contraindication to pharmacological prophylaxis (LMWH or UFH) and if patients have no contraindication for the use of mechanical thromboprophylaxis (conditional recommendation; low-quality evidence) for adult patients with EVD. The committee suggests the use of pharmacological prophylaxis for patients with additional risk factors for the development of VTE, provided that ICH is ruled out or stabilized (conditional recommendation, low-quality evidence).

CONCLUSIONS

Pharmacological prophylaxis requires assessment for the risk of bleeding *a priori* and whenever the clinical situation changes, the risks for bleeding and thromboembolism should be reassessed. Sequential compression devices are recommended for patients undergoing neurosurgery, whereas UFH or LMWH are suggested to be used in high-risk patients. However, it should be highlighted that it is crucial to determine the method for thromboprophylaxis according to the underlying pathology.

REFERENCES

1. Nyquist P, Bautista C, Jichici D, et al. Prophylaxis of venous thrombosis in neurocritical care patients: An evidence-based guideline: a statement for healthcare professionals from the Neurocritical Care Society. *Neurocrit Care* 2016;24:47–60.

2. Goldhaber SZ. Evolving concepts in thrombolytic therapy for pulmonary embolism. *Chest* 1992;101(Suppl 4): 183S–5S.

3. Patel R, Cook DJ, Meae MO, et al. Burden of illness in venous thromboembolism in critical care: a multicenter observational study. *J Crit Care* 2005;20(4):341–7.

4. Attia J, Ray JG, Cook DJ, Douketis J, Ginsberg JS, Geerts WH. Deep vein thrombosis and its prevention in critically ill adults. *Arch Intern Med* 2001;161(10):1268–79.

5. Raslan AM, Fields JD, Bhardwaj A. Prophylaxis for venous thrombo-embolism in neurocritical care: A clinical appraisal. *Neurocrit Care* 2010;12:297–309.

6. Brandes AA, Scelzi E, Salmistraro G, et al. Incidence of risk of thromboembolism during treatment of high-grade gliomas: a prospective study. *Eur J Cancer* 1997;33(10):1592–6.

7. Dhami MS, Bona RD, Calogero JA, Hellman RM. Venous thromboembolism and high-grade gliomas. *Thromb Haemost* 1993;70(3):393–6.

8. Bleau N, Patenaude V, Abenhaim HA. Risk of venous thromboembolic events in pregnant patients with autoimmune diseases: a population-based study. *Clin Appl Thromb Hemost* 2016 Apr;22(3):285–91.

9. Elkind MS. Inflammatory mechanisms of stroke. *Stroke* 2010;41(Suppl 10):S3–S8.

10. NICE guideline. Venous thromboembolism: reducing the risk for patients in hospital. Available from: https://www.nice.org.uk/guidance/cg92.

11. Wright JD, Hershman DL, Shah M, et al. Quality of perioperative venous thromboembolism prophylaxis in gynecologic surgery. *Obstet Gynecol* 2011;118(5):978–86.

12. Geerts WH, Bergqvist D, Pineo GF, et al. Prevention of venous thromboembolism: American College of Chest Physicians. Evidence-based clinical practice guidelines (8th edition). *Chest* 2008;133(suppl 6):381S–453S.

13. Nurmohamed MT, van Riel AM, Henkens CM, et al. Low molecular weight heparin and compression stockings in the prevention of venous thromboembolism in neurosurgery. *Thromb Haemost* 1996;75(2):233–8.

14. Zacharia BE, Youngerman BE, Bruce SS, et al. Quality of postoperative venous thromboembolism prophylaxis in neuro-oncologic surgery. *Neurosurg* 2016:1–9.

15. Danish S, Burnett M, Ong J, et al. Prophylaxis for deep venous thrombosis in craniotomy patients: a decision analysis. *Neurosurgery* 2005;56:1286–94.

16. Collen JF, Jackson JL, Shorr AF, Moores LK. Prevention of venous thromboembolism in neurosurgery: a meta-analysis. *Chest* 2008:134;237–49.

17. Agnelli G, Piovella F, Buoncristiani P, et al. Enoxaparin plus compression stockings compared with compression stockings alone in the prevention of venous thromboembolism after elective neurosurgery. *N Engl J Med* 1998;339:80–85.

18. Dickinson L, Miller L, Patel C, et al. Enoxaparin increases the incidence of postoperative intracranial hemorrhage when initiated preoperatively for deep venous thrombosis prophylaxis in patients with brain tumors. *Neurosurgery* 1998;43:1074–9.

19. Kurtoglu M, Yanar H, Bilsel Y, et al. Venous thromboembolism prophylaxis after head and spinal trauma: intermittent pneumatic compression devices versus low molecular weight heparin. *World J Surg* 2004;28:807–11.

20. Goldhaber S, Dunn K, Gerhard-Herman M, et al. Low rate of venous thromboembolism after craniotomy for brain tumor using multimodality prophylaxis. *Chest* 2002;122:1933–7.

21. Macdonald RL, Amidei C, Baron J, et al. Randomized, pilot study of intermittent pneumatic compression devices plus dalteparin versus intermittent pneumatic compression devices plus heparin for prevention of venous thromboembolism in patients undergoing craniotomy. *Surg Neurol* 2003;59:363–72, discussion 372–4.

22. Guyatt GH, Norris SL, Schulman S, et al. Methodology for the development of antithrombotic therapy and prevention of thrombosis guidelines: Anti-thrombotic therapy and prevention of thrombosis, 9th ed. American College of Chest Physicians evidence-based clinical practice guidelines. *Chest* 2012;141(Suppl 2):53S–70S.

23. Salmaggi A, Simonetti G, Trevisan E, et al. Perioperative thromboprophylaxis in patients with craniotomy for brain tumors: a systematic review. *J Neurooncol* 2013;113(2):293–303.

24. Kuderer NM, Khorana AA, Lyman GH, Francis CW. A meta-analysis and systematic review of the efficacy and safety of anticoagulants as cancer treatment: impact on survival and bleeding complications. *Cancer* 2007;110(5):1149–61.

25. Marras LC, Greets WH, Perry JR. The risk of venous thromboembolism is increased throughout the course of malignant glioma. *Cancer* 2000;89:640–6.

26. Semrad TJ, O'Donnell R, Wun T, et al. Epidemiology of venous thromboembolism in 9489 patients with malignant glioma. *J Neurosurg* 2007;106:601–8.

27. Treasure T, Hill J. NICE guidance on reducing the risk of venous thromboembolism in patients admitted to hospital. *J R Soc Med* 2010;103(6):210–12.

28. Gould MK, Garcia DA, Wren SM, et al. Prevention of VTE in nonorthopedic surgical patients: antithrombotic therapy and prevention of thrombosis, 9th ed. American College of Chest Physicians Evidence-based Clinical Practice Guidelines. *Chest* 2012;141(suppl 2):e227S–e277S.

29. Getlach R, Scheuet T, Beck J, Woszczyk A, Seifert V, Raabe A. Risk of postoperative hemorrhage after intracranial surgery after early nadroparin administration: results of a prospective study. *Neurosurgery* 2003;53(5):1028–34; discussion 1034–35.

30. Carmen T, Kanner A, Barnett G, et al. Prevention of thromboembolism after neurosurgery for brain and spinal tumors. *South Med J* 2003;96:17–22.

31. Turpie AG, Hirsh J, Gent M, et al. Prevention of deep vein thrombosis in potential neurosurgical patients. A randomized trial comparing graduated compression

stockings alone or graduated compression stockings plus intermittent pneumatic compression with control. *Arch Intern Med* 1989;149:679–81.

32. Bucci MN, Papadopoulos SM, Chen JC, et al. Mechanical prophylaxis for venous thrombosis in patients undergoing craniotomy; a randomized trial. *Surg Neurol* 1989;32: 285–8.

33. Wauthrecht JC, Macquaire V, Vandesteene A, et al. Prevention of deep vein thrombosis in neurosurgical patients with brain tumors: a controlled, randomized study comparing graded compression stockings alone and with intermittent sequential compression. Correlation with pre- and post-operative fibrinolysis. Preliminary results. *Int Angiol* 1996;15(3)(Suppl 1):5–10.

34. Constantini S, Kornowski R, Pomeranz S, et al. Thromboembolic phenomena in neurosurgical patients operated upon for primary and metastatic brain tumors. *Acta Neurochir (Wien)* 1991;109(3–4):93–7.

35. Brandes AA, Scelzi E, Salmistraro E, et al. Incidence and risk of thromboembolism during treatment of high-grade gliomas: a prospective study. *Eur J Cancer* 1997;33:1592–6.

36. Iorio A, Agnelli G. Low-molecular weight and unfractionated heparin for prevention of venous thromboembolism in neurosurgery: a meta-analysis. *Arch Intern Med* 2000;160:2327–32.

37. Robins HI, O'Neill A, Gilbert M, et al. Effect of dalteparin and radiation on survival and thromboembolic events in glioblastoma multiforme: a phase II ECOG trial. *Cancer Chemother Pharmacol* 2008;62(2):227–33.

38. Dennis M, Sandercock P, Reid J, et al. The effect of graduated compression stockings on long-term outcomes after stroke: the CLOTS trials 1 and 2. *Stroke* 2013;44(4): 1075–9.

39. Sherman DG, Albers GW, Bladin C, et al. The efficacy and safety of enoxaparin versus unfractionated heparin for the prevention of venous thromboembolism after acute ischemic stroke (PREVAIL Study): an open-label randomized comparison. *Lancet* 2007;369(9570): 1347–55.

40. Kawase K, Okazaki S, Toyoda K, et al. Sex difference in the prevalence of deep-vein-thrombosis in Japanese patients with acute intracerebral hemorrhage. *Cerebrovasc Dis* 2009;27(4):313–9.

41. Ogata T, Yasaka M, Wakugawa Y, Inoue T, Ibayashi S, Okada Y. Deep venous thrombosis after acute intracerebral hemorrhage. *J Neurol Sci* 2008;272(1–2):83–86.

42. Paciaroni M, Agnelli G, Venti M, Alberti A, Acciarresi M, Caso V. Efficacy and safety of anticoagulants in the prevention of venous thromboembolism in patients with acute cerebral hemorrhage: a meta-analysis of controlled studies. *J Thromb Haemost* 2011;9(5):893–8.

43. Lansberg MG, O'Donnell MJ, Khatri P, et al. Antithrombotic and thrombolytic therapy for ischemic stroke: antithrombotic therapy and prevention of thrombosis, 9th ed. American College of Chest Physicians

evidence-based clinical practice guidelines. *Chest* 2012; 141(Suppl 2):e601S–36S.

44. Kshettry VR, Rosenbaum BP, Seicean A, Kelly ML, Schiltz NK, Weil RJ. Incidence and risk factors associated with in-hospital venous thromboembolism after aneurysmal subarachnoid hemorrhage. *J Clin Neurosci* 2014;21(2):282–6.

45. Kamphuisen PW, Agnelli G, Sebastianelli M. Prevention of venous thromboembolism after acute ischemic stroke. *J Thromb Haemost* 2005;3(6):1187–94.

46. Nathans AB, McMurray MK, Cuschieri J, et al. The practice of venous thromboembolism prophylaxis in the major trauma patient. *J Trauma* 2007;62(3):557–62.

47. Reiff DA, Haricharan RN, Bullington NM, Griffin RL, McGwin G Jr, Rue LW 3rd. Traumatic brain injury is associated with the development of deep vein thrombosis independent of pharmacological prophylaxis. *J Trauma* 2009;66(5):1436–40.

48. Miranda AR, Hassouna HI. Mechanisms of thrombosis in spinal cord injury. *Hematol Oncol Clin North Am* 2000;14(2):401–16.

49. Aito S, Pieri A, D'Andrea M, MArcelli F, Cominelli E. Primary prevention of deep venous thrombosis and pulmonary embolism in acute spinal cord injured patients. *Spinal Cord* 2002;40(6):300–3.

50. Wilson JT, Rogers FB, Wald SL, Shackford SR, Ricci MA. Prophylactic vena cava filter insertion in patients with traumatic spinal cord injury: preliminary results. *Neurosurgery* 1994;35(2):234–9.

51. Khansarinia S, Dennis JW, Veldenz HC, Butcher JL, Hartland L. Prophylactic Greenfield filter placement in selected high-risk trauma patients. *J Vasc Surg.* 1995;22(3):231–5.

52. Rogers FB, Shackfor SR, Ricci MA, Wlson JT, Parsons S. Routine prophylactic vena cava filter insertion in severely injured trauma patients decreases the incidence of pulmonary embolism. *J Am Coll Surg* 1995;180(6): 641–7.

53. Fried HI, Nathan BR, Rowe AS, et al. The insertion and management of external ventricular drains: An evidence-based consensus statement. A statement for health-care professionals from the Neurocritical Care Society. *Neurocrit Care* 2016;24:61–81.

54. Bratton SL, Chestnut RM, Ghajar J, et al. Guidelines for the management of severe traumatic brain injury. VII. Intracranial pressure monitoring technology. *J Neurotrauma* 2007;24(Suppl 1):S45–54.

55. Hemphill JC 3rd, Greenberg SM, Anderson CS, et al. Guidelines for the management of spontaneous intracerebral hemorrhage: a guideline for healthcare professionals from the American Heart Association/American Stroke Association. *Stroke* 2015;46:2032–60.

56. Nathens AB, Cryer HG, Filders J. The American College of Surgeons Trauma Quality Improvement Program. *Surg Clin N Am* 2012;92:441–54,x–xi.

Part XI

Endocrinal Care

Editor: Konstantin Popugaev

44

Endocrine Care

K. A. Popugaev, A. Yu. Lubnin, S. A. Gracheva,
M. V. Zabelin, and A. S. Samoilov

ABSTRACT

Cerebral catastrophe and critical illness can both lead to endocrine abnormalities. Different types of endocrinopathies had been previously described in neurocritical care patients with traumatic brain injury (TBI), subarachnoid haemorrhage (SAH), ischaemic stroke, and intracerebral haemorrhage (ICH). Hormonal replacement therapy is absolutely indicated in cases with endocrinopathy. This approach is obvious from the pathogenetic point of view. However, meticulous assessment of critically ill neurological patients with regard to endocrinopathy and its correction are still beyond the scope of current national and international guidelines and recommendations. Moreover, the modern concept of management of endocrinal abnormalities in critically ill patients does not provide for the approach, alternative to classic endocrinological approach generally accepted for stable patients without vital organ disturbances. The present chapter is dedicated to endocrinal disturbances in neurocritically ill patients.

KEYWORDS

Adrenal dysfunction; thyroid dysfunction; pancreatic dysfunction; pituitary dysfunction; diencephalon dysfunction; glucose control; insulin therapy; neurocritical care.

INTRODUCTION

Nervous and endocrine systems are closely interrelated and both play a crucial role in the homoeostasis.[1] Neurological pathology can result in different endocrinopathies and vice versa. Some endocrinopathies lead to encephalopathy.[2] In acute phase of neurological catastrophes, the endocrine system is obviously involved. However, features of endocrinopathies in neurocritical patients are still not distinctly defined because their symptoms are nonspecific and are frequently masked with consequences of severe brain injury, systemic infection, aggressive therapy, or iatrogenic complications. Consequently, commonly accepted diagnostic criteria of endocrinopathies associated with neurocritical illnesses and therapeutic algorithms for their corrections are absent.[3] Simultaneously, looking over acute endocrinopathies can become an immediate cause of unfavourable outcomes in neurocritical patients.[2] Otherwise, prompt and adequate correction of endocrine dysfunction might stabilize a patient's condition, shorten the length of stay in both the intensive care unit and hospital, and improve outcomes.[4] Therefore, neurointensivists urgently need a systemic approach to assessment of endocrine status and treatment algorithms for correction of endocrinopathies, if diagnosed.

ADRENAL DYSFUNCTION

Cortisol, a glucocorticoid hormone, maintains normal vascular tone, and has anti-inflammatory and immunosuppressive effects.[5] It is secreted by the adrenal gland and regulated by adrenocorticotropin hormone (ACTH), the hormone of anterior lobe of pituitary gland. In turn, secretion of ACTH is regulated by corticotropin-releasing factor, the hormone of hypothalamus nuclei,[6] that is the hypothalamo-pituitary-adrenal axis (HPAA), which is activated during any stress, including acute illness.[6]

Adequate response of HPAA is an obligatory prerequisite for surviving. Otherwise dysfunction of HPAA in neurocritical patients leads to worsening outcomes and even death.[7] The physiological secretion of cortisol is pulsatile and circadian, and this rhythm is disturbed during both critical illness and brain injury.[8–10] Normal daily cortisol secretion amounts to 40–80 mmol, and enteral administration of 15–30 mg of hydrocortisone covers diurnal requirement.[11] More than 80% of plasma cortisol is bound with a cortisol-binding-globulin—transcortin. The biological effects are provided by free cortisol. The binding capacity of transcortin is limited, and if cortisol exceeds 700 nmol/L, free cortisol increases dramatically.[12]

Adrenal insufficiency (AI) is a life-threatening condition and a well-established phenomenon in neurocritical settings. It can be either primary (adrenal), secondary (pituitary), or tertiary (hypothalamic). A clinical picture of AI as well as laboratory data are non-specific and include fever, weakness, fatigue, abdominal pain, arterial hypotension, hyponatraemia, normal potassium, leucocytosis, and increased C-reactive protein (CRP).[13] Adrenal insufficiency was described in the acute phase of traumatic brain injury (TBI), subarachnoid haemorrhage (SAH), ischaemic stroke, spinal injury, and many others neurological emergencies.[14–21] Different groups report various rates of AI. For instance, in TBI, rate of AI varies from 25% to 100%, depending on the used diagnostic criteria.[14] Thus timely diagnosis of AI during neurocritical illness is a crucial issue and simultaneously difficult and controversial.

Several diagnostic approaches exist. Investigation of plasma total cortisol is the simplest test, but has very low sensitivity and specificity.[22–25] In critically ill patients cortisol varies from 218 to 11,040 nmol/L, and there are no correlations between cortisol and outcomes.[22,25] Increased cortisol means that HPAA has responded to stress, but it is not clear whether functional activity of the axis is adequate or not. Two ways for increasing diagnostic value of cortisol investigation were suggested. First is the assessment of free cortisol.[26] This test has the same limitations as compared to the total cortisol investigation, albeit it better reflects the physiological mechanisms of cortisol action. Determination of free cortisol did not become the routine test for AI diagnosis in critical care due to both the limitations described above, and its expensiveness. A second way of increasing diagnostic value of total plasma cortisol investigation is an approach introduced by MS Cooper and PM Stewart in 2003 for critically ill patients.[13] Adrenal insufficiency is ruled out if cortisol is above 940 nmol/L, and diagnosed if cortisol is less than 415 nmol/L. If cortisol is between 414 and 938 nmol/L, then a stimulation test is recommended. This approach can really help in making a decision regarding hydrocortisone administration in critically ill patients, and this concept is used in some centres, albeit it did not receive widespread adoption, the reason may be due to significant cortisol variation during critical care illnesses.

Stimulation tests include Synacthen® (tetracosactide) and insulin tests. Synacten (tetracosactide) is a synthetic analogue of ACTH. This test has two variations – high (250 µg) and low (1 µg) dose, and there are some discrepancies between them. High dose of Synacthen leads to ACTH concentration 100-fold greater than during physiological circumstances.[27] Low-dose Synacthen models are used more for a physiological situation and that is a gold standard for diagnosis of primary AI.[28,29] However, cortisol might be stable in spite of Synacthen, if initial cortisol is greater than 500 nmol/L.[30] Several trials assessed the value of Synacthen test for AI diagnosis in neurocritical care patients, and they concluded that neither high dose nor low dose test can be used for making a decision regarding the necessity of hydrocortisone administration.[31] These results can be explained by the fact that neurocritical patients might simultaneously have primary, secondary, and tertiary AI.

The insulin test consists of assessment of differences in concentrations of ACTH and cortisol in response to decrease of glucose below 2.2 mmol/L.[32] This test uniquely evaluates the function of the whole HPAA. However, the test is extremely dangerous in critically ill patients, especially in neurocritical patients who require plasma glucose between 7 and 10 mmol/L for avoidance of cerebral metabolic crisis.[33,34] Thus insulin test should not be used in neurocritical care.

Today neurointensivists do not have reliable diagnostic tools for identification of AI as the clinical picture is non-specific and many critical conditions are able to mimic AI. In spite of these difficulties, the only way of timely AI diagnosis is scrupulous surveillance of the patient. In any case AI in neurocritical settings should be considered as a clinical diagnosis. Combination of arterial hypotension, hyponatraemia, normal or increased level of potassium, especially with fever, and increased inflammatory markers should push an intensivist for the suspicion or identification of AI. High alertness could help in time to fix patients who might have AI. Simultaneously, any attempts at interpretation of plasma cortisol can confuse an intensivist and mislead in taking a wrong decision to refuse starting hydrocortisone. Glucocorticoids should be administered immediately after suspicion of AI. Moreover, a positive response of the patient to hydrocortisone, especially haemodynamic stabilization, is one the most sensitive and specific marker of AI in critical care.[4,20] The standard intravenous daily dose of hydrocortisone is 150–200 mg.[35,36] Sometimes in cases with arterial hypotension refractory to vasopressors, the dose of hydrocortisone can be increased up to 800 mg or even greater. Some patients require the addition of mineralocorticoids, which showed weak benefits in a few trials.[35,36]

THYROID DYSFUNCTION

Thyrotropic hormone is synthesized in the anterior lobe of the pituitary and regulated by thyrotropin-releasing hormone (TRH), the hypothalamic hormone. Thyroxine (T4) is regulated by thyrotropic hormone, and T4 suppresses the synthesis and secretion of TRH. Thyroxine is biologically inactive and converted into triiodothyronine (T3), a biologically active hormone in many tissues, especially in the liver and kidney.[37,38] Thyroxine and T3 are mostly bound with globulins and only their free fractions take part in biological processes. Conversion of T4 to T3 is impaired with cytokines, malnutrition, and many medications, for example, dopamine or glucocorticosteroids.[39–41] Simultaneously, conversion of T4 into biologically inactive forms (reverse T3–rT3) is increased during critical illnesses. These mechanisms lead to low-T3 syndrome, which is characterized by low T3, increased rT3, normal or slightly low thyrotropic hormone. Synonymous terms are euthyroid sick syndrome or nonthyroidal illness syndrome.[37,41] If T4 is decreased, it is classified as low-T4 syndrome. In neurocritical care patients, secondary or tertiary thyroid insufficiency can develop in addition to low-T3 and low-T4 syndromes, peculiar for general critical patients.

A clinical picture of acute hypothyroidism consists of hypothermia, bradycardia, ileus, polyserositis, and respiratory acidosis. Low-T3 syndrome and low-T4 syndrome rarely have a clear clinical picture. Some authors consider that the pathophysiological meaning of these states guide in decreasing metabolic demands for surviving in critical illness.[42] It is still debated whether to administrate or not to start replacement of thyroid hormones in such patients. The situation is different in neurocritical care patients with secondary or tertiary thyroid insufficiency. For example, in patients with sellar region tumours and complicated postoperative period thyroid insufficiency, it can be extremely severe, and these patients obviously require replacement therapy of thyroid hormones.[43] Also hypothyroidism is described in patients with TBI, stroke, aneurysmal SAH, and many others neurological emergencies.[2,16,39,44]

The cornerstone issue is the criteria of diagnosis of thyroid insufficiency in neurocritical patients. Isolated low levels of total T3, T4, and their free fractions are non-specific and non-sensitive diagnostic criteria.[37,39,41] Partly it can be explained by methodological errors when biologically inactive molecules, for instance, rT3, are counted in the total level of T3.[45] A decreased level of thyrotropic hormone adds both sensitivity and specificity for the diagnosis of hypothyroidism, albeit it is still an incorrect practice to guide thyroid hormone therapy for neurocritically ill patients with these laboratory data only. A clinical picture should be the main criteria of thyroid insufficiency in neurocritical care, whereas levels of total T3, T4, their free fractions, and thyrotropic hormone should play an ancillary diagnostic role.

Brain dead potential donors are a separate and special group of neurocritical patients, who frequently receive thyroid hormones.[46,47] A majority of the guidelines recommend T4, T3, or both for brain dead donors, especially in cases with unstable haemodynamics.[48] However, recent meta-analyses did not confirm benefits of such a therapy.[49,50] The main reason of these negative results is selection bias. The matter is trials inclusion criteria. Both haemodynamically stable and unstable patients and both patients with clinical picture of hypothyroidism and without these signs were included in the trials.[50] Thus thyroid hormones should still be administered in brain dead potential donors in cases with a clinical picture of thyroid insufficiency.

The medication of choice for thyroid replacement therapy is T4 in a dose of 2–3 µg/kg/day.[7] T3 can be used too. It has a shorter half-time and its dose is 0.5–1 µg/kg/day.[51] Administration of a combination of T4 and T3 is controversial. Starting replacement therapy with this combination is not justified, albeit this therapeutic strategy might be appropriate in cases with hypothyroidism resistant to initial T4 therapy.[52–54]

Therefore making a decision regarding thyroid hormone administration in a neurocritical patient should be primarily based on the clinical picture of hypothyroidism, which first of all includes bradycardia, ileus, and hypothermia, or normothermia in an infectious patient. Justified and timely administered replacement therapy with thyroid hormone is able to stabilize the patient's condition and improve results of treatment. The intensivist's alertness would help in correct treatment, whereas excessive support to the level of plasma thyrotropic hormone, T3, and T4 could confuse and hamper diagnostics of thyroid insufficiency. This approach is in line with the concept of diagnostics and correction of AI in neurocritical care settings.

PANCREATIC DYSFUNCTION

Two crucial neurocritical care issues will be covered below. The first issue is pancreatic dysfunction developed due to acute brain injury, and the second – conception of glucose management in neurocritical care patients.

In contrast to the adrenal or thyroid glands, direct hypothalamo-pituitary-pancreatic axis does not exist. Consequently, it is a commonly accepted point of view that neurological emergencies could not be an immediate cause of pancreatic dysfunction. However, there are very few clinical researches determining brain-pancreas interactions. The most prominent research deserved to be discussed is a study of Sanchez de Toledo and co-authors.[55] Authors defined pancreatic dysfunction as pancreatitis or increase of serum concentrations of pancreatic enzymes. It was shown that 40% of children with TBI developed pancreatic dysfunction in a delayed fashion. It occurred in 24 hours after trauma without blunt abdominal trauma. Intracranial hypertension and intracranial haemorrhage were independent risk factors of pancreatic dysfunction, which increased the length of stay in both the intensive care unit and hospital. The most probable causes of pancreatic dysfunction in brain-injured patients are: (1) imbalance of autonomic nervous system with excessive vagal stimulation; (2) central cholecystokinin release.[56–58]

The second important neurocritical care issue is glucose management. The rate of hyperglycaemia in brain-injured patients is extremely high.[59–64] Hyperglycaemia is strongly associated with severity of brain damage and the patient's condition during critical illness, length of stay in the intensive care unit (ICU) and hospital, and with outcomes in patients with almost all neurocritical care pathologies.[59–70] However, it is not clarified whether hyperglycaemia is a cause of all these phenomena or it is an epiphenomenon only. The causes of hyperglycaemia in neurological emergencies are increase of interleukins, cytokines, stress hormones, massive catecholamine release, and resistance to insulin.[71,72] Hyperglycaemia leads to brain damage, and the main mechanisms are neurotoxicity, exitotoxicity, oxidative stress, inflammation, mitochondrial damage, and dysfunction.[73–76] Therefore, hyperglycaemia should be controlled.

Adequate glucose management is extremely important for the neurocritical care patient. Two main strategies of glucose management are adopted in critical care. First is tight or intensive insulin therapy and the other is liberal insulin therapy. Van den Bergh with co-authors created the conception of tight glucose control for septic patients in 2001.[77] The matter of conception is the maintenance of glucose less than 6.08 mmol/L. This conception did not find a confirmation of its efficacy in later studies.[78–81] Moreover, in neurocritical illness it can be dangerous because of the high probability of hypoglycaemia, which leads to zero glucose levels in the brain interstitial fluid in some situations.[33,34] Patients with co-morbid diabetes mellitus are especially sensitive to hypoglycaemia.

Therefore, neurointensivists should be aware regarding a possibility of direct interactions between the brain and pancreas in neurocritical care patients. Glucose abnormalities are a very common phenomenon in neurological emergencies. Neurointesivists should choose a liberal strategy with glucose maintenance between 7.0 and 10.0 mmol/L.[63]

PITUITARY AND DIENCEPHALON DYSFUNCTION

A clinical picture of pituitary dysfunction consists of a combination of damage to the anterior pituitary lobe resulting in panhypopituitarism (two, or more secondary hormonal insufficiencies—secondary AI, hypothyroidism, hypogonadism) and posterior lobe of the pituitary predominantly leading to diabetes insipidus. Acute neurological deficit is not a criterion of pituitary dysfunction. In neurocritically ill patients isolated pituitary dysfunction develops extremely rarely. It can be caused by pituitary apoplexy or elective pituitary surgery, which is extremely precise.[82,83] Absolutely another situation occurs in patients with TBI, stroke, aneurysmal SAH, and in complicated postoperative periods in case of sellar region tumours involving not only the pituitary but also other parts of the diencephalon, especially the floor of the third ventricle (craniopharyngioma, meningioma). These patients have a complicated and confused clinical picture due to the involvement of other structures of the diencephalon.[43]

Diencephalon damage results in several consequences. First of all, different variants of consciousness alterations occur. Spectrum of such disturbances range from agitation and psychotic syndromes to depressed levels of consciousness, coma, or primary generalized status epilepticus.[43,84,85] Secondly, diencephalon injury results in somatic organ dysfunctions. Cardiovascular, respiratory dysfunctions, and ileus are the most frequent types of organ dysfunction in patients with diencephalon dysfunction. However renal, hepatic, and haematological dysfunctions were also described.[85] Thirdly, diencephalon damage leads to water-electrolyte disturbances, primarily dysnatraemia (hyponatraemia or hypernatremia), which is the most typical electrolyte disturbance in TBI, SAH, and patients with a sellar region.[86–91] Possible causes of dysnatraemia are injury of the pituitary gland, pituitary stalk, or hypothalamic nuclei. Mechanisms of dysnatraemia are secondary or tertiary AI, cerebral salt-wasting syndrome (CSWS), syndrome of inappropriate secretion of antidiuretic hormone (SIADH), and diabetes insipidus.

Therefore, diagnosis of diencephalon dysfunction in a neurocritical care patient should be primarily based on the clinical picture which is much wider than classical pituitary dysfunction. Our group coined the term diencephalon dysfunction syndrome, which consists of a combination of dysnatraemia, alterations in consciousness, and at least one somatic organ dysfunction.[85] More organ dysfunctions mean more severe patient condition and worse outcome.

CONCLUSIONS

Endocrinopathies in neurocritical patients are a well-established phenomena, which worsen the patient's condition and outcome. Timely and adequate correction of endocrinal dysfunctions can really improve outcomes. In spite of clearness and common acceptance of these assumptions, endocrinopathies during neurocritical care are still under-diagnosed and missed. This is happening due to a low level of the intensivist's alertness and excessive belief in the diagnostic value of laboratory data, especially plasma hormones. Adrenal and thyroid dysfunction in neurocritical care should be considered as a primary clinical diagnosis.

Neurointensivists should be aware that brain injury could be an immediate cause of pancreatic dysfunction and the strategy of tight glucose control has to be avoided.

Isolated pituitary dysfunction is an extremely rare condition in neurocritical patients. While diencephalon damage occurs frequently in neurocritical care, this calls for creation of a new conception for neurocritical care, which would describe brain injury, manifested with neurological deficit, endocrinopathies, and somatic organ dysfunction. Recently our group coined a new conception of diencephalon dysfunction syndrome in neurocritical care which consisted of dysnatraemia, consciousness alterations, and at least one organ dysfunction. It should be tested in further research.

REFERENCES

1. Ashley NT, Demas GE. Neuroendocrine-immune circuits, phenotypes, and interactions. *Horm Behav* 2016;17(87):25–34.
2. Vespa PM. Hormonal dysfunction in neurocritical patients. *Curr Opin Crit Care* 2013;19:107–12.
3. Parenti G, Cecchi PC, Ragghianti B, et al. Evaluation of the anterior pituitary function in the acute phase after spontaneous subarachnoid hemorrhage. *J Endocrinol Invest* 2011;34:361–5.
4. Bernard F, Outtrim J, Lynch AG, et al. Hemodynamic steroid responsiveness is predictive of neurological outcome after traumatic brain injury. *Neurocrit Care* 2006;5:176–9.
5. Lamberts SW, Bruining HA, de Jong FH. Corticosteroid therapy in severe illness. *N Engl J Med* 1997;337:1285–92.
6. Lamberts SW, de Herder WW, van der Lely AL. Pituitary insufficiency. *Lancet* 1998;352:127–34.
7. Sakharova OV, Inzucchi SI. Endocrine assessment during critical illness. *Crit Care Clin* 2007;23:467–90.
8. Annane D. Time for a consensus definition of corticosteroid insufficiency in critically ill patients. *Crit Care Med* 2003;31:1868–9.
9. Manglik S, Flores E, Lubarsky L, et al. Glucocorticoid insufficiency in patients who present to the hospital with severe sepsis: a prospective clinical trial. *Crit Care Med* 2003;31:1668–75.
10. Schroeder S, Wichers M, Klingmüller D, et al. The hypothalamic pituitary-adrenal axis of patients with severe sepsis: altered response to corticotropin-releasing hormone. *Crit Care Med* 2001;29:310–16.
11. Weitzman ED, Fukushima D, Nogeire C, et al. Twenty-four hour pattern of the episodic secretion of cortisol in normal subjects. *J Clin Endocrinol Metab* 1971;33:14–22.
12. Burchard K. A review of the adrenal cortex and severe inflammation: quest of the "eucorticoid" state. *J Trauma* 2001;51:800–14.
13. Cooper MS, Stewart PM. Corticosteroid insufficiency in acutely ill patients. *N Engl J Med* 2003;348:727–34.
14. Bernard F, Outtrim J, Menon DK, Matta BF. Incidence of adrenal insufficiency after severe traumatic brain injury varies according to definition used: clinical implications. *Br J Anaesth* 2006;96:72–6.
15. Vergouwen MD, van Geloven N, de Haan RJ, et al. Increased cortisol levels are associated with delayed cerebral ischemia after aneurysmal subarachnoid hemorrhage. *Neurocrit Care* 2010; 12:342–5.
16. Dimopoulou I, Kouyialis AT, Orfanos S, et al. Endocrine alterations in critically ill patients with stroke during the early recovery period. *Neurocrit Care* 2005;3:224–9.
17. Weant KA, Sasaki-Adams D, Kilpatrick M, Hadar EJ. Relative adrenal insufficiency in patients with acute spinal cord injury. *Neurocrit Care* 2008;8:53–56.
18. Savaridas T, Andrews PJ, Harris B. Cortisol dynamics following acute severe brain injury. *Intensive Care Med* 2004;30:1479–83.
19. Dimopoulou I, Tsagarakis S, Kouyialis AT, et al. Hypothalamic pituitary-adrenal axis dysfunction in critically ill patients with traumatic brain injury: incidence, pathophysiology, and relationship *Neurocrit Care* 2011;15:365–8.

20. Weant KA, Sasaki-Adams D, Dziedzic K, Ewend M. Acute relative adrenal insufficiency after aneurysmal subarachnoid hemorrhage. *Neurosurgery* 2008;63:645–9.

21. Poll EM, Bostrom A, Burgel U, et al. Cortisol dynamics in the acute phase of aneurysmal subarachnoid hemorrhage: associations with disease severity and outcome. *J Neurotrauma* 2010;27:189–95.

22. Schein RM, Sprung CL, Marcial E, et al. Plasma cortisol levels in patients with septic shock. *Crit Care Med* 1990;18:259–63.

23. Moran JL, Chapman MJ, O'Fathartaigh MS, et al. Hypocortisolaemia and adrenocortical responsiveness at onset of septic shock. *Intensive Care Med* 1994;20: 489–95.

24. Jarek MJ, Legare EJ, McDermott MT, et al. Endocrine profiles for outcome prediction from the intensive care unit. *Crit Care Med* 1993;21:543–50.

25. Jurney TH, Cockrell JL Jr, Lindberg JS, et al. Spectrum of serum cortisol response to ACTH in ICU patients. Correlation with degree of illness and mortality. *Chest* 1987;92:292–5.

26. Hamrahian AH, Oseni TS, Arafah BM. Measurements of serum free cortisol in critically ill patients. *N Engl J Med* 2004;350:1629–38.

27. Darmon P, Dadoun F, Frachebois C, et al. On the meaning of low-dose ACTH (1–24) tests to assess functionality of the hypothalamic-pituitary-adrenal axis. *Eur J Endocrinol* 1999;140:51–5.

28. Beishuizen A, van Lijf JH, Lekkerkerker JF, Vermes I. The low dose (1 microg) ACTH stimulation test for assessment of the hypothalamo-pituitary-adrenal axis. *Neth J Med* 2000; 56:91–99.

29. Tordjman K, Jaffe A, Trostanetsky Y, et al. Low-dose (1 microgram) adrenocorticotrophin (ACTH) stimulation as a screening test for impaired hypothalamo-pituitary-adrenal axis function: sensitivity, specificity and accuracy in comparison with the high-dose (250 microgram) test. *Clin Endocrinol (Oxf)* 2000;52:633–40.

30. Briegel J, Schelling G, Haller M, et al. A comparison of the adrenocortical response during septic shock and after complete recovery. *Intensive Care Med* 1996;22:894–9.

31. Wijesurendra RS, Bernard F, Outtrim B. Low-dose and high-dose synacthen tests and the hemodynamic response to hydrocortisone in acute traumatic brain injury. *Neurocrit Care* 2009;11:158–64.

32. Arlt W, Allolio B. Adrenal insufficiency. *Lancet* 2003;361:1881–93.

33. Vespa PM, McArthur D, O'Phelan K, et al. Persistently low extracellular glucose correlates with poor outcome 6 months after human traumatic brain injury despite a lack of increased lactate: a microdialysis study. *J Cereb Blood Flow Metab* 2003;23(7):865–77.

34. Helbok R, Schmidt JM, Kurtz P, et al. Systemic glucose and brain energy metabolism after subarachnoid hemorrhage. *Neurocrit Care* 2010;12(3):317–23.

35. Annane D, Sebille V, Charpentier C, et al. Effect of treatment with low doses of hydrocortisone and fludrocortisone on mortality in patients with septic shock. *JAMA* 2002;288:862–71.

36. Annane D. Time for a consensus definition of corticosteroid insufficiency in critically ill patients. *Crit Care Med* 2003;31:1868–9.

37. Kelly GS. Peripheral metabolism of thyroid hormones: a review. *Altern Med Rev* 2000;5:306–33.

38. Rosendale JD, Kauffman HM, McBride MA, et al. Aggressive pharmacologic donor management results in more transplanted organs. *Transplantation* 2003;75: 482–7.

39. Farwell AP. Sick euthyroid syndrome. *J Intensive Care Med* 1997;12:249–60.

40. Sugimoto T, Sakano T, Kinoshita Y, et al. Morphological and functional alterations of the hypothalamic-pituitary system in brain death with long term bodily living. *Acta Neurochir* 1992;115:31–6.

41. Umpierrez GE. Euthyroid sick syndrome. *South Med J* 2002;95:506–13.

42. Stathatos N, Levetan C, Burman KD, et al. The controversy of the treatment of critically ill patients with thyroid hormone. *Best Pract Res Clin Endocrinol Metab* 2001;15:465.

43. Popugaev KA, Savin IA, Goriachev AS, Kadashev BA. Hypothalamic injury as a cause of refractory hypotension after sellar region tumor surgery. *Neurocrit Care* 2008;8(3):366–73.

44. Takala R, Katila AJ, Sonninen P, Perttilä J. Panhypopituitarism after traumatic head injury. *Neurocrit Care* 2006;4:21–24.

45. Chopra IJ. An assessment of daily production and significance of thyroidal secretion of 3,3′,5′-triiodothyronine (reverse T3) in man. *J Clin Invest* 1976;58:32–40.

46. Mi Z, Novitsky D, Collins JF, Cooper DK. The optimal hormone replacement modality selection for multiple organ procurement from brain-dead organ donors. *Clin Epidemiol* 2015;7:17–27.

47. Wood K, Becker B, McCartney J, et al. Care of the potential organ donor. *N Engl J Med* 2004;351:2730–9.

48. Zaroff JG, Rosengard BR, Armstrong WF, et al. Consensus conference report: maximizing use of organs recovered from the cadaver donor: cardiac recommendations, March 28–29, 2001, Crystal City, VA. *Circulation* 2002; 13: 836–41.

49. Rech TH, Moraes RB, Crispim D, et al. Management of the brain-dead organ donor: a systematic review and meta-analysis. *Transplantation* 2013;95:966–74.

50. Macdonald PS, Aneman A, Bhonagiri D, et al. A systematic review and meta-analysis of clinical trials of thyroid hormone administration to brain dead potential organ donors. *Crit Care Med* 2012; 40:1635–44.

51. Goarin JP, Cohen S, Riou B, et al. The effects of triiodothyronine on hemodynamic status and cardiac

function in potential heart donors. *Anesth Analg* 1996;83:41–7.

52. Appelhof BC, Fliers E, Wekking EM, et al. Combined therapy with levothyroxine and liothyronine in two ratios, compared with levothyroxine monotherapy in primary hypothyroidism: a double-blind, randomized, controlled clinical trial. *J Clin Endocrinol Metab* 2005;90:2666–74.

53. Slawik M, Klawitter B, Meiser E, et al. Thyroid hormone replacement for central hypothyroidism: A randomized controlled trial comparing two doses of thyroxine (T4) with a combination of T4 and triiodthyronine. *J Clin Endocrinol Metab* 2007;92:4115–22.

54. Walsh JP, Shiels L, Mun Lim EE, et al. Combined thyroxine/Liothyronine treatment does not improve well-being, quality of life, or cognitive function compared to thyroxine alone: A randomized controlled trial in patients with primary hypothyroidism. *J Clin Endocrinol Metab* 2003;88:4543–50.

55. Sanchez de Toledo J, Adelson PD, Watson RS, et al. Relationship between increases in pancreatic enzymes and cerebral events in children after traumatic brain injury. *Neurocrit Care* 2009;11:322–9.

56. Liu KJ, Atten MJ, Lichtor T, et al. Serum amylase and lipase elevation is associated with intracranial events. *Am Surg* 2001;67:215–19.

57. Ulloa L. The vagus nerve and the nicotinic anti-inflammatory pathway. *Nat Rev Drug Discov* 2005;4:673–84.

58. Nelson M, Debas H, Mulvihill S. Vagal stimulation of rat exocrine pancreatic secretions occurs via multiple mediators. *Gastroenterology* 1993;105:221–8.

59. Badjatia N, Topcuoglu MA, Buonanno FS, et al. Relationship between hyperglycemia and symptomatic vasospasm after subarachnoid hemorrhage. *Crit Care Med* 2005;33:1603–9.

60. Frontera JA, Fernandez A, Claassen J, et al. Hyperglycemia after SAH: predictors, associated complications, and impact on outcome. *Stroke* 2006;37:199–203.

61. Jeremitsky E, Omert LA, Dunham CM, et al. The impact of hyperglycemia on patients with severe brain injury. *J Trauma* 2005;58:47–50.

62. Garg R, Chaudhuri A, Munschauer F, Dandona P. Hyperglycemia, insulin, and acute ischemic stroke: a mechanistic justification for a trial of insulin infusion therapy. *Stroke* 2006;37(1):267–73.

63. Godoy DA, Pinero GR, Svampa S, et al. Hyperglycemia and short-term outcome in patients with spontaneous intracerebral hemorrhage. *Neurocrit Care* 2008;9:217–29.

64. Fogelholm R, Murros K, Rissanen A, et al. Blood glucose and short term survival in primary intracerebral haemorrhage: a population based study. *J Neurol Neurosurg Psychiatry* 2005;76(3):349–53.

65. Godoy DA, Pinero GR, Svampa S, et al. Hyperglycemia and short-term outcome in patients with spontaneous intracerebral hemorrhage. *Neurocrit Care* 2008;9:217–29.

66. Kimura K, Iguchi Y, Inoue T, et al. Hyperglycemia independently increases the risk of early death in acute spontaneous intracerebral hemorrhage. *J Neurol Sci* 2007;255:90–4.

67. Fogelholm R, Murros K, Rissanen A, Avikainen S. Admission blood glucose and short term survival in primary intracerebral haemorrhage: a population based study. *J Neurol Neurosurg Psychiatry* 2005;76:349–53.

68. Passero S, Ciacci G, Ulivelli M. The influence of diabetes and hyperglycemia on clinical course after intracerebral hemorrhage. *Neurology* 2003;61:1351–6.

69. Gray CS, Hildreth AJ, Alberti GK, O'Connell JE. Poststroke hyperglycemia: natural history and immediate management. *Stroke* 2004;35:122–6.

70. Williams LS, Rotich J, Qi R, et al. Effects of admission hyperglycemia on mortality and costs in acute ischemic stroke. *Neurology* 2002;59(1):67–71.

71. Chrousos GP. The hypothalamic–pituitary–adrenal axis and immune-mediated inflammation. *N Engl J Med* 1995;332:1351–62.

72. Barth E, Albuszies G, Baumgart K, et al. Glucose metabolism and catecholamines. *Crit Care Med* 2007;35:S508–18.

73. Tomlinson DR, Gardiner NJ. Glucose neurotoxicity. *Nat Rev Neurosci* 2008;9:36–45.

74. Higashi Y, Noma K, Yoshizumi M, Kihara Y. Endothelial function and oxidative stress in cardiovascular diseases. *Circ J* 2009;73:411–18.

75. Kamada H, Yu F, Nito C, Chan PH. Influence of hyperglycemia on oxidative stress and matrix metalloproteinase-9 activation after focal cerebral ischemia/reperfusion in rats: relation to blood–brain barrier dysfunction. *Stroke* 2007;38:1044–9.

76. Clausen T, Khaldi A, Zauner A, et al. Cerebral acid–base homeostasis after severe traumatic brain injury. *J Neurosurg* 2005;103:597–607.

77. van den Bergh, Wouters P, Weekers F, et al. Intensive insulin therapy in the critically ill patients. *N Engl J Med* 2001;345:1359–67.

78. Brunkhorst FM, Engel C, Bloos F, et al. Intensive insulin therapy and pentastarch resuscitation in severe sepsis. *N Engl J Med* 2008;358:125–39.

79. Arabi YM, Dabbagh OC, Tamim HM, et al. Intensive versus conventional insulin therapy: a randomized controlled trial in medical and surgical critically ill patients. *Crit Care Med* 2008;36:3190–7.

80. Griesdale DE, de Souza RJ, van Dam RM, et al. Intensive insulin therapy and mortality among critically ill patients: a meta-analysis including NICESUGAR study data. *CMAJ* 2009;180:821–7.

81. Treggiari MM, Karir V, Yanez ND, et al. Intensive insulin therapy and mortality in critically ill patients. *Crit Care* 2008;12:R29.

82. Glezer A, Bronstein MD. Pituitary apoplexy: pathophysiology, diagnosis and management. *Arch Endocrinol Metab* 2015; 59:259–64.

83. Boellis A, di Napoli A, Romano A, Bozzao A. Pituitary apoplexy: an update on clinical and imaging features. *Insights Imaging* 2014;5:753–62.

84. Brodal P. Autonomic nervous system. In: Broadal P, editor. *The Central Nervous System. Structure and Function.* 4th ed. New York: Oxford University Press; 2010. pp. 409–58.

85. Popugaev KA, Lubnin AU. Postoperative care in neurooncology. In: Wartenberg KE, Shukri Kh, Abdelhak T, eds. *Neurointensive Care: A Clinical Guide to Patient Safety.* Switzerland: Springer; 2015:95–123.

86. Tomida M, Muraki M, Uemura K, Yamasaki K. Plasma concentrations of brain natriuretic peptide in patients with subarachnoid hemorrhage. *Stroke* 1998;29:1584–7.

87. Tung PP, Olmsted E, Kopelnik A, et al. Plasma B-type natriuretic peptide levels are associated with early cardiac dysfunction after subarachnoid haemorrhage. *Stroke* 2005;36:1567–9.

88. Berendes E, Walter M, Cullen P, et al. Secretion of brain natriuretic peptide in patients with aneurysmal subarachnoid haemorrhage. *Lancet* 1997;349:245–9.

89. Rabinstein AA, Bruder N. Management of hyponatremia and volume contraction. *Neurocrit Care* 2011;15:354–60.

90. Hasan D, Lindsay KW, Wijdicks EF, et al. Effect of fludrocortisone acetate in patients with subarachnoid hemorrhage. *Stroke* 1989;20:1156–61.

91. Mori T, Katayama Y, Kawamata T, Hirayama T. Improved efficiency of hypervolemic therapy with inhibition of natriuresis by fludrocortisone in patients with aneurysmal subarachnoid hemorrhage. *J Neurosurg* 1999;91:947–52.

Part XII

Neuromuscular Care

Editor: Nicola Latronico

45

Critical Illness Polyneuropathy and Myopathy

N. Latronico and F. A. Rasulo

ABSTRACT

Critical illness polyneuropathy (CIP) and critical illness myopathy (CIM) are the most common neuromuscular disorders acquired in the intensive care unit (ICU) affecting between a third and half of the most severely critically ill patients. Critical illness polyneuropathy and CIM often coexist and are associated with profound muscle weakness of the limbs and respiratory muscles. This ICU-acquired weakness (ICUAW) may present with tetraparesis or tetraplegia and difficulty or failure to wean from the ventilator, and is associated with prolonged mechanical ventilation, protracted ICU stay, and increased ICU, hospital, and 1-year mortality. Diagnosis of CIP and CIM requires electrophysiological investigations of peripheral nerves and muscles as well as clinical detection of limb and respiratory muscle weakness. Sepsis, immobilization, mechanical ventilation, and hyperglycaemia are key risk factors. Pathophysiology is multifactorial, and includes micro-circulatory, cellular, and metabolic mechanisms. There are no specific treatments for ICUAW, but early ICU rehabilitation and control of hyperglycaemia can reduce short-term physical impairments.

KEYWORDS

Muscle weakness; muscle wasting; rehabilitation; physical impairment; long-term outcome.

INTRODUCTION

Muscle weakness in the intensive care unit (ICU) is as common as arterial hypotension.[1] The causes can be many, and can be divided into pre-existing conditions, previously undiagnosed or new onset conditions, and conditions acquired during the ICU stay as complications of critical illness.[2] In the ICU, differential diagnosis includes concurrent complications, such as electrolyte abnormalities, rhabdomyolysis, nerve compression or entrapment, status epilepticus, surgery, or use of drugs.[3] This chapter focuses on ICU-acquired muscle weakness (ICUAW) caused by pathological processes involving one or more components of the motor unit comprising the motor neuron with its axon and myelin sheath, the neuromuscular transmission, and all the muscle fibres it innervates. The chapter also describes the impact of

ICUAW on short-term outcomes, including limb muscle weakness and paralysis, neuromuscular respiratory failure and prolonged dependency on mechanical ventilation, and long-term outcomes, including physical impairments and mortality.

HISTORICAL BACKGROUND

In 1984, Charles Bolton and his colleagues[4] first described acute polyneuropathy in critically ill patients who could not be weaned from the ventilator. Patients had suffered from acute respiratory distress syndrome (ARDS); pleural empyema complicating surgery; pneumonia; and lung abscesses. Despite the resolution of critical illness, 'the patient could not tolerate a reduction in the frequency of mandatory mechanical ventilation' and was unable to breathe spontaneously. Some clinical signs suggested polyneuropathy. Spontaneous limb movements were weak. The muscles were flaccid and deep tendon reflexes were absent but grimacing of facial muscles was induced by painful stimulation. Electrophysiological study (EPS) of peripheral nerves and muscles performed after several weeks provided 'early and definitive evidence of the polyneuropathy'. EPS and necropsy findings defined the nature of this polyneuropathy to be axonal degeneration. The authors described five patients in four years, so it seemed a very rare condition possibly due to 'either a toxin or nutritional deficiency affecting only the peripheral nervous system'. The authors presented their results at several meetings with virtually no audience.[5] Experts of neuromuscular diseases thought that these patients had a Guillain-Barré syndrome. In 1986, Bolton and team[6] demonstrated that 'critically ill polyneuropathy', how the condition was called at that time, was a distinct entity from Guillain-Barré syndrome. In 1987, Bolton and his colleagues[7] published their seminal paper in *Brain* and proposed the term 'critical illness polyneuropathy' (CIP) to characterize an axonal, sensory-motor polyneuropathy complicating sepsis and multiple organ failure (MOF). CIP was no longer considered as an isolated event but rather the dysfunction of the peripheral nervous system within a more complex syndrome of multiple organ dysfunctions and failures, caused by 'a fundamental, yet unknown defect'. A coexisting myopathy was also documented in four patients at necropsy; however, the relevance of myopathic changes were overlooked at that time. In 1995, Leijten[8] first demonstrated that critically ill patients developing CIP in the ICU were at increased risk for severe and persisting disability after hospital discharge.

The story of critical illness myopathy (CIM) probably started in 1977 when MacFarlane and Rosenthal reported the case of a young asthmatic woman developing diffuse muscle weakness after an acute respiratory failure requiring mechanical ventilation and large dose steroids.[9] After 8 days the patient was unable to breathe spontaneously and lift her limbs against gravity. Cranial nerves, deep tendon reflexes, and sensation were normal. Diagnosis of myopathy was based on electromyography. Muscle biopsy was not performed and the cause was attributed to large doses of corticosteroids used to treat asthma. In 1979, Sher reported the first case of acute myopathy with extensive and selective loss of myosin (thick) filaments, which is now considered a common muscle biopsy finding in mild CIM.[10] In 1985 and then in 1991, Op de Coul and colleagues[11,12] described a series of 22 patients of whom 16 had EPS revealing neurogenic changes in 11 patients and myogenic changes

in 5. As nerve and muscle abnormalities coexisted in 3 patients, these authors proposed the term critical illness polyneuromyopathy to describe the syndrome. In 1991, Helliwell[13] described muscle necrosis as a characteristic finding of the more severe forms of CIM and Witt[14] showed that hyperglycaemia together with hypoalbuminaemia and prolonged ICU stay strongly correlated with the development of CIP. A few years later in 2001, research on intensive insulin treatment showed a substantial reduction of CIP in patients treated with high doses of insulin aiming at normoglycaemia.[15,16] In 1996, Latronico[17] showed that combined CIP and CIM were the most common finding explaining tetraparesis and tetraplegia in acutely ill neurologic patients. In 22 patients, EPS indicated CIP that was confirmed at nerve biopsy in 8 cases; 14 patients had normal nerve histology suggesting that nerve dysfunction can precede structural nerve degeneration.[18,19] In 23 patients, muscle biopsy showed acute myopathy with muscle necrosis being the most prominent finding (50%), a result that has been confirmed in a recent series.[20] In 2002, De Jonghe[21] demonstrated that ICU-acquired paresis diagnosed using simple bedside clinical criteria was common and had an impact on prolongation of mechanical ventilation.

CRITICAL ILLNESS POLYNEUROPATHY AND CRITICAL ILLNESS MYOPATHY

Critical illness polyneuropathy is an acute distal axonal polyneuropathy affecting both motor and sensory nerves.[22] EPS features include abnormal reduction in the amplitude of motor and sensory nerve action potential with maintained nerve conduction velocity.[22] Nerve biopsy shows axonal degeneration with decreased density of myelinated fibres, while surviving fibres maintain their normal myelin sheath (Figure 45.1, part e).[23] Both limb and respiratory muscles are affected while facial muscles are usually spared. Muscle weakness is symmetrical, most prominent in the lower extremities and can be severe enough to cause tetraparesis or tetraplegia. When less severe, muscle weakness is usually more pronounced distally than proximally. Critical illness polyneuropathy has worse long-term prognosis than CIM[24,25] and may cause persistent limb muscle wasting, weakness, and ventilator dependency. Milder disabilities such as reduced or absent deep tendon reflexes, stocking and glove sensory loss, muscle atrophy, painful hyperaesthesia, and foot drop are common.[26]

Critical illness myopathy is an acute primary myopathy that is not secondary to muscle denervation.[22]

However, CIP and CIM often coexist, and hence, the muscle suffers twice: firstly because it is the site of an acute myopathic process and secondly because it is denervated by concurrent CIP. EPS features include abnormal reduction in the amplitude of the compound muscle action (motor) potential with normal sensory action potential and myopathic motor unit potentials on needle electromyography.[22] Muscle membrane can be inexcitable in some cases (Figure 45.1, part d). Muscle biopsy shows selective loss of myosin filaments (Figure 45.1, parts a and c), varying degrees of fibre necrosis (Figure 45.1, part b) as well as muscle fibre atrophy (Figure 45.1, part c). Early fibre IIa atrophy is predominant in patients with altered muscle membrane excitability and may coexist with selective loss of myosin filaments.[27] Clinical features of CIM are similar to CIP, but sensory function is intact.

Definite diagnosis of CIP and CIM require that both clinical and EPS criteria are fulfilled;[22] however, a probable diagnosis can be established based on EPS alone.[22] Simplified EPS studies can be used in the ICU,[18,19,28] and, if altered can predict long-term physical dysfunction and mortality.[8,29]

Intensive Care Unit Acquired Muscle Weakness

Muscle weakness acquired in ICU is a generalized symmetrical reduction of limb and respiratory muscle strength developing as a complication of critical illness.[3,30] It is estimated that 25% of patients who require prolonged mechanical ventilation develop global and persistent weakness.[31] Based on this, more than 75,000 patients in the United States and up to 1 million worldwide may develop ICUAW.[31] The key risk factors are sepsis, mechanical unloading of limbs (immobilization), and diaphragm (controlled mechanical ventilation), and hyperglycaemia.[31–33] Drugs such as steroids, neuromuscular blocking agents (NMBA) and opioids, which are commonly used in critically ill patients are not consistently associated with development of ICUAW.[34–36] Acute myopathy is well demonstrated in experimental rat models of high-dose steroids and muscle denervation, but direct evidence of an acute steroid myopathy in critically ill patients is lacking. Prolonged neuromuscular transmission block can be observed after protracted infusion of non-depolarizing NMBA in patients with hepatic or renal insufficiency, but muscle weakness commonly lasts a few hours.

ICUAW may cause flaccid tetraparesis and tetraplegia, and is associated with prolonged mechanical ventilation and ICU stay, resulting in increased ICU, hospital, and 1-year mortality.[21,29,37,38] Diaphragm dysfunction can be more frequent than limb muscle weakness and is significantly associated with subsequent weaning failure and mortality.[39]

The diagnosis of ICUAW is established clinically by testing 12 specified muscle groups using the Medical Research Council sum-score (MRC-SS) or handgrip or handheld dynamometry. With MRC-SS, scores below 48[21] and below 36[40] indicate, respectively, significant weakness (i.e., ICUAW) and severe weakness, while the average strength is limited to movement against gravity and partial resistance. With handgrip dynamometry, cut-off scores of less than 11 kilograms (interquartile range (IQR) 10–40) in males and less than 7 kg (IQR 0–7.3) for females indicate ICUAW.[41] Handgrip dynamometry can be used as a screening tool: if normal, ICUAW can be excluded, no further testing is required.[42] Difficulty in weaning the patient from ventilator is a major criterion for diagnosing CIP, CIM, and ICUAW after non-neuromuscular causes such as heart and lung disease have been excluded.[22] Specific cut-off values for respiratory muscle weakness are not required for diagnosing ICUAW; however, maximal inspiratory pressure (MIP) values > -30 cm H_2O and maximal expiratory pressures (MEP) <40 cm H_2O (MIP, MEP) predict neuromuscular respiratory failure needing mechanical ventilation.[2] MRC-SS, dynamometry, MIP, and MEP are volitional tests. They can be assessed only in awake and cooperative patients. Sedation, delirium, and coma preclude early participation in volitional testing of muscle strength. Moreover, MRC-SS scoring at seven days post-awakening, as in the original study,[21] can be remarkably less useful considering current trends towards earlier ICU discharge, as most patients are already discharged by this time.[43,44] Electrical and magnetic neuromuscular twitch stimulation are non-volitional tests that may serve as an alternative to assess muscle strength. Ulnar nerve supramaximal stimulation for the adductor pollicis muscle or peroneal nerve for ankle dorsiflexor muscles can provide measures of muscle function independent of the patient's cooperation.[45] Endotracheal tube pressure induced by bilateral phrenic nerve stimulation during airway occlusion can be used to estimate the capacity of diaphragm to generate pressure. Patients with pressures below 11 cm H_2O are considered to have diaphragm weakness.[39]

At long-term follow-up, recovery of muscle strength can be faster than recovery of physical dysfunction.[46–48] Persisting physical impairments can be detected using dynamic tests such as 6-Minute Walk Distance Test or 4-Meter Gait Speed Test.[49]

PATHOPHYSIOLOGY

The main defect leading to CIP and CIM during MOF is unknown. In a rat model of long-term mechanical ventilation, deep sedation, and muscle unloading, mechanical silencing, i.e., the complete loss of mechanical stimuli in skeletal muscles, triggers CIM through perturbation of genes that regulate mitochondrial dynamics.[50] Passive mechanical loading prevents these changes, which may explain the beneficial effects of early ICU mobilization. A puzzling aspect of CIP and CIM is their rapid onset and potentially rapid reversibility.[22] Nerve histology can be normal at an early stage of critical illness[17] and muscles can show only minimal alterations despite evidence of severe muscle weakness and paralysis, which suggest that the defect can be functional. Since CIP and CIM are part of the MOF syndrome, it is likely that the microcirculatory, cellular, and metabolic pathophysiological mechanisms leading to MOF also cause CIP and CIM. Muscle and nerve microcirculations can be impaired during critical illness thus favouring ischaemic hypoxia.[22,51] In nerves, endothelial cell and leucocyte activation, increased cytokine production, hyperglycaemia and hypoalbuminaemia can lead to altered microvascular permeability and endoneural oedema formation.[52] At a cellular level, mitochondrial function can be impaired favouring cytopathic hypoxia.[53] Acquired sodium channelopathy, impaired calcium release by the sarcoplasmic reticulum and satellite muscle cell dysfunction are other potentially relevant mechanisms operating at the cellular level.[32,35,53–55] In mice, dysfunction of satellite cells can be long-lasting, durably impairing muscle regeneration and replacing a fully functional muscle with a huge fibrotic area.[53] At a metabolic level, reduced protein synthesis and increased protein catabolism, altered glucose utilization and dysfunctional mitochondrial autophagy favour muscle wasting and weakness.[14–16,20,32,33,56] Metabolic adaptation to limit ischaemic damage includes reducing or abolishing the generation of the action potential, a costly energetic process;[17–19] however, with persisting ischaemic deficit, structural alterations ensue. Recently, early dysfunction of alpha motor neurons during repetitive firing has been identified as a novel mechanism leading to ICUAW in a rat model of sepsis.[57] Interestingly, no abnormalities indicating CIP or CIM were found suggesting that reduced central nervous system neuron excitability could be an important contributor to loss of motor unit activity and mechanical silencing.

TREATMENT

No specific treatment reduces the incidence and severity of CIP and CIM. Electrolyte abnormalities that alter nerve, neuromuscular transmission or muscle function such as hypomagnesaemia, hypokalaemia, hyperkalaemia, and hypophosphatemia should be corrected rapidly.[2] In patients at high risk of developing CIP, CIM, and ICUAW, drugs such as steroids, NMBA, some antibiotics (aminoglycosides, polymyxin B, clindamycin), drugs with anaesthetic-like action (lidocaine, procainamide, quinidine, phenytoin), calcium channel blockers, magnesium, beta-blockers, diuretics, and quinolones should be used with caution. Propofol infusion syndrome (PRIS) is a rare but potentially lethal condition of severe metabolic acidosis, kidney and liver failure, rhabdomyolysis, hyperkalaemia, renal failure, hyperlipidaemia, and rapidly progressing cardiac failure arising as a side effect of high-dose propofol.[58] No specific treatment exists. Recognition at an early stage can be vital for discontinuing propofol and preventing more serious complications.

Intensive insulin therapy to maintain normal blood glucose concentrations (80 to 110 mg/dL; 4.4 to 6.1 mmol/L) reduces the incidence of electrophysiologically-proven CIP in adult ICU patients and the duration of mechanical ventilation,[36] but increases mortality and is not recommended.[59]

Avoiding excessive hyperglycaemia remains a sensible therapeutic target with specific blood glucose thresholds that should be adapted to the local ICU context.[60]

Neuromuscular electrical stimulation can be used at the bedside and may be an effective treatment for muscle weakness in adults with advanced progressive disease but effectiveness in critically ill patients remains unproven.[61,62] Early physical rehabilitation in the ICU has an impact on short-term outcomes shortening the ICU length of stay and duration of delirium, and improving patients' functional mobility at hospital discharge,[63,64] but the effects on long-term outcome are unknown.[65]

FUTURE DIRECTIONS

Pathophysiological mechanisms leading to CIP and CIM as well as mechanisms leading to ICUAW by disrupting repetitive firing of the central nervous system motor neurons need to be better defined. Impact of treatments aimed at restoring impaired functions, such as the use of mesenchymal stem cells to improve satellite muscle cell function and muscle fibre regeneration needs investigations in clinical settings.[53] Future studies of adequate power should evaluate the impact of early rehabilitation on long-term physical impairments in survivors of critical illness.

CONCLUSIONS

Critical illness polyneuropathy and CIM are commonly encountered neuromuscular disorders in the ICU. It is frequently labelled as ICU-acquired profound muscle weakness that complicates the course of intensive care admission. It is believed to be a multifaceted pathognomonic process. The treatment of this disorder is targeted at symptomatic management with no single specific treatment currently known to reduce incidence and severity of this disorder. However, efforts are being invested in unveiling the impact of early rehabilitation on outcomes in critically ill patients.

REFERENCES

1. Eikermann M, Latronico N. What is new in prevention of muscle weakness in critically ill patients? *Intensive Care Med* 2013;39(12):2200–3.
2. Latronico N, Fagoni N. Neuromuscular disorders and acquired neuromuscular weakness. In: Smith Martin M. CG, Kofke Andrew W, eds. *Oxford Textbook of Neurocritical Care*. Oxford, England: Oxford University Press; 2016.
3. Sharshar T, Citerio G, Andrews PJD, et al. Neurological examination of critically ill patients: a pragmatic approach. Report of an ESICM expert panel. *Intensive Care Medicine* 2014;40(4):484–95.
4. Bolton CF, Gilbert JJ, Hahn AF, Sibbald WJ. Polyneuropathy in critically ill patients. *J Neurol Neurosurg Psychiatry* 1984;47(11):1223–31.
5. Bolton CF. The discovery of critical illness polyneuropathy: a memoir. *Can J Neurol Sci* 2010;37(4):431–8.
6. Bolton CF, Laverty DA, Brown JD, Witt NJ, Hahn AF, Sibbald WJ. Critically ill polyneuropathy: electrophysiological studies and differentiation from Guillain-Barre syndrome. *J Neurol Neurosurg Psychiatry* 1986;49(5):563–73.
7. Zochodne DW, Bolton CF, Wells GA, et al. Critical illness polyneuropathy. A complication of sepsis and multiple organ failure. *Brain* 1987;110(Pt 4):819–41.
8. Leijten FS, Harinck-de Weerd JE, Poortvliet DC, de Weerd AW. The role of polyneuropathy in motor convalescence after prolonged mechanical ventilation. *JAMA* 1995;274(15):1221–5.
9. MacFarlane IA, Rosenthal FD. Severe myopathy after status asthmaticus. *Lancet* 1977;2(8038):615.
10. Sher JH, Shafiq SA, Schutta HS. Acute myopathy with selective lysis of myosin filaments. *Neurology* 1979;29(1):100–6.

11. Op de Coul AA, Lambregts PC, Koeman J, van Puyenbroek MJ, Ter Laak HJ, Gabreels-Festen AA. Neuromuscular complications in patients given Pavulon (pancuronium bromide) during artificial ventilation. *Clin Neurol Neurosurg* 1985;87(1):17–22.
12. Op de Coul AA, Verheul GA, Leyten AC, Schellens RL, Teepen JL. Critical illness polyneuromyopathy after artificial respiration. *Clin Neurol Neurosurg* 1991;93(1):27–33.
13. Helliwell TR, Coakley JH, Wagenmakers AJ, et al. Necrotizing myopathy in critically-ill patients. *J Pathol* 1991;164(4): 307–14.
14. Witt NJ, Zochodne DW, Bolton CF, et al. Peripheral nerve function in sepsis and multiple organ failure. *Chest* 1991;99(1):176–84.
15. van den Berghe G, Wouters P, Weekers F, et al. Intensive insulin therapy in critically ill patients. *N Engl J Med* 2001;345(19):1359–67.
16. Hermans G, Wilmer A, Meersseman W, et al. Impact of intensive insulin therapy on neuromuscular complications and ventilator dependency in the medical intensive care unit. *Am J Respir Crit Care Med* 2007;175(5): 480–9.
17. Latronico N, Fenzi F, Recupero D, et al. Critical illness myopathy and neuropathy. *Lancet* 1996;347(9015): 1579–82.
18. Latronico N. Critical illness polyneuropathy and myopathy 20 years later. No man's land? No, it is our land! *Intensive Care Med* 2016;42(11):1790–3.
19. Latronico N, Bertolini G, Guarneri B, et al. Simplified electrophysiological evaluation of peripheral nerves in critically ill patients: the Italian multi-centre CRIMYNE study. *Crit Care* 2007;11(1): R11.
20. Puthucheary ZA, Rawal J, McPhail M, et al. Acute skeletal muscle wasting in critical illness. *JAMA* 2013;310(15):1591–600.
21. De Jonghe B, Sharshar T, Lefaucheur JP, et al. Paresis acquired in the intensive care unit: a prospective multicenter study. *JAMA* 2002;288(22):2859–67.
22. Latronico N, Bolton CF. Critical illness polyneuropathy and myopathy: a major cause of muscle weakness and paralysis. *Lancet Neurol* 2011;10(10):931–41.
23. Latronico N, Tomelleri G, Filosto M. Critical illness myopathy. *Curr Opin Rheumatol* 2012;24(6):616–22.
24. Guarneri B, Bertolini G, Latronico N. Long-term outcome in patients with critical illness myopathy or neuropathy: the Italian multicentre CRIMYNE study. *J Neurol Neurosurg Psychiatry* 2008;79(7):838–41.
25. Koch S, Wollersheim T, Bierbrauer J, et al. Long-term recovery in critical illness myopathy is complete, contrary to polyneuropathy. *Muscle Nerve* 2014;50(3): 431–6.
26. Latronico N, Shehu I, Seghelini E. Neuromuscular sequelae of critical illness. *Current Opinion in Critical Care* 2005;11(4):381–90.

27. Bierbrauer J, Koch S, Olbricht C, et al. Early type II fiber atrophy in intensive care unit patients with nonexcitable muscle membrane. *Crit Care Med* 2012;40(2):647–50.

28. Latronico N, Nattino G, Guarneri B, et al. Validation of the peroneal nerve test to diagnose critical illness polyneuropathy and myopathy in the intensive care unit: the multicentre Italian CRIMYNE-2 diagnostic accuracy study. *F1000Res* 2014;3:127.

29. Hermans G, Van Mechelen H, Bruyninckx F, et al. Predictive value for weakness and 1-year mortality of screening electrophysiology tests in the ICU. *Intensive Care Med* 2015;41(12):2138–48.

30. Stevens RD, Marshall SA, Cornblath DR, et al. A framework for diagnosing and classifying intensive care unit-acquired weakness. *Crit Care Med* 2009;37(Suppl. 10): 299–308.

31. Fan E, Cheek F, Chlan L, et al. An official American Thoracic Society Clinical Practice guideline: the diagnosis of intensive care unit-acquired weakness in adults. *Am J Respir Crit Care Med* 2014;190(12):1437–46.

32. Friedrich O, Reid MB, Van den Berghe G, et al. The Sick and the Weak: Neuropathies/Myopathies in the Critically Ill. *Physiol Rev* 2015;95(3):1025–109.

33. Farhan H, Moreno-Duarte I, Latronico N, Zafonte R, Eikermann M. Acquired muscle weakness in the surgical intensive care unit: nosology, epidemiology, diagnosis, and prevention. *Anesthesiology* 2016;124(1):207–34.

34. Murray MJ, DeBlock H, Erstad B, et al. Clinical practice guidelines for sustained neuromuscular blockade in the adult critically ill patient. *Crit Care Med* 2016;44(11): 2079–2103.

35. Dos Santos C, Hussain SN, Mathur S, et al. Mechanisms of chronic muscle wasting and dysfunction after an intensive care unit stay. a pilot study. *Am J Respir Crit Care Med* 2016;194(7):821–30.

36. Hermans G, De Jonghe B, Bruyninckx F, Van den Berghe G. Interventions for preventing critical illness polyneuropathy and critical illness myopathy. *Cochrane Database Syst Rev* 2014;1:CD006832.

37. Ali NA, O'Brien JM, Jr., Hoffmann SP, et al. Acquired weakness, handgrip strength, and mortality in critically ill patients. *Am J Respir Crit Care Med* 2008;178(3): 261–8.

38. Hermans G, Van Mechelen H, Clerckx B, et al. Acute outcomes and 1-year mortality of intensive care unit-acquired weakness. A cohort study and propensity-matched analysis. *Am J Respir Crit Care Med* 2014;190(4):410–20.

39. Dres M, Dube BP, Mayaux J, et al. Coexistence and impact of limb muscle and diaphragm weakness at time of liberation from mechanical ventilation in medical icu patients. *Am J Respir Crit Care Med* 2016.

40. Hermans G, Clerckx B, Vanhullebusch T, et al. Interobserver agreement of Medical Research Council sum-score and handgrip strength in the intensive care unit. *Muscle Nerve* 2012;45(1):18–25.

41. Latronico N, Gosselink R. A guided approach to diagnose severe muscle weakness in the intensive care unit. *Rev Bras Ter Intensiva* 2015;27(3):199–201.

42. Parry SM, Berney S, Granger CL, et al. A new two-tier strength assessment approach to the diagnosis of weakness in intensive care: an observational study. *Crit Care* 2015;19:52.

43. Hough CL, Lieu BK, Caldwell ES. Manual muscle strength testing of critically ill patients: feasibility and interobserver agreement. *Crit Care* 2011;15(1):R43.

44. Connolly BA, Jones GD, Curtis AA, et al. Clinical predictive value of manual muscle strength testing during critical illness: an observational cohort study. *Crit Care* 2013;17(5):R229.

45. Bittner EA, Martyn JA, George E, Frontera WR, Eikermann M. Measurement of muscle strength in the intensive care unit. *Crit Care Med* 2009;37(Suppl 10):S321–30.

46. Herridge MS, Tansey CM, Matte A, et al. Functional disability 5 years after acute respiratory distress syndrome. *N Engl J Med* 2011;364(14):1293–304.

47. Needham DM, Wozniak AW, Hough CL, et al. Risk factors for physical impairment after acute lung injury in a national, multicenter study. *Am J Respir Crit Care Med* 2014;189(10):1214–24.

48. Herridge MS, Chu LM, Matte A, et al. The RECOVER Program: Disability risk groups and 1-year outcome after 7 or more days of mechanical ventilation. *Am J Respir Crit Care Med* 2016;194(7):831–44.

49. Latronico N, Herridge M, Hopkins RO, et al. The ICM research agenda on intensive care unit-acquired weakness. *Intensive Care Med* 2017 Sep;43(9):1270–81.

50. Kalamgi RC, Salah H, Gastaldello S, et al. Mechano signaling pathways in an experimental intensive critical illness myopathy model. *J Physiol* 2016;594(15): 4371–88.

51. Vellinga NA, Boerma EC, Koopmans M, et al. International study on microcirculatory shock occurrence in acutely ill patients. *Crit Care Med* 2015;43(1):48–56.

52. Fenzi F, Latronico N, Refatti N, Rizzuto N. Enhanced expression of E-selectin on the vascular endothelium of peripheral nerve in critically ill patients with neuromuscular disorders. *Acta Neuropathol (Berl)* 2003;106(1):75–82.

53. Rocheteau P, Chatre L, Briand D, et al. Sepsis induces long-term metabolic and mitochondrial muscle stem cell dysfunction amenable by mesenchymal stem cell therapy. *Nat Commun* 2015;6:101–45.

54. Llano-Diez M, Cheng AJ, Jonsson W, et al. Impaired Ca(2+) release contributes to muscle weakness in a rat model of critical illness myopathy. *Crit Care* 2016;20(1):254.

55. Koch S, Bierbrauer J, Haas K, et al. Critical illness polyneuropathy in ICU patients is related to reduced motor nerve excitability caused by reduced sodium permeability. *Intensive Care Med Exp* 2016;4(1):10.

56. Hermans G, Casaer MP, Clerckx B, et al. Effect of tolerating macronutrient deficit on the development of intensive-care

unit acquired weakness: a subanalysis of the EPaNIC trial. *Lancet Respir Med* 2013;1(8):621–9.

57. Nardelli P, Vincent JA, Powers R, Cope TC, Rich MM. Reduced motor neuron excitability is an important contributor to weakness in a rat model of sepsis. *Exp Neurol* 2016;282:1–8.

58. Vasile B, Rasulo F, Candiani A, Latronico N. The pathophysiology of propofol infusion syndrome: a simple name for a complex syndrome. *Intensive Care Med* 2003;29(9):1417–25.

59. Finfer S, Chittock DR, Su SY, et al. Intensive versus conventional glucose control in critically ill patients. *N Engl J Med* 2009;360(13):1283–97.

60. Gunst J, Van den Berghe G. Blood glucose control in the ICU: don't throw out the baby with the bathwater! *Intensive Care Med* 2016;42(9):1478–81.

61. Parry SM, Berney S, Granger CL, Koopman R, El-Ansary D, Denehy L. Electrical muscle stimulation in the intensive care setting: a systematic review. *Crit Care Med* 2013;41(10):2406–18.

62. Jones S, Man WD, Gao W, Higginson IJ, Wilcock A, Maddocks M. Neuromuscular electrical stimulation for muscle weakness in adults with advanced disease. *Cochrane Database Syst Rev* 2016;10:CD009419.

63. Schweickert WD, Pohlman MC, Pohlman AS, et al. Early physical and occupational therapy in mechanically ventilated, critically ill patients: a randomised controlled trial. *Lancet* 2009;373(9678):1874–82.

64. Schaller SJ, Anstey M, Blobner M, et al. Early, goal-directed mobilisation in the surgical intensive care unit: a randomised controlled trial. *Lancet* 2016;388(10052):1377–88.

65. Tipping CJ, Harrold M, Holland A, Romero L, Nisbet T, Hodgson CL. The effects of active mobilisation and rehabilitation in ICU on mortality and function: a systematic review. *Intensive Care Med* 2017 Feb;43(2): 171–83.

Part XIII

Gastrointestinal Care

Editor: Swagata Tripathy

46

Gastrointestinal Bleeding in Neurocritical Care

G. Kakkar

ABSTRACT

The incidence of gastrointestinal (GI) bleeding in critical care has declined over the years and the incidence within neurocritical care remains within the same boundaries. These are as a result of better clinical practices, adherence to guidelines, and evolving practices involving care bundles. A clinically oriented definition is required in critical care to classify and manage the disease. Gastrointestinal bleeding in aspects of critical care should be defined as either overt or clinically significant. Specific interventions such as early enteral feeding, use of proton pump inhibitors (PPIs)/ H2 receptor antagonists, Helicobacter treatment, and endoscopy screening have all helped to reduce the disease burden. However, the small percentage of critical care patients where GI bleeding still happens require prompt diagnosis, assessment, and aggressive resuscitation. Treatment should involve multiple hospital specialities including critical care, gastroenterology, general surgery, intervention radiology, haematology, and optimum use of modern technological advances.

KEYWORDS

Neurointensive care; gastrointestinal bleed; haematemesis; enteral feed; haematochezia.

INTRODUCTION

The frequency of damage to the intestinal mucosa in critically ill patients is quite high. The subsequent gastrointestinal (GI) bleeding from the resultant damaged mucosa leads to adverse outcomes, especially in critically ill patients.[1,2] This holds true for neurocritical care patients as well who undergo the same severe physiological and metabolic changes during the neurological disease process. Most of the published literature on gastrointestinal bleeding in critical care patients is based on patients suffering from medical and general surgical illnesses. Precise mechanisms of injury are still unknown. Furthermore, there remains paucity of both knowledge and data about GI bleeding in critically ill patients suffering from neurological diseases.[1] Treatment of these patients remains a challenge, especially in the presence of neurological pathologies like raised intracranial pressure (ICP), subarachnoid haemorrhage (SAH), stroke, spinal cord injury (SCI), and neuromuscular disorders.

DEFINITION

Gastrointestinal bleeding is described in medical texts and literature with respect to its origin in relation to the ligament of Treitz. Bleeding occurring proximal to the ligament of Treitz is termed upper GI bleeding whilst bleeding occurring distally is called lower GI bleeding.[3] However, in critical care medicine, a more treatment-based definition assumes more relevance. It is defined as either overt or clinically significant,[4] and these two ways are described as follows:

Overt GI bleeding[4,5] is defined as GI bleeding with at least one of the parameters: Haematemesis, coffee ground emesis, melena, haematochezia, and bloody nasogastric aspirate.

Clinically significant GI bleeding[4,5] is defined as overt bleeding along with at least one of the following parameters:

- Decrease in blood pressure of at least 20 mmHg;
- Start/increase of vasopressor of at least 20%;
- Decrease in haemoglobin of at least 2 g/dL; and
- Transfusion of at least two units of red blood cells (RBCs) during bleeding.

INCIDENCE AND PREVALENCE

The prevalence of neurological stress ulcers is embedded and remarked in early medical literature. In 1841, Carl Rokitansky, a Bohemian physician proposed a neuronal basis for stress ulcers.[6] Further in 1932, Harvey Cushing reported 11 cases of stress ulcers in patients with elevated intracranial pressure. Together it was called Rokitansky–Cushing syndrome.

The true incidence of GI bleeding in neurocritical care remains unknown. Most of the GI bleeding is upper GI and lower GI bleed remains uncommon.[7] Among the lower GI bleeds intestinal bleed is further rarer and most of the lower GI bleeds are from either colon or local anal pathology. By one North American estimate the incidence of upper GI bleed is around 40–150 per 100,000 population whilst the incidence of lower GI bleed is around 20–30 per 100,000 population. In critically ill population, the incidence should be measured against overt or clinically significant bleeding.[5] The incidence of such bleeding in the intensive care unit (ICU) has decreased over the last 3–4 decades. The reported incidence of upper GI bleed in burns patients in the ICU was once reported as 30%. Since then, the use of guidelines in overall intensive care like correction of haemodynamic deficits, ventilatory insufficiency, and risk prophylaxis has brought the incidence down. The incidence of occult or overt bleeding may be around 5%–25% and most of this is usually self-limiting. The incidence of clinically significant bleeding in ICU admissions is around 1.5%–2% as confirmed by recent studies.[1,4]

AETIOLOGY

The most common aetiologies of upper GI bleeding include: duodenal ulcers (28%), gastric ulcers (26%), gastritis (13%), varices (12%), and oesophagitis (8%).[3,8] Gastrointestinal bleeding due to oesophageal or gastric varices and peptic ulceration carry the highest mortality. The most common causes of lower GI bleed under the age of 60 is from local anorectal causes like haemorrhoids but beyond that age the commonest causes are diverticular

disease and colonic pathologies. The various causes of both upper and lower GI bleed are given in Table 46.1.

PATHOPHYSIOLOGY

Gastrointestinal bleeding in critical care is usually a stress-related mucosal disorder. This results from predisposing clinical conditions that have the potential to alter local mucosal protective barriers, such as mucus, bicarbonate, blood flow, and prostaglandin synthesis, e.g., hypersecretion of acid, Zollinger–Ellison syndrome, defects in gastric glycoprotein mucous, increased refluxed bile salts or presence of uraemic toxins.[9] Ischaemia from shock, sepsis, and trauma can lead to impaired perfusion of the gut. Long-term use of non-steroidal anti-inflammatory drugs (NSAIDs) inhibit cyclooxygenase, decrease mucosal prostaglandin synthesis and lead to impaired mucosal defenses.[10]

In variceal disease, pathophysiology stems from consequences of portal hypertension. The initial factor in portal hypertension is the increase in vascular resistance to portal blood flow which leads to structural distortion and active contraction of portal/septal cells and hepatic myofibroblasts in the portal venules. This leads to the development of porto-systemic collaterals possibly from the influence of angiogenic factors and cause shunting of blood around the liver.

In ulcer-related upper GI bleeding, peptic ulcer disease is strongly associated with *Helicobacter pylori* (*H. pylori*) infection.[11] It causes disruption of the mucous barrier and has a direct inflammatory effect on gastric and duodenal mucosa. As the ulcer burrows deeper into the gastroduodenal mucosa, weakening and necrosis

Table 46.1 Causes of GI bleeding

Upper GI bleeding	Lower GI bleeding
Duodenal ulcers	Diverticular disease
Gastric ulcers	Ischaemic colitis
Gastritis	Vascular ectasia
Oesophageal/Gastric varices	Haemorrhoids
Oesophagitis	Rectal varices
Infections	Drug induced
Aorto-oesophageal fistula	Inflammatory bowel disease
AV malformations	Malignancy
Drug induced	Infections

Source: (1) Manning-Dimmitt LL, Dimmitt SG, Wilson GR. Diagnosis of gastrointestinal bleeding in adults. *Am Fam Physician* 2005;71:1339–46. (2) Lucas CE, Sugawa C, Riddle J, et al. Natural history and surgical dilemma of 'stress' gastric bleeding. *Arch Surg* 1971;102:266–73.

Neurointensive Care

452

of the arterial wall happens and there is development of a pseudo-aneurysm. The weakened wall ruptures and results in haemorrhage.

Although 10%–15% of hospital GI bleeds are from Mallory–Weiss syndrome, they are usually infrequent in critical care. It results from a tear in the mucosa of the gastric cardia as a consequence of forceful vomiting, retching, coughing, or straining. These actions create a rapid increase in the gradient between intragastric and intrathoracic pressures causing gastric mucosal tear from the forceful distension of the gastro-oesophageal junction.[12]

SPECIFIC AND GENERAL RISK FACTORS FOR GASTROINTESTINAL BLEEDING

General Risk Factors

Medications

One of the commonest causes of GI bleeding is drug induced due to either reversible or irreversible pharmacological agents. Numerous studies have illustrated the risk of GI bleeding and GI perforation with NSAID use.[13] As the incidence of GI bleeding in elderly patients using NSAIDs is up to 1 in 7 persons, NSAID use is responsible for about 30% of GI bleed hospitalizations and mortality.[14] Multiple locations including gastric, duodenal, and pre-pyloric areas may be affected. Aspirin is associated with about a 4-time increased risk of GI bleeding. The combined use of drugs like asprin, warfarin, and clopidogrel together for conditions like endovascular stents, etc., result in a greater risk of bleeding.

Comorbidities

Increasing age is amongst the leading risk factors with age >65 bringing the highest risk for GI bleeding.[14–16] Alcoholic liver disease, male gender, overall frailty, peptic ulcer disease, and malignancy are other risk factors. Re-bleeding causing septic shock and malnutrition are other indicators of poor prognosis.

Helicobacter Pylori Infection

H. pylori infection is an established risk factor for upper GI bleeding in the ICU. According to a cohort study which involved both medical and surgical ICUs, an increase in anti-H. pylori IgA concentration was predictive of active infection and risk of GI bleeding.[17] The presence of infection also increased the mortality by about 34%.[17]

Infections

Viral infections of the liver like hepatitis B and hepatitis C are associated with increased risk of GI bleeding secondary to decompensation of liver disease. Other risk factors are diarrhoeal diseases caused by infectious organisms like E. coli, Clostridium difficile, Shigella, Salmonella, and Campylobacter jejuni.[18]

Diverticular Disease

One of the leading causes of lower GI bleed in the intensive care setting (and otherwise) is diverticular bleeding. Up to about 40% cases of lower GI bleed are from diverticular disease and its risk factors are increasing age. They do need a high index of suspicion due to their painless and subacute nature on presentation.[19]

Specific Risk Factors

- Coagulation disorders: There is data to suggest that ICU patients admitted with coagulopathy are at increased risk of GI bleeding. These patients develop significant bleeding in the absence of prompt correction.[5,20]
- Mechanical ventilation: More than 48 hours of mechanical ventilation in critical care for respiratory failure is found to be linked to increased GI bleeding.[5,20]
- One of the most common risk factors for significant GI bleed is decompensated liver disease. Variceal bleeding as a result of portal hypertension is the commonest cause of mortality in cirrhotic liver disease which can be as high as 20%–25%.[21] Clinical tools such as risk prediction scores are of invaluable use in such circumstances. Common high risk predicting factors include the presence of varices, international normalized ratio (INR) >1.2, viral aetiology, alcoholic liver disease, and serum cholinesterase level <2.25 kU/L.[22]
- The other major risk factors in critical care population are sepsis and renal failure.

MORTALITY TRENDS

There is overall decline in the true incidence of upper GI bleeding due to protocol-driven treatments like that of H. pylori and the use of drugs like proton pump inhibitors (PPIs). However, the incidence of the same is increasing in certain subsets like those with oesophageal variceal bleeds.[23] Although they comprise less than 10% of the overall causes of GI bleeding, oesophageal varices remain a high mortality condition with a mortality rate of around 10% on initial admission which increases to about 60% by one year.[23,24] The re-bleeding rate could be as high as 70%

with a mortality increase of about 30% for every episode of re-bleed. Considering the size, smaller varices like those less than 0.5 cm have a 7% chance of bleeding at 2 years compared to varices more than 0.5 cm which have a 30% chance of bleeding at the end of the same period.[25,26] Variceal bleeding requiring surgical interventions for haemorrhage control have a very high mortality rate. Co-existing cardiopulmonary or renal damage, or host defense dysfunction can significantly increase the mortality by about 30%–60%.[25,26]

Although the incidence of lower GI bleeding from anorectal causes and occult blood is increasing, their morbidity and mortality is still less than that compared with upper GI bleeding.[27,28]

PRINCIPLES OF MANAGEMENT

Risk Assessment and Resuscitation

There should be a formal risk assessment for all patients with acute upper GI bleeding. This should be done with the Blatchford Score at first assessment (Table 46.2) and Rockall score at completion of endoscopy[29] (Table 46.3). Most GI bleeds in the ICU are self-limiting but a small number would actually be significant. These significant bleeds are the usual ones that result in high morbidity and mortality. Prompt recognition with quick assessment and initiation of primary resuscitation is key to reduce the morbidity burden.[29,30] With advances in technology and modern healthcare systems, early referrals should be sought from sub-specialties. These should include gastroenterology, general or GI surgery, haematology, and interventional radiology. The airway should be secured as a priority in the primary survey where necessary as aspiration of gastric contents occurs in up to 12% of the cases. Immediate intravenous access should be ensured (if already not in-situ) with large bore peripheral catheters

for volume resuscitation with crystalloids until the availability of blood products. Given that it lacks oxygen-carrying capacity and does not replenish clotting factors, the role of crystalloid fluid for volume resuscitation should

Table 46.2 Glasgow–blatchford score

Admission risk marker	Score component value
Blood urea (mmol/L)	
6.5–8.0	2
8.0–10.0	3
10.0–25	4
>25	6
Haemoglobin (g/dL) for men	
12.0–12.9	1
10.0–11.9	3
<10.0	6
Haemoglobin (g/dL) for women	
10.0–11.9	1
<10.0	6
Systolic blood pressure (mmHg)	
100–109	1
90–99	2
<90	3
Other markers	
Pulse ≥100 (per min)	1
Presentation with melena	1
Presentation with syncope	2
Hepatic disease	2
Cardiac failure	2

Reprinted with permission from: Blatchford O, Murray WR, Blatchford M. A risk score to predict need for treatment for upper-gastrointestinal haemorrhage. *Lancet* 2000; 356(9238):1318–21.

Table 46.3 Rockall score

Variable	Score 0	Score 1	Score 2	Score 3
Age	<60	60–79	>80	
Shock	No shock	Pulse >100 BP >100 Systolic	SBP <100	
Comorbidity	Nil major		CHF, IHD, major morbidity	Renal failure, liver failure, metastatic cancer
Diagnosis	Mallory-Weiss	All other diagnoses	GI malignancy	
Evidence of bleeding	None		Blood, adherent clot, spurting vessel	

Reprinted with permission from: Rockall TA, Logan RF, Devlin HB, Northfield TC. Risk assessment after acute upper gastrointestinal haemorrhage. *Gut* 1996;38(3):316–21.

ideally be restricted to this early phase of resuscitation in a bleeding patient. In cirrhotic patients with suspected variceal haemorrhage, excessive crystalloid resuscitation may be particularly harmful due to their susceptibility to extravascular fluid shifts in the setting of underlying low intravascular oncotic pressure.[31] Other measures to support vital organs should be instituted simultaneously whilst resuscitation is attempted. These include invasive monitoring and access, intravenous infusions, ventilatory support, laboratory markers and activation of local protocols to secure blood products. For acute blood loss anaemia with signs of hypovolaemic shock, O-negative packed red blood cells (PRBCs) (or O-positive PRBCs in women past childbearing age and in men) can be given until type-specific cross-matched blood is available.[29–31]

Correction of Coagulopathy

The optimal haemoglobin level in critically ill patients has been a consistent topic of debate. Recent studies associate a liberal haemoglobin transfusion trigger of 10 g/dL to be associated with higher mortality than a restrictive trigger of 7 g/dL.[32] An exception to this rule exists in the elderly and patients with coronary artery disease. The British Society for Haematology guidelines recommend maintenance of haemoglobin levels between 7–9 g/dL.[33] However, there are no randomized controlled trials to suggest an exact haemoglobin goal for transfusion. Target haemoglobin levels should be individualized for each patient and should be based upon the suspected aetiology of bleeding (i.e., variceal vs nonvariceal haemorrhage) as well as patient comorbidities. In the setting of ongoing massive bleeding, the recommended haemoglobin level of 7 to 8 g/dL should not be considered to be an endpoint of resuscitation. Instead, a mean arterial pressure (MAP) of >60 mmHg and evidence of adequate end-organ perfusion should be the target.[33,34] Endoscopy should be performed as soon as the patient is clinically stable and can be performed even during transfusion.[25] Blood products like fresh frozen plasma (FFP), platelets, and cryoprecipitate should be transfused at the earliest signs of major haemorrhage to prevent coagulopathy.[26] Considering the evidence from military literature on blood transfusion, a 1:1:1 or 2:1:1 ratio should be maintained for each unit of packed cell transfused to that of FFP and platelets.[20] Other sources disagree on the exact ratio, citing a lack of specific survival benefit to a higher PRBC to FFP ratio.[35] Many large western centres have massive transfusion protocols that allow the rapid release of blood products in varying ratios. While the

survival benefit remains unclear, most of these protocols have PRBC:FFP:platelet ratios near 1:1:1. Where possible it is recommended to use a point of care testing like TEG® (Thromboelastography) or ROTEM® (Rotational Thromboelastography) to ensure judicious and optimal use of blood products.[29]

Remember that the transfusion will have metabolic complications such as depletion of intravascular cations due to chelation by the sodium citrate used to anticoagulate blood components during storage. Citrate is primarily metabolized by the liver, so in cirrhotic patients receiving massive transfusion, this effect may be more profound. Consider giving calcium replacement (calcium gluconate 1–2 g IV or calcium chloride 0.5–1 g IV per 500 ml of transfused blood).[36,37]

Drug-induced GI bleeding is more commonly seen with the use of oral anti-coagulation drugs than with any other category of pharmacological agents. The newer oral anti-coagulants are also known to predispose to GI bleeding.[38] The problem is further accentuated in renal failure where the qualitative action of platelets is affected. These agents should be used with caution in GI bleed patients and even stopped when the risk of their administration outweighs the benefits.[38] Such scenarios should be handled with the involvement of sub-speciality teams and through the use of local protocols such as the use of haematology and blood bank services to aid reversal of anticoagulation and achieve source control in a timely fashion.

Endoscopy and Source Control

Upper GI Endoscopy

Upper GI endoscopy should be performed as soon as the patient is clinically stable and can be done even during blood transfusion. If the INR is >3, endoscopy should be deferred until the coagulation profile normalizes. This would require the use of FFP and administration of vitamin K and sub-speciality discussion with haematology.

Evidence of peptic ulcer disease should prompt the use of a PPI whilst in cases of liver cirrhosis or variceal bleeding, terlipressin infusion should be commenced.[39]

The risk of re-bleeding is maximal in patients with active bleeding, a visualized ulcer at the base, an adherent clot and an ulcer greater than 2 cm in size. Endoscopic interventions such as cautery, injection, or clipping are effective in achieving haemostasis. Early endoscopy has shown to improve outcome and reduce both length of stay and rate of re-bleed. Delay in endoscopy of suspected patients increases the risk of re-bleed, surgery, and also increases the length of stay in both the intensive care and hospital.[39]

Nasogastric lavage remains controversial and is not routinely recommended due to poor yield and risk of aspiration.[40] Computed tomography (CT) angiography and radionuclide scans can also be used for diagnostic purposes but are actually useful only in cases with active bleeding. High-risk patients should be given a proton pump infusion for at least 3 days after the procedure to prevent any further bleeding.[39,40]

Lower GI Endoscopy

For the diagnosis of lower GI bleeding, colonoscopy has a higher sensitivity of near 90% compared to angiography which is about 40% sensitive to diagnose active bleeding. Also, colonoscopy helps in achieving haemostasis in more number of cases and is shown to reduce the length of stay.[9]

For more occult bleeds and diagnostic failures, more complex options are available like barium contrast with small bowel follow-through, Meckel's scan, technetium-99 scan, and capsule enteroscopy.[3] Nuclear studies like technetium-99 scan are useful for cases which have a slow bleeding rate of 0.1–0.4 ml/min. For bleeding rates more than 0.5 L/min and for actively bleeding cases, angiography has a better diagnostic yield. Although it helps in immediate treatment via embolization, the sensitivity is poor compared to colonoscopy and it also introduces the risk of contrast-induced nephropathy.[41]

Capsule endoscopy is reserved for small bowel lesions which are beyond the ligament of Treitz.[3] The advantages of capsule endoscopy include higher sensitivity and a pain-free and non-invasive procedure. However, there is no option of taking a biopsy if required. Surgical exploratory laparotomy is the last option for cases with ongoing haemorrhage, clinical instability, or negative diagnostic yield.[3]

Special Measures for Variceal Bleeding

In patients with variceal bleeding or liver cirrhosis, prompt terlipressin infusion should be used.[14,29] Terlipressin is the recommended drug in variceal bleeding with a bolus of 2 mg followed by 1 mg every 6 hours until definitive treatment or 5 days. Combined pharmacotherapy and endoscopic management yields the best results. Prophylactic antibiotic therapy should be used at presentation for patients with suspected or confirmed variceal bleeding.

For oesophageal varices, band ligation with rubber rings helps control bleeding in patients who are sensitive to beta-blockade, but the portal pressures are not affected. Transjugular intrahepatic portosystemic shunting (TIPS) when initiated in the first three days improves the 2-year survival in portal hypertension reduces the rate of re-bleeding, and also reduces the risk of hepatic encephalopathy. Balloon tamponade carries the risk of oesophageal injury and is reserved for haemostasis only in patients with massive bleeding.

Endoscopic injection of varices with N-butyl-2-cyanoacrylate is also used failing which TIPS is then recommended. Complete liver transplantation remains the definitive treatment for recurrent variceal bleeding in liver cirrhosis.[41]

Role of Prophylaxis

A majority of critically ill patients will develop stress-related mucosal disorder (SRMD) or ulcerative disorder in the first few days of ICU admission due to ischaemia and increased acid production. Key prophylaxis is to start drugs that decrease gastric acid production like histamine 2 (H2) antagonists or PPIs. Studies combining early enteral feeding and H2 antagonists have shown lower upper GI bleeding rates in patients who are mechanically ventilated.[42] Stress ulcers can be prevented if the gastric pH (acidity level) is kept >4, but to prevent bleeding or re-bleeding, the pH must be kept >6. This can be achieved with both H2 antagonists as well as PPIs but the latter are more commonly used.[20] According to some case reports, H2 antagonists may cause encephalopathy, interact with anticonvulsant drugs, and increase the rates of nosocomial pneumonia, but its causation is not proved and remains controversial.[43]

Overall, clinically significant GI bleeding is rare in critically ill patients and thus stress ulcer prophylaxis should be initiated only if the patient has specific risk factors such as coagulopathy or mechanical ventilation.[20]

CONCLUSIONS

Most of the published data on gastrointestinal bleeding in critical care is based on heterogeneous patient groups in general critical care and very limited number of studies currently exist specific to gastrointestinal bleeding in neuro-critical care patients. However still, the overall risk of gastrointestinal bleeding has considerably reduced over the years in critical care patients, especially due to the prophylactic use of stress ulcer prophylaxis. This holds true for neuro-critical care patients as well

Short summary of NICE guideline CG:141 on management of acute upper gastrointestinal bleeding[29]

- A Blatchford Score should be done before endoscopy. If the score is zero, then discharge could be considered.
- The timing of Rockall score should be after endoscopy. This helps in planning post endoscopy management and logistical disposal.
- Patients who have massive haemorrhage should be transfused as per local guidelines. Care should be taken to avoid both surplus and under-transfusion.
- Platelets should only be given if the count is below 50,000.
- Fresh frozen plasma to be transfused if INR >1.5 and cryoprecipitate if the fibrinogen is <1 g/L.
- For patients on Coumarin derivatives like warfarin, Prothrombin Complex Concentrate (PCC) can be considered.
- Factor VIIa should be reserved as a tool of last resort.
- Endoscopy can be done for acute haemorrhages immediately post resuscitation or as soon as deemed stable.
- There is no role of PPI in non-variceal bleed unless an ulcer (or evidence of recent bleed) is demonstrated on endoscopy.
- Embolization of the offending vessels in the Interventional Suite is also extremely helpful for all re-bleeds and failed endoscopic management. TIPS should also be considered for such cases.
- Terlipressin is recommended for at least 5 days in variceal bleeding.
- All variceal bleeding patients should receive prophylactic antibiotics according to local protocols.

who could be at a higher risk than other general critical care patients which could be due to the increased stress response seen in patients with severe neurological diseases like traumatic brain injury, subarachnoid haemorrhage, intracerebral haemorrhage, etc.[44,45] Amongst these, acute thrombotic stroke predisposes an extra risk due to the presence or commencement of anti-platelet or anticoagulant medications.[46] Despite these evolving differences, the diagnostic and management principles of gastrointestinal bleeding in neuro-critical care remain the same and are based on prompt diagnosis, aggressive resuscitation, and multi-speciality treatment. Targeted prophylaxis for specific

risk factors should help in preventing significant GI bleeds and every unit should have a tailored approach to manage such cases.

REFERENCES

1. Cook DJ, Griffith LE, Walter SD, et al. The attributable mortality and length of intensive care unit stay of clinically important gastrointestinal bleeding in critically ill patients. *Crit Care* 2001;5:368–75.
2. Beejay U, Wolfe MM. Acute gastrointestinal bleeding in the intensive care unit. The gastroenterologist's perspective. *Gastroenterol Clin North Am* 2000;29:309–36.
3. Manning-Dimmitt LL, Dimmitt SG, Wilson GR. Diagnosis of gastrointestinal bleeding in adults. *Am Fam Physician* 2005;71:1339–46.
4. Cook DJ, Witt LG, Cook RJ, Guyatt GH. Stress ulcer prophylaxis in the critically ill: a meta-analysis. *Am J Med* 1991;91:519–27.
5. Cook DJ, Fuller HD, Guyatt GH, et al. Risk factors for gastrointestinal bleeding in critically ill patients. *N Engl J Med* 1994;330:377–81.
6. Cushing H. Peptic ulcer and the interbrain. *Surg Obst* 1932;55:1–34.
7. Czaja AJ, McAlhany JC, Pruitt BA, Jr. Acute gastroduodenal disease after thermal injury. An endoscopic evaluation of incidence and natural history. *N Engl J Med* 1974;291:925–9.
8. Lucas CE, Sugawa C, Riddle J, et al. Natural history and surgical dilemma of 'stress' gastric bleeding. *Arch Surg* 1971;102:266–73.
9. Stollman N, Metz DC. Pathophysiology and prophylaxis of stress ulcer in intensive care unit patients. *J Crit Care* 2005 Mar;20(1):35–45.
10. Imdahl A. Genesis and pathophysiology of lower gastrointestinal bleeding. *Langenbecks Arch Surg* 2001;386:1–7.
11. Norton L, Greer J, Eiseman B. Gastric secretory response to head injury. *Arch Surg* 1970;101(2):200–4.
12. Watts CC, Clark K. Gastric acidity in the comatose patient. *J Neurosurg* 1969;30(2):107–9.
13. Gutthann SP, Garcia Rodriguez LA, Raiford DS. Individual nonsteroidal antiinflammatory drugs and other risk factors for upper gastrointestinal bleeding and perforation. *Epidemiology* 1997;8:18–24.
14. Bhatt DL, Scheiman J, Abraham NS, et al. ACCF/ACG/AHA 2008 expert consensus document on reducing the gastrointestinal risks of antiplatelet therapy and NSAID use: a report of the American College of Cardiology Foundation Task Force on Clinical Expert Consensus Documents. *J Am Coll Cardiol* 2008;52:1502–17.
15. Pitchumoni CS, Brun A. *Geriatric Gastroenterology.* Springer, New York; 2012.
16. Pimentel M, Roberts DE, Bernstein CN, Hoppensack M, Duerksen DR. Clinically significant gastrointestinal bleeding

in critically ill patients in an era of prophylaxis. *Am J Gastroenterology* 2000;95:2801–6.

17. Ellison RT, Perez-Perez G, Welsh CH, et al. Risk factors for upper gastrointestinal bleeding in intensive care unit patients: role of helicobacter pylori. Federal Hyperimmune Immunoglobulin Therapy Study Group. *Crit Care Med* 1996;24:1974–81.

18. Guerrant RL, Van Gilder T, Steiner TS, et al. Practice guidelines for the management of infectious diarrhea. *Clin Infect Dis* 2001;32:331–51.

19. Schuetz A, Jauch KW. Lower gastrointestinal bleeding: therapeutic strategies, surgical techniques and results. *Langenbecks Arch Surg* 2001;386:17–25.

20. Cook D, Heyland D, Griffith L, et al. Risk factors for clinically important upper gastrointestinal bleeding in patients requiring mechanical ventilation. Canadian Critical Care Trials Group. *Crit Care Med* 1999;27:2812–17.

21. Ashkenazi E, Kovalev Y, Zuckerman E. Evaluation and treatment of esophageal varices in the cirrhotic patient. *Isr Med Assoc J* 2013;15:109–15.

22. Tacke F, Fiedler K, Trautwein C. A simple clinical score predicts high risk for upper gastrointestinal hemorrhages from varices in patients with chronic liver disease. *Scand J Gastroenterol* 2007;42:374–82.

23. Sharara AI, Rockey DC. Gastroesophageal variceal hemorrhage. *N Engl J Med* 2001;345:669–81.

24. Grace ND, Groszmann RJ, Garcia-Tsao G, et al. Portal hypertension and variceal bleeding: an AASLD single topic symposium. *Hepatology* 1998;28:868–80.

25. Bosch J, Abraldes JG, Groszmann R. Current management of portal hypertension. *J Hepatol* 2003;38(Suppl 1):S54–S68.

26. De Franchis R, Primignani M. Natural history of portal hypertension in patients with cirrhosis. *Clin Liver Dis* 2001;5:645–63.

27. Vorobioff J, Groszmann RJ, Picabea E, et al. Prognostic value of hepatic venous pressure gradient measurements in alcoholic cirrhosis: a 10-year prospective study. *Gastroenterology* 1996;111:701–9.

28. Ahmed Mahmoud El-Tawil. Trends on gastrointestinal bleeding and mortality: Where are we standing? *World J Gastroenterol* 2012 Mar 21;18(11):1154–8.

29. NICE Guidelines. Acute upper gastrointestinal bleeding in over 16s: management. [cited 2016 Aug] Available from: http://guidance.nice.org.uk/CG141/NICEGuidance/pdf/English (Guideline).

30. Scottish Intercollegiate Guidelines Network (SIGN). Management of acute upper and lower gastrointestinal bleeding. A national clinical guideline. Edinburgh (Scotland): Scottish Intercollegiate Guidelines Network (SIGN); 2008 Sep. (SIGN publication; no. 105). (Guideline)

31. Edelman DA, Sugawa C. Lower gastrointestinal bleeding: a review. *Surg Endosc* 2007;21:514–20.

32. Conrad SA. Acute upper gastrointestinal bleeding in critically ill patients: causes and treatment modalities. *Crit Care Med* 2002;30:S365–8.

33. Retter A, Wyncoll D, Pearse R, et al. British Committee for Standards in Haematology. Guidelines on the management of anaemia and red cell transfusion in adult critically ill patients. *Br J Haematol* 2013;160: 445–64. doi:10.1111/bjh.12143.

34. Hubert PC, Wells G, Blajchman MA, et al. A multicenter, randomized, controlled clinical trial of transfusion requirements in critical care. Transfusion Requirements in critical care investigators, Canadian Critical Care Trials Group. *N Engl J Med* 1999;340:409–17.

35. Villanueva C1, Colomo A, Bosch A, et al. Transfusion strategies for acute upper gastrointestinal bleeding. *N Engl J Med* 2013;368:11–21.

36. Hunt BJ, Allard S, Keeling D, Norfolk D, Stanworth SJ, Pendry K. The British Committee for Standards in Haematology. A practical guideline for the haematological management of major haemorrhage. *Br J Haematol* 2015;170:788–803. doi:10.1111/bjh.13580.

37. Kollef MH, O'Brien JD, Zuckerman GR, Shannon W. BLEED: a classification tool to predict outcomes in patients with acute upper and lower gastrointestinal hemorrhage. *Crit Care Med* 1997;25:1125–32.

38. Lanas A, Bajador E, Serrano P, et al. Nitrovasodilators, low-dose aspirin, other nonsteroidal antiinflammatory drugs, and the risk of upper gastrointestinal bleeding. *N Engl J Med* 2007;343:834–9.

39. Hwang JH, Fisher DA, Ben-Menachem T, et al. The role of endoscopy in the management of acute non-variceal upper GI bleeding. *Gastrointest Endosc* 2012;75:1132–8.

40. Cuellar RE, Gavaler JS, Alexander JA, et al. Gastrointestinal tract hemorrhage. The value of a nasogastric aspirate. *Arch Intern Med* 1990;150:1381–4.

41. Tacke F, Fiedler K, Trautwein C. A simple clinical score predicts high risk for upper gastrointestinal hemorrhages from varices in patients with chronic liver disease. *Scand J Gastroenterol* 2007;42:374–82.

42. Fennerty MB. Pathophysiology of the upper gastrointestinal tract in the critically ill patient: rationale for the therapeutic benefits of acid suppression. *Crit Care Med* 2002;30:S351–55.

43. Schirmer CM, Kornbluth J, Heilman CB, Bhardwaj Anish. Gastrointestinal prophylaxis in neurocritical care. *Neurocritical Care* 2012;16:184. doi:10.1007/s12028-011-9580-1.

44. Liu B, Liu S, Yin A, Siddiqi J. Risks and benefits of stress ulcer prophylaxis in adult neurocritical care patients: a systematic review and meta-analysis of randomized controlled trials. *Critical Care* 2015;19:409. doi:10.1186/s13054-015-1107-2.

45. Yang, Tie-Cheng Shi, Hong-Mei, et al. Gastrointestinal bleeding after intracerebral hemorrhage: a retrospective review of 808 cases. *Am J Med Sci* 2013;346(4):279–82.

46. Ogata T, Kamouchi M, Matsuo R, et al. Gastrointestinal bleeding in acute ischemic stroke: recent trends from the fukuoka stroke registry. *Cerebrovascular Diseases Extra* 2014;4(2):156–64. doi:10.1159/000365245.

47

Gastrointestinal Dysfunction and Ileus in Neurointensive Care

V. P. Nair

ABSTRACT

Gastrointestinal dysfunction in the intensive care has not taken priority in the myriad of problems an intensive care patient faces, though it contributes a great deal to morbidity and mortality. It ranges from being a mild self-limiting condition to ileus, bowel ischaemia, abdominal compartment syndrome, and other life-threatening conditions. The prevalence is higher in neuro-intensive care patients owing to the incident cause, as well as the longer duration of mechanical ventilation and sedation. There should be a dedicated dietician team and protocol management of enteral nutrition and bowel care in all units. The principal aim should be the prevention of gastric dysfunction and its early diagnosis and management.

KEYWORDS

Gastrointestinal dysfunction; ileus; Ogilvie's syndrome; intra-abdominal pressure (IAP); abdominal compartment syndrome.

INTRODUCTION

The development of gastric motility disturbances in critical care contributes to the failure to wean, prolongs the number of ventilation days, and increases intensive care as well as hospital bed days. The incidence of gastric dysfunction in general intensive care varies from 50% to 83%.[1,2] The incidence in neurointensive care is bound to be higher if one considers the predisposing factors for ileus—trauma, sedation, and prolonged mechanical ventilation—in combination with traumatic brain injury (TBI).

There is a lack of consensus in defining gastric dysfunction and failure in the intensive care. In 2012, the Working Group on Abdominal Problems (WGAP) of the European Society of Intensive Care Medicine (ESICM) made recommendations for the terminology, definitions, and management of gastrointestinal function in intensive care patients.[3] It defined gastric dysfunction occurring in critical care as 'acute gastric injury' (AGI) and described four grades.

Grade I is a self-limiting transient condition such as postoperative nausea and vomiting or decreased bowel motility following shock. Judicious fluid management, enteral feeding, and limiting the use of drugs slowing gastric motility helps limit the condition.

Grade II is when the patient develops actual gastric dysfunction and is not able to digest or absorb nutrients and fluids adequately. Gastroparesis with high residue and intra-abdominal pressures (IAP) of 12–15 mmHg (classified as Grade I intra-abdominal hypertension [IAH]) come under this category. The aim would be to prevent progression of this condition to grade III, by attempts to reverse the gastroparesis with prokinetics and persisting with enteral feeds at a lower rate.

Grade III is when the above measures have failed and the patient is in GI failure. Despite treatment, feeding intolerance persists with high gastric residue and worsening bowel dilatation. The IAH progresses to Grade II – IAP of 16–20 mmHg. Parenteral nutrition might have to be commenced along with regular enteral feed challenges. IAP should be monitored and drugs that affect GI motility adversely should be stopped or minimized.

Grade IV is when the GI failure has progressed to cause multi-organ failure and is fast becoming a life-threatening condition. Bowel ischaemia, abdominal compartment syndrome, and other similar conditions need immediate interventions and laparotomy may be required as a life-saving measure.

The WGAP also divides AGI into primary and secondary where the former is due to a primary pathology and the latter is the response to a critical illness in the absence of a primary bowel pathology.

The WGAP defines ileus as the inability of the bowel to pass stool due to impaired peristalsis—AGI Grade III. It is the non-mechanical inhibition of gastrointestinal motility that can cause arrest of intestinal peristalsis. There is obstruction and sequestration of the bowel contents.

PATHOPHYSIOLOGY

Normal gastrointestinal motility is controlled by the enteric neuronal system and the autonomic system. The enteric neuronal system consists of the myenteric (Auerbach's) plexus which regulates gut motility and the submucosal (Meissner's) plexus that regulates mucosal processes including mucus secretion, fluid and electrolyte secretions, blood flow, and neuroimmune reactions.[4,5] Excitatory motor neurons secrete acetylcholine and substance P while the inhibitory motor neurons secrete nitric oxide, vasoactive intestinal peptide, and adenosine triphosphate. Overactivity of the inhibitory neurons or suppression of the excitatory neurons leads to dysmotility and intestinal palsy. The autonomic nervous system has a role as well, with the sympathetic system being inhibitory and the parasympathetic system being excitatory.

The GI motility wave begins with peristalsis in the oesophagus as food is swallowed. Motility in the stomach and small intestine is divided into two patterns—an interdigestive pattern and a digestive pattern. The interdigestive pattern begins a couple of hours after a meal. It has three phases repeated every two hours. The first is a quiet phase followed by irregular contractions and then a regular forward propulsive force. When a meal is ingested this pattern is replaced by an accommodative phase which is then followed by stationary contractions. This digestive phase aids in adequate mixing of the food with gastrointestinal secretions and absorption of nutrients through the luminal walls. The next phase is propulsive peristalsis that pushes the contents forward.

This normal pattern that accounts for digestion and absorption of nutrients can be disrupted by a wide range of factors. In critical care, especially in neurointensive care, the factors are multiple. The initial insult which caused the patient to be in critical care, electrolyte and fluid imbalances, drugs administered such as catecholamines, sedatives and opiates, mechanical ventilation, sepsis, and any pre-existing patient comorbidities all contribute to this disruption. The incidence of feeding intolerance (more than 1000 ml/day gastric residual volume [GRV]) in the TBI patient is high and persists for a few weeks after the initial injury.[6,7] The actual mechanism here is not well understood. Motility abnormalities, mucosal ulceration and inflammation, and increased bowel wall permeability have been observed. One theory postulated is that TBI decreases the activity of intestinal tight junction proteins, thus increasing intestinal permeability and bacterial translocation. This also contributes to sepsis and multi-organ dysfunction[8] which in turn aggravates gastrointestinal dysfunction.

The incidence of gastric dysfunction in spinal cord injury (SCI) patients is higher than in the other critical care patients, with the highest rates being in upper SCI. In the acute stage, the patient goes into a state of spinal shock with loss of all autonomic and reflex activities. This can last for up to several weeks after the initial injury. Acute gastric dilatation and ileus occurs, which in most cases resolves within the first week. Early enteral nutrition should be established ideally within 24 to 48 hours of the injury.[9]

The incidence of ileus in the intensive care can be up to 50%–80%[10] and in neurocritical care this will be towards the higher end. The main factors leading to ileus is the critical illness itself, with sepsis, mechanical ventilation, and renal failure all contributing. The various drugs used including catecholamines, narcotics, and anticholinergics play an important role. Another causative factor is metabolic derangements such as electrolyte imbalances—hypokalaemia, hypomagnesaemia, acidosis, hypoxaemia, and fluid imbalances. Inflammatory causes include sepsis and peritonitis. Ileus might also be a part of generalized multi-organ dysfunction.[5]

In neurocritical care, the increased use of catecholamines to maintain adequate cerebral perfusion pressures, the longer duration of sedation and mechanical ventilation, and the inflammatory response to TBI increases the incidence of gastrointestinal dysfunction and makes it a very difficult condition to treat. Spinal cord injury would also be a significant contributing factor. As ileus progresses, intestinal dilatation occurs leading to abdominal distension, IAP, delayed gastric emptying, increased GRV, and increased risk of aspiration. The worrying point at this stage is the development of acute colonic pseudo-obstruction (ACPO) also termed Ogilvie's syndrome—acute dilatation of the colon in the absence of an anatomic lesion that obstructs the flow of intestinal contents.[11]

Signs and symptoms of gastric dysfunction are difficult to detect and elicit. Increasing GRV and feeding intolerance may be the first sign of impaired peristalsis. In critical care patients, the incidence of delayed gastric emptying and high GRV has been reported to vary from 5% to 30%.[12] High GRV is defined as volumes between 150 ml to 500 ml in various studies, however, the study protocols differ in how frequently residual volume is checked and whether it is discarded or replaced. Raising the definition of high GRV to 500 ml has not been found to increase the rate of complications such as pulmonary aspiration and ileus.[13]

High GRV is not in itself an indication to stop enteral feeding but a warning sign of impending ileus. In most cases this improves with enteral feeding and prokinetics. Critical care units should have formal enteral feeding regimens. The protocol followed in our unit is shown in the form of an algorithm in Figure 47.1. The feeding protocol is to measure GRV every four hours and if higher than 350 ml, twice consecutively to commence metoclopramide intravenously. If it persists after another 4 hours, erythromycin is added. Aspirates up to 250 ml are replaced and the rest discarded. If the aspirates persist at these high volumes, it is clinically co-related with other symptoms and signs and abdominal girth and IAP are monitored. Careful attention is paid to the history in the past 48 hours including hypovolaemia, fluid balance, vomiting, absent or abnormal bowel sounds, and other warning signs.

Abdominal distension is an important red flag to monitor for, as ileus develops. Increasing abdominal girth might be due to oedema, ascites, ileus, or haemorrhage. Abdominal girth should be measured at the same site, usually at the level of the umbilicus—once daily or more if concerned. Bowel sounds and bowel movements might be absent. It is essential that critical care units have a protocol for monitoring bowel function (Figure 47.2) and take early remedial action. The incidence of constipation in the intensive care can be as high as 83%.[2] It delays progress of the patient, prolongs mechanical ventilation, and hospital and critical care stay. It also hides ACPO or Ogilvie's syndrome.

Ogilvie's syndrome develops due to disruption of the autonomic nervous system leading to suppression of the parasympathetic system and over-activity of the sympathetic system. This leads to impaired colonic motility and accumulation of contents and gas leading to colonic dilatation. Mechanoreceptors on the wall of the colon are activated by the distension and they in turn activate the colo-colonic reflex that further inhibits colonic motility.[11] The colonic wall is stretched compromising blood supply and this vascular insufficiency leads on to colonic ischaemia.

Intra-abdominal pressures start increasing and this is multifactorial in origin. Gastroparesis, ileus, and ACPO as well as capillary leak increase the intraluminal and extraluminal content. Diminished abdominal wall compliance also plays a role. IAP should be monitored in any patient in whom ileus is suspected to progress or not resolve within 24 hours. Normal IAP level is 5–7 mmHg. It is affected by the volume of visceral contents, visceral oedema, pathological collections of fluid-pus, blood, ascites, compliance of the abdominal wall, and mechanical ventilation. Intra-abdominal hypertension is defined as IAP more than 12 mmHg confirmed by at least two readings 6 hours apart.[14,3] It is graded from 1–4 (Table 47.1).

Intra-abdominal pressure is measured transvesically via the urinary catheter. The catheter is connected to a pressure transducer through a three-way tap. Purpose-built devices using the same principle are available as well. The zero point is the iliac crest at the mid axillary line and it should be measured with the patient supine (IAP increases by 2 mmHg for every 20-degree head-up tilt) and at end expiration.[14] Regular measurements are taken at 4–6-hour intervals and treatment plans adjusted accordingly. Intra-abdominal perfusion pressure is calculated from the mean arterial pressure (MAP) and IAP. This mean arterial pressure should be higher than 60 mmHg to maintain organ function. It has been shown to be a better marker of resuscitation efficacy than others commonly used such as arterial pH, base deficit, and urine output.[15]

If ileus and distension progress, IAH increases, and vascular compromise and ischaemia results leading to abdominal compartment syndrome. This can be life-threatening and requires immediate intervention.

Table 47.1 Grading of intra-abdominal hypertension

Grade	Pressure in mmHg
I	12–15 mmHg
II	16–20 mmHg
III	21–25 mmHg
IV	>25 mmHg

INVESTIGATIONS

Blood tests such as full blood count, renal function, and liver function tests help diagnose developing gastrointestinal failure. Worsening acidosis and increasing serum lactate levels are red flags denoting a worsening condition. This combined with increasing residual gastric volumes, absent bowel sounds, abdominal distension, abdominal hypertension, and decreasing urine output warrant urgent surgical referral.

Plain X-ray of abdomen can show gas under the diaphragm as well as fluid levels, abnormal distribution of gas, calibre of the bowel wall, and distension and displacement of the bowel. In paralytic ileus, fluid and gas accumulates showing multiple fluid levels and dilatation of both small and large bowel (3–5 cm and >5 cm, respectively). Computed tomography (CT) of the abdomen with either oral or intravenous iodinated contrast provides a definitive diagnosis. Perforation, obstruction, and colonic ischaemia are diagnosed with a high level of sensitivity and specificity. Findings from CT scan in colonic ischaemia can be classified as wet, dry, and pneumatosis coli. It is described as wet when there is loss of colonic haustra with pericolic streakiness, correlating to reperfusion injury of the ischaemic bowel and dry when there is mild mural thickening with minimal pericolic streakiness denoting progression of ischaemic damage without reperfusion. The third group is pneumatosis coli or air in the colonic wall and portomesenteric venous gas which denotes colonic necrosis and impending death if not treated immediately.[16]

MANAGEMENT

Prevention of the condition is the main objective. Protocolized management of enteral nutrition and bowel management (Figure 47.2) should be the standard in all critical care units. The services of a dedicated dietician team are essential. Regular review of patients with all the above in place and a high index of suspicion for gastric dysfunction aids in detecting and preventing its further progression.

In neurocritical care, the use of catecholamines tend to be higher as we aim for higher mean arterial pressures to maintain cerebral perfusion pressures of at least 60 mmHg. Earlier use of cardiac output monitors to optimise the use of inotropes might help avoid invariable mesenteric vasoconstriction and colonic ischaemia that inotropes can cause. There is no evidence that renal and hepato-splanchnic blood flows are compromised in patients treated with noradrenaline.[17] It may actually improve microvascular flow and oxygenation. Dopamine, noradrenaline, and adrenaline all affect splanchnic blood flows in a similar fashion in moderate septic shock. In severe septic shock, adrenaline reduces the splanchnic blood flow compared to noradrenaline. The evidence for dopexamine improving splanchnic flow is equivocal and may only occur in some patient groups.[18] Dobutamine is equally effective as dopexamine in maintaining splanchnic blood flow.

Monitoring fluid balance daily to avoid over-hydration as well as dehydration aids in minimising ileus. Sedation requirements should be evaluated daily, opiates should be tailored off as required. Bowel movements should be monitored and constipation avoided.

Once gastric dysfunction and ileus are suspected, abdominal girth and intra-abdominal pressures should be measured at least once in 6 hours. Early surgical referral, radiological confirmation of diagnosis, and definitive treatment should be started. Parenteral nutrition might be required in the short term but must be reviewed daily and enteral nutrition should be restarted as soon as possible.

Medical management with neostigmine is recommended only if all mechanical factors are excluded. Continuous infusion of neostigmine 0.4–0.8 mg/hr promotes defecation in critical care patients with colonic ileus without significant adverse effects.[19–21] There are case reports of intravenous lignocaine infusions being used in resolving ACPO in SCI patients.[22]

Decompression of the distended bowel using a flatus tube might help. Surgical decompression by laparotomy improves mortality in patients at imminent risk of perforation, colonic necrosis, and abdominal compartment syndrome. The abdomen is left open—a plastic membrane is stitched to the wound edges thus increasing intra-abdominal space. Intra-abdominal pressures should be monitored daily and closure considered after five days.

CONCLUSIONS

Prevention of gastric dysfunction and early diagnosis and management should be one of the mainstays of intensive care management. The mnemonic—FAST HUG (feeding, analgesia, sedation, thromboembolic prophylaxis, head of bed elevation, ulcer prophylaxis, and glycaemic control)—was suggested by Jean-Louis Vincent, to help in daily reviews of critical care patients.[23] To this Moses Chikungwa[24] suggested adding FAITH—fluid balance, aperients, investigations and results, therapies, and hydration status. This is of particular significance in limiting gastric dysfunction and the acute abdomen in the patient in neurocritical care.

REFERENCES

1. Fruhwald S, Kainz J. Effect of ICU interventions on gastrointestinal motility. *Current Opinion in Critical Care* 2010 Apr 1;16(2):159–64.

2. Mostafa SM, Bhandari S, Ritchie G, Gratton N, Wenstone R. Constipation and its implications in the critically ill patient. *British Journal of Anaesthesia* 2003 Dec 1;91(6): 815–9.

3. Blaser AR, Malbrain ML, Starkopf J, et al. Gastrointestinal function in intensive care patients: terminology, definitions and management. Recommendations of the ESICM Working Group on Abdominal Problems. *Intensive Care Medicine* 2012 Mar 1;38(3):384–94.

4. Fruhwald S, Holzer P, Metzler H. Intestinal motility disturbances in intensive care patients pathogenesis and clinical impact. *Intensive Care Medicine* 2007 Jan 1;33(1): 36–44.

5. Aderinto-Adike AO, Quigley EM. Gastrointestinal motility problems in critical care: a clinical perspective. *Journal of Digestive Diseases* 2014 Jul 1;15(7):335–44.

6. Krakau K, Omne-Pontén M, Karlsson T, Borg J. Metabolism and nutrition in patients with moderate and severe traumatic brain injury: a systematic review. *Brain Injury* 2006 Jan 1;20(4):345–67.

7. Tan M, Zhu JC, Yin HH. Enteral nutrition in patients with severe traumatic brain injury: reasons for intolerance and medical management. *British Journal of Neurosurgery* 2011 Feb 1;25(1):2–8.

8. Olsen AB, Hetz RA, Xue H, et al. Effects of traumatic brain injury on intestinal contractility. *Neurogastroenterology and Motility* 2013 Jul 1;25(7):593–e463.

9. Wing PC. Early acute management in adults with spinal cord injury: a clinical practice guideline for health-care providers. Who should read it? *The Journal of Spinal Cord Medicine* 2008 Jan 1;31(4):360.

10. Caddell KA, Martindale R, McClave SA, Miller K. Can the intestinal dysmotility of critical illness be differentiated from postoperative ileus? *Current Gastroenterology Reports* 2011 Aug 1;13(4):358–67.

11. Saunders MD, Kimmey MB. Systematic review: Acute colonic pseudo-obstruction. *Alimentary Pharmacology and Therapeutics* 2005;22:917–25.

12. Blaser AR, Starkopf J, Malbrain ML. Abdominal signs and symptoms in intensive care patients. *Anaesthesiology Intensive Therapy* 2015;47(4):379–87.

13. Montejo JC, Minambres E, Bordeje L, et al. Gastric residual volume during enteral nutrition in ICU patients: the REGANE study. *Intensive Care Medicine* 2010 Aug 1;36(8):1386–93.

14. Berry N, Fletcher S. Abdominal compartment syndrome. Continuing education in anaesthesia. *Critical Care and Pain* 2012 Mar 8:mks006.

15. Cheatham ML, White MW, Sagraves SG, Johnson JL, Block EF. Abdominal perfusion pressure: a superior parameter in the assessment of intra-abdominal hypertension. *Journal of Trauma and Acute Care Surgery* 2000 Oct 1;49(4): 621–7.

16. Stoker J, van Randen A, Laméris W, Boermeester MA. Imaging patients with acute abdominal pain. *Radiology* 2009 Oct;253(1):31–46.

17. Reinelt H, Radermacher P, Fischer G, et al. Effects of a dobutamine-induced increase in splanchnic blood flow on hepatic metabolic activity in patients with septic shock. *The Journal of the American Society of Anesthesiologists* 1997 Apr 1;86(4):818–24.

18. Renton MC, Snowden CP. Dopexamine and its role in the protection of hepatosplanchnic and renal perfusion in high-risk surgical and critically ill patients. *British Journal of Anaesthesia* 2005 Apr 1;94(4):459–67.

19. Abeyta BJ, Albrecht RM, Schermer CR, Senagore AJ, Linz D. Retrospective study of neostigmine for the treatment of acute colonic pseudo-obstruction/Discussion. *The American Surgeon* 2001 Mar 1;67(3):265.

20. Paran H, Silverberg D, Mayo A, Shwartz I, Neufeld D, Freund U. Treatment of acute colonic pseudo-obstruction with neostigmine. *Journal of the American College of Surgeons* 2000 Mar 31;190(3):315–18.

21. Valle RG, Godoy FL. Neostigmine for acute colonic pseudo-obstruction: a meta-analysis. *Annals of Medicine and Surgery* 2014 Sep 30;3(3):60–64.

22. Baumann A, Audibert G, Klein O, Mertes PM. Continuous intravenous lidocaine in the treatment of paralytic ileus due to severe spinal cord injury. *Acta Anaesthesiologica Scandinavica* 2009 Jan 1;53(1): 128–30.

23. Vincent JL. Give your patient a fast hug (at least) once a day. *Critical Care Medicine* 2005 Jun 1;33(6):1225–9.

24. Chikungwa M. Extend 'FAST HUG' with 'FAITH'. *Journal of the Intensive Care Society* 2010;11(1):69–70.

48

Nutritional Requirements in Neurocritical Care

V. Davies and S. Tripathy

ABSTRACT

Critical illness is associated with a profound hypermetabolic response that predisposes individuals to impaired macronutrient metabolism. An exaggerated systemic inflammatory response together with the catabolism of lean body mass can lead to significant nutritional losses which have been linked to poor patient outcomes. As a consequence, nutritional therapy has become an important treatment strategy in the neurointensive care unit (NICU) and has been the focus of much research during the last three decades.

The provision of nutritional support in the NICU is both highly complex and challenging. Methods for determining nutritional requirements in critically ill patients with neurological insult or injury remain hotly debated and continue to evolve. Appropriate energy, protein, and micronutrient replacement are key priorities with the route and timing of nutritional delivery being important considerations.

Swallowing difficulties are common amongst patients presenting with neurological injury and dysphagia has been observed in almost two-thirds of those who have required a prolonged period of mechanical ventilation. Adequate nutritional provision often relies on tolerance to artificial nutritional support in the form of enteral feeding, especially during the acute phase of illness where requirements for intensive sedation and respiratory support are increased. Parenteral nutrition is normally reserved for those who develop or present with a non-functioning or inaccessible gastrointestinal (GI) tract and therefore close monitoring of GI parameters is essential for optimising nutritional care.

The fundamental principles staying the same certain subgroups of patients in the ICU may have special nutritional requirements. Close monitoring for complications related to the type, route, and nature of the feed is important.

KEYWORDS

Nutrition; neurocritical care; caloric calculation; enteral feed; parenteral feed.

INTRODUCTION

After an initial and brief state of hypometabolism that is observed during resuscitation, critical illness is associated with a profound hypermetabolic response that is characterised by abnormal regulation of endocrine, nervous, and inflammatory systems to provide an adequate supply of substrates for cellular energy and repair.[1,2] Increased production of pro-inflammatory cytokines including tumour necrosis factor alpha (TNFα), interleukin-1β (IL-1β), and interleukin-6 (IL-6),[3,4] and increased circulation of counter-regulatory hormones such as cortisol, glucagon, and catecholamines are common metabolic adaptations. These disturbances may be further exaggerated in individuals with direct injury or insult to the brain, the major organ responsible for internal regulation and homoeostasis.[1]

Disruption of internal regulation predisposes critically ill patients to impaired macronutrient metabolism.

Combined influences, including an increased reliance on anaerobic glycolytic metabolism, impaired mitochondrial function, increased oxidative stress, and increased endogenous glucose production precipitate hyperglycaemia. Further, it has been hypothesised that increased lactate shuttling during gluconeogenesis, particularly following trauma to the brain, is an adaptive mechanism for glucose production to support nutritive needs, promoting lactate as an alternative substrate during 'energy crisis'.[5]

Catabolism, whether from injury or infection, is observed alongside an exaggerated systemic inflammatory response and is characterised by an increase in nitrogen excretion and consequent negative nitrogen balance.[6–8] Increased muscle proteolysis and resistance to anabolic signals leads to loss of lean body mass and impaired muscle function.[9] Alongside the increases in substrate metabolism, undernutrition, and weight loss are likely to be more profound in acute critical illness than in uncomplicated starvation.[10] During the last three decades nutrition therapy has evolved to become an important treatment strategy in the intensive care unit (ICU) for attenuating metabolic adaptations to stress, positively influencing immune responses, and maintaining homoeostasis.[11]

NUTRITIONAL SUPPORT

The provision of nutritional support in the NICU is both highly complex and challenging. Determination of optimal energy, protein and micronutrient requirements, and the timing and route of delivery remains hotly debated. Nutritional support is commonly used to treat pre-existing malnutrition and minimise the loss of lean body mass that is associated with a hypermetabolic state, and has the potential to improve patient outcomes including length of stay, functional outcomes, morbidity, and mortality.[12–14]

Unfortunately, many critically ill patients do not receive appropriate nutrition during their ICU stay. In a study of 213 mechanically ventilated patients only 25% received energy provision within 10% of their caloric goal.[15] More recently, a large prospective multicentre study involving 26 countries found that only 26% of critically ill patients received greater than 80% of their predicted energy target.[16] Whilst hypocaloric feeding has been proposed to be beneficial during the acute phase of illness,[17] increasing nutritional deficits have been linked to poor outcomes, particularly for underweight or obese individuals.[18,19] Those identified as being at high nutritional risk are most likely to benefit from nutritional intervention[20] and use of an appropriate nutritional

screening tool can be useful for directing nutritional therapy towards those in greatest need.[21] Improved assessment of nutritional requirements, determination of optimal nutritional replacement, and strategies to improve nutritional delivery are key priorities within the intensive care setting.

ENERGY EXPENDITURE

Estimates of total energy expenditure (TEE) incorporate five components; basal metabolic rate (BMR), degree of metabolic stress, physical activity, thermic effects of food intake, and growth.[22] In adult intensive care, the latter contributes negligible amounts and therefore will not be considered further here. However, the remaining four factors can be highly variable, with significant differences observed between individuals with similar diagnoses and clinical pathologies.[11] These parameters must be closely evaluated in order to form an appropriate assessment of energy expenditure that will facilitate optimal energy replacement.

Basal Metabolic Rate

Basal metabolic rate represents the energy required to maintain cell membrane processes (namely ionic gradients), molecular metabolism, and involuntary muscular contractions. Basal energy expenditure has been noted to change according to body size and composition as well as other factors including age, sex, and genetics.[22] Losses in fat-free mass over time are associated with an age-related decline in BMR, which may be accelerated or attenuated by hormonal shifts and routine physical activity, respectively.[23,24] Fatty acid profiles within cell membranes are also thought to affect basal energy expenditure as part of the 'membrane-pacemaker' theory where a higher concentration of polyunsaturated fatty acids is thought to be associated with increased metabolic activity.[22] To date, there is insufficient research to conclude that membrane profiles significantly influence metabolic rate in humans.

Resting Metabolic Rate

An estimate of resting metabolic rate (RMR) can be produced by adding the BMR to the energy expended as a result of metabolic stress. As previously noted, critical illness is often accompanied by a hypermetabolic response, the degree of which can vary dramatically between individuals. Hypermetabolism is defined as the ratio of measured (m) to predicted (p) RMR. An mRMR greater than 110%

of pRMR indicates a hypermetabolic state, with severe hypermetabolism defined as mRMR >130%.[6]

In patients with traumatic brain injury (TBI), the degree of hypermetabolism is believed to be proportional to the severity of injury[25] and mRMR has been observed to reach 116%–200% in patients without paralysis, barbiturate-induced coma or sedation.[26] However, the use of these treatments may blunt the metabolic effects of brain injury, with mRMR ranging from just 80%–123% when they are utilized.[8,26–29] Patients with haemorrhagic stroke have been found to have a similar mRMR to those with TBI that does not decrease with sedation, suggesting that those with non-traumatic head injuries may be at greater risk of nutritional depletion during a sustained and refractory hypermetabolic state.[30] Few studies have explored RMR in acute spinal cord injury (SCI); however, there is some agreement that the metabolic response in patients with SCI is reduced in comparison to those with TBI.[31,32] Larger studies are needed to confirm these observations.

Patients with paroxysmal sympathetic hyperactivity (PSH) following TBI may have nutritional requirements that exceed their estimated needs despite adjustment for injury.[33] PSH, also known as 'autonomic storming' refers to the impact TBI can have on the autonomic nervous system resulting in a hyper stress response that affects the regulation of digestion, perspiration, breathing, temperature, and heart rate.[34] Whilst the precise contribution that PSH makes to energy expenditure is currently unknown, early diagnosis is important in preventing long-term organ dysfunction which may facilitate closer approximation of energy expenditure.

THERMIC EFFECTS OF FOOD INTAKE

The energy cost of digestion and assimilation of nutrients is dependent on substrate type and mode of delivery that either inhibits or permits substrate shifts between pre- and post-prandial states.[35] Diet-induced thermogenesis (DIT) can approximate 10% in conscious patients but falls during sedation.[36] Due to impairment in sympathetic function and reductions in lean body mass following SCI, it is thought that thoracic injury at T6–7 may decrease the thermic response to food intake, potentially contributing to the lower TEE observed in these patients.[37] Continuous feeding that maintains an intraprandial state to meet maintenance requirements may preclude DIT, which has been observed to increase during overfeeding.[36] Therefore, dose and administration needs to be considered when assessing the thermic effects of nutritional support.

PHYSICAL ACTIVITY

Estimations of TEE need to be accounted for any physical activity performed. Weighing, repositioning, and chest physiotherapy have been found to increase metabolic rate by 36%, 31%, and 20%, respectively and are important considerations when assessing the critically ill patient.[38] Further, adjustments in oxygen support and weaning from mechanical ventilation can have a significant impact on energy expenditure. In non-sedated patients, physiological presentations associated with neurological conditions including dyskinesia and muscular rigidity may also make important contributions to energy expenditure.[39]

Shivering induced by therapeutic cooling in head injury patients has been associated with a hypermetabolic response.[40] However, in those who are sedated and paralysed, moderate reduction in body temperature is associated with a significant decrease in TEE.[41] Conversely, pyrexia may be associated with significant increases in energy expenditure and therefore, in addition to body size and minute ventilation, temperature is a significant contributory factor for energy expenditure and has been shown to account for much of the variation observed between clinical populations.[30]

MEASURING ENERGY EXPENDITURE

Several methods can be employed to determine energy expenditure in critically ill patients and include direct calorimetry, indirect calorimetry, bicarbonate dilution, doubly labelled water, and body composition analysis. Of these, indirect calorimetry (IC) is considered the gold standard method for use during the early phase of critical illness and has been used as the criterion measure in research studies.[11,42–45] However, there are a number of impracticalities and contraindications that restrict the routine use of IC within the clinical setting, including the cost of the equipment and the time required to conduct the assessment. In view of this, predictive equations are commonly used.

Predictive Equations

There are three methods of estimating energy requirements in critically ill patients. The first involves a simplistic calculation of kilocalories per kilogram of actual body weight, producing a reference range of 20–25 kcal/kg for the majority of patients during the acute phase, with just 11–14 kcal/kg recommended for obese individuals with a body mass index (BMI) 30–50 kg/m^2.[10,11,45,46] For patients with a BMI >50 kg/m^2, 22–25 kcal/kg of ideal body weight (IBW) is recommended.[11] The second method requires calculation of healthy BMR that is adjusted for metabolic stress according to diagnosis and severity of illness.[47] The third approach utilizes a regression equation that incorporates determinants of healthy BMR and clinical indicators of illness and metabolic stress, such as temperature and respiration. Despite the numerous equations available, few have been clinically validated against IC.[48]

A systematic review of the most commonly used predictive equations for critically ill patients concluded that the Penn State University (PSU) equation[43] had the highest degree of accuracy according to IC measurements reaching 79% for non-obese patients (BMI <30 kg/m^2) with an overall predictive accuracy of 71%.[17] Both simplistic weight-based equations (kcal/kg) and those incorporating stress factors have been deemed inappropriate for use in critically ill patients and pose greater risks of either under- or over-feeding.[49–51] However, the PSU can only be used in those patients who are receiving mechanical ventilation and there is little guidance as to which method should be employed during later stages of recovery.

To date, there are no predictive formulas available that are designed to specifically estimate energy expenditure following neurological injury or illness. Whilst previous validation data has included head injured patients, the PSU has not been tested in patients with SCI.[48] Use of IC over predictive equations to determine energy requirements for these individuals is recommended due to the individual variability in RMR.[32,52] It is hoped that future technological advances will permit more routine use of IC devices to enable individualized patient care

and improve treatment outcomes for all patients within the NICU.[44]

ENERGY REPLACEMENT

Inadequate energy replacement in critically ill patients may exaggerate depletion of lean body mass, increase the risk of infectious complications, and impede survival.[53] Conversely, overfeeding energy can negatively affect organ function through hypercapnia, hyperglycaemia, azotaemia, hypertonic dehydration, and metabolic acidosis.[54] Whilst methods may be available to closely predict energy expenditure in critically ill patients, the optimal amount that should be replaced, particularly during the acute phase, remains controversial.

Observational research has revealed a relationship between increased energy provision and improved patient outcomes, including more ventilator-free days and reductions in 60-day mortality.[12,18] However, several randomised controlled trials have demonstrated an opposite effect, with underfeeding compared to full feeding during the first week of illness being of no observable detriment.[55–57] Patients identified at high risk of re-feeding syndrome (Table 48.1) may have a more positive response to hypocaloric, as opposed to isocaloric, delivery but this was not accounted for in these trials. A number of other factors, including the different methods used to calculate energy requirements and the discrepancies between clinical populations under investigation means that the results of studies investigating energy replacement must be interpreted with caution.

In view of the altered macronutrient metabolism that is likely in the acute phase, consideration may need to

Table 48.1 Criteria for assessing risk of re-feeding syndrome

Risk type	Body mass index	Unintentional weight loss (last 3–6 months)	Oral intake	Serum potassium, magnesium and phosphate levels	Other factors
Low risk	≥20 kg/m^2	Nil	Adequate	All in normal range	–
Medium risk	18.5–19.9 kg/m^2	0–9.9%	Little or none for 0–5 days	Only one below normal range	–
High risk	16–18.4 kg/m^2	10–14.9%	Little or none for 5–10 days	Only two below normal range	History of substance misuse, alcohol abuse or drugs including antacids, insulin, diuretics or chemotherapy
Very high risk	<16 kg/m^2	>15%	Little or none for >10 days	All three below normal range	–

be given to the source of energy in early feedings. Use of IC can determine the respiratory quotient (RQ) which is associated with macronutrient utilization. In a study of 27 patients with TBI, preferential utilization of fat and protein was observed with a RQ of 0.74, whereas a RQ of 0.84 favoured the use of carbohydrate.[58] At present, it is unclear whether continued adjustment of macronutrient profiles in line with the RQ throughout the course of critical illness would incur additional benefits. Use of alternative substrates, such as lactate, is also an important consideration. Administration of hypertonic sodium lactate (Na$^+$ 1000 mmol/L and lactate 1000 mmol/L) in 24 patients with severe TBI was found to have a cerebral glucose-sparing effect in patients with impaired cerebral oxidative metabolism and improve cerebral energetics.[59] However, assessment techniques such as cerebral microdialysis are currently required to identify individuals who would benefit from lactate administration and this method is not currently used in routine clinical practice. Further research is required to determine optimal macronutrient profiles and use of alternative energy substrates as part of individualised nutritional prescriptions.

Having considered the available evidence, clinical practice guidelines recommend replacing around 80% of energy requirements during the acute phase of illness, rising to 100% during the anabolic phase.[11] It is unfortunate that robust criteria for distinguishing the 'acute' from the 'anabolic' phase is yet to be defined for the purposes of nutrition therapy, however, it is generally accepted that the acute phase of critical illness falls within the first 7–9 days of admission. After this time the requirement for intensive sedation, inotropic support, and ventilation has typically reduced for the majority of patients and energy provision can increase in line with predicted energy requirements.[19]

NITROGEN REPLACEMENT

The inflammatory state observed during critical illness is associated with catabolism of muscle protein to provide amino acids, particularly glutamine and alanine, to maintain vital organ function and synthesis of proteins that facilitate immune function and cellular repair. Reduction in muscle mass is typically between 15% and 20% with increased losses observed in those with multi-organ as opposed to single-organ failure.[60] Oxidation of the branched chain amino acids (BCAA) leucine, isoleucine, and valine from skeletal muscle compensates for the increased energy expenditure and glutamine consumption.[61] Oxidation of BCAA can increase by

up to 20% in highly catabolic states and, if prolonged, will exceed the capability for protein synthesis, leading to increased nitrogen losses.[61]

Nitrogen requirements during critical illness may be determined by assessment of nitrogen balance through measurement of urinary urea nitrogen (UUN). Negative nitrogen balance is commonly observed during the acute phase and is considered to reflect the degree of catabolism during the hypermetabolic state. Patients with TBI appear to experience similar levels of protein catabolism to those with other traumatic injuries[62] and nitrogen losses have been observed in head injured patients at levels of up to 30 g/day with SCI patients losing up to 28.5 g/day.[6,52] However, unlike in TBI, the increase in nitrogen excretion following SCI may not be the result of a hypermetabolic response. Despite both groups exhibiting comparable urinary nitrogen losses, energy expenditure in SCI has been found to be significantly lower than that observed in TBI patients.[31] Alternative mechanisms for the catabolism observed following SCI may relate to mitochondrial dysfunction, oxidative stress, and reduced cell signalling within the skeletal muscle that results in accelerated loss of previously neuroactive tissue.[4]

Prolonged negative nitrogen balance has been associated with poor clinical outcomes[61] whereas achievement of nitrogen balance has been associated with survival.[63] However, attaining nitrogen equilibrium or positive nitrogen balance is challenging. A study of head injured patients found that higher rates of nitrogen replacement were associated with improved nitrogen balance but this was not consistent amongst all patients receiving the higher dose.[62] Whilst >2.0 g nitrogen per kilogram of body weight may increase the rate of protein synthesis, total nitrogen requirements may be much higher for some individuals.[62]

Increases of 30 g protein per day alongside increased energy provision have been associated with decreased mortality in septic patients, challenging previous recommendations from the Surviving Sepsis Campaign, which recommended restriction of nutritional intake during the acute phase of illness.[12] Increased protein provision without adequate energy can exacerbate nitrogen losses but outcomes are improved when protein targets are met alongside those of energy.[64,65] Therefore, high protein requirements must be considered as part of total energy intake to reduce the risks of under- or over-feeding.[54]

Clinical practice guidelines for the Provision and Assessment of Nutrition Support Therapy in the Adult Critically Ill Patient: Society of Critical Care Medicine (SCCM) and American Society for Parenteral and Enter Nutrition (ASPEN) recommend high dose protein provision that meets the minimum reference range of 1.2–2.0 g/kg of actual body weight per day.[11] Due to the increased adiposity in obese individuals, adjustments according to IBW are recommended, providing 2.0–2.5 g/kg/IBW/day. Though the quality of evidence behind these recommendations is acknowledged to be poor, the achievement of a positive nitrogen balance through provision of high protein may still be beneficial and should be a key priority until more well-designed studies are conducted.[60]

INITIATION OF FEEDING

A number of clinical guidelines recommend early initiation of enteral feeding within 24–48 hours in critically ill patients who are haemodynamically stable.[10,11,66] However, in the absence of specific criteria that can be used consistently to define 'haemodynamic stability', determining the optimal time to introduce nutrition for individual cases is challenging. There are emerging theories suggesting that maintaining a fasting state during the initial phase of illness can be beneficial by facilitating innate cell-survival mechanisms.

Autophagy, or 'self-eating', is an evolutionary, catabolic process that involves cellular degradation of damaged or unnecessary proteins. It is thought to play a role in the innate and adaptive immune system and programmed cell death, and may be a cell-survival mechanism during prolonged periods of cell starvation.[67] Interest in the role of autophagy during the acute phase of critical illness has gathered pace in recent years. However, several meta-analyses have demonstrated positive effects of early (within 48 hours) compared to delayed (after 48 hours) enteral nutrition, including reduced infectious morbidity, hospital length of stay, and mortality.[42] Based on research evidence to date, withholding nutritional support to promote autophagy is not recommended due to the potentially deleterious effects associated with underfeeding, and nutrition should be introduced within 24–48 hours once patients are resuscitated and haemodynamic stability is achieved.[68]

ROUTES FOR DELIVERY OF NUTRITION

The route of nutritional delivery to patients in the NICU will depend on many factors including the clinical presentation, severity of illness or injury, Glasgow Coma Scale (GCS) score, access to and function of the GI tract, swallow function, and other underlying comorbidities. Most patients who are unable to maintain volitional intake within the first 24–48 hours of admission will require artificial nutritional support during the acute phase before weaning to oral diet and fluids as tolerated during the recovery period.[11,19]

Enteral Feeding

Enteral nutrition (EN) is the preferred method for nutritional provision in patients who are unable to meet their nutritional needs orally. Enteral nutrition is thought to maintain the functional integrity of the gut by maintaining gut-associated lymphoid tissue and stimulating blood flow, gastric motility, and secretion of bile, digestive hormones, and immunoprotective agents. Increased intestinal permeability is associated with bacterial translocation and alteration of the microbiome, which may preclude the development of systemic infection.[69–71]

Placement of a nasogastric tube to provide gastric feedings is the most common mode of nutritional delivery. Access via the nasal canal can be contraindicated in some patients with craniofacial trauma or skull base fractures and there is risk of malpositioning into the intracranial cavity.[72] Under these circumstances, placement of an orogastric tube may be a suitable alternative in sedated patients requiring early nutritional support. Intolerance to gastric feedings and delayed gastric emptying has been reported to affect up to 80% of patients with brain injury[73] and post-pyloric enteral feeding via a nasojejunal tube may be beneficial.

Parenteral Nutrition

Parenteral nutritional support is primarily reserved for patients who present with, or who develop, a non-functioning or inaccessible GI tract, as well as those who are unable to achieve nutritional targets through enteral feeding. Unlike EN, early initiation of parenteral nutrition (PN) is not a key priority unless there is a high nutritional risk, as benefits relating to the maintenance of gut integrity will be obsolete. On the contrary, delivery of PN is often more successful as it is not influenced by GI tolerance or fasting requirements and higher doses are generally achieved.

The CALORIES trial conducted in 2014 found no significant differences in clinical outcomes between early EN and PN suggesting that administration of PN is no more harmful or beneficial than EN.[74] However, the impact of achieving full nutritional dose via either route was not investigated in this study. The benefits of EN over PN have been documented in other randomized controlled trials and include reductions in infectious complications and length of stay.[11] Hyperalimentation and hyperglycaemia have been identified as key contributory factors to the increased incidence of infections in those receiving PN and were found to be dose-dependent.[75] In the CALORIES trial, both groups failed to meet their full nutritional targets suggesting that underfeeding may have protected patients receiving PN from any adverse effects. A recent meta-analysis confirms the position that EN is the preferred route to PN, however, in those identified to have high nutritional risk, early PN may be beneficial if EN is contraindicated.[76] The importance of determining appropriate doses for energy and nitrogen replacement cannot be overstated and is fundamental to confirming the safest and most appropriate route for nutritional delivery during the acute phase of illness.

Oral Nutritional Support

Observational research has found that many patients will commence oral intake before discharge from the critical care setting. However dysphagia is extremely prevalent, particularly in patients who have received prolonged oral endotracheal intubation and those with neurologic injury.[19] Post-extubation dysphagia has been observed in up to 62% of patients requiring prolonged mechanical ventilation and is associated with increased risk of aspiration pneumonia following extubation.[77] In a small study of 22 patients with polyneuropathy, objective swallow assessments found 91% to have swallowing difficulties and, of all the consistencies trialled, liquids and saliva resulted in the highest rates of aspiration.[78] Dysphagia has a significant impact on hospital length of stay and mortality. Therefore, early assessment and appropriate management is imperative to prevent secondary complications.[79] Greater nutritional deficits will occur in patients who wean from artificial nutritional support too early during the recovery phase and who are not achieving adequate amounts of nutrition orally. In patients who are able to swallow safely, frequent monitoring of nutritional input with use of supplementary artificial nutrition and hydration is required until volitional intake can be restored.

Dietary Management in Special Circumstances

Certain patients in the NICU need specific tailoring of their nutrition to suit their physiological needs.[80–83]

Patients in renal failure who are not on dialysis will require a calorie-rich diet (2 kcal/ml) to allow for fluid restriction. Diet will also need to have limited quantity of phosphorous, potassium, magnesium, and proteins; those on continuous renal replacement therapy, however,

will not need any such modification.[81] In patients with liver disease, current recommendations call for calculating protein requirements in the same manner as for the general ICU patient. It is recommended to use dry weight for cirrhotic patients for calculations.[82] The role of BCAA on restriction of lipids is not clear in this group.[83]

In patients with respiratory failure—acute respiratory distress syndrome—overfeeding can exert metabolic effects that may lead to difficulty weaning from ventilation. Controlled calorie and macronutrient intake is recommended.

Up to 10% of patients in the ICU become chronically critically ill and repeated episodes of admission to the ICU in the course of hospital stay punctuated with sepsis, shock, infections, and malabsorption lead to a picture of adult kwashiorkor-like malnutrition. Early screening and treatment of at-risk NICU population is an important responsibility of the neurointensivist; a multidisciplinary approach is solicited from a team of the intensivist, dietician, and endocrinologist.[84]

COMPLICATIONS RELATED TO FEEDING

Initiation of feeding in the NICU may be associated with various complications (Tables 48.2 and 48.3) and close monitoring is required in patients on parenteral nutrition (Table 48.4).

Table 48.2 Complications of enteral feeding

Tube related	• Damage to cartilage and surrounding soft tissue, sinusitis • Misplacement of nasogastric tube into the cranium/trachea, causing trauma and infection • Misplacement of gastrostomy or jejunostomy tube causing peritonitis, necrotising fasciitis • Blockage of tube, resulting in inadequate feeding • Tube coiling in the lower oesophagus causing regurgitation
Feed related	• Osmotic diarrhoea, constipation, malabsorption • Intolerance to feed causing cramps, bloating, and discomfort • Hyperglycaemia, volume overload, electrolyte disturbances, etc. • Under- or over-feeding with associated problems
Clinical condition related	• Aspiration of feeds in patients with poor airway protection reflex

Table 48.3 Complications of parenteral nutrition

Mechanical complications	• During placement of central catheter-hemo/pneumothorax, arrhythmias • Venous thrombosis • Loss of guidewire (rare)
Central line-related blood stream infection	May occur in up to 50% cases. Preventable with aseptic insertion and handling techniques
Metabolic complications (early)	Volume overload, hyperglycaemia, re-feeding syndrome, hypokalaemia, hypomagnesaemia, hypophosphataemia, hyperchloraemic metabolic acidosis, coagulopathy, hypertriglyceridaemia, acalculous cholecystitis, acute pancreatitis
Metabolic complications (late)	Deficiency of vitamins and trace minerals, hepatic cholestasis, fatty liver, bone disease (e.g., osteoporosis, osteomalacia)
Adverse reactions to lipid emulsions	Dizziness, seating, dyspnoea, cutaneous reactions, headache, and backache

Table 48.4 Monitoring of a patient on parenteral nutrition

Investigation	Frequency
Electrolytes, Urea and Creatinine	Daily until stable, then 3 times per week
Complete Blood Counts	2–3 times a week/on clinical indication
Serum Triglycerides	Weekly
PT, PTT	Weekly
Glucose	3 times/day to keep <200 mg% consistently
Weight	Daily/weekly as appropriate
I and O (Input/Output monitoring)	Daily
Nitrogen Balance	PRN
Liver Function Tests	3 times a week
CRP	Baseline, 3 times a week/once a week as appropriate
Haematinics	Baseline and monthly thereafter

CONCLUSIONS

Identification of patients at a high risk of malnutrition and intervention to correct it may improve patient outcome in the ICU. Early initiation of feeding and 'using the gut when available' to provide adequate calories, proteins, and micronutrients is important. Further studies are needed to standardise the best feeding practices for special patient groups, special feeds, immunonutrition, and antioxidants. A close watch on patients who are on nutritional support for complications related to the device, route, or agent is mandatory.

REFERENCES

1. Agha A, Rogers B, Mylotte D, et al. Neuroendocrine dysfunction in the acute phase of traumatic brain injury. *Clin Endocrinol* 2004;60(5):584–91.
2. Ghirnikar RS, Lee YL, Eng LF. Inflammation in traumatic brain injury: role of cytokines and chemokines. *Neurochem Res* 1998;23(3):329–40.
3. Charrueau C, Belabed L, Besson V, Chaumeil J-C, Cynober L, Moinard C. Metabolic response and nutritional support in traumatic brain injury: evidence for resistance to renutrition. *J Neurotrauma* 2009 Nov;26(11):1911–20.
4. O'Brien LC, Gorgey AS. Skeletal muscle mitochondrial health and spinal cord injury. *World J Orthop* 2016;7(10):628–37.
5. Glenn TC, Martin NA, McArthur DL, et al. Endogenous nutritive support after traumatic brain injury: peripheral lactate production for glucose supply via gluconeogenesis. *J Neurotrauma* 2015;32(11):811–19.
6. Krakau K, Hansson A, Karlsson T, de Boussard CN, Tengvar C, Borg J. Nutritional treatment of patients with severe traumatic brain injury during the first six months after injury. *Nutrition* 2007;23(4):308–17.
7. Young AB, Ott LG, Beard D, Dempsey RJ, Tibbs PA, McClain CJ. The acute-phase response of the brain-injured patient. *J Neurosurg* 1988;69(3):375–80.
8. Clifton GL, Robertson CS, Grossman RG, Hodge S, Foltz R, Garza C. The metabolic response to severe head injury. *J Neurosurg* 1984;60(4):687–96.
9. Padilla FP, Martínez G, Vernooij RWM, Cosp XB, Alonso-Coello P. Nutrition in critically ill adults: A systematic quality assessment of clinical practice guidelines. *Clin Nutr* 2016;35(6):1219–25.
10. Kreymann KG, Berger MM, Deutz NEP, et al. ESPEN Guidelines on enteral nutrition: Intensive care. *Clin Nutr* 2006;25(2):210–23.
11. McClave SA, Taylor BE, Martindale RG, et al. Guidelines for the provision and assessment of nutrition support therapy in the adult critically ill patient: Society of Critical Care Medicine (SCCM) and American Society for Parenteral and Enteral Nutrition (A.S.P.E.N.). *JPEN J Parenter Enteral Nutr* 2016;40(2):159–211.
12. Elke G, Wang M, Weiler N, Day AG, Heyland DK. Close to recommended caloric and protein intake by enteral nutrition is associated with better clinical outcome of critically ill septic patients: secondary analysis of a large international nutrition database. *Crit Care* 2014;18(1):R29.

13. Nicolo M, Heyland DK, Chittams J, Sammarco T, Compher C. Clinical outcomes related to protein delivery in a critically ill population: a multicenter, multinational observation study. *JPEN J Parenter Enteral Nutr* 2016;40(1):45–51.

14. Ferrie S, Allman-Farinelli M, Daley M, Smith K. Protein requirements in the critically ill: a randomized controlled trial using parenteral nutrition. *JPEN J Parenter Enteral Nutr* 2016;40(6):795–805.

15. McClave SA, Lowen CC, Kleber MJ, et al. Are patients fed appropriately according to their caloric requirements? *JPEN J Parenter Enteral Nutr* 1998;22(6):375–81.

16. Heyland DK, Dhaliwal R, Wang M, Day AG. The prevalence of iatrogenic underfeeding in the nutritionally 'at-risk' critically ill patient: Results of an international, multicenter, prospective study. *Clin Nutr* 2015;34(4): 659–66.

17. Frankenfield D, Hise M, Malone A, Russell M, Gradwell E, Compher C. Prediction of resting metabolic rate in critically ill adult patients: results of a systematic review of the evidence. *J Am Diet Assoc* 2007;107(9):1552–61.

18. Alberda C, Gramlich L, Jones N, et al. The relationship between nutritional intake and clinical outcomes in critically ill patients: results of an international multicenter observational study. *Intensive Care Med* 2009;35(10):1728–37.

19. Chapple LS, Deane AM, Heyland DK, et al. Energy and protein deficits throughout hospitalization in patients admitted with a traumatic brain injury. *Clin Nutr* 2016;35(6):1315–22.

20. Kondrup J, Rasmussen HH, Hamberg O, Stanga Z. Nutritional risk screening (NRS 2002): a new method based on an analysis of controlled clinical trials. *Clin Nutr* 2003;22(3):321–36.

21. Heyland DK, Dhaliwal R, Jiang X, Day AG. Identifying critically ill patients who benefit the most from nutrition therapy: the development and initial validation of a novel risk assessment tool. *Crit Care* 2011;15(6):R268.

22. Hulbert AJ, Else PL. Membranes and the setting of energy demand. *J Exp Biol* 2005;208(9):1593–9.

23. Svendsen OL, Hassager C, Christiansen C. Age- and menopause-associated variations in body composition and fat distribution in healthy women as measured by dual-energy X-ray absorptiometry. *Metabolism* 1995;44(3): 369–73.

24. van Pelt RE, Dinneno FA, Seals DR, Jones PP. Age-related decline in RMR in physically active men: relation to exercise volume and energy intake. *Am J Physiol Endocrinol Metab* 2001;281(3):E633–9.

25. Fruin AH, Taylon C, Pettis MS. Caloric requirements in patients with severe head injuries. *Surg Neurol* 1986;25(1):25–8.

26. Foley N, Marshall S, Pikul J, Salter K, Teasell R. Hypermetabolism following moderate to severe traumatic acute brain injury: a systematic review. *J Neurotrauma* 2008;25(12):1415–31.

27. Bruder N, Raynal M, Pellissier D, Courtinat C, François G. Influence of body temperature, with or without sedation, on energy expenditure in severe head-injured patients. *Crit Care Med* 1998;26(3):568–72.

28. Saito T, Sadoshima J. Energy expenditure in children after severe traumatic brain injury. *HSS Public Access* 2016;116(8):1477–90.

29. Piek J, Zanke T, Sprick C, Bock WJ. Resting energy expenditure in patients with isolated head injuries and spontaneous intracranial haemorrhages. *Clin Nutr* 1989; 8(6):347–51.

30. Frankenfield DC, Ashcraft CM. Description and prediction of resting metabolic rate after stroke and traumatic brain injury. *Nutrition* 2012;28(9):906–11.

31. Kolpek JH, Ott LG, Record KE, et al. Comparison of urinary urea nitrogen excretion and measured energy expenditure in spinal cord injury and nonsteroid-treated severe head trauma patients. *JPEN J Parenter Enteral Nutr* 1989;13(3):277–80.

32. Nevin AN, Steenson J, Vivanti A, Hickman IJ. Investigation of measured and predicted resting energy needs in adults after spinal cord injury: a systematic review. *Spinal Cord* 2016;54(4):248–53.

33. Caldwell SB, Smith D, Wilson FC. Impact of paroxysmal sympathetic hyperactivity on nutrition management after brain injury: a case series. *Brain Injury* 2014;28(3): 370–3.

34. Meyer K. Understanding paroxysmal sympathetic hyperactivity after traumatic brain injury. *Surg Neurol Int* 2014;5(14):490.

35. Heymsfield SB, Casper K. Continuous nasoenteric feeding: bioenergetic and metabolic response during recovery from semistarvation. *Am J Clin Nutr* 1988;47(5):900–10.

36. Carlson GL. Nutrient induced thermogenesis. *Baillieres Clin Endocrinol Metab* 1997;11(4):603–15.

37. Asahara R, Yamasaki M. The thermic response to food intake in persons with thoracic spinal cord injury. *J Phys Ther Sci* 2016;28(4):1080–5.

38. Swinamer DL, Phang PT, Jones RL, Grace M, King EG. Twenty-four hour energy expenditure in critically ill patients. *Crit Care Med* 1987;15(7):637–43.

39. Markus HS, Cox M, Tomkins AM. Raised resting energy expenditure in Parkinson's disease and its relationship to muscle rigidity. *Clin Sci* 1992;83(2):199–204.

40. Badjatia N, Strongilis E, Gordon E, et al. Metabolic impact of shivering during therapeutic temperature modulation: the bedside shivering assessment scale. *Stroke* 2008;39(12):3242–7.

41. Bardutzky J, Georgiadis D, Kollmar R, Schwarz S, Schwab S. Energy demand in patients with stroke who are sedated and receiving mechanical ventilation. *J Neurosurg* 2004;100(2):266–71.

42. Cook AM, Peppard A, Magnuson B. Nutrition considerations in traumatic brain injury. *Nutr Clin Pract* 2008;23(6):608–20.

43. Frankenfield D, Smith JS, Cooney RN. Validation of 2 approaches to predicting resting metabolic rate in critically ill patients. *JPEN J Parenter Enteral Nutr* 2004;28(4): 259–64.

44. Haugen HA, Chan L-N, Li F. Indirect calorimetry: a practical guide for clinicians. *Nutr Clin Pract* 2007; 22(4):377–88.

45. Wichansawakun S, Meddings L, Alberda C, Robbins S, Gramlich L. Energy requirements and the use of predictive equations versus indirect calorimetry in critically ill patients. *Appl Physiol Nutr Metab* 2015;40(2):207–10.

46. Mogensen KM, Andrew BY, Corona JC, Robinson MK. Validation of the society of critical care medicine and American society for parenteral and enteral nutrition recommendations for caloric provision to critically ill obese patients: A pilot study. *JPEN J Parenter Enteral Nutr* 2016;40(5):713–21.

47. Henry CJ. Basal metabolic rate studies in humans: measurement and development of new equations. *Public Health Nutr* 2005;8(7a):1133–52.

48. Frankenfield DC, Coleman A, Alam S, Cooney RN. Analysis of estimation methods for resting metabolic rate in critically ill adults. *JPEN J Parenter Enteral Nutr* 2009;33(1):27–36.

49. Koukiasa P, Bitzani M, Papaioannou V, Pnevmatikos I. Resting energy expenditure in critically ill patients with spontaneous intracranial hemorrhage. *JPEN J Parenter Enteral Nutr* 2015;39(8):917–21.

50. Kross EK, Sena M, Schmidt K, Stapleton RD. A comparison of predictive equations of energy expenditure and measured energy expenditure in critically ill patients. *J Crit Care* 2012;27(3):321.e5–12.

51. Rousing ML, Hahn-Pedersen MH, Andreassen S, Pielmeier U, Preiser J-C. Energy expenditure in critically ill patients estimated by population-based equations, indirect calorimetry and CO2-based indirect calorimetry. *Ann Intensive Care* 2016;6(1):16.

52. Barco KT, Smith RA, Peerless JR, Plaisier BR, Chima CS. Energy expenditure assessment and validation after acute spinal cord injury. *Nutr Clin Pract* 2002;17(5):309–13.

53. Hoffer LJ, Bistrian BR. Nutrition in critical illness: a current conundrum. *F1000 Research* 2016;5(0):1–10.

54. Klein CJ, Stanek GS, Wiles CE. Overfeeding macronutrients to critically ill adults: metabolic complications. *J Am Diet Assoc* 1998;98(7):795–806.

55. Rice TW, Wheeler AP, Thompson BT, et al. Initial trophic vs full enteral feeding in patients with acute lung injury: the EDEN randomized trial. *JAMA* 2012;307(8):795–803.

56. Rice TW, Mogan S, Hays MA, Bernard GR, Jensen GL, Wheeler AP. Randomized trial of initial trophic versus full-energy enteral nutrition in mechanically ventilated patients with acute respiratory failure. *Crit Care Med* 2011;39(5):967–74.

57. Arabi YM, Tamim HM, Dhar GS, Al-Dawood A, Al-Sultan M, Sakkijha MH KS, R. B. Permissive underfeeding and intensive insulin therapy in critically ill patients: a randomized controlled trial. *Am J Clin Nutr* 2011;93: 569–77.

58. Maxwell J, Gwardschaladse C, Lombardo G, et al. The impact of measurement of respiratory quotient by indirect calorimetry on the achievement of nitrogen balance in patients with severe traumatic brain injury. *Eur J Trauma Emerg Surg* 2017;43(6): 775–82.

59. Quintard H, Patet C, Zerlauth J-B, et al. Improvement of neuroenergetics by hypertonic lactate therapy in patients with traumatic brain injury is dependent on baseline cerebral lactate/pyruvate ratio. *J Neurotrauma* 2016;33(7):681–7.

60. van Zanten ARH. Should we increase protein delivery during critical illness? *JPEN J Parenter Enter Nutr* 2016;40(6):756–62.

61. Choudry HA, Pan M, Karinch AM, Souba WW. Branched-chain amino acid-enriched nutritional support in surgical and cancer patients. *J Nutr* 2006;136(1):314S–318.

62. Dickerson RN, Pitts SL, Maish GO, et al. A reappraisal of nitrogen requirements for patients with critical illness and trauma. *J Trauma Acute Care Surg* 2012;73(3):549–57.

63. Frankenfield D. Energy expenditure and protein requirements after traumatic injury. *Nutr Clin Pract* 2006;21(5):430–7.

64. Weijs PJM, Stapel SN, de Groot SDW, et al. Optimal protein and energy nutrition decreases mortality in mechanically ventilated, critically ill patients: a prospective observational cohort study. *JPEN J Parenter Enteral Nutr* 2012;36(1):60–8.

65. Hoffer LJ. Protein and energy provision in critical illness. *Am J Clin Nutr* 2003;78(5):906–11.

66. Bullock MR, Povlishock JT. Guidelines for the management of severe traumatic brain injury. Editor's Commentary. *J Neurotrauma* 2007; 2 p preceding S1.

67. Marik PE. Is early starvation beneficial for the critically ill patient? *Curr Opin Clin Nutr Metab Care* 2016;19(2): 155–60.

68. McClave SA, Weijs PJM. Preservation of autophagy should not direct nutritional therapy. *Curr Opin Clin Nutr Metab Care* 2015;18(2):155–61.

69. Jabbar A, Chang W-K, Dryden GW, McClave SA. Gut immunology and the differential response to feeding and starvation. *Nutr Clin Pract* 2003;18(6):461–82.

70. Kang W, Kudsk KA. Is there evidence that the gut contributes to mucosal immunity in humans? *JPEN J Parenter Enter Nutr* 2007;31(3):246–58.

71. Patel JJ, Rosenthal MD, Miller KR, Martindale RG. The gut in trauma. *Curr Opin Crit Care* 2016;22(4):339–46.

72. Chandra R, Kumar P. Intracranial introduction of a nasogastric tube in a patient with severe craniofacial trauma. *Neurol India* 2010;58(5):804–5.

73. Kao CH, ChangLai SP, Chieng PU, Yen TC. Gastric emptying in head-injured patients. *Am J Gastroenterol* 1998;93(7):1108–12.

74. Harvey SE, Parrott F, Harrison DA, et al. Trial of the route of early nutritional support in critically ill adults. *N Engl J Med* 2014;371(18):1673–84.

75. Gramlich L, Kichian K, Pinilla J, Rodych NJ, Dhaliwal R, Heyland DK. Does enteral nutrition compared to parenteral nutrition result in better outcomes in critically ill adult patients? A systematic review of the literature. *Nutrition* 2004;20(10):843–8.

76. Elke G, van Zanten ARH, Lemieux M, et al. Enteral versus parenteral nutrition in critically ill patients: an updated systematic review and meta-analysis of randomized controlled trials. *Crit Care* 2016;20(1):117.

77. Kim MJ, Park YH, Park YS, Song YH. Associations between prolonged intubation and developing post-extubation dysphagia and aspiration pneumonia in non-neurologic critically ill patients. *Ann Rehabil Med* 2015;39(5):763–71.

78. Ponfick M, Linden R, Nowak DA. Dysphagia—a common, transient symptom in critical illness polyneuropathy: a fiberoptic endoscopic evaluation of swallowing study. *Crit Care Med* 2015;43(2):365–72.

79. Altman KW, Yu G-P, Schaefer SD. Consequence of dysphagia in the hospitalized patient: impact on prognosis and hospital resources. *Arch Otolaryngol Head Neck Surg* 2010;136(8):784–9.

80. Tripathy S. Nutrition in the neurocritical care unit. *J Neuroanaesthesiol Crit Care* 2015;2:88–96.

81. Chan LN. Nutritional support in acute renal failure. *Curr Opin Clin Nutr Metab Care* 2004;7:207–12.

82. Patel JJ, McClain CJ, Sarav M, Hamilton-Reeves J, Hurt RT. Protein requirements for critically ill patients with renal and liver failure. *Nutr Clin Pract* 2017 Apr;32 (1_suppl):101S–111S.

83. Sato S, Watanabe A, Muto Y, et al. Clinical comparison of branched-chain amino acid (l-leucine, l-isoleucine, l-valine) granules and oral nutrition for hepatic insufficiency in patients with decompensated liver cirrhosis (LIV-EN study). *Hepatol Res* 2005;31:232–40.

84. Nelson JE, Cox CE, Hope AA, Carson SS. Chronic critical illness. *Am J Respir Crit Care Med* 2010;182(4): 446–54.

49

Immunonutrition

E. SH. Ng. and N. W. Loh

ABSTRACT

Immunonutrition refers to the modulation of the immune system by providing certain dietary nutrients. This chapter explores the role of immunonutrition in the care of critically ill neurological patients. It covers omega-3 and -6 fatty acids, glutamine, arginine, antioxidants, and trace elements. Evidence for immunonutrition appears to be conflicting in nature with a paucity of studies conducted specifically in the neurocritical care population. Most of the evidence is from studies conducted on general critical care patients. The use of omega-3 fatty acids and gamma-linolenic acid appear to have potential benefits in neurocritical care patients, however, further studies need to be done in order to support stronger recommendations.

KEYWORDS

Immunonutrition; neurocritical care; omega-3 fatty acids; glutamine; arginine; antioxidants; trace elements.

INTRODUCTION

Immunonutrition refers to the modulation of the immune system by providing certain dietary nutrients. These include fatty acids (omega-3 fatty acids such as docosahexaenoic acid, eicosapentaenoic acid, omega-6 fatty acid, and gamma-linolenic acid), amino acids (arginine, glutamine), antioxidants (Vitamin C, E, and A), trace elements (selenium, zinc) and nucleotides.[1]

Neurological patients in critical care are a complex group of patients to manage. As the brain regulates many metabolic processes, injury results in a host of metabolic derangements involving endocrine dysfunction, catabolism, and inflammatory processes. These result in immune dysfunction involving all host defence mechanisms.[2] In addition, neurocritical care patients can develop acute respiratory distress syndrome (ARDS), sepsis, and multi-organ failure.

This chapter explores the role of immunonutrition in the care of critically ill neurological patients.

GLUTAMINE

Glutamine is the most abundant amino acid found in the body.[3] It is a non-essential alpha amino acid synthesized by glutamine synthetase. Glutamine is mainly produced in skeletal muscle and the liver.[4]

Glutamine plays an important role in cell metabolism. It not only serves as a substrate for protein synthesis and gluconeogenesis, but is also a precursor for nucleotide and neurotransmitter production. It is involved in acid-base regulation, urea metabolism in the liver, and is an energy source for cells of the immune system.[3,5,6] In critically ill patients, glutamine attenuates inflammatory responses, prevents cellular injury, and preserves cellular metabolic function.[7] As a precursor of glutathione, it also functions as an antioxidant.

In normal physiological conditions, the body produces adequate amounts of glutamine. However, under stress, it is postulated that the body is unable to produce enough glutamine to meet its needs.[8] Moreover, muscles release large amounts of glutamine during states of stress and catabolism. It has been observed that around 30% of critically ill patients are deficient in glutamine on admission to the intensive care.[9] Patients at higher risk of glutamine depletion include those who have prolonged critical illness, burns patients, and those who require parenteral nutrition. Data shows that severity of glutamine deficiency on admission to intensive care is associated with increased mortality.[9,10] This gives rise to the theory that glutamine is a conditionally essential amino acid in times of physiological stress.

Early studies have observed that glutamine supplementation in the critically ill have reduced infectious morbidity and hospital mortality. These studies mostly included patients who received low doses of glutamine requiring parenteral nutrition (PN) and who commenced glutamine supplementation with PN later in their intensive care unit (ICU) stay. They excluded patients with renal or hepatic failure.[11] The apparent potential benefits of glutamine supplementation prompted further studies in the critically ill population.

Results of these studies are mixed. A systematic review done by Wischmeyer et al. including 26 randomized controlled trials on parenteral supplementation of glutamine showed a significant reduction in hospital mortality and length of stay.[11] On the other hand, a systematic review done by van Zanten et al. including 11 randomized controlled trials examining enteral glutamine supplementation showed no benefit on hospital mortality, infectious morbidity, and ICU length of stay. However, there was a significant reduction in hospital length of stay. Analysis of a small group of burns patients revealed a significant reduction in hospital mortality with enteral glutamine supplementation.[12]

With respect to traumatic brain injury (TBI) patients, there was some concern that parenteral glutamine supplementation will increase intracerebral glutamate concentrations which will result in neuronal swelling and raised intracranial pressure (ICP). However, a study by Berg A showed unaffected cerebral glutamate concentrations despite parenteral glutamine supplementation.[13]

A concern over the safety of glutamine has been raised after two large scale, multi-centre general ICU trials (REDOXS and Metaplus), which indicated increased mortality with high-dose glutamine supplementation.[14,15]

In conclusion, the benefits of glutamine supplementation appears to be limited, while it could potentially cause harm in the general ICU population. Therefore, we cannot recommend glutamine supplementation in neurocritical care patients.

ARGININE

Arginine is a conditionally essential amino acid which plays an important role in both cellular and humoral immunity. It is vital for macrophage and lymphocyte activity and metabolism. In addition, it is essential for nitrogen transport, excretion, and ammonia metabolism. Arginine is also required for synthesis of many compounds

such as urea, ornithine, creatine, bioamines, and nitric oxide.[16] It also promotes mucosal barrier function and prevents bacterial translocation. It is broken down by either nitric oxide synthase or arginase into different end-products which have different physiological effects.[16] Metabolism of arginine by nitric oxide synthase results in production of nitric oxide, which is a double-edged sword in the critically ill patient. On one hand, the vasodilatation caused by nitric oxide worsens haemodynamic stability.[17] At the same time, vasodilation can increase oxygen and nutrient delivery to cells.[18] Furthermore, nitric oxide is utilized by the body's defences in the killing of pathogens. In critically ill patients, arginine levels are low because of poor nutrition, decreased synthesis, and increased metabolism.[19,20]

The safety of arginine supplementation has been a subject of controversy as it is postulated that increased nitric oxide worsens hypotension and shock in critically ill patients[21] (particularly as nitric oxide synthase is up-regulated in critically ill patients). However, a randomized controlled trial which studied the effects of nitric oxide synthase inhibitor administration in patients with septic shock showed increased mortality in the treatment.[17]

Arginine supplementation has been mainly studied as part of an immune-modulating formula rather than as a single agent. A study conducted by Luiking on eight patients with septic shock showed that intravenous infusion of arginine increased de novo production of arginine, nitric oxide, and reduced protein breakdown without negatively affecting haemodynamic parameters (stroke volume increased and arterial lactate decreased).[22]

Arginine supplementation in combination with omega-3 fatty acids appear to have a synergistic effect in improving clinical outcomes. A meta-analysis conducted by Drover using 35 trials on elective surgical patients showed reduced infectious morbidity and length of hospital stay with arginine and omega-3 fatty acid supplementation.[23] A meta-analysis performed by Osland showed similar reductions in infection and length of stay.[24] There was no significant effect seen on mortality. The American Society for Parenteral and Enteral Nutrition (ASPEN) recommends routine administration of an immune modulating formula containing both arginine and omega-3 fatty acids in postoperative patients.[25]

There have been no studies on arginine monotherapy in neurocritical care specifically.

ANTI-OXIDANTS

Under normal physiological conditions, the body is able to counter oxidative stress with a functioning antioxidant network. During critical illness, there is an increase in oxidative stress, resulting in excess reactive oxygen species (ROS) and reactive nitrogen species (RNS), and a diminished ability of the antioxidant network to counter these free radicals.[26]

Production of ROS and RNS occurs in normal cell physiology.[27] During oxidative phosphorylation, oxygen receives electrons from other molecules to generate adenosine triphosphate. In so doing, it is reduced to water. However, in a small percentage of reactions, incomplete reduction of oxygen occurs, resulting in ROS formation.[28] Generation of ROS and RNS is also important in the host response to infection. Immune cells such as activated phagocytes produce free radicals which kill bacteria.[28] The key enzyme complexes which produce free radicals include nicotinamide adenine dinucleotide phosphate (NADPH) oxidase complexes, xanthine oxidase, and nitric oxide synthase.[27]

Free radicals exert damage to cells by reacting with other molecules such as proteins, DNA, and lipids. This results in DNA strand damage and modification, lipid peroxidation, and enzyme inactivation.[29]

During a critical illness such as neurological injury, sepsis, and ARDS, there is an increase in production of free radicals.[26,30] Moreover, free radicals play a vital role in the pathophysiology of these conditions. After a period of ischaemia (e.g., ischaemic stroke), large amounts of free radicals released results in reperfusion injury, which in turn causes neuronal injury. In patients with intracranial haemorrhage, iron released by haemolysed red cells catalyse reactions in which highly reactive hydroxyl radicals are produced.[26] In sepsis, activated immune cells generate large amounts of free radicals, which increase the inflammatory response and give rise to the clinical manifestations of sepsis,[28,31] e.g., increased vascular permeability and reduced response to catecholamines.

At the same time, during critical illness, it has been shown that there is a reduction in antioxidants such as selenium, zinc, and vitamins A, C, and E. This is due to increased losses, redistribution, and dysfunctional regulatory mechanisms.[29]

With this background, it has been postulated that antioxidant supplementation in critically ill patients will improve their outcomes.

SELENIUM

Selenium is a component of selenoproteins, many of which have antioxidant properties. It has been found that plasma selenium levels are low in ICU patients, particularly in patients with systemic inflammatory response and sepsis.

Several studies have correlated low selenium levels with poor outcomes.[32,33]

Studies examining the effects of selenium supplementation in the critically ill have yielded conflicting results. A meta-analysis performed by Huang et al. showed a significant reduction in mortality with high doses of selenium supplementation.[34] This is generally supported by a meta-analysis conducted by Manzanares et al. on the effects of antioxidant supplementation which included a subgroup analysis on selenium monotherapy. This study showed that there was a trend towards reduced infections and mortality with selenium monotherapy.[35]

Subsequently, the REDOXS study showed no benefit and potential harm with antioxidant administration.[14] In addition, the MetaPlus study showed increased mortality with extra-enteral glutamine and selenium supplementation.[15]

Recently, ASPEN conducted a meta-analysis involving nine studies (1,888 patients) which showed that parenteral supplementation of selenium did not reduce mortality, length of stay, or duration of mechanical ventilation. Hence, they concluded that a recommendation for selenium supplementation cannot be made at this point.[25]

ZINC

Zinc does not directly interact with free radicals, however, it plays an important role in the antioxidant network as it functions as a cofactor of antioxidant enzymes and inhibits pro-oxidant enzymes.[36] It is also essential for wound healing and serves as a cofactor for transcription and replication factors. Plasma zinc levels are low in critically ill patients due to a combination of factors: leakage from vessels with increased permeability, increased demand by immune cells, and for formation of acute phase reactants, increased urinary excretion, and poor nutrition. Low zinc levels have adverse effects on the immune system, such as impaired maturation of B and T cells and poor function of natural killer cells and phagocytes.[36]

A randomized controlled trial by Young et al. comparing the effects of supplemental zinc versus standard zinc therapy on neurological recovery in patients with severe closed head injury showed that supplemental zinc was associated with improved Glasgow Coma Scale (GCS) scores.[37]

A study conducted on rats explored whether zinc supplementation increased the resilience of the brain to anxiety post TBI. It was found that zinc supplementation prior to brain injury decreased the development of anhedonia in the rats post injury. Moreover, the rats who were given zinc supplementation appeared to have better preserved cognitive function post injury.[38]

There has been concern that high concentrations of free zinc is neurotoxic.[39] However, a subsequent study conducted on rats with TBI failed to demonstrate a relation between post injury zinc supplementation and neuronal cell death.[40]

To date, four randomized trials have been conducted evaluating the effect of zinc supplementation in critically ill patients. Aggregated data from these four studies did not show a significant reduction in mortality with zinc supplementation.[36] Hence, there is insufficient evidence to recommend routine zinc supplementation in critically ill patients.

VITAMINS A, C, AND E

Vitamin A refers to fat-soluble retinoids and carotenoids. Alpha-, beta-, and gamma-carotene are retinol precursors. Vitamin A has many functions in the body including maintaining a healthy immune system, cell proliferation, and vision. Vitamin A, in particular, beta-carotene is an antioxidant. It acts by reacting with free radicals and binding with transition metals which catalyse reactions producing ROS and RNS.[28]

Vitamin C is a water soluble antioxidant. It mops up free radicals such as hydroxyl, superoxide, peroxyl, and nitroxide radicals. In addition, it prevents their production by inhibiting pro-oxidant enzymes such as NADPH oxidase. Vitamin C enhances the immune response to infection by improving chemotaxis, neutrophil phagocytic activity, and by supporting the production of lymphocytes and interferon.[41,42]

Vitamin E is a fat-soluble vitamin. It comprises a group of tocopherols and tocotrienoles. It also plays a vital role in functioning of the immune system and maintaining membrane stability.[43,44]

Vitamin supplementation has more frequently been studied as part of an antioxidant cocktail, rather than individual vitamin supplementation. Few studies evaluating the effects of vitamin monotherapy have been performed. A study on retinol monotherapy in patients undergoing coronary artery bypass graft showed reduced mortality and length of stay in the group who received supplementation.[45] Yet, another study performed on serum vitamin A levels in ICU patients showed no association between vitamin A levels and mortality.[46] A trial performed by Lassnigg et al. investigated the effects of intravenous vitamin E supplementation on elective cardiac surgery patients. Vitamin E supplementation demonstrated no effect on clinical outcome.[47] A phase I trial of intravenous vitamin C in patients with severe sepsis (involving 24 patients) showed a reduction in Sequential

Organ Failure Assessment (SOFA) scores, procalcitonin, and C-reactive protein levels.[48]

The effects of antioxidant cocktail therapy have been studied and appears to be promising. A meta-analysis done by Manzanares[35] examining 21 randomized controlled trials (RCTs) found a significant reduction in mortality and duration of ventilator days with antioxidant micronutrient supplementation. There was a trend towards reduction in infectious complications but no effect on hospital length of stay. ASPEN recommends that antioxidant therapy, in safe doses, be provided to critically ill patients as this may improve patient outcome. Aggregated data from 15 trials showed a significant reduction in mortality. However, there was no significant effect on length of stay and infectious morbidity. Of note, there was a lack of dose standardization of supplementation, route of administration, duration and frequency of therapy.[25]

The REDOXS trial brought into question the safety of antioxidant supplementation as 28-day mortality rate was higher in the antioxidant supplementation arm compared to placebo. Antioxidants also appeared to cause more harm in patients with renal impairment.[14,15] Baseline renal dysfunction should be taken into account when administering antioxidant supplementation.

OMEGA-3 FATTY ACIDS (FISH OIL) AND GAMMA-LINOLENIC ACID

Omega-3 fatty acids are long chain polyunsaturated fatty acids of which alpha-linolenic acid is the parent 18 carbon fatty acid.[49] The human body is unable to produce omega-3 fatty acids de novo. However, it is able to synthesize eicosapentaenoic acid (EPA) and docosahexaenoic acid (DHA) from alpha-linolenic acid.[49] EPA and DHA are omega-3 fatty acids which are metabolized to produce less pro-inflammatory mediators (compared to arachidonic acid, a fatty acid which is metabolized to inflammatory mediators such as leukotrienes and prostaglandins).[49]

There has been much interest in the role of omega-3 fatty acids in preventing cardiovascular diseases, diabetes, stroke, and arthritis. It is required for normal growth and development. It also functions in stabilizing cell membranes. Omega-3 fatty acids also have an anti-inflammatory effect.[50] This is postulated to be due to: replacement of arachidonic acid in membranes of immune cells thereby ameliorating the production of inflammatory mediators, and providing competition for enzymes cyclooxygenase and lipoxygenase, hence reducing the metabolism of arachidonic acid to inflammatory mediators.[51] The neuroprotective effects of omega-3 fatty acids have been studied in animal models. These have demonstrated that they improved cognitive ability and reduced neuronal damage after traumatic brain injury.[52] Eicosapentaenoic acid and DHA also give rise to protectins and resolvins which are neuroprotective.[53]

Many studies on the effects of omega-3 fatty acids include gamma linolenic acid (omega-6 fatty acid), which similarly is broken down to less pro-inflammatory mediators and hence exerts its anti-inflammatory effect in the same way.

A recent meta-analysis performed by Glenn showed that continuous administration of omega-3 fatty acids together with antioxidants produced a reduction in length of ICU stay, ventilator days, and mortality in patients with ARDS/acute lung injury (ALI), with no apparent effect on infectious morbidity.[54]

Observational studies have been performed which suggest that increased fish and omega-3 fatty acid consumption reduces ischaemic stroke risk.[55,56] Yoneda et al. conducted a prospective non-randomized study on 101 patients who underwent clipping of aneurysm after subarachnoid haemorrhage. This study showed a significant reduction in the incidence of vasospasm in the group treated with omega-3 fatty acids. The treated group of patients also had a higher percentage with good outcomes (defined as being independent, with moderate disability).[57]

ASPEN recommends the use of either arginine containing immune enhancing formula or standard formula with omega-3 supplement in patients with traumatic brain injury.[25]

The use of omega-3 fatty acids and gamma-linolenic acid appear to have potential benefits in neurocritical care patients. Further studies need to be conducted to evaluate the clinical benefits and adverse effects of supplementation in order to support stronger recommendations.

IMMUNONUTRITION IN TRAUMATIC BRAIN INJURY

The brain regulates many metabolic processes in the body. When there is brain injury, the body experiences dysfunction in many systems and this is sometimes complicated by our treatment. In particular, patients with TBI experience an intense inflammatory response[58] and hypermetabolic state.[59] The immune system is adversely affected[60] and this is compounded by prolonged immobility, presence of invasive lines, and increased aspiration risk, which all predispose to infection. There can also be endocrine disturbances resulting in hyperglycaemia which impedes wound healing. The gastrointestinal (GI) tract also takes a hit as there is increased mucosal permeability hence increasing the risk

of bacterial translocation, ileus, and gastric ulceration.[61] Induced barbiturate coma to manage raised ICP further weakens immunity,[62] predisposing the patient to infectious morbidity.

An early study done on 30 patients by Chendrasekkhar A et al. which was published in abstract form demonstrated a lower incidence of infections in patients given immune enhancing formula compared to standard formula. Lymphocyte studies were also done showing increased total lymphocyte count in patients who received immune-enhancing formula. However, details of the study are not available, rendering it difficult to assess its validity.[63]

Painter et al. conducted a retrospective study on 240 TBI patients comparing the effects of immune-enhancing nutrition formula versus standard formula. The group of patients who received immune-enhancing formula demonstrated an increase in pre-albumin levels and a decrease in bacteraemia rates. The increase in pre-albumin levels could suggest improved nutrition, however, pre-albumin levels can also vary significantly with stress and inflammation. There was no effect on pneumonia, urinary tract infection, and mortality. In fact, patients who received immune-enhancing formula had increased length of ICU stay and ventilated days.[64]

A small trial on 40 patients with brain injury showed decreased infections and reduced ICU length of stay with the use of immune-enhancing formula.[65] ASPEN recommends the use of either arginine-containing immune modulating formulations or EPA/DHA supplement with standard formula for TBI patients based on an expert consensus.[25]

Theoretically, immune-enhancing formula may benefit patients with neurological injury, particularly with respect to reduction of infection. Also, zinc supplementation has been shown in a study to improve GCS scores in brain injury patients.[37] However, data on immune-enhancing formula in neurological patients is limited; there have been no large randomized controlled trials demonstrating benefit in this population of patients. Immune-enhancing formula does appear to be well-tolerated in this group of patients; there has been no significant evidence demonstrating adverse effects of immune-enhancing formula in patients with neurological injury.

IMMUNONUTRITION IN CRITICAL CARE

Marik et al. conducted a systematic review (including 24 studies) evaluating the effect of immunonutrition in critical care patients. The review included ICU patients (medical and surgical), trauma, and burns patients. Different combinations of immune-enhancing formula were used—fish oil, glutamine, glutamine plus fish oils, arginine, arginine plus glutamine, arginine plus fish oils, and all three nutrients together. Most formulae contained selenium in varying amounts. The formulae used also contained different amounts of nucleic acids, antioxidants, and micronutrients. The review demonstrated a reduction in infections with immune-enhancing formula, but no effect on mortality or length of stay. Formulae containing fish oils produced a significant reduction in mortality, infections, and length of stay.[66]

SEPSIS AND ACUTE RESPIRATORY DISTRESS SYNDROME

A randomized controlled trial involving 176 patients was conducted to examine the effect of immune-enhanced formula (containing arginine, nucleic acids, fish oil) on septic patients. Mortality and bacteraemia rates were reduced in the treatment group. However, the mortality benefit was most significant in patients with APACHE II scores between 10 and 15. This limits the generalization of results to septic patients.[67]

Beale et al. demonstrated faster organ function recovery in patients receiving immune-enhanced formula as assessed by SOFA score.[68]

ASPEN conducted a meta-analysis of 20 RCTs which showed no clear benefit in the medical ICU population (of which a significant proportion of patients were septic). Hence, it does not recommend immune-enhanced formula in MICU patients or patients with sepsis.[25]

Aggregated data from randomized controlled trials conducted in patients with ARDS and acute lung injury failed to demonstrate any outcome benefit with immune-enhanced formula.[69–72]

CONCLUSION

Evidence for immunonutrition appears to be conflicting in nature with a paucity of studies conducted, specifically in the neurocritical care population. Based on current studies, there is a suggestion that immunonutrition may reduce infective complications, but with no effect on mortality or length of stay. Animal studies have shown promising effects of omega-3 fatty acids in neuronal healing but there is a lack of good quality human studies in the neurocritical care population. The current ASPEN guidelines have recommended the use of arginine and EPA/DHA supplements based on expert consensus. Arginine and EPA formulas can be started in neurocritical care patients.

REFERENCES

1. Robert FG. Basics in clinical nutrition: Immunonutrition —Nutrients which influence immunity: Effect and mechanism of action. *e-SPEN* 2009;4:e10–e13.
2. Cook AM, Peppard A, Magnuson B. Nutrition considerations in traumatic brain injury. *Nutr Clin Pract* 2008;23:608–20.
3. Roth E. Nonnutritive effects of glutamine. *Journal of Nutrition* 2008;138(10):2025S–2031S.
4. Kuhn KS, Stehle P, Fürst P. Quantitative analyses of glutamine in peptides and proteins. *Journal of Agricultural and Food Chemistry* 1996;44(7):1808–11.
5. Newsholme P, Procopio J, Ramos Lima MM, Pithon-Curi TC, Curi R. Glutamine and glutamate—their central role in cell metabolism and function. *Cell Biochemistry and Function* 2003;21(1):1–9.
6. Curi R, Lagranha CJ, Doi SQ, et al. Molecular mechanisms of glutamine action. *Journal of Cellular Physiology* 2005;204(2):392–401.
7. Wischmeyer PE. Glutamine: role in critical illness and ongoing clinical trials. *Curr Opin Gastroenterol* 2008;24:190–7.
8. Fürst P, Stehle P. Gluta mine and glutamine containing dipeptides. In: Cynober L ed. *Metabolic and Therapeutic Aspects of Amino Acids in Clinical Nutrition*. Boca Raton, FL:CRC Press, 2004; pp. 613–32.
9. Oudemans-van Straaten HM, Bosman RJ, Treskes M, van der Spoel HJ, Zandstra DF. Plasma glutamine depletion and patient outcome in acute ICU admissions. *Intensive Care Med* 2001;27:84–90.
10. Rodas PC, Rooyackers O, Hebert C, Norberg A, Wernerman J. Glutamine and glutathione at ICU admission in relation to outcome. *Clin Sci* 2012;122:591–7.
11. Wischmeyer PE, Dhaliwal R, McCall M, Ziegler TR, Heyland DK. Parenteral glutamine supplementation in critical illness: a systematic review. *Critical Care* 2014;18:R76.
12. van Zanten AR, Dhaliwal R, Garrel D, Heyland DK. Enteral glutamine supplementation in critically ill patients: a systematic review and meta-analysis. *Critical Care* 2015;19:294.
13. Berg A, Bellander BM, Wanecek M, et al. Intravenous glutamine supplementation to head trauma patients leaves cerebral glutamate concentration unaffected. *Intensive Care Med* 2006 Nov;32(11):1741–6.
14. Heyland D, Muscedere J, Wischmeyer PE, et al. A randomized trial of glutamine and antioxidants in critically ill patients. *N Engl J Med* 2013 Apr 18;368(16):1489–97.
15. van Zanten AR, Sztark F, Kaisers UX, et al. High-protein enteral nutrition enriched with immune-modulating nutrients vs standard high-protein enteral nutrition and nosocomial infections in the ICUA randomized clinical trial. *JAMA* 2014;312(5):514–24.

16. Peranzoni E, Marigo I, Dolcetti L, et al. Role of arginine metabolism in immunity and immunopathology. *Immunobiology* 2007;212:795–812.

17. Watson D, Grover R, Anzueto A, et al. Cardiovascular effects of the nitric oxide synthase inhibitor NG -methyl-L-arginine hydrochloride (546C88) in patients with septic shock: Results of a randomized, double-blind, placebo-controlled multicenter study (study no. 144-002). *Crit Care Med* 2004 Jan;32(1):13–20.

18. Zhou M, Martindale RG. Arginine in the critical care setting. *J Nutr* 2007;137:1687S–92S.

19. Barbul A. Arginine: biochemistry, physiology, and therapeutic implications. *JPEN J Parenter Enteral Nutr* 1986;10:227–38.

20. Castillo L, Yu YM, Marchini JS, et al. Phenylalanine and tyrosine kinetics in critically ill children with sepsis. *Pediatr Res* 1994;35:580–8.

21. De Werra I, Jaccard C, Corradin SB, et al. Cytokines, nitrite/nitrate, soluble tumor necrosis factor receptors, and procalcitonin concentrations: comparisons in patients with septic shock, cardiogenic shock, and bacterial pneumonia. *Crit Care Med* 1997;25:607–13.

22. Luiking YC, Poeze M, Deutz NE. Arginine infusion in patients with septic shock increases nitric oxide production without haemodynamic instability. *Clin Sci (Lond)* 2015 Jan;128(1):57–67.

23. Drover JW, Dhaliwal R, Weitzel L, Wischmeyer PE, Ochoa JB, Heyland DK. Perioperative use of arginine-supplemented diets: a systematic review of the evidence. *J Am Coll Surg* 2011;212(3):385–99.

24. Osland E, Hossain MB, Khan S, Memon MA. Effect of timing of pharmaconutrition (immunonutrition) administration on outcomes of elective surgery for gastrointestinal malignancies: a systematic review and metaanalysis. *JPEN J Parenter Enteral Nutr* 2014;38(1):53–69.

25. Taylor BE, McClave SA, Martindale RG, et al. Guidelines for the provision and assessment of nutrition support therapy in the adult critically ill patient: Society of Critical Care Medicine (SCCM) and American Society for Parenteral and Enteral Nutrition (ASPEN). *Crit Care Med* 2016 Feb;44(2):390–438.

26. Hanafy KA, Selim MH. Antioxidant strategies in neurocritical care. *Neurotherapeutics* 2012 Jan;9(1):44–55.

27. Di Meo S, Reed TT, et al. Role of ROS and RNS sources in physiological and pathological conditions. *Oxid Med Cell Longev* 2016:1245–9.

28. Koekkoek WA, van Zanten AR. Antioxidant vitamins and trace elements in critical illness. *Nutr Clin Pract* 2016 Aug;31(4):457–74.

29. Bulger EM, Maier RV. Antioxidants in critical illness. *Arch Surg* 2001 Oct;136(10):1201–7.

30. Alonso de Vega JM, Díaz J, Serrano E, Carbonell LF. Oxidative stress in critically ill patients with systemic inflammatory response syndrome. *Crit Care Med* 2002; 16:1782–6.

31. Victor VM, Rocha M, De la Fuente M. Immune cells: free radicals and antioxidants in sepsis. *Int Immunopharmacol* 2004 Mar;4(3):327–47.

32. Forceville X, Vitoux D, Gauzit R, et al. Selenium, systemic immune response syndrome, sepsis and outcome in critically ill patients. *Crit Care Med* 1998;26:1536–44.

33. Sakr Y, Reinhart K, Bloos F, et al. Time course and relationship between plasma selenium concentrations, systemic inflammatory response, sepsis, and multi-organ failure. *Br J Anaesth* 2007;98:775–84.

34. Huang TS, Shyu YC, Chen HY, et al. Effect of parenteral selenium supplementation in critically ill patients: a systematic review and meta-analysis. *PLoS One* 2013; 8(1):e54431.

35. Manzanares W, Dhaliwal R, Jiang X, Murch L, Heyland DK. Antioxidant micronutrients in the critically ill: a systematic review and meta-analysis. *Crit Care* 2012 Dec 12;16(2):R66.

36. Heyland DK, Jones N, Cvijanovich NZ, Wong H. Zinc supplementation in critically ill patients: a key pharmaconutrient? *JPEN J Parenter Enteral Nutr* 2008 Sep–Oct;32(5):509–19.

37. Young B, Ott L, Kasarskis E, et al. Zinc supplementation is associated with improved neurologic recovery rate and visceral protein levels of patients with severe closed head injury. *J Neurotrauma* 1996 Jan;13(1):25–34.

38. Cope EC, Morris DR, Scrimgeour AG, VanLandingham JW, Levenson CW. Zinc supplementation provides behavioral resiliency in a rat model of traumatic brain injury. *Physiol Behav* 2011 Oct 24;104(5):942–7.

39. Yeiser EC, Lerant AA, Casto RM, Levenson CW. Free zinc increases at the site of injury after cortical stab wounds in mature but not immature rat brain. *Neurosci Lett* 1999 Dec 24; 277:75–78.

40. Yeiser EC, Vanlandingham JW, Levenson CW. Moderate zinc deficiency increases cell death after brain injury in the rat. *Nutr Neurosci* 2002 Oct;5(5):345–52.

41. Oudemans-van Straaten HM, Spoelstra-de Man AM, de Waard MC. Vitamin C revisited. *Crit Care* 2014;18(4):460.

42. Berger MM, Oudemans-van Straaten HM. Vitamin C supplementation in the critically ill patient. *Curr Opin Clin Nutr Metab Care* 2015;18(2):193–201.

43. Traber MG, Atkinson J. Vitamin E, antioxidant and nothing more. *Free Radic Biol Med* 2007;43(1):4–15.

44. Azzi A. Molecular mechanism of alpha-tocopherol action. *Free Radic Biol Med* 2007;43(1):16–21.

45. Matos AC, Souza GG, Moreira V, Ramalho A. Effect of vitamin A supplementation on clinical evolution in patients undergoing coronary artery bypass grafting, according to serum levels of zinc. *Nutr Hosp* 2012;27(6):1981–6.

46. Corcoran TB, O'Neill MP, Webb SA, Ho KM. Inflammation, vitamin deficiencies and organ failure in critically ill patients. *Anaesth Intensive Care* 2009;37(5):740–7.

47. Lassnigg A, Punz A, Barker R, et al. Influence of intravenous vitamin E supplementation in cardiac surgery on oxidative

stress: a double blinded, randomized, controlled study. *Br J Anaesth* 2003;90(2):148–54.

48. Fowler AA 3rd, Syed AA, Knowlson S, et al. Phase I safety trial of intravenous ascorbic acid in patients with severe sepsis. *J Transl Med* 2014 Jan 31;12:32.

49. Martin JM, Stapleton RD. Omega-3 fatty acids in critical illness. *Nutr Rev.* 2010 Sep;68(9):531–50.

50. Simopoulos AP. Essential fatty acids in health and chronic disease. *Am J Clin Nutr* 1999;70(Suppl):S560.

51. Calder PC: n-3 polyunsaturated fatty acids, inflammation, and inflammatory diseases. *Am J Clin Nutr* 2006; 83 (Suppl 6): 1505S–1519S.

52. Wu A, Ying Z, Gomez-Pinilla F. Dietary omega-3 fatty acids normalize BDNF levels, reduce oxidative damage, and counteract learning disability after traumatic brain injury in rats. *J Neurotrauma* 2004 Oct;21(10):1457–67.

53. Serhan CN, Petasis NA. Resolvins and protectins in inflammation resolution. *Chem Rev* 2011;111(10): 5922–43.

54. Glenn JO, Wischmeyer PE. Enteral fish oil in critical illness: perspectives and systematic review. *Curr Opin Clin Nutr Metab Care* 2014 Mar;17(2):116–23.

55. Hu FB, Bronner L, Willett WC, et al. Fish and omega-3 fatty acid intake and risk of coronary heart disease in women. *JAMA* 2002;287(14):1815–21.

56. Mozaffarian D, Longstreth WT Jr, Lemaitre RN, et al. Fish consumption and stroke risk in elderly individuals: the cardiovascular health study. *Arch Intern Med* 165; 200–6.

57. Yoneda H, Shirao S, Kurokawa T, Fujisawa H, Kato S, Suzuki M. Does eicosapentaenoic acid (EPA) inhibit cerebral vasospasm in patients after aneurysmal subarachnoid hemorrhage? *Acta Neurol Scand* 118, 54–59.

58. Corrigan F, Mander KA, Leonard AV, et al. Neurogenic inflammation after traumatic brain injury and its potentiation of classical inflammation. *J Neuroinflammation* 2016 Oct 11;13(1):264.

59. Foley N, Marshall S, Pikul J, et al. Hypermetabolism following moderate to severe traumatic acute brain injury: a systematic review. *J Neurotrauma* 2008 Dec;25(12): 1415–31.

60. Hazeldine J, Lord JM, Belli A. Traumatic brain injury and peripheral immune suppression: primer and prospectus. *Front Neurol* 2015 Nov 5;6:235.

61. Bansal V, Costantini T, Kroll L, et al. Traumatic brain injury and intestinal dysfunction: Uncovering the neuro-enteric axis. *J Neurotrauma* 2009 Aug;26(8):1353–9.

62. Stover JF, Stocker R. Barbiturate coma may promote reversible bone marrow suppression in patients with severe isolated traumatic brain injury. *Eur J Clin Pharmacol* 1998 Sep;54(7):529–34.

63. Chendrasekkhar A, Fagerli JC, Prabhakar G, et al. Evaluation of an enhanced diet in patients with severe closed head injury. *Crit Care Med* 1997;25:A80.

64. Painter TJ, Rickerds J, Alban RF. Immune enhancing nutrition in traumatic brain injury—A preliminary study. *Int J Surg* 2015 Sep;21:70–4.

65. Falcao de Arruda IS, de Aguilar-Nascimento JE. Benefits of early enteral nutrition with glutamine and probiotics in brain injury patients. *Clin Sci (Lond)* 2004;106(3):287–92.

66. Marik PE, Zaloga GP. Immunonutrition in critically ill patients: a systematic review and analysis of the literature. *Intensive Care Med* 2008 Nov;34(11):1980–90.

67. Galban C, Montejo JC, Mesejo A, et al. An immune-enhancing enteral diet reduces mortality rate and episodes of bacteremia in septic intensive care unit patients. *Crit Care Med* 2000;28(3):643–8.

68. Beale RJ, Sherry T, Lei K, et al. Early enteral supplementation with key pharmaconutrients improves sequential organ failure assessment score in critically ill patients with sepsis: outcome of a randomized, controlled, double-blind trial. *Crit Care Med* 36:131–44.

69. Rice TW, Wheeler AP, Thompson BT, et al. Enteral omega-3 fatty acid, gamma-linolenic acid, and antioxidant supplementation in acute lung injury. *JAMA* 2011;306(14):1574–81.

70. Inger P, Theilla M, Fisher H, Gibstein L, Grozovski E, Cohen J. Benefit of an enteral diet enriched with eicosapentaenoic acid and gamma-linolenic acid in ventilated patients with acute lung injury. *Crit Care Med* 2006;34(4):1033–8.

71. Grau-Carmona T, Moran-Garcia V, Garcia-de-Lorenzo A, et al. Effect of an enteral diet enriched with eicosapentaenoic acid, gamma-linolenic acid and anti-oxidants on the outcome of mechanically ventilated, critically ill, septic patients. *Clin Nutr* 2011;30(5):578–84.

72. Stapleton RD, Martin TR, Weiss NS, et al. A phase II randomized placebo-controlled trial of omega-3 fatty acids for the treatment of acute lung injury. *Crit Care Med* 2011;39(7):1655–62.

Part XIV

Psychological Care

Editor: Ashima Nehra

50

Neuropsychological Assessment in the Neurointensive Care Setting: A Time-Based Approach

S. Bajpai and A. Nehra

ABSTRACT

Neurointensive care encompasses highly advanced care of patients suffering from acute and life-threatening diseases of the nervous system which requires a close monitoring of neurological functions and physiological parameters. In such a scenario, the role of neuropsychologists becomes multifaceted and has to be precisely defined from cognitive to psychosocial aspects. This chapter covers four aspects of neuropsychology which should be followed, especially in the neurointensive care setting. Firstly, what is the rationale and the need of neuropsychological assessment in such crunch scenarios; secondly, the basic assumptions and principles of neuropsychological testing; thirdly, the types of cognitive tests that could be used in neurointensive care which depends completely on the patient's alertness and neurointensive care procedures such as sedation, paralysis, monitoring techniques, etc. Lastly, the chapter concludes with a few major limitations and challenges of neuropsychological testing which are sometimes avoidable in such critical care situations.

KEYWORDS

Neuropsychological testing; neurologic patients; neurointensive care; Mini Mental State Examination (MMSE); Montreal Cognitive Assessment (MOCA); Dementia Assessment by Rapid Test (DART); Neuropsychological Evaluation Screening Tool (NEST).

INTRODUCTION

Neurocritical care specialists endeavour to improve health and clinical outcomes in patients with life-threatening neurological illnesses such as traumatic brain injury (TBI), spinal cord injury (SCI), cerebrovascular accidents, epilepsy, ruptured aneurysms, and neurological infections that require immediate medical and/or surgical intervention. Thus, it is typically undertaken by a collaboration of trained specialities, including neurosurgeons, neurologists, anaesthesiologists, and neurointensivists.[1] However, the role of neuropsychologists in such situations becomes multifaceted that has to be very precisely defined. It is

undeniable that such circumstances become a source of stress (including anxiety, depression, and pessimism) for the ill person, his or her family, and for the health personnel. It is therefore, the neuropsychologist who needs to have personal and professional skills that enable him/her to interact with people in special conditions, different to those commonly found in other professional fields. Likewise, he/she must integrate his/her knowledge of neuropsychological assessment in such a way that it suits the need of the other working professionals in the intensive care unit (ICU). This section briefly covers the need for neuropsychological assessments in the critical care settings; basic assumptions required for testing in such settings, few commonly used tests; and last but not the least, the limitations of neuropsychological testing.

NEED FOR NEUROPSYCHOLOGICAL ASSESSMENT IN THE NEUROINTENSIVE CARE SETTING

Neuropsychological assessment circumscribes clinical and psychometric testing procedures that objectively measure the effects of cerebral damage on cognition, social, emotional, and behavioural functioning.

In the last decade, researchers have become increasingly interested in the relationship between critical neurological illness and social-emotional-cognitive outcomes. For example, in one cohort study, 80% of survivors of acute respiratory distress syndrome (ARDS) had impaired memory, attention, or processing speed a year after hospital discharge,[2] and in another report, approximately 25% had mild cognitive impairment 6 months post ICU discharge.[3] However, there are no prospective reports describing neuropsychological impairment in the neurointensive setting. Thus, such researches depict a demanding need for neuropsychological testing not only to assess the current cognitive status of the patient, but also to track the level of cognitive stability, improvement, or impairment following discharge. Besides this, it also helps in planning for better prognosis in the patient through neuropsychological rehabilitation, thereby improving their quality of life.

BASIC ASSUMPTIONS OF NEUROPSYCHOLOGICAL TESTING IN NEUROINTENSIVE CARE

As neurointensive care has standard principles[4] to follow, neuropsychological testing too follows a pragmatic approach where the patient's current cognitive status plays a crucial role in planning cognitive prognosis for the long term.[5] Few of the assumptions are as follows:

- The patient has to be fully oriented, alert, awake, and conscious to the reality.
- The patient should not be under the influence of sedatives that hamper the cognitive status under evaluation.
- The patient's physical mobility also plays an important role—whether the patient is bedridden, wheelchair bound or attached to any electrophysiological and intracranial physiological monitoring indices— and whether that limits the performance ability of cognitive tasks.
- Damage to verbal ability, handedness, or movement too becomes challenging. Although clinical scales/ functional outcomes in such cases comes in handy.

- Above this, availability of the indigenous tests which are free from any education or culture bias (one of the major limitations of the Indian medical setup) plays a crucial role in assessing the cognitive status of the patient accurately.

COMMON TESTS USED IN THE NEUROINTENSIVE CARE SETTING

Cognitin is a broad term, which comprises a number of mental processes. These processes help an individual acquire, store, and process the information to make decisions and solve problems. These cognitive/mental abilities can be assessed by two means depending upon the assumptions mentioned above. If the patient is alert, conscious, and has no physical constraints, an objective cognitive test can be directly administered on the patient whereas if the patient has some physical or verbal limitation, relevant functional outcomes should be administered to the caregivers to know the best ability of the patient (Table 50.1). Each cognitive test and functional outcome scales are described briefly in three aspects in the subsequent section (Figure 50.1).

Neurointensive care and neuropsychology follows an antagonist time-based approach where the degree of time is limited at the neurointensive end whereas the neuropsychological testing is extensive on time. Thus, to suit the need of neurocritical care, three aspects of neuropsychological testing has to be considered: (1) identifying the target cognitive function; (2) the administration time (which has the utmost importance in neurocritical care settings); and (3) the applicability of the test (age, education, and gender specific relevance). After adjusting the above three aspects, the degree of time will be justified for any neurointensive care conditions.

Mini Mental Status Examination/Hindi Mental Status Examination

The Mini Mental Status Examination (MMSE)[6] is an assessment tool that has worldwide use as it is quite economical with respect to time and training required to administer. It is one of the cognitive tests which assesses multiple cognitive functions in a brief time period. This test includes domains of:

- Orientation to time and place
- Registration
- Attention and calculation
- Recall
- Language (receptive and expressive)
- Visuospatial construction

Besides its brevity and comprehensiveness, ample literature supports its use in various neurointensive conditions owing to its sensitivity. For e.g., a cut-off of 23 generally is used to differentiate normal functioning from cognitive impairment[7,8] with age and education specific norms. In an Indian context, considering the literacy and language factor, this scale was modified as Hindi Mental Status Examination (HMSE)[9] which comes out with good sensitivity and specificity.

Montreal Cognitive Assessment

The Montreal Cognitive Assessment (MOCA) is another substitute to the MMSE, which is more sensitive than the MMSE in discriminating impairment from normal functioning.[10] The MOCA places greater importance on assessing attention and executive functions as compared to the MMSE, although it includes slightly more difficult memory tasks in comparison with the MMSE. A maximum score of 30 can be obtained on the MOCA and a score below 26 is indicative of impairment.[11]

Dementia Assessment by Rapid Test

Dementia Assessment by Rapid Test (DART) is a recent indigenous screening tool developed in India that is administered directly to the patient. It has been developed as a quick screening tool for the clinician to not only have an instant perception of the patient's probable cognitive status but also to rule out the need for further evaluation.[10] It is a very brief tool at par to MMSE where multiple domains can be assessed without any applicability issues. The domains assessed include:

- Registration and recent memory
- Verbal fluency
- Delayed memory
- Visuo-spatial ability
- Executive functioning

The scoring of DART follows 'all or none' principle, i.e., each item is either scored 0 (correct) or 1 (incorrect). The range of scores is 0–4 which follows the interpretation of 'lower the score, less likelihood of cognitive impairment and higher the score, there is more likelihood of cognitive impairment'. Considering its sensitivity of 95.5% against MMSE, it is now widely used in various centres of India.[12]

Recently, in the Indian Scenario, newer scales such as Preliminary Aphasia Screening Test (PAST) are being devised, which are specifically targeted towards regional patient needs.

Neuropsychological Evaluation Screening Tool (NEST)

It is a quick, culture and education-free 6-item cognitive screening tool developed in India evaluating memory, executive functioning, attention, and visuo-spatial ability domains. This tool can be used on literates as well as the illiterate population. A cut-off of 3 holds 95.3% of sensitivity and 47.6% specificity against HMSE for detecting cognitive impairment.[13]

Neurobehavioural Cognitive Status Examination

The Neurobehavioural Cognitive Status Examination (NCSE, now known as Cognistat) is considered to be more comprehensive in nature than the MMSE or MOCA. The Cognistat was found to be more sensitive than the MMSE.[11] The domains assessed include:

- Level of consciousness
- Orientation
- Language (speech, comprehension, repetition, and naming)
- Memory
- Constructional ability
- Calculations
- Reasoning (similarities and judgement)

The Cognistat[14,15] takes approximately 10–20 minutes to administer. The interesting feature of this test is that it has a difficult screen item which is typically more difficult than the items that follow which are termed as the metric section. If the patient passes the screen item, the metric items in that section may be skipped bringing down the testing time to 5 minutes. The scores are also represented on a profile sheet highlighting the position of the score in comparison with an average making for easy interpretation and understanding.[7,11] Besides this, it has an Indian adaptation as well where the 'screen and metric' approach of assessment was eliminated. Despite that, the psychometric properties hold good value as it had very high internal consistency (Cronbach's alpha = 0.94).[16]

TESTS OF FUNCTIONAL STATUS

In a physically or cognitively constraint situation such as coma, the functional status rating scales could be used to estimate the current status of the patient.

Glasgow Outcome Scale and Extended Glasgow Outcome Scale

The Glasgow Outcome Scale (GOS)[17] has been frequently used with conditions such as TBI, stroke, etc.

The GOS assesses five levels of functional outcome and is regarded as the basis of the Extended Glasgow Outcome Scale (GOS-E)[18] as well as the Disability Rating Scale (DRS).[19] The GOS-E has three additional outcome category results in comparison to the GOS. The categories include:

- Dead
- Vegetative state
- Lower severe disability
- Upper severe disability
- Lower moderate disability
- Upper moderate disability
- Lower good recovery
- Upper good recovery

The E-GOS is frequently used as an outcome measure in neurosurgical studies while the DRS is generally the more popular choice in neuropsychological studies.[7]

Disability Rating Scale

The DRS[18] is a popular measure which includes eight items and four categories. Patients can observe a maximum score of 29 (indicative of extreme vegetative state) and a minimum of 0 (indicative of no disability). The DRS could be self-administered or rated by interviewing the patient, relative or caregiver. However, the scale is not very sensitive for high functioning patients with mild deficits.[7,20]

The Everyday Abilities Scale for India

The Everyday Abilities Scale for India (EASI) is an 11 item activities of daily living scale developed for the illiterate elderly population in the Ballabgarh rural area in North India which takes 5 minutes to administer. This study was conducted on people over 55 years of age and suggested an operational cut-off point of 3, yielding a sensitivity of 62.5% and specificity of 89.7%. Besides this, it has also been validated against MMSE, which showed 81.3%, and 89.7% of sensitivity and specificity, respectively. Thus, this tool is not just education and culture bias free but also holds good psychometric properties.[21]

Barthel Index

The Barthel Index assesses a patient's activities of daily living as well as their mobility. The original scale published in 1965 contained a 100-point evaluation of independence in 10 activities of daily living which can be assessed in 5–7 minutes.[22] These include: feeding, bathing, grooming, dressing, bowel, bladder, toilet use, transfers, mobility, and stairs.

Functional Independence Measure

The functional independence measure (FIM) is a detailed assessment that looks at various performance and behavioural variables. The rating assesses the individual in an attempt to understand the patient's level of dependence. Each domain is assessed on a 7-point scale with 7 being total independence and 1 being total assistance. The FIM assesses 18 items, grouped into 2 subscales—motor and cognition.[23] The motor subscale includes: eating, grooming, bathing, dressing (upper body and lower body), toileting, bladder management, bowel management, transfers to bed/chair/wheelchair, transfers to toilet, bath/shower, walk/wheelchair, and climbing stairs, while the cognition subscales include comprehension, expression, social interaction, problem solving, and memory.

Short Form-36 Health Survey (SF-36) and Short Form-12 Health Survey (SF-12)

The Short Form-36 Health Survey (SF-36) was developed by RAND Corporation as a part of a Medical outcomes study and comprises of 36 items that assess 8 domains of well-being which include vitality, physical functioning, bodily pain, general health perceptions, physical role functioning, emotional role functioning, social role functioning, and mental health.[24] It has the easiest scoring where the lowest score interpreted higher disability quotient.

The Short Form-12 Health Survey (SF-12)[25] as the name suggests is a shorter version of the SF-36. The SF-12 also assesses 8 domains but has fewer items in each domain. Although the shorter version is not as comprehensive as the SF-36, the SF-12 has been found to be a good tool. This is especially true if time is limited or if several other measures are also being used to assess the patient.[7]

The World Health Organization Quality of Life Scale and WHOQOL-BREF

The World Health Organization (WHO) Quality of Life (WHOQOL) scale is a quality of life assessment tool which consists of 100 items. It was developed by the WHO quality of life group with the aim of creating a quality of life measure that could be used across different cultures. The study was carried out in 15 international field centres simultaneously. The WHOQOL-BREF is a shortened version of the WHOQOL-100. It was developed by the WHO in 1996.

It consists of 26 items, which measure four broad domains:[26]

- Psychological health
- Physical health
- Social relationships
- Environment

The brief version was developed for convenience in larger research studies or clinical trials. The higher the score, the greater the estimation of good quality of life rated. This scale has an Indian adaptation too.[27]

Sickness Impact Profile

The Sickness Impact Profile (SIP)[28] is a behaviour measure to assess the health status. It assesses two major domains (physical and psychological) which are spread across 12 categories namely: sleep and rest, eating, work, home management, recreation and pastimes, ambulation, mobility, body care and movement, social interaction, alert behaviour, emotional behaviour, and communication.

The results are represented as a total score, two domain scores and 12 category scores. It consists of 136 items and can either be self-administered or administered by a professional. The test-retest reliability and internal consistency of the scale was found to be high. It is generally considered to be a long measure but is extremely detailed and comprehensive and is therefore widely used.[7]

Besides the above mentioned tests, there are other scales too which are commonly used in the neurointensive care settings such as COMBI (Centre for Outcome Measurement in Brain Injury), ImPACT concussion assessment test scales and many more.

LIMITATIONS OF NEUROPSYCHOLOGICAL ASSESSMENT IN THE NEUROINTENSIVE CARE

Neuropsychological assessment is laden with practical difficulties when it comes to critical illnesses where the test has to be chosen with specific physical and cognitive need per se. Sometimes, we get restricted due to neurointensive care which includes sedation, paralysis, monitoring techniques, etc., but nevertheless, as stated earlier, it is a time-based approach which is antagonistic in both the disciplines. Hence in such cases, the functional scales are the only approach to follow. However, the only caution in following this approach is interpreting the results as it takes great skill and expertise to interpret these results in light of the circumstances particular to the neurointensive care setting.

Table 50.1 Summary of neuropsychological tests based on the time taken to administer in neurointensive care centres

Domain	Test	Time taken (minutes)
Cognitive	MMSE/HMSE*	10
	MOCA**	10
	DART*	5
	PAST*	15
	NEST*	10
	Cognistat**	20
Functional Status	GOS/E-GOS	5
	DRS	10
	EASI*	5
	Barthel Index	10
	FIM	15
	SF-36/SF-12	20
	WHOQOL/WHO-BREF**	20
	SIP	10

*Tests developed in India.
**International tests adapted in India.

CONCLUSIONS

Neuropsychological assessment comprises clinical and psychometric testing procedures that objectively measure the effects of cerebral damage on cognition, social, emotional, and behaviour functioning. Since neurointensive care and neuropsychology follow an antagonist time-based approach where the time span is limited at the neurointensive care end while neuropsychological testing is extensive on time. Therefore, it is advisable to use short screening neuropsychological tests that are sensitive enough to provide a provisional cognitive report for undertaking the primary care of action. Nevertheless, post discharge, a full-fledged neuropsychological testing is mandatory for planning better prognosis.

REFERENCES

1. Suarez, Jose I. Outcome in neurocritical care: advances in monitoring and treatment and effect of a specialized neurocritical care team. *Critical Care Medicine* 2006; 34(9):S232–S238.
2. Hopkins R, Weaver L, Pope D, et al. Neuropsychological sequelae and impaired health status in survivors of severe acute respiratory distress syndrome. *Am J Respir Crit Care Med* 1999;160(1):50.
3. Jackson JC, Hart RP, Gordon SM, et al. Six-month neuropsychological outcome of medical intensive care unit patients. *Crit Care Med* 2003;31(4):1226.
4. Grant IS, Andrews PJ. ABC of intensive care: neurological support. *BMJ* 1999;319(7202):110.

5. Evans JJ. Basic concepts and principles of neuropsychological assessment. *Handbook of Clinical Neuropsychology*. 2003: 15–26.

6. Folstein MF, Folstein SE, McHugh PR. Mini-mental state. A practical method for grading the cognitive state of patients for the clinician. *Journal of Psychiatric Research* 1975;12(3):189–98.

7. Daroff, Robert B, Joseph Jankovic, John CM, Scott LP, editors. *Bradley's Neurology in Clinical Practice*. London: Elsevier Health Sciences, 2015; pp. 511–27.

8. Brambrink, Ansgar M, Jeffrey RK. *Essentials of Neurosurgical Anesthesia and Critical Care: Strategies for Prevention, Early Detection, and Successful Management of Perioperative Complications*. London: Springer Science and Business Media, 2011,109; pp. 731–40.

9. Ganguli, Mary, Graham Ratcliff, et al. A Hindi version of the MMSE: the development of a cognitive screening instrument for a largely illiterate rural elderly population in India. *International Journal of Geriatric Psychiatry* 1995; 10(5):367–77.

10. Nasreddine ZS, Phillips NA, Bedirian V, et al. The Montreal Cognitive Assessment, MoCA: a brief screening tool for mild cognitive impairment. *Journal of the American Geriatrics Society* 2005;53(4):695–9.

11. Le Roux PD, Levine JM, Kofke WA. *Monitoring in Neurocritical Care*. Philadelphia, PA: Elsevier/Saunders; 2013. [Cited 2018 Jun 21] Available from: https://www.clinicalkey.com/dura/browse/bookChapter/3-s2.0-C20090386158.

12. Swati B, Sreenivas V, Manjari T, Ashima N. Dementia Assessment by Rapid Test (DART): An Indian screening tool for dementia. *J Alzheimers Dis Parkinsonism* 2015; 5:198.

13. Chopra S, Kaur H, Pandey RM, Nehra A. Development of neuropsychological evaluation screening tool: An education-free cognitive screening instrument. *Neurology India* 2018 Mar 1;66(2):391.

14. Schwamm LH, Van Dyke C, Kiernan RJ, Merrin EL, Mueller J. The neurobehavioral cognitive status examination: comparison with the cognitive capacity screening examination and the mini-mental state examination in a neurosurgical population. *Annals of Internal Medicine* 1987;107(4):486–91.

15. Kiernan RJ, Mueller J, Langston JW, Van Dyke C. The neurobehavioral cognitive status examination: a brief but quantitative approach to cognitive assessment. *Annals of Internal Medicine* 1987;107(4):481–5.

16. Gupta A, Kumar NK. Indian adaptation of the Cognistat: Psychometric properties of a cognitive screening tool for patients of traumatic brain injury. *The Indian Journal of Neurotrauma* 2009;6(2):123–32.

17. Wilson JTL, Laura ELP, Graham MT. Structured interviews for the Glasgow Outcome Scale and the extended Glasgow Outcome Scale: guidelines for their use. *Journal of Neurotrauma* 1998;15(8):573–85.

18. Weir J, Steyerberg EW, Butcher I, et al. Does the extended Glasgow Outcome Scale add value to the conventional Glasgow Outcome Scale? *Journal of Neurotrauma* 2012; 29(1):53–8.

19. Bellon K, Wright J, Jamison L, Kolakowsky-Hayner S. Disability Rating Scale. *The Journal of Head Trauma Rehabilitation* 2012;27(6):449–51.

20. Fillenbaum GG, Chandra V, Ganguli M. Development of an activities of daily living scale to screen for dementia in an illiterate rural older population in India. *Age and Ageing* 1999;28:161–8.

21. Raina SK, Chander V, Raina S, Kumar D. Feasibility of using everyday abilities scale of India as alternative to mental state examination as a screen in two-phase survey estimating the prevalence of dementia in largely illiterate Indian population. *Indian J Psychiatry* 2016;58: 459–61.

22. Mahoney FI, Barthel DW. Functional Evaluation: The Barthel Index. *Maryland State Medical Journal* 1965;14: 61–5.

23. Linacre, John Michael, Allen WH, Benjamin DW, Carl VG, Byron BH. The structure and stability of the functional independence measure. *Archives of Physical Medicine and Rehabilitation* 1994;75(2):127–32.

24. Ware Jr, John E, Cathy Donald Sherbourne. The MOS 36-item short-form health survey (SF-36): I. Conceptual framework and item selection. *Medical Care* 1992: 473–83.

25. Jenkinson C. A shorter form health survey: can the SF-12 replicate results from the SF-36 in longitudinal studies? *Journal of Public Health Medicine* 1997;19(2):179–86. PMID 9243433.

26. Skevington SM, Lotfy M, O'Connell KA, Group W. The World Health Organization's WHOQOL-BREF quality of life assessment: psychometric properties and results of the international field trial. A report from the WHOQOL group. *Quality of Life Research: An International Journal of Quality of Life Aspects of Treatment, Care and Rehabilitation* 2004;13(2):299–310.

27. Saxena S, Chandiramani K, Bhargava R. WHOQOL-Hindi: A questionnaire for assessing quality of life in health care settings in India. World Health Organization Quality of Life. *Natl Med J India* 1998;11:160–5.

28. Bergner M, Bobbitt RA, Carter WB, Gilson BS. The sickness impact profile: development and final revision of a health status measure. *Medical Care* 1981;19(8): 787–805.

51

Assessment and Management of Delirium in Medical Practice

S. Grover and N. Kate

ABSTRACT

Delirium is a reversible neuropsychiatric syndrome, which is highly prevalent in medically and surgically ill patients. It is characterized by the acute onset of symptoms with a fluctuating course and clinical characteristics in the form of altered level of consciousness, disturbance in attention, and other cognitive functions (i.e., disorientation, disturbance in memory, visuospatial abilities, etc.), thought disturbances, perceptual abnormalities, and behavioural problems. Delirium is associated with high mortality rate, cognitive decline and development of dementia, prolonged hospital stay, need for institutional care, poor functionality, and cost of treatment distress to the patient and family. Due to these adverse outcomes, it is important to detect and manage delirium. This chapter provides an overview of the risk factors, aetiopathogenesis, clinical features, nosology, assessment, differential diagnosis, management, prevention, and prognosis of delirium.

KEYWORDS

Delirium; assessment; clinical features; risk factors; management.

INTRODUCTION

Delirium is a reversible neuropsychiatric syndrome seen quite frequently in medically ill patients. Considering the fact that the clinical syndrome is seen in different medical surgical settings, it is referred with different names by physicians from different disciplines. Some of the commonly used terms include acute confusional state, acute brain failure, intensive care unit (ICU) psychosis, hepatic encephalopathy, metabolic encephalopathy, and toxic psychosis.[1] It is characterized by acute onset of symptoms, with a fluctuating course and clinical characteristics in the form of altered level of consciousness, disturbance in attention span and other cognitive functions (i.e., disorientation, disturbance in memory, visuospatial abilities, etc.), thought disturbances, perceptual abnormalities, and behavioural problems. The alteration in the mental status in delirium is considered to be on a continuum between normal wakefulness and alertness at one extreme end and coma and stupor at the other end.[1]

Delirium is associated with high mortality rate, cognitive decline and development of dementia, prolonged hospital stay, need for institutional care, poor functionality, and cost of treatment distress to the patient and family.[2] Hence it is important to detect and manage delirium to reduce the emergent morbidity, mortality, and associated distress among patients and caregivers.[2]

EPIDEMIOLOGY: PREVALENCE AND INCIDENCE

Prevalence of delirium has varied across different studies with generally higher rates reported for patients admitted to various ICUs. According to a review, which included data from mostly prospective studies, incidence of delirium varies from 3% to 42%, and the prevalence varies from 5% to 44% in hospitalized patients.[3] The prevalence and incidence among various studies is influenced by the study setting (ICU setting, medical/surgical ward, postoperative patients, consultation-liaison psychiatry services), population assessed, and method used for identification (screening instrument and diagnostic instrument). In general, it is seen that delirium is more often encountered among patients of older age, those with cognitive impairment/dementia, certain medical or surgical problems (infections, renal impairment, fracture of the neck of femur, etc.), and admission to the ICU.[3] Recent studies, which have focused on a whole period of hospital stay have come up with prevalence figures of as high as 82%.[4,5] It is further noted that 20%–50% of subjects with less severe physical problems admitted to the ICU develop delirium whereas those requiring mechanical ventilation have prevalence of delirium in the range of 50%–80%. Further, in a small proportion of cases (10%), delirium persists at discharge.[4–9] Studies evaluating the incidence of delirium suggest that ICU delirium usually starts after 2 ± 1.7 days of ICU stay and usually lasts 4.2 ± 1.7 days.[6–8,10] Data from India suggest that prevalence and incidence of delirium are 53.57% and 24.41%, respectively, among patients admitted to the respiratory intensive care unit. The prevalence was higher (64%) among those on mechanical ventilation and in the elderly (95.83%).[11] A study evaluated patients admitted to the Coronary Care Unit (CCU) and reported prevalence and incidence to be 18.77% and 9.27%, respectively.[12] A study which evaluated the prevalence and incidence among patients admitted to the general ICU reported prevalence of 68.2% and incidence of 59.6%.[13]

NOSOLOGY

There have been minor modifications in the criteria used to define delirium. The Diagnostic and Statistical Manual of Mental Disorders (DSM-III)[14] laid emphasis on 'clouding of consciousness with reduced capacity to shift, focus, and sustain attention' to be the core feature. DSM-III-R[15] moved the emphasis from 'clouding of consciousness' to 'reduced attentiveness' and 'disorganized thinking', each as a major criterion and the term 'clouding of consciousness' was dropped. The DSM-IV[16] again maintained the emphasis on 'disturbance in consciousness and inattention' as one of the major criteria and described five types of delirium depending on the aetiology. The DSM-5[17] again changed the emphasis to disturbance in attention (i.e., reduced ability to direct, focus, sustain, and shift attention) and awareness (reduced orientation to the environment). However, this approach of DSM-5 has been questioned by some of the authors.[18] A study which evaluated the concordance between DSM-IV and DSM-5 criteria for delirium reported that the concordance rate varied significantly depending on the interpretation of criteria. Further the authors noted that if someone tries

to use the DSM-5 criteria very strictly, then the number of cases diagnosed with delirium will reduce, whereas, use of a more relaxed approach yields comparable rates to DSM-IV.[18]

The DSM-5 criteria for delirium is:[17]

1. Disturbance in attention (i.e., reduced ability to direct, focus, sustain, and shift attention) and awareness (reduced orientation to the environment).
2. The disturbance has developed over a short period of time (usually hours to a few days), represents a change from baseline attention and awareness, and tends to fluctuate in severity during the course of a day.
3. An additional disturbance in cognition (e.g., memory deficit, disorientation, language, visuospatial ability, or perception).
4. The disturbances in Criteria (1) and (3) are not better explained by a pre-existing, established, or evolving neurocognitive disorder and do not occur in the context of a severely reduced level of arousal, such as coma.
5. There is evidence from the history, physical examination, or laboratory findings that the disturbance is a direct physiological consequence of another medical condition, substance intoxication or withdrawal, or exposure to a toxin, or is due to multiple aetiologies.

The World Health Organization's (WHO) International Classification of Diseases (ICD) (10th revision)[19] describes disturbance in cognition manifested by both 'impairment of immediate recall and recent memory' and 'disorientation to time, place, and person.' Additionally, the ICD-10 also provides criteria for 'disturbance in sleep–wake cycle', 'psychomotor disturbances', and 'emotional disturbances'. Further, ICD-10 specifies the upper limit of duration of delirium to 6 months, hence it does not allow inclusion of cases with chronic delirium. Occasional studies which have evaluated the concordance between DSM-IV and ICD-10 suggest that DSM-IV is more sensitive than ICD-10 for the diagnosis of delirium.[20]

CLINICAL FEATURES OF DELIRIUM

The clinical features of delirium encompass a constellation of physical, biological, and psychological disturbances. However, it is important to note that all the symptoms are not seen in all patients and most of the studies which have reported symptoms included patients in non-ICU settings. The frequency of different symptoms vary across different studies and the commonly reported symptoms include inattention, disturbance in sleep–wake cycle, and change in the motor activity (hypoactive/hyperactive), which are considered as core features of delirium.[21]

Symptoms of delirium can broadly be divided into cognitive and non-cognitive. The cognitive symptoms comprise disturbances in the domains of attention, memory, orientation, comprehension, vigilance, visuo-spatial abilities, and executive functioning. Among these, inattention is the most consistent feature and is considered as an important diagnostic criterion. Impairment of attention in patients with delirium involves all aspects, i.e., difficulty in mobilizing, shifting, and sustaining attention. Memory disturbances include both short- and long-term memory with particular disruption of recent memory. Disorientation to time, place, and person is also common. Visuo-spatial disturbances are also common and impair the functionality of patients in a clinical setting.[2] The non-cognitive symptoms of delirium include speech and language disturbances, sleep–wake cycle disturbances, and psychotic symptoms. Sleep–wake cycle disturbances range from napping and nocturnal disruptions to severe disintegration of the normal circadian cycle. Other symptoms include psychotic features and affective lability. In terms of symptoms, data in general suggests that the symptom profile does not differ much across different age groups, i.e., among children and adolescents, adults, and elderly.[2]

Based on the psychomotor activity, delirium is subtyped as hyperactive, hypoactive, and mixed.[1] In general, studies which have evaluated referred patients of delirium seen in a consultation-liaison psychiatry setup report hyperactive delirium to be the most common subtype whereas studies from the ICU or those which have screened inpatients for delirium report hypoactive delirium as the most common subtype of delirium.[2] Studies which have evaluated the outcome of delirium suggest that those with hypoactive delirium have higher mortality rates.[11,12]

Many factor analytic studies have tried to delineate the symptom clusters of delirium. These studies in general suggest that symptoms of delirium load onto two to three factors with minor differences in composition of symptoms across different factors. In most of the factor analytic studies, the cognitive symptoms load together onto one factor, the motor and psychotic symptoms load together, and the third factor consists of language disturbances, abnormality in the thought process, and diagnostic items. In general the motor and psychotic symptom factors have been reported to have better consistency across different studies.[22–26] Studies conducted in ICUs have in general come up with two-factor models.[27,28]

RISK FACTORS FOR DELIRIUM

In general delirium is considered to be multi-factorial in origin.[1,29,30] Certain factors are considered to predispose a person to develop delirium and other factors have been shown to be associated with development of delirium. Accordingly various authors have categorized these factors as risk factors/predisposing factors and aetiological/precipitating factors. However, it is important to note that there is some overlap in these factors. *Predisposing factors* are those factors which reflect the underlying vulnerability of the individual to delirium and are often present prior to admission to the hospital. In contrast, *precipitating factors* are those noxious insults or hospital-related factors which contribute to the development of delirium. In general predisposing risk factors are considered to have relatively greater contribution than the precipitating factors for the onset of delirium.[1] It is important to note that the predisposing and precipitating factors also vary according to treatment setting, for example, the predisposing and precipitating factors associated with delirium seen in the cardiac ICU, respiratory ICU, and medical inpatient setting vary. Among all the risk factors, higher age, pre-existing cognitive impairment, severe co-existing illnesses, and exposure to medication are considered as 'robust risk factors'.[1] According to a recent review, the commonly associated risk factors for delirium among the elderly in acute hospital medical units include dementia, older age, co-morbid illness, higher severity of medical illness, infection, use of 'high-risk' medications, diminished activities of daily living, immobility, sensory impairment, presence of urinary catheter, raised urea levels, electrolyte imbalance, and malnutrition. Among these factors, which were shown to be significantly associated with delirium in the pooled analyses, dementia, higher severity of illness, presence of visual impairment, presence of urinary catheter, low serum albumin level, and longer duration of hospital stay had statistically significant association with delirium.[29]

Predisposing Factors

The predisposing factors for delirium are:[1,29,30]

- Cognitive decline/dementia
- Visual or hearing impairment
- Poorer functionality/immobility
- Older age
- Male gender
- Severity of illness, elevated APACHE II score
- Brain disorders like Parkinson's disease, tumours
- Co-morbid illnesses

- Alcohol abuse
- Use of medications (prescribed or non-prescribed)
- Urinary catheterization, presence of intravenous lines, bladder catheters, physical restraints
- History of hypertension
- Vascular disease/history of stroke
- History of alcohol abuse, substance abuse, or smoking
- Past history of delirium
- Perioperative: course of postoperative period, type of surgery (e.g., hip replacement), emergency surgery, longer duration of surgery, type of anaesthetic, postoperative pain, intraoperative blood loss
- Social isolation
- Immobility

Precipitating Factors

The precipitating factors for delirium are:[1,29,30]

- Malnutrition
- Any iatrogenic event during hospitalization
- Use of physical restraints
- Use of more than three newly prescribed medications
- High number of procedures during early hospitalization (X-rays, blood tests, etc.)
- Intensive care treatment
- Prolonged waiting time before surgery
- Dehydration
- Metabolic disturbances: electrolyte imbalance, anaemia, acid-base imbalance, hypoglycaemia
- Acute renal or hepatic failure
- Sleep disturbances
- Withholding visual or hearing aids
- Hypoxia
- Postoperative pain and poor pain management
- Infection
- Alcohol and benzodiazepine withdrawal
- Congestive cardiac failure, acute myocardial infarction
- Use of drugs with high anticholinergic activity, opiates, benzodiazepines, corticosteroids, psychotropic medications, antihistamines, anti-parkinsonian medications, anti-epileptics

AETIOPATHOGENESIS OF DELIRIUM

From an aetiopathogenesis point of view, factors which lead to delirium can be broadly divided into two distinct classes, i.e., those that cause direct brain insults (dysfunction and damage) and those which elicit aberrant stress response. The factors which are considered to act directly on the brain include hypoxia and various metabolic disturbances. Other precipitating factors such as severe illness, surgery,

and trauma are considered to induce immune activation and physical stress which leads to increased activity of the hypothalamo-pituitary-adrenocorticoid axis and changes in the permeability of the blood-brain barrier. This leads to elevated levels of cortisol (in cerebrospinal fluid [CSF] but not in serum), which is considered to precipitate and maintain delirium. Predisposing factors like ageing leads to changes in the blood–brain barrier (BBB) permeability, neuronal loss, alteration in stress management neurotransmitters, reduced vascular density, and changes in intracellular signal transmission systems. Based on the understanding of these factors, multiple hypotheses have been proposed to understand the underlying aetiopathogenesis of delirium. These include neuro-inflammatory hypothesis, neuronal ageing hypothesis, oxidative stress hypothesis, neurotransmitter deficiency hypothesis, neuroendocrine hypothesis, diurnal dysregulation hypothesis, and network disconnectivity hypotheses. It is important to understand that most of these hypotheses are not independent and rather these are complementary to each other. The basic understanding is that a host of factors considered in these hypotheses ultimately lead to a common pathway which involves disturbance in neurotransmitters. The neurotransmitters commonly implicated in the pathogenesis of delirium include reduction in the acetylcholine levels and increase in dopamine levels. Other neurotransmitter abnormalities which have been described include alteration in the level of norepinephrine, glutamate, gamma-aminobutyric acid (GABA), serotonin, and melatonin (Figure 51.1).[31] It is also important to understand that delirium is not just an interaction of acetylcholine and dopamine, but these systems also interact with glutamate, GABA, and opioids.

DIFFERENTIAL DIAGNOSIS

The most common differential diagnosis of delirium is dementia, especially among the elderly patients. Other diagnoses which are often confused with delirium include primary psychiatric disorders like depression and psychosis/schizophrenia.[32,33] It is important to remember that dementia is also a risk factor for delirium and many elderly patients can have delirium superimposed on dementia and the phenomenology of delirium occurring in the background of dementia is not different from delirium seen in patients without premorbid cognitive disturbances.[34] In contrast to delirium, dementia often has insidious onset, progressive downhill course, and cognitive symptoms are seen in the absence of altered levels of consciousness. The presence of persistent sadness of mood and morning worsening of symptoms are characteristics of depression, whereas delirium is characterized by lability of mood and evening worsening of symptoms. Patients of delirium more often have visual and tactile hallucinations, whereas auditory hallucinations are predominant in patients of schizophrenia. Further, cognitive disturbances are not as prominent as delirium in patients with schizophrenia.[1]

MANAGEMENT OF DELIRIUM

It is very important to identify delirium at the earliest and treat the same adequately because delirium is associated with significantly increased risk of mortality, longer hospitalization, and medical complications (falls, infection, bed sores), even after controlling for confounders. The management of delirium should focus on identification and correction or removal of the aetiological factors and treatment of specific symptoms of delirium, including:

- Identifying, monitoring, and treating the underlying cause
- Medications associated with delirium: discontinuing or reducing the dose of causative agent
- Identifying and eliminating other contributory factors for delirium
- Using specific antidotes in poisoning or toxic conditions
- Using non-pharmacological measures
- Using pharmacological agents for management of delirium

Before starting treatment, it is important that the diagnosis of all medical conditions, including neurological conditions must be clearly established, and the mental state and behaviour of the patient should be quantified through standardized assessment tools. The family members and caregiver should be involved in the care. They should be explained about the nature of the condition and their role in management in the form of providing regular reorientation cues, how to talk to the patient, and how to maintain the environment so as to reduce the confusion in the patient.[1]

The patient's treatment must be reviewed both for prescription and over the counter medications with special focus on recent addition of any new drug or an increase in dosage of medication. The offending agent must be removed in consultation with the primary treating team. Additionally, all non-required medications need to be stopped.[35] Delirium may be attributed to a medication when there is a temporal correlation between onset of delirium and starting of medication or change in the dose of medication. An important aspect of management is communication between the primary

treating team, family members, and the liaison mental health professionals. Many a times, because of the predominant psychiatric symptoms, the physicians and surgeons consider delirium to be a primary psychiatric disorder and request the mental health professionals to shift the patient to the psychiatric unit. In such a scenario, it is important to inform the primary team members that although the patient is having a clinical picture akin to primary psychiatric disorders like psychosis, delirium is a result of the underlying medical-surgical aetiology and is reversible. Similarly, anxiety of family members must also be allayed and they must be clearly explained about their role in management of delirium.

Management directed at symptoms specific for delirium can be broadly divided into non-pharmacological management and pharmacological management. These have been discussed in the following paragraphs.

Non-Pharmacological Treatment

Non-pharmacological treatment involves providing support and orientation, providing an unambiguous environment and maintaining competence. It is important to provide support in both environmental and social terms. It is critical that the environment is manipulated in such a way that it makes the patient comfortable.[34] Psychological care must not be limited to the symptomatic phase only, as even after recovery many patients report distress arising out of the whole experience of delirium.[35–37]

Support and orientation can be provided by:

- Frequently reorienting the patient (repeated reminders for the day, time and location, and identity of key individuals including team members treating the patient)
- Clear and concise communication—communication with the patient should be slow, simple, clear, and firm with frequent reminders
- Making eye contact, frequent touching, and using clear verbal instructions when talking to patients
- Providing clear markers/signs for patient's location
- Providing items such as a clock, a calendar, and a chart with the day's schedule in the patients room
- Keeping personal/familiar objects (photos, favourite blanket) from the patient's home in the room to enhance orientation and security
- Encouraging the patient to indulge in cognitively stimulating activities: many times a day (puzzle books, magazines, or video games, etc.)
- Avoiding frequent changes to attendant staff
- Using a television/radio/smartphone or other means for relaxation and to help the patient maintain contact

with the outside world—listening to light music can prevent under-stimulation while also buffering against noise extremes

- Avoiding physical restraints, if possible. If used, the restraints should be remove in a timely manner
- Involving family members/caregivers to encourage feelings of security and orientation

An *unambiguous environment* can be provided by:

- Removing unnecessary objects in the care area and having adequate space between beds
- If available, providing a single room to aid rest and avoid extremes of sensory experience. This reduces the disturbance caused by staff attending other patients in the same room
- Keeping the patient's bed at one place
- Avoiding using medical jargon in front of the patient as this may encourage paranoia
- Providing appropriate lighting to the time of day and minimal lighting at night may reduce disorientation (40–60 W night light reduces misperceptions)
- Reducing noise (use of vibrating pagers/phones rather than call bells, cut down on noise from staff, equipment, visitors with an aim of <45 decibels during the daytime and <20 decibels at night)
- Keeping the room's temperature between 21°C and 23.8°C

Competence can be maintained by:

- Identifying and correcting sensory impairments; ensuring that the patients have their glasses, hearing aid, and dentures
- Using an interpreter, if needed
- Encouraging self-care and participation in treatment (for example have the patient give feedback on pain)
- Scheduling treatment/interventions/IV fluids in such a way that the patient can have maximum periods of uninterrupted sleep (use a sleep protocol to promote quiet hours)
- Ambulating/mobilizing the patient at the earliest. If ambulation is not possible then encouraging full range of movements for at least 15 minutes three times a day
- Ensuring adequate nutrition
- Removing the urinary catheter, central line, IV line, etc. at the earliest
- Providing adequate skin care and measures to prevent a fall

Other ways of offering support include:

- Preventing hypoxia, electrolyte imbalance
- Management of severe pain
- Elimination of unnecessary medications

- Regulation of bowel/bladder
- Prevention, detection, and treatment of major postoperative complications

Importance should also be given to the psychological needs of the caregivers as they can play an important role in the re-integration of the patient, both cognitively and socially. Providing adequate information about delirium is of paramount importance. In eastern countries like India, many a times, because of presence of psychotic symptoms, many caregivers attribute delirium to supernatural causes, a result of religious disobedience and attention-seeking behaviour.[38] Further, certain symptoms such as decreased sleep, raised motor activity, attempts to get out of bed, and attempts to remove intravenous lines and tubings are associated with severe or very severe distress.[39] Hence, it is important to understand the aetiological models and distress of caregivers. Clinicians and mental health professionals should help the caregivers understand the nature of the condition and specific needs of the patient. The caregivers must be clearly informed that delirium is a result of underlying severe physical illness, will be short-lasting and fluctuating in nature. Good therapeutic alliance with patients and caregivers is very useful. The prognosis of delirium with respect to the underlying physical illnesses, including neurological illness should be elucidated and explained in detail. The caregivers must be explained about the reorientation cues and what they can do to reduce the confusion of patients. Even after the symptoms of delirium recede, the caregivers must be encouraged to maintain follow-up for the psychiatric symptoms along with their existing condition, allowing for close monitoring to prevent further complications of the symptoms.

Pharmacological Treatment

Various pharmacological agents have been tried for the management of delirium. These include antipsychotics, cholinesterase medications, benzodiazepines, highly selective α-2 receptor agonist (dexmedetomidine), and melatonin.

- Antipsychotics: haloperidol, droperidol, risperidone, quetiapine, olanzapine, aripiprazole, zuclopenthixol, ziprasidone, perospirone
- Benzodiazepines: Lorazepam
- Cholinesterase inhibitors: Donepezil, physostigmine, rivastigmine
- Highly selective α-2 receptor agonist: dexmedetomidine
- Melatonin-based medications: ramelteon, melatonin

Among all these agents, antipsychotics are considered as the medication of choice in the treatment of delirium.[40]

Among the various antipsychotics, haloperidol is considered to be the most preferred agent. Haloperidol has the advantage of availability in different formulations (oral, intramuscular and intravenous) and lower chance of sedation and hypotension. It is usually initiated in the dose range of 1–2 mg, 2–4 hourly (0.25–0.50 mg, 4 hourly for elderly), with titration to higher doses, as needed. However, one major problem with haloperidol is the need for monitoring the electrocardiogram because of increased incidence of cardiac conduction defects such as prolongation of the QT interval and arrhythmias, which can further lead to torsade de pointes and ventricular fibrillation.[40] A recent review concluded that the use of haloperidol is associated with reduction in severity of symptoms of delirium and not associated with treatment-limiting side effects. However, the authors cautioned that few studies have systematically assessed adverse events.[41]

Over the years data has accumulated for risperidone, quetiapine, olanzapine, aripiprazole, zuclopenthixol, ziprasidone, and perospirone in the management of delirium.[42] However, multiple reviews suggest that data from randomized controlled trials (RCTs), especially double-blind RCTs is limited. Available data suggest that various atypical antipsychotics like olanzapine, risperidone, and quetiapine to be as efficacious as haloperidol in reducing the severity of delirium and improving the cognitive functions and have lower incidence of side effects when compared to haloperidol.[43,44] One double-blind, placebo-controlled trial showed that quetiapine reduces the severity of non-cognitive symptoms of delirium faster than placebo.[45] While using atypical antipsychotics, it is important to note that the mean doses required for control of symptoms of delirium are much lower than those used conventionally for the management of other psychiatric disorders. Accordingly, when used these must be started in low doses and then titrated upwards as per the need.[46] Regarding the duration of treatment, there is some consensus to suggest that these may be tapered off after one week of symptom-free period.[1]

Benzodiazepines are not the first line treatment for management of delirium as these can often worsen the cognitive functions and lead to excessive sedation. Use of benzodiazepines is generally limited to delirium, which is attributable to sedative or alcohol withdrawal or in patients with delirium associated with seizures. However, it is important to note that such cases of delirium more often are multifactorial and the use of antipsychotics along with benzodiazepines may be required. Among the various benzodiazepines, lorazepam is preferred because of its short half-life, lack of major active metabolites, and relatively

predictable bioavailability when given intramuscularly. As with antipsychotics when used, benzodiazepines must be used in lower doses in the elderly, those with respiratory or hepatic impairment, or those receiving medications which undergo extensive hepatic oxidative metabolism.[42] It is important to remember that in general benzodiazepines are contraindicated in delirium associated with hepatic encephalopathy as in this condition there is accumulation of glutamine, which is chemically related to GABA.[40] Further, if benzodiazepines are to be used in patients with hepatic insufficiency or those receiving other medications metabolized by the cytochrome P450 system, benzodiazepines which are primarily metabolized by glucuronidation (lorazepam, oxazepam, and temazepam) should be used. Other conditions in which benzodiazepines must be used with caution include those with respiratory insufficiency. While using benzodiazepine, lower doses must be used and the patient's condition must be serially monitored to titrate the doses.[40]

There are few reports on the use of combination of antipsychotics and benzodiazepines (haloperidol and lorazepam) and these suggest that the use of this combination may decrease the emergent side effects and may improve the clinical effectiveness (shorter duration of delirium, and less extrapyramidal symptoms) in special populations, like those with severely ill cancer and acquired immunodeficiency syndrome (AIDS).[40]

As delirium is considered to be an outcome of excess acetylcholine, cholinergic medications have also been evaluated among patients with delirium. Among these agents, physostigmine, which is a centrally active cholinesterase inhibitor has been most commonly evaluated, although few studies have also evaluated the usefulness of tacrine and donepezil. However, the evidence is very limited for this class of medications.[42]

Dexmedetomidine, which is a highly selective α-2 receptor agonist has also been evaluated in the management of delirium because it has sedating properties which are not mediated through GABA receptors, anxiolytics, and modest analgesic properties. These effects are associated with minimal respiratory depression. All these features have led to the use of this medication in delirium, especially among those in ICUs. A recent review, which included data from eight clinical trials, five of which were double-blind RCTs, although of small sample size concluded that dexmedetomidine may be useful in the treatment of delirium.[47]

Considering the role of melatonin in the aetiopathogenesis of delirium, some of the preliminary reports have reported the beneficial effect of ramelteon.[48–50]

Hyperactive delirium often leads to overexertion, fatigue, and hypercatabolic state. These further complicate the clinical picture by exacerbating hypoxia and metabolic abnormalities. Hence, when patients with hyperactive delirium do not respond to conventional pharmacological agents, paralytic agents along with mechanical ventilation are considered in the management of delirium in the ICU setting. Use of heavy sedation with morphine improves oxygenation and reduces skeletal muscle exertion. Further, morphine and other opioids are also useful in patients of delirium where pain is a precipitating or contributory factor.[40] However, it is important to remember that like benzodiazepines, opiates can also worsen or cause delirium, especially those with anticholinergic properties (i.e., meperidine and fentanyl).

Some authors suggest beneficial effect of electroconvulsive therapy (ECT) in the management of delirium. However, the limited data which is available mainly in the form of case reports is not sufficient to consider the use of ECT as a substitute of conservative and conventional treatments. The use of ECT must be limited to cases of delirium, such as those associated with neuroleptic malignant syndrome, who have not responded to other measures.[40]

PREVENTION OF DELIRIUM

Considering the negative impact of delirium on patient outcomes, it is better to prevent delirium by identifying the risk factors and those who are at high risk for development of delirium. As with treatment of delirium, preventive strategies for delirium also include removal of unnecessary medications, ensuring appropriate hydration and nutrition, adequate and appropriate pain management, minimizing sensory deprivation by correction of sensory deficits, ensuring adequate sleep and providing adequate cognitive stimulation.[1] Additionally, patient education and/or preparation prior to surgery can help in reducing the rate of delirium.[51] Evidence suggests that among elderly patients, preoperative mental health consultations in non-delirious patients followed by daily visits for the duration of hospitalization and targeted recommendations based on a structured protocol reduce the incidence of delirium.[52] Some of the steps that can help prevent delirium include:

- Adequate lighting
- Ensure adequate sleep
- Avoid room changes
- Limit exposure to medications which are more likely to cause delirium (anticholinergics) and use alternative agents if possible

- Adjust dose of medications in patients with impaired drug clearance
- Always weigh the risk and benefit of use of anticholinergics, opioids, and sedatives, especially in elderly and vulnerable subjects
- Avoid using high doses, especially while using polypharmacy
- Provide non-pharmacological support in the form of frequent reorientation, minimization of sensory deprivation (restoration of eyeglasses and hearing aids)
- Encourage normalization of sleep–wake cycles
- Appropriate cognitive stimulation
- Minimizing immobility
- Perform proper mental status examination to pick up the symptoms of delirium at the earliest

All the pharmacological agents used for the management of delirium (i.e., haloperidol, cholinesterase inhibitors—donepezil, benzodiazepines, dexmedetomidine, etc.) have also been evaluated for their role in prevention of delirium, especially in patients undergoing surgical procedures. In general, the evidence for prophylactic use of pharmacological agents in the prevention of delirium is inconclusive.[53]

A recent systematic review and meta-analysis suggested that antipsychotics reduce the incidence of postoperative delirium, mainly in persons undergoing orthopaedic surgery and those who are at higher risk for delirium. However, the authors noted that there is a lot of heterogeneity in the data.[54] Another review evaluated the usefulness of melatonin in prevention of delirium and concluded that melatonin leads to reduction in the incidence of delirium in elderly patients admitted to medical wards.[55] Data also suggests that the use of combination of benzodiazepines and an opioid during the postoperative period to improve sleep-wake cycle disorders helps in preventing delirium.[56] Studies which have evaluated the role of donepezil have generally come up with negative results.[53,57] A recent Cochrane review which evaluated the role of various treatments in prevention of delirium in hospitalized non-ICU patients concluded that supportive multi-component interventions have strong evidence base for prevention of delirium. However, currently available evidence for antipsychotics as well as melatonin and cholinesterase inhibitors do not suggest that these agents are effective in the prevention of delirium.[58]

PROGNOSIS

Delirium is considered to be a short-term condition with most cases resolving completely in 10–12 days.[40] However, in many cases, the symptoms may persist beyond two months.[59] Occasional studies have reported that one-third of patients remain symptomatic at six months.[60] Further, negative impact of delirium in the elderly includes persistent cognitive deficits even after symptomatic recovery and higher risk of developing dementia.[61–64] Delirium is also associated with increased risk of inpatient mortality and mortality at 6–12 months after delirium.[61,65,66]

CONCLUSIONS

Delirium is one of the most commonly encountered psychiatric syndromes among those admitted to medical-surgical wards and ICUs with severely compromised medico-surgical conditions. Delirium is associated with negative outcomes in the form of prolonged hospitalization, increased cost of care, morbidity, distress among patients and caregivers, cognitive decline, and dementia. Considering the fact that this condition can be largely prevented, clinicians across different specialities and settings need to be aware of its existence and management. Efforts must be made to prevent delirium and whenever a patient develops delirium, treatment (both pharmacological and non-pharmacological) needs to be instituted at the earliest.

REFERENCES

1. Mattoo SK, Grover S, Gupta N. Delirium in general practice. *Indian Journal of Medical Research* 2010;131:387–98.

2. Grover S, Kate N. Delirium Research: Contributions from India. In: Savita Malhotra, Subho Chakrabarti, eds. *Developments in Psychiatry in India: Clinical, Research and Policy Perspectives*. Springer (India) Pvt. Ltd., 2015; pp. 463–92.

3. Fann JR. The epidemiology of delirium: a review of studies and methodological issues. *Semin Clin Neuropsychiatry* 2000;5:64–74.

4. Ely EW, Shintani A, Truman B. Delirium as a predictor of mortality in mechanically ventilated patients in the intensive care unit. *JAMA* 2004a;291:1753–62.

5. Ely EW, Stephens RK, Jacson JC. Current opinions regarding the importance, diagnosis, and management of delirium in the intensive care unit: a survey of 912 healthcare professionals. *Crit Care Med* 2004b;32:106–12.

6. Ely EW, Gautam S, Margolin R, Francis J, May L, Speroff T. The impact of delirium in the intensive care unit on hospital length of stay. *Intensive Care Med* 2001a;27: 1892–1900.

7. Ely EW, Inouye SK, Bernard GR. Delirium in mechanically ventilated patients: validity and reliability of confusion assessment methods for the intensive care unit (CAM-ICU). *JAMA* 2001b;286:2703–10.

8. Ely EW, Margolin R, Francis J. Evaluation of delirium in critically ill patients: validation of the Confusion Assessment Method for the Intensive Care Unit (CAM-ICU). *Crit Care Med* 2001c;29:1370–79.

9. Kishi Y, Iwasaki Y, Takezawa K. Delirium in critical care unit patients admitted through an emergency room. *Gen Hosp Psychiatry* 1995;17:371–9.

10. McNicoll L, Pisani MA, Zhang Y, Ely EW, Siegel MD, Inouye SK. Delirium in the intensive care unit: occurrence and clinical course in older patients. *J Am Geriatr Soc* 2003;51:591–8.

11. Sharma A, Malhotra S, Grover S, Jindal SK. Incidence, prevalence, risk factor and outcome of delirium in intensive care unit: a study from India. *Gen Hosp Psychiatry* 2012;34:639–46.

12. Lahariya S, Grover S, Bagga S, Sharma A. Delirium in patients admitted to a cardiac intensive care unit with cardiac emergencies in a developing country: incidence, prevalence, risk factor and outcome. *Gen Hosp Psychiatry* 2014;36:156–64.

13. Grover S, Sarkar S, Yaddanapudi LN, Ghosh A, Desouza A, Basu D. Intensive Care Unit delirium: A wide gap between actual prevalence and psychiatric referral. *J Anaesthesiol Clin Pharmacol* 2017 Oct–Dec;33(4):480–6.

14. American Psychiatric Association. *Diagnostic and Statistical Manual of Mental Disorders*. 3rd ed, (DSM-III). Washington, DC, American Psychiatric Association, 1980.

15. American Psychiatric Association. *Diagnostic and Statistical Manual of Mental Disorders*. 3rd ed, revised (DSM-III-R). Washington DC: American Psychiatric Association, 1987.

16. American Psychiatric Association. *Diagnostic and Statistical Manual of Mental Disorders*. 4th ed, text revision (DSM-IV). Washington DC: American Psychiatric Association, 1994.

17. American Psychiatric Association. *Diagnostic and Statistical Manual of Mental Disorders*. 5th ed. VA: Arlington, 2013.

18. Meagher DJ, Morandi A, Inouye SK, et al. Concordance between DSM-IV and DSM-5 criteria for delirium diagnosis in a pooled database of 768 prospectively evaluated patients using the delirium rating scale-revised-98. *BMC Med* 2014;12:164.

19. World Health Organization. *The ICD-10 Classification of Mental and Behavioural Disorders—Clinical Descriptions and Diagnostic Guidelines*. Geneva, 1992.

20. Laurila J, Pitkala K, Strandberg T, Tivilis R. Impact of different diagnostic criteria on prognosis of delirium: a prospective study. *Dement Geriatr Cogn Disord* 2004;18:240–4.

21. Gupta N, de Jonghe J, Schieveld J, Leonard M, Meagher D. Delirium phenomenology: what can we learn from the symptoms of delirium? *J Psychosom Res* 2008;65:215–22.

22. Jain G, Chakrabarti S, Kulhara P. Symptoms of delirium: an exploratory factor analytic study among referred patients. *Gen Hosp Psychiatry* 2011;33:377–85.

23. Grover S, Chakrabarti S, Shah R, Kumar V. A factor analytic study of the delirium rating scale-revised-98 in untreated patients with delirium. *J Psychosomatic Res* 2011;70:473–8.

24. Grover S, Kate N, Aggarwal M, et al. Delirium in elderly: A study from a psychiatric liaison service in North India. *International Psychogeriatrics* 2012;24:117–27.

25. Mattoo SK, Grover S, Chakravarty K, Trzepacz P, MeagherDJ, Gupta N. Symptom profile and etiology of delirium in a referral population in northern India: factor analysis of the DRS-R98. *Journal of Neuropsychiatry and Clinical Neurosciences* 2012;24:95–101.

26. Grover S, Agarwal M, Sharma A, et al. Symptoms and etiology of delirium: A comparison of elderly and adult patients. *East Asian Archives of Psychiatry* 2013;23: 56–64.

27. Shyamsundar G, Raghuthaman G, Rajkumar AP, Jacob KS. Validation of memorial delirium assessment scale. *J Crit Care* 2009;24:530–4.

28. George C, Nair JS, Ebenezer JA, et al. Validation of the intensive care delirium screening checklist in non-intubated intensive care unit patients in a resource-poor medical intensive care setting in South India. *J Crit Care* 2011;26:138–43.

29. Ahmed S, Leurent B, Sampson E. Risk factors for incident delirium among older people in acute hospital medical units: a systematic review and meta-analysis. *Age Ageing* 2014;43:326–33.

30. Vasilevskis E, Han JH, Hughes CG, Ely EW. Epidemiology and risk factors for delirium across hospital settings. *Best Pract Res Clin Anaesthesiol* 2012;26:277–87.

31. Maldonado JR. Neuropathogenesis of delirium: Review of current etiologic theories and common pathways. *Am J Geriatr Psychiatry* 2013;21:1190–1222.

32. Gleason OC. Delirium. *Am Fam Physician* 2003;67: 1027–34.

33. Meagher D. Delirium: the role of psychiatry. *Advances in Psychiatric Treatment* 2001;7:433–43.

34. Grover S, Chakrabarti S, Avasthi A. Influence of preexisting cognitive deficits on symptom profile and motoric subtypes of delirium. *J Geriatr Ment Health* 2015;2:83–9.

35. Grover S, Shah R. Distress due to delirium experience. *Gen Hosp Psychiatry* 2011;33:637–9.

36. Grover S, Ghosh A, Ghormode D. Experience in delirium: is it distressing? *J Neuropsychiatry Clin Neurosci* 2015;27:139–46.

37. Meagher D. Delirium: optimising management. *BMJ* 2001;322:144–9.

38. Grover S, Shah R. Perceptions among primary caregivers about the etiology of delirium: a study from a tertiary care centre in India. *Afr J Psychiatry (Johannesbg)* 2012;15: 193–5.

39. Grover S, Shah R. Delirium-related distress in caregivers: a study from a tertiary care centre in India. *Perspect Psychiatr Care* 2013;49:21–9.

40. Trzepacz P, Breitbart W, Franklin J, Levenson J, Martini DR, Wang P. American Psychiatric Association practice guidelines for the treatment of patients with delirium. *Am J Psychiatry* 1999;156:1–20.

41. Schrijver EJ, de Graaf K, de Vries OJ, Maier AB, Nanayakkara PW. Efficacy and safety of haloperidol for in-hospital delirium prevention and treatment: A systematic review of current evidence. *Eur J Intern Med* 2016;27:14–23.

42. Grover S, Mattoo SK, Gupta N. Usefulness of atypical antipsychotics and choline esterase inhibitors in delirium: A review. *Pharmacopsychiatry* 2011;44:43–54.

43. Grover S, Kumar V, Chakrabarti S. Comparative efficacy study of haloperidol, olanzapine and risperidone in delirium. *J Psychosomatic Res* 2011;71:277–81.

44. Grover S, Mahajan S, Chakrabarti S, Avasthi A. Comparative effectiveness of quetiapine and haloperidol in delirium: A single blind randomized controlled study. *World J Psychiatry* 2016;6:365–71.

45. Tahir TA, Eeles E, Karapareddy V, et al. A randomized controlled trial of quetiapine versus placebo in the treatment of delirium. *J Psychosom Res* 2010;69:485–90.

46. Meagher D, Leonard M. The active management of delirium: improving detection and treatment. *Advances in Psychiatric Treatment* 2008;14:292–301.

47. Mo Y, Zimmermann AE. Role of dexmedetomidine for the prevention and treatment of delirium in intensive care unit patients. *Ann Pharmacother* 2013;47:869–76.

48. Miura S, Furuya M, Yasuda H, Miyaoka T, Horiguchi J. Novel therapy with ramelteon for hypoactive delirium: a case report. *J Clin Psychopharmacol* 2015t;35:616–8.

49. Tsuda A, Nishimura K, Naganawa E, Otsubo T, Ishigooka J. Ramelteon for the treatment of delirium in elderly patients: a consecutive case series study. *Int J Psychiatry Med* 2014;47:97–104.

50. Kimura R, Mori K, Kumazaki H, Yanagida M, Taguchi S, Matsunaga H. Treatment of delirium with ramelteon: initial experience in three patients. *Gen Hosp Psychiatry* 2011;33:407–9.

51. Trzepacz PT, Meagher DJ. Delirium. In: Yudofsky S, Hales R, eds. *Textbook of Neuropsychiatry* (5th edn). Washington DC: American Psychiatric Press; 2007: pp. 445–517.

52. Marcantonio ER, Flacker JM, Wright RJ, Resnick NM. Reducing delirium after hip fracture: a randomized trial. *J Am Geriatr Soc* 2001;49:516–22.

53. Sampson EL, Raven PR, Ndhlovu PN, et al. A randomized, double-blind, placebo-controlled trial of donepezil hydrochloride (Aricept) for reducing the incidence of postoperative delirium after elective total hip replacement. *Int J Geriatr Psychiatry* 2007;22:343–9.

54. Fok MC, Sepehry AA, Frisch L, et al. Do antipsychotics prevent postoperative delirium? A systematic review and meta-analysis. *Int J Geriatr Psychiatry* 2015;30:333–44.

55. Chen S, Shi L, Liang F, et al. Exogenous melatonin for delirium prevention: a meta-analysis of randomized controlled trials. *Mol Neurobiol* 2016;53:4046–53.

56. Aizawa K, Kanai T, Saikawa Y, et al. A novel approach to the prevention of postoperative delirium in the elderly after gastrointestinal surgery. *Surg Today* 2002;32:310–14.

57. Liptzin B, Laki A, Garb JL, Fingeroth R, Krushell R. Donepezil in the prevention and treatment of post-surgical delirium. *Am J Geriatr Psychiatry* 2005;13: 1100–6.

58. Siddiqi N, Harrison JK, Clegg A, et al. Interventions for preventing delirium in hospitalised non-ICU patients. *Cochrane Database Syst Rev* 2016;3:CD005563.

59. Manos PJ, Wu R. The duration of delirium in medical and postoperative patients referred for psychiatric consultation. *Ann Clin Psychiatry* 1997;9:219–26.

60. Levkoff SE, Liptzin B, Evans D, et al. Progression and resolution of delirium in elderly patients hospitalized for acute care. *Am J Geriatr Psychiatry* 1994;2:230–8.

61. Rockwood K, Cosway S, Carver D, Jarrett P, Stadnyk K, Fisk J. The risk of dementia and death after delirium. *Age Ageing* 1999;28:551–6.

62. Jackson JC, Hart RP, Gordon SM, et al. Six-month neuropsychological outcome of medical intensive care unit patients. *Crit Care Med* 2003;31:1226–34.

63. Hopkins RO, Weaver LK, Collingridge D, Parkinson RB, Chan KJ, Orme JF Jr. Two-year cognitive, emotional, and quality-of-life outcomes in acute respiratory distress syndrome. *Am J Respir Crit Care Med* 2005;171:340–7.

64. Wacker P, Nunes PV, Cabrita H, Forlenza OV. Postoperative delirium is associated with poor cognitive outcome and dementia. *Dement Geriatr Cogn Disord* 2006;21:221–7.

65. Lin SM, Liu CY, Wang CH, et al. The impact of delirium on the survival of mechanically ventilated patients. *Crit Care Med* 2004;32:2254–9.

66. Ely EW, Shintani A, Truman B, et al. Delirium as a predictor of mortality in mechanically ventilated patients in the intensive care unit. *JAMA* 2004;291:1753–62.

52

Cognitive Dysfunctions in Psychiatric and Neurological Conditions

K. Srivastava, P. S. Bhat, G. Joshi, and A. Nehra

ABSTRACT

Cognitive dysfunction often accompanies various psychiatric and neurological conditions. Major disorders having cognitive dysfunction associated as a major symptom are depression, schizophrenia, bipolar disorder, anxiety disorders, and delusion disorders amongst psychiatric conditions. Neurological disorders such as dementia, epilepsy, traumatic brain injury (TBI), and other forms of acquired brain injuries along with autoimmune and infectious disorders also have dysfunction in cognition in the areas of attention, memory, perception, visuomotor functioning, language, and executive functions. The pathogenesis of cognitive dysfunction in psychiatric and neurological conditions is often chronic and progressive. They can be reversed and the progression of cognitive decline can be impeded with the use of neurocognitive rehabilitation in the form of traditional cognitive enhancement therapy along with more modern contemporary approaches such as neurobiofeedback and computer-based neuropsychological rehabilitation. The benefit of neurocognitive rehabilitation has been empirically proven and is widely accepted in the reintegration of patients and the affected families. It is highly important to ensure that the patients in the neurointensive care receive adequate specialized post hospice counselling and facilities for family liaison of patients is made available to provide expert, compassionate, and personalized support to patients and their families throughout the continuum of care in both inpatient and outpatient facilities.

KEYWORDS

Cognitive dysfunction; neurological patients; neurointensive care; cognitive functions; depression; anxiety disorders; schizophrenia; alcohol dependence; epilepsy; cerebrovascular diseases.

INTRODUCTION

Cognition refers to thinking skills or intellectual abilities used for perceptions, acquiring, understanding, and responding to information presented to a person. Thinking, memory, perception, skilled movements, and language are essential aspects of cognitive functions. Cognitive functions such as learning and memory are part of the neural circuitry within the hippocampus, dealing mainly in perceptual and intellectual aspects of mental functioning.

The adequacy of cognitive domain is assessed on the basis of performance on orientation, ability to solve problems and make judgements. Retention of information and recall of information are other aspects.[1]

Cognitive dysfunction is the impairment of these functions and abilities that can affect a person's thoughts, memories, and reasoning capabilities. It can be seen across various neurological/psychiatric disorders. Some of the disorders which show evidence of having dysfunctions are depression, schizophrenia, bipolar mood disorder, anxiety disorders, alcohol dependence syndrome, delusional disorders, and neurological conditions such as stroke, traumatic brain injury, and other neurodegenerative and autoimmune disorders such as dementia and multiple sclerosis. Some of the cognitive dysfunctions are reversible or improve over time as the disease or disorder begins to improve. In a few cases cognitive dysfunction can also worsen without improvement at all. The research in cases of schizophrenia and depression has highlighted serious implications of these deficits. Employability, adjustment, and role performance are some of the direct implications of research in these disorders. The understanding of this disorder will provide importance in outcome and management of cases as well.

COGNITIVE DEFICITS IN PSYCHIATRIC CONDITIONS

These are illustrated through Figure 52.1, and discussed in the following paragraphs.

Depression

Impairment in attention in major depressive disorder (MDD) has been noted in various studies, and the primarily affected areas are processing speed and selective attention as part of executive functions.[2–5]

Attention, executive function (EF), and memory are some of the domains checked for cognitive deficits in mood disorders. Some of the dysfunctions are stable over a period of time even in the euthymic state suggesting a trait characteristic.[6] Some of the deficits in verbal memory, verbal fluency, and visuospatial ability are noted in the euthymic state of mood as well. This finding indicates the possibility of trait characteristics affecting the cognitive functions of patients with mood disorder.[7–11]

Most of the evidence in context of cognitive functions pertains to cross-sectional evidence. It is equally important to answer whether these deficits are long-term or episodic, and if they are related with the phase of illness or improve with recovery.[12,13] Patients with depression have shown distinct patterns of cognitive impairment.[14] The cognitive deficits noted during the illness phase also continues to be in the remission phase and some of them last even after six months of recovery. The findings of a 2-year follow-up study indicated that improvement in mood symptoms is associated with improvement in cognitive functions also, indicating reversible aspects during remission.[15–17] Some of the cognitive functions namely attention and sustained attention continue to show deficits in the remission phase.[17]

In a meta-analysis study some interesting observations emerged. Attention and executive functioning were more like trait markers and psychomotor speed and memory functioning were indicative of state specific cognitive deficits in the first episode MDD.[18] The EF in depression determines the vocational performance and response to treatment. The presence of dysfunction is an indicator of vocational disability and poor response to treatment.[19] Research findings on patients with bipolar disorder in remission noted significant impairments in attention, EF, and memory in the study group compared with a matched control group of normal subjects. In fact, memory deficit pattern also did not differ in both unipolar and bipolar cases of depression.[20,21]

Anxiety Disorders

Generalized anxiety disorder (GAD) is characteristic of excessive worry, anxiety, and also shows a relation to impaired social and occupational functioning.[22] Identifying such impairments will be useful for making triage and treatment decisions in subjects with GAD.[23]

Schizophrenia

Characteristic deficits of schizophrenia include impairments in domains such as attention, memory, processing speed, problem-solving, and working memory. Abnormalities in abstraction, problem-solving, and other EFs are the core aspects of deficits in schizophrenia. They are crucial determinants of functional and vocational outcome and index of recovery. Neuropsychological tests have revealed that patients of schizophrenia do poor on tests of working memory and sustained attention.

The working memory serves as an important cognitive function of continuation and completion of tasks.[24,25] Other domains affected are visual learning, problem-solving, and social cognition along with speed of processing the information. Impairment in vigilance has a large consequence in day to day functioning as it may disrupt the ability to follow a social conversation and also follow important instructions; reading and television watching can become difficult for the person.[26]

Cognitive functions are catalysts to functional requirement of reintegration of patients in the society. In this background, functional capacity thus encompasses the capacity of an individual to perform the task of daily living.

Assessments of functional capacity will determine the daily skills in managing social conversation, public transport or taking medication without supervision. These learned skills are to be generalized in other domains of performance. The conclusion regarding community adaptation cannot be drawn based on limited information.[27]

Research evidence proves that cognitive assessment aids the prediction of later functional outcomes. It is understood that community functioning has a host of factors apart from cognition that are usually not considered in clinical trial studies (e.g., psychosocial rehabilitation and educational/vocational opportunities), which affect the outcome of adaptation of patients in day to day living.[28,29]

Management of Cognitive Deficits in Schizophrenia

Atypical neuroleptics have shown neurocognitive advantages over conventional neuroleptics in the management of cognitive deficits in schizophrenia.[30] Adjunctive pharmacological interventions with some reported effectiveness include tandospirone,[31] donepezil,[32] and N-methyl-D-aspartate (NMDA)-receptor stimulating agents.[33] However, efforts to improve cognition should be both pharmacological and psychological.

Alcohol Dependence Syndrome

Impairments in cognitive domains due to alcohol consumption affect EF, memory, and visuospatial functions. These cognitive impairments disrupt efficacy of management and hampers the prognosis. It also interferes in everyday management of these patients. Cognitive recovery and abstinence are an interdependent process. Early identification of cognitive impairment can go a long way in the intervention of these deficits.

Cerebral atrophy in the brains of chronic alcohol patients is supported by neurological findings.[34] Decreased frontal lobe glucose utilisation along with reduced cerebral blood flow (CBF) has been reported using functional imaging studies. Frequent relapses and detoxifications in alcohol dependence cases lead to greater degree of cognitive impairment.[35,36] Repeated withdrawal leads to 'kindling effect' and associated brain damage.[37] Alcohol dependence cases are noted to be having cognitive deficits in working memory and EF. Progressive cognitive function disturbances are also corroborated by neuropsychological findings. Decision-making and complex problem-solving abilities are also impaired in them.[38,39]

Patients of alcohol dependence and normal controls were compared on neuropsychological tests after one year of abstinence. Cognitive deficits were noted in 37 patients. The comparison was done with a control group of healthy subjects on Wisconsin card sorting test and N back test for assessment of working memory and EF.[40] It was found that those with alcohol dependence had significant disturbances in working memory and EF compared to normal controls. These cognitive deficits were irrespective of short-term and long-term abstinence. Duration of alcohol drinking had a negative impact on cognitive functions. The findings are suggestive of core central cognitive deficits often noted in disturbance of prefrontal cortex of patients with alcohol dependence.[40] Alcohol dependents demonstrated significant impairment of abstract ability, error utilization, and persuading goal directed behaviour.[38–40]

Management of Cognitive Dysfunction in Psychiatric Disorders

As has been discussed above, many of the psychiatric disorders have some amount of cognitive deficits that can be assessed by detailed neurocognitive evaluation. Most of the time, these deficits are clinically not apparent. Also, currently there is no definite evidence that primary psychiatric disorders increase the risk for future dementia. Research on specific pharmacological interventions so far have also not suggested any definitive role for them in the management of cognitive deficits in psychiatric disorders.

However, many times clinicians face problems in managing these cases in ICU settings when admitted with co-morbid medical conditions. These patients are more vulnerable to develop acute confusional states or frank delirium, in view of preexisting cognitive deficits and impaired mental faculty due to the primary psychiatric disorders. Such cases need to be managed energetically with low doses of neuroleptics, followed up more frequently, and medicines to be tapered off at the earliest. Many times the doses of medicines used in primary psychiatric disorders also may require downward titration temporarily. More importantly, continuous reorientation strategies work effectively and hence are to be implemented vigorously.[41,42]

Neuropsychological studies have yielded consistent evidence of cognitive dysfunction impairment in psychiatric disorders. Neuropsychological assessment is widely carried out on Wisconsin card sorting test, problem solving, vigilance test, attention and concentration tests, and intelligence tests. Indian studies also concur the findings of the same nature. In the ICU setting, cognitive deficits have a huge implication. The need of understanding such co-morbid disorders cannot be overemphasized.

COGNITIVE DYSFUNCTION IN NEUROLOGICAL CONDITIONS

In the field of neurointensive care, the patients are either at risk of or have had severe nervous system injury. A fundamental aspect of neurointensive care is a standardized protocol of care for critically ill patients. Adopting best practice evidence-based guidelines to optimize the outcomes and providing continued care with a consistent, unified approach is the need of the hour.

Patients in this unit often suffer from debilitating cognitive deficits and severe loss of functioning leading to decrease in quality of life of the patient and the caregiver. The rehabilitation, both psychological and physical, is often a long journey for these families. Figure 52.2 illustrates cognitive dysfunction in neurological conditions.

Therefore, it requires a coordinated effort of multidisciplinary clinicians and amalgamation of sophisticated monitoring techniques in order to increase the chances of survival and provide a chance for the patient to regain the levels of independence which was not possible 10 years ago. It has become increasingly important to have services specialized for family liaison of patients to provide expert, compassionate, and personalized support to patients and their families throughout the continuum of care in both inpatient and outpatient facilities. Figure 52.3 presents the various problems faced by survivors of neurological conditions.

Cognitive Impairment in Cerebrovascular Accidents (CVA)

The risk for post-stroke cognitive decline ranges from 20% to 80% depending on demographic factors such as age, occupation, education, and other vascular factors such as the type of stroke, location of the lesion, etc.[43] Strokes are the second most prevalent cause of death leading to rising burden of stroke in low and middle-income countries.[44] A prospective study shows the prevalence of cognitive impairment to be 20% during the post-stroke period.[45]

In stroke patients, typically multiple domains are affected ranging from lower order to higher order functions. Memory, visuoconstructional, and EF are found to be most commonly impaired.[46] The activities of daily living is most commonly impaired and patients may face personality[47] and behavioural changes post ictus with increased irritability, aggression, apathy, impulsivity, and disinhibition; and may also present with affective changes including increased anxiety and depressive symptoms.[48]

Dementia

In India, the latest data suggests that India was home to 4.1 million people living with dementia, second only to China (9.5 million) and the USA (4.2 million).[49] The prevalence of Alzheimer's disease is 60% in developing countries, while 20% to 30% of the elderly population with dementia suffer from vascular or mixed vascular dementia.[50,51] Dementia is a form of neurodegenerative disease which is marked by impairment in memory, and at least one domain of cognitive functioning such as visuospatial ability, comprehension, language, and EF, which affect the occupational and social aspects of functioning of the patient, severely affecting their quality of life.[52]

The pathophysiological hallmarks of cognitive decline in Alzheimer's dementia are well-defined as the neurofibrillary tangles and plaques leading to reduced

ability to cope with everyday activities[53] and behavioural alterations are other features marked by mood disorder and hallucination. Neuropsychiatric co-morbidities such as depression, psychosis, and bipolar affective disorder are common in the course of the illness.[54]

A systematic review of computerized cognitive training (CCT) in older adults studied the effect on overall cognition in 17 trials and found that CCT had a moderate effect size across all trials; with small to moderate effects for global cognition, attention and concentration, working memory, immediate and delayed memory, and auditory and verbal learning ability along with psychosocial functioning, including depressive symptoms.[55]

Epilepsy

Epilepsy is marked by structural changes in the brain, but its functional repercussions remains unclear and less explored. Most studies do not reveal any significant adverse effects, but a sub-group of 10%–20% of patients show significant intellectual decline and cognitive impairments, clinically. Patients with generalized seizures, high antiepileptic drug use and early onset, appear to be at higher risks, with psychosocial and economic factors playing an important role with the prognosis of illness.[56]

The cognitive and behavioural problems can have multiple causes ranging from brain lesions, epileptic dysfunction, and treatment effects of antiepileptic drugs. These problems can range from being static and irreversible to more dynamic and reversible symptoms, such as those originating due to treatment. Active epilepsy or treatment often interferes with critical phases of brain development; under certain conditions, severe epilepsy can cause mental decline affecting all areas of cognitive functioning.[57]

Traumatic Brain Injury

Traumatic brain injury (TBI) often results in permanent disability, particularly due to cognitive decline. Survivors often are young, having near-normal life expectancy, thereby increasing the burden on public health. The most commonly affected domains are memory, executive function, and processing speed. Disturbance of cognitive domains such as attention, executive functioning, and memory are more prevalent in the post-TBI cognitive sequelae, in all levels of severity. Disruption of these domains causes additional disturbances of communication, activities of daily living, exacerbating the effects of cognitive decline in the global quality of life of patients and the caregivers.[58]

Due to the high rates of other symptoms post TBI, psychological, neurological and physical, psychometric assessment should be thoroughly carried out in order to plan the treatment for cognitive impairment.

Autoimmune and Infectious Diseases

NMDA-receptor encephalitis is an autoimmune disorder with psychiatric changes including anxiety, epileptic seizures, and cognitive decline.[59] The cognitive changes can persist after recovery with alterations in the levels of consciousness.

Mild cognitive impairment often precedes the autoimmune limbic encephalitis (ALE). In addition to memory impairment, clinical features that might suggest this disorder include personality changes, agitation, insomnia, alterations of consciousness, and seizures.[60]

Cognitive impairment has a prevalence rate of 40%–65% in patients with multiple sclerosis (MS) and affects the domains of attention, speed of information processing, episodic memory, and executive functioning. It can be seen in clinically isolated syndrome, all phases of clinical MS, and subclinical radiologically isolated syndrome.[61]

Multiple sclerosis is determined by the disease duration, its subtypes, and demographic factors such as race, gender, and the cognitive reserve of an individual. The progressive subtypes have greater prevalence of cognitive decline.[60] Patients with MS also have compromised attention span and face cognitive deficits ranging from mild to moderate severity.[61,62]

Also, a considerable impairment in the multitasking ability is present. As the patient may not have appropriate mental status to carry out a detailed evaluation of functioning and start rehabilitation, it is imperative that the patient and the caregiver should have a well-established therapeutic relationship with the clinician in order to provide continued interventional guidance post discharge.

Management of Cognitive Dysfunction in Neurological Conditions in Neurointensive Care

Wilson[63] describes the core components of neuropsychological rehabilitation principles to be practiced, which are elucidated further. It is firmly believed that one must address what needs to rehabilitated, then plan an appropriate rehabilitative course for those deficits and have continuous evaluations done in order to determine the response to rehabilitation (Figure 52.4).[63]

Neuropsychological rehabilitation can primarily be divided into those involving interval strategies such as the use of mnemonics, imagery, and other forms of remembering such as the use of rhymes, acronyms, and systematic queuing.[64] Another category is dependent on external resources such as a personal assistant device, a diary, and any other technique to compensate for memory and organizational skills. The objective is to alleviate the impediment and handicap caused by the deficits. Cognitive retraining and computer-based cognitive therapy can be administered on the patients once they stabilize. It is important to have home-based tasks assigned to the patients in order to target their deficits in a continued manner, besides the lab-based therapies.[65] For example, patients with aphasia post stroke or brain injury should be started immediately on speech therapy in order to ameliorate the symptoms and increase the chances of recovery[66] (Figure 52.4).

Similarly, for neurocognitive deficits, specific cognitive retraining can be started which should be a bottoms-up approach, starting with the most basic cognitive functions such as attention and concentration, and proceeding to higher order functioning such as executive functioning and problem solving.[63,65] A clinical neuropsychologist should be involved in order to plan and monitor the rehabilitative process of retraining.

CONCLUSIONS

Cognitive dysfunctions are noted in both psychiatric disorders and neurological disorders. Neuropsychological assessment is the primary step towards neurocognitive rehabilitation. In the backdrop of neurointensive care, it is important to simplify the process and make it deliverable to the patients. This necessitates a basic understanding of the nature of these deficits in patients and integration through neuropsychological rehabilitation. The importance of neuropsychological rehabilitation cannot be overemphasized.

REFERENCES

1. Campbell RJ. *Campbell's Psychiatric Dictionary*. 8th ed. New York: Oxford: Oxford University Press; 2004. p. 131.
2. Cohen R, Lohr I, Paul R, Boland R. Impairments of attention and effort among patients with major affective disorders. *J Neuropsychiatry Clin Neurosci* 2001;13(3):385–95.
3. Pardo JV, Pardo PJ, Humes SW, Posner MI. Neurocognitive dysfunction in antidepressant-free non–elderly patients with unipolar depression: alerting and convert orienting of visuospatial attention. *J Affect Disord* 2006;92:71–78.
4. Egeland J, Rund BR, Sundet K, et al. Attention profile in schizophrenia compared with depression: differential effects of processing speed, selective attention and vigilance. *Acta Psychiatr Scand* 2003;108:276–84.
5. Simons CJP, Jacobs N, Derom C, et al. Cognition as a predictor of current and follow up depressive symptoms

in the general population. *Acta Psychiatr Scand* 2009;120: 45–52.

6. Cherie LM, Sergio Paradiso. Cognitive and neurological impairment in mood disorders. *Psychiatr Clin North Am.* 2004 Mar;27(1):19–viii.

7. Ferrier IN, Stanton BR, Kelly TP, Scott J. Neuropsychological function in euthymic patients with bipolar disorder. *Br J Psychiatry* 1999;175:246–51.

8. Clark LD, Iversen SD, Goodwin G. Sustained attention deficit in bipolar disorder. *Br J Psychiatry* 2002;180:313–9.

9. Van Gorp WG, Altshuler L, Theberge DC, Mintz J. Declarative and procedural memory in bipolar disorder. *Biol Psychiatry* 1999;46:525–31.

10. El-Badri SM, Ashton CH, Moore PB, Marsh VR, Ferrier IN. Electrophysiological and cognitive function in young euthymic patients with bipolar affective disorder. *Bipolar Disord* 2001;3:79–87.

11. Denicoff KD, Ali SO, Mirsky AF, et al. Relationship between prior course of illness and neuropsychological functioning in patients with bipolar disorder. *J Affect Disord* 1999;56:67–73.

12. Gruber S, Rathgeber K, Braunig P, Gauggel S. Stability and course of neuropsychological deficits in manic and depressed bipolar patients compared to patients with major depression. *J Affect Disord* 2007;104:61–71.

13. Nakano Y, Baba H, Maeshima H, et al. Executive dysfunction in medicated, remitted state of major depression. *J Affect Disord* 2008;111:46–51.

14. Srivastava K, Ryali VSSR, Prakash J, Bhat PS, Shashikumar R, and Khan S. Neuropsychophysiological correlates of depression. *Ind Psychiatry J* 2010 Jul–Dec; 19(2):82–89.

15. Airakinsen E, Wahlin Å, Larsson M, Forsell Y. Cognitive and social functioning in recovery from depression: results from a population-based three-year follow-up. *J Affect Disord* 2006;96:107–10.

16. Lahr D, Beblo T, Hartje W. Cognitive performance and subjective complaints before and after remission of major depression. *Cogn Neuropsychiatry* 2007;12:25–45.

17. Biringer E, Lundervold A, Stordal KI, et al. Executive function improvement upon remission of unipolar major depression. *Eur Arch Psychiatry Clin Neurosci* 2005;255: 373–80.

18. Weiland-Fiedler P, Erickson K, Waldeck T, et al. Evidence for continuing neuropsychological impairments in depression. *J Affect Disord* 2004;82:253–8.

19. Rico SC Lee, Daniel F Hermens, Melanie A Porter, Antoinette Redoblado Hodge M. A meta-analysis of cognitive deficits in first-episode major depressive disorder. *Journal of Affective Disorders* 2012;140(2):113–24.

20. Must A, Szabo Z, Bodi N, Szasz A, Janka Z, Keri S. Neuropsychological assessment of the prefrontal cortex in major depressive disorder. *Psychiatr Hung* 2005;20:412–16.

21. Taj M, Padmavati R. Neuropsychological impairment in bipolar affective disorder. *Indian J Psychiatry* 2005;47:48–50.

22. Bearden CE, Glahn DC, Monkul ES, et al. Patterns of memory impairment in bipolar disorder and unipolar major depression. *Psychiatry Res* 2006;142:139–50.

23. Johnsen GE, Asbjornsen AE. Consistent impaired verbal memory in PTSD: a meta-analysis. *J Affect Disord* 2008; 111(1):74–82.

24. Dickinson D, Ramsey ME, Gold JM. Overlooking the obvious: A meta-analytic comparison of digit symbol coding tasks and other cognitive measures in schizophrenia. *Arch Gen Psychiatry* 2007;64:532–42.

25. Lee J, Park S. Working memory impairments in schizophrenia: a meta-analysis. *J Abnorm Psychol* 2005;114:599–611.

26. Green MF1, Kern RS, Heaton RK, Heaton C. Longitudinal studies of cognition and functional outcome in schizophrenia: implications for MATRICS. *Schizophrenia Research* 2004;72:41–51.

27. Patterson TL, Goldman S, McKibbin CL, Hughs T, Jeste DV. UCSD performance-based skills assessment: development of a new measure of everyday functioning for severely mentally ill adults. *Schizophrenia Bulletin* 2001;27:235–45.

28. Michael F Green, Robert S Kern, Robert K Heaton. Longitudinal studies of cognition and functional outcome in schizophrenia: implications for MATRICS. *Schizophrenia Research* 2004;72(1):41–51.

29. Yingxue Yang, Xiating Zhang, Yu Zhu, Yakang Dai, Ting Liu, Yuping Wang. Cognitive impairment in generalized anxiety disorder revealed by event-related potential N270. *Neuropsychiatr Dis Treat* 2015;11:1405–11.

30. Keefe RSE, Silva SG, Perkins DO, et al. The effects of atypical antipsychotic drugs on neurocognitive impairment in schizophrenia: A review and metaanalysis. *Schizophr Bull* 1999;25:201–22.

31. Sumiyoshi T, Matsui M, Yamashita I, et al. The effect of tandospirone, a serotonin (1A) agonist, on memory function in schizophrenia. *Biol Psychiatry* 2001;49:861–8.

32. Buchanan RW, Summerfelt A, Tek C, et al. An open labeled trial of adjunctive donepezil for cognitive impairments in patients with schizophrenia. *Schizophr Res* 2003;59:29–33.

33. File SE, Fluck E, Fernandes C. Beneficial effects of glycine (bioglycine) on memory and attention in young and middle aged adults. *J Clin Psychopharmacol* 1999;19:506–12.

34. Moselhy HF, Georgiou G, Kahn A. Frontal lobe changes in alcoholism. *Alcohol* 2001;36:357–68.

35. Buhler M, Mann K. Alcohol and the human brain: A systematic review of different neuroimaging methods. *Alcoholism: Clinical and Experimental Research* 2011;35(10): 1771–93.

36. Nowakowska K, Jabłkowska K, Borkowska A. Cognitive dysfunctions in patients with alcohol dependence. *Archives of Psychiatry and Psychotherapy* 2008;10(3):29–35.

37. Rosenbloom MJ, O'Reilly A, Sassoon SA, Sullivan EV, Pfefferbaum A. Persistent cognitive deficits in community-treated alcoholic men and women volunteering for research: limited contribution from psychiatric comorbidity. *J Stud Alcohol* 2005;66:254–65.

38. Blume AW, Schmaling KB, Marlatt GA. Memory, executive cognitive function, and readiness to change drinking behavior. *Addict Behav* 2005;30:301–14.

39. Katarzyna Nowakowska, Karolina Jabłkowska, Alina Borkowska. Cognitive dysfunctions in patients with alcohol dependence. *Archives of Psychiatry and Psychotherapy* 2008;3:29–35.

40. Manisha Jha, Vinod Kumar Sinha. Conceptual abilities of alcohol dependent patients—An analysis of WCST profile. *Delhi Psychiatry Journal* 2015;18(1):77–85.

41. Kalisvaart KJ, de Jonghe JF, Bogaards MJ, et al. Haloperidol prophylaxis for elderly hip-surgery patients at risk for delirium: a randomized placebo-controlled study. *J Am Geriatr Soc* 2005;53:1658–66.

42. Girard TD, Pandharipande PP, Wesley EE. Delirium in the intensive care unit. *Crit Care* 2008;12(Suppl 3):S3. doi: 10.1186/cc6149.

43. Sun J-H, Tan L, Yu J-T. Post-stroke cognitive impairment: epidemiology, mechanisms and management. *Ann Transl Med* [Internet]. 2014 Aug [cited 2017 Feb 6];2(8). Available from: http://www.ncbi.nlm.nih.gov/pmc/articles/PMC4200648/.

44. Strong K, Mathers C, Bonita R. Preventing stroke: saving lives around the world. *Lancet Neurol* 2007 Feb;6(2):182–7.

45. Das S, Paul N, Hazra A, et al. Cognitive dysfunction in stroke survivors: a community-based prospective study from Kolkata, India. *J Stroke Cerebrovasc Dis* Off of J Natl Stroke Assoc. 2013 Nov;22(8):1233–42.

46. Jokinen H, Melkas S, Ylikoski R, et al. Post-stroke cognitive impairment is common even after successful clinical recovery. *Eur J Neurol* 2015 Sep;22(9):1288–94.

47. Stone J, Townend E, Kwan J, Haga K, Dennis MS, Sharpe M. Personality change after stroke: some preliminary observations. *J Neurol Neurosurg Psychiatry* 2004 Dec 1; 75(12):1708–13.

48. Emotional and personality changes after stroke fact sheet—Stroke Foundation - Australia. [Internet] [cited 2017 Feb 6]. Available from: https://strokefoundation.org.au/About-Stroke/Help-after-stroke/Stroke-resources-and-fact-sheets/Emotional-and-personality-changes-after-stroke-fact-sheet.

49. Prince M, Wilmo A, Guerchet M, Ali G, Wu Y, Prina M. World Alzheimer Report 2015. The Global impact of dementia. An analysis of prevalence, incidence, cost and trends. Alzheimer's Disease International. 2015. Available from: https://www.alz.co.uk/research/WorldAlzheimerReport2015.pdf.

50. Mathuranath PS, George A, Ranjith N, et al. Incidence of Alzheimer's disease in India: A 10 years follow-up study. *Neurol India* 2012 Nov 1;60(6):625.

51. Rizzi L, Rosset I, Roriz-Cruz M. Global epidemiology of dementia: Alzheimer's and vascular types. *BioMed Research International* 2014;1–8. doi:10.1155/2014/908915.

52. Introduction—Screening for Dementia—NCBI Bookshelf [Internet]. [cited 2017 Feb 7]. Available from: https://www.ncbi.nlm.nih.gov/books/NBK42775/.

53. De-Paula VJ, Radanovic M, Diniz BS, Forlenza OV. Alzheimer's disease. *Subcell Biochem* 2012;65:329–52.

54. Alzheimer's disease associated with psychiatric comorbidities [Internet]. [cited 2017 Feb 7]. Available from: http://www.scielo.br/scielo.php?script=sci_arttext&pid=S0001-37652015000301461.

55. Hill NTM, Mowszowski L, Naismith SL, Chadwick VL, Valenzuela M, Lampit A. Computerized cognitive training in older adults with mild cognitive impairment or dementia: a systematic review and meta-analysis. *Am J Psychiatry* 2016 Nov 14. appi.ajp.2016.16030360.

56. Vingerhoets G. Cognitive effects of seizures. *Seizure* 2006 Jun;15(4):221–6.

57. Hermann B, Seidenberg M. Epilepsy and cognition. *Epilepsy Curr* 2007 Jan;7(1):1–6.

58. Arciniegas DB, Held K, Wagner P. Cognitive impairment following traumatic brain injury. *Curr Treat Options Neurol* 2002 Jan;4(1):43–57.

59. Vahter L, Kannel K, Sorro U, Jaakmees H, Talvik T, Gross-Paju K. Cognitive dysfunction during anti-NMDA-receptor encephalitis is present in early phase of the disease. *Oxf Med Case Rep* 2014(4):74–6.

60. Gross R, Davis J, Roth J, Querfurth H. Cognitive impairments preceding and outlasting autoimmune limbic encephalitis. *Case Rep Neurol Med* 2016 Jan 10;2016: e7247235.

61. Jongen PJ, Ter Horst AT, Brands AM. Cognitive impairment in multiple sclerosis. *Minerva Med* 2012 Apr;103(2):73–96.

62. Nabavi SM, Sangelaji B. Cognitive dysfunction in multiple sclerosis: Usually forgotten in the clinical assessment of MS patients. *J Res Med Sci* Off of J Isfahan Univ Med Sci. 2015 May;20(5):533–4.

63. Wilson BA. Neuropsychological rehabilitation. *Annu Rev Clin Psychol* 2008;4(1):141–62.

64. Wilson BA, Glisky EL. Memory rehabilitation: integrating theory and practice. New York, NY: Guilford Press; 2009.

65. Rajeswaran J. *Neuropsychological Rehabilitation: Principles and Applications.* Elsevier: London; 2009.

66. Allen L, Mehta S, Mcclure JA, Teasell R. Therapeutic interventions for aphasia initiated more than six months post stroke: a review of the evidence. *Topics in Stroke Rehabilitation* 2009;19(6):523–35. doi:10.1310/tsr1906-523.

Part XV

Ethical Care

Editor: Mike Souter

53

End-of-Life Care

M. J. Souter

ABSTRACT

The end-of-life care presents many challenges to the neurocritical care physician—which includes understanding the appropriate authority of decision-making, if the patient is incapable of communicating their desires and wishes, as is the case more often than not.

Communication and the creation of trusting relationships are key attributes of successful management of end-of-life situations. This facilitates transparency, together with the avoidance of frequently held concerns (of patients and families) for loss of control and dignity, alongside the suffering of unnecessary pain and distress.

Conflict in goals of care discussions can intrude at all levels and is best handled with compassion, patience, and an ability to consult ethical, palliative, and spiritual care experts to help in consistent messaging of facts on prognosis, while avoiding undue bias.

The withdrawal of invasive therapies is ethically permissible in these settings provided that it is consistent with previously expressed wishes of the patient or active family direction. Such steps should be accompanied, however, by active prophylaxis of any pain and distress initiated with the appropriate use of analgesic and anxiolytic medication, titrated to specific goals within pre-specified institutional protocols.

KEYWORDS

End of life; medical ethics; autonomy; beneficence; non-maleficence; substituted judgement; principle of double effect; futility.

INTRODUCTION

The neurologically impaired patient in the neurointensive care unit may present ethical challenges to the unprepared physician. The disease process effect upon their abilities in communication, comprehension, and consciousness can varyingly frustrate the clinician's ability to confidently pursue directions of care that align with the patient's wishes.

As such they are said to lack both *Capacity* (the ability to understand the situation) and *Competency* (the ability to make a decision to resolve the situation at hand).

Most cultures recognize an inherent right of the individual to control their own body—this forms the fundamental basis of *autonomy*. As such, patients would reasonably expect to be informed of associated risks and benefits and consent to procedures required for their care, except with circumstances of critical emergency. They would also expect to be able to participate in discussions around how far to extend treatment in cases of severe illness. In some cases, these decisions have been considered, made, and are delivered in the form of written instructions. Examples include the advance directive or 'living will', and the more proscriptive Physicians Orders for Life Sustaining Treatment (POLST).

A living will may do the following, either singly, or in combination with each other:

1. It can provide specific instructions towards healthcare systems to be undertaken should a particular event (normally disabling illness or disease) occur. This is usually an instruction to forego life-sustaining therapy in the event of anticipated death or non-recovery of autonomy.

2. It can nominate an authorized individual to make decisions on the patient's behalf, if again the patient is rendered incompetent by disabling disease or illness. This is often known as 'durable power of attorney for healthcare' or similar. This is not necessarily the same individual, as one instructed and qualified to make financial and fiduciary decisions on behalf of a patient, but is often chosen based on their sympathy for, and knowledge of, the patient's attitudes and quality of life goals. This authority can usually only be designated by an individual when they are competent.

3. In combination, both measures may provide direction to an authorized surrogate to make detailed medical decisions based on the state of injury/disease, consequent prognosis, and the expressed attitudes of the patient.

In contrast, the POLST structure provides actual orders for care (in applicable jurisdictions) for a physician or healthcare provider to satisfy, based on previously discussed attitudes and goals of the patient with their usual physician.

As such, this is really only appropriate for those seriously ill patients who are not expected to survive the forthcoming year.[1] Depending on local laws, providers may be bound to honour these orders, e.g., emergency responders avoiding inappropriate resuscitation if called to the patient's home and finding a POLST form. Depending on local laws again, POLST forms are expected to be carried with the patient to their health care destination, whereas advance directives remain the responsibility of the patient and/or family.

SURROGACY

In the absence of any such directions, recognizing that comatose patients lack the fundamental ability to provide informed consent, physicians consequently look for alternate decision-makers to exercise what is termed *substituted judgement*. This exercise of judgement and decision-making authority is similar to that afforded to the living will designee, but defaults to family members in the absence of specific instruction on the premise that they are most likely to have insight into the attitudes of the patient.

Many jurisdictions operate a graduated hierarchy of authority for surrogates in decision-making; e.g., authority starting with the spouse (or civil partner; again depends on the local laws), then descending to adult children, followed by parents, then siblings. As a general principle when more than one individual of equal authority is consulted (e.g., in the case of siblings), there should be a consensus on the decisions made.

Conflicts between equally ranked surrogates require careful discussion with the individuals concerned to re-examine the goals of decision-making and help them reach an agreement. If that agreement is still unattainable, then this may result in either no decisions being made, or in appropriate circumstances, a requirement to initiate legal processes to find court-appointed decision-makers.

Similarly, in the persistent absence of competency, but where no surrogates exist, a court may designate an appropriate individual to make decisions on behalf of the incompetent patient.

The exercise of substituted judgement is not to merely provide the ability for family members or guardians to decide what should happen to the patient, but is instead a responsibility conferred upon them to decide for the best interests of the patient. That decision should be informed by their knowledge of the patient and insights into what he/she would have wanted, were the patient able to participate in the discussion.

A useful concept in practice is to instruct family or surrogates to imagine the patient present at any discussion and voice what he or she might say.

The goal of substituted judgement decisions is to protect autonomy, but also seeks to serve two other important ethical principles, i.e., beneficence (taking actions to benefit that patient) and *non-maleficence* (the avoidance of harm to that patient through actions or omissions of care). These principles operate widely across healthcare to direct and inform the actions and decisions of care providers at all levels.

Decisions are even more challenging when considering end-of-life situations. Families may find it increasingly difficult to put aside their own attitudes and orient their decisions to the prior attitudes and goals of the patient. Palliative care services and hospital ethics committees can help resolve some of the complexity of decision-making at these times.

As a general rule, clarity of communication is eased by early consideration of the goals of care that should be considered for a patient.[2] This need not involve early prognostication but is simply an exercise in discovery, asking about what is important to the patient in the context of their acute illness. Listening to and understanding what is expected or anticipated by a family allows identification of any gaps in comprehension, as well as centring subsequent communication around how these goals are either being or likely to be met. This also provides an opportunity to reiterate to the family the importance in considering any expressed wishes of the patient that they know of, or attitudes to illness and disability that they can realistically extrapolate from.

Substituted decision-making is often difficult in circumstances of estrangement, distances of time and space, and limited interactions, and care must be taken to ensure that the decisions made actually serve that best interest goal as well as avoid harm.

FUTILITY

The concept of futility often intrudes in these discussions but should be used sparingly. True physiological futility indicates that no matter what interventions are performed or treatments introduced, the disease process has crossed a threshold of reversibility in progression towards inevitable death.[3] In other words, in these circumstances death may be a matter of hours, occasionally days, but a forecast of weeks raises concerns on accuracy.

A definite prediction of physiological failure is distinct from a physician offering subjective estimates of prognosis, which may unfortunately be erroneous.[4]

The accuracy of probabilistic assessments of outcomes depend on accumulated historical experience, the accuracy of matching that previous data to the current clinical situation, and the validity of conclusions drawn. There is an ethical duty of honesty towards examining the biases that may affect these assessments; e.g., limited experience, inappropriate matching of the patient to previous situations, and undue weighing of one consequence over another because of personal belief.

However, physicians do make errors of pessimism as well as the more common errors of optimism.[4,5] The former may be relatively more prevalent in cases of neurological dysfunction. The primary concern is that in over-emphasizing the probability of a negative outcome to surrogate decision makers, outcome may be translated into certainty by a consequent withdrawal of care in what is now a self-fulfilling prophecy of nihilism.[6]

Conversely, errors of optimism may have fundamental effects upon not just the patient (e.g., the extended induction of pain and discomfort without benefit), but can also have secondary consequences on patient families, as well as indirect effects upon the community.

An inability to admit the limitations of circumstance and skill puts the physician's goals ahead of those of the patient. While that may be seen as extending life (ordinarily a good goal in itself), the ethical doctrine of *Deontology* asks that we consider the worth of our actions

as well as the result. The ends can only be justified by the means, when the means themselves are morally appropriate.

Utilitarianism is an alternate ethical approach which asks that actions taken should be with an aim to have the greatest benefit. Benefit can be considered at the individual level, but can also be considered at the community level— 'social justice'.

Consideration of these principles may mean that it is ethically inappropriate to offer an over-optimistic prognosis where there are genuine family concerns of an overwhelming risk of outcomes that would not have been acceptable to the patient. Misplaced optimism may persuade them to continue treatment, which may risk those inappropriate outcomes.

This would be wrong from a deontological point of view and from both individual and community senses of utilitarianism where utilization of limited treatment resources may restrict the ability of others to receive appropriate care.

In navigating between the Scylla and Charybdis of therapeutic nihilism and misplaced optimism, the ethically responsible physician must retain objectivity in considering the strength of data along with transparency in admitting what is known and what is not known. This serves to engage authorized surrogates in the decision-making process with increased confidence that the patient's best interests are being served.[7]

Jonsen and colleagues have developed a useful construct to aid the identification and collation of this type of critical information, and the neurocritical care physician is advised to develop some awareness of the methodology of this approach.[3]

A series of detailed questions on the patient and their situation are asked within each of the four domains, each of which encapsulate key ethical principles:[3]

- Medical indications: the principles of beneficence and non-maleficence
- Patient preferences: the principle of respect for autonomy
- Quality of life: the principles of beneficence, non-maleficence, and respect for autonomy
- Contextual features: justice and fairness

In answering these questions, the clinical team and family members (occasionally in the same sitting) facilitate the construction of a summary of key issues to be subsequently referred to in discussion. The identification of these issues affords clarity in that and later discussions. It can expose biases and uncertainties that might otherwise have undue effect upon decision-making.

CONFLICTS

Although rare, family members may sometimes pursue decisions for their own personal advantage, e.g., financial gains or avoidance of costs, social inconvenience, and general disinterest in the patient's well-being. The clinical team is not duty bound to follow all orders from each of the surrogates, if they believe that in doing so, the patient may come to unexpected harm or disadvantage. However, this does not provide a platform for the healthcare team to unilaterally reject a direction towards end-of-life care when it may reasonably be deemed appropriate.

Instead, clinical teams should be able to seek objective review by the hospital ethics committee or similar agency so as to protect the patient against what may be perceived as adverse interests.

A more common scenario is that of persistent family or surrogate optimism towards outcome, which physicians and health providers feel is misplaced, and at odds with the patient's prognosis. This may happen, despite honest and candid self-assessment of practitioner biases and the possibility of therapeutic nihilism. It can derive from distrust of physicians based on previous experience. Race may also be a factor with concerns around trust for non-Caucasian families when dealing with Caucasian physicians.[8]

The invocation of faith (i.e., 'God will provide a miracle') adds significant further complexity and challenge.[9] If rejecting the possibility of divine intervention, the physician or care provider can be perceived as rejecting or attacking the faith of the family and/or patient. Careful exploration of the meaning and significance of a miracle, in a non-argumentative fashion, may help this situation,[9] and the advantages of enlisting the support of spiritual care services in this discussion cannot be overemphasized.

Even if the situation cannot be resolved and care is maintained in the face of a hopeless prognosis, there needs to be a careful but honest discussion of non-escalation of therapy.

While recognizing that futility may be subjective, physicians are not obliged to introduce care that will not improve outcome. That, in turn, does not mean that palliative interventions cannot be considered and used. Relief of suffering is a critical goal independent of curative prognosis. However, interventions that only briefly extend life must be thoroughly assessed for their risk of inducing accompanying pain and distress—such questions may require a specific ethics consult.[10]

MANAGEMENT OF END OF LIFE

If a decision is made to proceed to end-of-life care, based on either physiological futility or recognized inability to achieve an outcome based on the patient' attitudes and goals, it marks a profound shift of priorities from potential curative strategies towards the maintenance of comfort and freedom from adverse symptoms.

This decision should never be hurried nor inaccessible to appeal or requests of urgent ethical review. The practice of end-of-life care benefits from the use of protocols based on institutional consensus, which affords confidence and protection to individual physicians.[11]

Palliation of pain, anxiety, and distress are key goals that may require the use of medications such as benzodiazepines and opiates titrated for specific effect.

Concerns of both families and patients at this stage revolve around loss of control, autonomy, and dignity,[12] and much can be served in these respects by careful discussion around anticipated events and goals with the aim of providing knowledge and choice wherever possible. For example, patients may wish to forego certain sedative or analgesic regimens if they see these as obtunding their conscious state where clarity of mind is important for their communication with family and friends. Others may have more specific concerns on pain and anxiety that outweigh all other considerations. This latter aspect is usually mostly the case when dealing with the specifics of neurocritical care, given the frequency of pre-existing obtundation of consciousness and consequent constraints on communication.

Patients and families should be offered as much detail as they want on what precisely will happen. This information may extend to what devices will be removed, and how any attendant discomfort will be tended to. Alternatively, it may be enough to clearly establish what their goals are and leave specifics aside, with the understanding that these questions can be re-addressed, if situations or attitudes change.

It is ethically permissible to remove devices or treatments that will not bring about a beneficial change in outcome[13]—this can include (but is not restricted to) ventilators, external ventricular drains, extracorporeal oxygenation, pacemakers, circulatory assistance, and dialysis. The removal of feeding is generally considered as acceptable, as such medically-assisted nutrition is viewed as a medical intervention rather than basic comfort. It should also be remembered that both feeding tubes and nutrition can induce discomfort.[14] Palliative treatment for any concerns of hunger is easily provided, and most patients are anorexic in these situations.[15] Dehydration is more controversial and many authorities will provide basal fluid maintenance.

There is often tension around the treatment of pain and discomfort in the terminally ill patient amidst concerns that agents used for such can accelerate a patient's demise. In this setting, the principle of double effect can come into being. The maxim 'primum, non nocere' (firstly, do no harm) is well established in medical culture and training.[16] However, it may be permissible to perform an act (i.e., administer a treatment) that might ultimately accelerate the death of a patient, if it is for the purpose of relieving pain and distress, and does not directly cause death. Opiate and benzodiazepine infusions prescribed for analgesia and anxiolysis are classical examples of this approach. These should never be construed as euthanasia, as the intent is not to halt breathing or depress cardiovascular function, but rather allow titration to carefully defined end-points of relief from pain and agitation/anxiety. Neither by that perspective, can it be considered assisted suicide, given the difference in dosing targets.

Removal of the supportive devices listed above can frequently provoke distress and treatment should generally be initiated before their removal. As mentioned earlier, well-constructed institutional protocols afford significant advantages here such as the opportunity for pre-existing education of the whole clinical team as to methods and goals of care, and so the opportunity to avoid misperception and miscommunication of intent.[11]

CONCLUSION

End-of-life care presents many challenges to the clinician outside of their knowledge of physiology, pathology, pharmacology, and infectious disease. As such, the neurocritical care physician must understand and be fluent in concepts of communication, ethical practice, legal context, and the involvement and coordination of multidisciplinary care in mitigating pain and distress. Talking to patients and/or their families about end of life should be considered a medical intervention and requires no less skill than an operative procedure or a diagnostic manoeuvre.

Being unable to save life and recognizing the inevitability of death does not absolve our duty of care to the patient; rather it focuses our attention on listening, understanding, and facilitating what, for them, constitutes a good death.

REFERENCES

1. Moss AH, Ganjoo J, Sharma S, et al. Utility of the 'surprise' question to identify dialysis patients with high mortality. *Clin J Am Soc Nephrol* 2008;3(5):1379–84.

2. Rhodes A, Evans LE, Alhazzani W, et al. Surviving sepsis campaign: international guidelines for management of sepsis and septic shock 2016. *Intensive Care Medicine* 2017 Mar;43(3):304–77.

3. Jonsen AR, Siegler M, Winslade WJ. *Clinical Ethics: a Practical Approach to Ethical Decisions in Clinical Medicine.* 8th ed. New York: McGraw-Hill Education; 2015;6:244.

4. Christakis NA, Lamont EB. Extent and determinants of error in physicians' prognoses in terminally ill patients: prospective cohort study. *Western Journal of Medicine* 2000;172(5):310–13.

5. Navi BB, Kamel H, McCulloch CE, et al. Accuracy of neurovascular fellows' prognostication of outcome after subarachnoid hemorrhage. *Stroke* 2012;43(3):702–7.

6. Creutzfeldt CJ, Becker KJ, Weinstein JR, et al. Do-not-attempt-resuscitation orders and prognostic models for intraparenchymal hemorrhage. *Crit Care Med* 2011;39(1):158–62.

7. Lautrette A, Ciroldi M, Ksibi H, Azoulay E. End-of-life family conferences: rooted in the evidence. *Crit Care Med* 2006;34(Suppl 11):S364–72.

8. Welch LC, Teno JM, Mor V. End-of-life care in black and white: race matters for medical care of dying patients and their families. *Journal of the American Geriatrics Society* 2005;53(7):1145–53.

9. DeLisser HM. A practical approach to the family that expects a miracle. *Chest* 2009;135(6):1643–7.

10. Consensus statement of the Society of Critical Care Medicine's Ethics Committee regarding futile and other possibly inadvisable treatments. *Crit Care Med* 1997;25(5):887–91.

11. Pham TN, Otto A, Young SR, et al. Early withdrawal of life support in severe burn injury. *J Burn Care Res* 2012;33(1):130–5.

12. Steinhauser KE, Christakis NA, Clipp EC, McNeilly M, McIntyre L, Tulsky JA. Factors considered important at the end of life by patients, family, physicians, and other care providers. *JAMA* 2000;284(19):2476–82.

13. Lampert R, Hayes DL, Annas GJ, et al. HRS expert consensus statement on the management of cardiovascular implantable electronic devices (CIEDs) in patients nearing end of life or requesting withdrawal of therapy. *Heart Rhythm* 2010;7(7):1008–26.

14. Fine RL. Ethical issues in artificial nutrition and hydration. *Nutr Clin Pract* 2006;21(2):118–25.

15. Langhans W. Signals generating anorexia during acute illness. *The Proceedings of the Nutrition Society* 2007;66(3):321–30.

16. Smith CM. Origin and uses of primum non nocere—above all, do no harm! *Journal of Clinical Pharmacology* 2005;45(4):371–7.

54

Brain Death

M. J. Souter

ABSTRACT

Brain death is, in essence, the diagnosis of death by neurological criteria. It has been established as a concept for over half a century, consequent to technological innovations in cardiopulmonary critical care support, and is generally accepted across the world and its major religions. Diagnosis requires a history of cause, supportive imaging of neurological pathology, and detailed clinical neurological examination. Confounders must be carefully excluded. Alternatively, diagnosis may require the use of validated ancillary studies to support the examination in cases of induced uncertainty. Communication with families is crucial, in helping them understand a reality that may appear contradictory and is not intuitive. Compassion, sensitivity, and communication skills are key attributes for physicians to successfully manage these often sudden and tragic events.

KEYWORDS

Brain death; declaration of death by neurological criteria; Harvard criteria; apnoea test; ancillary study; cerebral blood flow (CBF); spinal reflexes.

INTRODUCTION

The concept of brain death is a relatively recent one consequent to advances in critical care in the latter half of the 20th century. The development of technology and capacity to provide a sustainable duration of positive pressure ventilation created a problem for neurologically devastated patients who would never previously have survived beyond hours of their crisis.

HISTORY

Whether by injury or disease, comatose patients were now being intubated (with an expectation of subsequent critical care), and their circulations supported with increasing availability of inotropes to survive variable durations thereafter in whatever critical care beds were available. Although Mollaret and Goulon were the authors of the more widely known paper identifying this clinical grouping of patients 'beyond coma',[1] Wertheimer and Jouvet were the earlier and more accurate reporters of 'death of the central nervous system [CNS]'.[2]

The absence of a medico-legal or ethical mechanism to inform or guide physicians towards the next steps led to scarce resources becoming occupied by patients who had no hope of recovery, but who could be maintained for days and weeks with appropriately attentive care. There were real concerns of liability for homicide if physicians decided to remove physiological support, especially in those patients who had been injured by the acts of others.

The concurrent development of immunology saw major advances in organ transplantation, with transplant surgeons subsequently turning their regard away from asystolic organ procurement towards an apparent source of perfused and functioning organs, with some attendant capacity for elective decision-making and preparation. Again, an absence of legal infrastructure led to challenges with uncontrolled approaches and declarations of brain death for the purposes of organ donation, with widespread concerns on conflict of interest.[3]

These apparent and potential conflicts led Henry Beecher, a Harvard ethicist and anaesthesiologist, to request the Dean of the Harvard Medical School to convene an ad hoc committee to determine criteria for the diagnosis of brain death. A group of neurologists, ethicists, neurosurgeons, public health physicians, and theologians were chaired by Beecher in the production of guidelines published in 1968.[4] These guidelines for management provided the objective criteria to determine irreversible loss of brain function associating that with brain death, but also identified an opportunity for organ procurement from these patients who could now be considered dead. As such this was the first appearance of what can be called the 'dead donor rule',[5] where it was also stated that living patients must not be harmed by removal of vital organs.

In that same year, the World Medical Assembly made the Declaration of Sydney, which identified death as a continuum from the death of a few cells, through death of tissues, organs and then of the organism itself.[6] It also identified that points of irreversibility exist on this continuum beyond which tissues, organs, or indeed the organism itself cannot survive, irrespective of treatment. Death of the brain was taken as a point of irreversibility, signifying the inevitable death of the patient.

The Harvard criteria were essentially prospectively validated by the national corroborative study[7] where 102 of the 503 patients admitted in apnoeic coma met the Harvard criteria. All these patients expired despite sustained management.

Finland was the first country in the world to legally codify brain death in 1971.[8] Subsequently, a President's Commission on Bioethics Report[9] recognized the need for a legal definition of death based on irreversible loss of function of the whole brain, which was codified by the Uniform Determination of Death Act.[10] In the UK, a joint report of the royal colleges proposed the criteria of brain death in 1976 along with details of an apnoea test, subsequently retitled to reflect the diagnosis of death of the brainstem.[11] In these and many other jurisdictions, the concept of death declared on neurological criteria is now widely recognized, whereas the details of criteria employed are left to prevailing medical standards with consequent variability of opinion and practice.[12]

NEUROLOGICAL EXAMINATION

As with any diagnostic process, the initial consideration of brain death must start with history. There should be a proximate and irreversible cause of injury and/or disease to explain sustained coma, supplemented by available imaging to demonstrate CNS pathological changes.

Following this, at the central core of most declarations based on neurological criteria, is an *irreversible* loss of neurological function, which, in turn, is defined as a persistent inability to evoke a *reflex* response on centrally delivered stimuli and that persistence should extend beyond the possible contribution of such transient factors like oedema or local mass effect, e.g., brainstem haemorrhages.

Testing a reflex arc highlights the concept of a functional pathway traversing the CNS. When receptor and effector pathway components are intact, subsequent deficit of function is interpreted as a loss of CNS integration. This capacity of *integrative* function is of critical importance in relating brain death to death of the individual.

The reflex arcs tested therein, lie within the mid-brain, pons, and medulla. The examples of neurological reflex testing are listed in Table 54.1.

CONFOUNDERS

The interpretation of the absence of these reflexes may be confounded by the presence of

a. Drug intoxication: whether that be iatrogenic or self-induced, including (but is not restricted to) analgesics, sedatives, and neuromuscular paralytics
b. Severe electrolyte abnormalities: e.g., hyponatraemia, hypokalaemia, hyperkalaemia, hypomagnesaemia, hypophosphataemia, uraemia, hyperammonaemia. Hypernatraemia is unlikely to be a cause of depressed neurological function, especially if iatrogenic, consequent to the use of hypertonic saline
c. Endocrinological abnormalities: e.g., hypothyroidism
d. Hypotension: e.g., blood pressure less than 100 mmHg systolic or 65 mmHg mean
e. Hypoxia: e.g., <90% saturation on pulse oximeter
f. Hypothermia: less than 36 degrees Celsius

Appropriate care should be devoted towards excluding these factors before starting any testing. This includes prior consideration and anticipation of their occurrence during a clinical examination. It would not be appropriate, for example, to start an apnoea test on a patient who was barely above acceptable blood pressure limits, and subsequently expect vasodilation induced by hypercarbia. Similar caveats apply to borderline oxygenation.

Therapeutic hypothermia has been implicated in delayed recovery of neurological function when accompanied by confounding medication agents.[13] It is difficult to see how accidental hypothermia in this context is any less confounding than deliberate hypothermia given that the physiology would appear independent of intent. A period of observation once the patient is normothermic appears prudent, but there is little to no data on exactly how long

Table 54.1 Examples of neurological reflex testing

Neurological test	Reflex arc components
Absence of pupillary response to light	Retina; optic nerve; pretectal nuclei (olive); Edinger-Westphal nucleus; oculomotor nerve; ciliary ganglion.
Absence of cough in response to laryngeal, carinal or bronchial stimulation	Mucosal sensory receptors; internal laryngeal nerve; superior laryngeal nerve; vagus nerve; upper medulla and pons; (1) nucleus ambiguus – > vagus; laryngeal muscles (2) nucleus retroambigualis – > phrenic + intercostal nerves; diaphragm and intercostal muscles
Absence of gag in response to palatal or posterior pharyngeal stimulation	Mucosal sensory receptors; glossopharyngeal nerve; nucleus ambiguus; glossopharyngeal + vagus + cranial accessory nerves; palatal and pharyngeal muscles
Absence of blinking or ocular movement in response to corneal stimulation (pressure or fluid drops)	Corneal sensory receptors; ciliary nerves; ophthalmic nerve; trigeminal nerve; trigeminal nucleus; reticular formation interneurons; facial nucleus; facial nerve (temporal branch); orbicularis oculi
Absence of eye movement in response to stimulation of the vestibular apparatus, either by temperature or movement	Sensory receptors of vestibular apparatus; vestibular nerve; vestibular nuclei; contralateral abducens nucleus; (1) Abducens nerve → lateral rectus (2) Medial longitudinal fasciculus → contralateral oculomotor nucleus → medial rectus
Absence of grimacing or similar responsiveness in response to noxious stimuli in the trigeminal nerve distributions	Ophthalmic/maxillary/mandibular nerves; trigeminal nerve; trigeminal nucleus; thalamo-cortical processing; facial nerve; facial muscles
Absence of induced respiratory drive upon presentation of a sufficiently elevated $PaCO_2$ challenge	(1) Central chemoreceptors respond to cerebrospinal fluid pH (elevated with hypercapnoea); (2) peripheral chemoreceptors in carotid and aortic bodies respond to elevated $PaCO_2$; respiratory centre; phrenic + intercostal nerves; diaphragm and intercostal muscles

a waiting period is required for confident assessment. Additional testing seems warranted (see ancillary test below).

It can be inferred from the above that the promotion and maintenance of physiological stability is an important component of a valid brain death assessment, and indeed for any neurological prognostication.[14] Essentially what is good for examining the brain death candidate is generally good for the survivor where the clinical situation is expected to improve.

CONDUCT OF TESTING

Prerequisites and diagnostic criteria and test to confirm brain death are elicited as follows:[15]

Prerequisites

- Confirm the presence of coma.
- Pre-oxygenate the patient with 100% oxygen.
- Ensure blood pressure is adequate.
- Check a baseline arterial blood gas (ABG).

Diagnostic criteria

- Pupillary light reflex: The pupils should be unresponsive ('fixed') to a bright light stimulus. Both eyes should be

tested for presence of direct and consensual constriction reflexes. The pupils need not be maximally dilated, and are often not, remaining in the midrange. Brain death removes both mydriatic as well as miotic tone. If in case of doubt, use a magnifier or pupilometer. Artificial eyes can be deceptively lifelike and embarrassing if missed.

- Cough reflex: A soft suction catheter should be directed down the endotracheal tube to ensure stimulation of the carina, which is the most sensitive area of the bronchial tree. The external larynx, chest, and abdomen should be watched carefully for movement. There should be none seen in brain death.

- Gag reflex: The palatal fauces should be directly stimulated (bilaterally) with a tongue depressor or rigid suction device. Look for palatal movement (e.g., stylopharyngeus).

- Corneal reflex: Press firmly on the temporal and nasal margins of the iris for each eye with a cotton bud. This is within the area of corneal innervation, but avoids abrading the central cornea and the risk of visual scarring or ulcer. Look for direct and consensual blink reflexes. They should be absent in brain death.

- Oculovestibular reflex: Incline the head of the bed to 30 degrees. Inspect the ear for plugs of blood or cerumen. With an assistant holding both eyes open, pass a soft cannula into the auditory canal, and direct 30–50 ml of ice-cold water (at least 10 degrees below ambient temperature) towards the tympanum over 45–60 seconds. Look for nystagmus with the fast component pointing away from the irrigated ear. There should be no response in brain death. Wait for 5 minutes, then repeat with the other ear. The presence of tympanic perforation generally renders the vestibular apparatus even more sensitive to temperature changes.[15] A gentle trickle of fluid may be used rather than forceful injection.

- Oculocephalic reflex: *After excluding the presence of spinal instability or injury*, the head should be rotated swiftly from right to left. The presence of eye movements should be assessed. If the patient is brain dead, the eyes are fixed in place and move with the head. If the patient is not brain dead but in coma, the eyes conjugately deviate opposite to the movement. The neck may also be flexed and extended, but care should be taken with flexion and the position of the endotracheal tube to avoid inappropriate progression down a bronchus.

- Noxious stimuli to the cranial nerve distributions: While avoiding areas of facial trauma, pain can be elicited by, (1) supraorbital pressure on the nerve as it exits the supraorbital notch at the junction of middle and medial thirds of the eyebrow, (2) forceful pressure with knuckles onto the temporomandibular joint, and (3) trapezius pinch. The presence of response to peripheral pain can also be elicited, but spinal reflexes may induce concern and confusion (see below).

- Apnoea test: After 10 minutes of pre-oxygenation have been accomplished (taken in performing the preceding tests), the baseline ABG should be reviewed. The patient's normal partial pressure of carbon dioxide ($PaCO_2$) would be indicated by a normal pH (acidity) (7.35 to 7.45) at that level, and ideally the patient should be managed close to that point, to abbreviate the apnoea period. The target for conclusion is 20 mmHg above baseline or greater than 60 mmHg, whichever is the *higher* of those two changes.

Hypocapnoeic (<40 mmHg) starting points can be entertained, but demand a longer period of apnoea to progress to over 60 mmHg.

The patient should be removed from the ventilator to remove any concern for cardiac impulse being perceived and supported as a breath. Use either:

1. A suction catheter with side port occluded and pass this down the endotracheal tube with opportunity for gas to exit the circuit and avoid barotrauma. A flow of around 8–10 litres per minute is ordinarily sufficient, as higher flows risk turbulence inducing CO_2 clearance.

2. A T-piece circuit with 8–10 litres per minute of oxygen and *partial* occlusion of the distensible reservoir bag sufficient to *partially* expand it, but not enough to fully do so (risking insensitivity to active signs of breathing as well as barotrauma). This partial expansion provides an indicator of breathing (bag deflation) as well as providing some continuous positive airway pressure, which inhibits alveolar collapse during the apnoea period.

A useful rule of thumb for the required duration of apnoea is to assume 6 mmHg change in $PaCO_2$ in the first minute and 3 mmHg for each subsequent minute. This assumes normal metabolic production of carbon dioxide at temperatures above 36°C. Having an adequately warmed patient again minimizes the apnoea period and reduces the risk of inadequate end-point and invalid test. The chest and abdomen (and reservoir bag, if used) should be watched during this period for any signs of respiratory activity. If any such occurs, the test is immediately stopped and the patient returned to the ventilator. Do not wait to sample blood gases. Some reduction in blood pressure is not uncommon over the course of the apnoea test, consistent with CO_2 inducing local vasodilation. Administration of 500–1000 ml of intravenous fluid often suffices to mitigate this.

If the patient becomes significantly hypotensive (less than 90 mmHg systolic) or hypoxic (less than 85% on pulse oximeter), an ABG should be quickly drawn to assess the $PaCO_2$ target while the patient is being returned to the ventilator.

With appropriate attention to stability of blood pressure and oxygenation, the apnoea test can be conducted safely without incident. For that reason alone, the physician should never leave the room during the conduct of this test, but the primary responsibility remains the correct diagnosis of death, entrusted to physicians by society, which cannot and should not be abdicated.

Different countries express varying opinions on the question of the most appropriate speciality to conduct brain death testing[12]—most identify *recent* neurological expertise as important. This does not exclude neurointensivists who should render themselves within that community by means of appropriate speciality training. The answers to questions on the number of tests required and requisite periods of time between observations vary considerably across the world.

ANCILLARY STUDIES

There are however consistent expectations that ancillary investigations should be used to reduce any uncertainty induced by the presence of confounders of examination. These investigations are based on either flow-based imaging (digital angiography, isotopic perfusion studies) or electroencephalographic correlates of function.

In circumstances where a comprehensive examination is not feasible, these ancillary studies are targeted towards supplementing those parts of the clinical examination which can be completed. Typical scenarios include pulmonary oedema precluding adequate performance of an apnoea test, as above, or trauma-induced facial oedema that renders the pupils inaccessible to clinical examination. Drug intoxication and hypothermia (especially when used for neurologic protection after anoxia) are also prevalent contributors of uncertainty and flow studies may be especially helpful.

However, a critically important principle is that these tests have their own incidence of error, and while being informative, cannot altogether *replace* a test of function. Illustrating that most physicians would not use a chest X-ray to independently diagnose deficits of gas exchange—the deficits may be inferred, but not confirmed. Consequently, ancillary studies should *accompany* and *supplement* the clinical exam, rather than be used as a means of avoiding appropriate clinical assessment.

Unvalidated modalities currently include computed tomography (CT) angiography and perfusion, magnetic resonance (MR) angiography, and positron emission tomography (PET) scanning. These possess insufficient accuracy for confident use and should not be used to either make or support a diagnosis of brain death.[16–18]

While there have been many publicized instances of 'miraculous' recovery, these have without exception arisen from the presence of a confounder or an imperfectly executed examination.

There are to date no instances of return of cerebral function following a properly conducted clinical examination in over 50 years of accumulated experience.[17] Examination must always be repeated or supplemented in circumstances of uncertainty.

SPINAL REFLEXES

One of the most distressing causes of uncertainty are spinally mediated reflexes independent of the brain, which can occur in up to 50% of neurologically deceased patients.[19] Central generators within the spinal cord function to maintain patterns of movement responses in a state of readiness, but are selectively inhibited by descending glycinergic pathways from the brain. The degree of activity seen in peripheral limbs tends to inversely correlate to the distance from the brain. This author has seen arms flailing, legs kicking, and truncal flexing— all in patients who manifested no response to detailed neurological testing by two independent examiners, and many instances accompanied by absence of any cerebral blood flow (CBF).

Families and caregivers should ideally be warned beforehand to expect these movements, with the aim of limiting induced confusion, falsely raised hopes, and subsequent distress.

COMMUNICATION

Pronouncement and communication of the diagnosis of brain death should have been preceded wherever possible by communication of the severity of the patient condition and anticipation of possible findings. Two examiner protocols separated by obligate time periods do allow presentation of the findings of the first examination, with confirmation by the second examination in what is essentially a staged presentation. In any circumstance, questions should be answered comprehensively and any opportunities for family presence during the examination should be utilized, as this often translates abstract concepts during discussion into an inescapable factual reality.

Families who were present for brain death examination demonstrated improved understanding of brain death, and reported no adverse emotional or psychological consequences—indeed recommending that this should be extended to other family members.[20]

Families may often manifest denial as a part of acute grief reactions to communication of the diagnosis. These deaths are often precipitated and there is rarely an opportunity to be prepared for the worst. Sensitivity, compassion, and repetition are key attributes in helping them come to terms with the tragic situation. Second opinions may be furnished as necessary, as equating death with ongoing pulse, ventilation, and warm extremities is not an easy step for many families to make.

Spiritual care services are often very helpful in mitigating the degree of grief and distress felt, and aid the handling of desperate arguments for miracles, etc. (see Chapter 53, 'End-of-Life Care'). There are some very specific religious exemptions from discontinuation of support after a diagnosis of brain death,[3] but these are limited to certain beliefs, countries, and areas, and local hospital protocols should be evolved for this contingency.

The important consistent message overall is that their loved one has died—in essence, brain death is the final common pathway of all modes of dying, including cardiopulmonary arrest.

CONCLUSIONS

Diagnosis of death by neurological criteria mandates attention to detail with no room for compromise in fact or circumstance. To do otherwise is a disservice to patients, families, and society as a whole.

REFERENCES

1. Mollaret P, Goulon M. [The depassed coma (preliminary memoir)]. *Rev Neurol (Paris)* 1959;101:3–15.

2. Wertheimer P, Jouvet M, Descotes J. [Diagnosis of death of the nervous system in comas with respiratory arrest treated by artificial respiration]. *Presse Med* 1959;67(3):87–8.

3. Souter M, Van Norman G. Ethical controversies at end of life after traumatic brain injury: defining death and organ donation. *Crit Care Med* 2010;38(Suppl 9):S502–9.

4. A definition of irreversible coma. Report of the ad hoc committee of the Harvard Medical School to examine the definition of brain death. *JAMA* 1968;205(6):337–40.

5. Robertson JA. The dead donor rule. *Hastings Cent Rep* 1999;29(6):6–14.

6. Gilder SS. Twenty-second world medical assembly. *Br Med J* 1968;3(5616):493–4.

7. An appraisal of the criteria of cerebral death. A summary statement. A collaborative study. *JAMA* 1977;237(10): 982–6.

8. Randell TT. Medical and legal considerations of brain death. *Acta Anaesthesiol Scand* 2004;48(2):139–44.

9. President's Commission for the Study of Ethical Problems in Medicine and Biomedical and Behavioral Research. Defining death: a report on the medical, legal and ethical issues in the determination of death. Washington DC;1981.

10. Uniform Determination of Death Act, 1980. Available from: http://www.lchc.ucsd.edu/cogn_150/Readings/death_act.pdf

11. Criteria for the diagnosis of brain stem death. Review by a working group convened by the Royal College of Physicians and endorsed by the Conference of Medical Royal Colleges and their faculties in the United Kingdom. *J R Coll Physicians Lond* 1995;29(5):381–2.

12. Wahlster S, Wijdicks EF, Patel PV, et al. Brain death declaration: Practices and perceptions worldwide. *Neurology* 2015;84(18):1870–9.

13. Webb AC, Samuels OB. Reversible brain death after cardiopulmonary arrest and induced hypothermia. *Crit Care Med* 2011;39(6):1538–42.

14. Souter MJ, Blissitt PA, Blosser S, et al. Recommendations for the critical care management of devastating brain injury: prognostication, psychosocial, and ethical management: a position statement for healthcare professionals from the Neurocritical Care Society. *Neurocrit Care* 2015;23(1):4–13.

15. Machado C. Diagnosis of brain death. *Neurology International* 2010;2(1):e2.

16. Taylor T, Dineen RA, Gardiner DC, Buss CH, Howatson A, Pace NL. Computed tomography (CT) angiography for confirmation of the clinical diagnosis of brain death. *Cochrane Database Syst Rev* 2014(3):CD009694.

17. Wijdicks EF, Varelas PN, Gronseth GS, Greer DM. American Academy of N. Evidence-based guideline update: determining brain death in adults: report of the quality standards subcommittee of the American Academy of Neurology. *Neurology* 2010;74(23):1911–8.

18. Luchtmann M, Bernarding J, Beuing O, et al. Controversies of diffusion weighted imaging in the diagnosis of brain death. *J Neuroimaging* 2013;23(4):463–8.

19. Saposnik G, Basile VS, Young GB. Movements in brain death: a systematic review. The Canadian journal of neurological sciences. *Le Journal Canadien Des Sciences Neurologiques* 2009;36(2):154–60.

20. Tawil I, Brown LH, Comfort D, et al. Family presence during brain death evaluation: a randomized controlled trial. *Crit Care Med* 2014;42(4):934–42.

55

Organ Donation

M. J. Souter

ABSTRACT

Advances in immunology have rendered organ transplantation as a viable treatment for organ failure. Organs are procured from three different sources: (1) living donation, (2) donation from a deceased donor with a beating heart, and (3) donation from a deceased donor without a beating heart.

Despite this diversity, the available pool is inadequate to meet the demand with more patients added to the waiting list every year than there are available donors with consequent mortality. Attention is therefore focused on maximizing the deceased donor pool by challenging pre-existing dogma on organ 'rule-outs'. Concurrently, addressing the respective inflammatory and ischaemic consequences arising from brain death or cardiac arrest may improve the functional quality of available organs. In the brain dead, operating principles of critical care can focus on targeted physiological support of the donor with the aim of mitigating secondary/tertiary insults while facilitating recovery. Organs sourced from donors without a beating heart are being increasingly identified as possible sources of allograft for not just liver and kidneys, but now lungs, and possibly even hearts. Donors previously considered 'marginal' may now have organs transplanted into elderly recipients in attempts to match function to expectations of requisite viability. The use of paired as opposed to single donations may also contribute meaningful function from a single previously unconsidered donor and transform recipient quality of life. At the same time, extracorporeal perfusion is beginning to offer possibilities for selective reconditioning and functional organ resuscitation.

KEYWORDS

Organ donation; transplantation; living donors; brain death; donation after death declared by circulatory criteria; Maastricht Protocol; catecholamines; hormonal resuscitation; extracorporeal perfusion.

INTRODUCTION

Developments in immunology and pharmacotherapy have transformed the practice of organ donation to the extent that it has now passed from the realm of the exceptional into relatively commonplace practice. Insights into Human Leukocyte Antigen (HLA) donor–recipient interactions has progressed from a dependency on identical haplotypes to now allowing more efficient matching of the dominant HLA-antigen D Related (DR) and B antigens, recognizing that the A antigen has little impact.[1] At the same time, development of the interleukin (IL)-2 antagonist, tacrolimus has provided significant reduction in the rates of acute graft rejection.[2]

The consequent effect is that transplantation is now a realistic option for patients experiencing terminal organ failure. This also means that more patients are on the waiting list for transplantation than ever before. The gap between organ availability and need has worsened rather than improved with 22 patients dying each day on the waiting list in the United States, but only 3 in every 1000 of the general public dying in a way that allows organ donation after death.[3]

While up to eight individuals may possibly receive a transplanted organ from a single deceased donor, both the disease/injury causing death and those pathophysiological changes induced by death can impair organ function (especially heart and lungs), precluding successful transplantation. This is prior to consideration of any existing co-morbidities. Consequently, the average number of organs transplanted per donor (OTPD) is around 3.07.[4] This limited number is a provocation to continually assess opportunities to improve donor organ function.

LIVING ORGAN DONATION

The first successful organ transplant was the donation of a kidney between living identical twin brothers, and living donation remains a significant part of organ transplantation. By avoiding the physiological insults associated with injury and death, living donor organs demonstrate the best function after transplantation. While 40% of donors in the US are living donors, the donated organs constitute around 20% of total transplants.[3] This difference is explainable on the basis of living donors being able to donate a single paired organ or a single lobe of liver or lung.

The central ethical doctrine operating throughout all organ donations is related to the 'do no harm' principle, i.e., organ procurement should not cause death or injury. Consequently, single vital organs can only be procured from the dead—not the living. This is known as 'the dead donor rule'.[5]

Consequently, there are rigorous screening and counselling processes surrounding living donation with extensive opportunities for reconsideration and a high standard of informed consent. There are known implications to later health, including consequent reduced functional reserve, as well as the risks of the surgical procedure itself. Nonetheless, many individuals persist—perhaps related to the fact that 75% of these donations are between family members.[6]

DONATION AFTER DEATH

Most transplantation worldwide is from organs donated after death. Ensuring that diagnosis is correct and independent of any secondary consideration of transplantation is fundamental to maintaining the public trust in organ donation.

Living individuals may authorize donation after their death in a manner analogous to making a will. This can be considered as an instruction for the disposition of their body—in this case, their organs. In the United States, this donation falls under laws governing gifts and does not require detailed informed consent as the subjects are deceased. Many countries have similar provisions.

Mechanisms for donating organs after death differ significantly depending on the criteria used to declare death. Essentially, death can be declared by either neurological or circulatory criteria.

Donation after Death Declared by Neurological Criteria (Brain Death)

After verification of death, if there is no prior authorization, it is ethically permissible to make a direct request of surrogate decision makers to consider organ donation based on what they know of the deceased's attitudes and wishes.

Such requests are best done by suitably trained staff as they enjoy a higher positive response than untrained requestors.[7] The Joint Commission (an accrediting body in the USA) makes using a trained requester a condition of participation for hospitals receiving accreditation.[8] This does not mean that medical staff cannot make that request; simply that they must be trained how to do so. In the author's experience, many physicians prefer that separation in order to present an appearance of acting purely for the donor, without perceptions of secondary gain or conflict of interest.

After a decision to donate has been made, the clinical team should clarify the bounds of intervention; for example, whether it is appropriate to perform manual cardiopulmonary resuscitation (CPR) on a potential donor following brain death. There is no ethical barrier to doing so, and the main issue is the pragmatic question of organ viability in the face of additional hypotensive or anoxic insults. Hearts that have experienced recent CPR can be transplanted successfully.[9,10] In these situations, some degree of judgement is required, and if there is no rapid return of spontaneous circulatory activity within an acceptable time period, then attempts at resuscitation can be discontinued.

Minimizing risk to the recipient requires careful evaluation of both organ function and the possibility of infectious or neoplastic transmission, but must be considered in the light of their possible mortality while on the waiting list.

The risk–benefit equation for transplant varies significantly between possible recipients depending on the gravity of their condition and urgency of need. Donor hospitals should generally not make decisions on donor candidacy based on their perceptions of donor suitability.

However, in contrast to historical practices geared towards rushing to the operating room, careful management of the deceased donor can offer opportunities for recovery of organ function and increase the number of organs procured especially where management goals are clearly targeted towards correcting deficits of blood pressure, circulatory volume, and oxygenation.[11,12]

Time and effort spent in optimizing donors also improves the function of transplanted kidneys for the recipient.[13] This is best accomplished by understanding the pathophysiological changes occurring after death.

Pathophysiology

The sequence of primary injury initiating brain death, accompanying trauma, and the subsequent inflammatory consequences of cerebral ischaemic injury initiate cytokine release and complement activation with diverse effects on organ systems in what has been termed a 'double-hit'.[14–16]

The cardiopulmonary system usually experiences the worst of this, being first in line for cerebral venous effluent and the associated inflammatory dysfunction.[14,17–19] Dysfunction is often aggravated by the sympathetically mediated hypertension of herniation.[20]

Preceding treatment of intracranial hypertension and cerebral ischaemia can induce additional iatrogenic insult, e.g., hypovolaemia following mannitol or increased cardiac work secondary to inotropes targeted at improving cerebral blood flow.

Once the brain has died, these insults are further compounded by disruption of central homoeostasis and the sympathetic nervous system with consequent vasoplegia, reduction in myocardial chronotropy and contractility, and frequent diabetes insipidus. Around 80% of patients require treatment to maintain stable physiology.[20] While 30% of adults will have reduced ejection fraction on echocardiography,[21] so will 38% of children,[22] suggesting that such depressed function is less a consequence of chronic atherosclerotic disease, and more the result of acute metabolic stress, in a mechanism similar to Takotsubo cardiomyopathy.[23] This suggestion is supported by recovery of function over the next few days. Without intervention, the resulting hypotension and reduction in cardiac output give rise to peripheral ischaemia and acidosis—an end result which, in many ways, is very similar to the shock state.

Even with targeted treatment to augment blood pressure and cardiac output, 25% of possible donors remain hypotensive with subsequent organ dysfunction and loss of viability.[19]

As may be expected, the lungs do not escape lightly, with decreased pulmonary vascular resistance and increased blood flow,[24] associated with increased lung water[25] and impaired gas exchange.[17]

It should be remembered, however, that as for any intensive care unit (ICU) patient, lungs of the brain dead are just as vulnerable to the frequently encountered dysfunction induced by passive atelectasis and infection—this latter may arise from aspiration at the time of injury or hypostasis associated with immobility and postural limitation.[26,27]

Hypoxic and hypotensive insults are well recognized causes of liver and kidney dysfunction. Contrast computed tomography (CT) studies used for preceding diagnosis may also worsen renal function, especially when accompanied by hypovolaemia of diabetes insipidus or mannitol osmotherapy.[16,28] Hypernatraemia consequent to these last two conditions may also impair hepatic graft function, although this is increasingly being argued.[29]

Hyperglycaemia and electrolyte abnormalities are common,[30,31] although these are usually corrected to facilitate brain death diagnosis. They may recur subsequently though. Decreased adrenal[32] and thyroid function are common hormonal deficits with concern that anaerobic metabolism caused by the latter further depletes high energy phosphates depressing myocardial contractility.[31]

Management

Treatment of the such pathologies are based on correction of deficits and management to targeted physiological goals correcting hypovolaemia, supporting contractility with inotropes, and the vasoplegic circulation with pressors. These are primary skills of critical care physicians and consequently, it is not surprising that their involvement in management of the potential donor improves available organ recovery,[33] evidenced by decreased risks of delayed graft function with increased ICU time spent managing younger donors after brain death.[13]

Simple maintenance of physiological stability permits the demonstration of cardiac function recovery,[21,22] while optimization guided by output measurement increases the number of heart(s) procured.[34]

The use of vasopressors and inotropes is associated with increased OTPD and improved graft function.[35,36] However, restricting these agents to circumstances of definite need is also associated with improvement in OTPD.[37] Norepinephrine and vasopressin are preferred to epinephrine or dopamine on the basis of reduced frequency of arrhythmias.[38]

Vasopressin has an array of actions governed by its differing receptors. Vasoconstriction and platelet aggregation are stimulated by the action of the V1 receptor, whereas the V2 receptor has an antidiuretic effect on the distal collecting duct, stimulating water resorption. Activation of V2 receptors on endothelial cells induce the release of Factor VIII and von Willebrand factor (vWf).[39]

By infusion, it will increase mean arterial pressure and reduce catecholamine requirements,[40,41] although there are differing viewpoints on its role in correcting vasoplegia.[41,42] Higher doses may induce intestinal ischaemia,[43] and care should be exercised in circumstances of critical visceral perfusion.

Its use, when combined with glucorticoid and thyroid hormone was associated with improving cardiac function to the extent that initially unsuitable hearts could be transplanted.[44,45] A large case series associated such combination use with increased function in hearts, lungs, livers, and kidneys after transplant, although the treatment group may have been biased by a reduced burden of comorbidities.[46,47]

Steroids are not used for anti-inflammatory effect, but more likely to facilitate the effectiveness of catecholamines.[48] Given the inflammatory storm accompanying brain death, it is unlikely that subsequent pharmacologic modulation has any real effect. They reduce prostacyclin production, increase the population of alpha-adrenoceptors, and inhibit nitric oxide,[49] which together with intracellular signalling actions enhances cyclic adenosine monophosphate (AMP) and serves to promote vasoconstriction.[50]

The use of steroids in patients experiencing brain death is associated with a reduction in catecholamine requirements,[51] but systematic reviews have failed to confirm this, with positive effects seen in observational studies that have not been supported by randomized controlled trials.[52]

Thyroid hormones increase calcium entry into the sarcoplasmic reticulum with consequent enhancement of heart rate and contractility.[53] In clinical studies, however, beneficial effects are concentrated within case series and are uncorroborated by randomized trials.[54]

The use of insulin is more controversial with concerns that its use decreased organ procurement, but these associations are based on a historical cohort analyses.[55] There is no evidence to support any donor nutritional strategy at present.

Fluid resuscitation should avoid the use of hydroxyethyl starch, which is associated with impaired renal function in critical illness.[56–60] There is little evidence to indicate further specificity of choice of fluids, although there is a reported association in critical illness between hyperchloraemia and an increased requirement for renal replacement therapy.[61]

Transfusion targets should be based on those used in general critical care given concerns for lung injury associated with red cell transfusion.[62] Albumin has been used to promote volume expansion, however, there

Table 55.1 Donor management goals

Physiological target	Donor management goal
1. Mean Arterial Pressure (MAP)	60–110 mmHg
2. Central Venous Pressure (CVP)	4–12 mmHg
3. Ejection Fraction (EF)	>50%
4. Vasopressor Use	≤1 and low dose
5. Arterial Blood Gas pH	7.3–7.5
6. PaO_2:FiO_2 (P:F)	>300 on PEEP = 5
7. Serum sodium (Na)	<155 mEq/L
8. Blood Glucose	<150 mg/dL
9. Urine Output (averaged over 4 hours)	>0.5 cc/kg/hr

Reprinted with permission from: Malinoski DJ, Patel MS, Ahmed O, et al. The impact of meeting donor management goals on the development of delayed graft function in kidney transplant recipients. *American Journal of Transplantation* 2013;13(4):993–1000.

are some theoretical concerns of caveolin-1 induced hyperpermeability across the alveolar membrane of transplanted lungs,[63] although no clinically significant evidence has as yet come to light.

Fluids should be titrated to resuscitation targets indicating adequate vascular filling balanced against an effect on donor lungs. The use of such 'donor management goals' (Table 55.1) is associated with increased organ procurement, despite the inclusion of more marginal and older donors,[11,64–66] and avoids excesses of loading. Dynamic circulatory assessments are increasingly preferred to static pressure measurement in critical care patients.[67,68]

Lung procurement has been relatively low, in comparison to abdominal organs, with only 20% of donor lungs being used, most probably for all the reasons of infectious risk and atelectatic changes described above, with high bars for age, pressure of arterial oxygen (PaO_2)/ fraction of inspired oxygen (FiO_2) ratio, and smoking history. These criteria have been increasingly questioned given that they arose from observations of a relatively small case series. [27] Aggressive interventions can increase the availability of suitable lungs.[69–71] Protocols for diuresis, fluid management, and recruitment manoeuvres can all improve lung function, and have translated initially rejected lungs into transplantable organs for selected recipients.[72] This would seem to indicate possible options for widening the donor pool, but many surgeons remain highly selective.

Other possibilities for improving marginal organs include the use of temperature management, as a recent study suggested better graft function in recipients receiving kidneys from donors randomized to moderate hypothermia versus those managed to normothermia.[73]

Combining marginal kidneys from less optimal donors into a single recipient is proving successful in expanding the donor pool. One of these kidneys as a single transplant may have proven inadequate, but in combination they achieve sufficient quality of renal function and excellent medium term outcomes, especially in older recipients.[74]

Perhaps the most striking example of changing boundaries is the now frequent transplantation of hepatitis C infected organs with eradication of the virus in the recipient. This principle has now been further extended towards removal of what was, in the United States, a federal prohibition against procurement of organs from HIV infected donors. This is now permitted for transplantation into HIV infected recipients as directed by the HIV Organ Policy Equity (HOPE Act).[75]

Assessment for infection is a continued concern throughout given the recipient risks of transmitted infection while immunosuppressed.[26] Thought should be given to aggressive and broad prophylactic coverage wherever suspicion of infection is present, given that the time course does not allow the normal evaluation process of species and sensitivities used for infectious evaluation in the critical care unit.[76]

Given the beneficial effects of critical-care-oriented intervention on continued physiological stability and subsequent graft function, there is an ethical mandate for physicians to maintain duty of care to the donor after death, increasing the opportunity for procurement and improving the outcome afforded by the donors wishes.

Donation after Death Declared by Circulatory Criteria (Cardiopulmonary Death)

Non-heart-beating donors were the mainstay of organ donation in the years prior to the introduction of legislation recognizing brain death. Although attention was focused on heart-beating donors for some time, the continued deficit in supply of organs encouraged a return to consideration of donors after death by circulatory criteria. While these organs may suffer an ischaemic insult at the time of death, this may be mitigated by a reduction in the inflammatory activation initiated by brain death. Certainly, explanted livers from donors declared by neurological criteria have increased inflammatory expression and leukocyte infiltration as opposed to those livers from donors after circulatory death.[77]

The Maastricht protocol initially identified opportunities for rapid donation after cardiac arrest, but is now categorized to include such uncontrolled presentations alongside the more commonplace controlled withdrawals of care.[78,79]

Maastricht Category III patients are those in whom circulatory death is *anticipated as a consequence of withdrawal of life-sustaining therapies*. Typical examples include patients with terminal neurological, cardiac, or respiratory disease where there has been a considered decision that the expected quality of life is not consistent with the patient's goals or wishes. If the patient is incompetent or incapable, then family or appointed individuals may exercise substituted judgement, as outlined in Chapter 53.

Patients wishing to donate their organs after death may have already identified their intent, and in the United States, hospitals are mandated to refer any patient who is critically ill to their local organ procurement organization (OPO) for consideration in the event that they proceed to end-of-life care.[8] Hospitals are similarly instructed to partner with OPO's to create carefully structured protocols for the management of such situations.

This does not entitle the OPO to make an approach to a dying patient, but is simply giving notice of a patient so that questions of suitability for donation can be addressed in advance, improving the logistics of preparation, screening and assessment, thus maintaining the option to donate if end of life care proceeds rapidly. This has directly facilitated an increased procurement of kidneys, liver, pancreas, and recently lungs. Hearts are also now being considered in this setting, supported by extracorporeal perfusion devices.

The key principle supporting ethical behaviour is that a decision to let death occur *must* have been made before *any* mention of organ donation can take place.

The development of institutional protocols for the practice of donation after death declared by circulatory criteria is strongly recommended and requires significant education, discussion, and review thereafter.[80] There are several key ethical principles that *do not permit compromise* and that involved physicians must have knowledge of.[81]

- Approaches to either patient or their surrogates can only be made after a decision has been made to move to end-of-life care.
- The patient's treating physician cannot be directly involved in any part of the procurement process.
- Procurement or transplant staff cannot be involved in the management of end-of-life care. This includes sedation, anxiolysis, and removal of life-supporting therapies.
- Pre-mortem procedures directly involving the patient (e.g., bronchoscopy, cannula insertion) require informed consent from the patient and/or their surrogates.
- Protocols should be devised to account for the likelihood of refusal of such procedures and that refusal should not inhibit proceeding with donation.

- Families should be permitted to be in attendance up until declaration of death and escorted away with support staff subsequently.

Successful graft function is dependent upon the burden of hypoxia suffered prior to death and the degree of what is entitled 'warm ischaemia' after death. Consequently, there are practical limits to the time window for viable donation. Removal of life-sustaining therapy can occur in an operating room environment or closely adjacent area to minimize inappropriate delays.

The time window extends from removal of life support to circulatory arrest. These limits are institutionally variable, but may extend up to 2 hours for kidneys, 1 hour for lungs, and 20–30 minutes for liver. Patients who do not expire within these periods should be transferred to a nursing environment elsewhere for continued end-of-life care.[80] The clinical team may be asked for a prediction of time till death. This is not an unusual question from relatives in this situation, and actually aids appropriate care of the patient by avoiding ill-placed attempts to donate if a more gradual deterioration of function is anticipated, as opposed to swift arrest of cardiopulmonary function. It also aids the efficiency and utilization of procurement resources, which may be needed for other donors elsewhere.

Death is declared on irreversible cessation of circulatory activity, usually characterized by pulselessness. Significant concerns arose around the optimal period of time required to determine irreversibility, with fear of spontaneous return of cardiac activity (i.e., auto-resuscitation) if that time were too short, but very real concerns on graft viability from warm ischaemia if there were inappropriate extension of the duration of observation. Those concerns have been addressed in North America by using a minimum period of pulselessness of 2 minutes and a maximum of 5 minutes before declaring death.[80,82] Surgical site disinfection and draping are permissible, prior to death, so long as they do not exclude family presence.

If lung procurement is planned in this setting, reintubation after death will be required with re-inflation, recruitment, and transient ventilation.[83] Anaesthesia staff should be involved in the formulation of protocols for lung procurement ahead of time—this may include specific prohibitions on involvement in prior withdrawal of life-sustaining therapy, as by intubating they are now considered a member of the procurement team.

As mentioned above, extracorporeal perfusion and reconditioning of organs is being performed with a goal of increasing both heart and lung utilization,[84] although heart perfusion is still experimental. Perfusion devices are currently used for extension of renal viability.

CONCLUSIONS

Donation of organs after death can bring comfort to bereaved and grieving family members if done well. This requires appropriate communication, compassion, and sensitivity. It is difficult to see how relief of family distress in such circumstances would not be in keeping with patient goals and principles of family-based care. If performed poorly, however, organ donation can amplify the distress for family members, with the risk of extension of that distress into the community.[85] The subsequent effects may extend well beyond the circumstances of individual cases, in biasing the public against being organ donors after their death. This in turn imperils the lives of other patients currently awaiting organ transplantation. The duty of care towards clinical conduct that supports and facilitates organ donation is evident and pressing.

REFERENCES

1. Opelz G. Correlation of HLA matching with kidney graft survival in patients with or without cyclosporine treatment. *Transplantation* 1985;40(3):240–3.
2. Haddad EM, McAlister VC, Renouf E, Malthaner R, Kjaer MS, Gluud LL. Cyclosporin versus tacrolimus for liver transplanted patients. *Cochrane Database Syst Rev* 2006;(4):CD005161.
3. U.S. Department of Health and Human Services. Organ donation statistics 2016. [cited 2017]. Available from: https://www.organdonor.gov/statistics-stories/statistics.html.
4. Association of Organ Procurement Organizations. Data on donation and transplantation 2016. [cited 2017 Jan 30]. Available from: http://www.aopo.org/related-links-data-on-donation-and-transplantation/.
5. Robertson JA. The dead donor rule. *Hastings Cent Rep* 1999;29(6):6–14.
6. International Association of Living Organ Donors I. Living Donors Online! 2016. [cited 2017 Jan 30]. Available from: http://www.livingdonorsonline.org/kidney/kidney2.htm.
7. von Pohle WR. Obtaining organ donation: who should ask? *Heart Lung* 1996;25(4):304–9.
8. Joint Commission on Accreditation of Healthcare Organizations. Strategies for narrowing the organ donation gap and protecting patients. Health care at the crossroads. [document on the Internet]. 2005. [cited 2016 Dec 28]. Available from: https://www.jointcommission.org/assets/1/18/organ_donation_white_paper.pdf.
9. Quader MA, Wolfe LG, Kasirajan V. Heart transplantation outcomes from cardiac arrest-resuscitated donors. *The Journal of Heart and Lung Transplantation* 2013;32(11):1090–5.
10. Orioles A, Morrison WE, Rossano JW, et al. An under-recognized benefit of cardiopulmonary resuscitation: organ transplantation. *Critical Care Medicine* 2013;41(12):2794–9.

11. Patel MS, Zatarain J, De La Cruz S, et al. The impact of meeting donor management goals on the number of organs transplanted per expanded criteria donor: a prospective study from the UNOS region 5 donor management goals workgroup. *JAMA Surg* 2014;149(9):969–75.

12. Abuanzeh R, Hashmi F, Dimarakis I, et al. Early donor management increases the retrieval rate of hearts for transplantation in marginal donors. *European Journal of Cardiothoracic Surgery* 2015;47(1):72–7; discussion 7.

13. Nijboer WN, Moers C, Leuvenink HG, Ploeg RJ. How important is the duration of the brain death period for the outcome in kidney transplantation? *Transplant International* 2011;24(1):14–20.

14. Barklin A. Systemic inflammation in the brain-dead organ donor. *Acta Anaesthesiol Scand* 2009;53(4):425–35.

15. Watts RP, Thom O, Fraser JF. Inflammatory signalling associated with brain dead organ donation: from brain injury to brain stem death and posttransplant ischaemia reperfusion injury. *J Transplant* 2013;2013:521369.

16. Dictus C, Vienenkoetter B, Esmaeilzadeh M, Unterberg A, Ahmadi R. Critical care management of potential organ donors: our current standard. *Clin Transplant* 2009; 23(Suppl 21):2–9.

17. Busl KM, Bleck TP. Neurogenic pulmonary edema. *Critical Care Medicine* 2015;43(8):1710–15.

18. Mierzewska-Schmidt M, Gawecka A. Neurogenic stunned myocardium—do we consider this diagnosis in patients with acute central nervous system injury and acute heart failure? *Anaesthesiology Intensive Therapy* 2015;47(2):175–80.

19. Wood KE, Coursin DB. Intensivists and organ donor management. *Curr Opin Anaesthesiol* 2007;20(2):97–9.

20. Cooper DK, Novitzky D, Wicomb WN. Hemodynamic and electrocardiographic responses. *Transplant Proc* 1988 Oct;20,5(Suppl 7):25–28.

21. Borbely XI, Krishnamoorthy V, Modi S, et al. Temporal changes in left ventricular systolic function and use of echocardiography in adult heart donors. *Neurocrit Care* 2015;23(1):66–71.

22. Krishnamoorthy V, Borbely X, Rowhani-Rahbar A, Souter MJ, Gibbons E, Vavilala MS. Cardiac dysfunction following brain death in children: prevalence, normalization, and transplantation. *Pediatr Crit Care Med* 2015;16(4):e107–12.

23. Berman M, Ali A, Ashley E, et al. Is stress cardiomyopathy the underlying cause of ventricular dysfunction associated with brain death? *The Journal of Heart and Lung Transplantation* 2010;29(9):957–65.

24. Bittner HB, Kendall SW, Chen EP, Craig D, Van Trigt P. The effects of brain death on cardiopulmonary hemodynamics and pulmonary blood flow characteristics. *Chest* 1995;108(5):1358–63.

25. Venkateswaran RV, Dronavalli V, Patchell V, et al. Measurement of extravascular lung water following human brain death: implications for lung donor assessment and transplantation. *European Journal of Cardio-Thoracic Surgery* 2013;43(6):1227–32.

26. Ruiz I, Gavaldà J, Monforte V, et al. Donor-to-host transmission of bacterial and fungal infections in lung transplantation. *American Journal of Transplantation* 2006; 6(1):178–82.

27. Van Raemdonck D, Neyrinck A, Verleden GM, et al. Lung donor selection and management. *Proceedings of the American Thoracic Society* 2009;6(1):28–38.

28. Mundt HM, Yard BA, Krämer BK, Benck U, Schnülle P. Optimized donor management and organ preservation before kidney transplantation. *Transplant International* 2016 Sep;29(9):974–84.

29. Kaseje N, McLin V, Toso C, Poncet A, Wildhaber BE. Donor hypernatremia before procurement and early outcomes following pediatric liver transplantation. *Liver Transplantation* 2015;21(8):1076–81.

30. Rhoney DH, Parker D, Jr. Considerations in fluids and electrolytes after traumatic brain injury. *Nutrition in Clinical Practice* 2006;21(5):462–78.

31. Novitzky D, Cooper DK, Rosendale JD, Kauffman HM. Hormonal therapy of the brain-dead organ donor: experimental and clinical studies. *Transplantation* 2006; 82(11):1396–401.

32. Dimopoulou I, Tsagarakis S, Anthi A, et al. High prevalence of decreased cortisol reserve in brain-dead potential organ donors. *Critical Care Medicine* 2003;31(4):1113–17.

33. Singbartl K, Murugan R, Kaynar AM, et al. Intensivist-led management of brain-dead donors is associated with an increase in organ recovery for transplantation. *American Journal of Transplantation* 2011;11(7):1517–21.

34. Venkateswaran RV, Steeds RP, Quinn DW, et al. The haemodynamic effects of adjunctive hormone therapy in potential heart donors: a prospective randomized double-blind factorially designed controlled trial. *Eur Heart J* 2009; 30(14):1771–80.

35. Schnuelle P, Berger S, de Boer J, Persijn G, van der Woude FJ. Effects of catecholamine application to brain-dead donors on graft survival in solid organ transplantation. *Transplantation* 2001;72(3):455–63.

36. Schnuelle P, Gottmann U, Hoeger S, et al. Effects of donor pretreatment with dopamine on graft function after kidney transplantation: a randomized controlled trial. *JAMA* 2009; 302(10):1067–75.

37. Franklin GA, Santos AP, Smith JW, Galbraith S, Harbrecht BG, Garrison RN. Optimization of donor management goals yields increased organ use. *Am Surg* 2010;76(6): 587–94.

38. Dellinger RP, Levy MM, Carlet JM, et al. Surviving sepsis campaign: International guidelines for management of severe sepsis and septic shock: 2008. *Critical Care Medicine* 2008;36(1):296–327.

39. Sharman A, Low J. Vasopressin and its role in critical care. Continuing Education in Anaesthesia. *Critical Care & Pain* 2008;8(4):134–7.

40. Chen JM, Cullinane S, Spanier TB, et al. Vasopressin deficiency and pressor hypersensitivity in hemodynamically

unstable organ donors. *Circulation* 1999;100(Suppl 19): II244–6.

41. SerpaNeto A, Nassar AP, Cardoso SO, et al. Vasopressin and terlipressin in adult vasodilatory shock: a systematic review and meta-analysis of nine randomized controlled trials. *Crit Care* 2012;16(4):R154.

42. Polito A, Parisini E, Ricci Z, Picardo S, Annane D. Vasopressin for treatment of vasodilatory shock: an ESICM systematic review and meta-analysis. *Intensive Care Med* 2012;38(1):9–19.

43. Russell JA. Bench-to-bedside review: Vasopressin in the management of septic shock. *Crit Care* 2011;15(4):226.

44. Novitzky D, Cooper DK, Reichart B. Hemodynamic and metabolic responses to hormonal therapy in brain-dead potential organ donors. *Transplantation* 1987;43(6): 852–4.

45. Wheeldon DR, Potter CD, Oduro A, Wallwork J, Large SR. Transforming the 'unacceptable' donor: outcomes from the adoption of a standardized donor management technique. *The Journal of Heart and Lung Transplantation* 1995;14(4):734–42.

46. Rosendale JD, Kauffman HM, McBride MA, et al. Hormonal resuscitation yields more transplanted hearts, with improved early function. *Transplantation* 2003;75(8):1336–41.

47. Rosendale JD, Kauffman HM, McBride MA, et al. Aggressive pharmacologic donor management results in more transplanted organs. *Transplantation* 2003;75(4): 482–7.

48. Nicolas-Robin A, Barouk JD, Amour J, Coriat P, Riou B, Langeron O. Hydrocortisone supplementation enhances hemodynamic stability in brain-dead patients. *Anesthesiology* 2010;112(5):1204–10.

49. Suzuki T, Nakamura Y, Moriya T, Sasano H. Effects of steroid hormones on vascular functions. *Microsc Res Tech* 2003;60(1):76–84.

50. Taylor DR, Hancox RJ. Interactions between corticosteroids and beta agonists. *Thorax* 2000;55(7):595–602.

51. Pinsard M, Ragot S, Mertes PM, et al. Interest of low-dose hydrocortisone therapy during brain-dead organ donor resuscitation: the CORTICOME study. *Crit Care* 2014;18(4):R158.

52. Dupuis S, Amiel JA, Desgroseilliers M, et al. Corticosteroids in the management of brain-dead potential organ donors: a systematic review. *Br J Anaesth* 2014;113(3):346–59.

53. Klein I, Ojamaa K. Thyroid hormone and the cardiovascular system. *The New England Journal of Medicine* 2001;344(7):501–9.

54. Macdonald PS, Aneman A, Bhonagiri D, et al. A systematic review and meta-analysis of clinical trials of thyroid hormone administration to brain dead potential organ donors. *Critical Care Medicine* 2012;40(5):1635–44.

55. Novitzky D, Mi Z, Videla LA, Collins JF, Cooper DK. Thyroid hormone therapy and procurement of livers from brain-dead donors. *Endocr Res* 2016;41(3):270–3.

56. Giral M, Bertola JP, Foucher Y, et al. Effect of brain-dead donor resuscitation on delayed graft function: results of a monocentric analysis. *Transplantation* 2007;83(9): 1174–81.

57. Robert R, Guilhot J, Pinsard M, et al. A pair analysis of the delayed graft function in kidney recipient: the critical role of the donor. *J Crit Care* 2010;25(4):582–90.

58. Cittanova ML, Leblanc I, Legendre C, Mouquet C, Riou B, Coriat P. Effect of hydroxyethylstarch in brain-dead kidney donors on renal function in kidney-transplant recipients. *Lancet* 1996;348(9042):1620–2.

59. Reinhart K, Perner A, Sprung CL, et al. Consensus statement of the ESICM task force on colloid volume therapy in critically ill patients. *Intensive Care Med* 2012; 38(3):368–83.

60. Hokema F, Ziganshyna S, Bartels M, et al. Is perioperative low molecular weight hydroxyethyl starch infusion a risk factor for delayed graft function in renal transplant recipients? *Nephrol Dial Transplant* 2011;26(10):3373–8.

61. Zhang Z, Xu X, Fan H, Li D, Deng H. Higher serum chloride concentrations are associated with acute kidney injury in unselected critically ill patients. *BMC Nephrol* 2013;14:235.

62. Kahn JM, Caldwell EC, Deem S, Newell DW, Heckbert SR, Rubenfeld GD. Acute lung injury in patients with subarachnoid hemorrhage: incidence, risk factors, and outcome. *Critical Care Medicine* 2006;34(1):196–202.

63. Maniatis NA, Kardara M, Hecimovich D, et al. Role of caveolin-1 expression in the pathogenesis of pulmonary edema in ventilator-induced lung injury. *Pulmonary Circulation* 2012;2(4):452–60.

64. Malinoski DJ, Daly MC, Patel MS, Oley-Graybill C, Foster CE, 3rd, Salim A. Achieving donor management goals before deceased donor procurement is associated with more organs transplanted per donor. *J Trauma* 2011;71(4):990–5; discussion 6.

65. Malinoski DJ, Patel MS, Ahmed O, et al. The impact of meeting donor management goals on the development of delayed graft function in kidney transplant recipients. *American Journal of Transplantation* 2013;13(4):993–1000.

66. Marshall GR, Mangus RS, Powelson JA, Fridell JA, Kubal CA, Tector AJ. Donor management parameters and organ yield: single center results. *J Surg Res* 2014;191(1):208–13.

67. Al-Khafaji A, Elder M, Lebovitz DJ, et al. Protocolized fluid therapy in brain-dead donors: the multicenter randomized MOnIToR trial. *Intensive Care Med* 2015;41(3):418–26.

68. Rhodes A, Evans LE, Alhazzani W, et al. Surviving sepsis campaign: International guidelines for management of sepsis and septic shock: 2016. *Intensive Care Med* 2017; 43(3):304–77.

69. Bhorade SM, Vigneswaran W, McCabe MA, Garrity ER. Liberalization of donor criteria may expand the donor pool without adverse consequence in lung transplantation. *The Journal of Heart and Lung Transplantation* 2000; 19(12):1199–204.

70. Gabbay E, Williams TJ, Griffiths AP, et al. Maximizing the utilization of donor organs offered for lung transplantation. *Am J Respir Crit Care Med* 1999;160(1):265–71.

71. Angel LF, Levine DJ, Restrepo MI, et al. Impact of a lung transplantation donor-management protocol on lung donation and recipient outcomes. *Am J Respir Crit Care Med* 2006;174(6):710–6.

72. Zych B, Garcia Saez D, Sabashnikov A, et al. Lung transplantation from donors outside standard acceptability criteria—are they really marginal? *Transplant International* 2014;27(11):1183–91.

73. Niemann CU, Feiner J, Swain S, et al. Therapeutic hypothermia in deceased organ donors and kidney-graft function. *The New England Journal of Medicine* 2015;373(5):405–14.

74. Stratta RJ, Farney AC, Orlando G, et al. Dual kidney transplants from adult marginal donors successfully expand the limited deceased donor organ pool. *Clin Transplant* 2016;30(4):380–92.

75. Durand CM, Segev D, Sugarman J. Realizing HOPE: The ethics of organ transplantation from HIV-positive donors. *Annals of Internal Medicine* 2016;165(2):138–42.

76. Powner DJ, Allison TA. Bacterial infection during adult donor care. *Progress in Transplantation* (Aliso Viejo, Calif) 2007;17(4):266–74.

77. Xu J, Sayed BA, Casas-Ferreira AM, et al. The impact of ischemia/reperfusion injury on liver allografts from deceased after cardiac death versus deceased after brain death donors. *PloS One* 2016;11(2):e0148815.

78. Sanchez-Fructuoso AI, Prats D, Torrente J, et al. Renal transplantation from non-heart beating donors: a promising alternative to enlarge the donor pool. *J Am Soc Nephrol* 2000;11(2):350–8.

79. Thuong M, Ruiz A, Evrard P, et al. New classification of donation after circulatory death donors definitions and terminology. *Transplant International* 2016;29(7):749–59.

80. The Institute of Medicine, Committee on Non-Heart-Beating Transplantation II. *Non-Heart-Beating Organ Transplantation: Practice and Protocols*. Washington, DC: National Academies Press; 2000.

81. Manara AR, Murphy PG, O'Callaghan G. Donation after circulatory death. *British Journal of Anaesthesia* 2012;108(suppl 1):i108–i21.

82. Ethics Committee ACoCCM, Society of Critical Care M. Recommendations for non-heart-beating organ donation. A position paper by the Ethics Committee, American College of Critical Care Medicine, Society of Critical Care Medicine. *Critical Care Medicine* 2001;29(9):1826–31.

83. Dunne K, Doherty P. Donation after circulatory death. *Continuing Education in Anaesthesia, Critical Care & Pain* 2011;11(3):82–6.

84. Vogel T, Brockmann JG, Coussios C, Friend PJ. The role of normothermic extracorporeal perfusion in minimizing ischemia reperfusion injury. *Transplantation Reviews* 26(2):156–62.

85. Merchant SJ, Yoshida EM, Lee TK, Richardson P, Karlsbjerg KM, Cheung E. Exploring the psychological effects of deceased organ donation on the families of the organ donors. *Clin Transplant* 2008;22(3):341–7.

Part XVI

Palliative Care

Editor: Mhoira Leng

Part XIII

PRINCIPLE DATA

56

Palliative Care in Neurology

M. E. F. Leng, C. Venkateswaran, and C. Singh

ABSTRACT

Palliative care which focuses on the holistic needs and quality of life for those living with chronic illness should be integrated into the management of chronic neurological illness. Prior to a neurointensive care admission palliative care interventions may improve decision-making and communication and allow for a more informed choice regarding intensive management, especially at the end of life. Following neurointensive care admission, recognising and assessing palliative needs can be supported with tools and practice-based protocols. Interventions will include excellent symptom control including pain management, support for ethical decision-making, establishing goals of care, improved communication, family support, and advanced care planning including end of life care. Integrated training with agreed core competencies and clinical pathways for specialist advice is essential including awareness of the need to care for healthcare providers.

KEYWORDS

Neurological patients; palliative care; terminal illness; neurointensive care.

INTRODUCTION

The World Health Organization (WHO) defines palliative care as 'an approach that improves the quality of life of patients and their families facing problems associated with life-threatening illness, through the prevention and relief of suffering by means of early identification and impeccable assessment and treatment of pain and other problems, physical, psychosocial, and spiritual'.[1] Historically, palliative care was thought of as a treatment for specific illnesses such as cancer and human immunodeficiency virus (HIV)/acquired immune deficiency syndrome (AIDS) and only applicable at the end of life. It is now well-recognized that this approach to care should be widened to include all chronic illnesses and must address the growing prevalence of non-communicable disease.[2] The management of chronic neurological conditions should include a palliative care approach and increasing evidence for early palliative care intervention and multidisciplinary care. We will explore the context for palliative care in neurointensive care, advance care planning, care in a neurointensive care setting, end-of-life care, and support for caregivers.

CONTEXT FOR PALLIATIVE CARE IN NEUROINTENSIVE CARE

The UK National Service Framework for Long Term Conditions mentions palliative care as a quality requirement for treating pain, other symptoms, and providing emotional and social support.[3] The 2017 National Health Policy for India[4] states the aim to 'improve health status through concerted policy action in all sectors and expand preventive, promotive, curative, palliative, and rehabilitative services provided through the public health sector with focus on quality'.

EARLY INTEGRATED PALLIATIVE CARE

This drive towards early identification of those living with chronic life-limiting illness who need palliative care interventions alongside other treatments is important when it comes to considering neurointensive care management. We should be thinking of the holistic needs of patients and their carers long before an admission to neurointensive care in addition to post-admission care.[5,6]

Some of the neurological conditions where palliative care may have a role include:

- Sudden onset conditions, e.g., acquired brain injury of any cause including stroke, and spinal cord injury (SCI), infections including malaria, cryptococcal meningitis, rabies, and tetanus[7,8]
- Intermittent conditions, e.g., severe chronic epilepsy
- Progressive conditions, e.g., motor neuron disease, multiple sclerosis (MS), Parkinson's disease and other neurodegenerative disorders, muscular dystrophies, malignancy, Alzheimer's disease and other dementias, infections such as HIV/AIDS, Creutzfeld-Jacob disease, subacute sclerosing panencephalitis
- Stable conditions with or without age-related degeneration, e.g., polio or cerebral palsy

Guidelines and practice support frameworks backed by increasing evidence show the importance and benefits of early, integrated palliative care for chronic neurological conditions.[9–11] This support should include symptom control such as pain relief but also social, psychological, and spiritual support which is person-centred and includes the family or carer networks.[12] There are particular challenges for this patient group including potential long duration of disease with fluctuating course, possibility of sudden deterioration such as an aspiration pneumonia and the presence of comorbidities, all of which makes both prognostication as well as the recognition of the end stage or dying phase difficult.[13–15] In addition, managing symptoms may be complex, especially if neuropsychiatric symptoms are present. There is also the need for multidisciplinary and intra-professional involvement requiring coordination and excellent communication. Finally, there is significant caregiver burden which will include financial and social implications of the existing illness prior to the neurointensive care admission.

PATHWAYS FOR INTEGRATING PALLIATIVE CARE

The 'UK End-of-Life Care in Long-Term Neurological Conditions: A Framework for Implementation' outlines a pathway for neurological disease:[11]

- *Diagnosis of the neurological condition*: Involves palliative and supportive care, as well as holistic measures
- *Future care discussions*: Discussion of cognitive status; ethical considerations; proactive management plans; and wishes and preferences and advance decisions

- *Generic triggers which show a decline in physical status including swallowing difficulties, weight loss, recurring admissions, and frequent infection*: Considerations include identifying a key worker and contacting the relevant palliative care service; detailing a needs assessment; an assessment for continuing healthcare; and assessing a person's decision-making/mental capacity. Clinicians also need to consider what may be the specific triggers showing that the end of life may be approaching
- *End-of-life care discussions and care in the last days of life*: Encompasses diagnosis and review of current medications, and ethical decision-making, along with support for carers
- *Care after death*: Includes bereavement support and supporting information

This integrated approach does not imply every patient should be seen by a specialist palliative care physician but rather a palliative care approach should be part of all chronic neurological and neurointensive care management with interventions by the neurointensive team and clear referral networks to specialist palliative care for complex problems as part of the multidisciplinary care.[16] Integration within training and continuing medical education is therefore essential and should include cross-disciplinary competencies for neurology, internal medicine, critical care, and anaesthesia, rehabilitation, oncology, care of the elderly, paediatrics, primary care as well as palliative care.[17]

ADVANCED CARE PLANNING

Many patients being admitted to neurointensive care have had little or no support to plan for their care and make the best choices for themselves and their family. Despite evidence that this can improve patient and carer satisfaction and support clinical decision-making, we all too often find communication has been inadequate combined with a lack of clear documentation leaving the patient, family, and clinical teams with little option other than an intensive care unit (ICU) admission.[18]

Some of the characteristics of patients who may be admitted to the ICU and yet have the goals of care for less-intensive management have been described as follows:[19]

- Patients who have an acute illness before understanding the outcome or patient's wishes
- Patients who require a high level of nursing/care
- Patients who may require medications, e.g., sedation which may not be possible in a ward
- Difficult symptom control

An innovative approach being modelled in India shows the benefits of early multidisciplinary assessment including palliative care, establishment of a hospital ethics committee to support clinical decision-making and introduction of 'allow natural death' orders that support good communication, information, and support for the patient, family, and medical team to make choices that avoid futile and expensive ICU admissions at the end of life.[20]

Advanced care planning also includes those who will be discharged to home after a neurointensive care admission and will heavily rely on effective rehabilitation and coordination of care as well as agreeing changing goals of care and support systems.

CARE IN A NEUROINTENSIVE CARE SETTING

The needs of patients in an intensive care are different from those with chronic neurological conditions. These patients need acute medical care but also have holistic needs including a huge burden of symptoms and emotional needs. In addition, there is uncertainty about prognosis and long-term recovery.[6]

IDENTIFYING PALLIATIVE CARE NEED

The most effective way to identify need is by ensuring a thorough holistic assessment is completed using a team approach whose members have competencies for palliative care and who have clear pathways for referral to specialist palliative care expertise.

The triggers for palliative care referral have been identified and these may support decision-making but also may be context-specific. These include:[17,21,22]

- Age (over 80 years)
- Length of stay (more than 10–14 days)
- Presence of number of life-threatening co-morbidities
- Status post cardiac arrest or advanced malignancy
- Poor pre-existing functional status
- Interventions such as tracheostomy or dialysis
- Request from patient or family

Effective referrals may also be hampered by poor understanding of palliative care, fear from the clinical team of seeming failure, poor communication skills, unrealistic expectations from family, and the overall challenges of managing the transition from curative focused care to palliative focused care. This has been described as a change from futility to utility.[23,24]

Focusing more on need rather than referral is the 4-item Palliative Care Needs Screening Tool (PNST) developed as part of the Improving Palliative Care in the ICU project.[25]

- Does the patient have distressing physical or psychological symptoms?
- Are there specific support needs for the patient and family?
- Are treatment options matched with patient-centred goals?
- Are there disagreements among teams and family?

This tool identified 62% of the studied ICU population with unmet palliative care needs irrespective of the level of consciousness at diagnosis. The most frequent need was for social support (53%) followed by goals of care (28%) and symptom control (12%). Perhaps this is a more appropriate way to offer an integrated approach as needs can be identified and interventions started by the ICU team, which may in turn lead to a specialist palliative care referral.

SUPPORTING PALLIATIVE CARE INTERVENTIONS

The actual pathway or model of care will be different according to the setting and resources available but the common principle should be a smooth transition between care providers with pathways based on need.[26,27]

- *Generalist*: Palliative care interventions are part of regular neurointensive care practice as well as other parts of the critical illness pathway. Guidelines are in place to support interventions with integrated training and regular updates.
- *Specialist*: Multidisciplinary specialist palliative care colleagues are invited to support the specific needs of a patient, family, or the ICU team. This can be individual consultations or as part of a neurointensive care multidisciplinary team. This may include complex problems such as difficult symptom control, family distress, ethical dilemmas, end-of-life care or discharge support.

COMMUNICATION

Perhaps the single most important skill in offering effective palliative care is effective communication. This is both within the health care teams in order to coordinate care as well as with the patient and family. It is a crucial skill in assessment and management, goal-setting discussions and managing expectations to achieve agreement and ensure congruence between patient and family understanding and treatment interventions.[28]

Communication is a skill that requires judgement to be used effectively. Understanding, practicing, and modelling effective communication is also needed to maintain effective communication. Active listening, verbal and non-verbal skills underpin this approach and should be combined with an awareness of the setting and adherence to core values such as mutual respect, dignity, and good ethical practice.

We can use simple steps to help in the actual communication scenario such as those outlined in the SPIKES protocol:[29,30]

- SETTING up the interview should involve avoiding interruptions and ensuring privacy
- Assessing the person's PERCEPTION including their understanding of the illness, expectations, and concerns
- Obtaining the person's INVITATION is important as not everyone wants or is ready for the same level of information
- Giving KNOWLEDGE and INFORMATION avoiding the use of jargon and at an appropriate pace
- Addressing the person's EMOTIONS and concerns
- Agreeing to a STRATEGY and SUMMARY for the way forward and checking mutual understanding.

Challenges in communication may reflect lack of skill,[31] but also difficulties in handling uncertainty,[32] a focus on medical models of care which are disease-focused rather than person-centred, pressure on resources or lack of team working such that the team members most often in contact with the family are unsure of what information to share. One particularly challenging area is the discussion regarding futility and end of life care.[15] Interventions to improve communication skills can be effective.[33]

DECISION-MAKING AND GOALS OF CARE

Communication with the patient may be hampered by the neurological illness and current neurointensive care setting. Sensory aphasias, altered consciousness, delirium, and dementias may mean the patient does not have the capacity for decision-making. Frameworks for deciding capacity and decision-making need to respect the ethical principles and legal context and this has been covered in Chapter 53, 'End-of-Life Care'. This however does not mean the patients should be excluded from communication. We continue to communicate as effectively as possible in an open, timely way making use of any advanced care planning information that is available. However, the family will often be the main avenue for communication and it will require a clear understanding of the decision-making roles and responsibilities and avoidance of hidden agendas and collusion. Forming a therapeutic team with the family ensures we avoid most of the areas where disagreements and dissatisfaction can arise. A focus on the quality of neurointensive care is essential and is responsive to change intervention.[34]

A neurointensive care admission often follows a sudden, even catastrophic deterioration, with uncertainties regarding the overall prognosis and the likely outcome of significant disability and rehabilitation needs if discharge is achieved. Families are trying to adjust to the new reality and are often distressed and struggling to adjust even if they have had sufficient information.

Family meetings are an important tool in agreeing goals of care and have been used in many settings including in the ICU.[35,36] Early agreed goals of care can results in more effective palliative care interventions and facilitate changes in management including withdrawal of ventilation, end of life care and issues of organ transplantation. Patients and families do not just require information but also time, presence, empathy, realistic reassurance, and hope. While uncertain prognosis may make hope for a full recovery unrealistic, achievable goals of care can maintain hope, foster trust with mutual involvement, and help adjustment.[37] This may also support the process of bereavement.[38,39]

One of the outcomes of improved goal setting may be a better use of resources and in particular an awareness of the huge financial burden placed on the family members[40] and the wider society. This applies in low, middle, and high income settings where care at the end of life and in particular intensive care, consumes a disproportionate and rising amount of resources. One initiative looked at choices in critical care settings which may support appropriate use of resources.[41]

Choosing wisely

(1) Do not order diagnostic tests at regular intervals (such as every day), but rather in response to specific clinical questions; (2) do not transfuse red blood cells in haemodynamically stable, nonbleeding ICU patients with a Hb concentration greater than 7 g/dl; (3) do not use parenteral nutrition in adequately nourished critically ill patients within the first 7 days of an ICU stay; (4) do not deeply sedate mechanically ventilated patients without a specific indication and without daily attempts to lighten sedation; and (5) do not continue life support for patients at high risk for death or severely impaired functional recovery without offering patients and their families the alternative of care focused entirely on comfort.

SYMPTOM CONTROL

Pain Assessment and Management

Pain is common in patients in the ICU[42] and remains under-recognized and therefore under-treated. The effects of pain are immediate with impact on cardiovascular and immune function but also have an impact on chronic pain neurophysiology. Perhaps most importantly, the impact of uncontrolled pain and distress lives on in the memory of those patients discharged from the ICU. It can lead to chronic insomnia, anxiety, and a form of post-traumatic stress disorder.[43] As with pain in all settings, prevention, then early recognition and prompt intervention is essential with a patient-centred approach.

Several guidelines exist including an excellent, evidenced-based review, and recommendations from the American College of Critical Medicine.[44]

Pain is often multifactorial occurring at rest,[45] during routine care, and during interventions. It may be due to underlying pathology such as malignancy or trauma due to mobilisation or coughing but is commonly related to procedures including respiratory suction,[46] dressing changes, cannulations, surgery, and mechanical ventilation.

The first step to effective assessment is recognizing the problem and then adopting a multidisciplinary approach including the use of appropriate pain assessment tools. The common barrier includes fears of causing sedation, communication inadequacies or lack of agreed protocols.[47] The best measurements use the patient's own ratings and the commonly used is a 0–10 visual analogue scale.[48] For patients who are unable to self-report, there are several behavioural tools available with the Critical-Care Pain Observation Tool (CPOT)[49] and the Behavioural Pain Scale (BPS)[50] recommended as valid and reliable.[51] Vital signs may be less useful but can still help to trigger a full pain assessment.

Pain management should include pharmacological and non-pharmacological approaches and should be considered pre-emptively. Management principles follow the principles of WHO guidelines for chronic pain[52] with a stepwise approach using a combination of opiates, non-opiates, and adjuvant medications that are given regularly to prevent and alleviate pain. The route should be the most appropriate for the setting which in neurointensive care will be intravenous (IV) though other routes including spinal and enteral may be useful. The choice of analgesic should take into account the pharmacokinetics and pharmacodynamics as well as the pathophysiology of the causal mechanism. Bolus administration allows control of pain or pre-emptive analgesia and it is then followed by continuous infusion titrated against need.

For pain that is not neuropathic, the first choice should be an opiate such as:

- morphine, dose 2–4 mg IV q1–2 hrs 2–30 mg/hr; onset of analgesia after 5–10 min and elimination after 3–4 hr

- fentanyl, dose 0.35–0.5 µg/kg IV q0.5–1 hr 0.7–10 µg/kg/hr; onset of analgesia after 1–2 min and elimination after 2–4 hr
- equi-analgesic dose of morphine to fentanyl in 10 to 0.1

Non-opiates can improve pain control and allow for a lower opiate use.[53] Non-steroidal anti-inflammatory medications should be used with caution and may be contraindicated especially with renal failure or platelet dysfunction. These can be:

- acetaminophen 325–1000 mg every 4–6 hr; max dose ≤4 g/day
- ibuprofen 400–800 mg IV every 6 hr infused over >30 mins; max dose = 3.2 g/day

In case of pain that has a neuropathic element, use the opiate and non-opiate combination as above and consider adding an adjuvant such as gabapentin, via the enteral route, with a starting dose of 100 mg orally three times daily, and a maintenance dose of 900–3600 mg/day in three divided doses.

Alongside analgesia attention should be paid to skin care, positioning, management of muscle spasm, and cough. These and the management of agitation and delirium are described in other chapters.

END-OF-LIFE CARE

The ethical issues relating to withdrawal of treatment have been covered in Chapter 53. Applying ethical principles in a clinical context needs particular attention to be given to the context. Where the legal framework is not clear agreed guidelines can offer support and can also ensure palliative care interventions including referral for end of life care.[54]

CARE FOR THE CAREGIVERS

Healthcare providers in a neurointensive care setting are experiencing ongoing stress[55] and loss as they care for patients and families, seek to communicate with empathy and compassion, and to hold the balance between utility and futility in decision-making.

Formal support mechanisms include effective multidisciplinary working, opportunities to debrief[56] and raise concerns, using guidelines and protocols,[57] ensuring safe working practices including staff capacity,[58] and regular appraisal and feedback. More formal psychological care may be offered for group or one-to-one support. Addressing areas of conflict, involving staff in research, and ensuring end of life care is well-managed when all contribute to avoiding burnout. Informal support will be offered by a healthy team but a culture of mutual support, recognition and value, and celebrating significant events. Attention should be given to the needs of the health care staff and systems put in place to foster informal and formal support and ensure a resilient[59] and satisfied workforce that offers excellent care.

CONCLUSIONS

The most effective approach is to ensure that palliative care focuses on the holistic needs and quality of life for those living with chronic illness and integrate it into the complete management of chronic neurological illness. Prior to a neurointensive care admission palliative care interventions may improve decision-making and communication and allow for a more informed choice regarding intensive management, especially at the end of life. Following a neurointensive care admission, recognising and assessing palliative needs can be supported with tools and practice-based protocols. These interventions will include excellent symptom control including pain management, support for ethical decision-making, establishing goals of care, improved communication, family support, and advanced care planning including end of life care and managing uncertainty. However, neurointensive care staff need support which includes integrated training with agreed core competencies to give them the skills to integrate palliative care. There will also need to be clinical pathways for specialist advice when needed and those palliative care specialists also need core competency training in critical care and intensive care management. Finally, caring for patients in neurointensive care settings is a demanding and at times stressful role for staff and planning such services must also include awareness of the need to care for the healthcare providers.

REFERENCES

1. World Health Organization. WHO Definition of Palliative Care. 2017. Available at: http://www.who.int/cancer/palliative/definition/en/ [accessed on 2017 Mar 29].

2. United Nations. Strengthening of palliative care as a component of comprehensive care throughout the life course. 67th World Health Assembly. WHA 67/19. 2014. Available at http://apps.who.int/medicinedocs/en/d/Js21454ar/.

3. DH Long-term Conditions NSF Team. The National Service Framework for Long-term Conditions. 10 March 2005. Available at https://www.gov.uk/government/publications/quality-standards-for-supporting-people-with-long-term-conditions.

4. Government of India. National Health Policy for India 2017. Ministry of Health and Family Welfare www.mohfw.nic.in.

5. Turner-Stokes L, Sykes N, Silber E. Long-term neurological conditions: management at the interface between neurology, rehabilitation and palliative care. *Clin Med (Lond)* 2008 Apr;8(2):186–91.

6. Gofton TE, Jog MS, Schulz V. A palliative approach to neurological care: a literature review. *Canadian Journal of Neurological Sciences/Journal Canadien des Sciences Neurologiques* 2009;36(3):296–302.

7. Marsden S, Cabanban C. Rabies: a significant palliative care issue. *Progress in Palliative Care* 2006;14(2):62–7.

8. Firth PG, Solomon JB, Roberts LL, Gleeson TD. Airway management of tetanus after the Haitian earthquake: new aspects of old observations. *Anesth Analg* 2011 Sep; 113(3):545–7.

9. Borasio GD. The role of palliative care in patients with neurological diseases. *Nat Rev Neurol* 2013 May;9(5): 292–5.

10. Oliver DJ, Borasio GD, Caraceni A, et al. A consensus review on the development of palliative care for patients with chronic and progressive neurological disease. *Eur J Neurol* 2016 Jan;23(1):30–38.

11. Palliative Care Australia (PCA) and the Neurological Alliance Australia (NAA). Palliative care and neurological conditions position statement. 2017. [accessed on 2017 Mar 29]. Available from: http://www.palliativecare.org.au/policy-and-publications/position-statements.

12. The National Council for Palliative Care, The Neurological Alliance, National End of Life Care Programme. End of life care in long term neurological conditions: a framework for implementation. 2011. [cited 2017 Mar 29]. Available at https://www.nai.ie/assets/98/E29C88A6-9CA5-06B3-E74D285E3C0695A2_document/End_20life_20care_20long_20term_20neuro_20conditions.pdf.

13. Edmonds P, Hart S, Wei Gao, et al. Palliative care for people severely affected by multiple sclerosis: evaluation of a novel palliative care service. *Mult Scler* 2010 May;16(5):627–36.

14. Higginson IJ, McCrone P, Hart SR, et al. Is short-term palliative care cost-effective in multiple sclerosis? A randomized phase II trial. *J Pain Symptom Manage* 2009 Dec;38(6):816–26.

15. Veronese S, Gallo G, Valle A, et al. Specialist palliative care improves the quality of life in advanced neurodegenerative disorders: NE-PAL, a pilot randomised controlled study. *BMJ Support Palliat Care* 2017 Jun;7(2):164–72.

16. Mohamed ZU, Muhammed F, Singh C, Sudhakar A. Experiences in end-of-life care in the Intensive Care Unit: A survey of resident physicians. *Indian J Crit Care Med* 2016;20(8):459–64.

17. Weafer J. The palliative care needs of people with advancing neurological disease in Ireland. Dublin. Irish Hospice Foundation, 2014. Available from: http://hospicefoundation.ie/wp-content/uploads/2015/

05/IHF-Neurology-Roundtable-Report-Website-Version. pdf.

18. Isaac M, Curtis JR. Palliative care: Issues in the intensive care unit in adults. UpToDate. 24 June 2016. [accessed on 2017 Mar 29]. Available from: http://www.uptodate.com/contents/palliative-care-issues-in-the-intensive-care-unit-in-adults.

19. Singh C, Venkateswaran C. Integrating palliative care within intensive care units (ICU) in a tertiary referral teaching hospital—our experience. Presentation at 22nd conference of the Indian Association for Palliative care. IAPCON 2015 Hyderabad.

20. Nelson JE, Curtis JR, Mulkerin C, et al. Choosing and using screening criteria for palliative care consultation in the ICU: A report from the Improving Palliative Care in the ICU (IPAL-ICU) Advisory Board. *Crit Care Med* 2013;41(10):2318–27.

21. Norton SA, Hogan LA, Holloway RG, Temkin-Greener H, Buckley MJ, Quill TE. Proactive palliative care in the medical intensive care unit: Effects on length of stay for selected high-risk patients. *Crit Care Med* 2007;35(6): 1530–5.

22. Kaur J, Mohanti BK. Transition from curative to palliative care in cancer. *Indian Journal of Palliative Care* 2011;17(1):1–5.

23. Creutzfeldt CJ, Engelberg RA, Healey L, et al. Palliative care needs in the neuro-ICU. *Crit Care Med* 2015 Aug; 43(8):1677–84.

24. Advisory Board and the Center to Advance Palliative Care. *Crit Care Med* 2015 Sep;43(9):1964–77.

25. Sleeman KE. End-of-life communication: let's talk about death. *J R Coll Physicians Edinb* 2013;43(3):197–9.

26. Frontera JA, Curtis JR, Nelson JE, et al. Integrating palliative care into the care of neurocritically ill patients: a report from the improving palliative care in the ICU project.

27. Braus N, Campbell TC, Kwekkeboom KL, et al. Prospective study of a proactive palliative care rounding intervention in a medical ICU. *Intensive Care Med* 2016 Jan;42(1):54–62.

28. Shaw DJ, Davidson JE, Smilde RI, Sondoozi T, Agan D. Multidisciplinary team training to enhance family communication in the ICU. *Crit Care Med* 2014 Feb; 42(2):265–71.

29. Boersma I, Miyasaki J, Kutner J, Kluger B. Palliative care and neurology: Time for a paradigm shift. *Neurology* 2014;83(6):561–7.

30. Baile WF, Buckman R, Lenzi R, Glober G, Beale EA, Kudelka AP. SPIKES-A six-step protocol for delivering bad news: Application to the patient with cancer. *Oncologist* 2000;5(4):302–11.

31. Accreditation Council for Graduate Medical Education. Neurology program requirements. Available from: http://www.acgme.org.

32. The American Academy of Neurology Ethics and Humanities Subcommittee. Palliative care in neurology. *Neurology* 1996;46:870–2.

33. Scheunemann LP, McDevitt M, Carson SS, et al. Randomized, controlled trials of interventions to improve communication in intensive care: a systematic review. *Chest* 2011;139(3):543–54.

34. Kon AA, Davidson JE, Morrison W, et al. Shared decision-making in intensive care units. Executive summary of the American College of Critical Care Medicine and American Thoracic Society policy statement. *Am J Respir Crit Care Med* 2016;193:1334.

35. Black MD, Vigorito MC, Curtis JR, et al. A multifaceted intervention to improve compliance with process measures for ICU clinician communication with ICU patients and families. *Crit Care Med* 2013 Oct;41(10):2275–83.

36. Lilly CM, De Meo DL, Sonna LA, et al. An intensive communication intervention for the critically ill. *Am J Med* 2000 Oct 15;109(6):469–75.

37. Widera AU, Rosenfeld KE, Sulmasy DP, Arnold RM. Approaching patients and family members who hope for a miracle. *J Pain Symptom Manage* 2011 Jul;42(1):119–25.

38. Lautrette A, Darmon M, Megarbane B, et al. A communication strategy and brochure for relatives of patients dying in the ICU. *N Engl J Med 2007* Feb 1; 356(5):469–78.

39. Nelson JE, Puntillo KA, Pronovost PJ, et al. In their own words: patients and families define high-quality palliative care in the intensive care unit. *Crit Care Med* 2010 Mar; 38(3):808–18.

40. Jayaram R, Ramakrishnan N. Cost of intensive care in India. *Indian Journal of Critical Care Medicine* 2008;12(2):55–61.

41. Halpern SD, Becker D, Curtis JR, et al. An official American Thoracic Society/American Association of Critical-Care Nurses/American College of Chest Physicians/Society of Critical Care Medicine policy statement: the Choosing Wisely® Top 5 list in Critical Care Medicine. *Am J Respir Crit Care Med* 2014 Oct 1;190(7):818–26.

42. Chanques G, Jaber S, Barbotte E, et al. Impact of systematic evaluation of pain and agitation in an intensive care unit. *Crit Care Med* 2006;34:1691–9.

43. Granja C, Gomes E, Amaro A, et al. JMIP Study Group: Understanding posttraumatic stress disorder-related symptoms after critical care: The early illness amnesia hypothesis. *Crit Care Med* 2008;36:2801–09.

44. Barr J, Gilles L, Fraser GL, Puntillo K, et al. Clinical practice guidelines for the management of pain, agitation, and delirium in adult patients in the Intensive Care Unit. *Crit Care Med* 2013; Jan 41(1):263–306.

45. Chanques G, Sebbane M, Barbotte E, et al. A prospective study of pain at rest: Incidence and characteristics of an unrecognized symptom in surgical and trauma versus medical intensive care unit patients. *Anesthesiology* 2007; 107:858–60.

46. Arroyo-Novoa CM, Figueroa-Ramos MI, Puntillo KA, et al. Pain related to tracheal suctioning in awake acutely and critically ill adults: A descriptive study. *Intensive Crit Care Nurs* 2008;24:20–7.

47. Baithia AM. Pain management barriers in critical care units: A qualitative study. *Int J Adv Nursing Studies* 2013;1:1–5.

48. Chanques G, Viel E, Constantin JM, et al. The measurement of pain in intensive care unit: Comparison of 5 self-report intensity scales. *Pain* 2010;151:711–21.

49. Arbour C, Gélinas C, Michaud C. Impact of the implementation of the Critical-Care Pain Observation Tool (CPOT) on pain management and clinical outcomes in mechanically ventilated trauma intensive care unit patients: A pilot study. *J Trauma Nurs* 2011;18:52–60.

50. Merkel, Voepel-Lewis, Shayevitz, Malviya. The FLACC: A behavioural scale for scoring postoperative pain in young children. *Pediatric Nursing* 1997;23(3):293–7.

51. Li D, Puntillo K, Miaskowski C. A review of objective pain measures for use with critical care adult patients unable to self-report. *J Pain* 2008;9:2–10.

52. Cancer pain control. 2nd ed. WHO 1996. Available from: http://www.who.int.

53. Memis D, Inal MT, Kavalci G, et al. Intravenous paracetamol reduced the use of opioids, extubation time, and opioid-related adverse effects after major surgery in intensive care unit. *J Crit Care* 2010;25:458–62.

54. Mani RK, Amin R, Chawla, et al. Guidelines for end-of-life and palliative care in Indian intensive care units: ISCCM consensus ethical position statement. *Indian J Crit Care Med* 2012 Jul-Sep;16(3):166–81.

55. Poncet MC, Toullic P, Papazian L, et al. Burnout syndrome in critical care nursing staff. *Am J Respir Crit Care Med* 2007 Apr;175(7):698–704.

56. Khot S, Billings M, Owens D, Longstreth WT. Coping with death and dying on a neurology inpatient service: death rounds as an educational initiative for residents. *Arch Neurol* 2011 Nov;68(11):1395–7.

57. Higgenson IL, Koffman J, Hopkins P, et al. Development and evaluation of the feasibility and effects of staff, patients and families of a new tool, the psychological and communication evaluation (PACE) to improve communication and palliative care in intensive care and during clinical uncertainty. *BMC Med* 2013;11:213.

58. Neuraz A, Guérin C, Payet C, et al. Patient mortality is associated with staff resources and workload in the ICU: A multicenter observational study. *Crit Care Med* 2015; 43(8):1587–94.

59. Mealer M, Jones J, Newman J, McFann KK, Rothbaum B, Moss M. The presence of resilience is associated with a healthier psychological profile in ICU nurses: Results of a national survey. *International Journal of Nursing Studies* 2012;49(3):292–9.

Part XVII

Nursing Care and Physiotherapy

Editor: Lena Nyholm

57

Nursing Care

L. Nyholm

ABSTRACT

Neurointensive care patients are vulnerable, in a stressful situation, and at the mercy of the personnel. Therefore all care has to be performed with integrity. All nursing interventions are performed with the aim of preventing complications and to offer comfort. On the other hand, nursing interventions can cause increased intracranial pressure (ICP) in a patient with exhausted intracranial adaptive capacity. Thus, the balance between performing nursing interventions to prevent possible future secondary insults and avoiding secondary insults directly related to nursing interventions is essential to achieve the best possible outcome for the patients. This chapter covers hygienic interventions, skincare management, surgery wound management, airways, maintenance of therapeutic milieu, and next-of-kin care.

KEYWORDS

Nursing care; hygienic interventions; skincare management; surgery wound management; airway management; maintenance of therapeutic milieu; next-of-kin care.

INTRODUCTION

Both the patient admitted to a neurointensive care unit (NICU) and their next of kin are in a vulnerable situation and at the mercy of the personnel in the NICU. All care of the patient has to be done with great integrity. Due to sedation and unconsciousness of NICU patients, it is rarely possible to communicate through normal means with them. Therefore, nurses have to make decisions about how to give the best possible care to patients by considering monitored data and analysing possible physiological reactions.

Neurointensive care unit patients have a primary injury which causes cellular damage, and the outcome partially depends on the degree of primary cell death as a result of that injury. It is well-known that cell death will continue to occur several days after the primary injury and that this is caused by two different things: Destructive biochemical and inflammatory processes and secondary clinical insults. Secondary insults can be both systemic (e.g., hypoxia, hypercapnia, and hypotension) and intracranial (e.g.,

intracranial hypertension, seizures, and vasospasm).[1,2] The degree of secondary injury will strongly influence the patients' outcomes. There have been several clinical trials with neuroprotective drugs that have failed[3] and prevention of secondary insults is still a cornerstone in the management of NICU patients.

Patients at an NICU are frequently cared for in different ways around the clock. The nurses' responsibilities can be divided into four categories:[4]

- *Neurophysiological interventions*: e.g., monitoring general and neurophysiological parameters, administration of medicines, ventilator management, and monitoring fluid status; all with the purpose of avoiding secondary brain injury.
- *Injury prevention interventions or preventing complications*: e.g., turning/repositioning, hygienic measures, reorienting the patient, and fall prevention.
- *Maintaining therapeutic milieu*: limit stimuli, e.g., light, noise, visitors, and space nursing activities.
- *Psychological intervention*: e.g., family support.

All nursing interventions are performed with the aim of benefiting the patient; for example, oral care and endotracheal suction is done in order to prevent lung failure. A nursing intervention can halt an ongoing secondary intracranial pressure (ICP) insult. For example, when a patient is coughing and a nurse performs endotracheal suction making it possible for the patient to rest again, or when repositioning a patient to a better position in the bed (head elevated by 30° and neck stretched). On the other hand, when caring for patients at an NICU, nursing interventions can also lead to secondary ICP insult, due to, among others, stress, head rotation, and/or a flat position in the bed. It is the nurse's responsibility to monitor and observe whether a secondary insult occurs and to stop its progression adequately.[5] When caring for NICU patients it is important to consider that a nursing intervention can result in unwanted side effects such as high ICP and therefore a holistic approach is necessary. The timing of nursing interventions influences the risk for secondary insults.[6] It is the nurses' obligation to achieve a balance between prevention of secondary insults and performing nursing interventions. This balance gives the patient the best chance of recovery.[7] One way to reduce the risk for secondary insults in connection with nursing interventions is to allow enough time between each intervention so that the patients return to their baseline ICP.[8]

When planning a nursing intervention it is helpful to have an idea about the patient's intracranial adaptive capacity (ability to compensate for added intracranial volume), i.e., intracranial compliance in order to avoid a rise in ICP. This can be done by reviewing the experience from earlier nursing interventions with that particular patient and by evaluating their computed tomography (CT) scans. If the adaptive capacity is exhausted, a nursing intervention may cause an elevation of ICP. If the adaptive capacity is increased, the risk of ICP elevation associated with a nursing intervention is decreased. In order to prevent the development of high ICP during these kinds of interventions, the nurse could try to increase the adaptive capacity at the same time by giving extra sedation and/or using a therapeutic body position with a raised head and stretching the neck to avoid venous stasis.[9,10]

A DECISION-MAKING TOOL

Nurses at a NICU continuously make decisions about which nursing interventions should be performed. They have to consider both the positive effects that the intervention could have for the patient and the risk that the patient could develop a secondary insult related to

the nursing intervention. A clinical tool to predict each patient's risk for developing a secondary ICP insult related to a nursing intervention can be helpful in daily practice (Figure 57.1).[11,12]

If the patient's ICP is less than 15 mmHg, all kind of nursing interventions should be performed to prevent possible future secondary insults. Patients should be made comfortable during the intervention. For patients with ICP 15–20 mmHg, nursing interventions should be performed in a way that minimizes the probability of secondary insults. Only the most important interventions should be chosen and the intervention should be well planned. For example, care should be taken to correct the body position (head elevated by 30° and neck stretched) for optimal venous outflow. Extra sedation/pain relief should be considered. When ICP is >20 mmHg, only nursing interventions that could stop an ongoing secondary insult should be performed, e.g., suction in an endotracheal tube if the patient is coughing. Extra sedation and pain relief should be given. In some instances, a nursing intervention has to be performed regardless of elevated ICP. If this occurs with a patient at risk for developing a secondary insult, the intervention should be done with great care and attention, with qualified personnel and extra sedation, pain relief, and necessary equipment nearby to ensure a smooth and swift intervention.[12]

One way to provide education and improve quality of patient care is to organise nursing rounds. The round should be managed by a senior well-educated nurse who discusses all patients special needs; for example risk for infections, fall prevention, pressure ulcers, delirium, and pain treatment.[13]

HYGIENIC INTERVENTIONS

Patients at an NICU need help with all their personal hygiene. In order to do this, a nurse has to show great respect to the patient. Being cleaned and dressed provides the patient with dignity. Washing a patient is also a way to show concern for them. When performing hygienic interventions, a nurse has an opportunity to assess the patient and in particular their skin. Daily bed baths are routine in most NICUs. The timing of hygienic interventions should be chosen so as to not disturb the patient's sleep. This also applies to sedated patients. A nurse should also be aware of the risk that the patient could become hypothermic during the bed bath.

The Australian Wound Management Association states that alkaline soaps should be avoided as they can irritate skin. They can also affect the water-holding capacity of the skin. Other studies recommend daily washing with chlorhexidine to reduce pathogen transmission.[14] The washing should be performed as follows:

- Wash with soap
- Rinse with water
- Dry the skin
- Moisturize the skin with cream

Start the procedure by washing the face, followed by the upper body, legs and feet, and the genitals last. Hygienic interventions also include shaving, combing and, if necessary, braiding hair and cutting nails.

ORAL CARE

Oral care is important as it decreases the risk for developing ventilator-associated pneumonia (VAP) and even bacteraemia and organ dysfunction.[15,16] It is also important because a clean and moisturised mouth offers the patient comfort and dignity, although the procedure can be perceived inconvenient. In many ways, critically ill patients are exposed to threats to their oral health. For example, medication, tachypnoea, breathing with an open mouth, stress, intubation, fever, and inability to drink can result in xerostomia. In addition, patients with an endotracheal tube and/or oral feeding tube have reduced access to the oral cavity.

Oral care has no effect on ICP among traumatic brain injury (TBI) patients[17,18] and tooth brushing manually or by an electric toothbrush will have a similar effect on ICP to one another.[19]

Oral care, in order to prevent VAP, is well-known and there are numerous articles about oral care, but no established guideline on how to perform oral care in practice. The Cochrane library concludes that chlorhexidine mouthwash reduces the risk of VAP and that there is no strong evidence that using a toothbrush as a compliment to chlorhexidine mouthwash reduces the risk for VAP further.[20]

Dental plaque is accumulation of microorganisms on the tooth surface. In critical care patients this can cause bacteraemia and organ dysfunction and, as previously mentioned, VAP. The best way to reduce dental plaque is by using a small, soft toothbrush and non-foaming toothpaste.[15,21,22] Foam or cotton swabs are not effective at removing plaque, but with water they can provide moisture.[22] Foam swabs with lemon and glycerol may result in xerostomia and decalcification of tooth enamel.[15] As mouth rinses go, chlorhexidine 0.1%–0.2% is the most recommended and most effective antiplaque agent.[16,23] Saliva provides mechanical removal of plaque and microorganisms.[16] Xerostomia is common in intensive

care patients and therefore salivary substitutes or water are important agents for moisturising the mouth.[22] Adding moisture to the oral cavity prevents development of oral candidiasis. Even the tongue, gum, and lips have to be cleaned and moisturised. Figure 57.2 shows the necessary oral care devices.

In order to increase the quality of oral care in an NICU, nurses need education, sufficient time to perform oral care and the right equipment.[23–25]

EYE CARE

The incidence of iatrogenic ophthalmologic complications (e.g., microbial keratitis, corneal ulcer, and keratopathy) during intensive care is 3%–60%.[26] The main reasons are that blinking and eyelid closure do not occur properly in sedated and/or unconscious patients. Intensive care patients often suffer from capillary leakage that can cause conjunctival oedema (ventilator eye).[27] Intensive care unit patients with eye infection are often colonized by bacteria from the respiratory tract.[27] Nurses have to inspect at a minimum of every day if the patients' eyes are properly closed and if there are signs of iatrogenic ophthalmologic complications. All intensive care patients who are sedated should have their eyes cleaned with saline soaked gauze and specific eye lubricant administered twice daily. Incomplete eye closure is the main risk factor for eye complications. Interventions to maintain corneal moisture reduces this risk for complications.[26] Moisture chambers are more effective than lubrication in maintaining corneal moisture.[28,29] Using an eye care protocol prevents iatrogenic ophthalmologic complications.[27] These complications can result in poor vision, which affects the quality of life after intensive care.[27,30]

SKIN CARE MANAGEMENT

Patients at an NICU are at risk of developing pressure ulcers and/or incontinence-associated dermatitis. Both can result in severe suffering and delayed rehabilitation for patients. These conditions also are very costly to society. Fortunately, both are preventable.[31,32]

Pressure Ulcers

The prevalence of pressure ulcers in Europe is reported to be between 4%–49% in adult intensive care patients.[33] In an NICU, the incidence rate has been reported to be at 12%.[34] Pressure ulcers are caused by local ischaemia and/or hypoxia in the affected tissue. Therefore, pressure ulcers are usually localized over bony prominences and are most common in the heels and sacrum, but can also develop in the elbows, shoulders, ears, buttocks, and knees.[31,33]

In patients with a bandage on their head, pressure ulcers can easily develop on the ears. Pressure ulcers can also occur because of shearing force and friction, in those cases the blood vessels are stretched or bent and that can cause ischaemia.[35] Shearing occurs for example when the patient's head is raised in bed and then the patient slides down. In the intensive care, pressure ulcers can also result from tubes and catheters burrowing into skin folds. Figure 57.3 shows how to fixate a nasogastric tube in a way that reduces the risk for pressure ulcer inside the nose. Obese patients have an increased risk for this kind of pressure ulcer.[36] The known risk factors are listed in Table 57.1. Patients with barbiturate-induced coma treatment often have several of these risk factors.

Prevention

Several studies have been done looking at assessment scales for detection of patients at risk for developing presser ulcers. Two of the most mentioned scales for assessment of risk of developing pressure ulcers are the Norton scale and the Braden scale, but they have not been adapted to intensive care patients.[31] There is one scale developed for patients in intensive care and it is called the Critical care Pressure Ulcer Assessment made Easy (CALCULATE).[37,38] The Cochrane library concludes that there is no evidence that the occurrence of pressure ulcers decreases if such assessment scales are used.[39] Patients in intensive care

are at high risk for developing pressure ulcers and their entire skin surface should be inspected regularly and signs of developing pressure ulcers must be treated and documented. In order to be able to do this properly, nurses need adequate education.

Pressure-release intervention is the most effective way to prevent and treat pressure ulcers. Repositioning should be performed approximately every third hour.[40] Patients with a high risk of developing pressure ulcers should have special mattresses with the aim of relieving pressure and distributing the surface pressure more evenly. Mattresses with alternating pressure are the most effective at reducing the risk.[41]

There are studies showing that five-layer soft silicone bordered dressings placed at the sacrum, buttocks, and heels reduce the risk for pressure ulcers in high-risk patients.[42,43]

Well-conducted hygienic interventions and taking care of the skin decrease the risk for pressure ulcers. The bed should be dry and the bedsheets stretched, no hard items or equipment should touch the patient and unnecessary plastic should be avoided. The skin has to be dry at all times, cleaned gently, and moisturized regularly.

Several studies have described the increased risk for developing pressure ulcers in patients with malnutrition and this increased risk also applies to skinny patients.[34,37,38] The Cochrane library states that there is no evidence that any particular nutritional intervention could prevent or treat pressure ulcers.[44]

Table 57.1 Risk factors resulting in pressure ulcers

Risk factor	Examples
Impaired circulation[*,$]	Vasopressor infusion, barbiturate coma treatment, cooling blanket for reducing fever, previous cigarette smokers.
Underweight[#,@]	BMI 19–24 kg/m^2 is considered normal.
Immobility[@]	Unconsciousness and/or sedation.
Patients that are difficult to turn or mobilize[*]	Unstable ICP, spinal cord injury, multiple fractures, continuous veno-venous dialysis.
Malnutrition[*]	Periods without nutrition or with inadequate nutrition.
Faecal incontinence[*,@]	Faecal incontinence and/or diarrhoea. Diarrhoea increases the risk more than an ordinary stool.
Mechanical ventilation[*]	Mechanical ventilation required.
Long surgery[*]	The duration in the operating theatre determines the risk. The risk increases after 4 hours, and after 8 hours the risk is extremely high.

*Richardson A, Barrow I. Part 1: Pressure ulcer assessment—the development of Critical Care Pressure Ulcer Assessment Tool made Easy (CALCULATE). *Nurs Crit Care* 2015;20(6):308–14.

$Smit I, Harrison L, Letzkus L, Quatrara B. What Factors Are Associated With the Development of Pressure Ulcers in a Medical Intensive Care Unit? *Dimens Crit Care Nurs* 2016;35(1):37–41.

#Fife C, Otto G, Capsuto EG, Brandt K, Lyssy K, Murphy K, et al. Incidence of pressure ulcers in a neurologic intensive care unit. *Critical Care Medicine* 2001;29(2):283–90.

@Kirby JP, Gunter OL. Prevention and treatment of pressure ulcers in the surgical intensive care unit. *Curr Opin Crit Care* 2008;14(4):428–31.

Treatment

Pressure-release intervention is the first and most important step in treating pressure ulcers. Avoid positioning the patients on areas with reddened or broken skin. The sore has to be cleaned and then treated in accordance with how deep it is. If there are signs of infection, antibiotics should be considered. Pressure ulcers can be painful and the patient may need analgesics. There are different ways to classify pressure ulcers. The European Pressure Ulcer Advisory Panel (EPUAP) has made a classification system that is widely used (see Table 57.2).[40,45]

Incontinence-Associated Dermatitis

Incontinence-associated dermatitis is defined as 'erythema and oedema of the surface of the skin, sometimes accompanied by bullae with serous exudate, erosion, or secondary cutaneous infection'.[46] This kind of skin damage is caused by exposure to stool or/and urine and histopathological analysis reveals inflammation of the upper dermis.[47] Differences in characteristics between incontinence-associated dermatitis and pressure ulcer are shown in Table 57.3.

Prevention and treatment

A strict skincare regimen is the best way to prevent incontinence-associated dermatitis. The regimen should include four interventions:

- Interventions to minimise exposure to stool or/and urine, for example, using a urinary catheter and faecal management system.
- Gentle cleaning with a product pH 5.4–5.9.
- Moisturising to repair and increase the skin's moisture barrier.
- Applying a skin protectant to prevent skin breakdown.[47,48]

Treatment of this condition has the same components as for the regimen and, if needed, antifungal products can also be used.[47]

Table 57.2 The European National Pressure Ulcer Advisory Panel (EPUAP) classification system

Category/Stage I	Non-blanchable erythema
Category/Stage II	Partial thickness skin loss
Category/Stage III	Full thickness skin loss
Category/Stage IV	Full thickness tissue loss
Unstageable	Depth unknown
Suspected deep tissue injury	Depth unknown

Table 57.3 Characteristics in incontinence-associated dermatitis and pressure ulcers

Characteristic	Incontinence-associated dermatitis	Pressure ulcer
Aetiology	On skin exposed to urine, stool and perspiration	Skin exposed to pressure and/or shear forces
Pathophysiology	Inflammation	Ischaemia and tissue destruction
Colour	Bright red	Dark red
Location	Areas where skin is exposed to urine, stool, and perspiration	Mostly over bony prominences
Depth	Epidermis and dermis	Variable death, could extend to underlying muscle, fascia, and bone

Source: Stausberg J, Kiefer E. Classification of pressure ulcers: a systematic literature review. *Stud Health Technol Inform* 2009;146:511–15.

POST-SURGERY WOUND MANAGEMENT

Postoperative wound infections occurs in 0%–7% of neurosurgery patients.[49] Patients with a healthy immune system have the lowest risk of postoperative wound infection. If preoperative bathing or showering with an antiseptic skin wash product is performed, skin bacteria are reduced and the risk for infections decreases.[50] However, there is no evidence as to which antiseptic skin product is best. Also there is no clear evidence that preoperative showering or bathing with chlorhexidine decreases the number of surgical site infections.[51]

Preoperative scalp shaving probably increases the risk of developing postoperative wound infection.[49] Many studies show that hair removal does not decrease the infection rate and if hair has to be removed, hair clipping is the best alternative.[50,52] Hair removal can allow for better visualization of the wound and the dressing can be easier to apply without hair. On the other hand, hair removal can be a psychologically traumatic experience.[49,53] The use of chlorhexidine as a preoperative skin disinfectant has no additional risk and is more effective than alcohol.[53]

Surgical Site Infections

General risk factors for surgical site infections are: age, underlying illness, malnutrition, obesity, smoking, length and complexity of the procedure, steroids, and presence of surgical drains.[50,54]

The clinical signs of local wound infection are increased or new pain, excessive or increased serous exudate, localised erythema, swelling, delayed healing, strong malodour, itching, and, sometimes, fever.

Dressings and Sutures

If possible the dressing from the operation room should remain intact and unchanged for at least 48 hours postoperatively.[54] The optimal dressing material controls exudate without desiccating the wound, acts as a bacterial barrier and allows atraumatic removal. The dressing must remain dry.[55] If necessary, the wound should be cleaned with sterile sodium chloride (NaCl), alcohol or chlorhexidine.[54] Historically, chlorhexidine was never used in neurosurgical wounds because of its neurotoxicity. Recent studies, however, recommend chlorhexidine because it is more effective than alcohol and if there is no entrance into the cerebral fluid and nerve cells it is considered safe.[53] Dressing changes should be performed by trained personnel and should occur once or twice a week or when needed (if it is wet or has become dislodged). When a dressing change is performed, strict aseptic technique should be followed and sterile gloves, mask, gown, and cap should be used.[53,55]

If there is a leakage of cerebrospinal fluid (CSF), it must be noticed immediately due to the increased risk for meningitis and because of the risk of compromised ventricles and in worst case herniation.

A bandage is used to hold the dressings, drains, and ICP, and other measurement devices in place and to protect the wound from bacteria and other contamination.[56] Disadvantages of a bandage could be hidden bleeding and leakage of CSF, missed signs of wound infection, patient discomfort, and expenses.[56] An outline of how to apply a bandage is shown in Figure 57.4a–d.

Sutures after neurosurgery should generally be removed after 8–10 days. Some patients may have delayed wound healing. In those cases, every other suture could be taken out after 10–14 days and after another 2–3 days the rest could be removed. Risk factors for post-surgery wound rupture are listed below.

- Haemicraniectomy
- Barbiturate coma treatment
- Signs of surgical site infections
- Intracranial hypertension (I)
- Reoperated patients
- Patient treated with radiation therapy

MANAGEMENT OF EXTERNAL VENTRICULAR DRAINS TO REDUCE THE OCCURRENCE OF MENINGITIS

The incidence of infections related to external ventricular drains is reported to be 10%–17%.[53] Insertion of an external ventricular drain is performed by a physician, often in the operating room. After insertion, there is still a risk for contamination and infections, and the external ventricular drain has to be managed with a high level of skill.[57] Aseptic technique is recommended when handling an external ventricular drain. Sampling should be done from the distal port but only when clinically indicated. A bio-occlusive dressing is recommended and it should be changed weekly with aseptic technique. The dressing has to remain dry. The external ventricular drain should be labelled and separated from other devices, such as intravenous tubing and airway devices. This decreases the risk of developing an infection.[53]

There are studies reporting decreased rate of external ventricular drain infections by using a chlorhexidine patch over the insertion site and antibiotic-coated or silver catheters.[53,58]

AIRWAYS

Neurointensive care unit patients who do not respond to commands should be intubated and artificially ventilated in order to secure oxygen delivery.[59] Artificial ventilation is also needed in patients receiving sedative agents in order to reduce ICP.

Patients who are sedated and unconscious are often unable to adequately cough up secretions. Endotracheal suctioning is therefore a common procedure in an NICU. Performing endotracheal suction increases the risk for secondary ICP insults, but this risk can be reduced if the patient is properly sedated.[60] When studying planned endotracheal suction in adults with severe head injuries, Gemma et al. concluded that it can be done without risk for secondary insults if the patients have a level of sedation that precludes moving or coughing.[60]

Endotracheal suction should only be performed when necessary or at least every 8 hours. Indications for suction are: cough, visible or audible secretion, coarse or absent respiratory sounds, increased airway pressure, desaturation or increased respiratory work.[61] In order to protect both staff and patients, aseptic technique should be used and gloves should be worn.[61] A suction catheter that is occluding half or less than half of the lumen of the endotracheal tube should be used with as low possible suction pressure (80–120 mmHg).[61] The catheter should not be inserted further than the carina and the suction procedure should last a maximum of 15 seconds.[61] There are both open and closed tracheal suction systems in the market. There is no strong evidence that one system is better than the other in preventing VAP and mortality.[62] Bench and animal studies have shown that closed tracheal suction systems decrease alveolar collapse.[63]

The use of endotracheal tubes with subglottic secretion drainage has shown a significant decrease of VAP.[64,65]

The inspired gases from a ventilator have to be humidified by artificial means and there are two ways to perform that, either by a heat and moisture exchanger or by a heated humidification device. There is some evidence that the heat and moisture exchanger decreases the risk for VAP, but on the other hand, the risk for obstruction events are increased.[66,67]

Both tracheal tubes and tracheostomy tubes decrease the ability of the patient to communicate verbally. Some patients are able to communicate with lip reading, an alphabet, picture, or writing board.[68] There are techniques to assist vocalization in patients with tracheostomy tubes.[69] For example, patients who can breathe without help, a speaking valve can be used to facilitate communication.

Tracheal Tube Care

Tube fixation can be done with several different commercial devices or with adhesive tape (Figure 57.5a–b), and no method has been found more secure than any other.[70] A pressure ulcer can develop in the corner of the mouth. In order to avoid this, the tracheal tube should be placed on different sides each day.

Unplanned extubation is a dangerous incident in an NICU. The known risk factors are altered level of consciousness, agitation, use of analgesia and/or sedation, physical restraints, increased nursing workload, delirium, inadequate tube fixation, and delayed ventilator weaning.[71,72]

Tracheostomy Care

The indications for a tracheotomy are the need for ventilation, airway obstruction, airway protection, and secretion.[73] Due to the risk for secondary insults while performing a tracheotomy, the patient should have stable vital signs and especially stable ICP. Two serious risks with a tracheostomy tube are that it could be displaced or acutely occluded. Supplies to replace/change a tracheostomy tube should always be nearby and all personnel must know how to handle such a situation.[73] If the tracheostomy tube is occluded and no air can come through, the first step is to try to perform tracheal suction and call for help.

If the catheter cannot pass through the tube, the cuff has to be deflated and the patient needs to be ventilated with a bag-valve-mask by the mouth. If that does not work, the tracheostomy tube has to be removed and the patient ventilated with bag-valve-mask by the mouth. Be aware that in this circumstance, air can slip out from the tracheostomy. If that happens, something should be put over the stoma to force the air into the lungs.[68] There are tubes with an inner cannula that can easily be changed to prevent and treat tube blockages.[68] Patients with a tracheostomy tube need humidification, filtration, and warming of inspired air. Another risk is bleeding at the stoma site or into the trachea. The stoma should be clean and the skin around it dry to avoid skin irritation. The tracheostomy tube is usually fixed with a tracheostomy tie. When changing the tie, one person should hold the tube in place and one should perform the change.[68,73] Most tracheostomy tubes have a cuff to provide a closed system and to allow effective ventilation. The cuff pressure should be 20–25 cm H_2O.[68,73] The common causes of high cuff pressure are small tube or poor positioning of the tube.[69]

MAINTAINING THE THERAPEUTIC MILIEU

The first person describing the physical environment and how it influenced the patients was Florence Nightingale.[74] Her book, *Notes on Nursing: What It Is, and What It Is Not*, describes for example how light and noise can disturb the patient and impair recovery.

In order to maintain patient safety, the rooms at an NICU should be standardized, offer visibility of the patient, have access to medicines, devices, and other supplies and be easy to clean. For the patients' well-being, the room should offer privacy, a view from a window, daylight, reduction of noise, and the possibility to store personal items.[75]

Neurointensive care units often have a high level of noise related to staff conversation, treatments, and medical devices.[76] The same noise can be disturbing for one patient and safe and comforting for another.

Some sounds have been described as positive and those create a feeling of safety, security, and familiarity. Negative sounds create feelings of fear, helplessness, and anxiety.[76]

The circadian rhythm depends on light, preferably daylight, with daytime being light and night time dark. Light during night time is one of the most reported reasons for sleep deprivation in intensive care.[77,78] It should also be noted that there are patients that feel more secure in a light room even during the night and staff do need some light to be able to work and observe the patients.[78]

SLEEP

There are many reasons that patients suffer from sleep disruption and even sleep deprivation in an NICU. For example, the NICU environment exposes patients to light, noise, treatment, and nursing activities at all hours. Even the situation itself, with things such as anxiety, pain, discomfort, loss of physical activity, and loss of circadian rhythms is threatening to sleep.[77–79] Several of the drugs used in an NICU are also a potential cause of sleep disturbance.[80] Sleep deprivation causes, amongst other things, reduced immune function, increased capacity in the inspiration muscles, induced catabolism and is a risk factor for delirium.[77] Fortunately, it is possible to arrange changes in the environment and in the patient's surroundings to promote better opportunities for sleep.

PSYCHOLOGICAL INTERVENTION

A nurse has to give the next of kin the experience of being seen, confirmed, and accepted as they are.[81]

All the next of kin of a patient admitted to an NICU have different needs, but there is always a need for accurate and understandable information. The information has to be repeated several times in different ways and it has to be factual, while also providing a glimmer of hope.[80] Sometimes the need for hope and reassurance is greater than the need for accurate information. The next of kin often want to be near their loved one. Thus, as well as all examinations and nursing activities, nurses have to facilitate the visits for the next of kin regularly.[82] Even the next of kin's practical problems must be managed in order for them to have a feeling of comfort and security. Example of arrangements are offering food and a place to rest, lending a phone or computer, financial help, and whatever needed.[82]

The high-tech environments are often overwhelming for the next of kin. The nurses can help the next of kin feel safe and secure in the NICU by explaining all equipment, putting something on the wall to look at, creating some privacy with curtains or screens and placing some personal things near to the patient.[83]

When the next of kin are present during an acute emergency situation, such as a resuscitation, they come away with a real sense of the severity of their loved one's situation and they often remember the incident/s as valuable experiences in understanding the situation their loved one find themselves in. The recommendation is that the next of kin should be given the choice to stay with their loved one if they want to in such a situation. A designated nurse should escort the next of kin, explain the interventions, provide information, and give support.[84]

The next of kin can give the caregivers information about the patient, which can then result in more individualized care. They also give the patient the strength to continue and feelings of safety which can help their recovery.[85]

CONCLUSIONS

To conclude, neurointensive care patients are vulnerable and a multidisciplinary care team is important to handle the complex situation. With a proper balance between nursing interventions and prevention of secondary insults, patients have good potential to recover from their severe injury with a minimum of complications.

REFERENCES

1. Maas AI, Dearden M, Servadei F, Stocchetti N, Unterberg A. Current recommendations for neurotrauma. *Curr Opin Crit Care* 2000;6(4):281–92.
2. Reilly PL, Graham DI, Adams JH, Jennett B. Patients with head injury who talk and die. *Lancet* 1975;2(7931):375–7.
3. Narayan RK, Michel ME, Ansell B, et al. Clinical trials in head injury. *Journal of Neurotrauma* 2002;19(5):503–57.
4. McNett MM, Gianakis A. Nursing interventions for critically ill traumatic brain injury patients. *The Journal of Neuroscience Nursing* 2010;42(2):71–7.
5. Walleck CA. Preventing secondary brain injury. *AACN Clin Issues Crit Care Nurs* 1992;3(1):19–30.
6. Olson DM, Graffagnino C. Consciousness, coma, and caring for the brain-injured patient. *AACN Clinical Issues* 2005;16(4):441–55.
7. Chamberlain DJ. The critical care nurse's role in preventing secondary brain injury in severe head trauma: achieving the balance. *Australian Critical Care* 1998;11(4):123–9.
8. Tume LN, Baines PB, Lisboa PJ. The effect of nursing interventions on the intracranial pressure in paediatric traumatic brain injury. *Nurs Crit Care* 2011;16(2):77–84.
9. Fan JY, Kirkness C, Vicini P, Burr R, Mitchell P. An approach to determining intracranial pressure variability capable of predicting decreased intracranial adaptive capacity in patients with traumatic brain injury. *Biological Research for Nursing* 2010;11(4):317–24.
10. Mitchell PH. Decreased adaptive capacity, intracranial: a proposal for a nursing diagnosis. *The Journal of Neuroscience Nursing* 1986;18(4):170–5.
11. Rauch ME, Mitchell PH, Tyler ML. Validation of risk factors for the nursing diagnosis decreased intracranial adaptive capacity. *The Journal of Neuroscience Nursing* 1990;22(3):173–8.
12. Nyholm L, Howells T, Enblad P. Predictive factors that may contribute to secondary insults with nursing interventions in adults with traumatic brain injury. *The Journal of Neuroscience Nursing* 2017;49(1):49–55.

13. Mahanes D, Quatrara BD, Shaw KD. APN-led nursing rounds: an emphasis on evidence-based nursing care. *Intensive and Critical Care Nursing* 2013;29(5):256–60.

14. Coyer FM, O'Sullivan J, Cadman N. The provision of patient personal hygiene in the intensive care unit: a descriptive exploratory study of bed-bathing practice. *Australian Critical Care* 2011;24(3):198–209.

15. Berry AM, Davidson PM, Masters J, Rolls K. Systematic literature review of oral hygiene practices for intensive care patients receiving mechanical ventilation. *American Journal of Critical Care* 2007;16(6):552–62.

16. Munro CL, Grap MJ. Oral health and care in the intensive care unit: state of the science. *American Journal of Critical Care*: an official publication, American Association of Critical Care Nurses. 2004;13(1):25–33.

17. Prendergast V, Hallberg IR, Jahnke H, Kleiman C, Hagell P. Oral health, ventilator-associated pneumonia, and intracranial pressure in intubated patients in a neuroscience intensive care unit. *American Journal of Critical Care* 2009;18(4):368–76.

18. Szabo CM. The effect of oral care on intracranial pressure: a review of the literature. *The Journal of Neuroscience Nursing* 2011;43(5):E1–E9.

19. Prendergast V, Hagell P, Hallberg IR. Electric versus manual tooth brushing among neuroscience ICU patients: is it safe? *Neurocritical Care* 2011;14(2):281–6.

20. Hua F, Xie H, Worthington HV, Furness S, Zhang Q, Li C. Oral hygiene care for critically ill patients to prevent ventilator-associated pneumonia. *The Cochrane Database of Systematic Reviews* 2016;10:CD008367.

21. Pearson LS, Hutton JL. A controlled trial to compare the ability of foam swabs and toothbrushes to remove dental plaque. *J Adv Nurs* 2002;39(5):480–9.

22. Berry AM, Davidson PM. Beyond comfort: oral hygiene as a critical nursing activity in the intensive care unit. *Intensive and Critical Care Nursing* 2006;22(6):318–28.

23. Hillier B, Wilson C, Chamberlain D, King L. Preventing ventilator-associated pneumonia through oral care, product selection, and application method: a literature review. *AACN Advanced Critical Care* 2013;24(1):38–58.

24. Allen Furr L, Binkley CJ, McCurren C, Carrico R. Factors affecting quality of oral care in intensive care units. *J Adv Nurs* 2004;48(5):454–62.

25. Ross A, Crumpler J. The impact of an evidence-based practice education program on the role of oral care in the prevention of ventilator-associated pneumonia. *Intensive and Critical Care Nursing* 2007;23(3):132–6.

26. Marshall AP, Elliott R, Rolls K, Schacht S, Boyle M. Eyecare in the critically ill: clinical practice guideline. *Australian Critical Care* 2008;21(2):97–109.

27. Alansari MA, Hijazi MH, Maghrabi KA. Making a difference in eye care of the critically ill patients. *Journal of Intensive Care Medicine* 2015;30(6):311–7.

28. Zhou Y, Liu J, Cui Y, Zhu H, Lu Z. Moisture chamber versus lubrication for corneal protection in critically ill patients: a meta-analysis. *Cornea* 2014;33(11):1179–85.

29. Rosenberg JB, Eisen LA. Eye care in the intensive care unit: narrative review and meta-analysis. *Critical Care Medicine* 2008;36(12):3151–5.

30. Azfar MF, Khan MF, Alzeer AH. Protocolized eye care prevents corneal complications in ventilated patients in a medical intensive care unit. *Saudi J Anaesth* 2013;7(1):33–6.

31. Cox J. Predictors of pressure ulcers in adult critical care patients. *American Journal of Critical Care* 2011;20(5):364–75.

32. Coyer F, Campbell J. Incontinence-associated dermatitis in the critically ill patient: an intensive care perspective. *Nurs Crit Care* 2017 Dec 20.

33. Shahin ES, Dassen T, Halfens RJ. Pressure ulcer prevalence and incidence in intensive care patients: a literature review. *Nurs Crit Care* 2008;13(2):71–9.

34. Fife C, Otto G, Capsuto EG, et al. Incidence of pressure ulcers in a neurologic intensive care unit. *Critical Care Medicine* 2001;29(2):283–90.

35. Campbell C, Parish LC. The decubitus ulcer: facts and controversies. *Clin Dermatol* 2010;28(5):527–32.

36. Gallagher S. The challenges of obesity and skin integrity. *Nurs Clin North Am* 2005;40(2):325–35.

37. Richardson A, Barrow I. Part 1: Pressure ulcer assessment —the development of critical care pressure ulcer assessment tool made easy (CALCULATE). *Nurs Crit Care* 2015;20(6):308–14.

38. Kirby JP, Gunter OL. Prevention and treatment of pressure ulcers in the surgical intensive care unit. *Curr Opin Crit Care* 2008;14(4):428–31.

39. Moore ZE, Cowman S. Risk assessment tools for the prevention of pressure ulcers. *The Cochrane Database of Systematic Reviews* 2014(2):CD006471.

40. Gillespie BM, Chaboyer WP, McInnes E, Kent B, Whitty JA, Thalib L. Repositioning for pressure ulcer prevention in adults. *The Cochrane Database of Systematic Reviews* 2014(4):CD009958.

41. McInnes E, Jammali-Blasi A, Bell-Syer SE, Dumville JC, Middleton V, Cullum N. Support surfaces for pressure ulcer prevention. *The Cochrane Database of Systematic Reviews* 2015(9):CD001735.

42. Clark M, Black J, Alves P, et al. Systematic review of the use of prophylactic dressings in the prevention of pressure ulcers. *Int Wound J* 2014;11(5):460–71.

43. Black J, Clark M, Dealey C, et al. Dressings as an adjunct to pressure ulcer prevention: consensus panel recommendations. *Int Wound J* 2015;12(4):484–8.

44. Langer G, Fink A. Nutritional interventions for preventing and treating pressure ulcers. *The Cochrane Database of Systematic Reviews* 2014(6):CD003216.

45. Stausberg J, Kiefer E. Classification of pressure ulcers: a systematic literature review. *Stud Health Technol Inform* 2009;146:511–5.

46. Flanagan M. *Wound Healing and Skin Integrity: Principles and Practice.* 2013.

47. Gray M, Beeckman D, Bliss DZ, et al. Incontinence-associated dermatitis: a comprehensive review and update. *J Wound Ostomy Continence Nurs* 2012;39(1):61–74.

48. Gray M. Optimal management of incontinence-associated dermatitis in the elderly. *Am J Clin Dermatol* 2010;11(3):201–10.

49. Sebastian S. Does preoperative scalp shaving result in fewer postoperative wound infections when compared with no scalp shaving? A systematic review. *The Journal of Neuroscience Nursing* 2012;44(3):149–56.

50. Walcott BP, Redjal N, Coumans JV. Infection following operations on the central nervous system: deconstructing the myth of the sterile field. *Neurosurgical Focus* 2012;33(5):E8.

51. Webster J, Osborne S. Preoperative bathing or showering with skin antiseptics to prevent surgical site infection. *The Cochrane Database of Systematic Reviews* 2015(2): CD004985.

52. Tanner J, Norrie P, Melen K. Preoperative hair removal to reduce surgical site infection. *The Cochrane Database of Systematic Reviews* 2011(11):CD004122.

53. Hepburn-Smith M, Dynkevich I, Spektor M, Lord A, Czeisler B, Lewis A. Establishment of an external ventricular drain best practice guideline: the quest for a comprehensive, universal standard for external ventricular drain care. *The Journal of Neuroscience Nursing* 2016;48(1):54–65.

54. Gillespie BM, Chaboyer W, Kang E, Hewitt J, Nieuwenhoven P, Morley N. Postsurgery wound assessment and management practices: a chart audit. *Journal of Clinical Nursing* 2014;23(21–22):3250–61.

55. Hill M, Baker G, Carter D, et al. A multidisciplinary approach to end external ventricular drain infections in the neurocritical care unit. *The Journal of Neuroscience Nursing* 2012;44(4):188–93.

56. Winston KR, McBride LA, Dudekula A. Bandages, dressings, and cranial neurosurgery. *Journal of Neurosurgery* 2007;106:450–4.

57. Camacho EF, Boszczowski Í, Freire MP, et al. Impact of an educational intervention implanted in a neurological intensive care unit on rates of infection related to external ventricular drains. *PloS One* 2013;8(2):e50708.

58. Flint AC, Rao VA, Renda NC, Faigeles BS, Lasman TE, Sheridan W. A simple protocol to prevent external ventricular drain infections. *Neurosurgery* 2013;72(6): 993–9.

59. Maas AI, Dearden M, Teasdale GM, et al. EBIC-guidelines for management of severe head injury in adults. European Brain Injury Consortium. *Acta Neurochir* 1997;139(4):286–94.

60. Gemma M, Tommasino C, Cerri M, Giannotti A, Piazzi B, Borghi T. Intracranial effects of endotracheal suctioning in the acute phase of head injury. *J Neurosurg Anesthesiol* 2002;14(1):50–4.

61. Pedersen CM, Rosendahl-Nielsen M, Hjermind J, Egerod I. Endotracheal suctioning of the adult intubated patient—what is the evidence? *Intensive and Critical Care Nursing* 2009;25(1):21–30.

62. Subirana M, Sola I, Benito S. Closed tracheal suction systems versus open tracheal suction systems for mechanically ventilated adult patients. *The Cochrane Database of Systematic Reviews* 2007(4):CD004581.

63. Reissmann H, Bohm SH, Suarez-Sipmann F, et al. Suctioning through a double-lumen endotracheal tube helps to prevent alveolar collapse and to preserve ventilation. *Intensive Care Medicine* 2005;31(3):431–40.

64. Hubbard JL, Veneman WL, Dirks RC, Davis JW, Kaups KL. Use of endotracheal tubes with subglottic secretion drainage reduces ventilator-associated pneumonia in trauma patients. *J Trauma Acute Care Surg* 2016;80(2):218–22.

65. Muscedere J, Rewa O, McKechnie K, Jiang X, Laporta D, Heyland DK. Subglottic secretion drainage for the prevention of ventilator-associated pneumonia: a systematic review and meta-analysis. *Critical Care Medicine* 2011;39(8):1985–91.

66. Kelly M, Gillies D, Todd DA, Lockwood C. Heated humidification versus heat and moisture exchangers for ventilated adults and children. *The Cochrane Database of Systematic Reviews* 2010(4):CD004711.

67. Gross JL, Park GR. Humidification of inspired gases during mechanical ventilation. *Minerva Anestesiologica* 2012;78(4):496–502.

68. Dawson D. Essential principles: tracheostomy care in the adult patient. *Nurs Crit Care* 2014;19(2):63–72.

69. Hess DR, Altobelli NP. Tracheostomy tubes. *Respiratory Care* 2014;59(6):956–71; discussion 71–3.

70. Gardner A, Hughes D, Cook R, Henson R, Osborne S, Gardner G. Best practice in stabilisation of oral endotracheal tubes: a systematic review. *Australian Critical Care* 2005;18(4):60–5, 158.

71. King JN, Elliott VA. Self/unplanned extubation: safety, surveillance, and monitoring of the mechanically ventilated patient. *Crit Care Nurs Clin North Am* 2012;24(3): 469–79.

72. Kiekkas P, Aretha D, Panteli E, Baltopoulos GI, Filos KS. Unplanned extubation in critically ill adults: clinical review. *Nurs Crit Care* 2013;18(3):123–34.

73. Morris LL, Whitmer A, McIntosh E. Tracheostomy care and complications in the intensive care unit. *Critical Care Nurse* 2013;33(5):18–30.

74. Nightingale F. *Notes on Nursing: What it is, and What it is Not.* London: Harrison & Son. 1860.

75. Evans J, Reyers E. Patient room considerations in the intensive care unit: caregiver, patient, family. *Crit Care Nurs Q* 2014;37(1):83–92.

76. Johansson L, Bergbom I, Waye KP, Ryherd E, Lindahl B. The sound environment in an ICU patient room—a content analysis of sound levels and patient experiences. *Intensive and Critical Care Nursing* 2012;28(5):269–79.

77. Pulak LM, Jensen L. Sleep in the intensive care unit: a review. *Journal of Intensive Care Medicine* 2016;31(1): 14–23.

78. Engwall M, Fridh I, Johansson L, Bergbom I, Lindahl B. Lighting, sleep and circadian rhythm: An intervention study in the intensive care unit. *Intensive and Critical Care Nursing* 2015;31(6):325–35.

79. Drouot X, Cabello B, d'Ortho MP, Brochard L. Sleep in the intensive care unit. *Sleep Med Rev* 2008;12(5):391–403.

80. Bourne RS, Mills GH. Sleep disruption in critically ill patients—pharmacological considerations. *Anaesthesia* 2004;59(4):374–84.

81. Johansson I, Fridlund B, Hildingh C. What is supportive when an adult next-of-kin is in critical care? *Nurs Crit Care* 2005;10(6):289–98.

82. Verhaeghe S, Defloor T, Van Zuuren F, Duijnstee M, Grypdonck M. The needs and experiences of family members of adult patients in an intensive care unit: a review of the literature. *Journal of Clinical Nursing* 2005;14(4):501–9.

83. Olausson S, Ekebergh M, Lindahl B. The ICU patient room: views and meanings as experienced by the next of kin: a phenomenological hermeneutical study. *Intensive and Critical Care Nursing* 2012;28(3):176–84.

84. Ardley C. Should relatives be denied access to the resuscitation room? *Intensive and Critical Care Nursing* 2003;19(1):1–10.

85. Engstrom A, Soderberg S. Close relatives in intensive care from the perspective of critical care nurses. *Journal of Clinical Nursing* 2007;16(9):1651–9.

86. Smit I, Harrison L, Letzkus L, Quatrara B. What factors are associated with the development of pressure ulcers in a medical intensive care unit? *Dimens Crit Care Nurs* 2016;35(1):37–41.

58

Physiotherapy

A. Thelandersson

ABSTRACT

Intensive care treatment along with critical illness/trauma, immobility, and bed rest causes great changes with a diversity of complications in many bodily systems such as the respiratory, circulatory, and musculoskeletal systems as well as in mental health. Some of these complications can lead to long-lasting morbidities and even death. Physiotherapy in intensive care is aimed at physical deconditioning, neuromuscular and musculoskeletal complications, and prevention and treatment of respiratory conditions. Physiotherapy often starts with passive interventions followed by more active ones when the patient is able. Passive interventions used are, among others, positioning, range of motion, continuous passive motion, and stretching. Active interventions are strengthening exercises, mobilization, and ambulation. Before commencing any physiotherapy, the patient's neurological, circulatory, and respiratory status has to be checked and a risk assessment has to be made. It is also very important that every treatment is individually adjusted for that specific patient.

KEYWORDS

Physiotherapy; positioning; range of motion (ROM); continuous passive motion (CPM); stretching; neuromuscular electrical stimulation (NMES); mobilization; respiratory physiotherapy.

INTRODUCTION

Physical inactivity is one of the leading risk factors for mortality and its incidence is rising in many countries. Physical inactivity is defined as 'an activity level insufficient to meet present recommendations',[1] i.e., the recommendations of the World Health Organization (WHO) for physical activity.

Physical activity for adults as recommended by the WHO are:[2]

- At least 150 minutes of moderate-intensity physical activity throughout the week, or do at least 75 minutes of vigorous-intensity physical activity throughout the week, or an equivalent combination of moderate- and vigorous-intensity activity
- For additional health benefits adults should increase their moderate-intensity physical activity to 300 minutes per week, or equivalent
- Muscle strengthening activities should be done involving major muscle groups on two or more days a week

Patients who are critically ill and/or injured and admitted to an intensive care unit (ICU) spend most of their time in bed and a large part of the day alone.[3] This inactivity along with their critical illness and treatment can lead to changes in many bodily systems, such as the respiratory, circulatory, and musculoskeletal systems as well as mental health. Bed rest, immobility, mechanical ventilation, and anaesthesia cause great changes in the respiratory system such as displacement of the diaphragm which leads to decreased functional residual capacity, the development of atelectasis and ventilation/perfusion mismatch. This along with the underlying cause of admission to intensive care may also lead to ventilator-associated pneumonia and acute respiratory distress syndrome, the latter of which has a mortality rate of 40%–50%. In the circulatory system, changes such as increased heart rate, decrease in stroke volume, loss of cardiac muscle mass, decrease in blood volume, and orthostatic intolerance can be seen. Due to bed rest and immobility along with the intensive care treatments, reduced strength and endurance in skeletal muscles and tendons, bone loss, and degeneration of cartilage and joint contractures can also be seen in the musculoskeletal system.[4–6] A stay in an ICU is also a great mental stress for the patients and many ICU survivors suffer from post-traumatic stress disorder and depression which can be seen in 33% of patients up to one year after discharge from the hospital.[7]

Patients in the neurointensive care unit (NICU) are more often on mechanical ventilation than other ICU patients. They are also mechanically ventilated for longer time periods, more often have a tracheostomy, have longer ICU and hospital stay, and a higher mortality rate than other ICU patients.[8]

From a physiotherapy point of view, one can divide the NICU stay into three phases. The acute phase when the patient is often sedated/unconscious and the physiotherapy treatments are completely passive, such as positioning and passive range of motion (ROM). In this phase the patient may also be so unstable with regards to intracranial pressure and other circulatory variables that physiotherapists do nothing. The second stage is the subacute stage when many of the complications of ICU care develop and physiotherapy is aimed at preventing these complications by treatments such as positioning, ROM, continuous passive motion (CPM), stretching, and splinting. The third and final phase during an NICU admission is the phase where the patients are starting their ICU rehabilitation with more active ROM and strengthening exercises for the whole body, active motion, active respiratory physiotherapy, and mobilization.

PHYSIOTHERAPY

Physiotherapists have been a part of the multi-professional teams caring for critically ill patients reducing morbidity and enhancing survival rates since the first ICUs were developed in the 1950s.[9] Several important areas for physiotherapists working in the ICUs were identified by the European Respiratory Society and European Society of Intensive Care Medicine Task Force in 2008.[10] These areas were physical deconditioning, neuromuscular and musculoskeletal complications, prevention and treatment of respiratory conditions, and emotional problems and communication.[10]

Most studies about exercise and physiotherapy are done in the ICUs but more and more studies are published from research done in NICUs. For patients in an NICU, the same physiotherapy treatments are used as for patients in a regular ICU. They are, however, often started later in the NICU.

In order to describe the physiotherapy interventions in ICUs different terms are used, the most common are mobilization, mobility, exercise, activity, and rehabilitation, and some of these terms are used for both active and passive interventions.[11–15] The treatment often starts with passive interventions and then when the patients are able to, more and more active interventions are used. Passive interventions used are positioning, passive ROM, stretching, CPM, neuromuscular electrical stimulation (NMES), and splinting. The active interventions are, for example, active limb exercises, actively turning in bed, sitting on the edge of the bed or out of bed, standing and walking. The first reports of ambulating ICU patients during mechanical ventilation were published in the 1970s, but the real breakthrough for mobilization in the ICU first came in 2007.[11,12,16–21] Since 2007, an increasing number of research papers about the positive effects of early mobilization, as well as its safety have been reported. Some of the reported positive effects of early mobilization in ICUs are enhanced muscle strength, shorter time of delirium, improved functional outcome, decreased hospital-acquired infections, more ventilator-free days, decreased ICU and hospital length of stay, and reduced costs.[22,23] The lack of early ICU mobility is a factor associated with readmission and death during the first year after ICU admission.[24] Safety and feasibility during early mobilization of patients in an ICU has also been described several times suggesting that it is safe to mobilize patients even when they are on mechanical ventilation, with femoral catheters, during continuous renal replacement therapy (CRRT) and extracorporeal membrane oxygenation. Very few adverse events occur during early mobilization, and the most common are patient–ventilator asynchrony and agitation.[13,25–28]

Historically, physical activity for patients that are critically ill due to severe brain injury or stroke has been restricted to a minimum due to the eventual risks for complications and adverse events. Recently an increasing number of reports of physical activity's feasibility have been published concluding that the positive effects of early physiotherapy interventions outweigh the potential adverse events.[15,29]

Physiotherapy interventions can be complicated to perform due to the patients' critical circulatory and respiratory conditions, invasive monitoring, and necessary medications. An ICU patient's condition can rapidly deteriorate and it is therefore of utmost importance during physiotherapy to monitor the patient's vital parameters. Before the physiotherapist can start any treatments she/he has to make a risk assessment where the patient is screened for potential absolute and relative contraindications.[30] There are a lot of important variables to consider before commencing and during the physiotherapy session for critically ill patients and the most common ones are listed in Table 58.1. These variables are to be considered before and during physiotherapy. They do not mean that it is an absolute contraindication if a patient presents with them. Every patient has to be assessed individually.

Physiotherapy is more complicated for patients in an NICU with a range of specific considerations. Cerebral autoregulation can be impaired in the acute phase after a brain injury or stroke, and as a result cerebral ischaemia may arise due to a decrease in blood pressure (BP), and an increase in BP could raise the intracranial pressure (ICP) due to an increase in cerebral blood volume (CBV).[31] After an aneurysmal subarachnoid haemorrhage, there is also the risk of re-bleeding, seizure, and vasospasm.[32,33]

Table 58.1 Most important variables to consider before and during physiotherapy in a critically ill patient when admitted to an intensive care unit

Neurologic instability	Intracranial pressure ≥20 cm H_2O
Circulation	Heart rate <40 and >130 beats per minute; Recent myocardial ischaemia; Mean arterial blood pressure <60 and >110 mmHg
Respiration	Oxygen saturation <90%; Respiratory rate >40 breaths/minute; Fraction of inspired oxygen ≥0.6; Positive end-expiratory pressure ≥10 cm H_2O
Level of consciousness	Richmond agitation sedation scale −4, −5, 3, 4
Inotropic support	Dopamine ≥10 µg/kg/min; Nor/adrenaline ≥0.1 µg/kg/min
Body temperature	≤36°C and ≥38.5°C
Clinical view	Decreased level of awareness/consciousness; Abnormal face colour; Sweating; Pain; Fatigue
Others	Unstable fractures; Presence of lines that make mobilization unsafe

Adapted from: Sommers J, Engelbert RH, Dettling-Ihnenfeldt D, et al. Physiotherapy in the intensive care unit: an evidence-based, expert driven, practical statement and rehabilitation recommendations. *Clin Rehabil* 2015;29(11):1051–63.

Many patients in a NICU also present with cognitive impairments, hemiparesis, and hemiplegia and this can also be a risk for the patients themselves, as well as staff.[34]

PHYSIOTHERAPY INTERVENTIONS

A suggestion for a simplified model for the progression of physiotherapy interventions for the critically ill patient in an NICU is presented in Table 58.2.

Positioning

For patients that are comatose/sedated and/or paralysed, it is of utmost importance how they are positioned in bed. The complications of bad positioning and/or handling of these patients include pressure ulcers, peripheral nerve and vessel damage, compartment syndrome, joint dislocation, contractures, and a rise in ICP.[35–37] For patients with severe brain injuries, there are also risks for abnormal posturing due to spasticity, flexor or extensor synergies, and primitive reflexes. These abnormal postures could very easily be triggered by stimuli such as sudden movements and unexpected light or touch and in turn raise ICP, therefore how these patients are handled is very important.[37]

When placing a patient suffering from head injuries or stroke in bed, the head should be in a neutral position and not allowed to be extended or fall forward, as this could lead to raised ICP and increased tone. When placed in the supine position, the arms should be supported by pillows so that they are placed straight and with the palm

Table 58.2 A simplified model for the progression of physiotherapy in an NICU

Stage	Intervention	Activity
1	Passive interventions in bed	Changing position in bed; Head of bed elevation; Passive ROM; Passive CPM; Respiratory physiotherapy
2	Active interventions in bed	Moving in bed; Active ROM exercises; Active motion (as bed cycling); Sitting in bed; Sitting on the edge of bed; Respiratory physiotherapy
3	Activities out of bed	Stand beside of the bed; Stand and pivot to chair
4	Ambulating	Walking with assistance; Walking without assistance

of the hands facing up. The legs should be supported so that they do not rotate out at the hips and the knees should be slightly flexed for relaxation. When sitting up, on the other hand the arms should be placed on a pillow to avoid the shoulders from dropping and the palms of the hand should be facing downwards. It is also important to place the wrists in a neutral position and the fingers extended to avoid the hand from closing into a grip position. When laying on the left or right side, the body weight should be on the flat of the shoulder blade and the upper arm supported on a pillow. The leg lying against the bed should be placed in line with the body and the knee slightly bent; the upper leg should be placed forward to prevent the patient from rolling onto his/her back and flexed at the hip and the knee and placed on a pillow.[35–37] These positions could be, and mostly are, used for all patients in an ICU when they are comatose and/or sedated and thus unable to actively move on their own. By using these positions and changing the patient position every second hour, the risks for pressure, nerve and vessel damage as well as the risk for compartment syndrome are reduced.[35]

It is also possible to turn the patients to a prone position, but it requires multiple staff, is difficult, and makes nursing duties difficult to administer. Therefore the prone position is mostly used in an ICU when the patients have severe lung complications with a high oxygen demand. There are two different positions frequently used and they are a semi-prone position with different angles and a total prone position. In the semi-prone position, soft pillows are used to place the patients in a good position and in the total prone position specialized pillows or beds can be used.[38–39] Studies have shown that prone position is safe to use in critically ill patients in an NICU without any deleterious effects on the circulatory and intracranial variables and with great respiratory effects.[39] The prone position is also a great position to stretch the hip flexors in order to avoid contractures and to minimize abnormal posturing.[37,40]

Range of Motion

There are four main themes for the physiotherapist when doing passive ROM exercises or having the patient doing active ROM exercises and they are: assessment, prevention, maintenance, and restoration.[19] Assessed are the range of motion, muscle tone, pain, and neurological function.[10,19] Prevention, maintenance, and restoration are aimed at joint range of motion, soft tissue extensibility, muscle strength and function, prevention of thromboembolism and oedema.[19,41] Passive ROM is used

for patients that are unable to move their arms and legs on their own due to sedation, coma or paralyses and is mostly performed by physiotherapists. Passive ROM performed early during NICU admission has been proven to be safe regarding circulatory and intracranial variables.[42] Unfortunately, there are not many studies evaluating the effects of passive ROM exercises. However, what is known is that longer periods of passive exercise have positive effects on muscle fibres, pain, and oedema.[43–45] One study though established that bilateral passive ROM for patients suffering from acute stroke while in the intensive care could improve the function of upper extremities and activities of daily living.[46]

Continuous Passive Motion

Continuous passive motion has mostly been used after trauma to or surgery in a joint, or after implantation of prostheses in joints that are prone to stiffness such as the knees and elbows. The rationale for using CPM after joint surgery or trauma is to avoid stiffness in the joint. Joint stiffness has four stages; bleeding, oedema, granulation tissue, and fibrosis. Continuous passive motion could be effective in pumping fluid away from the affected area and thereby avoiding stiffness and reduced ROM.[45] When used in intensive care, CPM is mostly used for the lower extremities and one device that can be used is a bedside cycle ergometer. There are bedside cycles that can be used for both passive and active exercise and patients can change back and forth between them. When used for passive exercise, the bedside cycle is adjusted for revolutions per minute and in case of active cycling different gears can be used. Adding an extra session of bedside cycling to the ordinary physiotherapy schedule for critically ill patients has been proven to improve functional exercise capacity, muscle force, and perceived functional status at hospital discharge in ICU patients.[11] Whether this effect is applicable to patients in an NICU still remains to be seen. Still, very early exercise with a bedside cycle ergometer has been proven to be safe according to circulatory and intracranial variables in patients when admitted to an NICU.[47] Continuous passive motion might also be of great use in the NICU for patients that are restricted to the bed, but are still very restless and/or motorically disturbed to calm them down and for patients with high muscle tone to relax their muscles.

Stretching and Splinting

Stretching and splinting is used in patients with spasticity or great flexor or extensor tone in their extremities in order to prevent them from building up contractures though its usefulness is debated. Stretching induces an increase in tissue extensibility due to viscous deformation but this increase is transient and contracture management needs more long-lasting tissue extensibility. Stretching can be self-administered or manually administered by others, with positioning or with different splints or casts. The duration of stretch varies based on whether it is administered manually or, for example, with casts. A manual stretch is performed a few minutes at a time and with casts the stretch could be for days or even weeks.[20]

Neuromuscular Electrical Stimulation

Neuromuscular electrical stimulation is used to activate inactive, weak, or paralysed muscles mostly in the lower extremities with quadriceps femoris being the most common muscle stimulated. Without input from the central nervous system, NMES causes muscle contractions in the stimulated muscles. No consensus has yet been established on the most effective NMES parameters to be used. Most studies use a biphasic symmetrical setting, frequencies used are between 35–100 Hz, pulse width 200–400 μs, stimulation intensities 15–150 mA and a duration of 30–60 minutes per day, i.e., a wide range in settings are used making it very difficult to interpret its use in ICU practice. Neuromuscular electrical stimulation however has been reported to increase muscle strength and show potential benefit for joint range of motion and activity limitations. No major adverse events or complications have been reported when using NMES in the setting for critically ill patients and it does not seem to interfere with monitoring equipment.[21]

Mobilization

In the NICU setting early mobilization, out of bed activities, and ambulation have been restricted to a minimum due to the potential risks of patient deterioration. Early mobilization for patients in an NICU have however been shown to give the patients higher mobility levels, fewer days in restraint (not used everywhere), decreased NICU and hospital length of stay, decreased infections, fewer hospital acquired pressure ulcers, lower anxiety rates, and patients were more likely to be discharged home.[15,34] For patients suffering from subarachnoid haemorrhage, bed rest has traditionally been prescribed due to the fear of decreased cerebral perfusion, due to head elevation, which could lead to cerebral ischaemia. Mobilization is/was also thought to enhance the risk of re-bleeding and negatively affect the development of cerebral vasospasm.[48] Lately, a few articles have been published

describing the safety and feasibility of early mobilization for patients suffering from subarachnoid haemorrhage. A few adverse events occurred and they were mean arterial blood pressure or heart rate below or above the criteria set by the researchers.[29,48] One report even stated that early mobilization probably increases the chance of a good functional outcome in patients with poor-grade aneurysmal subarachnoid haemorrhage.[48]

Early mobilization with protocols ranging from passive in-bed activities to ambulation in the ward has been proven to be an effective way to increase mobility levels in patients admitted to an NICU. It is also important that the entire staff knows that the protocol is standard care and not to view the protocol as an exception. A protocol is most effective if the patients are screened for their personal highest mobility level every day.[15,34]

Limited mobility progression is a factor associated with poorer clinical outcome for patients in the intensive care. Patient factors associated with less mobility are being female, mechanical ventilation, and higher Acute Physiology and Chronic Health Evaluation (APACHE) score.[49]

Respiratory Physiotherapy

Different deep breathing techniques with or without different devices are used to enhance pulmonary function, to prevent pulmonary complications such as atelectasis and pneumonia, to evacuate secretions after surgery and for persons with pulmonary or neurological disorders.[50,51]

Positive expiratory pressure (PEP), i.e., breathing against an expiratory pressure is used to increase lung volume, reduce hyperinflation, and improve airway clearance. Indications for the treatment are acute or chronic ventilator failure due to surgery, neurological or musculoskeletal dysfunctions, old age, and immobility. Positive expiratory pressure can be reached with different techniques such as pursed lips breathing or with different devices that are either flow or pressure regulated. Either a mouthpiece or a mask is placed on the device; some of the devices can also be placed right on the tracheostomy. Positive expiratory pressure breathing has been reported to increase lung volumes, gas exchange, and decrease atelectasis in patients as well as healthy subjects. The technique used is to get the patient to reach a mid-expiratory pressure of 10–20 cm H_2O, and the duration, number of treatment sessions, and breaths per session is individually prescribed. Resistance on inspiration can also be used, a so-called inspiratory resistance – positive expiratory pressure (IR-PEP).[51]

Positive expiratory pressure can also be used as an airway clearance technique during infection, postoperatively or for patients with impaired mucociliary clearance or coughing ability. Different breathing techniques can also be used in combination with positioning to make use of the effect of gravity. The only known absolute contraindication for PEP is an undrained pneumothorax.[51]

In the intensive care setting mechanical in-exsufflation (M I-E) technique could be used for airway clearance as well as weaning from mechanical ventilation and tracheostomy. For patients with impaired breathing due to pulmonary disease, weakness of pulmonary muscles or central nervous system disease it is a great aid to facilitate removal of secretions. The M I-E starts with a gradual insufflation of the lungs with positive pressure followed by an immediate change to negative pressure which leads to an exhalation (exsufflation) that simulates a cough which moves the secretions upward. Pressures of +40/−40 cm H_2O have been found to be optimal in adults in most studies. A session of M I-E consists of 3–5 cycles of I-E followed by a short rest and then repeated until the secretion has been sufficiently removed. The device could be used in either manual or automatic mode and the I-E could be delivered via a mask or tracheostomy.[52]

Manually assisted cough (MAC) could be used on its own or in combination with other treatments as M I-E to improve cough flow in order to remove secretions from the airways. Manually assisted cough starts with a full insufflation followed by an abdominal thrust or a thoracic squeeze to augment the patient's cough. When using this technique it is important to be careful not to injure abdominal organs or to cause a reflux by pressure on gastric contents.[52,53]

CONCLUSIONS

Intensive care treatment has tremendous impact on respiratory, circulatory, musculoskeletal, and mental health of the patients. For prevention and treatment of physical deconditioning of neuromuscular and musculoskeletal complications, physiotherapy constitutes an important aspect of management. There are a lot of physiotherapy treatments to use for patients admitted to an ICU, the most common ones being positioning, range of motion, mobilization, and respiratory physiotherapy. Since 2007, an increasing number of research papers about the positive effects of early mobilization as well as its safety have been reported. Some of the reported positive effects of early mobilization in the ICUs are enhanced muscle strength, shorter time of delirium, improved functional outcome, decreased hospital-acquired infections, more ventilator free days, decreased ICU and hospital length of stay, and reduced costs.

Physiotherapy could be started early after admission but before commencing any physiotherapy, the patient's neurological, circulatory, and respiratory status has to be checked and a risk assessment made. It is also very important that every treatment is individually adjusted for that specific patient.

REFERENCES

1. Lee IM, Shiroma EJ, Lobelo F, Puska P, Blair SN, Katzmarzyk PT. Effect of physical inactivity on major non-communicable diseases worldwide: an analysis of burden of disease and life expectancy. *Lancet* 2012;380(9838):219–29.
2. World Health Organization. Fact sheet N385: Physical activity. January 2015. Available from: http://www.who.int/mediacentre/factsheets/fs385/en/.
3. Berney SC, Rose JW, Bernhardt J, Denehy L. Prospective observation of physical activity in critically ill patients who were intubated for more than 48 hours. *J Crit Care* 2015;30(4):658–63.
4. Topp R, Ditmyer M, King K, Doherty K, Hornyak J 3rd. The effect of bed rest and potential of prehabilitation on patients in the intensive care unit. *AACN Clin Issues* 2002;13(2):263–76.
5. Karcz M, Papadakos PJ. Respiratory complications in the postanesthesia care unit: A review of pathophysiological mechanisms. *Can J Respir Ther* 2013;49(4):21–9.
6. Froese AB, Bryan AC. Effects of anesthesia and paralysis on diaphragmatic mechanics in man. *Anesthesiology* 1974;41(3):242–55.
7. Jackson JC, Pandharipande PP, Girard TD, et al. Depression, post-traumatic stress disorder, and functional disability in survivors of critical illness in the BRAIN-ICU study: a longitudinal cohort study. *Lancet Respir Med* 2014;2(5):369–79.
8. Pelosi P, Ferguson ND, Frutos-Vivar F, et al. Management and outcome of mechanically ventilated neurologic patients. *Crit Care Med* 2011;39(6):1482–92.
9. Kelly FE, Fong K, Hirsch N, Nolan JP. Intensive care medicine is 60 years old: the history and future of the intensive care unit. *Clin Med (Lond)* 2014;14(4):376–9.
10. Gosselink R, Bott J, Johnson M, Dean E, et al. Physiotherapy for adult patients with critical illness: recommendations of the European Respiratory Society and European Society of Intensive Care Medicine Task Force on Physiotherapy for Critically Ill Patients. *Intensive Care Med* 2008;34(7):1188–99.
11. Burtin C, Clerckx B, Robbeets C, et al. Early exercise in critically ill patients enhances short-term functional recovery. *Crit Care Med* 2009;37(9):2499–505.

12. Bailey P, Thomsen GE, Spuhler VJ, et al. Early activity is feasible and safe in respiratory failure patients. *Crit Care Med* 2007;35(1):139–45.

13. Damluji A, Zanni JM, Mantheiy E, Colantuoni E, Kho ME, Needham DM. Safety and feasibility of femoral catheters during physical rehabilitation in the intensive care unit. *J Crit Care* 2013;28(4):535.e9–15.

14. Engel HJ, Tatebe S, Alonzo PB, Mustille RL, Rivera MJ. Physical therapist-established intensive care unit early mobilization program: quality improvement project for critical care at the University of California San Francisco Medical Center. *Phys Ther* 2013;93(7):975–85.

15. Titsworth WL, Hester J, Correia T, et al. The effect of increased mobility on morbidity in the neurointensive care unit. *J Neurosurg* 2012;116(6):1379–88.

16. Stiller K. Physiotherapy in intensive care: an updated systematic review. *Chest* 2013;144(3):825–47.

17. Morris PE. Moving our critically ill patients: mobility barriers and benefits. *Crit Care Clin* 2007;23(1):1–20.

18. Burns JR, Jones FL. Letter: Early ambulation of patients requiring ventilatory assistance. *Chest* 1975;68(4):608.

19. Stockley RC, Morrison J, Rooney J, Hughes J. Move it or lose it? A survey of the aims of treatment when using passive movements in intensive care. *Intensive Crit Care Nurs* 2012;28(2):82–7.

20. Katalinic OM, Harvey LA, Herbert RD. Effectiveness of stretch for the treatment and prevention of contractures in people with neurological conditions: a systematic review. *Phys Ther* 2011;91:11–24.

21. Burke D, Gorman E, Stokes D, Lennon O. An evaluation of neuromuscular electrical stimulation in critical care using the ICF framework: a systematic review and meta-analysis. *Clin Respir J* 2016;10(4):407–20.

22. Winkelman C, Johnson KD, Hejal R, et al. Examining the positive effects of exercise in intubated adults in ICU: a prospective repeated measures clinical study. *Intensive Crit Care Nurs* 2012;28(6):307–18.

23. Cameron S, Ball I, Cepinskas G, et al. Early mobilization in the critical care unit: A review of adult and pediatric literature. *J Crit Care* 2015;30(4):664–72.

24. Morris PE, Griffin L, Berry M, et al. Receiving early mobility during an intensive care unit admission is a predictor of improved outcomes in acute respiratory failure. *Am J Med Sci* 2011;341(5):373–7.

25. Pohlman MC, Schweickert WD, Pohlman AS, et al. Feasibility of physical and occupational therapy beginning from initiation of mechanical ventilation. *Crit Care Med* 2010;38(11):2089–94.

26. Wang YT, Haines TP, Ritchie P, et al. Early mobilization on continuous renal replacement therapy is safe and may improve filter life. *Crit Care* 2014;18(4):R161.

27. Abrams D, Javidfar J, Farrand E, et al. Early mobilization of patients receiving extracorporeal membrane oxygenation: a retrospective cohort study. *Crit Care* 2014;18(1):R38.

28. Schweickert WD, Pohlman MC, Pohlman AS, et al. Early physical and occupational therapy in mechanically ventilated, critically ill patients: a randomised controlled trial. *Lancet* 2009;373(9678):1874–82.

29. Olkowski BF, Devine MA, Slotnick LE, et al. Safety and feasibility of an early mobilization program for patients with aneurysmal subarachnoid hemorrhage. *Phys Ther* 2013;93(2):208–15.

30. Sommers J, Engelbert RH, Dettling-Ihnenfeldt D, et al. Physiotherapy in the intensive care unit: an evidence-based, expert driven, practical statement and rehabilitation recommendations. *Clin Rehabil* 2015;29(11):1051–63.

31. Kocan MJ, Lietz H. Special considerations for mobilizing patients in the neurointensive care unit. *Crit Care Nurs Q* 2013;36(1):50–5.

32. Diringer MN. Management of aneurysmal subarachnoid hemorrhage. *Crit Care Med* 2009;37(2):432–40.

33. Levine JM. Critical care management of subarachnoid hemorrhage. *Curr Treat Options Neurol* 2009;11(2):126–36.

34. Klein K, Mulkey M, Bena JF, Albert NM. Clinical and psychological effects of early mobilization in patients treated in a neurologic ICU: a comparative study. *Crit Care Med* 2015;43(4):865–73.

35. Griffiths H, Gallimore D. Positioning critically ill patients in hospital. *Nurs Stand* 2005;19(42):56–64.

36. De D, Wynn E. Preventing muscular contractures through routine stroke patient care. *Br J Nurs* 2014;23(14):781–6.

37. Palmer M, Wyness MA. Positioning and handling: important considerations in the care of the severely head-injured patient. *J Neurosci Nurs* 1988;20(1):42–9.

38. Guérin C, Reignier J, Richard JC, et al. Prone positioning in severe acute respiratory distress syndrome. *N Engl J Med* 2013;368(23):2159–68.

39. Thelandersson A, Cider A, Nellgård B. Prone position in mechanically ventilated patients with reduced intracranial compliance. *Acta Anaesthesiol Scand* 2006;50(8):937–41.

40. Skalsky AJ, McDonald CM. Prevention and management of limb contractures in neuromuscular diseases. *Phys Med Rehabil Clin N Am* 2012;23(3):675–87.

41. Stiller K. Physiotherapy in intensive care: towards an evidence-based practice. *Chest* 2000;118(6):1801–13.

42. Thelandersson A, Cider Å, Volkmann R. Cerebrovascular and systemic haemodynamic parameters during passive exercise. *Advances in Physiotherapy* 2010;12:58–63.

43. Amidei C, Sole ML. Physiological responses to passive exercise in adults receiving mechanical ventilation. *Am J Crit Care* 2013;22(4):337–48.

44. Llano-Diez M, Renaud G, Andersson M, et al. Mechanisms underlying ICU muscle wasting and effects of passive mechanical loading. *Crit Care* 2012;16(5):R209.

45. O'Driscoll SW, Giori NJ. Continuous passive motion (CPM): theory and principles of clinical application. *J Rehabil Res Dev* 2000;37(2):179–88.

46. Kim HJ, Lee Y, Sohng KY. Effects of bilateral passive range of motion exercise on the function of upper extremities and activities of daily living in patients with acute stroke. *J Phys Ther Sci* 2014;26(1):149–56.

47. Thelandersson A, Nellgård B, Ricksten SE, Cider Å. Effects of early bedside cycle exercise on intracranial pressure and systemic hemodynamics in critically ill patients in a neurointensive care unit. *Neurocrit Care* 2016 May 23. [Epub ahead of print].

48. Karic T, Røe C, Nordenmark TH, Becker F, Sorteberg A. Impact of early mobilization and rehabilitation on global functional outcome one year after aneurysmal subarachnoid hemorrhage. *J Rehabil Med* 2016;48:676–82.

49. Mulkey M, Bena JF, Albert NM. Clinical outcomes of patient mobility in a neuroscience intensive care unit. *J Neurosci Nurs* 2014;46(3):153–61.

50. Bodin P, Kreuter M, Bake B, Olsén MF. Breathing patterns during breathing exercises in persons with tetraplegia. *Spinal Cord* 2003;41:290–5.

51. FagevikOlsén M, Lannefors L, Westerdahl E. Positive expiratory pressure—Common clinical applications and physiological effects. *Respir Med* 2015;109(3):297–307.

52. Homnick D. Mechanical insufflation-exsufflation for airway mucus clearance. *Respir Care* 2007;52(10):1296–305.

53. Finder JD. Airway clearance modalities in neuromuscular disease. *Paediatr Respir Rev* 2010 Mar;11(1):31–4.

Part XVIII

Clinical Procedures in Neurointensive Care Unit

Editor: Avinash Bhargava

59

Venous and Arterial Access

R. Neeley

ABSTRACT

This chapter describes the various insertion sites of venous and arterial cannulations and placement of central venous catheters. The anatomical landmarks have been illustrated with the accompanying video, as given in the DVD.

KEYWORDS

Arterial line; central line; anatomical landmarks; peripheral line; procedure.

VENOUS ACCESS

Intravenous (IV) access has become synonymous with hospital admission. Presumably the patient is getting an IV in order to receive therapy that can only be administered intravenously or in a hospital setting. In the US, hospitals purchase approximately 150 million intravascular devices for the delivery of fluids, medications, blood products, parenteral nutrition, or to monitor haemodynamics or provide haemodialysis.[1] Commonly, even if the patient is receiving minimal to no IV therapy, the IV remains as an emergency measure. If by some chance the patients were to experience an in-hospital catastrophic event, it would be used to deliver emergency medications.

There are many modalities for obtaining venous access, from the most common, a peripheral IV (PIV), to central venous catheters (CVC), or a peripherally inserted central catheter (PICC). The reason to choose one over the other depends primarily on its purpose. For the administration of most IV fluids and basic IV medications, any PIV is sufficient. Peripheral IVs come in many sizes, from 14–24 gauge. The flow rate is dependent on the diameter of the angiocatheter[4] (Table 59.1).

If the primary need is for rapid resuscitation of the patient, a larger bore IV is necessary. If it is only being used for simple medication administration, smaller ones are sufficient. Larger gauge ones can increase the risk of thrombophlebitis.[2] However, some medications such as high potency vasopressors, hypertonic fluids,

Table 59.1 Flow rate of IV fluid, based on the gauge size of the angiocatheter

Gauge	Flow rate (ml/min)
14	330
16	220
18	105
20	65
22	35
24	20

Adapted from: Sommers J, Engelbert RH, Dettling-Ihnenfeldt D, et al. Physiotherapy in the intensive care unit: an evidence-based, expert driven, practical statement and rehabilitation recommendations. *Clin Rehabil* 2015;29(11):1051–63.

or total parenteral nutrition (TPN) require central venous access. Alternatively, as patients get older or have more comorbidities, gaining PIV access may become increasingly difficult,[3] and they may require central venous access.

The choice of the type of central venous access depends on the purpose for which it is needed. Patients who require large volume resuscitations would benefit more from large bore access, either a double lumen line, introducer sheath, or multi-access catheter (MAC) compared to a triple lumen catheter (TLC) or PICC line. For the critically ill patient who requires multiple ongoing infusions for which many access points are required, a TLC would be optimal. Generally, a PICC line is reserved in instances when patients require a prolonged course of antibiotics, TPN, or have had a history of difficult IV access in which case it is more humane to place a PICC line compared to the many attempts it may take to gain PIV access (which may require replacement in the next hours to couple of days regardless).

Since IV access is considered as a surgical procedure there is a risk of developing complications. Complications include IV infiltration and extravasation, thrombophlebitis, central-line-associated blood stream infection (CLABSI), deep venous thrombosis (DVT), sepsis, and pneumothorax. Approximately 250,000 CLABSI are reported in the US annually, with a significant percentage leading to deaths.[5,6]

The proceduralist also faces certain risks primarily related to needlestick injury and blood exposure such as Hepatitis C or human immunodeficiency virus (HIV) transmission. The estimated amount of needlestick injuries is 384,000/year, with an estimated cost of $120 million to $590 million.[7] The U.S. Centers for Disease Control recommends changing PIVs every 72–96 hours to reduce the patients' risk of infection. However, it is debatable as some reviews have shown no benefit in this practice.[8] Certain institutions do not replace PIVs in their paediatric population because of the difficulty in gaining IV access unless it becomes clinically indicated.

Method

Peripheral Intravenous Insertion

Procedure

- An appropriate site is chosen and flexural creases or lower extremities are avoided if possible. It is recommended to start distally and move proximally.
- A tourniquet is placed above the insertion site.
- Cleaned with alcohol-based surgical prep solutions.
- Traction is placed on the skin to stabilize the vessel.
- The needle is inserted at approximately 30–40° angle.
- Once a flash of blood appears, the angle of the needle is lowered and advanced to 1–2 mm.
- The angiocatheter is advanced off the needle.
- The IV tubing is connected and tourniquet removed. The IV is opened to ensure it is free-flowing.
- The sterile dressing is secured.
- The needle is disposed in an appropriate sharps container.

Central Line Insertion[9]

Indications

- Administration of venotoxic agents (vasopressors, hypertonic solutions, i.e., 3% NS or TPN)
- Chemotherapeutic agents
- Inability to get PIV access

Sites

- Internal jugular vein
- Subclavian vein
- Femoral veins

Recent data shows that there is not a significant difference in infection rates between the sites.[10]

Procedure

- In possible cases, informed consent from patient or surrogate is obtained and documented prior to placement.
- A 'Time Out' should be performed when possible prior to CVC insertion, assisted by a bedside nurse. It includes:
  a. Assuring the correct patient;
  b. Locating site of insertion;
  c. Confirming if the patient is on a blood thinner;
  d. Confirm that there is no coagulopathy or thrombocytopenia; and
  e. Ensuring sterile preparation and equipment.
- Hand hygiene, assessment, or dressing change of the catheter exit site is completed prior to insertion.
- Insertion site is cleaned with >0.5% chlorhexidine and alcohol.
- Systemic antimicrobial prophylaxis is not indicated.
- Maximum sterile barrier precautions must be used during insertion, including cap, mask, sterile gown, sterile gloves, and a sterile full-body drape.
- An insertion site should be selected that is not contaminated or potentially contaminated (e.g., burned or infected skin, inguinal area, adjacent to tracheostomy or open surgical wound).
- When clinically appropriate and feasible, central venous access in the neck or chest should be performed with the patient in the Trendelenburg position, and in the reverse Trendelenburg position for femoral access.
- A central venous catheter should be used with the minimum number of lumens required for patient care.
- Static ultrasound imaging should be used in elective situations before prepping. Use of real-time ultrasound guidance has shown best results in terms of fewer complications and fewer needle passes before insertion.[11]
- Confirm placement of needle/catheter.
  a. Ultrasound, manometry, pressure-waveform analysis, or venous blood gas measurement.
  b. Blood colour or absence of pulsatile flow should not be relied upon for confirming that the catheter or thin-wall needle resides in the vein.
- Confirm wire placement: Surface ultrasound, transoesophageal echocardiography, continuous

electrocardiography (identification of narrow-complex ectopy), or fluoroscopy.

- After final catheterization and before use, residence of the catheter in the venous system must be confirmed as soon as clinically appropriate.
- Using either (or in combination) chest radiography, fluoroscopy, or continuous electrocardiography.

ARTERIAL ACCESS

The placement of an arterial catheter is a common procedure performed in the perioperative and critical care setting. It is strictly a monitoring device and provides beat-to-beat reporting of blood pressure, easy access for blood gas analysis or collection of other laboratory data.[12] It should never be used for administration of medications.

Indications

Operative procedures in which the physician suspects haemodynamic liability and the possible need for vasoactive medications, inability to get reliable non-invasive blood pressure (NIBP) monitoring (i.e., morbid obesity), severity of patient's comorbidities, the need for frequent blood gas or other lab analysis indications are the reasons for choosing to place an arterial line. Other factors that play a role in choosing to place an arterial line include predictability of the anatomy, accessibility, and low complication rate.

Sites

Site options for arterial cannulation include radial, axillary, brachial, femoral, or dorsalis pedis artery. The radial artery (RA) is most commonly chosen because it is easily accessed and has a lower complication rate.[13] One study noted a rate of severe nerve or vascular injury approximately 3.5 per 10,000 lines placed[14] in over 60,000 patients. Complications during arterial catheterization include injury to nerves, or vessels, thrombosis, limb ischaemia, bleeding, or infection.

The RA comes off of the brachial artery as it proceeds towards the styloid process of the radius. Variations have been noted, but these are more commonly found proximally compared to distally where A-line insertion occurs and thus should have minimal impact on insertion. However, with the advent of ultrasound guidance, it may not matter. Ultrasound guidance has shown reduction in number of insertion attempts, time to successful insertion, and haematoma formation compared to palpation.[15]

Method

Radial Artery Catheterization

Procedure

- There should be a discussion with and consent of the patient or their family prior to insertion, if time or circumstances permit.
- Radial artery pulse should be palpated:
  a. The site should be chosen based on patient or procedure requirements.
  b. Sufficient palmar collateral blood flow must be assessed by Modified Allen's Test (Figure 59.1).
- Rest the patient's forearm on a table with rolled surgical towel or bandage rolls under the wrist in a supinated position. Tape the hand to the table to provide mild hyperextension.
- Wrist must be cleaned with chlorhexidine gluconate and isopropyl alcohol or other alcohol-based solution.
- Drape the area with sterile towels or paper drape.
- At minimum, sterile gloves and equipment should be used. Hat, mask, and gown may be used as per institutional policy.
- Distally begin to palpate the pulse gently.
- Local anaesthesia should be used to infiltrate the area in case the patient is alert/awake.
- An angiocatheter 20 g and 5 cm is inserted at a 30–45° angle into the RA as distally as possible. If additional attempts are required, one can move proximally.
- Once a flash of blood is obtained, the angle is lowered and guide wire inserted if blood return continues.
- Alternatively:
  i. If not using a guide wire, the angiocatheter should be advanced over the needle.
  ii. Trans-arterial: After blood return, the needle should be advanced through the vessel. The needle and wire are to be removed. Angiocatheter to be withdrawn until pulsatile blood return is observed. The guidewire is then inserted and angiocatheter advanced over guidewire.
  iii. For femoral artery catherization, one may want to use 20 g (or 18 g) 12 cm angiocatheter.
- Angiocatheter is advanced over guide wire into the vessel.
- Troubleshooting: If there is no blood return and angiocatheter is advanced, the angiocatheter must be gently withdrawn until pulsatile blood return is seen, then passing the wire is attempted, and re-advanced over the wire.
- A transducer should be connected to observe pulsatile waveform; sterile dressing must be used for securing the site (suture in place depending on practice or patient factors).

- It is important to ensure that the arterial line is clearly labelled to prevent accessing it for medication delivery.
- Arterial catheter should be removed as soon as it is no longer needed for patient care.

RISK FACTORS FOR LIMB ISCHAEMIA[16]

The following factors may lead to limb ischaemia:

- Patient-related
  - Documented incomplete hand collateralization
  - Anatomical limitations: small RA diameter
  - Anatomical variations: absent ulnar artery (UA)
  - Pre-existing atherosclerosis, e.g., elderly diabetic smoker with peripheral artery disease
  - Disease states: scleroderma, Raynaud's disease
- Catheter and technique-related risks
  - Inexperienced operator
  - Haematoma at puncture site
  - Vasospasm
- Surgery and hospital course-related risks
  - Anticipated need for prolonged arterial cannulation
  - High risk for profound circulatory failure
  - High risk for prolonged perioperative hypotension
  - Anticipated need for prolonged or high-dose vasopressor therapy
  - High risk for thrombosis and/or digital emboli, e.g., preoperative hypercoagulable state
  - Direct injection of vaso-caustic medications (e.g., promethazine)
- Factors with limited or conflicting evidence
  - Number of puncture attempts
  - Large indwelling catheters (>20 g)
  - Polypropylene catheter (compared to polytetrafluoroethylene)
  - Female gender
  - Infiltration of local anaesthetics
- Factors not associated with increased frequency of RA occlusion
  - Transfixation cannulation technique (compared to direct puncture cannulation technique)
  - Recannaluation of previously cannulated RA
  - Reversing the direction of the cannula

CONCLUSIONS

Intravenous and arterial cannulations have become an integral part of management of patients admitted to hospitals. Medications and IV fluids are administered through the veins. Arterial cannulations help in noting beat-to-beat variations in the blood pressure.

REFERENCES

1. Mermel LA, Allon M, Bouza E, et al. Clinical practice guidelines for the diagnosis and management of intravascular catheter-related infection: 2009. Updated by the Infectious Diseases Society of America. *Clin Infect Dis* 2009;49:1–45.
2. Tagalakis V, Kahn SR, Libman M, Blostein M. The epidemiology of peripheral vein infusion thrombophlebitis: a critical review. *Am J Med* 2002;113:146–51.
3. Dychter SS, Gold DA, Carson D, Haller M. Intravenous therapy: a review of complications and economic considerations of peripheral access. *J Infus Nurs* 2012; 35:84–91.
4. Royer T. Maximum flow rates achievable through peripherally inserted central catheters using standard hospital infusion pumps. *J of the Assoc for Vasc Access* 2012; 17:78–83.
5. Mermel LA. Prevention of intravascular catheter-related infections. *Ann Int Med* 2000;132:391–402.
6. O'Grady NP, Alexander M, Burns LA, et al. and the Healthcare Infection Control Practices Advisory Committee (HICPAC). Guidelines for the prevention of intravascular catheter-related infections. Centers for Disease Control and Prevention. [Accessed 2011 Sep 29]. Available from: https://www.cdc.gov/hai/pdfs/bsi-guidelines-2011.pdf.
7. Saia M, Hofmann F, Sharman J, et al. Needlestick injuries: incidence and cost in the United States, United Kingdom, Germany, France, Italy, and Spain. *Biomedicine International* 2010;1:41–9.
8. Webster J, Osborne S, Rickard CM, New K. Clinically-indicated replacement versus routine replacement of peripheral venous catheters. *Cochrane Database of Systematic Reviews* Issue 8, 2015. CD007798. DOI: 10.1002/14651858.CD007798.pub4.
9. Rupp SM, Apfelbaum JL, Blitt C, et al. American Society of Anesthesiologists task force on central venous access. Practice guidelines for central venous access: a report by the American Society of Anesthesiologists Task Force on Central Venous Access. *Anesthesiology* 2012;116:539–73.
10. Marik PE, Flemmer M, Harrison W. The risk of catheter-related bloodstream infection with femoral venous catheters as compared to subclavian and internal jugular venous catheters: A systematic review of the literature and meta-analysis. *Crit Care Med* 2012;40:2479–85.
11. Troianos CA, Hartman GS, Glas KE, et al. Guidelines for performing ultrasound guided vascular cannulation: recommendations of the American Society of Echocardiography and the Society of Cardiovascular Anesthesiologists. *J Am Soc Echocardiogr* 2011;24: 1291–318.
12. Clark VL, Kruse JA. Arterial catheterization. *Crit Care Clin* 1992;8:687–97.
13. Scheer B, Perel A, Pfeiffer UJ et al. Clinical review: complications and risk factors of peripheral arterial

catheters used for haemodynamic monitoring in anesthesia and intensive care medicine. *Crit Care* 2002;6: 198–204.

14. Nuttall G, Burckhardt J, Hadley A, et al. Surgical and patient risk factors for severe arterial line complications in adults. *Anesthesiology* 2016;124:590–7.

15. Gu WJ, Liu JC. Ultrasound-guided radial artery catheterization: a meta-analysis of randomized controlled trials. *Intensive Care Med* 2014;40:292–3.

16. Brzezinski M, Luisetti T, London MJ. Radial artery cannulation: a comprehensive review of recent anatomic and physiologic investigations. *Anesth Analg* 2009;109:1763–81.

60

Fibreoptic Bronchoscopy and Bronchoalveolar Lavage

C. P. Henson

ABSTRACT

This chapter discusses the indications, uses, and techniques for flexible fibreoptic bronchoscopy in the management of critically ill patients. From evaluation of airway anatomy and diagnosis of pneumonia to treatment of luminal obstruction, bronchoscopy has become a significant part of the intensive care armamentarium. It covers contraindications as well as specific procedural points of emphasis. Special consideration is given to equipment preparation, patient sedation and topicalization, technique, and the performance of bronchoalveolar lavage for the appropriate microbiologic sample.

KEYWORDS

Bronchoscopy; fibreoptic bronchoscopy; bronchoalveolar lavage.

INTRODUCTION

Rigid bronchoscopy has been in use for well over a century, but the more portable flexible bronchoscope is a relatively new invention and the video bronchoscope has only been available for 30 years.[1] As technology has allowed for increased miniaturization, further refinements have been made to the size and scope of the tool. Currently, we have a device with the capability to perform precise interventions on small areas, guided by world-class optics, which provides us the opportunity to evaluate and treat conditions of the airway with remarkable ease and precision.

Bronchoscopy remains the primary diagnostic and treatment modality of interventional pulmonology that is useful in assessing obstructing lesions, parenchymal diseases, and cellular pathology. The ease of use, manoeuvrability, and practicality provide for excellent visualization and sampling, and modern day instruments are safer and less traumatic to the soft tissues. Advances in imaging technology have allowed for miniaturization of components and smaller devices. This reduces the risk of

trauma and accidental injury to the airway structures and allows for greater portability of the device.

As a result of critical illness, surgery or systemic disease, patients often alter their respiratory pattern due to pain, weakness, or altered mental status, and may develop hypoxaemia or respiratory acid-base abnormalities. Inflammation associated with primary lung injury, infection, or other systemic process may also negatively affect the pulmonary system. Patients requiring mechanical ventilation are at greater risk of pneumonia and other pulmonary complications, and many of these may require advanced diagnostic and therapeutic interventions including bronchoscopic evaluations and bronchoalveolar lavages.

APPLIED ANATOMY/PHYSIOLOGY

In a patient with a natural airway, the entrance to the lungs is via the glottis, which includes the vocal cords. These structures provide a natural barrier to aspiration in most settings. The larynx connects this with the trachea, bounded by cartilaginous rings anteriorly and a membranous portion posteriorly and this provides a conduit into the true lungs. In patients intubated with either an endotracheal tube or tracheostomy, the glottis and larynx are bypassed.

The trachea divides into two primary bronchi at the carina, approximately 10–15 cm from the vocal cords, creating a functional separation point of the right from left lung. The airway at this region is approximately 15–25 mm in diameter, narrowing to 5–10 mm in diameter as we divide into the mainstem bronchi. Further division occurs rapidly, with the first several divisions of the airway being conductive, not participating in gas exchange. The conducting airways are responsible for maintaining a reservoir of air and sufficient luminal pressure to keep the structure and opening of the airway system intact. This is considered the anatomic dead space of the lungs, and normally accounts for about 30% of a normal breath or tidal volume.[2]

As the diameter of the airways shrink to about 5 mm and smaller, the wall thickness decreases sufficiently to allow for gas exchange across the surface and into the matched pulmonary capillaries, which provide deoxygenated blood high in carbon dioxide (CO_2). Proper gas exchange allows for the delivery of oxygenated blood to tissues and promotes a normal acid-base status through clearance of CO_2. Alveoli, the terminal segments of the pulmonary tree, are the thinnest and shortest airway structures, and it is here that most of the gas exchange takes place. It is fitting that their total surface area in orders of magnitude is greater than any of the previous segments, while the luminal diameter is often 0.5 mm or less at this point.

Gas exchange at the alveolar membrane occurs along a gradient of oxygen and CO_2, and is dependent upon airway patency, capillary blood flow, haemoglobin concentration, and oxygen binding capacity. Many conditions affect the transfer of gases and the loading and unloading of haemoglobin, such as critical illness, acidosis, temperature extremes, and haemoglobinopathies, as well as obstructive conditions that occur at the blood/lung interface such as pulmonary oedema, acute respiratory distress syndrome (ARDS), and chronic obstructive pulmonary disease. Pulmonary embolism causes occlusion of a segment of pulmonary blood flow, and increases pathologic dead space ventilation. Bronchoscopic evaluation and therapy may aid in the diagnosis and treatment of these intrapulmonary processes.

When performing bronchoscopy, it is reasonable to expect to be able to evaluate down to the 3rd or 4th division of the bronchus. This is still well within the conducting portion of the airways; therefore, we are unable to directly evaluate the alveoli with this technique. Given that many

of the problems seen on imaging or clinically that present the need for bronchoscopy are either global or confined to a discrete segment of the lung, we can usually perform focused regional evaluation without direct evaluation of the lower segments of the airway. Foreign material causing obstruction, source of haemorrhage and infection can be assessed from this position in the secondary or tertiary bronchi.

INDICATIONS FOR BRONCHOSCOPY

The indications for bronchoscopy have not changed significantly in the last 40 years. Some of the common indications are outlined in Table 60.1.

From a practical perspective, bronchoscopy is most often used to assess for airway patency in patients with gas exchange abnormalities, as well as to provide diagnostic and therapeutic intervention to those with abnormal findings on imaging or clinical exam, such as consolidation on chest X-ray or diminished breath sounds in someone with copious pulmonary secretions. Many pulmonary pathologies fit into these characteristic findings, and as such, you can feel justified in utilizing fibreoptic bronchoscopy to the limits of your abilities when confronted with focal areas of concern. Bronchoscopy is unlikely to help in cases of severe pulmonary oedema or inflammation, except in cases where a microbiological diagnosis needs to be made or when secretions are significant enough to cause obstruction.

CONTRAINDICATION

Perhaps the only true contraindication to performing diagnostic or therapeutic bronchoscopy is refusal of consent, either from the patient or their surrogate. Relative contraindications vary, depending on patient cooperation and presence of endotracheal tube, and the clinician's best

Table 60.1 Indications for bronchoscopy

Common indications for bronchoscopy	Additional ICU-specific indications
Chronic cough of unclear aetiology	Acute inhalational injury
Abnormal chest imaging	Assessment of airway oedema
Haemoptysis (blood in sputum)	Evaluation and clearance of pulmonary secretions
Unresolved pneumonia	Foreign body assessment
Diffuse chronic lung disease	Acute respiratory distress syndrome
Biopsy of mass lesion	

judgement should be used in the presence of an expert (Table 60.2).

While the potential exists for bronchoscopy to relieve some of these situations, such as hypoxaemia and obstruction, consideration should be given to whether the patient will tolerate the procedure without further optimization. In cases of recent severe cardiopulmonary injury, significant bleeding or raised intracranial pressure (ICP), it may be prudent to delay bronchoscopy in non-urgent situations. When patient condition can be stabilized, bronchoscopy can usually be performed safely; however, emergency equipment should be available in the event of cardiac arrest or decline in status might be provoked by procedural complications such as bleeding or pneumothorax.[3]

EQUIPMENT

The components of a flexible bronchoscope are fairly uniform and include a controls section, complete with insertion ports, camera switches, and levers to manipulate the distal end of the scope, as well as an insertion tube with enough length to navigate the distal airways and a hollow centre for suction and instrumentation. Optics are provided either by direct magnified visualization or through connection to a video monitor. Most commonly, the bronchoscope is powered by and transmits through a universal cord connected to a light source and video monitor, but some devices allow for portable battery power and visualization through direct viewing.

The bronchoscope is capable of three-dimensional steering through the use of internal mechanical components such as levers and wires, controlled at the base of the device that results in a tool that can be advanced or withdrawn as well as rotated 360 degrees and flexed/extended to between 90 and 180 degrees.

Table 60.2 Contraindications to bronchoscopy

Contraindications to bronchoscopy
Refusal of consent (absolute)
Diffuse coagulopathy (relative)
Moderate-to-severe hypoxaemia and/or hypercarbia (relative)
Recent myocardial infarction (relative)
Partially obstructing tracheal lesion (relative)
High PEEP on mechanical ventilation (>10 cm H$_2$O) (relative)
Elevated intracranial pressure (relative)
Morbidly obesity and/or sleep apnoea in the non-intubated patient (relative)

Internal channels allow for passage of smaller accessory instruments as well as for suctioning of secretions and samples. During bronchoscopy, additional equipment may be needed, including:

- Swivel adapter for the endotracheal tube
- Biopsy suction valves
- Sterile suction tubing
- Wall or portable suction device
- Sterile sample containers/suction traps (Lukens trap or similar equipment)
- Sterile basin
- Normal saline, or other non-bacteriostatic sterile fluid
- Lubricating jelly
- Cotton fluffs
- Sterile gown
- Sterile gloves
- Eye protection
- 4% lidocaine solution
- Bite block
- Sterile towels
- Full body drape

PRE-PROCEDURE PREPARATION

Assessment of the patient's underlying status should be a priority. Patients who are awake and do not require intubation may still need sedation and/or topicalization of the airway to tolerate the procedure, and care should be taken to ensure that they are appropriate candidates for this. Medical allergies should be confirmed as well as patient history. Nil per os (NPO; nothing by mouth) status of at least 6 hours for solid foods and 2 hours for liquids should be confirmed. Patient's informed consent should be obtained.

Many techniques exist for sedation and topical anaesthesia, including use of oral medications such as midazolam or diazepam, or intravenous sedation with ketamine, dexmedetomidine, or propofol.[4] Oral or intravenous opioids can be used as well, but they are more likely to depress respiratory drive and should be administered cautiously, especially when in conjunction with other sedating agents. Topicalization of the airway is best achieved with concentrated lidocaine nebulization of the supraglottic structures and carina using either an atomizer or the bronchoscope directly.[5,6] The posterior tongue and palate may also be topicalized if the gag reflex is pronounced. The provider should be aware of the cumulative dose of lidocaine and care should be taken to avoid crossing the threshold of 5 mg/kg (i.e., 300–350 mg in a 75 kg patient or approximately 7–9 cc of 4% solution).[6]

While the same techniques apply to patients on mechanical ventilation, they may also have the procedure performed without topicalization, although these patients may require more intravenous sedation. Regardless of the respiratory status, careful monitoring of vital signs should be in place to observe for changes in heart rate, blood pressure, and systemic oxygenation through the use of 3- or 6-lead electrocardiography (ECG), pulse oximetry, and noninvasive blood pressure (BP) monitoring at a minimum (Table 60.3).

TECHNIQUE

- Gather necessary tools, including fibreoptic bronchoscope, power source/cart, and disposable items (suction, basin, syringes, etc).
- A bedside nurse should be present to monitor patient vitals and assist with administration of medications and performance of procedure, if able.
- **Sedation/neuromuscular blockade**
  - For patients who are intubated, consider whether sedation can be used. Propofol, midazolam, and fentanyl are all reasonable choices for this patient population.
  - Chemical paralysis with rocuronium, vecuronium, or cisatracurium may allow for less patient interaction during the procedure; however, use of these agents can prolong the need for mechanical ventilation and potentially worsen myopathic syndromes.
- **Ventilator settings**
  - Place the patient on 100% oxygen if they are intubated and some form of high-flow oxygen support (nasal cannula, non-rebreather mask, etc.) if they are not.

Table 60.3 Pre-procedure setup

Precautions	Topicalization	Common sedating agents
3- or 6-lead ECG	Nebulized lidocaine, 1% or 2%	Diazepam (oral or IV)
Continuous oxygen source		Midazolam (oral or IV)
Blood pressure monitoring		Ketamine (oral or IV)
Audible pulse oximetry		Propofol (IV)
		Dexmedetomidine (IV)
		Fentanyl (IV)

- For patients on mechanical ventilation, the ventilator should be set to deliver volume control breaths as pressure control breathing may allow for hypoventilation during the procedure.
- For intubated patients who are spontaneously breathing and in whom chemical paralysis is not chosen, they may remain on a supportive mode of ventilation.
- Overall, mechanical ventilation will be less effective during the procedure and care should be taken to ensure adequate ventilation with the use of frequent procedural breaks.
- Assistance from respiratory therapist during the procedure is recommended, if available.
- **Topicalization**
  - Airway topicalization may be useful for patients who are not intubated and/or those who are easily stimulated during the procedure. This may manifest through coughing, agitation, and haemodynamic instability.

    Topicalization should be strongly considered in those patients where coughing or haemodynamic changes might not be well-tolerated (elevated intracranial pressure, unsecured vascular aneurysm or dissection, haemodynamic instability, etc.)
  - In the intubated patient, consider aerosolization of lidocaine (1–2%) at the carina and further down, should the patient exhibit these signs.
  - In the patient who is not intubated, topicalization of the oropharynx with viscous solutions of lidocaine, as well as aerosolization of the glottic aperture and the carina may help alleviate these symptoms.
  - Take note of and do not exceed the maximal dose of lidocaine (around 5 mg/kg or 300–350 mg total in a 75 kg patient).
- **Sterility of procedure**
  - The proceduralist should employ universal personal protective protocols including gloves, gown, and eye protection.[7]
  - For maintenance of procedure sterility and of gathered samples, it is recommended to use sterile suction tubing and syringes, saline, and sample collection tubes.
  - Use of sterile gown and gloves for the proceduralist and maintenance of sterile field and technique is recommended for quality of sample collected and prevention of contamination of the patient's respiratory tract with new pathogens.
- **Procedure**
  - Insert the fibre-optic bronchoscope through either the endotracheal tube (via introducer or the tube

directly), or the bite block airway. A small amount of lubricating jelly near the distal end of the scope may be helpful, with care being taken to avoid the camera end of the scope.

- In patients who are not intubated, the proceduralist will need to navigate past the tongue and supraglottic structures to visualize the vocal apparatus (epiglottis, arytenoids, and vocal cords may be seen). In patients with endotracheal tubes, the first structure seen as the scope leaves the tube should be the trachea.
- Upon entering the trachea, reorientation may be necessary depending on position of the proceduralist. It is important to remember that the anterior aspect of the trachea will have cartilaginous rings for support, whereas the posterior aspect will have tissue with a softer appearance.
- At the carina, approximately 20–25 cm from the scope insertion point, the trachea will divide into the right and left mainstem bronchi. The anterior position of the cartilaginous rings is maintained through the carina, but these become circumferential as the airway divides into the mainstem and smaller bronchi.
- The entrance of the left mainstem bronchus will allow for visualization of the left upper/superior and lower/inferior lobe bronchi.
- The entrance of the right mainstem bronchus will allow for visualization of the right upper/superior, middle, and lower/inferior lobe bronchi.
- Secretions or foreign material may be encountered at any point along the way, and suction may be used to remove these. For mass lesions or haemorrhagic lesions, it may be prudent to defer manipulation of these and consult an interventionalist.
- Pulmonary secretions can be thin or thick, and may be copious or strongly adherent to the bronchial wall. Infusion of sterile saline solution through the infusion port may aid in mobilization of mucous secretions to allow for removal via suction.
- Intermittent withdrawal of the scope may be necessary to clear the suction port or clean the camera.

- **Bronchoalveolar lavage**
  - Steps are recommended to ensure quality of the sample when a bacteriologic diagnosis is required.
  - Removal of proximal secretions, if copious, should be done prior to collecting the sample.
  - Position the distal tip of the bronchoscope at the entrance to a secondary bronchus or deeper, if able.

  - Lavage with 20–50 cc of normal saline and remove via syringe or external suction.
  - Attach sterile suction trap and repeat 20–50 cc lavage and suction, up to four times.
  - Remove sterile suction trap and seal for laboratory analysis.
  - If a specific segment of the pulmonary tree is suspected (i.e., right middle lobe), a sample should be taken from that side. One sample from the opposite lung should also be taken.
  - Ensure adequate airway patency, removing proximal obstructions as able. It is not necessary to clear all secretions from the pulmonary tree, as this may not be possible, and excessive suction should be avoided.

- Withdraw the bronchoscope, inspecting for evidence of trauma or new proximal obstruction.
- Verify endotracheal tube position if it is in place (should be approximately 4–6 cm above the carina).
- Clean the scope as per hospital and unit policy.

POST-PROCEDURE CARE

Continue regular monitoring of vital signs after the procedure. Patients who have been administered intravenous sedation should be carefully monitored until the sedative effects have clearly worn off. Patients receiving topical anaesthesia to the upper airway should be observed for return of airway reflexes. The ability to swallow and cough, as well as use of the vocal apparatus should be assessed.

If a chemical paralytic was used, continue mechanical ventilation and intravenous sedation until you have confirmed the absence of residual paralytic effect. Check neuromuscular train of four if possible, and consider pharmacological reversal of the paralytic agent if medically appropriate. Patients receiving chemical paralysis for bronchoscopy are likely to remain intubated for a longer period of time.

It is reasonable to defer acquiring a chest radiograph in the intensive care unit (ICU) patient following uneventful bronchoscopy, as the incidence of pneumothorax is very low.[8,9] Some reasons to consider post-procedural chest radiograph include:

- Copious secretions requiring frequent suctioning
- Possibility of trauma from excessive suctioning or tissue biopsy
- Clinical decompensation during or immediately after the procedure

Evaluation of improvement following therapeutic bronchoscopy (i.e., for proximal obstruction/collapsed lung segments).

COMPLICATIONS/PROBLEMS

Complications following bronchoscopy are typically minor, self-limiting, and are usually related to the underlying patient condition. Irritability of the pulmonary tree and vocal apparatus may result in bronchospasm or stridor and may need treatment. Nausea and vomiting or mild alteration in sensorium may be associated with administration of sedatives. Cardiac compromise may occur due to the stress of the procedure and the underlying condition and should be managed based on the needs of the patient.[6,8,10]

Hypoxaemia and hypoventilation from sedation and manipulation of the airways is common, and is usually addressed by titrating ventilator settings or by supporting the unintubated patient with increased inspired oxygen. Patients may ultimately require intubation or non-invasive positive pressure ventilation.

The production of pulmonary secretions may be increased following bronchoscopy. This may be due to increased production as part of the natural disease process or it may be due to mobilization from therapeutic bronchoscopy. Regardless, clearing of secretions may be necessary to maintain patency of the airway and care should be taken to ensure that this is adequate.

Elevations in intrathoracic and intracranial pressure should be anticipated during and possibly following fibreoptic bronchoscopy. Elevating the head of the bed and adequate topicalization and/or sedation and paralysis may minimize coughing and haemodynamic changes associated, and use of these measures should be strongly considered in patients for whom these changes would be a problem. With patients in whom the neurologic status is dynamic and those who require frequent neurologic checks, deep sedation should be avoided and fast-acting agents such as dexmedetomidine, remifentanil or propofol may be preferred over benzodiazepines.[10]

Airway bleeding is very rare following uncomplicated flexible bronchoscopy and is usually related to underlying coagulopathy or excessive suction. Care should be taken to avoid directly applying suction to the wall of the airway at any point for any extended period of time. Massive bleeding from biopsy of a lesion of iatrogenic complication may require surgical intervention and consult should not be delayed if the aetiology is in question. Pulmonary arteriography or computed tomography (CT) scan may help differentiate source.[8]

Pneumothorax following flexible bronchoscopy is rare, especially in the absence of tissue biopsy, and occurs in about 0.2% of cases.[8,9] It should be considered and ruled out when patients exhibit distress after the bronchoscopic procedure. The spectrum of presentation may vary, depending on the condition of the patient prior to the procedure and the presence of mechanical ventilation, which may cause smaller pneumothoraces to become large and create intrathoracic compromise.

Tension pneumothorax physiology can occur and the affected patient is likely to demonstrate classical physical exam signs and symptoms, including hypotension, tachycardia, decreased oxygen saturation, increased jugular venous distension, and absence of breath sounds on the affected side. Treatment may require urgent needle decompression and thoracostomy. Smaller pneumothoraces with no tension pathophysiology may be managed conservatively in patients without distress. The optimal time for a radiograph to rule out pneumothorax following bronchoscopy is between one and four hours post-procedure and can reasonably be deferred in patients without clinical symptoms.[9]

Breaks in sterile technique may be a source of secondary infection, as well as contamination of samples taken from the patient. Antibiotic stewardship may be impacted as the initial infectious source may be invalid and further contamination may delay recovery.

CONCLUSIONS

Fibreoptic bronchoscopy is an important part of intensive care management, especially in patients who require prolonged mechanical ventilation. It is important to have an understanding of the equipment preparation, patient sedation and topicalization, technique, and performance of bronchoalveolar lavage for appropriate sampling.

REFERENCES

1. Yarmus L, Feller-Kopman D. Bronchoscopes of the twenty-first century. *Clin Chest Med* 2010;31(1):19–Contents.
2. Levitzky M. *Pulmonary Physiology*. 8th ed. The Mcgraw-Hill Companies Inc. USA; 2013:1–264.
3. Ernst A. *Introduction to Bronchoscopy*. 1st ed. New York: Cambridge University Press; 2009:1–178.
4. José RJ, Shaefi S, Navani N. Sedation for flexible bronchoscopy: current and emerging evidence. *Eur Respir Rev* 2013;22(128):106–16.
5. Dreher M, Cornelissen CG, Reddemann MA, Müller A, Hübel C, Müller T. Nebulized versus standard local application of lidocaine during flexible bronchoscopy: a randomized controlled trial. *Respiration* 2016;92(4):266–73.
6. Tai DYH. Bronchoscopy in the intensive care unit (ICU). *Ann Acad Med Singapore* 1998; 27:552–9.

7. National Institutes of Health. Bronchoscopy assistance. critical care therapy and respiratory care section. July 2002:1–18. [Accessed 2018 Jan 13]. Available from: https://clinicalcenter.nih.gov/ccmd/cctrcs/cctrcs.html.

8. Pue CA, Pacht ER. Complications of fiberoptic bronchoscopy at a university hospital. *Chest* 1995 Feb;107(2):430–2.

9. Boskovic T, Stojanovic M, Stanic J, et al. Pneumothorax after transbronchial needle biopsy. *J Thorac Dis* 2014; 6(Suppl 4):S427–S434.

10. Stahl DL, Richard KM, Papadimos TJ. Complications of bronchoscopy: A concise synopsis. *Int J Crit Illn Inj Sci* 2015;5(3):189–95.

61

Intraparenchymal Intracranial Pressure Catheter Insertion

F. A. Rasulo, R. Bertuetti, and N. Latronico

ABSTRACT

This chapter briefly describes the placement of intraparenchymal intracranial pressure (ICP) monitoring catheter insertion. This is a procedure commonly performed in the neurointensive care unit (NICU). The various indications and precautions followed during the procedure are enumerated. The stepwise approach to perform this procedure has been discussed and accompanied by a video provided in the DVD.

KEYWORDS

Neurointensive care; intracranial pressure (ICP); monitoring; parenchymal catheter.

INTRODUCTION

Monitoring and treatment of intracranial pressure (ICP), also necessary for cerebral perfusion pressure (CPP) calculation, has been adopted into clinical practice not only for severe traumatic brain injury (TBI) management, but also for other types of brain injuries such as stroke and spontaneous intracerebral and aneurysmal subarachnoid haemorrhage since intracranial hypertension following acute brain injury is associated with poor outcome.[1–3] Since ICP measurement helps determine the interventions necessary to prevent secondary brain injury, guidelines recommending ICP monitoring for these forms of acute brain injury have been published.[3]

A variety of techniques can be used to monitor ICP including clinical examination, brain imaging, and both invasive and non-invasive techniques.[4] However the gold standard remains invasive monitoring by insertion of intracerebral catheters through cranial burr holes.

The most accurate invasive method for ICP monitoring is through insertion of a cerebral intraventricular catheter. However, this later is associated with a relatively high risk of catheter-related infection leading to meningitis. There are several advantages with intraparenchymal catheter insertion, such as the low infection rate associated with

this type of monitoring. Due to its low complication rate, intraparenchymal catheter insertion for ICP monitoring is being frequently applied by non-neuro-operators. Few recent studies have demonstrated that bedside insertion of an ICP monitor performed by intensive care physicians is a safe procedure with a complication rate comparable to other series published by neuro-operators.[5–9] The overall morbidity rate is comparable to or even lower than that caused by central vein catheterization.

PROCEDURE

Most cranial access kits are disposable and contain the basic items necessary during each step of the cranial access procedure.

Cranial Access Material

- Lidocaine (1%, 1:200,000 epinephrine)
- Syringe and 25-G needle
- Scalpel
- Periostium scraper
- Drill (hand operated or battery powered), plus a 2.7 mm drill bit with stop and wrench
- Mosquito forceps

- Adison forceps
- Suture scissors
- Suture

Drape

Sterile drapes should be placed to define the extent of the surgical field. The area where the incision will be performed is shaved, cleansed, and prepped with an iodine-based antiseptic solution.

Landmark for Incision and Bolt Insertion

It is preferable to perform the bolt screw insertion on the right side, since the motor cortex is usually found on the left. If the right side is not accessible, then the left side can be chosen. The landmark for the skin incision and bolt insertion is called the Kocher's point, and can be located in the following manner (see Figure 61.1): the point which is derived from the intersection of the mid-pupillary line (2–4 cm lateral to the midline) and a line which passes 2–3 cm anterior to the coronal suture. If it is not possible to palpate the coronal suture, its location can be estimated by following a line up midway between the lateral canthus and the external auditory meatus.

The operator should stand at the head end of the bed, which can be elevated as desired, and with the patient supine and facing forward. The head may be held in place either with tape running along the forehead or with two bed rolls positioned laterally. However, it may sometimes be necessary for an assistant to hold the head of the patient during the drilling.

Analgesia/Sedation

The patient should be sufficiently sedated in order to avoid further increases in ICP, however, effort should be made in trying to avoid excessive reductions in systemic blood pressure; for example, avoiding or treating hypovolaemia or scalp infiltration with local anaesthesia such as lidocaine (1%, 1:200,000 epinephrine) prior to incision and drilling.

Skin Incision and Skull Exposure

The skin incision should be performed antero-posteriorly for roughly 2–3 cm in length and should be deep enough to incise the subcutaneous tissues and reach the periosteum.

- Divaricate with the mosquito forceps in order to retract the skin and subcutaneous tissue.
- The skin should be retracted and the periosteum scraped off in order for the skull, corresponding to the Kocher's point to be exposed.

Alternatively, it is possible to perform an even smaller incision (1 cm) without divarication. Following incision, the tip of the scapula is used to scrape off a small amount of periosteum, followed by direct placement of the bit on the skull bone and trepanation. However, after drilling is performed, skill derived from experience is necessary in order to maintain access with the burr hole in order to insert the bolt screw (Figure 61.2).

Drilling Procedure

Select the appropriate drill bit. Use the 2.7 mm drill bit for subdural, epidural, and intraparenchymal bolt insertion procedures. Larger bits are usually necessary if double or triple bolts for multimodality monitoring are to be placed.

Place the drill bit into the vice and tighten by turning the chuck anticlockwise. This later can be further tightened or loosened by using the hex wrench. Once the appropriate skull depth is estimated and determined, slide the white guide towards the tip of the bit until this depth is reached.

The operator should be aware that several layers of soft and bony tissue must be crossed to reach the intracranial space. Going from superficial to deep, the layers are: the scalp (composed of the skin, connective tissue-dense, aponeurosis, and loose connective tissue), skull bone, dura mater, arachnoid, pia mater, and the brain.

When drilling, the hole should be irrigated with sterile saline in order to lubricate and avoid overheating of the drill area. The drilling procedure must be performed with the drill held in a perpendicular position to the skull so as to avoid damage to the bone caused by pressure strain fractures. When reaching a sufficient depth, the operator should be cautious while perforating the dura and avoid excessive introduction of the bit within the brain parenchyma. A small stylet or needle-like probe (usually included with the cranial access kit) should be used to verify if the dura is open. The stylet can be then used in order to clear the passage for the transducer-tipped catheter, which will later be placed through the bolt.

Bolt Screw Insertion

Following the drilling, the bolt is manually screwed into the skull bone to a depth corresponding to roughly 3–6 mm for the neonatal and paediatric age group and 5 mm to 1 cm for the adult age group (Figure 61.3). The bolt should be then filled with saline after checking for cerebrospinal fluid (CSF) leakage out of the bolt. It is also always worthy to note if CSF does leak, at what pressure.

Great care should be taken when applying sutures to catheters, and over-tightening of bolt screws could result in catheter occlusion, breakage, or skull bone damage.

Zeroing

The most commonly used ICP monitoring devices are provided with catheters that have the transducer at one extremity (must remain sterile), and the socket that is to be attached to the monitor itself at the other. Depending on the monitoring device, the zeroing is performed either by simply holding the transducer tip in air or in sterile saline solution until the zero reading appears on the monitor, after which the transducer is inserted inside the bolt and the screw tightened. The ICP value can then be read. Again, it is important to note the first ICP reading after the catheter is inserted. A few seconds may be necessary until this first value can be read with accuracy.

COMPLICATIONS

Although very rare, the most clinically relevant complications were infection, intracranial hemorrhage, and device failure.

Infection

The risk of infection is greater with external ventricular drains (EVDs) (5%–20%) than parenchymal monitors (0%–1%). The incidence may depend on definitions, i.e., contamination, colonization, or infection. The consequences of an infection, however, are greater with an EVD than parenchymal monitors.[10]

Cerebral Haemorrhage

The risk of intracranial haemorrhage (ICH) associated with parenchymal monitors is less than 2.5%. Patients who require an ICP monitor may have abnormal coagulation parameters. Insertion is justified in the presence of an international normalized ratio (INR) ≤1.6, and a platelet count >100,000.

Device Failure

Once inserted, except for the pneumatic Spiegelberg ICP parenchymal monitors, the device cannot be recalibrated. Technical complications, e.g., drift, breakage, or dislodgement, are observed with the use of intraparenchymal devices. Most occur during patient transport or when a patient is moved for nursing.

CONCLUSIONS

Monitoring ICP is a routine protocol in many NICU. It is important to understand the equipment as much as its use and care. Intensivists must be aware of all possible complications that can occur with the use of ICP monitoring devices.

REFERENCES

1. Karnchanapandh K. Effect of increased intracranial pressure on cerebral vasospasm in SAH. *Acta Neurochir Suppl* 2008;102:307–10.
2. Qureshi AI, Palesch YY, Martin R, et al. Effect of systolic blood pressure reduction on hematoma expansion, perihematomal edema, and 3-month outcome among patients with intracerebral hemorrhage: results from the antihypertensive treatment of acute cerebral hemorrhage study. *Arch Neurol* 2010 May;67(5):570–6.
3. Carney N, Totten MA, O'Reilly C, et al. Guidelines for the management of severe traumatic brain injury. 4th ed. Brain Trauma Foundation 2016. BTF 2016 Guidelines. [Accessed on 2016 Dec 19]. Available from: https://braintrauma.org/uploads/07/04/Guidelines_for_the_Management_of_Severe_Traumatic.97250__2_.pdf.
4. Rasulo FA, Bertuetti R, Robba C, et al. The accuracy of transcranial Doppler in excluding intracranial hypertension following acute brain injury: a multicenter prospective pilot study. *Crit Care* 2017 Feb 27;21(1):44.
5. Bochicchio M, Latronico N, Zappa S. Bedside burr hole for intracranial pressure monitoring performed by intensive care physicians. A 5-year experience. *Intensive Care Med* 1996;22:1070–4.
6. Harris CH, Smith RS, Helmer SD. Placement of intracranial pressure monitors by non-neurooperators. *Am Surg* 2002;68:787–90.
7. Ko KM, Conforti A. Training protocol for intracranial pressure monitor placement by non neurooperators: 5-year experience. *J Trauma Injury Infect Crit Care* 2003;55:480–3.
8. Latronico N, Marino R, Rasulo FA, Stefini R, Schembari M, Chandiani A. Bedside burr hole for intracranial pressure monitoring performed by anaesthetist intensive-care physicians: extending the practice to the entire team. *Minerva Anestesiol* 2003;69:159–68.
9. Stefini R, Rasulo FA. Intracranial pressure monitoring. *European Journal of Anaesthesiology* 2008 Feb;25:192–5.
10. Soavi L, Rosina M, Stefini R, et al. Post-neurosurgical meningitis: Management of cerebrospinal fluid drainage catheters influences the evolution of infection. *Surg Neurol Int* 2016 Dec 5;7(Suppl 39):S927–S934.

62

External Ventricular Drainage Systems

L. He, S. M. Weaver, and K. D. Weaver

ABSTRACT

External ventricular drainage systems are commonly placed for cerebrospinal fluid (CSF) diversion, can be life-saving interventions, and are now some of the most commonly performed neurosurgical procedures in the neurocritical care setting. These drains have both diagnostic and therapeutic functions and there are very few contraindications to their placement. In this chapter we discuss the relevant anatomy, indications, and contraindications for placement, procedural steps, post-procedural care, and complications associated with the drain and its management.

KEYWORDS

External ventricular drain (EVD); cerebrospinal fluid diversion (CSF); hydrocephalus; intracranial hypertension (ICH); intraventricular; Kocher's point; intracranial pressure (ICP).

INTRODUCTION

The placement of an external ventricular drain (EVD) or ventriculostomy is often a life-saving procedure performed in many neurosurgical clinical scenarios such as hydrocephalus and refractory intracranial hypertension (ICH) requiring cerebrospinal fluid (CSF) diversion. The procedure involves creating a small burr hole through the skull and then passing a silastic catheter into the frontal horn of the ventricle. The catheter is then connected to a closed CSF collection system. The greatest benefit of EVD placement over other forms of continuous CSF diversion (mainly lumbar drainage) is that it also allows for the accurate measurement of intracranial pressure (ICP).[1]

Initially described in the 1740s,[2] EVD placement is now one of the most commonly performed bedside neurosurgical procedures. It is usually performed by junior residents.[3,4] Its use, both as a diagnostic tool for ICP measurement and to improve outcomes in subarachnoid haemorrhage (SAH) and traumatic brain injury (TBI), is well documented.[5,6] The common indications for placement of EVDs are listed in Table 62.1.

Table 62.1 Indications for EVD placement

Hydrocephalus
• Subarachnoid haemorrhage
• Intraventricular haemorrhage
• Infection
• Cerebrospinal fluid obstruction (tumour, aqueductal stenosis, etc.)
Traumatic brain injury
Tension pneumocephalus
Cerebrospinal fluid rhinorrhoea/otorrhoea*

*In particular, those thought to be due to a large anterior skull base defect where there is concern that cerebrospinal fluid diversion via lumbar drain may precipitate pneumocephalus and neurologic sequelae.

ANATOMY

The cerebral ventricular system is a connected series of four cavities filled with CSF: right and left lateral ventricles; the third ventricle; and the fourth ventricle. Spinal fluid freely flows within this system and exits the fourth ventricle into the cisterna magna where it communicates with the cortical subarachnoid space, and also with the spinal canal.

The lateral ventricles are two mirror image C-shaped cavities deep within the cerebral hemispheres and are divided into the frontal horn, body, atrium, occipital (posterior) horn, and the temporal (inferior) horn.[7] The target of the distal catheter tip is most commonly the anterior horn of the lateral ventricle (Figure 62.1).

The most commonly used landmark for insertion of an EVD is Kocher's point (Figure 62.2), which is located 1–2 cm anterior to the coronal suture in the mid-pupillary line.[2,8]

This point is anterior enough to avoid the motor strip and lateral enough to avoid bridging lateral veins and the superior sagittal sinus. When passing the ventriculostomy catheter, the tip is aimed at the medial canthus in the medial-lateral plane and the tragus/external auditory canal (EAC) in the anterior–posterior plane. Cerebral spinal fluid is encountered at a depth of 5–7 cm from the scalp surface.

INDICATIONS AND CONTRAINDICATIONS

The indications for placement of an EVD are generally related to processes requiring CSF diversion and ICP monitoring (see again Table 62.1). Occasionally, intrathecal antibiotics may be required for cases of ventriculitis/cerebritis.[9,10] In cases of tension pneumocephalus, large anterior skull base defects or rhinorrhoea/otorrhoea requiring CSF diversion, external ventricular drainage is the preferred CSF diversion modality, as it is less likely to precipitate air entrainment with CSF drainage.

Absolute contraindications to EVD placement include frank coagulopathy with elevated international normalized ratio (INR), partial thromboplastin time (PTT) or thrombocytopenia; and overlying scalp infection. While there is a paucity of data regarding ideal coagulation levels prior to placement,[11] the general practice is to maintain an INR less than 1.7, platelet count above 100,000/uL and PTT less than 40 sec.

Relative contraindications to EVD placement include mass effect from subdural/epidural haemorrhage (concern that CSF diversion may worsen the mass effect) and recent use of antiplatelet/anticoagulant medications (should be appropriately reversed prior to EVD insertion). The authors recognize that in some situations, EVD placement is thought to be life-saving and that may proceed prior to full reversal of coagulopathy. In these scenarios, the risk of haemorrhage should be discussed.

EQUIPMENT

The majority of EVD placements occur emergently at the bedside. As such, several companies have developed cranial access kits that include all the necessary tools for EVD placement, which include hand twist drill with bit, scalpel, pickups, needle drivers, antiseptic agents, markers, rulers, and drape, in addition to the catheter and CSF collection system. Additional equipment suggested to be obtained prior to the procedure based on kit availability and personal preference, include local anaesthetics, sterile towels, and suture. The proceduralist will need sterile gown and gloves, and everyone in the room should have a mask and cap.

PRE-PROCEDURE PREPARATION

- Obtain routine laboratory samples for complete blood chemistry (CBC), INR, PTT.
- Obtain appropriate pre-procedural antibiotics.
- Obtain cranial access kit, EVD catheter, CSF collection bag, all sterile towels/drapes/gloves and masks and caps, sutures, antiseptic for skin preparation.
- Take pre-procedure timeout to verify consent, laboratory results, anticoagulation status, and need for blood products.
- Discuss the need for sedation (if not performed in the operating room [OR]).
- Review imaging to assess skull thickness, midline shift, and ventricular size.

TECHNIQUE

- Clip hair and mark the midline, then mark Kocher's point.
  - Prepare aseptic skin.
  - Place sterile draping with appropriate towels and drapes. Transparent drapes can assist with using landmarks for trajectory.
- Perform local infiltration to the incision site.
- Make a small 1–2 cm incision at Kocher's point to the depth of the scalp.
- Use the hand twist drill bit to drill through the skull to the dura [use the medial canthus and external auditory canal to guide trajectory]. The drill will encounter three layers: a harder outer table; the softer cancellous bone; and finally a harder inner cortical table.
- Fenestrate the dura appropriately with a needle and remove any bone ledges.
- Place the EVD 6–7 cm from the skin aiming medial to lateral at the medial canthus, and anterior to posterior at the EAC. This should place the tip of the

EVD catheter within the lateral ventricle and near the foramen of Monro.

- Once CSF is obtained, estimate the opening pressure using the length of the drain catheter as a manometer.
- Tunnel the EVD catheter out at a distal site. Suture the incision and EVD exit site and place additional staples or sutures as necessary to 'loop coil' the EVD to help minimize dislodging the catheter.
- Place a sterile adhesive dressing over insertion/exit sites.
- Change the dressing as per institutional protocol.
- Monitor for any leakage from the initial incision or EVD exit site. CSF leak increases risk of infection.
- Connect EVD to the CSF collection bag maintaining the sterile conditions.
- Zero the drain at the EAC, adjust the 'pop-off' pressure as appropriate, and connect to the patient monitor for ICP monitoring.

POST-PROCEDURE CARE

Immediately post-procedure, the nurse should adjust the ICP transducer of the CSF collection system at the level of the tragus/EAC. This sets the zero point for ICP monitoring at the foramen of Monro[12,13] From here, the responsible physician will select the appropriate pop-off pressure.

It should be noted that the ICPs on the patient monitor are reported in units of 'mmHg' while on the CSF drainage system, there is both 'mmHg' and 'cmH$_2$O' scales to designate the level of drainage. Institutional standard convention should be consistently used and clearly documented to avoid confusion.

From a nursing standpoint, every hour the ICP, CSF output, and also patient neurological status should be assessed.[14,15] Additionally, nurses should monitor for any changes in the neurological examination and/or any sustained ICPs greater than 20 mmHg for more than 5 minutes. As the patient's position changes (sitting, supine), the zero of the EVD system will also need to be adjusted as necessary. From a safety standpoint, the EVD should be clamped for all transport, changes in position prior to re-zeroing, working with physical therapy, imaging, or procedures.

The EVD cranial site dressing should also be monitored, changed according to institutional protocol, and generally kept sterile. Care should also be taken to monitor for any leakage of CSF or blood from the EVD tunnelled exit site or cranial burr hole site, as this can make ICP monitoring inaccurate and also predispose it to infection.

Depending on the institutional protocols, it is at the discretion of the physician managing the EVD as

to when appropriate venous thromboembolism (VTE) prophylaxis can be started. This is generally within 24 hours of EVD placement, if there are no concerns for haemorrhage.[16] For therapeutic anticoagulation, there are no clear guidelines about timing of anticoagulation and the risk–benefit ratio must be weighed judiciously against potential devastating haemorrhagic complication. There is a paucity of data to guide best practice determinations of when to start VTE prophylaxis or therapeutic anticoagulation.[11]

COMPLICATIONS

Obstruction of the catheter, preventing drainage of CSF, and/or dampened ICP waveforms is quite common. This is thought to be caused by cellular debris (blood clots or tissue). Additional structural failures (tube kinking, unintentional clamping), inadvertent EVD dislodgement or collapsed ventricles may also contribute to this phenomenon.[14] Briefly lowering the EVD to provoke spontaneous flow of CSF is often enough to ascertain whether the EVD tip is still within the ventricle. If a proximal EVD catheter obstruction is suspected, the general practice entails obtaining cranial imaging to ensure that the EVD tip has not migrated, and if stable, careful irrigation proximally and distally is often enough to dislodge any debris.[13] This manoeuvre should only be performed by a practitioner capable of replacing the catheter in the case of failure. If cranial imaging reveals dislodgement of the EVD from the ventricle, replacement is warranted.

The reported rates of infection associated with EVD placement range from 0%–22%.[12–14] Potential risk factors that have been associated with increased infection rate include: systemic infection; additional cranial injury; lack of EVD tunnelling; CSF leak; catheter irrigation; and frequency of CSF sampling.[11,12,14,17] Aside from peri-procedural administration of antibiotics, there is no evidence to support any additional benefit from scheduled antibiotics.[11] The use of antibiotics or silver impregnated ventriculostomy catheters shows mixed results in literature, with some studies reporting decreased rates of infection[18–20] while others show no difference,[21,22] likely due to study heterogeneity and varying definitions of CSF infection. There is a general consensus, though, that antibiotic impregnated catheters have a longer time to onset of positive CSF cultures.[11,18,21,22]

The incidence of haemorrhagic complications range from 5%–41%,[4,23,24] with the vast majority of them being asymptomatic.[11,23,24] With regard to VTE prophylaxis, two studies have shown that the use of prophylactic doses of subcutaneous heparin or enoxaparin did not increase the risk of symptomatic haemorrhage and reduced the risk of pulmonary embolism or deep vein thrombosis (DVT) significantly in patients with EVDs.[16,25] There is, unfortunately, no data to guide the initiation or restarting of full anticoagulation in the setting of a patient with an EVD.[11]

CONCLUSIONS

An EVD is one of the most common, life-saving procedures performed in cranial neurosurgery, not only for its ICP monitoring capabilities, but also for CSF diversion. Care should be taken to ensure aseptic technique and handling of the catheter, both during insertion and post-procedurally to minimize sequelae from infection. Although there are always risks associated with invasive procedures, appropriate risk–benefit assessment is prudent to ensure the safest outcome.

CONFLICTS OF INTEREST

The authors have no conflicts of interest.

FUNDING SOURCES

Departmental funds only.

REFERENCES

1. Lundberg N. Continuous recording and control of ventricular fluid pressure in neurosurgical practice. *Acta Psychiatr Scand Suppl* 1960;36(149):1–193.
2. Srinivasan VM, O'Neill BR, Jho D, Whiting DM, Oh MY. The history of external ventricular drainage. *J Neurosurg* 2013;120(1):228–36.
3. Sekula RF, Cohen DB, Patek PM, Jannetta PJ, Oh MY. Epidemiology of ventriculostomy in the United States from 1997 to 2001. *Br J Neurosurg* 2008;22(2):213–18.
4. Kakarla UK, Kim LJ, Chang SW, Theodore N, Spetzler RF. Safety and accuracy of bedside external ventricular drain placement. *Neurosurgery* 2008 Jul;63(Suppl 1):ONS162–166; discussion ONS166–7.
5. Kusske JA, Turner PT, Ojemann GA, Harris AB. Ventriculostomy for the treatment of acute hydrocephalus following subarachnoid hemorrhage. *J Neurosurg* 1973 May;38(5):591–5.
6. Narayan RK, Kishore PR, Becker DP, et al. Intracranial pressure: to monitor or not to monitor? A review of our experience with severe head injury. *J Neurosurg* 1982 May;56(5):650–9.
7. Gray, Henry. IX. Neurology. 4c. The Fore-brain or Prosencephalon. *Anatomy of the Human Body*. 1918.

[cited 2019 Jan 2]. Available at https://www.bartleby.com/107/189.html.
8. Mortazavi MM, Adeeb N, Griessenauer CJ, et al. The ventricular system of the brain: a comprehensive review of its history, anatomy, histology, embryology, and surgical considerations. *Childs Nerv Syst* 2014 Jan;30(1):19–35.
9. Remeš F, Tomáš R, Jindrák V, Vaniš V, Setlík M. Intraventricular and lumbar intrathecal administration of antibiotics in postneurosurgical patients with meningitis and/or ventriculitis in a serious clinical state. *J Neurosurg* 2013 Dec;119(6):1596–602.
10. Ng K, Mabasa VH, Chow I, Ensom MHH. Systematic review of efficacy, pharmacokinetics, and administration of intraventricular vancomycin in adults. *Neurocrit Care* 2014 Feb;20(1):158–71.
11. Fried HI, Nathan BR, Rowe AS, et al. The insertion and management of external ventricular drains: an evidence-based consensus statement: a statement for healthcare professionals from the Neurocritical Care Society. *Neurocrit Care* 2016 Feb;24(1):61–81.
12. Dey M, Jaffe J, Stadnik A, Awad IA. External ventricular drainage for intraventricular hemorrhage. *Curr Neurol Neurosci Rep* 2012 Feb;12(1):24–33.
13. Muralidharan R. External ventricular drains: Management and complications. *Surg Neurol Int* 2015 May 25;6 (Suppl 6):S271–4.
14. Woodward S, Addison C, Shah S, Brennan F, MacLeod A, Clements M. Benchmarking best practice for external ventricular drainage. *Br J Nurs* Mark Allen Publ. 2002 Jan 10;11(1):47–53.
15. Care of the patient undergoing intracranial pressure monitoring/external ventricular drainage or lumbar drainage. National Guideline Clearinghouse. [Internet] [cited 2016 Sep 9]. Available from: https://www.guideline.gov/summaries/summary/34438/care-of-the-patient-undergoing-intracranial-pressure-monitoringexternal-ventricular-drainage-or-lumbar-drainage.
16. Tanweer O, Boah A, Huang PP. Risks for hemorrhagic complications after placement of external ventricular drains with early chemical prophylaxis against venous thromboembolisms. *J Neurosurg* 2013 Aug 30;119(5): 1309–13.
17. Wong FWH. Cerebrospinal fluid collection: a comparison of different collection sites on the external ventricular drain. *Dynamics Pemb Ont* 2011;22(3):19–24.
18. Cui Z, Wang B, Zhong Z, et al. Impact of antibiotic- and silver-impregnated external ventricular drains on the risk of infections: A systematic review and meta-analysis. *Am J Infect Control* 2015 Jul 1;43(7):e23–32.
19. Root BK, Barrena BG, Mackenzie TA, Bauer DF. Antibiotic impregnated external ventricular drains: meta and cost analysis. *World Neurosurg* 2016 Feb;86:306–15.
20. Wang X, Dong Y, Qi X-Q, Li Y-M, Huang C-G, Hou L-J. Clinical review: Efficacy of antimicrobial-impregnated

catheters in external ventricular drainage—a systematic review and meta-analysis. *Crit Care Lond Engl* 2013; 17(4):234.

21. Mikhaylov Y, Wilson TJ, Rajajee V, et al. Efficacy of antibiotic-impregnated external ventricular drains in reducing ventriculostomy-associated infections. *J Clin Neurosci* 2014 May;21(5):765–8.

22. Shekhar H, Kalsi P, Dambatta S, Strachan R. Do antibiotic-impregnated external ventriculostomy catheters have a low infection rate in clinical practice? A retrospective cohort study. *Br J Neurosurg* 2016; 30(1):64–9.

23. Gardner PA, Engh J, Atteberry D, Moossy JJ. Hemorrhage rates after external ventricular drain placement. *J Neurosurg* 2009 Jan 16;110(5):1021–5.

24. Maniker AH, Vaynman AY, Karimi RJ, Sabit AO, Holland B. Hemorrhagic complications of external ventricular drainage. *Neurosurgery* 2006 Oct;59(4 Suppl 2):ONS419–424; discussion ONS424–425.

25. Zachariah J, Snyder KA, Graffeo CS, et al. Risk of ventriculostomy-associated hemorrhage in patients with aneurysmal subarachnoid hemorrhage treated with anticoagulant thromboprophylaxis. *Neurocrit Care* 2016 Feb;29:1–6.

63

Lumbar Drainage Systems

L. He, S. M. Weaver, and K. D. Weaver

ABSTRACT

Lumbar drainage systems are commonly used for cerebrospinal fluid (CSF) diversion in the absence of the need for direct intracranial pressure (ICP) monitoring. Placement is generally a safe and well-tolerated intervention with a host of indications in the otolaryngology, neurosurgery, and vascular surgery arenas. We will review relevant anatomy, indications, and contraindications for drain placement, procedural steps, along with post-procedural care and complication management/avoidance.

KEYWORDS

Lumbar drain (LD); cerebrospinal fluid diversion (CSF); hydrocephalus; intracranial pressure (ICP); rhinorrhoea; otorrhoea.

INTRODUCTION

Lumbar drain (LD) placement for cerebrospinal fluid (CSF) diversion has long been described in the otolaryngology, neurosurgery, and vascular surgery literature.[1-5] The procedure involves the placement of a silastic catheter into the subarachnoid space in the lumbar cistern via access through a large-bore Tuohy needle.[3,6] The common indications for LD placement are listed in Table 63.1.

Table 63.1 Common indications for lumbar drain placement in the neurosurgical population

Intracranial pressure control
• Infection
• Idiopathic
• Peri-operative
Cerebrospinal fluid fistula
• Peri-operative (spinal or cranial surgery)
Cerebrospinal fluid rhinorrhoea/otorrhoea*

*In cases of rhinorrhoea/otorrhoea thought to be due to a large anterior skull base defect (in particular, where there is concern that CSF diversion via lumbar drain may precipitate pneumocephalus and neurologic sequelae), supratentorial external ventricular drainage may be warranted.

ANATOMY

The lumbar approach to the subarachnoid CSF space is similar to that for lumbar punctures.[7] Midline spinous processes should be identified and carefully marked. Care should be taken in patients with larger body habitus as the natural crease in the back is not often overriding the actual bony midline. The orthogonal line drawn from the top of the iliac crest to the midline (intercristal line) generally marks the L3/4 interspinous space, although the exact level may vary with body habitus[8] (Figure 63.1). The subarachnoid space is safely accessed at the L3/4 or L4/5 interspaces.

Layers that will be traversed by the Tuohy needle from superficial to deep include: the epidermal and dermal skin layers; subcutaneous adipose; fascia/supraspinous ligament; interspinous ligament; ligamentum flavum; epidural space; dura and arachnoid mater; followed by the CSF-filled subarachnoid space (Figure 63.2). There are generally two points with more palpable resistance (the fascia and ligamentum flavum) prior to the 'pop' commonly reported once the subarachnoid space is entered. This is not to be confused with the 'loss of resistance' commonly used for directing access to the epidural space.

Given that a silastic catheter will be left in place for CSF diversion, the median and paramedian approaches avoiding the interspinous ligament and midline interspinous process are often favoured to prevent kinking or shearing of the catheter after placement.

INDICATIONS AND CONTRAINDICATIONS

The common indications for LD placement versus other methods (mainly ventriculostomy) arise when there is need for CSF diversion without an absolute need for direct intracranial pressure (ICP) monitoring. As such, LDs have since long been described in the treatment of spontaneous or acquired CSF fistulas (postoperative or traumatic), treatment of CSF rhinorrhoea or otorrhoea, perioperative CSF diversion for ICP management, and CSF diversion in the diagnosis or treatment of idiopathic intracranial hypertension (IH) or normal pressure hydrocephalus.[2–5,9] Vascular surgeons have also used LDs in an effort to decrease risk of paraplegia secondary to spinal cord ischaemia after thoraco-abdominal aortic aneurysm repair, although its exact efficacy is debated.[1,10]

Absolute contraindications to the placement of a LD include: non-communicating hydrocephalus (e.g., posterior fossa masses, aqueductal stenosis, trapped ventricle, and intraventricular haemorrhage) given the concern for potential herniation of the infratentorial space without diversion of supratentorial CSF fluid; and large supratentorial space-occupying lesions (e.g., tumour, subdural haematoma, epidural haematoma) where CSF diversion inferiorly may worsen shift of intracranial contents and increase the risk of herniation. In these patients, intracranial supratentorial diversion via ventriculostomy may be a better choice.

Caution prior to LD placement should also be taken in patients with frank coagulopathy, including elevated international normalized ratio (INR), elevated partial thromboplastin time (PTT), use of non-reversible direct thrombin inhibitor anticoagulants, and/or thrombocytopenia. The use of antiplatelet agents is a relative contraindication and often transfusion of platelets is done just prior to the procedure. Absolute risk of haemorrhagic complication (subdural or epidural haematoma, retroperitoneal haematoma, etc.) is poorly quantified in literature, but is estimated to be approximately 3%.[1,9]

Other relative contraindications to bedside LD placement include: spinal curvature abnormalities from either scoliosis, prior surgery, or significant degenerative spine disease; and obesity.[11,12] In these patients, normal anatomical landmarks may be difficult to palpate or are significantly distorted. Placement of the Tuohy needle into the CSF space may be easily achieved using imaging guidance in these situations.[12–14]

EQUIPMENT

Most LD kits commonly include a 14- or 16-gauge Tuohy needle, a lumbar catheter, connector cap for the CSF collection system, and various forms of anchoring devices to prevent accidental removal. Differences that can be found in these kits include: variable lengths or diameters of the Tuohy needle; inner guide wire; and radio-opacity of the catheter. In addition to the LD kit, a CSF collection system will need to be obtained. In many hospitals this is the same CSF collection system used for the ventriculostomy systems which is used to measure ICPs as well, and creates a closed sterile system for collection.

Additional necessary equipment include sterile towels; drapes; gloves for the proceduralist; mask and cap for individuals helping with the procedure; and local anaesthesia should also be at the bedside. Non-absorbable suture is suggested for securing the LD after placement to prevent inadvertent dislodgement.

PRE-PROCEDURE PREPARATION

- Obtain routine laboratory parameters including complete blood chemistry (CBC), INR, PTT and assess anticoagulation status.
- Obtain appropriate pre-procedural antibiotics.
- Obtain LD kit, CSF collection bag, all sterile towels/ drapes/gloves/masks/hats, and sutures.
- Pre-procedure timeout should be performed to verify consent, laboratory results, anticoagulation status, and need for blood products.
- Depending on the patient's mental status and tolerability, discussion with a sedation provider may be necessary.

TECHNIQUE

- The patient should lie in the lateral decubitus position with as much hip flexion as possible to open the interlaminar space.
- The midline based on the spinous processes should be marked, along with the intersection of the intercristal line and midline.
- The skin should be prepped by institutional standards.
- Local anaesthetic should be administered along the entire tract that the Tuohy needle will traverse, with additional subcutaneous injections at the planned securement.

- Using either a median or paramedian approach, gradually insert the Tuohy needle through the skin and fascial layer.
- At the location of the laminar bone, small adjustments to the trajectory may need to be performed to find the interlaminar space and pierce the ligamentum flavum.
- Advance the Tuohy needle slowly until there is loss of resistance through the ligamentum; some describe subsequent entry into the subarachnoid space as a 'pop'-like sensation. Frequently remove the inner stylet to check for CSF flow.
- Measure the opening pressure using a standard sterile manometer.
- Direct the bevel cranially or caudally to facilitate threading of the LD in parallel with the subarachnoid space.
- A gentle twirling motion of the catheter can be utilized to advance within the space. If resistance is met, attempt to subtly change the direction of the Tuohy or the angle of the bevel.
- Never pull the catheter out of the Tuohy once it has been advanced past the needle tip, given the risk of shearing off a portion of the catheter.
  - Removal of both the catheter and needle should be performed together.
  - Prior knowledge of the Tuohy needle's length is prudent, as this can be compared to the length of the catheter advanced (most Tuohy needles and lumbar catheters have length markers measured in centimetres).
- After the catheter has been passed into the thecal space, continue to pass it until at least 15 cm from the skin to prevent migration into the epidural space.
- Carefully remove the Tuohy needle over the LD catheter.
- Connect the LD catheter to the cap and secure it in place to prevent dislodgement.
  - Insert a purse string stitch at the exit site to prevent CSF leak.
  - Placing a strain relief loop, kept in place with non-absorbable suture, is also common practice.
- Use a clear adhesive dressing without any gel or antibiotic impregnation to cover the catheter insertion site.
- Connect to the CSF collection system.

POST-PROCEDURE CARE

Management of the LD catheter involves a goal volume of CSF to be diverted per hour, generally 5–15 ml/hr. Two commonly used techniques for LD management include: (1) leaving the drain open with careful adjustment of the patient bed or LD to obtain gradual CSF drainage that amounts to the goal volume per hour; or (2) initial adjustment of the patient or LD height to quickly drain the goal for the hour, then leaving the LD clamped for the remainder of the hour. Patients should be reminded that they should avoid any abrupt changes in position of their head relative to the lumbar spine to avoid inadvertent dumping of CSF with changes in position. Furthermore, patients, nurses, and family members should take care to avoid having the LD catheter and CSF collection tubing become snagged or caught on barriers, which could lead to inadvertent disconnection. Bedside nursing staff should be trained to troubleshoot the drain, such as when CSF output slows or stops draining (look for kinks and tubing clamps). They should also be aware that no ICP is transduced and that LD management is based upon hourly CSF goals. Neurological examination should be performed routinely per unit protocol. Physicians should be notified immediately if any of the following are noted: CSF leakage; disconnected tubing; altered mental status; cranial neuropathy; and/or weakness/sensory changes—the latter being signs that there has been under- or over-drainage of CSF, in addition to other more ominous post-procedural complications, such as ICH.

COMPLICATIONS

Minor complications are reported to be as high as 59%, and include: low pressure or spinal headache; nausea/vomiting; and spinal nerve root irritation.[9,15] Fluid resuscitation, analgesia, and symptom management are generally enough to alleviate these symptoms. Occasionally, a temporary hiatus from CSF drainage or decreased volume per hour may be necessary.

Major complications have an incidence of 3%–12%, and include: cranial nerve palsy; downward transtentorial herniation; subdural haematoma; tension pneumocephalus; and spinal cord compression.[9,15–19] Acute management includes immediate clamping of the LD. Significant mental status changes may necessitate intubation for airway protection. Positioning the patient flat or in slight Trendelenberg position have been reported to improve the CSF's buoyant effect on the brain.[16,18] Serial imaging may be warranted to monitor for appropriate improvement.

In cases where anterior skull base defects (traumatic or acquired via surgery) are present and a LD is placed for treatment of CSF rhinorrhoea, it is prudent to avoid application of positive pressure via bag mask, bi-level positive airway pressure (BiPAP), or continuous positive airway pressure (CPAP), as this can cause, exacerbate, or worsen pneumocephalus. In the case of tension pneumocephalus, immediate intubation is commonly employed.[15] In extreme scenarios, emergent craniotomy or ventriculostomy placement may be necessary to relieve the compressive effect of the pneumocephalus.

Infectious complications from LD have been reported in the 1.7%–5% range.[9,19] Common pathogens include common skin flora and usually present with signs and symptoms of meningitis within 24 hours of LD placement. Appropriate sterile technique and pre-procedure antibiotics should be sufficient for protection against infectious complication, and concomitant prophylactic antibiotic administration is not warranted.[19]

Additional minor complications include LD system disconnection if the tubing or catheter should become stretched or sheared. In these scenarios, immediately clamping the most proximal port of the catheter to prevent uncontrolled loss of CSF is mandatory. Following this, a decision will have to be made about removal of the LD system versus replacement with a new sterile system. Although rare, there is a risk of internal shearing of the catheter. Such cases require urgent imaging, as well as possible surgical exploration, for localization and removal of the distal catheter tip, as migration deep into the ligamentum flavum is possible.

The use of automated, programmable, gravity-driven CSF drainage monitoring systems is becoming more commonplace in both the neurosurgical and vascular surgery populations.[20–21] These have the potential to remove traditional disadvantages such as over-drainage as well as the need for continuous repositioning/levelling to set reference points.

CONCLUSIONS

Lumbar drainage is in general a safe and well-tolerated procedure for CSF diversion that can be used to treat a variety of pathologies. Adequate training on the management of CSF output volume, troubleshooting of the device, as well as the need for routine neurological examination is warranted. Neurological decline may be a sign of CSF over-drainage, which can be a harbinger of a potentially serious complication.

CONFLICTS OF INTEREST

The authors have no conflicts of interest.

FUNDING SOURCES

Departmental funds only.

REFERENCES

1. Weaver KD, Wiseman DB, Farber M, Ewend MG, Marston W, Keagy BA. Complications of lumbar drainage after thoracoabdominal aortic aneurysm repair. *J Vasc Surg* 2001 Oct;34(4):623–7.

2. McCallum J, Maroon JC, Jannetta PJ. Treatment of postoperative cerebrospinal fluid fistulas by subarachnoid drainage. *J Neurosurg* 1975 Apr;42(4):434–7.

3. Hood RS, Boyd HR. Technique for intraoperative cerebrospinal fluid drainage. *J Neurosurg* 1975 Feb; 42(2):239.

4. Findler G, Sahar A, Beller AJ. Continuous lumbar drainage of cerebrospinal fluid in neurosurgical patients. *Surg Neurol* 1977 Dec;8(6):455–7.

5. Kitchel SH, Eismont FJ, Green BA. Closed subarachnoid drainage for management of cerebrospinal fluid leakage after an operation on the spine. *J Bone Joint Surg Am* 1989 Aug;71(7):984–7.

6. Post KD, Stein BM. Technique for spinal drainage. *Neurosurgery* 1979 Mar;4(3):255.

7. Sakula A. A hundred years of lumbar puncture: 1891–1991. J R Coll Physicians Lond. 1991 Apr;25(2):171–5.

8. Margarido CB, Mikhael R, Arzola C, Balki M, Carvalho JCA. The intercristal line determined by palpation is not a reliable anatomical landmark for neuraxial anesthesia. *Can J Anaesth* 2011 Mar;58(3):262–6.

9. Governale LS, Fein N, Logsdon J, Black PM. Techniques and complications of external lumbar drainage for normal pressure hydrocephalus. *Neurosurgery* 2008 Oct;63(4) (Suppl 2):379–84; discussion 384.

10. Coselli JS, LeMaire SA, Schmittling ZC, Köksoy C. Cerebrospinal fluid drainage in thoracoabdominal aortic surgery. *Semin Vasc Surg* 2000 Dec;13(4):308–14.

11. Boddu SR, Corey A, Peterson R, et al. Fluoroscopic-guided lumbar puncture: fluoroscopic time and implications of body mass index—a baseline study. *Am J Neuroradiol* 2014 Aug 1;35(8):1475–80.

12. Chee CG, Lee GY, Lee JW, Lee E, Kang HS. Fluoroscopy-guided lumbar drainage of cerebrospinal fluid for patients in whom a blind bedside approach is difficult. *Korean J Radiol* 2015;16(4):860–5.

13. Stiffler KA, Jwayyed S, Wilber ST, Robinson A. The use of ultrasound to identify pertinent landmarks for lumbar puncture. *Am J Emerg Med* 2007 Mar;25(3):331–4.

14. Gold MM, Miller TS, Farinhas JM, Altschul DJ, Bello JA, Brook AL. Computed tomography–guided lumbar drain placement. *J Neurosurg Spine* 2008 Sep 24;9(4):372–3.

15. Roland PS, Marple BF, Meyerhoff WL, Mickey B. Complications of lumbar spinal fluid drainage. *Otolaryngol Head Neck Surg* 1992 Oct;107(4):564–9.

16. Bloch J, Regli L. Brain stem and cerebellar dysfunction after lumbar spinal fluid drainage: case report. *J Neurol Neurosurg Psychiatry* 2003 Jul;74(7):992–4.

17. Açikbaş SC, Akyüz M, Kazan S, Tuncer R. Complications of closed continuous lumbar drainage of cerebrospinal fluid. *Acta Neurochir (Wien)* 2002;144(5):475–80.

18. Graf CJ, Gross CE, Beck DW. Complications of spinal drainage in the management of cerebrospinal fluid fistula. *J Neurosurg* 1981 Mar;54(3):392–5.

19. Coplin W, Avellino A, Kim D, Winn H, Grady M. Bacterial meningitis associated with lumbar drains: a retrospective cohort study. *J Neurol Neurosurg Psychiatry* 1999 Oct;67(4):468–73.

20. Linsler S, Schmidtke M, Steudel WI, et al. Automated intracranial pressure-controlled cerebrospinal fluid external drainage with LiquoGuard. *Acta Neurochir* 2013;155(8): 1589–95.

21. Leopardi M, Tshomba Y, Kahlberg A, et al. Automated lumbar drainage for the control of the cerebrospinal fluid pressure during surgery for thoracoabdominal aortic aneurysms. *Annals Vasc Surg* 2015;29(6):1050.

64

Subdural Evacuating Port System (SEPS) Placement for Chronic Subdural Haematoma Evacuation

M. Miles and H. Bow

ABSTRACT

Drilling a cranial burr hole and attaching a suction drain is a commonly performed procedure in the neurological and neurointensive care unit (NICU) for the evacuation of chronic subdural haematomas. This bedside procedure is performed to evacuate the liquid haematoma. This chapter discusses the stepwise technique of performing this procedure. The various clinical indications, management, and complications are also discussed.

KEYWORDS

Subdural haemorrhage; bedside evacuation; haematoma; neurointensive care unit (NICU); burr hole; raised intracranial pressure (ICP); technique; complications; neurointensive care.

INTRODUCTION

A chronic subdural haematoma is a collection of haemolysed blood between the brain and the dura. Due to its mass effect on the brain and cortical irritation, it is associated with seizures, decreased mental status, and potentially death.[1,2] Specifically, chronic subdural haematomas are associated with a 13% risk of death and a 20% risk of poor outcomes.[1] Chronic subdural haematomas are frequently encountered in the elderly population, secondary to falls or other trauma that occurred in the recent past. Due to the growing population of the elderly, chronic subdural haematomas are increasing in incidence and may become the most common neurosurgical condition in the near future.[3]

Significant predictors of death include age, admission Glasgow Coma Scale (GCS), and hospital length of stay (LOS) (P<0.05). The length of stay in the intensive care unit (ICU) was inversely correlated with disposition (P<0.01). Furthermore, ICU and hospital LOS were significant predictors of treatment cost (P<0.05).

Several methods exist for evacuating chronic subdural haematomas. One method involves placing the patient under general anaesthesia and drilling burr holes to drain the haematoma. Another method also involves placing the patient under general anaesthesia but involves temporarily removing a portion of the skull to evacuate the haematoma. The method of using burr holes has been found to improve outcomes.[4] However, the risks of general anaesthesia increase the risks of this procedure. In this chapter, we discuss a variant of burr holes that can be performed under conscious sedation at the bedside. The procedure involves use of the subdural evacuating port system (SEPS).

Placement of SEPS is advantageous in several ways: it can help to reduce hospital length of stay, allow faster treatment, and reduce overall cost to the patient while maintaining equal efficacy as burr hole placement.[5] SEPS placement is commonly done in the ICU under conscious sedation, obviating the risks of general anaesthesia. The SEPS applies suction to the subdural space. It does not involve any object entering this space, such as a catheter. It also does not involve irrigation.

The disadvantages of the SEPS procedure include a trend towards slightly higher failure rates in some studies.[6] If the SEPS procedure requires general anaesthesia, the advantage of reduction in length of stay is diminished.[7]

APPLIED ANATOMY AND PHYSIOLOGY

A subdural haematoma is a collection of blood between the dura and arachnoid, and can usually be classified as acute, subacute, and chronic. Acute subdural haematoma usually occurs after significant trauma and is generally associated with other injuries. Chronic subdural haematoma, on the other hand, is commonly seen in the elderly, and is associated with insignificant to no trauma. The peak incidence is observed around 70–85 years.[8] These subdural haematomas occur secondary to damaged bridging veins between the dura and arachnoid, which then cause bleeding into the subdural space.[9]

Adhiyaman et al. outlined the common presentation of chronic subdural haematomas as altered mental status, neurologic deficit, headache, unsteadiness resulting in falls, and seizures.[9]

INDICATIONS

After a chronic subdural haematoma (Figure 64.1) is diagnosed it is appropriate to pursue definitive treatment if the patient is symptomatic. Conservative management is an option available as well to those patients who have mild symptoms or for whom operative risks are high.[8]

CONTRAINDICATIONS

The SEPS system should be used to treat acute subdural haematoma or if the patient is on anticoagulation therapy that has not been reversed.

EQUIPMENT

- SEPS kit
- Lidocaine 1% or 2%
- Sterile towels
- Chlorhexidine gluconate skin preparation

PRE-PROCEDURE PREPARATION

First, as for any procedure, informed consent should be obtained. Risks such as bleeding, infection, and damage to surrounding structures as well as more specific risks related to this procedure should be outlined. Please see the 'Complications' section for further detail.

A computed tomography (CT) scan should be completed before beginning the procedure to determine where to begin the approach. Of note, hypodense subdural collections are more amenable to the SEPS drain compared to collections with mixed density.[10]

Monitors should be applied and the nurse or other assisting staff should monitor the patient's vital signs.

TECHNIQUE

- Shave the area for the procedure.
- Determine the area for incision and burr hole based on pre-procedure CT scans. Mark the location with marking pen.
- As per institutional protocol, the chosen site should be prepared and draped in a sterile manner.
- Infiltrate the skin and deeper tissues with local anaesthetic agent.
- Make a 5 mm linear incision on the marked spot down to the level of the periosteum.
- Attach the safety stop collar to the drill. The stop can be adjusted by the user by loosening the set crews, moving the stop to the correct position and re-tightening the screws. The hex wrench needed to do this is provided in the kit.
- In the standard manner, create a hole through the skull with the twist drill.
- Incise the dura with a spinal needle. At this time, a fluid with the colour and consistency of motor oil should exit from the burr hole site.
- Insert the metal evacuating port by twisting it into place in the drilled hole. The port should not stick below the level of the inner table of the skull.
- Apply the suction tubing and suction bulb to the port.
- Close the wound around the port and apply a sterile dressing.

POST-PROCEDURE CARE

A head CT can be obtained on postoperative day 1 to evaluate the success of the procedure and whether any complications have occurred. If the evacuation was successful, the SEPS system can be removed. Magnetic resonance imaging (MRI) is contraindicated due to the metal in the SEPS system. The patient should be monitored continuously, ideally in the ICU, for any changes in neurological status.

COMPLICATIONS

As with any procedure there is risk of bleeding, infection, reaction to materials used, or damage to the surrounding structures. Further complications include seizures, pneumocephalus, stroke, occlusion of the system by various biological materials and even death.[11] These should all be discussed with the patient or with their appropriate surrogate.

With this procedure there is a risk that the SEPS may not evacuate the subdural haematoma adequately. Some studies have shown subdural collections that present as mixed density have a higher rate of failure and may require further intervention than those that present as hypodense collections.[10] However, other studies have shown the rate of re-intervention to be very similar between SEPS and burr hole placement.[7]

If the SEPS port becomes occluded and if further drainage is needed, needle aspiration may be required. Please see the Medtronic SEPS Cranial Access Kit manual for this procedure.[11] If the port fails and aspiration either fails or is not an option, the patient may need to undergo burr hole or craniotomy for definitive treatment.[11]

In some studies the SEPS device has not been as successful as an open burr hole procedure. However benefits of the SEPS system include a faster time to procedure, lower cost of stay, and shorter length of stay.[6] Other studies have shown equal efficacy and safety in subdural haematoma evacuation.[7] However, not all studies have supported these advantages,[12] therefore both advantages and risks of the bedside procedure should be weighed against the traditional open procedure. The ability to avoid a trip to the operating room and avoid general anaesthesia could be a great advantage for the tenuous patient or one with significant co-morbidities.

CONCLUSIONS

Chronic subdural haematomas are associated with poor outcomes and even death. The placement of a drain at the bedside called the Medtronic SEPS can relieve these lesions and help improve outcomes while avoiding the dangers of the operating room and general anaesthesia.

CONFLICTS OF INTEREST

None.

REFERENCES

1. Frontera JA, de los Reyes K, Gordon E, et al. Trend in outcome and financial impact of subdural hemorrhage. *Neurocrit Care* 2011;14(2):260–6.
2. Ivan ME, Nathan JK, Manley GT, Huang MC. Placement of a subdural evacuating port system for management of iatrogenic hyperacute subdural hemorrhage following intracranial monitor placement. *J Clin Neurosci* 2013; 20(12):1767–70.
3. Kudo H, Kuwamura K, Izawa I, Sawa H, Tamaki N. Chronic subdural hematoma in elderly people: present status on Awaji Island and epidemiological prospect. *Neurol Med Chir (Tokyo)* 1992;32(4):207–9.
4. Borger V, Vatter H, Oszvald Á, Marquardt G, Seifert V, Güresir E. Chronic subdural haematoma in elderly patients: a retrospective analysis of 322 patients between the ages of 65–94 years. *Acta Neurochir (Wien)* 2012;154(9):1549–54.
5. Balser D, Rodgers SD, Johnson B, Huang JH, Tabak E, Samadani U. A cost analysis of bedside subdural evacuating port system (SEPS) versus burr holes for the treatment of chronic subdural hematoma. Preprint. 2010.
6. Balser D, Rodgers SD, Johnson B, Shi C, Tabak E, Samadani U. Evolving management of symptomatic chronic subdural hematoma: experience of a single institution and review of the literature. *Neurol Res* 2013;35(3):233–42.
7. Rughani AI, Lin C, Dumont TM, Penar PL, Horgan MA, Tranmer BI. A case-comparison study of the subdural evacuating port system in treating chronic subdural hematomas. *J Neurosurg* 2010;113(3):609–14.
8. Santarius T, Kirkpatrick PJ, Kolias AG, Hutchinson PJ. Working toward rational and evidence-based treatment of chronic subdural hematoma. *Clin Neurosurg* 2010;57:112–22.
9. Adhiyaman V, Asghar M, Ganeshram KN, Bhowmick BK. Chronic subdural haematoma in the elderly. *Postgrad Med J* 2002;78(916):71–5.
10. Kenning TJ, Dalfino JC, German JW, Drazin D, Adamo MA. Analysis of the subdural evacuating port system for the treatment of subacute and chronic subdural hematomas. *J Neurosurg* 2010;113(5):1004–10.
11. Medtronic. Medtronic subdural evacuating port system cranial access kit. 2001. Available from: http://manuals.medtronic.com/content/dam/emanuals/st/18912COM-1D.pdf
12. Safain M, Roguski M, Antoniou A, Schirmer CM, Malek AM, Riesenburger R. A single center's experience with the bedside subdural evacuating port system: a useful alternative to traditional methods for chronic subdural hematoma evacuation. *J Neurosurg* 2013;118(3):694–700.

65

Percutaneous Tracheostomy

N. N. Saied

ABSTRACT

Tracheostomy is a long-term airway often required by few critically ill patients. Percutaneous insertion of tracheostomy tubes has become the method of choice and compares favourably to open tracheostomy in the intensive care setting. Many techniques have been developed as well as many commercially available kits are available in the market. Percutaneous dilatational tracheostomy (PDT) is a very safe and effective method if proper patient selection, preparation, and training is exercised. In addition, it is a cost-effective and time-saving technique.

KEYWORDS

Percutaneous; tracheostomy; respiratory failure; complication; techniques.

INTRODUCTION

Patients with neurological diseases, compared to other critically ill patients, may suffer even more from impaired swallowing, airway reflexes, and lose the ability to maintain a patent airway. Tracheostomy tubes offer an easier access to the airway, facilitate needed respiratory care, and provide some protection against aspiration.[1–5] The chapter focuses on indication, contraindication, and the various percutaneous techniques of insertion of tracheostomy tubes. In addition, it compares open surgical techniques of similar procedures and their short- and long-term complications.

APPLIED ANATOMY AND PHYSIOLOGY

Percutaneous dilatational tracheostomy (PDT) is performed at the level of 2nd to 4th tracheal ring. Landmarks of the location include, thyroid cartilage, cricoid cartilage (1st tracheal ring) and the cricothyroid membrane. While only skin and subcutaneous tissue overlay the cricothyroid membrane, the thyroid isthmus bridges over the upper few tracheal rings. Of note, the anterior jugular veins form at the level of the hyoid bone and descend paramedially on both sides to empty into the external jugular veins. A communicating vein is usually present at the suprasternal notch but may vary (Figure 65.1).

INDICATIONS AND CONTRAINDICATIONS

While PDT is becoming the default choice (gold standard) for performing tracheostomy in critically ill patients, few exceptions may require surgical tracheostomy. Table 65.1 outlines a shrinking list of contraindications to PDT. Relative contraindications are numerous and likely to depend on operator skills, experience, and knowledge of a specific technique. Antiplatelet therapy is not a

Table 65.1 Absolute and relative contraindications to percutaneous dilatational tracheostomy

Absolute	Relative
• Anatomic abnormalities	• Previous neck surgery or radiation
• Severe coagulopathy	• Morbid obesity, short neck
• Cervical spine instability	• Thyroid hyperplasia, neoplasm
• Infection at insertion site	• Tracheal disease or surgery
	• High ventilatory support requirement

contraindication to PDT and it is safe to perform the procedure without stopping it, especially if there is a strong indication for their continued use.

Timing

In general most patients who will require mechanical ventilation beyond 10–14 days are considered candidates for tracheostomy. The proposed benefits of tracheostomy over endotracheal tubes (ETT) are reduced sedation requirement, easier access to clear secretion, and facilitation of weaning. While some randomized studies were able to show decreased hospital length of stay, in-hospital mortality and incidence of pneumonia, others did not. While day-to-day care of tracheostomy tubes is easier than ETT, there is no strong evidence to support its impact on long-term patients' morbidity and mortality.[6] However, the timing of PDT in the neurointensive care unit (NICU) is more challenging due to many factors:

- *Intracranial hypertension (ICH)*: Many patients in the NICU have decreased intracranial compliance and elevated intracranial pressure (ICP). Invasive procedures are likely to aggravate ICP and will require close monitoring and management. Adequate levels of anaesthesia, muscle relaxation, and tight control of haemodynamics to avoid hypertension or hypotension is critical to ensure adequate cerebral perfusion pressure during tracheostomy procedures.[7]
- *Unpredictable disease state*: Patients with evolving stroke, those with intracranial pathology and an unpredictable course, neuromuscular disorders and combination of disease states (seizures, chronic obstructive pulmonary disease [COPD] among others) may make it difficult to predict the need for PDT, let alone when it is absolutely indicated. While clinicians may easily determine the need for PDT in many patients, in many others the decision is not as straightforward.

Equipment

Percutaneous dilatational tracheostomy can be performed safely as a bedside procedure in the intensive care unit (ICU). In addition, it is cost-effective and avoids patient-related complications during transport. There are many commercially available PDT kits and the choice of using a particular device is mainly dependent on the expertise and training of the operator. Percutaneous dilatational tracheostomy is relatively easy to learn by most physicians providing critical care from various backgrounds and with limited or no surgical training.

Pre-Procedure Preparation

Detailed medical and surgical history is an integral part of making appropriate patient selection. An adequate monitoring and anaesthesia care team or dedicated ICU nurse should administer anaesthesia, monitor the patient and treat haemodynamics and ICP throughout the procedure. Depending on the technique used, fibreoptic bronchoscopy equipment, ultrasound, and electrocautery may be needed at the bedside. Patients should be intubated, ventilated with 100% fraction of inspired oxygen (FiO_2), and full mechanical ventilatory support during the procedure.

Technique

Many techniques are used to insert PDTs and vary across practices, as the next few sections discuss.

Sequential Dilatational Tracheostomy

As described in the mid-1950s by Ciaglia, this technique gained popularity in the 1980s when many commercially available kits came to the market. The technique steps are outlined in Table 65.2.

Single Dilator Modification (Ciaglia Blue Rhino®)

The technique was introduced two decades later and became widely adopted. It represents the current practice of PDT placement today. A multistage dilator with hydrophilic coating (Figure 65.2) is used instead of multiple dilators. The safety and efficacy of both techniques has been compared and found to be equal in most studies.

In most current practices, the procedure is performed under continuous bronchoscopic guidance. Real-time bronchoscopy may assist with ETT withdrawal,

Table 65.2 Steps for sequential dilatational tracheostomy

1. Landmark identification: midline, thyroid, and cricoid cartilage
2. Injection of lidocaine with epinephrine (Figure 65.1)
3. ETT is withdrawn below the level of vocal cords
4. Needle is inserted into the trachea
5. The guide wire is advanced through the needle
6. 1.5 cm vertical incision of skin below cricoid cartilage
7. An 8F Teflon catheter guide is threaded over the guide wire
8. Serial dilators (12–28F) are introduced over the Teflon catheter at a 45-degree angle
9. Tracheostomy tube fitted onto an 18F dilator is introduced

confirmation of proper insertion point, wire placement, and visualization of the dilator and tracheostomy tube insertion.

PercuTwist

Designed as a single-step technique after placing the guide wire in the trachea, the PercuTwist dilator (Figure 65.3) creates a track by twisting it like a screw while advancing it into the airway. Upon entering the trachea, the dilator should elevate pulling the anterior tracheal wall away from posterior wall to prevent injury. Some studies comparing PercuTwist to the multi-dilators method showed higher incidence of complications, especially difficulty of insertion as well as higher incidence of posterior wall injury.[8–10]

Griggs' Guide Wire Dilating Forceps (GGWDF)®

A sharp-tipped forceps designed with a channel to accommodate a guide wire (Figure 65.4) is used to create a track for insertion of the tracheostomy tube. The forceps glides over the guide wire into the neck incision to reach the trachea. Opening the forceps in place dilates the track and allows for insertion of the tracheostomy tube.

Translaryngeal (Fantoni), balloon dilatational (Ciaglia Blue Dolphin®), and many others are proposed techniques for PDT placement but are less commonly utilized at the moment.

POST-PROCEDURE CARE

Patients are allowed to recover from the anaesthetic effect and mechanical ventilatory support is resumed to pre-procedure levels. A quick bronchoscopy is usually performed to ensure patency of the airways and remove blood and debris after the procedure. A chest X-ray is helpful in ruling out immediate postoperative complications such as pneumothorax and haemothorax as well as to confirm proper positioning of the tracheostomy tube tip.

COMPLICATIONS

Percutaneous dilatational tracheostomy is a safe procedure and compares favourably to surgical tracheostomy with about half the cost and similar or less incidence of major complications.[11–15] However, the incidence of complications vary considerably depending on the technique used, patient selection, and provider experience.[16–22] Table 65.3 lists the common intraoperative, early, and late complications of PDT as reported by many studies.

Table 65.3 Incidence of complications of percutaneous dilatational tracheostomy

Intraoperative complications	Incidence percentage
Hypoxaemia	3%–10%
Loss of airway requiring re-intubation	2%–15%
Arrhythmias	2%–7%
Technical difficulties	2%–28%
Tracheal ring fracture	2%–36%
Tracheal wall injury	1%–10%
Oesophageal perforation	2%–3%
Paratracheal insertion	1%–3%
Conversion to surgical tracheostomy	0.5%–23%
Early complications	
Pneumothorax	2%–4%
Subcutaneous emphysema	3%–10%
Late complications	
Bleeding	0.5%–43%
Infection	7%

CONCLUSIONS

Traditionally, patients requiring long-term mechanical ventilation often underwent surgical tracheostomy. With the introduction of percutaneous techniques, tracheostomy has become a safe procedure in experienced hands.

REFERENCES

1. Abouzgheib W, Meena N, Jagtap P, Schorr C, Boujaoude Z, Bartter T. Percutaneous dilational tracheostomy in patients receiving antiplatelet therapy: is it safe? *Journal of Bronchology & Interventional Pulmonology* 2013;20(4): 322–5.
2. Belanger A, Akulian J. Interventional pulmonology in the intensive care unit: percutaneous tracheostomy and gastrostomy. *Seminars in Respiratory & Critical Care Medicine* 2014;35(6):744–50.
3. Birbicer H, Doruk N, Yapici D, et al. Percutaneous tracheostomy: a comparison of PercuTwist and multi-dilators techniques. *Annals of Cardiac Anaesthesia* 2008; 11(2):131.
4. Gadkaree SK, Schwartz D, Gerold K, Kim Y. Use of bronchoscopy in percutaneous dilational tracheostomy. *JAMA Otolaryngology, Head & Neck Surgery* 2016;142(2): 143–9.
5. Guinot PG, Zogheib E, Petiot S, et al. Ultrasound-guided percutaneous tracheostomy in critically ill obese patients. *Critical Care (London, England)* 2012;16(2):R40.

6. Holevar M, Dunham JC, Brautigan R, et al. Practice management guidelines for timing of tracheostomy: the EAST Practice Management Guidelines Work Group. *Journal of Trauma-Injury Infection & Critical Care* 2009; 67(4):870–4.

7. Imperiale C, Magni G, Favaro R, Rosa G. Intracranial pressure monitoring during percutaneous tracheostomy 'percutwist' in critically ill neurosurgery patients. *Anesthesia & Analgesia* 2009;108(2):588–92.

8. Jackson LS, Davis JW, Kaups KL, et al. Percutaneous tracheostomy: to bronch or not to bronch—that is the question. *Journal of Trauma-Injury Infection & Critical Care* 2011;71(6):1553–6.

9. Jacobs JV, Hill DA, Petersen SR, Bremner RM, Sue RD, Smith MA. 'Corkscrew stenosis': defining and preventing a complication of percutaneous dilatational tracheostomy. *Journal of Thoracic & Cardiovascular Surgery* 2013;145(3):716–20.

10. Kilic D, Findikcioglu A, Akin S, Korun O, Aribogan A, Hatiboglu A. When is surgical tracheostomy indicated? Surgical 'U-shaped' versus percutaneous tracheostomy. *Annals of Thoracic & Cardiovascular Surgery* 2011;17(1):29–32.

11. Klein M, Agassi R, Shapira AR, Kaplan DM, Koiffman L, Weksler N. Can intensive care physicians safely perform percutaneous dilational tracheostomy? An analysis of 207 cases. Israel Medical Association Journal: *IMAJ* 2007;9(10):717–9.

12. Klotz R, Klaiber U, Grummich K, et al. Percutaneous versus surgical strategy for tracheostomy: protocol for a systematic review and meta-analysis of perioperative and postoperative complications. Systems Review. 2015;4:105. PubMed PMID: 26253532.

13. Louh IK, Freeman WD. Safety of percutaneous tracheostomy in NeuroICU patients with intracranial pressure monitoring. *Critical Care (London, England)* 2014; 18(3):432. PubMed PMID: 25043273.

14. Pilarczyk K, Haake N, Dudasova M, et al. Risk factors for bleeding complications after percutaneous dilatational tracheostomy: a ten-year institutional analysis. *Anaesthesia & Intensive Care* 2016;44(2):227–36.

15. Putensen C, Theuerkauf N, Guenther U, Vargas M, Pelosi P. Percutaneous and surgical tracheostomy in critically ill adult patients: a meta-analysis. *Critical Care (London, England)* 2014;18(6):544.

16. Siempos, II, Ntaidou TK, Filippidis FT, Choi AM. Effect of early versus late or no tracheostomy on mortality and pneumonia of critically ill patients receiving mechanical ventilation: a systematic review and meta-analysis. *The Lancet Respiratory Medicine* 2015 Feb;3(2):150–8.

17. Sollid SJ, Soreide E. Human factors play a vital role in the outcome of percutaneous dilatational tracheostomy. *Critical Care (London, England)* 2014;18(1):409.

18. Mirski MA, Pandian V, Bhatti N, et al. Safety, efficiency, and cost-effectiveness of a multidisciplinary percutaneous tracheostomy program. *Critical Care Medicine* 2012;40(6): 1827–34.

19. Maxwell BG, Ganaway T, Lighthall GK. Percutaneous tracheostomy at the bedside: 13 tips for improving safety and success. *Journal of Intensive Care Medicine* 2014; 29(2):110–15.

20. Flint AC, Midde R, Rao VA, Lasman TE, Ho PT. Bedside ultrasound screening for pretracheal vascular structures may minimize the risks of percutaneous dilatational tracheostomy. *Neurocritical Care* 2009;11(3): 372–6.

21. Alansari M, Alotair H, Al Aseri Z, Elhoseny MA. Use of ultrasound guidance to improve the safety of percutaneous dilatational tracheostomy: a literature review. *Critical Care (London, England)* 2015;19:229.

22. Cools-Lartigue J, Aboalsaud A, Gill H, Ferri L. Evolution of percutaneous dilatational tracheostomy—a review of current techniques and their pitfalls. *World Journal of Surgery* 2013;37(7):1633–46.

66

Percutaneous Endoscopic Gastrostomy in the Intensive Care Unit

R. D. Betzold and M. B. Patel

ABSTRACT

A durable enteral access option for intensive care unit (ICU) patients is the formal gastrostomy with the endoscopic percutaneous method first described in 1980 as a feeding access method for children with dysphagia. Some other options for surgical feeding access include an open gastrostomy, radiographically-guided percutaneous gastrostomy placement, laparoscopic gastrostomy, or jejunostomy placement using either open or minimally invasive methods. While there are many methods for gastrostomy placement, we discuss percutaneous endoscopic gastrostomy (PEG) as an ICU procedure.

KEYWORDS

Percutaneous endoscopic gastrostomy (PEG); feeding access; enteral feeding; tube feeding; endoscopy; ICU; critical care.

INTRODUCTION

Nutrition is a necessary component of recovery for the critically ill patient and the most physiological form of nutrition is the restoration of enteral feeding.[1] These ideas are generalizable to the neurocritical intensive care unit (NICU) with survival and neurologic recovery both improved after initiation of early enteral nutrition. Establishment of enteral access can be accomplished by both minimally invasive techniques and traditional open surgery.[2] The ideal non-invasive method is re-initiation of oral feeding, but often neurocritical care patients endure some oropharyngeal dysphagia related to their neurological disease or more commonly secondary to acute respiratory failure and endotracheal intubation. Nasoenteral feeding (e.g., nasogastric, nasojejunal) is another option, but the risks (discomfort, sinus infection, nasal skin breakdown, and dislodgement) all decrease the durability of this option and constrain transitions of care from acute care hospitalization.[3]

The more durable enteral access option is the formal gastrostomy with the endoscopic percutaneous method first described in 1980 as a feeding access method for children with dysphagia.[4] Some other options for surgical feeding access include an open gastrostomy, radiographically-guided percutaneous gastrostomy placement, laparoscopic gastrostomy, or jejunostomy placement using either open or minimally invasive methods.[2] Percutaneous endoscopic gastrostomy (PEG) is discussed as an ICU procedure in this chapter.

ANATOMY AND PHYSIOLOGY

The gastrostomy tube is placed into the body of the stomach anterior to the greater curvature. Externally, this corresponds to an area left of the midline 2 cm from the costal margin. A window above the colon and lateral to the liver is blindly and percutaneously accessed after full insufflation of the stomach is achieved. This allows for feeding of the stomach and utilization of the full surface area of the gastrointestinal tract for absorption.[5]

INDICATIONS AND CONTRAINDICATIONS

Candidates for this procedure include critically ill patients who need durable long-term feeding access and have swallowing difficulties that prevent maintenance of adequate nutrition. There are few absolute contraindications and these include the inability to visualize deflection and transillumination during gastrostomy placement, unfavourable anatomy, and coagulopathy. Other contraindications include ascites, gastric outlet or other bowel obstruction, poor gastric emptying, intolerance of enteral feeding, and excessive gastrooesophageal reflux. Should the patient have a gastric outlet obstruction or reflux, a feeding jejunostomy tube may be a more viable option if enteral feeding is a necessity.[5]

EQUIPMENT

There are multiple methods for performing the percutaneous endoscopic gastrostomy. In our practice, this procedure requires a gastroscope and a pull gastrostomy kit.

PRE-PROCEDURE PREPARATION

In preparation for the procedure, the first important step is performing a full history and physical examination to look for barriers to successful gastrostomy placement (e.g., prior abdominal surgical scars, prior head and neck disease), as well as moderate sedation and anaesthetic considerations. Any previous abdominal imaging is also reviewed and informed consent is obtained from the patient or their family. Once this is complete, the patient is positioned supine in the hospital bed. In many practices, knowing the clean-contaminated nature of this procedure, no preoperative antibiotics are given for percutaneous endoscopic gastrostomy tube placement. Once adequate sedation is achieved, the procedure is initiated.[5,6]

TECHNIQUE

Although supine positioning is standard, if possible, we prefer a reverse Trendelenburg position to facilitate any residual or abnormally positioned colon or bowel to drop as inferior as possible during the procedure. The abdomen is prepared and draped using sterile technique. The procedure is initiated after placing the endoscope into the oropharynx under visualization. The oesophagus is then intubated and the scope is passed through the oesophagus with gentle insufflation. The stomach is then entered and insufflation is performed. Once the stomach is adequately insufflated, deflection of the abdominal wall at an area

below the costal margin is performed. Visualization of this abdominal wall deflection on the mucosal side of the stomach is a necessary first-step for safe performance of this procedure. Then, the scope is used to transilluminate the stomach and external visualization of this light through the abdominal wall is observed. Visualization of transillumination is also necessary for safe performance of this procedure, but is sometimes problematic in those with thick abdominal walls.

After deflection and transillumination are confirmed, a modified Seldinger technique is used for gastrostomy placement. As an additional measure of protection, the 'safe tract' technique is used during gastric entry. A small incision is made in the skin 2 cm inferior to the costal margin. Under direct visualization, a 25-gauge needle on a syringe filled with local anaesthetic is inserted through the abdominal wall in this area into the stomach. On placement, the proceduralist vocalizes visualization of bubbling in the syringe while the endoscopist vocalizes the time of visualization of the needle in the stomach. When these times are congruent, a safe tract into the stomach (and not the colon or other structures) can be assumed but of course, never guaranteed.

From here, the catheter-tipped 14-gauge needle is similarly filled with local anaesthetic and the safe tract technique is repeated. The needle is removed, but the catheter sheath is left traversing the anterior abdominal wall and stomach. The long wire is passed through the catheter into the stomach. Intragastrically, the wire is snared with the endoscope and withdrawn through the mouth. Residual wire must be present in the catheter sheath traversing the anterior abdominal wall.

Externally, the gastrostomy tube is then looped and fixed to the wire. Utilizing the mnemonic 'the blue through,' the blue wire is placed through the metal loop on the gastrostomy tube and the gastrostomy tube is brought 'through the blue' to accomplish wire fixation. If possible, the snare can partially grab the gastrostomy tube disk, and the tube can be followed back into the stomach while the wire is withdrawn (a pitfall in this additional manoeuvre of disc snaring is the inability to de-snare the disc on completion of the PEG). In any case, the wire is withdrawn directly perpendicular from the abdominal wall. Steady force is required during the wire withdrawal process, particularly when the gastrostomy tube is exiting the abdominal wall. It is then secured in place with the gastrostomy tube disk approximately 4 cm at the skin level (highly variable based on abdominal wall thickness), taking care to prevent any significant indentation of the skin and ensuring that the tube rotates freely.

If the camera was able to return intragastrically, air is withdrawn to collapse the stomach, and the tube should freely rotate with the internal PEG bumper opposed to the stomach. The endoscope is then withdrawn, but sometimes, internal visual confirmation is not performed. Although many PEG kits contain suture for approximating the gastrostomy tube disk to the skin, and this was our historic practice, we have abandoned this practice for years as we feel it increases local wound complications and does not prevent PEG dislodgement.[4–6]

POST-PROCEDURE CARE

The gastrostomy tube is capped and can be used for medication administration during the first 24 hours. After that point, tube feedings are initiated and advanced to goal rates per hospital protocol. The tube is kept clean and dry.

Once the PEG is determined ready for removal because there is no clinical need for enteral feeding access (e.g., sustained adequate oral nutrition, achieved suitable nutrition parameters), it is simply removed with traction and the site is covered with dry gauze until the gastrocutaneous fistula is closed.[5] Refer to surgery if after 4 weeks, there is still gastric drainage from the fistula site or if the PEG cannot be removed. Percutaneous endoscopic gastrostomies indwelling longer than 12 months are more likely to have persistence of the gastrocutaneous fistula and could require operative surgical closure.[7]

COMPLICATIONS

This procedure is commonly performed in the ICU, but this is not a marker of safety for gastrostomy placement. In fact, it has up to a 50% complication rate as per some studies[8] and patients receiving a PEG have an increased in-hospital mortality.[9] Procedure-related complications include bleeding, misplacement of the tube into the colon or other intra-abdominal structure (Figure 66.1), inadvertent perforation of the oesophagus or stomach, tube dislodgement, feeding intolerance, necrotizing soft tissue infections, aspiration, or a cardiac event. Less serious, but perhaps more common problems relate to food leakage around the tube, late tube dislodgement requiring percutaneous or radiology-guided replacement,[10] and/or bleeding, painful granulation tissue needing silver nitrate therapy.[8]

One of the more feared complications in the immediate (<4 weeks) postoperative period is tube dislodgement. In this setting, the gastric wall is not fixed to the abdominal wall, so there is concern for free leakage of gastric contents into the peritoneal space.[5] Current recommendations vary, but in the immediate postoperative period, tube

dislodgement can be evaluated with oral contrast administration and plain films and/or computed tomography (CT) scan. If no gross leak is detected, this can be managed by careful observation and serial abdominal examinations.[11] In the absence of peritonitis, it could also be managed endoscopically by replacing the gastrostomy tube. Should peritonitis develop, however, at least a laparoscopic exploration should occur to washout the abdomen and evaluate the gastrotomy.[12] Ultimately, there are many complications that can occur after gastrostomy placement and a close relationship with the surgeons who place gastrostomy tubes can help mitigate some of the consequences of these complications.

CONCLUSIONS

The PEG tube technique has become the most prevalent permanent enteral access method in the modern ICU. It can easily be performed at the bedside in most patients, reducing unnecessary moves and costly operating room visits. While the operative technique is simple, the complications can be disastrous, so careful attention must be paid in the perioperative period.

REFERENCES

1. Chiang YH, Chao DP, Chu SF, et al. Early enteral nutrition and clinical outcomes of severe traumatic brain injury patients in acute stage: a multi-center cohort study. *J Neurotrauma* 2012;29:75–80.
2. Lord LM. Enteral access devices: types, function, care, and challenges. *Nutr Clin Pract* 2018;33:16–38.
3. Prabhakaran S, Doraiswamy VA, Nagaraja V, et al. Nasoenteric tube complications. *Scand J Surg* 2012;101: 147–55.
4. Gauderer MW, Ponsky JL, Izant RJ. Gastrostomy without laparotomy: a percutaneous endoscopic technique. *J Pediatr Surg* 1980;15:872–5.
5. Gore D. Percutaneous gastrostomy feeding tube placement. In: Townsend C, Evers, BM, eds. *Atlas of General Surgical Techniques*. 1st ed. Philadelphia, PA: Saunders Elsevier, 2010;1: pp. 253–60.
6. Ponsky JL, Gauderer MW, Stellato TA, Aszodi A. Percutaneous approaches to enteral alimentation. *Am J Surg* 1985;149:102–5.
7. Schulman AR, Aihara H, Thompson CC. Treatment of gastrocutaneous fistula after percutaneous gastrostomy placement. *Gastrointest Endosc* 2016;84:851–2.
8. Schrag SP, Sharma R, Jaik NP, et al. Complications related to percutaneous endoscopic gastrostomy (PEG) tubes. A comprehensive clinical review. *J Gastrointestin Liver Dis* 2007;16:407–18.
9. Muratori R, Lisotti A, Fusaroli P, et al. Severe hypernatremia as a predictor of mortality after percutaneous endoscopic

gastrostomy (PEG) placement. *Dig Liver Dis* 2017;49: 181–7.

10. Kim CY, Patel MB, Miller MJ, et al. Gastrostomy-to-gastrojejunostomy tube conversion: impact of the method of original gastrostomy tube placement. *J Vasc Interv Radiol* 2010;21:1031–7.

11. Marshall JB, Bodnarchuk G, Barthel JS. Early accidental dislodgement of PEG tubes. *J Clin Gastroenterol* 1994;18:210–12.

12. Mincheff TV. Early dislodgement of percutaneous and endoscopic gastrostomy tube. *J S C Med Assoc* 2007;103: 13–15.

67

Evaluation of Intracranial Pressure Using Bedside Ultrasonography: Estimation of Optic Nerve Sheath Diameter

S. Krishnan and A. B. Kumar

ABSTRACT

Measurements of the optic nerve sheath diameter (ONSD) have been shown to correlate with clinical and radiological signs of increased intracranial pressure (ICP). The ONSD can be measured at the bedside in a rapid, non-invasive, and reproducible manner using ultrasonography. This chapter outlines the considerations and methods to perform an effective measurement of the ONSD in the neurointensive care unit (NICU).

KEYWORDS

Ultrasonography; optic nerve sheath diameter (ONSD); intracranial pressure (ICP).

INTRODUCTION

The rapid detection of raised intracranial pressure (ICP) can be life-saving in the neurologically injured patient and failure to recognize raised ICP can lead to delays in treatment and interventions that can ultimately affect patient outcomes. The conventional methods of evaluating raised ICP have significant practical limitations (invasive, specialized monitors) making the rapid objective assessment more challenging. The widespread availability of bedside ultrasonography makes the surrogate assessment of raised ICP using optic nerve sheath (ONS) assessment very attractive to the bedside intensivist. In this chapter, we review the basics of ONSD to evaluate raised ICP.

OPTIC NERVE SHEATH ANATOMY

The subarachnoid space enveloping the optic nerve continues intracranially as the chiasmal cistern. The optic nerve and its sheath are not a uniform diameter tube-like structure. In fact, the intraorbital portion is about 25 mm and is approximately S-shaped. The diameters of the anterior and posterior segments are also not uniform. The variation of ONSD is due to the presence of other interlacing structures such as arachnoid trabeculae, septa, and stout pillars.[1]

As the ONS is distensible, changes in cerebrospinal fluid (CSF) pressures will dynamically affect the ONSD. The ONS itself has an average diameter of 4 mm with the subarachnoid compartment of 0.1 mm allowing for 0.1 ml of CSF. It is stated that under normal conditions, the CSF flows towards the bulbous and enlarged portion of the sheath and the movement of the globe reverses the flow of CSF allowing for a circulatory effect within the ONS.[2]

When the ICP rises, the CSF flow towards the perineural space increases and results in an increase in distension of the ONS and thus its diameter. The distension is more pronounced in the anterior region (i.e., 3 mm behind the optic disc [Figure 67.1]) compared to the posterior regions. Thus the measurements are completed in this segment of the ONS.

EVIDENCE FOR USING OPTIC NERVE SHEATH DIAMETER FOR NON-INVASIVE ESTIMATION OF INTRACRANIAL PRESSURE

In the present day, ICP is measured via a surgically inserted ICP monitor placed in the subdural, intra-parenchymal, or intra-ventricular space. The placement of an ICP monitor has become a fairly routine procedure in neurointensive care units worldwide. The procedures although safe in experienced hands carries a small but not insignificant rate of complications—most notably intracranial haemorrhage (ICH) and post-procedure infection.[3]

Transorbital ultrasound for the non-invasive estimation of increased ICP has gained ground over the past decade. The use of this technique has been supported based on a number of small studies in neurological aetiologies including traumatic brain injury (TBI), mass lesions, intracranial infections, and post-transplant reperfusion injury.[3–5] Geeraerts et al. studied the relationship between ONSD and invasively measured intra-parenchymal ICP in sedated neurocritical care patients and reported a strong correlation between elevated ICP >20 mmHg and concurrent changes in the ONSD.[4] Tayal et al. demonstrated in a study of 59 adult head injury patients that elevated ICP (as evidenced on computerized tomography [CT] scan[6]) could be accurately predicted by the changes in ONSD.

PRE-PROCEDURE CARE

Ultrasound Equipment

Since the structures to be imaged are superficial, a linear high frequency probe such as the 13–6 MHz linear-array probe can be used. Although ocular ultrasound specific probes are available, it may not be needed always and good quality imaging can be obtained using the vascular access probe commonly used in the intensive care unit (7–10/12 Hz).

The orbital imaging settings with a high-resolution optimization setting should be used on the machine. The orbital setting lowers the power on the ultrasound to decrease the potential injury to the vitreous humour and retina. Probes and ultrasound power settings specifically approved for ocular imaging are recommended.[7]

Contraindications

Open globe injury, retrobular haemorrhage or periorbital fractures can be considered true contraindications. This can be challenging to perform in a non-cooperative patient.[8]

TECHNIQUE

A sterile clear dressing is applied over the closed eye as shown in the video included in the DVD. The ultrasound gel goes over the clear dressing and never comes in direct contact with the eye.

The probe is placed on the superior and lateral aspect of the orbit against the closed upper eyelid and angled caudally and medially (Figure 67.2). This brings the optic nerve into view. The optic nerve is visualized as a linear hypoechoic finger-like structure with clearly defined margins posterior to the globe. The probe is always placed gently on the closed eyelid and never in direct contact with the cornea or sclera to avoid corneal abrasions. One must be cautious with the contact of the probe even with the eye closed and excess pressure is never directly applied on the globe with the probe as this can theoretically result in nausea/vomiting and a vagal bradycardic response.

The image seen in patients with normal intracranial dynamics is shown in Figure 67.2. The globe can be visualized with the lens anteriorly and the optic disc posteriorly. Magnification is not routinely performed and not usually indicated. The ONS appears as a linear hyper-echoic structure behind the optic disc.

The ONSD is measured 3 mm behind the retina (Figure 67.3). The widest perpendicular measurement 3 mm behind the globe is the ONSD. The measurements are ideally reviewed offline to minimize the ultrasound exposure time to the globe.

Measurements

There is a wide variation reported in the optimal cut-off values when ONSD was compared with invasive ICP monitoring ranging from 4.8 to 5.9 mm. The more current studies are in better agreement that an ONSD >6 mm correlates to an ICP >20 mmHg.[2,7]

Practical points to consider:

- Always perform at least three ultrasound evaluations of each eye and use the average measurements ignoring the outliers (similar to conventions with thermodilution cardiac output measurements).
- Exercise caution when the eyes are divergent following intracranial injury. This can add to the discrepancy of measurements with the ultrasound beam not being aligned parallel to the area of focus.
- Always turn the power down on the ultrasound machine to the ophthalmic ultrasound setting.
- Clinical correlation is the key.

POST-PROCEDURE CARE

The procedure does not require IV or local anaesthesia in a cooperative patient and can be performed in the emergency room, operating room, or ICU setting.

CONCLUSIONS

Optic nerve sonography may alert the intensivist to the presence of ICH and the need for other interventions (diagnostic or therapeutic). Estimation of ONSD using bedside ultrasonography is a safe and expeditious method of recognizing increased ICP and to help make clinical management decisions in the ICU.

CONFLICT OF INTEREST

The authors have no conflicts of interest.

REFERENCES

1. Moretti R, Pizzi B. Ultrasonography of the optic nerve in neurocritically ill patients. *Acta Anaesthesiologica Scandinavica* 2011;55(6):644–52.
2. Soldatos T, Chatzimichail K, Papathanasiou M, Gouliamos A. Optic nerve sonography: a new window for the non-invasive evaluation of intracranial pressure in brain injury. *Emergency Medicine Journal: EMJ* 2009;26(9):630–4.
3. Zeiler FA, Ziesmann MT, Goeres P, et al. A unique method for estimating the reliability learning curve of optic nerve sheath diameter ultrasound measurement. *Critical Ultrasound Journal* 2016;8(1):9.
4. Geeraerts T, Merceron S, Benhamou D, Vigue B, Duranteau J. Non-invasive assessment of intracranial pressure using ocular sonography in neurocritical care patients. *Intensive Care Medicine* 2008;34(11):2062–7.
5. Lee SU, Jeon JP, Lee H, et al. Optic nerve sheath diameter threshold by ocular ultrasonography for detection of increased intracranial pressure in Korean adult patients with brain lesions. *Medicine* 2016;95(41):e5061.
6. Bekerman I, Sigal T, Kimiagar I, Ben Ely A, Vaiman M. The quantitative evaluation of intracranial pressure by optic nerve sheath diameter/eye diameter computed tomographic measurement. *The American Journal of Emergency Medicine* 2016;34(12):2336–42.
7. Rajajee V, Vanaman M, Fletcher JJ, Jacobs TL. Optic nerve ultrasound for the detection of raised intracranial pressure. *Neurocritical Care* 2011;15(3):506–15.
8. Hsu JM, Joseph AP, Tarlinton LJ, Macken L, Blome S. The accuracy of focused assessment with sonography in trauma (FAST) in blunt trauma patients: experience of an Australian major trauma service. *Injury* 2007;38(1):71–5.

68

Echocardiography and Ultrasound in the Neuro ICU

S. Krishnan and A. B. Kumar

ABSTRACT

Over the last few decades, intensivists around the world have enthusiastically embraced the use of point-of-care ultrasound (POCUS) in the intensive care unit (ICU). Point-of-care ultrasound techniques have been proven to be widely applicable and easy to learn. Acquisition and interpretation of ultrasound images is performed by the bedside clinician, which enables rapid intervention. The patient's cardiopulmonary response to interventions can also then be easily followed with this technique. In this chapter, we describe some commonly acquired POCUS views, and discuss examples of pathologies frequently encountered on ultrasound evaluation in the neurointensive care unit (NICU).

KEYWORDS

Ultrasonography; echocardiography; point-of-care ultrasound (POCUS); neurointensive care; neurointensive care unit (NICU).

INTRODUCTION

Point-of-care ultrasound (POCUS) has become part of the routine evaluation of critically ill patients.[1,2] Using POCUS, the critical care physician can diagnose the cause of haemodynamic and respiratory compromise with a rapid, non-invasive, bedside evaluation. Further evaluations can be repeated as often as required to assess the patient's progress and the impact of therapy.

In this chapter, we describe common POCUS views and discuss common pathologies diagnosed with POCUS in neurocritical care patients. It is important to realize that the goal of POCUS is not to replace detailed evaluations by experts in various medical specialities, but rather to provide the bedside clinician with a rapid and repeatable assessment that can alter management while awaiting further consultation if necessary. In addition, the clinician's training, education, and experience, as well as factors pertaining to the patient, such as suboptimal positioning, subcutaneous emphysema, obesity, and the presence of drains or dressings, can impact the quality

of image acquisition and interpretation. As with all monitoring techniques, one should take the entire clinical picture into account while using POCUS to guide management.

COMMONLY USED PROBES

Point-of-care ultrasound machines usually come equipped with a high-frequency linear probe for vascular and other superficial evaluation, as well as a low-frequency phased array probe for deeper tissue evaluation, including cardiac exams (Figure 68.1). Occasionally, they might include a low frequency curved array probe.[1,2]

POINT-OF-CARE ULTRASOUND ECHOCARDIOGRAPHY

Introduction and Anatomy

Bedside evaluation of left and right ventricular systolic function and volume status with ultrasonography is highly beneficial in titrating haemodynamic support in critically ill patients. It is particularly important to perform POCUS evaluation of cardiac function in patients who continue to have signs of hypoperfusion despite fluid or vasopressor therapy.[1,2] While evaluating the response to changes in management, clinicians should use POCUS assessment in addition to conventional haemodynamic monitoring.

While the cardiac anatomy is complex, the operator must focus on pre-defined views (described below) while performing POCUS assessments of the heart. The convention on acquiring these views also includes pointing the marker on the probe in a specific direction, which helps develop image orientation.

Evidence for POCUS Echocardiography

Point-of-care ultrasound echocardiography is useful in determining the cause of shock and evaluating the response to therapy. Evaluating fluid status is needed to avoid fluid overload and hypovolaemia in critically ill patients. Point-of-care ultrasound can help identify patients with significantly low or high right atrial filling pressure.[3] In mechanically ventilated patients, a 15% variation in inferior vena cava (IVC) diameter can identify fluid responders from non-responders.[4] Evaluation of cardiac function can help identify left and right ventricular systolic dysfunction, which can often be unrecognized in critically ill patients.[5,6] Bedside ultrasound is particularly useful in identifying pericardial tamponade.[7] Finally, echocardiography is recommended for evaluation of a cardiac source of embolus in patients with acute ischaemic stroke.[8] However, this non-emergent evaluation is usually performed by cardiologists.

Technique

The cardiac transthoracic echocardiography probe (Figure 68.1) is used for the POCUS echocardiography exams. As it has a low frequency, this probe is useful for imaging deeper tissue, hence allowing for imaging of the entire heart. Commonly acquired views in basic POCUS assessment of cardiac function and volume are listed in Table 68.1. Probe placement for these views is described in Figures 68.2–68.6, and examples of normal cardiac function in these views are provided in videos 1–5. These figures and videos are described in the following points:

- Parasternal long axis view (Figure 68.2 and video 1): The probe is placed in the 3rd or 4th intercostal space on the left edge of the sternum with the marker pointed towards the right shoulder, and the ultrasound beam pointed posteriorly. The pericardium, right ventricle

Table 68.1 Commonly acquired point-of-care ultrasound views for assessment of cardiac function and volume

View	Probe placement	Marker position
Parasternal long axis view	3rd or 4th intercostal space on the left edge of the sternum	Towards the right shoulder
Parasternal short axis view	3rd or 4th intercostal space on the left edge of the sternum	Towards the left shoulder
Apical four-chamber view	At the cardiac apex	Towards the patient's left side
Subcostal four-chamber view	Inferior to the xiphoid	Towards the patient's left side
Subcostal IVC view	Inferior to the xiphoid	Cephalad direction

(RV), left ventricle (LV), and aortic and mitral valves can be evaluated in this view. The LV apex is usually not visualized in this view.

- Parasternal short axis view (Figure 68.3 and video 2): The probe is placed in the 3rd or 4th intercostal space, on the left edge of the sternum, with the marker pointed towards the left shoulder, and the ultrasound beam pointed posteriorly. The pericardium, RV, and LV can be evaluated in this view. The anterolateral and posteromedial papillary muscles of the LV are visualized within the LV cavity.

- Apical four-chamber view (Figure 68.4 and video 3): The probe is placed on the cardiac apex, with the marker pointed towards the patient's left side, and the ultrasound beam pointed medially and cephalad to acquire this view. The pericardium, RV, LV, and tricuspid and mitral valves can be evaluated in this view.

- Subcostal four-chamber view (Figure 68.5 and video 4): The probe is placed subcostally, inferior to the xiphoid process with the marker pointed towards the patient's left side, and the ultrasound beam pointed cephalad and towards the left at a shallow angle under the ribcage. The pericardium, RV, LV, and tricuspid and mitral valves can be evaluated in this view. Raising the marker edge of the probe anteriorly by a slight angle can help open up the LV apex for imaging.

- Subcostal IVC view (Figure 68.6 and video 5): The probe is placed subcostally inferior to the xiphoid process with the marker pointed towards the cephalad direction, and the ultrasound beam pointed posteriorly. The IVC can be evaluated in this view in long axis. One must differentiate the IVC from the aorta by visualizing the hepatic veins joining the IVC and the IVC subsequently joining the right atrium.[1,2]

The left lateral position is optimal for acquiring cardiac views. However, it is often difficult to position critically ill patients appropriately for ultrasound evaluation. In addition, lung hyperinflation might make cardiac imaging difficult.[1,2]

Evaluation of Haemodynamics

Left Ventricular Function

Hyperdynamic and poor LV systolic function can usually be visualized in the parasternal short axis view (videos 6–7). However, to evaluate the entire ventricle for regional wall motion abnormalities and to confirm the initial assessment, one should acquire all of the views mentioned in Table 68.1. Left ventricular function is assessed by a quantitative assessment in multiple views.

Right Ventricular Function

Failure and dilatation of RV might be visualized in the parasternal short axis view as an eccentric LV with a flattened septum (video 8). Systolic septal flattening represents RV pressure overload, while diastolic flattening represents RV volume overload. In the apical four-chamber view, an RV end-diastolic area larger than 60% of LV end-diastolic area suggests RV dysfunction (video 9). In patients with acute pulmonary embolism, RV pressure overload is often accompanied by a specific pattern of abnormal regional wall motion with akinesia of the mid free wall but normal motion at the apex. This pattern of RV dysfunction with apical sparing (McConnell's sign) has prognostic implications in patients with pulmonary embolism, though other aetiologies of acute RV dysfunction can cause a similar echocardiographic pattern.[9]

Preload Assessment

Hypovolaemia is evident on the parasternal short axis as the kissing papillary muscle sign (video 10). It should be noted that while this is a sensitive sign of hypovolaemia, its specificity for predicting a decreased preload is only 30%.[10] Assessment of the IVC size and respiratory variation allows for estimation of right-sided cardiac filling pressures reference (Table 68.2). In spontaneously breathing patients, a small IVC with inspiratory collapse suggests a low right atrial pressure (RAP), and fluid responsiveness (video 11). On the other hand, a dilated IVC with minimal respiratory variation indicates a high RAP (video 12). Assessment of IVC for RAP in mechanically ventilated patients and evaluation of RAP

Table 68.2 Estimated right atrial pressure based on inferior vena cava size and respiratory variation

Inferior vena cava diameter (cm)	% collapse with sniff	Estimated right atrial pressure (mmHg)
≤2.1 cm	>50	3
Intermediate values		8
>2.1 cm	<50	15

using IVC assessment is not well-validated, though a small and collapsed IVC still suggests hypovolaemia and the presence of respiratory variation predicts fluid responsiveness.[2]

Pericardial Effusion

Pericardial effusions can be visualized in all of the cardiac POCUS views (video 13). Right ventricular collapse during diastole suggests tamponade physiology.[2]

Stroke

Cardiac evaluation for an embolic source in patients with stroke, to look for the presence of atrial septal defect, patent foramen ovale, left atrial appendage thrombus or ascending aortic pathology is best done with transoesophageal echocardiography.[8]

Limitations

The limitations of POCUS echocardiography are:

- Suboptimal imaging due to inability to position the patient in a left lateral position and due to lung hyperinflation
- Inability to image due to dressings, tubes, and drains
- Varied user training, skill, knowledge, and experience[1,2]

Practical Points to Consider

- Correlate echocardiography findings with clinical condition before making management decisions.
- Repeat the echo examination after interventions or if the clinical condition changes to monitor improvement or worsening.
- Consult an expert if echocardiography findings are either very subtle or highly unexpected.
- Good imaging requires training under supervision and plenty of practice.
- Hand motions are often subtle. Stabilize the heel of your hand on the patient's chest.

ULTRASOUND FOR LUNG EVALUATION

Introduction and Anatomy

Point-of-care ultrasonography evaluation of lung pathology is limited by air in the lungs, which creates an acoustic mismatch with surrounding tissue, preventing the ability to image the lung parenchyma. Despite this limitation, various lung pathologies can be identified via lung ultrasound.

Evidence for Using Lung Ultrasound in the Intensive Care Unit

Lung ultrasound has been shown to be of benefit for recognition of fluid overload and pulmonary oedema.[11] The sensitivity and specificity of lung ultrasound for diagnosis of pneumothorax exceeds that of chest radiography.[12] Ultrasound performed by intensivists has been shown to have comparable or even better results than chest radiography for detection and estimation of size of pleural effusions.[13] Furthermore, using ultrasound during thoracocentesis has been shown to reduce the incidence of complications.[14] The diagnostic accuracy of ultrasound for lung consolidation exceeds 90%.[15]

Technique

Probe selection and placement: Surface ultrasound evaluation of the lungs can be performed using the linear or sector probes. Deeper evaluation of effusions and collapsed lung can require a low-frequency cardiac ultrasound probe or a curvilinear probe.

Probe placement is recommended on multiple areas on each side, both anteriorly and laterally, and when possible, posteriorly. As with auscultation of the lungs, the findings elucidated on examination provide information about the lung underneath the area of the chest wall.[12]

Views

Commonly, the probe is placed in the longitudinal orientation, with the marker pointed in a cephalad direction (Figure 68.7). Two ribs are visualized in cross-section on the screen. The ribs cast a sonographic shadow below. The intercostal space is visible between the ribs, and the pleural line is visible as a hyperechoic line 0.5–1 cm deeper than the ribs, perpendicular to the ultrasound beam.[12]

Recognition of Pathology

The presence of lung sliding (video 14) indicates normal motion of the visceral pleura against the parietal pleura. B-lines (video 15) are normal reverberation artifacts that occur due to the presence of sub-pleural fluid or collagen collections. Multiple B-lines in many intercostal spaces suggest the presence of pulmonary oedema. The presence of either lung sliding or B-lines rules out pneumothorax. The absence of both lung sliding and B-lines suggests that pneumothorax is possible (video 16). Lung sliding itself may be absent with endobronchial intubation of the contralateral lung, consolidation, atelectasis or contusion. Lung point refers to an area of transition between pleural line showing lung sliding and absent lung sliding, indicating the area of chest wall where inflated lung falls away because of pneumothorax.[12]

Pleural effusions appear as large echolucent areas on ultrasound, usually evident just above the diaphragm in the costophrenic angles (video 17). Often, a collapsed lung with compression atelectasis can be seen floating in the effusion. Visualization of size and location of pleural effusion by ultrasound is useful for guiding thoracocentesis procedures.[13]

Lung tissue with consolidation due to pneumonia would appear as a solid organ above the diaphragm (video 18), often with air bronchograms visible within the lung parenchyma.[15]

Limitations

The limitations of lung ultrasound are related to not being able to image deeper tissue because of the presence of air. In patients with subcutaneous emphysema, imaging is even more restricted, and often impossible. In patients with pneumothorax, the size of the pneumothorax cannot be diagnosed by lung ultrasound.[12]

Practical Points to Consider

- For aerated lung, ultrasound is useful only in evaluating the lung surface. Deeper pathology is not visualized by this technique.
- The probe must be placed on many spots on the chest bilaterally to perform a complete exam.
- Absence of lung sliding and B-lines suggests the presence of pneumothorax, but this should not be used as a diagnostic confirmation alone. Only lung point is diagnostic of pneumothorax.

ULTRASOUND FOR DEEP VEIN THROMBOSIS EVALUATION

Introduction and Anatomy

Point of care ultrasonography evaluation of the upper and lower extremity veins is useful for diagnosis of deep venous thrombosis (DVT). The presence of clots in these large veins points towards acute pulmonary thromboembolism as a cause for respiratory distress.[16] Vascular ultrasound of the carotids for evaluation of atheromatous disease and stenosis is usually performed by sonographers.

Evidence for Performing Deep Vein Thrombosis Evaluation

The focused ultrasound exam is the gold standard for DVT screening.[17] A multicentre study showed that intensivists performed favourably when compared to vascular technicians in diagnosing DVT, with real-time availability.[16]

Technique

Probe selection: The linear high-frequency probe is used for DVT evaluation.

Technique and views: The internal jugular, subclavian, common femoral, and popliteal veins are commonly examined. The probe is placed such that a short axis view of the vein is obtained along with the adjoining artery (Figure 68.8). It is important to consider usual anatomical orientation of the arteries and veins to allow for identification. At the same time, one must be aware of the possibility of aberrant anatomy.

Deep vein thrombosis is diagnosed[18] by direct visualization of the thrombus or an inability to completely compress the vein (videos 19 and 20).

Limitations

Deep vein thrombosis evaluation can be limited by the presence of dressings, drains, or vascular catheters. In obese patients, visualization of veins can be difficult because of increased depth needed for visualization.[19]

Practical Points to Consider

• Intensive care unit patients are at risk for DVT and pulmonary embolism because of immobility and hypercoagulability.
• Direct visualization of thrombus or inability to compress veins are signs of DVT.

CONCLUSIONS

POCUS is a non-invasive, non-ionizing method of rapid assessment for unstable critically ill patients. All clinicians taking care of neurocritical care patients should strive to achieve basic competency in performing rapid cardiac, lung, and DVT evaluations.

REFERENCES

1. Frankel HL, Kirkpatrick AW, Elbarbary M, et al. Guidelines for the appropriate use of bedside general and cardiac ultrasonography in the evaluation of critically ill patients-Part I: General Ultrasonography. *Crit Care Med* 2015 Nov;43(11):2479–502.
2. Levitov A, Frankel HL, Blaivas M, et al. Guidelines for the appropriate use of bedside general and cardiac ultrasonography in the evaluation of critically ill patients-Part II: Cardiac Ultrasonography. *Crit Care Med* 2016 Jun; 44(6):1206–27.
3. Rudski LG, Lai WW, Afilalo J, et al. Guidelines for the echocardiographic assessment of the right heart in adults: a report from the American Society of Echocardiography endorsed by the European Association of Echocardiography, a registered branch of the European Society of Cardiology and the Canadian Society of Echocardiography. *J Am Soc Echocardiogr* 2010 Jul;23(7): 685–713.
4. Feissel M, Michard F, Faller JP, Teboul JL. The respiratory variation in inferior vena cava diameter as a guide to fluid therapy. *Intensive Care Med* 2004 Sep;30(9):1834–7.
5. Vieillard-Baron A, Caille V, Charron C, Belliard G, Page B, Jardin F. Actual incidence of global left ventricular hypokinesia in adult septic shock. *Crit Care Med* 2008 Jun;36(6):1701–6.
6. Krishnan S, Schmidt GA. Acute right ventricular dysfunction: real-time management with echocardiography. *Chest* 2015 Mar;147(3):835–46.
7. Joseph MX, Disney PJ, Da Costa R, Hutchison SJ. Transthoracic echocardiography to identify or exclude cardiac cause of shock. *Chest* 2004 Nov;126(5):1592–7.
8. Saric M, Armour AC, Arnaout MS, et al. Guidelines for the use of echocardiography in the evaluation of a cardiac source of embolism. *J Am Soc Echocardiogr* 2016 Jan;29(1):1–42.
9. Casazza F, Bongarzoni A, Capozi A, Agostoni O. Regional right ventricular dysfunction in acute pulmonary embolism and right ventricular infarction. *Eur J Echocardiogr* 2005 Jan;6(1):11–14.
10. Leung JM, Levine EH. Left ventricular end-systolic cavity obliteration as an estimate of intraoperative hypovolemia. *Anesthesiology* 1994; 81:1102–9.
11. Picano E, Frassi F, Agricola E, Gligorova S, Gargani L, Mottola G. Ultrasound lung comets: a clinically useful sign of extravascular lung water. *J Am Soc Echocardiogr* 2006 Mar;19(3):356–63.
12. Lichtenstein DA, Mezière G, Lascols N, et al. Ultrasound diagnosis of occult pneumothorax. *Crit Care Med* 2005; 33:1231–8.
13. Rozycki GS, Pennington SD, Feliciano DV. Surgeon-performed ultrasound in the critical care setting: its use as an extension of the physical examination to detect pleural effusion. *J Trauma* 2001 Apr;50(4):636–42.

14. Gordon CE, Feller-Kopman D, Balk EM, Smetana GW. Pneumothorax following thoracentesis: a systematic review and meta-analysis. *Arch Intern Med* 2010 Feb 22;170(4):332–9.

15. Lichtenstein DA, Lascols N, Mezière G, Gepner A. Ultrasound diagnosis of alveolar consolidation in the critically ill. *Intensive Care Med* 2004 Feb;30(2):276–81.

16. Kory PD, Pellecchia CM, Shiloh AL, et al. Accuracy of ultrasonography performed by critical care physicians for the diagnosis of DVT. *Chest* 2011;139:538–42.

17. Lensing AW, Prandoni P, Brandjes D, et al. Detection of deep-vein thrombosis by real-time B-mode ultrasonography. *N Engl J Med* 1989;320:342–5.

18. Narasimhan M, Koenig SJ, Mayo PH. A whole-body approach to point of care ultrasound. *Chest* 2016 Oct; 150(4):772–6.

19. Modica MJ1, Kanal KM, Gunn ML. The obese emergency patient: imaging challenges and solutions. *Radiographics* 2011 May–Jun;31(3):811–23.

69

Cervical Spine Fixation with the Halo Brace

A. Yengo-Kahn and M. Miles

ABSTRACT

Cervical spine fractures due to either falls or motor vehicle collisions are exceedingly common, especially in the elderly and the incidence may be increasing as our world's population continues to age. Spine fractures are generally managed through either external fixation or surgically. External fixation may be preferable in young patients to preserve range of motion or in the elderly who may not tolerate a surgical procedure. The halo brace provides excellent external fixation for a variety of cervical spine injuries, most notably within the high cervical spine. For an experienced provider, the halo may provide quick and secure fixation while transitioning to surgery or as definitive treatment. This chapter details the indications and contraindications, placement, post-procedural care, and complications of the halo brace system.

KEYWORDS

Cervical fixation; external fixation; cervical spine fracture; neurointensive care unit (NICU); halo brace; traction; spinal stabilization.

INTRODUCTION

Cervical spine fractures are exceedingly common due to high-risk trauma mechanisms including motor vehicle collisions, fall from heights or even from ground level in the elderly. Current estimates place the incidence of cervical fracture at about 12/100,000/year.[1] Importantly, the incidence of cervical fracture has been increasing steadily in the geriatric (>65 years old) population.[2] Even without spinal cord injury (SCI), cervical fractures represent a source of increased morbidity for patients, especially the elderly, and require eventual surgical fixation in about 25% of cases.[3] However, more commonly, in about 70%, cervical spine fractures are managed with external fixation or bracing.

A variety of options exist for external fixation of the cervical spine. The basic options include soft collar, rigid collar, cervicothoracic orthosis (CTO), and the halo brace. Each method has specific advantages and disadvantages that must be weighed closely. In choosing a fixating device, the degree of fixation offered must be a primary consideration. The halo brace is preferred for inherently unstable injuries requiring a significant reduction in cervical spine motion. A halo can provide a 96% reduction in cervical flexion/extension and lateral bending as well as a 99% reduction in rotation. These reductions far exceed those obtained with a rigid collar or even a CTO.[4-6]

Significant reductions in motion resulting from the halo brace allow for fracture healing with preservation of range of motion at the conclusion of bracing. In contrast, surgical (internal) fixation and fusion of the cervical spine is likely to cause permanent decrements in cervical range of motion to varying degrees based on level.[3,7-10] Additional advantages to definitive treatment with external fixation include prevention of intra-operative injury to surrounding structures (i.e., vertebral artery) and anaesthesia risks associated with internal fixation.[11] Further, with simple modification of the halo ring, the halo brace allows the use of bedside traction for closed reduction of fractures, which is not possible with other forms of external fixation.[3] The disadvantages of halo brace utilization include: chance of malunion or non-union requiring subsequent surgical intervention, loss of alignment, risks of infection, skin breakdown, airway compromise, dysphagia, and increased morbidity and mortality in the elderly.[4,11–14]

While this chapter focuses on the application of the halo brace for traumatic cervical spine fractures, the brace may also be utilized in staged cervical spine procedures such as those to correct severe kyphotic deformities or basilar invagination of the dens.[15–17]

APPLIED ANATOMY AND PHYSIOLOGY

A basic understanding of cranial anatomy is required for successfully placing a halo brace, while limiting complications. As described further in the section 'Technique' the halo brace system (Figure 69.1) consists of a vest, a cranial ring, and four posts that anchor the ring to the vest. The ring is affixed to the head with four pins for adults (more pins often used for younger paediatric patients). The goal of pin placement is to minimize risk of skiving, slippage, and loosening as well as damage to a few critical structures.

In order to minimize slippage the pins should be placed perpendicular to the curvature of the skull with attention to avoid the slope of the forehead. Ideally, the ring will sit in line or just below with the equator of the head (Figure 69.2). For the two frontal pins, this is about 0.5 cm to 1 cm above the orbit, which also minimizes the risk of a pin slipping into the orbit during placement.[4] Often a computed tomography (CT) scan of the head is available to give the provider a more individualized understanding of the patient's anatomy. The frontal sinus should be avoided as a pin may easily fracture the outer table of the frontal sinus during tightening. The risk of violating the frontal sinus increases with more medial positioning of the frontal pins. Placing the pins too far lateral may result in the pin piercing the temporalis muscle superficially, which may lead to difficulty in control of bleeding or haematoma, especially in the coagulopathic trauma patient or those on anticoagulant medications. Deep to the temporalis muscle is the thin squamous portion of the temporal bone, which is also prone to fracture upon final tightening of the pins. Avoidance of both the frontal sinus and squamous temporal bone necessitates pin position roughly 0.5 cm to 1 cm superior to the lateral two-thirds of the eyebrow (Figure 69.2). This location may be considered safe from violation of neurovascular structures. The supratrochlear nerve and artery as well as the supraorbital nerve and artery exit the orbit within the medial third of the orbital ridge. Over-medialization of the frontal pins may place these structures at risk.[4]

The location of the posterior pins often will lie at about the 4 o'clock and 8 o'clock positions, superior and posterior to the pinna. The ring should sit about 1 cm above the pinna, as any contact may lead to skin breakdown over the course of treatment with the brace.[4]

INDICATIONS

In general, the halo brace is indicated for acute stabilization of an unstable high cervical spine fracture. Acute stabilization may serve simply as a transition to definitive surgical intervention, but in the correct patient, the halo may serve as a definitive treatment by itself. In the high cervical spine (occiput through C2), the halo is ideal for correcting fractures with angular and translation displacement about the fracture site (i.e., Type II/IIA Hangman's fracture of C2 or Type II dens fracture) while preserving rotational range of motion, compared with surgical fusion, following healing. Table 69.1 provides a summarization of the indications for halo brace use in the occipitoatlantoaxial spine.

Table 69.1 Summary of indications for halo bracing in the occipitoatlantoaxial spine

Atlanto-occipital junction	Atlanto-axial junction	C1	C2
Type III OCF*[8]	AA rotatory subluxation[15]	Fracture with disrupted TL[9]	Type II, IIA Hangman's fracture#[10]
AOD**[18]	Anterior AA subluxation[19]	Combined anterior and posterior arch fractures[9]	Type II or III odontoid fracture^[10]
		May be considered for combined C1/C2 fractures	
			Other unstable appearing C2 fracture with or without significant ligamentous injury

Abbreviations: OCF: occipital condyle fracture; *type III is associated with avulsion of transverse ligament; AOD: atlanto-occipital dislocation; **temporizing measure until fusion, primary management with high-risk mechanism, clinical suspicion and equivocal imaging findings; AA: atlanto-axial; TL: transverse ligament; #Type based on Levine grading;[3] ^grading on D'Alonzo and Anderson system,[20] surgery preferred if age >50 or severely displaced.

In the subaxial (C3–C7) cervical spine, the halo may be used again as temporary or definitive treatment in patients with a variety of injuries. However, surgical fixation may be preferred given a less severe loss of range of motion with subaxial fusion and a fairly significant quality of life burden for weeks to months (depending on the injury) in a halo brace. With that caveat, a halo ring may be used in traction to reduce unilateral or bilateral facet dislocation followed by fixation to the halo vest to maintain reduction prior to surgery. Primary management with the halo brace has been reported for unilateral facet dislocations, stable burst fractures, flexion-compression, and 'tear-drop' fractures.[4,21]

CONTRAINDICATIONS

The absolute contraindications to halo bracing include cranial fracture, extensive scalp lacerations or soft-tissue injury compromising pin placement and those who will likely require decompressive craniotomy or other cranial surgery necessitating halo removal without replacement.[4] Likewise, for those with recent craniotomies or synthetic bone plates, alternative management should be discussed thoroughly prior to placement of the halo.

Relative contraindications include barrel-chest habitus (related to chronic obstructive pulmonary disease or obesity), obesity, and imminent need for intubation. In those with SCI, loss of sensation over the chest and back may enhance skin breakdown as well as limit often diminished ability to fully expand the chest wall, increasing pulmonary complications.[4,12] In those aged greater than 65, the use of a halo brace should be weighed extensively against alternatives given the possibility of increased complications.[4,13,22,23]

EQUIPMENT

- Hair clippers
- Sterile collection cup
- Betadine solution
- Chlorhexidine gluconate skin preparation
- Lidocaine 1% or 2%
- Halo brace system (Figure 69.1)
- Calibrated torque wrench capable of 8- and 30-inch pounds settings

PRE-PROCEDURE PREPARATION

First, as for any procedure, informed consent should be obtained. Risks such as bleeding, infection, paralysis, and damage to surrounding structures should be outlined as well as more specific risks related to this procedure. Please see the Complications section for further detail.

A CT scan of the head should be completed before beginning the procedure to determine any areas of unexpectedly thin bone, lateral extents of the frontal sinus, and for confirmation of the absence of significant skull fractures or unexpected cranial findings which may alter pin placement. We recommend obtaining a CT scan of the cervical spine if the diagnosis of fracture was made on plain X-ray as the CT will provide further detail of fracture planes to assist in determining further course of treatment. If traction is planned and the patient is stabilized both haemodynamically and neurologically, we recommend magnetic resonance imaging of the cervical spine without contrast to locate potential extra-axial haematoma or intervertebral disc contents, which may impinge upon the spinal cord during fracture/dislocation reduction. A finding of extensive ligamentous damage may shift treatment paradigm towards surgical intervention rather than bracing.

The primary nurse for the patient should be informed of the procedure and present if able. Any staff that will be assisting with sedation as needed should also be present and prepared. Monitors should be applied and the nurse or other staff assisting should be monitoring the patient's vital signs. Additionally, the treating physician should consider advanced pre-procedure muscle relaxants including diazepam and/or cyclobenzaprine for any patient who is to undergo traction to relax the cervical musculature to improve the chance of reduction.

TECHNIQUE

Vest Placement

- Determine sizing of the vest based on either direct or estimated waist and chest at the xiphoid process and circumferences (sizes are brand-specific but based on these measurements). A well-fitted vest will have an antero-inferior border at the xiphoid process and postero-inferior border around T12.
- Place rods in posterior vest rod sockets and loosen prior to placing it under the patient.
- While maintaining cervical spine precautions log roll the patient, sliding the posterior vest as far as possible towards the opposite shoulder.
- Either log roll the patient in opposite direction as the previous step or simply pull the vest from under the patient such that it is at the centre with straps protruding at the shoulders and waist.

- Apply the anterior vest, inserting the white plastic bands into the associated plastic fasteners.
- Buckle the leather straps by counting holes such that waist buckles and shoulder buckles are symmetric.
- Ensure the vest is not over-tightened compromising pulmonary function; one should be able to fit a flat hand easily under the vest.[3,4]

Halo Ring Placement

- Determine pin sites—recall 0.5–1 cm above the lateral 2/3rd of the eyebrow, 4 and 8 o'clock positions posteriorly.
- Use hair clippers to clear the hair posteriorly (in patients with long hair, placing the hair in a pony-tail or braid will keep it out of the way of pin placement), otherwise wrap the pin in process of tightening.
- Place permanent pins in a sterile cup full of betadine solution.
- With chlorohexidine gluconate preparation swabs clean each pin site thoroughly (2–3 swabs).
- Pre-thread temporary pins into the halo ring.
- Position the halo ring such that it sits 0.5–1 cm above the brow line, 1 cm above the pinna and is close but below the equator of the head to minimize chance of slippage.
- Screw down temporary pins to hold in place.
- Inject local anaesthetic at planned permanent pin sites down to the periosteum.
- Have the patient close eyes tightly throughout permanent pin placement to prevent 'tacking-up' of the facial muscles with eyes open, leading to difficulty with eye closure post-procedure.
- Thread permanent pins to the skin; there should be very little resistance to threading. If resistance is encountered, reverse the direction and rethread (*do not force the pin*).
- Once all pins are against the skin, beginning posteriorly tighten with fingers until unable to thread further. Check frequently that the ring is maintaining a symmetric position about 1 cm off of skull, parallel to the axial plane, without contact of the pinna.
- Using the calibrated torque wrench set to 8-inch pounds, proceed in a crossed pin pattern (direction outlined by blue line in Figure 69.3) providing a 360-degree rotation at each pin until all are at 8-inch pounds (signified by clicking of the wrench).
- If one pin continues to turn/tighten 2–3 rotations after the remaining pins have clicked, stop. This may indicate that the screw has breached the skull, consider a CT scan to evaluate and determine whether to choose a new pin location or abort the procedure.
- Once all pins are torqued in place, tighten down nuts with finger strength.

Halo Ring Block and Rod Application

1. Use long block screws with washers to secure the blocks to the ring, do not fully tighten to allow for easier placement of rods (place only 1 screw on each side if planning traction).
2. If performing traction see steps 2a–c, if not skip to step 3:
   (a) Affix traction ring to halo ring through halo blocks using the remaining long block screw and washer such that both the blocks and traction ring are attached to the halo ring (Figure 69.4).
   (b) Set up traction apparatus pulley system to suspend weights.
   (c) Tie rope to the centre of halo traction ring, thread through the pulley and tie it to the weight carrying apparatus.
3. Thread rods through halo blocks and position head and spine to desired alignment.
4. Tighten halo block screws and rod set screws in place to 30-inch pounds. One may need to wait to tighten if performing traction with the goal of reduction, tighten as described when desired effect of traction is obtained to maintain alignment.

POST-PROCEDURE CARE

Immediate

Following the application of the halo, obtain anteroposterior (AP) and lateral cervical spine X-rays to assess alignment. Additionally, perform and document neurological examination in new alignment. Within 24–36 hours of halo placement the pins as well as the vest set screws should all be retorqued to 8- or 30-inch pounds, respectively. When doing this, it is imperative to loosen the nuts associated with each pin, retorque, and then retighten the nuts.

Pin Sites

On a daily basis the pin sites should be cleaned with soap (often we recommend baby shampoo), water, and q-tips. We recommend against the use of ointments, creams, and strong antiseptic washes at the pin sites. The patient will need significant help to shampoo and clean their hair. We recommend baby shampoo (or shampoo without perfumes, dyes or tints) and water, with specific attention to keeping the vest dry.

Vest Care

The patient should have a caregiver perform daily inspections underneath the waist straps, one at a time. At this time the area under the vest can be rinsed with plain water and dried well prior to refastening the straps. Do not ever loosen the shoulder straps. We recommend simply using a damp towel under the vest followed by a dry towel. The patient may wash in the bathtub as long as the water level stays below the vest. We recommend against using soaps, lotions, or powders under the vest as it often leads to skin irritation. The vest may need to be readjusted or switched out if the patient loses or gains a significant amount of weight during the course of treatment.

COMPLICATIONS

As with any procedure there is risk of bleeding, infection, reaction to materials used, or damage to the surrounding structures. Further complications can be categorized as immediate, late, and indirect.

Immediate

The most immediate complication that can be encountered is fracture or puncture of the skull with or without associated dural puncture in 1%–4% of cases.[4,24–26] This is often realized as one pin continues to turn well past where others became well seated. If this situation is encountered or there is a sudden loss of resistance to pin tightening, the pin should be removed and the tract investigated to assess for breach. A CT scan of the head may be obtained to assess the extent of probable fracture or puncture, which may need further evaluation and treatment. Depending on the extent of fracture, the pin may be relocated or the procedure may be aborted if no suitable alternative position exists or the fracture is extensive, requiring surgical intervention.[24] Puncture of the skull also puts the patient at risk for possible dural puncture, which may present as positional headache, cerebrospinal fluid rhinorrhoea, blurred vision, and/or nausea with or without vomiting.[4,24,26] Further, there may be leakage around the pin site. Careful review of the pre-procedure CT scan of the head and ensuring the torque wrench is set appropriately will help reduce the risk of this complication.

Immediate injury to the neurovascular structures can almost always be avoided with strict attention placing pins in the 'safe zones' as described previously. However,

at times aberrant anatomy is encountered or limited suitable pin sites exist due to extensive scalp injury and the more lateral supraorbital is injured (2%–3%) resulting in forehead and scalp numbness.[4,26] The patient should be counselled that this may be permanent but there is a small chance of recovery of sensation over the course of months to a year depending on the severity of the nerve injury.

Subacute to Late Complications

Pin loosening is the most common complication in adults occurring in 8% to 36% of patients.[14,26] The loose pin should be inspected for associated infection and retorqued if the alignment appears stable. In the event of multiple loose pins, alignment may need to be reassessed with plain films following retorque of the pins. We recommend routine clinic visits for patients using halo braces in order to ensure the pins are tight and can be retorqued if necessary.

Pin infections may occur in about 13%–20% of patients if metal pins are used.[14,26] Management of pin site infection is dependent on the depth and systemic signs. Local purulent drainage without cellulitis or systemic signs may be managed with daily cleaning and oral antibiotics, with or without pin removal depending on the clinician's judgement. If there is suspicion for pin site infection with associated cellulitis or systemic signs (fever, elevated white blood cell count), the pin must be removed and the patient started on intravenous antibiotics.[4] There should be a low threshold for cranial imaging, especially if associated meningitis or neurological signs exist, to assess for epidural abscess or subdural empyema.[27,28] A lumbar puncture may be required if there is high suspicion for the infected pin extending intracranially to assess for meningitis.

As discussed in post-procedure care, the skin contacted by the vest should be evaluated on a daily basis to avoid skin breakdown. Pressure necrosis related to the halo occurs in about 2% to 11% of cases and requires meticulous wound care.[4,26]

Indirect

Indirect complications are largely related to the alignment maintained by the halo and loss of subtle flexion and extension movement achieved by the occipitoatlantoaxial spine. If the patient does not have a protected airway prior to halo placement, the inpatient team will need to be prepared for a likely difficult intubation while fitting the halo brace. The patient will have nearly no ability to extend the neck and the additional hardware (rods and halo ring) can be daunting to the inexperienced intubating provider. A video laryngoscope or direct fibreoptic intubation cart's availability can be critical.[12,26]

Dysphagia is another often unanticipated complication that may occur in up to 11% of patients due to loss of subtle movements about the craniocervical junction required for normal swallowing mechanics.[12] These changes may predispose patients to aspiration and further pulmonary complications. Additional indirect complications include falls due to fixation of the patient's eyes in a position in which the ground cannot be visualized.

Overall, the use of the halo brace in elderly patients may encounter as much as a 3-fold increase in the number of complications leading to increased morbidity and mortality.[22] Sharpe and colleagues suggest this increased complication rate could be evident as early as 55 years old, given increased ICU days and greater mortality (13% vs. 0%).[13] The decision to pursue external rather than surgical fixation should be weighed heavily.[13,22,23]

CONCLUSIONS

Cervical spine fractures are increasingly managed by neurological and trauma intensive care units today. External fixation via the halo brace system provides an alternative to surgical fixation for a number of injuries. However, there are important nuances of placement, management, and complications to be aware of when using the halo system in practice. Becoming familiar with these nuances allows the intensive care provider to have an additional non-surgical method to provide a quick and secure external fixation of often critical cervical spine injuries prior to or in the absence of surgical fixation.

CONFLICTS OF INTEREST

There are no conflicts of interest.

REFERENCES

1. Fredo HL, Rizvi SA, Lied B, et al. The epidemiology of traumatic cervical spine fractures: a prospective population study from Norway. *Scand J Trauma Resusc Emerg Med* 2012;20:85.
2. Baidwan NK, Naranje SM. Epidemiology and recent trends of geriatric fractures presenting to the emergency department for United States population from year 2004–2014. *Public Health* 2017;142:64–9.
3. Greenberg MS. *Handbook of Neurosurgery*. 8th ed. New York: Thieme, 2016.
4. Bono CM. The halo fixator. *J Am Acad Orthop Surg* 2007;15(12):728–37.
5. Richter D, Latta LL, Milne EL, Varkarakis GM, Biedermann L, Ekkernkamp A, Ostermann PA. The stabilizing effects of different orthoses in the intact and unstable upper cervical spine: a cadaver study. *J Trauma* 2001;50(5):848–54.
6. Karimi MT, Kamali M, Fatoye F. Evaluation of the efficiency of cervical orthoses on cervical fracture: A review of literature. *J Craniovertebr Junction Spine* 2016;7(1):13–19.
7. Gelb DE, Aarabi B, Dhall SS, et al. Treatment of subaxial cervical spinal injuries. *Neurosurgery* 2013;72(Suppl 2):187–94.
8. Theodore N, Aarabi B, Dhall SS, et al. Occipital condyle fractures. *Neurosurgery* 2013;72(Suppl 2):106–13.
9. Ryken TC, Aarabi B, Dhall SS, et al. Management of isolated fractures of the atlas in adults. *Neurosurgery* 2013;72(Suppl 2):127–31.
10. Ryken TC, Hadley MN, Aarabi B, et al. Management of isolated fractures of the axis in adults. *Neurosurgery* 2013;72(Suppl 2):132–50.
11. Bransford RJ, Stevens DW, Uyeji S, et al. Halo vest treatment of cervical spine injuries: a success and survivorship analysis. *Spine (Phila Pa 1976)* 2009;34(15):1561–6.
12. Horn EM, Theodore N, Feiz-Erfan I, et al. Complications of halo fixation in the elderly. *J Neurosurg Spine.* 2006;5(1):46–9.
13. Sharpe JP, Magnotti LJ, Weinberg JA, et al. The old man and the C-spine fracture: Impact of halo vest stabilization in patients with blunt cervical spine fractures. *J Trauma Acute Care Surg* 2016;80(1):76–80.
14. Kraemer P, Lee MB, Englehardt H, et al. Infectious pin complication rates in halo vest fixators using ceramic versus metallic pins. *J Spinal Disord Tech* 2010;23(8):e59–62.
15. Govender S, Kumar KP. Staged reduction and stabilisation in chronic atlantoaxial rotatory fixation. *J Bone Joint Surg Br* 2002;84(5):727–31.
16. Nemani VM, Kim HJ, Bjerke-Kroll BT, et al. Preoperative halo-gravity traction for severe spinal deformities at an SRS-GOP site in West Africa: protocols, complications, and results. *Spine (Phila Pa 1976)* 2015;40(3):153–61.
17. Yang C, Wang H, Zheng Z, et al. Halo-gravity traction in the treatment of severe spinal deformity: a systematic review and meta-analysis. *Eur Spine J* 2017;26(7):1810–16.
18. Sears W, Fazl M. Prediction of stability of cervical spine fracture managed in the halo vest and indications for surgical intervention. *J Neurosurg* 1990;72(3):426–32.
19. Boakye M, Arrigo RT, Kalanithi PS, et al. Impact of age, injury severity score, and medical comorbidities on early complications after fusion and halo-vest immobilization for C2 fractures in older adults: a propensity score matched retrospective cohort study. *Spine (Phila Pa 1976)* 2012;37(10):854–9.
20. Majercik S, Tashjian RZ, Biffl WL, et al. Halo vest immobilization in the elderly: a death sentence? *J Trauma* 2005;59(2):350–6; discussion 356–8.

21. Cheong ML, Chan CY, Saw LB, et al. Pneumocranium secondary to halo vest pin penetration through an enlarged frontal sinus. *Eur Spine J* 2009;18(Suppl 2):269–71.

22. Menon KV, Al Rawi AE, Taif S, et al. Orbital roof fracture and orbital cellulitis secondary to halo pin penetration: case report. *Global Spine J* 2015;5(1):63–8.

23. Garfin SR, Botte MJ, Waters RL, et al. Complications in the use of the halo fixation device. *J Bone Joint Surg Am* 1986;68(3):320–5.

24. Botte MJ, Byrne TP, Abrams RA, et al. Halo skeletal fixation: techniques of application and prevention of complications. *J Am Acad Orthop Surg* 1996;4(1):44–53.

25. Goodman ML, Nelson PB. Brain abscess complicating the use of a halo orthosis. *Neurosurgery* 1987;20(1):27–30.

26. Horn EM, Feiz-Erfan I, Lekovic GP, et al. Survivors of occipitoatlantal dislocation injuries: imaging and clinical correlates. *J Neurosurg Spine* 2007;6(2): 113–20.

27. Dickman CA, Greene KA, Sonntag VK. Injuries involving the transverse atlantal ligament: classification and treatment guidelines based upon experience with 39 injuries. *Neurosurgery* 1996;38(1):44–50.

28. Anderson LD, D'Alonzo RT. Fractures of the odontoid process of the axis. *J Bone Joint Surg Am* 1974;56(8):1663–74.

Part XIX

Case Management

Editors: Charu Mahajan, Indu Kapoor, and Hemanshu Prabhakar

70

Adult Traumatic Brain Injury

G. S. Umamaheswara Rao

ABSTRACT

Traumatic brain injury (TBI) can be classified into primary injury that occurs at the time of accident and is not amenable to therapy and secondary brain injury that occurs as a result of systemic factors and intracranial epiphenomena. The course of secondary injury that ultimately culminates in cerebral ischaemia/hypoxia can be modified to some extent by intensive care management. The key components in intensive care management consists of good systemic care, rapid evacuation of significant mass lesions, identification and prompt management of raised intracranial pressure (ICP), optimization of cerebral blood flow (CBF) and cerebral oxygenation, and early identification and appropriate treatment of multisystem sequelae.

KEYWORDS

Head injury; adults; trauma; brain; contusions; closed injury; open injury; outcome.

CASE STUDY

A 45-year-old man met with a road traffic accident under the influence of alcohol. He had a brief period of unconsciousness from which he woke up. He was restless. He vomited twice and had a tonic-clonic seizure. He had right ear bleed. He was picked up by an ambulance. He received oxygen by mask during the transport.

In the emergency department, he had a Glasgow Coma Scale (GCS) score of E4, V4, and M5. His pupils were bilaterally normal in size and reacting to light. His blood pressure was 146/84 mmHg, pulse rate 96 bpm, and respiratory rate 28 breaths/min. His oxygen saturation on room air was 92%. The chest radiograph showed diffuse bilateral pulmonary congestion. A computed tomography (CT) scan of the head revealed a 2.5 cm extradural haematoma in the right temporoparietal region and a contusion in the left temporal region. As he was being prepared for a craniotomy, he became tachypnoeic and started to decerebrate. His right pupil dilated and became unresponsive to light. His trachea was immediately intubated and he was placed on a ventilator. He received 100 ml of 20% mannitol and 1.0 g of phenytoin. A right temporoparietal craniotomy was done and the extradural haematoma was evacuated. At the end of surgery, the brain was mildly tense and his right pupil still continued to be unreactive to light. His motor response improved to M3 on GCS and he was opening eyes to pain (E2 response). An intraventricular intracranial pressure (ICP) monitoring was started at the end of surgery. The initial ICP was 23 mmHg. Back in the intensive care unit (ICU), on the same pressure control level, as before surgery, his tidal volume dropped to 150 ml and he was very tachypnoeic. There was pink frothy secretion coming out of the endotracheal tube. On auscultation, there were extensive bilateral crepitations. An arterial blood gas (ABG) analysis revealed a pH of 7.501, PaO_2 of 42 mmHg, a $PaCO_2$ of 20 mmHg, and a HCO_3 of 17 mmol/L. An emergency chest radiograph showed bilateral pulmonary oedema. The positive end-expiratory pressure (PEEP) on the ventilator was increased to 10 cm H_2O and sedation increased to 100 µg/hr of fentanyl. The crepitations disappeared after 24 hours while the patient was on ventilator.

After 24 hours, the patient's GCS still remained E2, VT, and M3. His ICP was 24 mmHg. Another head CT scan showed a moderate increase in the size of the contusion in the left temporal region, a midline shift of 5 mm to the right and a hypodensity in the right posterior cerebral artery (PCA) territory. A left temporal craniotomy was done and the contusion decompressed. The bone flap was placed in the abdomen. With the decompression, the ICP came down to 18 mmHg, but the patient's neurological status remained unchanged.

INTRODUCTION

Head injury is a major cause of death among young adults and associated with a high degree of disability among the survivors. Head injury can occur in isolation or as a part of polytrauma. When it occurs as a part of polytrauma, the associated systemic effects can adversely affect the outcome of head trauma. Intensive management of these victims from the time of accident helps to decrease the preventable mortality and morbidity.[1]

PATHOLOGY

The pathological process that ensues subsequent to a traumatic injury is complex. The events that take place after trauma to the head may be broadly classified into *primary* and *secondary injury*. Primary injury is the injury to the brain and the other intracranial structures that occurs at the time of accident. The injury to the neurons that results from intracranial and extracranial events that follow primary injury is referred to as secondary injury.[2]

Primary Injury

The primary injury may take the form of a *diffuse injury*, which is characterized by the absence of any significant mass lesion on a CT scan, or a *focal injury*, which is characterized by the presence of mass lesions >25 ml on the CT scan.[3]

Diffuse Injury

Diffuse axonal injury (DAI) is the most common form of injury occurring in 56% of all head injuries. Of patients who die after a head injury, 90% have DAI. Any patient with traumatic coma lasting for more than 6 hours is considered to be having DAI. Mortality in this group of patients is about 24%.[4] Diffuse injuries are further classified into four categories based on the severity of injury to the brain as evaluated by the extent of midline shift and the patency of the basal cisterns on CT scan[5] (Table 70.1).

Table 70.1 Classification of diffuse injuries

	Type I	Type II	Type III	Type IV
Haematoma >25 ml	No	No	No	No
Compression of cisterns	No	No	Yes	Yes
Midline shift >5 mm	No	No	Yes	Yes
Incidence of intracranial hypertension	No	Variable	63%	100%
Mortality	10%	14%	34%	56%

Focal Injury

The common forms of focal lesions following head injury are extradural haematoma (EDH), subdural haematoma (SDH), and cerebral contusion.

Subdural haematoma

Subdural haematoma occurs in 24% of head injuries.[4] It is generally hyperdense on CT scan; 10% of these lesions may be isodense. Mortality in these patients was 50% if the clot measured more than 18 mm in thickness or caused more than 20 mm midline shift.[6]

Extradural haematoma

Extradural haematoma occurs less frequently than SDH; only 6% of patients of the traumatic coma databank (TCDB) had EDH.[4] The common sources of bleeding are skull fractures/arterial or venous injury. Mortality is nil in awake patients with EDH, 9% in obtunded patients, and 20% in patients with deep coma.[7]

Cerebral contusion

Cerebral contusion is seen in about 10% of head injuries.[4] The lesion is generally hyperdense on CT. It is common in frontal and temporal regions.

Secondary Injury

The epiphenomena that cause secondary injury may be intracerebral or extracerebral. The important intracranial causes of secondary injury are the biochemical changes that occur in the ischaemic brain, intracranial hypertension (IH) caused by brain oedema or brain swelling, cerebral vasospasm, seizures or intracranial infections. Hypoxia, hypotension, hypercapnia, hypocapnia, hyperthermia, electrolyte abnormalities, infection, and anaemia are some of the extracranial causes of secondary injury.[8]

PATHOPHYSIOLOGICAL CONSIDERATIONS

Some of the important intracranial pathophysiological events following head trauma are:

- Occurrence of delayed focal lesions such as EDH, SDH, and intracerebral haematomas and cerebral contusions
- Changes in cerebral metabolism
- Ischaemic/hyperaemic changes in CBF
- Elevation of ICP
- Cellular and molecular events

Delayed haematomas are known to occur in 1.5%–7% of patients up to two weeks following the injury. The majority of them occur within the first 48–72 hours.[9]

Cerebral metabolic rate of oxygen ($CMRO_2$) is decreased after head trauma. The extent of metabolic depression correlates well with the GCS.

Cerebral blood flow changes after head trauma can be divided into four phases:[10]

1. The first phase lasts up to 12 hours and is characterized by very low blood flow.
2. Next, within 24 hours, the blood flow increases rapidly to reach a hyperaemic level (absolute or relative). The hyperaemic phase lasts up to about 72 hours.
3. A phase of hypoperfusion then follows, lasting for about 15 days.
4. The delayed ischaemic phase is followed by a phase of recovery of CBF to values proportionate to the functional recovery of the brain.

The long-term neurological outcome of the patient depends on the degree of hypoperfusion during the early and delayed ischaemic phases. A variable degree of impairment of autoregulatory control of CBF also follows head trauma. The time course of autoregulatory impairment in head injury is not clearly understood. Vascular response to carbon dioxide (CO_2) is preserved till late in the course of head trauma. Loss of response to CO_2 predicts poor prognosis.

Raised ICP has been documented in 50%–70% of all severe head injuries.[11] Uncontrolled IH is responsible for 58% of mortality in head injuries. The common causes of raised ICP in head injury are: (1) mass lesions such as haematomas; (2) cerebral hyperaemia; (3) brain oedema—vasogenic and cytoxic; and (4) hydrocephalus due to blockade of cerebrospinal fluid (CSF) pathways in patients with posterior fossa haematomas or contusions.

The consequences of raised ICP are twofold: (1) Uncontrolled IH leads to cerebral ischaemia by decreasing cerebral perfusion pressure (CPP). (2) Differential pressure gradients in the various intracranial compartments lead to herniation of brain structures across the compartments leading to brainstem compression. The most common forms of herniation are: (1) transtentorial herniation of the uncus of the temporal lobe, (2) herniation of cerebellar tonsils through the foramen magnum, (3) subfalcine herniation of temporal lobe, and (4) herniation of the brain matter through open skull.[12]

Ischaemia after a TBI sets off a number of biochemical events that culminate in the death of neurons. Two important processes involved are necrosis that starts early and apoptosis that starts late but continues for a long time.[13]

INITIAL MANAGEMENT

The goals in initial management of a head-injured patient are to maintain adequate circulating blood volume, blood pressure (BP), oxygenation and ventilation, and to control ICP. Early post-injury episodes of hypotension and hypoxia have been correlated with poor outcome. Hypotension occurring at any point during the initial resuscitation or intensive care management is a powerful predictor of poor outcome.[14] Measures for reducing ICP, such as administration of mannitol and hyperventilation, are best reserved to patients who show evidence of herniation or rapid neurological deterioration.[15]

INTENSIVE CARE MANAGEMENT

The specific issues in the intensive care management of head injuries consists of:

- Optimization of extracranial organ function
- Control of IH
- Optimization of CPP
- Specific measures of cerebral protection
- Recognition and treatment of multi-system sequelae

Management of Extracranial Organ Function

Adequate management of extracranial organ function is essential to prevent secondary neuronal loss. This encompasses multisystem modalities.

Haemodynamic and Respiratory Management

Haemodynamic management in a head injured patient comprises maintaining normovolaemia and adequate mean arterial pressure (MAP) to achieve optimal CPP. Maintaining systolic blood pressure (SBP) at ≥100 mmHg for patients 50 to 69 years old or at ≥110 mmHg or above for patients 15 to 49 or over 70 years old may be considered to decrease mortality and improve outcomes.[15] Central venous pressure is ideally maintained around 5–10 mmHg. The injured brain is highly vulnerable to hypoxia. Both hypercapnia and hypocapnia are detrimental to injured neurons. Based on the evidence that cerebral ischaemia is responsible for poor outcome in head injury, measures that increase cerebral oxygen delivery have been tried to avert the ischaemic injury. Some publications showed a significant increase in brain tissue oxygen tension and decrease in brain tissue lactate concentration with hyperoxic (FiO$_2$ >0.6) ventilation in severe TBI.[16] Hyperoxia prevents cerebral oxygen desaturation caused by hyperventilation. Therefore, early during the course of management, it is logical to ventilate the patients with a high FiO$_2$, especially if hyperventilation is instituted.

Fluid Management

Many head-injured patients also have multisystem injuries that cause hypovolaemia. Vigorous fluid/blood resuscitation of these patients should not be withheld for the fear of enhancing brain oedema. Vigorous fluid resuscitation is not associated with any major adverse effect on either injured or uninjured brain.[17] Blood pressure should be maintained by transfusion of glucose-free, isotonic crystalloid solutions, albumin, blood, or blood products depending on the situation. Crystalloids, when used, should not be hypotonic; isotonic or hypertonic solutions alone should be used. Glucose-containing solutions should not be used during early resuscitation. Hypertonic solutions may have a role in resuscitation of a patient with haemorrhagic shock and head injury. Resuscitation with small volumes of hyperosmotic, hyperoncotic solutions has been shown to expand extracellular fluid volume, increase central venous pressure, and cardiac output without a significant rise in ICP. During intensive care management, excessive dehydration or overhydration must be avoided. Excessive urinary losses due to diuretics have to be replaced. If the serum sodium is higher than 140 mEq/L, 0.45% saline is used for maintenance therapy; if it is less than 140 mEq/L, isotonic saline is indicated. Potassium losses due to diuretic therapy need adequate replacement.[1]

Nutritional Support

The caloric requirement of critically ill patients is about 35–40 kcal/kg/day. Their protein requirement ranges from 1.5 to 2.0 g/kg/day. A caloric intake of 140% of metabolism in unparalysed patients and 100% in paralysed patients is recommended.[18]

Level IIA evidence of Brain Trauma Foundation (BTF) *Guidelines for the Management of Severe Traumatic Brain Injury* (hereafter BTF Guidelines), 4th Ed., recommends feeding patients to attain basal caloric replacement at least by the fifth day and at most by the seventh day post-injury to decrease mortality. Level IIB evidence suggests that transgastric or jejunal feeding is recommended to reduce the incidence of ventilator-associated pneumonia.[15]

Temperature Control

Hyperthermia is associated with an increase in CMRO$_2$. Therefore, normothermia should be targeted. Appropriate treatment of infections should be aimed. Symptomatic treatment of fever should consist of paracetamol use, cold saline infusion, and cooling blankets.[19]

Prophylaxis Against Thromboembolic Events

Level IIIA evidence of BTF Guidelines suggests that low molecular weight heparin (LMWH) or unfractionated heparin in a low dose may be combined with mechanical prophylaxis. The risk for expansion of intracranial haemorrhage exists with this regimen.[15]

Treatment of established pulmonary embolism with high-dose heparin is fraught with unacceptably high risk of intracranial haemorrhage at least for 7–14 days following head injury. A vena-caval filter is an alternative under such circumstances.

Seizure Prophylaxis

Post-traumatic seizures occur in a significant number of patients with severe head injury. These seizures may be classified as early (<7 days) and late (>7 days), the incidences of which are 4%–25% and 9%–42%, respectively. The risk factors for enhanced posttraumatic seizures are: GCS <10, cortical contusion, depressed skull fractures, SDH, EDH, intracerebral haematoma, penetrating injury, and seizures within 24 hours. Level IIA evidence from BTF Guidelines, Section 11 suggests that phenytoin or valproate given prophylactically is not recommended for preventing late post-traumatic seizures (PTS). Recommendation for phenytoin is only to decrease the incidence of early PTS occurring within 7 days of injury.

At the present time, there is insufficient evidence to recommend levetiracetam over phenytoin regarding efficacy in preventing early post-traumatic seizures and toxicity.[15]

Infection Prophylaxis

The major sources of infection in unconscious head-injured patients are respiratory tract, urinary tract, operative wounds, septicaemia, and meningitis. Antibiotic treatment must be based on appropriate microbiology reports.

Level IIA evidence from the BTF Guidelines Section 11 recommends early tracheostomy to reduce mechanical ventilation days. Early tracheostomy does not reduce the mortality or rate of nosocomial pneumonia. Oral care with povidone-iodine may cause an increased risk of acute respiratory distress syndrome and hence is not recommended. Level III evidence suggests that when external ventricular drainage is contemplated antimicrobial-impregnated catheters may be considered.[15]

Management of Intracranial Hypertension

Raised ICP is seen in 50%–70% of all patients with severe head injury. Evidence on the usefulness of routine ICP monitoring in severe head injury remains controversial. Level IIB evidence suggests mortality increases when ICP exceeds 22 mmHg and hence requires to be treated. At the same time level III evidence recommends that management decisions be made by a combination of ICP values as well as clinical and brain CT findings.[15] Contusions in temporal fossa or deep frontal region need to be treated even at a lower level because they may cause herniation even at a lower ICP level. The measures used to treat IH may be classified as general and specific.

General Measures

All extracranial parameters should be maintained within normal limits. Normovolaemia, adequate oxygenation (PaO_2 >90 mmHg), and ventilation ($PaCO_2$ ~ 32–35 mmHg) should be ensured. Fever increases ICP by several mmHg and needs to be treated rigorously. Head elevation by 15°–30° decreases ICP and also avoids ICP spikes by facilitating cerebral venous outflow. Before elevation of the head, normovolaemia should be ensured to prevent a decrease in MAP and CPP. The head should be maintained in a neutral position such that there is no pressure on the neck veins.

Seizure activity may increase ICP precipitously in a patient with raised ICP. The only indications of seizure activity in patients under pharmacologic paralysis are tachycardia, increased ICP, and fluctuation of BP. The most commonly used drug for seizure prophylaxis is phenytoin.[15]

Specific Measures
Hyperventilation

In the BTF Guidelines, Section 5 Level IIB evidence is available for this issue. Prolonged prophylactic hyperventilation with $PaCO_2$ of 25 mmHg is not recommended. Recommendations from the prior edition of BTF guidelines not supported by evidence meeting current standards are incorporated into the 4th ed. as well, which states that hyperventilation is recommended as a temporizing measure for the reduction of elevated ICP. Hyperventilation should be avoided during the first 24 hours after injury when CBF is often reduced critically. If hyperventilation is used, jugular venous oxygen saturation ($SjvO_2$) or brain tissue O_2 tension ($PbtO_2$) measurements are recommended to monitor cerebral oxygen delivery.[15]

Cerebrospinal fluid drainage

Only Level III evidence is available for this treatment, which recommends continuous drainage of CSF through an external ventricular drainage (EVD) system zeroed at the midbrain level. Intracranial pressure lowering may be considered by CSF drainage in patients with an initial GCS 6 during the first 12 hours after injury.[15]

Diuretics

Mannitol does not cross the intact blood–brain barrier (BBB). It is ideal if mannitol can be given under the control of ICP monitoring. In the absence of such monitoring, it may be administered only when the patients exhibits signs of herniation or progressive neurologic deterioration. Serum osmolality must be kept <320 mOsm/kg to avoid renal dysfunction associated with severe hyperosmolality. Euvolaemia should be maintained during mannitol administration.[15]

Sedatives and hypnotics

Level IIB evidence is available in BTF Guidelines, Section 6 for this subject. Burst suppression with barbiturates is not recommended. Intracranial hypertension refractory to maximum medical and surgical treatment can be attempted to be treated by high-dose barbiturate administration. Haemodynamic stability should be ensured during barbiturate therapy. Propofol controls ICP but caution is required as high-dose propofol can produce significant morbidity.[15]

Corticosteroids

Prompted by the results of a meta-analysis of 13 trials that indicated a marginal pooled risk reduction with steroids, a multicentre randomized controlled study of methyl prednisolone in acute severe head injury (the CRASH trial) was undertaken. An interim analysis after recruiting close to 10,000 patients showed increased mortality with the use of steroids.[20] Therefore, the current standard is that steroids are not recommended for improving outcome or reducing ICP in TBI.[15] At the same time, it is worth considering maintenance doses of hydrocortisone in patients having intractable hypotension despite adequate volume replacement and inotropes. Low circulating cortisol levels have been documented in some of these patients.[21]

Decompressive craniectomy

Where IH has not been amenable to maximum medical therapy, a decompressive craniectomy has been suggested to decrease the ICP. However, two major clinical trials have failed to show any beneficial effects on the outcome. The Decompressive Craniectomy [DECRA] trial reported an increase in mortality in the decompressed group compared to non-decompressed group, while the Randomised Evaluation of Surgery with Craniectomy for Uncontrollable Elevation of Intracranial Pressure (RESCUE-ICP) trial showed a decrease in mortality in the decompressed group, but an increased number of patients with severe disability.[22,23]

Evidence from Level IIA of the BTF Guidelines 4th ed. is available for this topic, which states that bifrontal decompressive craniectomy is not recommended to improve outcomes. However, this procedure reduces ICP and minimizes the days in the ICU. A large frontotemporoparietal craniectomy is recommended over a small craniectomy to decrease mortality and improve neurological outcomes.[15]

Management of Cerebral Perfusion Pressure

Cerebral perfusion pressure is defined as the difference between MAP and ICP. The lowest CPP that is adequate for a brain-injured patient remains controversial.

One strategy proposed by Rosner and colleagues suggested that CPP values higher than 70 mmHg improve outcome in adults. One clinical study by the group, where the CPP was maintained above 70 mmHg, reported 59% favourable outcome and 29% mortality.[24] The hypothesis that a CPP higher than 70 mmHg preserves CBF in the normal range is based on the assumptions that the lower limit of autoregulation is elevated in TBI and CPP is maintained in the autoregulatory range with rise in the BP. Both these assumptions are not founded on any strong evidence base. A second strategy proposed by a group of workers at Lund, Sweden, opposes maintenance of high CPP values, as CBF autoregulation and BBB are impaired in patients with TBI. Under these conditions, high MAP may increase brain oedema. Lower intravascular pressures are recommended by these workers to decrease brain oedema. Other therapeutic strategies suggested by the Lund group are: (1) to reduce capillary hydrostatic pressure by suppressing the stress response with metaprolol or clonidine, (2) to reduce cerebral blood volume with precapillary cerebral vasoconstrictors such as low dose thiopentone or dihydroergotamine, and (3) to preserve plasma colloid oncotic pressure by transfusing albumin. With this strategy, it was claimed that even lower CPP values (50 mmHg) are well tolerated with low mortality.[25]

In a study comparing the CBF-targeted management with ICP-targeted management, the CBF-targeted group had a lower incidence of secondary ischaemia but an increased risk of acute respiratory distress syndrome (ARDS). Thus the possible reduction of secondary ischaemia is offset by complications associated with maintenance of high BP.[26]

According to the BTF Guidelines, Level IIB, evidence suggests that a CPP value of 60 and 70 mmHg is necessary for survival and favourable outcomes. Whether 60 or 70 mmHg is optimal depends upon the patient's autoregulatory status. Level III evidence recommends that aggressive attempts to maintain CPP above 70 mmHg with fluids and pressors should be avoided as it entails the risk of ARDS.[15]

Cerebral Protective Interventions in Head Injury

All the specific protective therapies investigated have been uniformly disappointing. They include hypothermia,[27–29] selfotel, a competitive N-methyl-D-aspartate receptor (NMDA) blocker,[30] nimodipine[31] and free radical scavengers.[32,33] Level IIB evidence clearly states that hypothermia induced within 2.5 hours for 48 hours post injury does not improve outcomes in patients with diffuse injury.[15]

NEUROMONITORING IN HEAD INJURY

Intracranial Pressure Monitoring

The importance of raised ICP and measures to control it are discussed in the section management of IH. A randomized controlled trial conducted by a group of American researchers in Bolivia and Ecuador in 2012 showed that care focused on maintaining monitored ICP at 20 mmHg or less was not shown to be superior to care based on imaging and clinical examination.[34]

The BTF recommendations on ICP monitoring in head trauma are as follows: Level IIB evidence suggests that a reduction in in-hospital and 2-week post-injury mortality can be achieved by managing patients with information from ICP monitoring. Since there are no studies to support any new recommendation, the recommendations of the 3rd ed. are retained in the 4th ed. too. The following are the recommendations from the 3rd ed.:[35]

- ICP should be monitored in patients with a severe TBI (with post-resuscitation GCS of 3–8) and an abnormal CT scan which reveals haematomas, contusions, swelling, herniation, or compressed basal cisterns.
- In patients with a normal CT scan and severe TBI, ICP monitoring is indicated if two or more of the following features are present: age over 40 years, unilateral or bilateral motor posturing, or SBP <90 mmHg.[15]

A wide range of devices can be used to monitor ICP. The ventricular catheter connected to a pressure transducer is currently the most accurate, low-cost, and reliable monitor for ICP. Parenchymal ICP monitoring with fibreoptic or strain-gauge-tip catheter is comparable to ventricular pressure monitoring, but has a potential for drift after a few days. Subarachnoid, subdural, and epidural monitors are less accurate. As for the threshold for treatment of raised ICP, it is 22 mmHg.[15] Interpretation and treatment of ICP, based on any threshold should be corroborated with frequent clinical examination and cerebral perfusion data.

Jugular Venous Oximetry

Simultaneous monitoring of SjvO$_2$ and arterial oxygen saturation gives information on 'demand vs supply' of oxygen to the brain. Correction of the common causes of decrease in SjvO$_2$ (hypoxia, hypovolaemia, hypotension, anaemia, intracranial hypertension) helps to optimize cerebral oxygen delivery. It must, however, be remembered that SjvO$_2$ is only a global estimate of the adequacy of CBF and focal events cannot be detected by this technique.[36]

Transcranial Doppler

Transcranial Doppler (TCD) examination with a 2 MHz probe is a non-invasive technique for obtaining CBF velocities. Middle cerebral artery is commonly chosen for examination as it can be easily insonated and 75%–80% of ipsilateral carotid blood flows through it. In head-injured patients TCD is useful: (1) as a non-invasive monitor of CBF, (2) to diagnose post-traumatic vasospasm, and (3) for indirect estimation of ICP or CPP.

Changes in the morphology of flow velocity waveform with increasing ICP may be used for semi-quantitative assessment of ICP. With an increase in ICP, the diastolic velocity decreases and the pulsatility index (PI) increases. When the ICP is higher than the diastolic blood pressure but lower than the systolic pressure, a biphasic (oscillatory) pattern occurs followed later by a total disappearance of the waveform with intracranial circulatory arrest.[37]

Brain Tissue Oxygen Tension Monitoring

Direct monitoring of PbtO$_2$ with miniature probes placed into brain parenchyma is currently under investigation. One study reported that poor outcome in TBI is related to the duration for which the PbtO$_2$ was less than 15 mmHg or the occurrence of even a single episode of PbtO$_2$ less than 6 mmHg.[38] Another study reported a good correlation between SjvO$_2$ and PbtO$_2$ only in normal brain and not in the brain areas with pathology.[39]

MULTISYSTEMIC SEQUELAE OF HEAD INJURY

Head injury precipitates a number of multisystemic complications. Some of the important complications are described below.

Apart from hypertension and tachycardia, which are most commonly seen, sinus arrhythmia, atrial fibrillation, premature ventricular contraction, heart block, and ventricular tachycardia may also occur. Electrocardiography (ECG) changes of myocardial ischaemia such as depressed ST, inverted/flattened T, and peaked P, prolonged QT, and prominent U waves may also be evidenced in some patients. Supraventricular tachycardia has been correlated with elevated creatine kinase-muscle/brain (CK-MB) levels.

Hypoxaemia, which is commonly seen in head-injured patients and related to the depth of coma may have a diverse aetiology: (1) abnormal respiratory patterns, (2) respiratory infection, (3) altered V/Q relationships, and (4) neurogenic pulmonary oedema.

Hyponatraemia most frequently follows head injury. In turn, it also worsens the outcome of head injury. Hyponatraemia may be associated with normovolaemia, hypovolaemia or hypervolaemia. The commonest cause of normovolaemic hyponatraemia is the syndrome of inappropriate antidiuretic hormone secretion (SIADH) diagnosed by: (1) serum sodium <135 mmol/L, (2) serum osmolality <280 mOsm/kg, (3) urinary osmolality greater than serum osmolality, and (4) urinary sodium >40 mmol/L. Treatment of this condition consists of restriction of intake by 800–1000 ml/day. If the serum sodium is <120 mmol/L, correction by 0.9% or 3% sodium solution is indicated restricting the rate of rise of serum sodium to 1–2 mmol/L/hour until serum sodium reaches 130 mmol/L. Where fluid restriction is not possible, demeclocycline (300 mg oral every 6 hours) or fludrocortisone (0.1–0.2 mg oral/day) may be used. Hypovolaemic hyponatraemia is usually a result of cerebral salt wasting syndrome (CSWS). This syndrome is characterized by loss of both water and sodium through the kidney. Treatment of this condition consists of replacement of both water as well as sodium. Hypervolaemic hyponatraemia is not directly related to the trauma but is usually caused by cirrhosis, congestive heart failure, or renal failure. Hyponatraemia in these cases is usually dilutional and therapy should be directed at the underlying pathology.

Hypernatraemia in head-injured patients may be secondary to diabetes insipidus (DI) or severe dehydration. Central DI presents with polyuria, polydyspsia, hypernatraemia, hyperosmolality, and low urinary specific gravity. Treatment of DI consists of replacement of free water (hypotonic saline), aqueous vasopressin, or desmopressin as required.[40]

Hyperglycaemia in head injured patients is correlated with poor outcome.[41]

In patients with TBI, endothelial damage stimulates the intrinsic coagulation pathway. At the same time, release of thromboplastin from the injured brain also stimulates the extrinsic pathway. Both these processes might culminate in disseminated intravascular coagulation (DIC).

Gastric ulceration, gastroparesis, and swallowing disorders are common in patients with head injury. Gastric paresis may interfere with initiation and maintenance of enteral nutrition.[42]

THE IMPACT OF BRAIN TRAUMA FOUNDATION GUIDELINES (THIRD EDITION) ON THE OUTCOME OF TBI

The 4th edition of the BTF Guidelines was published in 2016. While it is interesting to see how these guidelines will affect the outcome of TBI in future, it is worthwhile to take a look at the reports of the effect of implementation of the 3rd ed. on the outcome of TBI.[35]

In patients with severe TBI treated for IH, the use of an ICP monitor was associated with significantly lower mortality when compared with patients treated without an ICP monitor. Based on these findings, the authors conclude that therapy in patients with severe TBI should be guided by ICP monitoring.[43] In another study, compliance with BTF ICP monitoring guidelines third edition was 46.8%. Patients managed according to the BTF ICP guidelines experienced significantly improved survival.[32] There was a significant reduction in TBI mortality between 2001 and 2009 in New York State. Increase in guidelines adherence occurred at the same time as the pronounced decrease in 2-week mortality and decreased rate of intracranial hypertension suggesting a causal relationship between guidelines adherence and improved outcomes.[33] Another study reported that patients with ICP monitoring based on BTF Guidelines experienced longer hospital length of stay, longer ICU stay, and more ventilator days compared with those without ICP monitors.[44] The time indices (the percentage of time for which the CPP was maintained at a given level) for CPP ≥70 and <50 mmHg were associated with decreased and increased mortality, respectively.[45] In another similar study, following adjustment for age, Abbreviated Injury Scale (AIS) head, and GCS motor score, patients with 55%–75% compliance and >75% compliance had reduced odds of mortality, as compared to <55% compliance to the BTF Guidelines. When the unadjusted rate of mortality was compared across the compliance spectrum, the odds of mortality decreased as compliance increased until 75%, and then reversed.[46]

There are also reports that suggest that there is a subset of patients meeting BTF criteria for ICP monitoring that do well without ICP monitoring.[47]

OUTCOME

Some of the powerful predictors of outcome are the age of the patient, GCS at admission, pupillary reactivity, CT findings, and co-existing systemic diseases. In a series of 202 patients provided intensive care in our hospital, mortality was 31%. Initial GCS, haemodynamic instability, and effacement of basal cisterns on CT scan were the independent predictors of mortality.[48] In another series of 127 patients who required surgical interventions, univariate analysis showed that age >40 years, preoperative GCS <8, bilateral absence of pupillary reactivity, subdural haematoma, tense brain at the end of surgery, and large volume of intraoperative fluid administration were the factors that had significant correlation with the poor outcome defined as lack of improvement or worsening of neurological status during the patient's hospital stay.[49]

CONCLUSION

In conclusion, management of head-injured patients comprises good systemic care, rapid evacuation of significant mass lesions, identification and prompt management of raised ICP, optimization of CBF and cerebral oxygenation, and early identification and appropriate treatment of multisystem sequelae. While the primary injury may not be amenable for therapeutic manipulation, secondary insults are eminently avoidable.

REFERENCES

1. Haddad SH, Arabi YM. Critical care management of severe traumatic brain injury in adults. *Scand J Trauma Resusc Emerg Med* 2012;20:12.

2. Werner C, Engelhard K. Pathophysiology of traumatic brain injury. *Br J Anaesth* 2007;99:4–9.

3. Moppett LK. Traumatic brain injury: assessment, resuscitation and early management. *Br J Anaesth* 2007;99:18–31.

4. Foulkes M, Eisenberg HM, Jane JA, et al. The traumatic coma data bank: Design, methods and baseline characteristics. *J Neurosurg* 1991;75(Suppl):S8–S13.

5. Marshall LF, Marshall SB, Klauber MR, et al. A new classification of head injury based on computerized tomography. *J Neurosurg* 1991;75:S14–S20.

6. Zumkeller M, Behrmann R, Heissler HE, et al. Computed tomographic criteria and survival rates for patients with acute subdural haematoma. *Neurosurgery* 1996;39:708–12.

7. Servadei F. Prognostic factors in severely head injured adult patients with epidural haematoma. *Acta Neurochir* 1997;139:273–8.

8. Reed AR, Welsh DG. Secondary injury in traumatic brain injury patients—a prospective study. *S Afr Med J* 2002 Mar;92:221–4.

9. Cooper PR. Post-traumatic intracranial mass lesions. In: Cooper PR, ed. *Head Injury*. 3rd Ed. Baltimore: Williams and Wilkins, 1993: pp. 275–329.

10. Doberstein C, Martin NA. Cerebral blood flow in clinical neurosurgery. In: Yoemens, ed. *Neurological Surgery*. 4th Ed. vol 1. Philadelphia: W.B. Saunders, 1996: pp. 519–69.

11. Miller JD, Butterworth JE, Gudeman SK, et al. Further experience in the management of severe head injury. *J Neurosurg* 1981;54:289–99.

12. Stevens RD, Shoykhet M, Cadena R. Emergency neurological life support: Intracranial hypertension and herniation. *Neurocrit Care* 2015;23(Suppl 2): S76–S82.

13. Mennel HD, El-Abhar H, Schilling M, Bausch J, Krieglstein J. Morphology of tissue damage caused by permanent occlusion of middle cerebral artery in mice. *Exp Toxicol Pathol* 2000 Oct;52(5):395–404.

14. Chestnut RM, Marshall LF, Klauber MR, et al. The role of secondary brain injury in determining the outcome of severe head injury. *J Trauma* 1993;34:216–22.

15. Guidelines for the management of severe TBI. 4th ed. [cited 2016 Dec 25]. Available from: https://braintrauma. org/guidelines/guidelines-for-the-management-of-severe-tbi-4th-ed#/.

16. Menzel M, Doppenberg EM, Zauner A, et al. Increased inspired oxygen concentration as a factor in improved brain tissue oxygenation and tissue lactate levels after severe head injury. *J Neurosurg* 1999;91:1–10.

17. Warner DS, Boehland LA. Effects of iso-osmolal intravenous fluid therapy on post-ischemic brain water content in the rat. *Anesthesiology* 1988;68:86–91.

18. Clifton GL, Robertson CS, Choi SC. Assessment of nutritional requirements of head-injured patients. *J Neurosurg* 1986 Jun;64(6):895–901.

19. Kilpatrick MM, Lowry DW, Firlik AD, Yonas H, Marion DW. Hyperthermia in the neurosurgical intensive care unit. *Neurosurgery* 2000 Oct;47(4):850–5.

20. Edwards P, Arango M, Balica L, et al. Final results of MRC CRASH, a randomised placebo-controlled trial of intravenous corticosteroid in adults with head injury-outcomes at 6 months. *Lancet* 2005;365:1957–9.

21. Cohan P1, Wang C, McArthur DL, et al. Acute secondary adrenal insufficiency after traumatic brain injury: a prospective study. *Crit Care Med* 2005 Oct;33(10):2358–66.

22. Cooper DJ, Rosenfeld JV, Murray L, et al. Decompressive craniectomy in diffuse traumatic brain injury. *N Engl J Med* 2011;364:1493–502.

23. Hutchinson PJ, Kolias AG, Timofeev IS, et al. Trial of decompressive craniectomy for traumatic intracranial hypertension. *N Engl J Med* 2016;375:1119–30.

24. Rosner MJ, Rosner SD, Johnson AH. Cerebral perfusion pressure: Management protocol and clinical results. *J Neurosurg* 1995;83:949–62.

25. Eker C, Asgeirsson B, Grande PO, et al. Improved outcome after severe head injury with a new therapy based on principles for brain volume regulation and preserved microcirculation. *Crit Care Med* 1998;26:1881–6.

26. Robertson CS, Valadka AB, Hannay HJ, et al. Prevention of secondary insults after severe head injury. *Crit Care Med* 1999;27:2086–95.

27. Clark RS, Kochanek PM, Marion DW, et al. Mild post-traumatic hypothermia reduces mortality after severe

controlled cortical impact in rats. *J Cereb Blood Flow Metab* 1996;16:253–61.

28. Clifton GL, Miller ER, Choi SC, et al. Lack of effect of induction of hypothermia after acute brain injury. *N Engl J Med* 2001;344:556–63.

29. Hutchison JS, Ward RE, Lacroix J, et al. Hypothermia therapy after traumatic brain injury in children. *N Engl J Med* 2008;358:2447–56.

30. Morris GF, Bullock R, Marshall SB, et al. Failure of the competitive N-methyl-D-aspartate antagonist Selfotel (CGS 19755) in the treatment of severe head injury results of two Phase III clinical trials. *J Neurosurg* 1999;91:737–43.

31. Harders A, Kakareika A, Braakman R. The German SAH study group: Traumatic subarachnoid haemorrhage and its treatment with nimodipine. *J Neurosurg* 1996;85:82–9.

32. Talving P, Karamanos E, Teixeira PG, et al. Intracranial pressure monitoring in severe head injury: compliance with Brain Trauma Foundation guidelines and effect on outcomes: a prospective study. *J Neurosurg* 2013;119:1248–54.

33. Gerber LM, Chiu YL, Carney N, Härtl R, Ghajar J. Marked reduction in mortality in patients with severe traumatic brain injury. *J Neurosurg* 2013;119:1583.

34. Chesnut RM, Temkin N, Carney N, et al. A trial of intracranial-pressure monitoring in traumatic brain injury. *N Engl J Med* 2012;367:2471–81.

35. Guidelines for the management of severe traumatic brain injury. 3rd ed. VI. Indications for Intracranial Pressure Monitoring. *J Neurotrauma* 2007;24(suppl 1):S1–S106.

36. Matta BF, Lam AM, Mayberg TS, Shapira Y, Winn HR. A critique of the intraoperative use of jugular venous bulb catheters during neurosurgical procedures. *Anesth Analg* 1994;79:745–50.

37. Hassler W, Steinmetz H, Gawlowski J. Transcranial Doppler ultrasonography in raised intracranial pressure and intracranial circulatory arrest. *J Neurosurg* 1988; 68:745–51.

38. Van den Brink WA, van Sant Brink, Steyerberg EW, et al. Brain oxygen tension in severe head injury. *Neurosurgery* 2000;46:868–76.

39. Gopinath SP, Valadka AB, Uzura M, et al. Comparison of jugular venous oxygen saturation and brain tissue PO2 as monitors of cerebral ischemia after head injury. *Crit Care Med* 1999;27:2337–45.

40. Bradshaw K, Smith M. Disorders of sodium balance after brain injury. *Continuing Education in Anaesthesia Critical Care & Pain* 2008;8:129–33.

41. Alvis-Miranda HR, Navas-Marrugo SZ, Velasquez-Loperena RA, et al. Effects of glycemic level on outcome of patients with traumatic brain injury: a retrospective cohort study. *Bull Emerg Trauma* 2014;2:65–71.

42. Tan M, Zhu JC, Yin HH. Enteral nutrition in patients with severe traumatic brain injury: reasons for intolerance and medical management. *Br J Neurosurg* 2011;25:2–8.

43. Farahvar A, Gerber LM, Chiu YL, et al. Increased mortality in patients with severe traumatic brain injury treated without intracranial pressure monitoring. *J Neurosurg* 2012;117:729–34.

44. Alkhoury F, Kyriakides TC. Intracranial pressure monitoring in children with severe traumatic brain injury: national trauma data bank-based review of outcomes. *JAMA Surg* 2014;149:544–8.

45. Griesdale DE, Örtenwall V, Norena M, et al. Adherence to guidelines for management of cerebral perfusion pressure and outcome in patients who have severe traumatic brain injury. *J Crit Care* 2015;30:111–5.

46. Lee JC, Rittenhouse K, Bupp K, et al. An analysis of Brain Trauma Foundation traumatic brain injury guideline compliance and patient outcome. *Injury* 2015;46:854–8.

47. Tang A, Pandit V, Fennell V, et al. Intracranial pressure monitor in patients with traumatic brain injury. *J Surg Res* 2015;194:565–70.

48. Santhanam R, Pillai SV, Sastry KVR, Umamaheswara Rao GS. Intensive care management of head injury patients without routine intracranial pressure monitoring. *Neurology India* 2007;55:349–54.

49. Basavaraj KG, Venkatesh HK, Umamaheswara Rao GS. A prospective study of demography and outcome in operated head injuries. *Indian J Anaesth* 2005; 49(1):24–30.

71

Paediatric Traumatic Brain Injury

G. S. Umamaheswara Rao

ABSTRACT

Primary injury that occurs at the time of an accident may or may not be amenable to therapy, but a lot can be done to avert secondary injury by attending to the cardiorespiratory parameters in time and good systemic management. Management of intracranial dynamics is more complex in children than in adults because age-specific targets for physiological parameters are not very clear. The Brain Trauma Foundation (BTF) has evolved guidelines for management of paediatric traumatic brain injury (TBI) in 2012 (2nd edition). There is literature to suggest that following these evidence-based guidelines improves the favourable outcomes and averts unfavourable outcomes.

KEYWORDS

Head injury; children; infants; trauma; brain; contusions; closed injury; open injury; outcome.

CASE STUDY

A 4-year-old child weighing 20 kg fell down from the first floor of the house. The child was restless for half an hour and then became unconscious and vomited twice. She developed a tonic-clonic seizure lasting for two minutes en route to the hospital. After an hour when she was in the emergency department of the hospital, her heart rate was 60 bpm, blood pressure (BP) 60/40 mmHg, respiratory rate was 45 breaths per minute and airway obstructed. Her systemic examination revealed a swollen right thigh. On neurological examination, she had a Glasgow Coma Scale (GCS) score of E1, V1, and M3. Her right pupil was 4 mm in size and not reacting to light and her left pupil was 3 mm in size and sluggishly reacting to light. Computed tomography (CT) scan of the brain revealed a thin subdural haematoma, gross oedema of the right cerebral hemisphere, a midline shift of 5 mm with effaced sulci, and basal cisterns. Her chest radiograph was normal and a radiograph of the right thigh revealed a closed fracture shaft of the femur. Her cervical spine radiograph was normal. The haemogram showed a haemoglobin concentration of 6 g/dL. Her blood glucose was 126 mg/dL, serum sodium 142 mmol/L, serum potassium 4.2 mmol/L, blood urea 30 mg/dL, and serum creatinine 0.8 mg/dL. Her liver function tests were within normal limits.

Two intravenous lines were established and 400 ml of normal saline was administered. Blood was sent for grouping and cross matching. In the meantime, airway was established with a 6-mm cuffed endotracheal tube after administering propofol 40 mg intravenously. Sedation was started with fentanyl 1.0 µg/kg/hr. The child was mechanically ventilated with an FiO_2 of 0.4 and the minute volume adjusted to achieve a $PaCO_2$ level of 35 mmHg. Mannitol was administered at a bolus dose of 50 ml. At this point of time the child was shifted to the neurosurgical intensive care unit.

In the intensive care unit (ICU), 400 ml of packed red blood cells (PRBCs) were transfused to correct anaemia. Immediately after shifting the child to the ICU an external ventricular drain (EVD) was established and it was connected to a pressure transducer placed at the level of the tragus to monitor the intracranial pressure (ICP). The initial ICP value was 19 mmHg which gradually increased to 25 mmHg over the next one hour. Cerebrospinal fluid (CSF) was drained through the EVD with which the ICP decreased to 15 mmHg. However, the ICP increased to 25 mmHg after half an hour. At this time, opening the EVD was not useful in decreasing the ICP to less than 20 mmHg. Fifty millilitres of 20% mannitol was administered and the ICP came down to 18 mmHg within

15 minutes, but the effect lasted only for one hour and again the ICP went up to 30 mmHg. Repeat doses of mannitol was not effective in decreasing the ICP. Her BP was stable and blood gases were normal. She was adequately sedated. A CT scan of the head was repeated which showed an increase in brain oedema and a small increase in the subdural haematoma. Since the ICP was refractory to the first line measures and also to mannitol, a decompressive craniectomy was carried out under general anaesthesia.

With decompressive craniectomy, the ICP decreased to 17 mmHg. The patient was shifted back to the ICU and ICP monitoring was continued. Her neurological status remained E2, VT, and M5, pupils were reacting to light, heart rate was 100 bpm, BP was 110/70 mmHg, and her blood gases were normal on the ventilator. The child went through an episode of meningitis and recovered to E4, V4, and M6 in three months' time.

INTRODUCTION

Paediatric head injury has some distinctive features which differentiate it from adult head injury. The mechanisms of injury are different. The pathophysiological features of the injured brain are influenced by unique characteristics of the paediatric brain. Injury may interfere with the normal growth of the child. Similarly, neuronal plasticity might influence the outcome. Furthermore, the immature brain seems more vulnerable to physiological insults.[1] However, there is paucity of literature on age-related specific physiological targets.

PATHOPHYSIOLOGY OF BRAIN TRAUMA IN CHILDREN

The chances of head deformability are higher in children owing to open fontanelles. The ICP buffering capacity is good in children before fontanelle closure. The volume of the brain is only 25% of the adult brain soon after birth, however, it reaches 75% of its adult size at the age of one year. Cerebral oxygen consumption is low at birth, but rises during development proportional to cerebral growth. In order to provide substrates necessary for the elevated energy metabolism, cerebral blood flow (CBF) in children is higher than in adults.[2]

In a child, the cisterns and ventricles are small, and the cortical sulci are tight, in proportion to the total intracranial volume. These reduced compensatory capabilities in the infant brain account for reduced intracranial compliance. The immature brain seems more vulnerable to insults, including trauma. The occurrence of brain swelling in children is greater than in adults.[3]

Different mechanisms of injury are predominant at specific ages. Diffuse axonal injury (DAI), for instance in the form of 'shaken baby syndrome' is more common in the first months of life while epidural haematomas due to falls are seen in the first years. In adolescents, the injuries are largely similar to those seen in adults where predominant findings include contusions and DAI.

Traumatic brain injury occurs in two phases: Primary injury that occurs at the site of accident and secondary injury that is caused by both intracranial epiphenomena including inflammatory and excitotoxic processes that lead to brain oedema and raised ICP. In addition, extracranial complications such as hypotension, hypertension, hypoxia, hypercapnia, hyperglycaemia, fluid and electrolyte disturbances, anaemia, fever, seizures, and intracranial infections also add insult to the primary injury. Primary injury is more or less irreversible. Therefore, the emphasis while managing the brain-injured patients in the hospital is on prevention of secondary insults.[4]

ASPECTS OF MANAGEMENT OF HEAD INJURY

Initial Care

Cervical Spine Care

Cervical spine injury must be ruled out in all head-injured patients. In young children, the cervical spine has the highest mobility at C1–C3 and after 12 years, the movement occurs at C5–C6. In infants under 6 months of age, the head and cervical spine should be immobilized using a spine board with tape across the forehead and towels around the neck. In children over 6 months of age, the head should be immobilized in the same manner or by using a rigid cervical collar.[5]

Airway Management

Children with a GCS score of 8 or less should have their trachea intubated. The anterior part of the rigid collar can be removed to facilitate cricoid pressure. Manual in-line stabilization is given by a trained medical assistant. The most common technique of establishing an airway is to administer preoxygenation, induce anaesthesia, and perform an orotracheal intubation. Nasotracheal intubation is contraindicated in patients with faciomaxillary injuries.[5]

Systemic and Cerebral Haemodynamics

In adults the impact of hypoxia and arterial hypotension has been documented in the last 20 years. Paediatric guidelines also confirm that these insults are associated with worse outcome in paediatric TBI.[6] Avoidance of hypoxia and hypotension is of paramount importance. Lower limit of systolic blood pressure for age may be estimated by the formula 70 mmHg + (2 × age in years). The exact cerebral perfusion pressure (CPP) to be maintained in a paediatric patient is not known. Maintaining a CPP of >50 mmHg in children aged over 6 years and >40 mmHg in children up to the age of 5 years seems to be reasonable. In a report of 188 children, no patient with a CPP less than 40 mmHg survived.[7]

Paediatric patients are more likely to survive if transported immediately to a paediatric trauma centre compared to any other type of centre.

Severity Assessment

The severity of injury can be assessed by a combination of clinical evaluation and a CT scan. For older children GCS is used. For smaller children various paediatric coma scales have been proposed. A combination of clinical, instrumental, and imaging data in prognosticating the outcome has been investigated. A combination of motor response, pupillary changes, age, and CT scan findings seem to be helpful in prognosticating the outcome. An early CT scan might miss mass lesions which might take some time to develop.[8]

Surgical Mass Lesions

Extradural haematomas are very common in falls, which is the commonest mode of injury in children. Subdural haematomas and cerebral contusions occur less frequently. Surgery should be carried out rapidly to save mortality and morbidity.

Intensive Care Management

Maintenance of normal oxygenation, arterial pressure, and normal laboratory values is the main objective of intensive care. Normoglycaemia has to be maintained. However, tight glycaemic control is associated with the risk of hypoglycaemic episodes. Hence, it is recommended to use a pragmatic approach in controlling blood glucose levels.[4]

Intracranial Pressure Monitoring and Control

Despite lack of studies providing unquestionable evidence, ICP monitoring has become the standard of care at least in the western ICUs. When children are at risk for intracranial hypertension (IH), the devastating consequences of raised

and sustained ICP should be balanced against the relatively low risks of ICP monitoring in experienced hands. Without measurement of ICP it becomes impossible to maintain CPP, optimize oxygen delivery, and prevent cerebral herniation. The thresholds for treatment of raised ICP are controversial for the paediatric age group. In children below the age of 2 years, ICP of 4–10 mmHg is considered as normal. After the age of 2 years, values of 20 mmHg are considered as threshold for therapy. Level III evidence from the Second Edition of Brain Trauma Foundation Guidelines (BTF Guidelines) 2012 advocates that the use of ICP monitoring may be considered in infants and children with severe TBI and treatment of ICP may be considered at a threshold of 20 mmHg.[9]

CPP Control

There is significant controversy regarding the CPP values at different ages. The BTF Guidelines suggest 40 mmHg for neonates. A value of 50 mmHg for patients below 5 years and 60 mmHg after this age may be appropriate.[10]

CSF Drainage

Level III evidence from the BTF Guidelines suggests that CSF through an EVD may be considered in the management of increased ICP in children with severe TBI. The addition of a lumbar drain may be considered in case of refractory IH with a functioning EVD, open basal cisterns, and no evidence of a mass lesion or shift on imaging studies.[11]

Hyperosmolar Therapy

Level II evidence suggests that hypertonic saline should be considered for the treatment of intracranial hypertension. Effective doses for acute use range between 6.5 and 10 ml/kg. Level III evidence indicates that hypertonic saline should be considered for the treatment of severe paediatric TBI associated with intracranial hypertension. Effective doses as a continuous infusion of 3% saline range between 0.1 and 1.0 ml/kg of body weight per hour administered on a sliding scale. The minimum dose needed to maintain ICP <20 mmHg should be used. Serum osmolarity should be maintained below 360 mOsm/L.[12]

Hyperventilation

Level III recommendation advocates avoidance of prophylactic severe hyperventilation up to a $PaCO_2$ <30 mmHg in the initial 48 hours after injury. If hyperventilation is used in the management of refractory ICP, advanced neuromonitoring for evaluation of cerebral ischaemia may be considered.[13]

Temperature Control

Temperature control to avoid hyperthermia has become an integral part of neuroprotection in children with TBI. Moderate hypothermia (32°–33°C) beginning early after severe TBI for only 24-hour duration should be avoided. Moderate hypothermia (32°–33°C) beginning within 8 hours after severe TBI for up to 48-hour duration should be considered to reduce ICH. If hypothermia is induced for any indication, rewarming at a rate >0.5°C/hr should be avoided.[14]

Antiseizure Medication

There is limited evidence to support the use of prophylactic anticonvulsants in severe TBI patients. However, a recommendation is made for their use to reduce early post-traumatic seizures.[15]

Advanced Neurological Monitoring

Monitoring of ICP and CPP has been discussed earlier. Monitoring and maintaining ICP and CPP may be too simplistic to prevent secondary insults. Several factors other than ICP and CPP are independently related to outcomes. Some of the monitored parameters are CBF, cerebral autoregulation, cerebral oxygenation, and metabolism.

CBF Autoregulation

In a normal brain CBF is maintained within normal limits in a wide range of blood pressures. This autoregulatory function is affected in TBI. The deranged autoregulation decides the CPP that has to be maintained in a given patient. One method to decide the autoregulatory function in an injured brain is to measure the pressure reactivity index. Pressure reactivity index (PRx) is a correlation coefficient between arterial blood pressure (ABP) and ICP.[16,17] By continuously studying cerebrovascular reactivity through PRx and plotting it against CPP, the CPP at which the vasculature is most reactive can be calculated. This CPP is the most optimal CPP that should be maintained.[18,19] The time that CPP stays above the optimum CPP has been shown to be associated with outcome.

Transcranial Doppler Ultrasonography

Transcranial Doppler (TCD) ultrasonography has emerged as a non-invasive method of CBF estimation. TCD measures the flow velocity. Middle cerebral artery is commonly insonated. It gives a non-quantitative estimate of CBF. The state of CBF autoregulation is estimated based on the assumption that the diameter of the vessels insonated is relatively constant. If the autoregulation is intact, the CBF velocity will remain the same in spite of changes in blood pressure. Various indices have been developed to interpret the state of CBF and autoregulation, CPP and ICP, and CO_2 reactivity by using TCD. Pulsatility index (PI) has been used to assess brain compliance and CPP, and has been shown to have an association with ICP.[20,21] Cerebrovascular resistance (CVR) is estimated by a ratio of mean arterial pressure (MAP) to the flow velocity measured by TCD. Estimated CVR is then used to calculate the autoregulation index.[22,23]

Brain Tissue Oxygen Tension Monitoring

Brain tissue oxygenation ($PbtO_2$) is monitored in a few paediatric TBI studies.[24,25] A level III recommendation suggests to keep $PbtO_2$ above 10 mmHg in paediatric TBI.[26] In focal injury, the sensor should be placed in the pericontusional area while in diffuse injuries, it is usually placed in the non-dominant hemisphere. A value of 20–30 mmHg is normal for the uninjured brain.[27] Oxygenation levels below 10 mmHg have been associated with poor outcome.

Jugular Venous Oxygen Saturation Monitoring (SjvO₂)

A retrograde catheter inserted into the jugular venous bulb measures continuous $SjvO_2$. There is no consensus for normal levels of $SjvO_2$ in children but in adults 50%–75% is considered normal. Values outside this range are considered abnormal and have been shown to be associated with poor outcome.[28]

Brain Metabolism and Chemistry

Markers of brain metabolism (glucose, lactate, and pyruvate), neurotransmitters (glutamate), and tissue damage (glycerol) can be measured by small amounts of interstitial fluid collected by the microdialysis catheter inserted into the brain parenchyma. There are established normal values for adults for some of these chemicals. Sustained elevations of lactate–pyruvate ratio (LPR) have been shown to be associated with poor outcome.[29] Similarly, brain glucose levels can be used to guide optimal threshold for blood glucose levels.[30]

Outcome

Adherence to the paediatric guidelines was associated with significantly higher discharge survival and improved discharge GCS.[31] Another study has shown that there is an association between Apolipoprotein E (APOE)-ε4 allele and outcome following paediatric TBI at six months.[32] Emotional symptoms were commonly reported among paediatric patients with sports-related concussion.[33] In a study, younger age, lower GCS score after resuscitation, lower revised trauma score, absent cisterns on imaging, associated subarachnoid haemorrhage (SAH) and intraventricular haemorrhage, and a lower Marshall score were associated with higher mortality.[34] In another study, there was a strong association between prehospital GCS scores and short-term outcomes in children with TBI.[35]

CONCLUSIONS

Primary injuries due to trauma may not be amenable to treatment, however, significant efforts can be directed towards prevention and management of secondary injury by prompt systemic intervention. The management is more complex in children compared to adults owing to physiological intricacies. A body of evidence exists that directs management of paediatric patients to avoid unfavourable results.

REFERENCES

1. Anderson V, Spencer-Smith M, Wood A. Do children really recover better? Neurobehavioural plasticity after early brain insult. *Brain* 2011;134(Pt 8):2197–221.

2. Muizelaar JP, Marmarou A, DeSalles AA, et al. Cerebral blood flow and metabolism in severely head-injured children. Part 1: Relationship with GCS score, outcome, ICP, and PVI. *J Neurosurg* 1989;71:63–71.

3. Zwienenberg M, Muizelaar JP. Severe pediatric head injury: the role of hyperemia revisited. *Journal of Neurotrauma* 1999;16:937–43.

4. Stocchetti N, Conte V, Ghisoni L, Canavesi K, Zanaboni C. Traumatic brain injury in pediatric patients. *Minerva Anestesiol* 2010;76:1052–9.

5. Hardcastle N, Benzon HA, Vavilala MS. Update on the 2012 guidelines for the management of pediatric traumatic brain injury – information for the anesthesiologist. *Paediatr Anaesth* 2014;24:703–10.

6. Adelson PD, Bratton SL, Carney NA, et al. Guidelines for the acute medical management of severe traumatic brain injury in infants, children, and adolescents. Chapter 4. Resuscitation of blood pressure and oxygenation and prehospital brain-specific therapies for the severe pediatric traumatic brain injury patient. *Pediatr Crit Care Med* 2003;4(Suppl 3):S12–S18.

7. Adelson PD, Bratton SL, Carney NA, et al. Guidelines for the acute medical management of severe traumatic brain injury in infants, children, and adolescents. Chapter 2: Trauma systems, pediatric trauma centers, and the neurosurgeon. *Pediatr Crit Care Med* 2003;4(Suppl 3): S5–S8.

8. Tepas JJ 3rd, Ramenofsky ML, Mollitt DL, Gans BM, DiScala C. The Pediatric Trauma Score as a predictor of injury severity: an objective assessment. *J Trauma* 1988;28:425–9.

9. Adelson PD, Bratton SL, Carney NA, et al. Guidelines for the acute medical management of severe traumatic brain injury in infants, children, and adolescents. Chapter 4: Threshold for treatment of intracranial hypertension. *Pediatr Crit Care Med* 2012;13(1)(Suppl.): S18–S23.

10. Adelson PD, Bratton SL, Carney NA, et al. Guidelines for the acute medical management of severe traumatic brain injury in infants, children, and adolescents. Chapter 5: Cerebral perfusion pressure thresholds. *Pediatr Crit Care Med* 2012;13(1)(Suppl.):S24–S29.

11. Adelson PD, Bratton SL, Carney NA, et al. Guidelines for the acute medical management of severe traumatic brain injury in infants, children, and adolescents. Chapter 10: Cerebrospinal fluid drainage. *Pediatr Crit Care Med* 2012;13(1)(Suppl.):S46–S48.

12. Adelson PD, Bratton SL, Carney NA, et al. Guidelines for the acute medical management of severe traumatic brain injury in infants, children, and adolescents. Chapter 8: Hyperosmolar therapy. *Pediatr Crit Care Med* 2012;13(1) (Suppl.):S36–S41.

13. Adelson PD, Bratton SL, Carney NA, et al. Guidelines for the acute medical management of severe traumatic brain injury in infants, children, and adolescents. Chapter 13: Hyperventilation. *Pediatr Crit Care Med* 2012;13(1) (Suppl.):S58–S60.

14. Adelson PD, Bratton SL, Carney NA, et al. Guidelines for the acute medical management of severe traumatic brain injury in infants, children, and adolescents. Chapter 9: Temperature control. *Pediatr Crit Care Med* 2012;13(1) (Suppl.):S42–S45.

15. Adelson PD, Bratton SL, Carney NA, et al. Guidelines for the acute medical management of severe traumatic brain injury in infants, children, and adolescents. Chapter 17: Antiseizure prophylaxis. *Pediatr Crit Care Med* 2012;13(1) (Suppl.):S72–S75.

16. Czosnyka M, Smielewski P, Kirkpatrick P, Laing RJ, Menon D, Pickard JD. Continuous assessment of the cerebral vasomotor reactivity in head injury. *Neurosurgery* 1997;41:11–17.

17. Budohoski KP, Czosnyka M, de Riva N, et al. The relationship between cerebral blood flow autoregulation and cerebrovascular pressure reactivity after traumatic brain injury. *Neurosurgery* 2012;71:652–60.

18. Kolias AG, Hutchinson PJ, Brady KM, Menon DK, Pickard JD, Smielewski P. Continuous determination of optimal cerebral perfusion pressure in traumatic brain injury. *Crit Care Med* 2012;40:2456–63.

19. Depreitere B, Güiza F, Van den Berghe G, et al. Pressure autoregulation monitoring and cerebral perfusion pressure target recommendation in patients with severe traumatic

brain injury based on minute-by-minute monitoring data. *J Neurosurg* 2014;120:1451–7.

20. Brandt L. Transcranial Doppler sonography pulsatility index (PI) reflects intracranial pressure (ICP). *Surg Neurol* 2004;62:45–51.

21. Splavski B, Radanović B, Vranković D, et al. Transcranial doppler ultrasonography as an early outcome forecaster following severe brain injury. *Br J Neurosurg* 2006;20:386–90.

22. Figaji AA, Zwane E, Fieggen AG, et al. Pressure autoregulation, intracranial pressure, and brain tissue oxygenation in children with severe traumatic brain injury. *J Neurosurg Pediatr* 2009;4:420–8.

23. Paulson OB, Strandgaard S, Edvinsson L. Cerebral autoregulation. *Cerebrovasc Brain Metab Rev* 1990;2:161–92.

24. Figaji AA, Zwane E, Thompson C, et al. Brain tissue oxygen tension monitoring in pediatric severe traumatic brain injury. Part 1: Relationship with outcome. *Childs Nerv Syst* 2009;25:1325–33.

25. Stippler M, Ortiz V, Adelson PD, et al. Brain tissue oxygen monitoring after severe traumatic brain injury in children: relationship to outcome and association with other clinical parameters. *J Neurosurg Pediatr* 2012;10:383–91.

26. Adelson PD, Bratton SL, Carney NA, et al. Guidelines for the acute medical management of severe traumatic brain injury in infants, children, and adolescents. Chapter 6: Advanced neuromonitoring. *Pediatr Crit Care Med* 2012;13(1)(Suppl.):S30–S32.

27. Maas AI, Fleckenstein W, de Jong DA, van Santbrink H. Monitoring cerebral oxygenation: experimental studies and preliminary clinical results of continuous monitoring of cerebrospinal fluid and brain tissue oxygen tension. *Acta Neurochir Suppl (Wien)* 1993;59:50–7.

28. Cormio M, Valadka AB, Robertson CS. Elevated jugular venous oxygen saturation after severe head injury. *J Neurosurg* 1999;90:9–15.

29. Timofeev I, Carpenter KL, Nortje J, et al. Cerebral extracellular chemistry and outcome following traumatic brain injury: a microdialysis study of 223 patients. *Brain* 2011;134:484–94.

30. Oddo M, Schmidt JM, Carrera E, et al. Impact of tight glycemic control on cerebral glucose metabolism after severe brain injury: a microdialysis study. *Crit Care Med* 2008;36:3233–8.

31. Vavilala MS, Kernic MA, Wang J, et al. Acute care clinical indicators associated with discharge outcomes in children with severe traumatic brain injury. *Crit Care Med* 2014;42:2258–66.

32. Kassam I, Gagnon F, Cusimano MD. Association of the APOE-ε4 allele with outcome of traumatic brain injury in children and youth: a meta-analysis and meta-regression. *J Neurol Neurosurg Psychiatry* 2016;87:433–40.

33. Ellis MJ, Ritchie LJ, Koltek M, et al. Psychiatric outcomes after pediatric sports-related concussion. *J Neurosurg Pediatr* 2015;16:709–18.

34. Ujjan B, Waqas M, Khan MB, Bakhshi SK, Bari ME. Paediatric traumatic brain injury: Presentation, prognostic indicators and outcome analysis from a tertiary care center in a developing country. *J Pak Med Assoc* 2016;66(Suppl 3)(10):S65–S67.

35. Nesiama JA, Pirallo RG, Lerner EB, Hennes H. Does a prehospital Glasgow Coma Scale score predict pediatric outcomes? *Pediatr Emerg Care* 2012;28:1027–32.

72

Hypoxic Ischaemic Encephalopathy

S. Rajan and S. Ahuja

ABSTRACT

Hypoxic ischaemic encephalopathy (HIE) is one of the most devastating neurological injuries. Advancement of medical knowledge in the area of resuscitation has led to a better understanding of the neurological outcomes after primary injury. Early intervention with an aim to achieve return of spontaneous circulation makes a huge difference in the prognosis ranging from complete recovery to even death. A thorough knowledge of brain circulation pathophysiology, ischaemia vulnerable zones along with effective measures to prevent secondary insults of brain injury has given a new dimension to the management of patients with brain injuries. Prognostication of individuals after the injury according to set neurological status prognostic parameters is helpful in limiting the tireless efforts of physicians and also resources. Meticulous search of reversible causes of inciting event and timely intervention to reverse the conditions cannot be overstressed. Conditions mimicking the signs and symptoms of hypoxic ischaemic damage must be acknowledged and managed accordingly. Supportive care in the intensive care unit (ICU) remains the mainstay of therapy. Targeted temperature management has proven survival benefits after neurological injury. Early introduction of therapeutic hypothermia with adequate monitoring is of utmost importance in the management of patients with brain injury. Non-reassuring response after adequate efforts should be considered for organ transplantation. Regular counselling of family members regarding the prognosis of patients is always helpful in making decisions.

KEYWORDS

Hypoxic ischaemic encephalopathy (HIE); cardiopulmonary resuscitation (CPR); pulseless electrical activity (PEA); ventricular tachycardia (VT); reticular activating system (RAS); Electroencephalogram (EEG); acute respiratory distress syndrome (ARDS); return of spontaneous circulation (ROSC); blood–brain barrier (BBB); continuous renal replacement therapy (CRRT); cerebral blood flow (CBF).

CASE STUDY

A 75-year-old female is found unresponsive and pulseless when the ambulance arrives. The initial electrocardiogram (ECG) confirms asystole. Cardiopulmonary resuscitation (CPR) with advanced cardiac life support is initiated, she is subsequently intubated, resuscitated, and transferred to emergent care in the hospital. Urgent computed tomography (CT) scan demonstrates 'hyperdense material within the subarachnoid space' consistent with subarachnoid haemorrhage (SAH). The comorbid conditions of the patient are hypertension, coronary artery disease, and congestive heart failure with low ejection fraction. On evaluation in the neurointensive care unit (NICU) on day 1, she is deeply comatose and unresponsive to any verbal and tactile stimuli. Her temperature is 98.6°F, blood pressure (BP) 135/85, and pulse rate (PR) 75/min. Pupils are dilated and fixed at 6 mm size. Absent cough reflexes are also noted by intensive care unit (ICU) nurses. Two days later the patient's condition remained same and the family members are very concerned and would like to know the prognosis of the patient.

INTRODUCTION

Hypoxic-ischaemic encephalopathy (HIE), also known as anoxic encephalopathy or po-cardiac-arrest syndrome, is defined as acute global brain injury resulting from critical reduction or loss of blood flow and/or supply of oxygen and nutrients. It comprises a complex constellation of pathophysiological, biochemical, and molecular injuries related to hypoxia, ischaemia or a combination of these conditions.[1] Despite major advances in the CPR practices, the overall prognosis remains poor. The most common cause (Table 72.1) includes cardiac arrest, respiratory arrest, near-drowning, near-hanging, and other forms of incomplete suffocation, and carbon monoxide (CO) and other poisonous gas exposures. The ischaemic-reperfusion vulnerable area of the brain primarily involves the grey matter which mostly contains the dendrites, basal ganglia, thalami, and cerebral cortex. It is also more metabolically active than white matter and therefore early to be involved in the excitotoxicity. In neonates, the relative immaturity of Purkinje cells (exquisitely sensitive to ischaemic damage) somehow shows positive protective effects on cerebellar cortex.[2]

Coma is defined as a state of unresponsiveness in which the individual is unaware of the surroundings. It depends largely on the area involved as previously mentioned, the cortex, cerebellum, and thalamus are more prone to anoxic injury than the brainstem and subcortical areas. The most common clinical presentations (Figure 72.1) include disorders of consciousness (i.e., coma or vegetative state), seizures, myoclonus, and loss of airway reflex and cardiovascular instability.

Resuscitation is successful in a third of hospital cardiac arrests. Factors such as prolonged resuscitation (more than 5 minutes), pace of onset, prodromal symptoms, duration of ventricular fibrillation (VF), bystander CPR, and circumstances of CPR in which resuscitation is done are detrimental in predicting outcomes.[3–5] Prior history of cardiac disease, cancer, sepsis, organ failure, prolonged CPR (>5 mins) are associated with decreased survival.[6] Prognostication of patient is important as it may help in essential decision-making of sustaining life supportive measures. There exists a relationship between the mechanism of the inciting event and the overall prognosis.[7,8] The inciting events caused by in-hospital events when initial rhythm is asystole/pulseless electrical activity (PEA), the prognosis is less than 10% and it jumps to 25%–40% when the cardiac arrest[9] is caused by VF. Haemodynamically unstable ventricular tachycardia (VT) has more favourable outcomes (up to 65%–70%).[10] More organized rhythms like monomorphic VT retains systemic perfusion which accounts for much better prognosis as compared to others.

CLINICAL PRESENTATIONS

Locked-in Syndrome

It is caused by injury to bilateral anterior pontine regions while sparing the ascending sensory and reticular activating system (RAS) pathways. Level of alertness, ability to blink, and vertical eye movements are generally preserved. There are medial and lateral gaze palsies, with no other voluntary movement. Here electroencephalography (EEG) and metabolism are normal.

Persistent Vegetative State

It is a condition in which the brainstem function is preserved with bilateral cortical damage. The patient has no speech or awareness and is unresponsive to physical stimuli. The EEG has polymorphic delta or theta waves, sometimes alpha.

Akinetic Mutism (coma vigile)

In this condition, the patient is partially or fully awake. The lesion is limited to the frontal lobes. The EEG shows diffuse slowing pattern.

Table 72.1 The mechanism and most common causes of anoxic encephalopathy

	Mechanism of hypoxia/ischaemia	Causes
1.	Cardiac arrest followed by respiratory depression	Massive blood loss, septic/traumatic shock, and heart disease, such as AMI or ventricular arrhythmia
2.	Respiratory failure followed by cardiac arrest with poor inspired oxygen	Tracheal compression/obstruction, drowning, strangulation, aspiration of gastric content, or during GA if the inspired gas is oxygen poor
3.	Respiratory muscle weakness	Guillain-Barre's syndrome, amyotrophic lateral sclerosis, myasthenia gravis or central nervous system injury (mainly spinal cord injury)
4.	Reduced oxygen carriage by the blood	Carbon monoxide poisoning
5.	Histotoxicity	Cyanide poisoning

Catatonia

In this condition, there is decreased motor activity, consciousness is preserved and body may be fixed to a posture with non-specific EEG patterns.

Minimally Conscious State

There is globally impaired responsiveness due to significant neuronal damage. The EEG shows theta and alpha waves.

Brain Death

It shows irreversible absence of all cerebral and brainstem functions including pupillary, oculocephalic, oculovestibular, corneal, gag, sucking, swallowing, and extensor posturing.

Post-Cardiac-Arrest Syndrome

The most common cause of poor prognosis after a cardiac arrest is post-cardiac-arrest syndrome.[11] Post-cardiac-arrest syndrome is a combination of processes involving post-cardiac-arrest brain injury, myocardial dysfunction, and systemic ischaemic reperfusion response.

PATHOGENESIS

The brain utilizes energy primarily from hydrolysis of adenosine triphosphate (ATP) and a majority of it is utilized by neurons to maintain resting membrane potential and restore ionic concentration. In fact, the brain does not have storage energy reserve of its own except a small amount of glycogen which is insufficient to meet its demand in crisis. Therefore, the brain depends on continuous supply of oxygen and glucose from the circulation. Depending on the selective vulnerability of cerebral regions to anoxic injury various patterns of cerebral insults have been defined. This impaired reflow can cause persistent ischaemia and small infarctions in some brain regions.

The areas more prone to hypoxic/ischaemic injury include areas supplied by distal branches of deep and superficial penetrating blood vessels, grey matter, zones between the major cerebral arteries 'watershed areas', regions of hippocampus, and neocortical layers 3, 4, and 5. Apart from head trauma, shock, and poisoning, the most characteristic insults leading to HIE are produced by cardiac arrest. Global ischaemia resulting from the causes mentioned earlier is the main reason for 'energy crisis' resulting in failure of electrochemical transmission ultimately leading to cellular death.[3,4]

Brain injury triggered by cardiac arrest and resuscitation are complex which includes the formation of free radicals, altered calcium homoeostasis, and activation of cell death signalling pathways. Circulatory arrest leads to oxygen and glucose deprivation in the brain tissues, accumulation of toxic metabolites which further causes ATP depletion and subsequent Na^+ and K^+ pump failure. Dysfunction of membranous ATP-dependent Na^+ and K^+ pumps leads to 'depolarization' of neuronal membrane which releases glutamate into the synaptic cleft. Glutamate causes excitotoxic injury that is mediated through N-methyl-D-aspartate (NMDA) receptors.[12,13] Opening of NMDA receptors allows calcium ions into the intracellular space. Raised intracellular calcium increases oxygen-free radicals via interaction with the mitochondrial oxidative enzymes leading to cellular death.[14] The neuropathology of HIE is the same regardless of the initial event.

After successful resuscitation, there is a brief period of hyperaemia followed by absence of flow which is attributed to the occlusion of brain microvasculature by thrombotic emboli, further exacerbating the condition by causing failure of autoregulation. During the initial hours after cardiac arrest, oxygen deprivation leads to endothelial activation and systemic response causing a spurting rise in inflammatory markers, cytokines which are primarily responsible for subsequent multi-organ failure and mortality.

DIAGNOSIS

The diagnosis of HIE is primarily clinical.[15] A knowledge of the inciting event is always helpful from a quick history given by a bystander. The potential cause may not be obvious in every situation. A quick physical examination may be helpful in documenting the current state and prioritizing the interventions. Physical assessment needs to be incorporated as the initial documentation should include: (1) spontaneous movements, (2) response to touch, pain, and verbal stimuli, (3) size of pupil, (4) cranial nerve examination, and (5) respiratory pattern. The GCS and the Coma Remission Scale (CRS) are used to measure the depth of coma. The CRS[16] is more detailed as compared to GCS. FOUR score (Full outline of unresponsiveness),[17] devised by Widjicks, also includes brainstem functions and respiration pattern in addition to eye and motor response. Various other validated scales (like Early Rehabilitation Index [ERI] and Barthel Index) are described in the medical literature to predict the neurological outcomes in hypoxic damage patients. A recent large multicentric trial compared[18] the validity of Early Rehabilitation Index (ERI)[19] and other validated scales like Barthel Index[20] and CRS with GCS and claimed significant correlation.

Basic investigations such as blood glucose and electrolyte levels, arterial blood gas (ABG) analysis, liver and renal test, osmolality check, blood film analysis, and full blood count are used to detect polycythemia or infection, and C-reactive protein to detect infection should be done in an unresponsive patient and almost every patient to exclude reversible causes.

A meticulous search is necessary to rule out potential confounders that are primarily reversible such as:

- Severe dyselectrolytaemia
- Effects of recent illicit drugs use or alcohol overdose
- Effects of therapeutic drugs (e.g., anticholinergic) used in resuscitation or sedative narcotics and hypnotics. The plasma concentration of the offending drug does not always correlate with therapeutic effects in critically ill brain-injured patients. Antagonists may be instituted as early as possible
- Severe hypothermia: core temperature should be >35°C and hypotension: (systolic blood pressure [SBP] should be >90, mean arterial pressure [MAP] >60).

There are no definitive tests or procedures specific to HIE, however, urgent neuroimaging is necessary in an unresponsive patient to rule out haemorrhage or stroke.

According to a recent study there are insufficient scientific evidences to support the use of neuroimaging[21] in the diagnosis of HIE. Diagnostic workup may be helpful in understanding the aetiology, severity, prognosis, and excluding any associated pathological processes.

NEUROIMAGING FEATURES OF HYPOXIC-ISCHAEMIC ENCEPHALOPATHY

The neuroimaging features in HIE vary according to age and severity and are not specific.[2] These include:

- Diffuse oedemas with effacement of the CSF-containing spaces.
- Decreased cortical grey matter attenuation with loss of normal grey-white differentiation.
- Reversal Sign: Reversal of the normal CT attenuation of grey and white matter demonstrated within the first 24 hours.
- White Cerebellum Sign: Diffuse oedema and hypo-attenuation of the cerebral hemispheres with sparing of the cerebellum and brainstem.

ANCILLARY TESTS HELPFUL IN PROGNOSTICATION

Electroencephalography

Electroencephalography is widely used for neurological prognostication in cardiac arrest to assess the level of consciousness.[22,23] The absence of detectable EEG activity, burst suppression pattern, delta waves, periodic post-anoxic lateralized diffuse epileptiform discharge (PLED or BiPLED),[24] and alpha coma (frontal predominant unresponsive rhythms with unwavering waves) indicate bad prognosis. EEG waves are easily influenced by metabolic derangements, sepsis, and sedating drugs. EEG is good in predicting the extremes of situations. Those with early resuscitation and normal EEG have fair chances of recovery whereas the outcome is less predictable when the waveforms are not extreme.[23]

Biochemical Markers

Biochemical markers such as neuron-specific enolase (NSE),[25] S-100,[26] and interleukin-8 (IL-8)[27] serve as predictors of neurological outcome in patients after cardiac arrest and return of spontaneous circulation.

Neuron-specific enolase is present in the cytoplasm of neurons and platelets. Its cut-off levels vary in small studies. Serum NSE levels >33 μg/L at days 1 to 3 post-CPR accurately predict poor outcome (recommendation level B). Other biomarkers that have been studied so far are brain creatine phosphokinase (CPK-BB), glutamate transaminase, lactate dehydrogenase, pyruvate (serum/CSF), IL-8, and glial fibrillary acidic protein (glial origin).

Evoked Potentials

Visual, brainstem, and somatosensory evoked potentials (SSEPs) test the integrity of neuroanatomical pathways. These tests have better prognostic value than clinical judgement in patients with hypoxic injury. Somatosensory evoked potentials are more accurate than EEG in prognostication and is less influenced by drugs, infections, and metabolic derangements.[28] Poor outcomes can be predicted by bilateral absence of cortical SSEP (N 20 response) between 1 and 3 days.[29] Table 72.2 represents key points in predicting the prognosis of a patient.

MANAGEMENT

The management of HIE requires multidisciplinary involvement that begins in the prehospital phase and continues throughout the emergency and intensive care. Coordination among the treating physicians and different teams is an essential component.

General Therapy

The goal is to restore normal cerebral function, stable cardiac rhythm, adequate organ perfusion, and quality of life. Supportive management and prevention of secondary insults remain the mainstay of therapy. It is important to establish cardiac and pulmonary function as early as possible. Ensure a clear airway, adequate oxygenation, and

Table 72.2 Rules predicting good and poor prognosis

Time after cardiac arrest	Good prognosis	Prognosis
Initial examination	Pupillary light reflex examination present and motor response flexor or extensor and spontaneous roving horizontal eye movements at 12 to 24 hours	Age >70 years, stroke or renal failure prior to admission Recent CHF No pupillary light reflex (rule out atropine administration) Prolonged CPR >15 minutes
1 day	1-day motor response withdrawal or better and 1-day eye opening improved at least two grades. Speech and comprehension within the first 48 hours	1-day motor response no better than flexor and 1-day spontaneous eye movements neither orienting nor roving conjugate No spontaneous limb movement (GCS <4), decelerate posture and no localization of pain stimuli Presence of myoclonic seizures
3 days	3-day motor response withdrawal or better and 3-day spontaneous eye movements normal	3-day motor response no better than flexor
1 week	1-week motor response obeying commands	1-week motor response not obeying commands and initial spontaneous eye movements neither orienting nor roving conjugate and 3-day eye opening not spontaneous
2 weeks	2-week oculocephalic response normal	2-week oculocephalic response not normal and 3-day motor response not obeying commands and 3-day eye opening not spontaneous and 2-week eye opening not improved at least two grades

Sources: (1) Levy DE, Caronna JJ, Singer BH, et al. Predicting outcome from hypoxic-ischemic coma. *JAMA* 1985;253(10):1420. doi:10.1001/jama.1985.03350340072020. (2) Saklayen M, Liss H, Markert R. In-hospital cardiopulmonary resuscitation. Survival in 1 hospital and literature review. Medicine (Baltimore). 1995;74(4):163–75. Available from: http://www.ncbi.nlm.nih.gov/pubmed/7623652. Accessed November 11, 2016. (3) Enohumah KO, Moerer O, Kirmse C, et al. Outcome of cardiopulmonary resuscitation in intensive care units in a university hospital. *Resuscitation* 2006;71(2):161–70. doi:10.1016/j.resuscitation.2006.03.013. (4) Berek K, Jeschow M, Aichner F. The prognostication of cerebral hypoxia after out-of-hospital cardiac arrest in adults. *Eur Neurol* 2008;37(3):135–45. (5) Mullie A, Verstringe P, Buylaert W, et al. Predictive value of Glasgow coma score for awakening after out-of-hospital cardiac arrest. Cerebral Resuscitation Study Group of the Belgian Society for Intensive Care. *Lancet* (London, England). 1988;1(8578):137–40. Available from: http://www.ncbi.nlm.nih.gov/pubmed/2892987. Accessed November 11, 2016.

ventilation. Maintenance of advanced airways gradually and tapering down the fraction of inspired oxygen (FiO_2) is needed to avoid hyperoxia. Hyperoxia itself has some delirious effects which are still under current research. A recent large multicentre study[30] identified hyperoxia as an independent factor associated with increased in-hospital mortality in post-resuscitated patients in the ICU. It is also important to avoid hypoxia, hypercapnia, hyperthermia, and hypotension. Insert a gastric tube to decompress the stomach and improve lung compliance. Secure the airway for transfer. Consider immediately extubating if the patient is breathing and conscious level improves quickly after return of spontaneous circulation (ROSC).

Routine ICU care is well explained by the acronym 'FAST HUGS BID',[31] which comprises **f**eeding/fluids, **a**nalgesia, **s**edation, **t**hromboprophylaxis, **h**ead-up position, **u**lcer prophylaxis, **g**lycaemic control, **s**pontaneous breathing trial, **b**owel care, **i**ndwelling catheter removal, **d**e-escalation of antibiotics if any.

After addressing the urgent issues, it is a wise strategy to prevent secondary insult (Figure 72.2).

The early post-arrest phase could be considered as the period between 20 minutes and 6 to 12 hours after ROSC. Reperfusion of areas after ROCS follows the opposite path of return of brainstem function first and cortical functions later.[6] Although resumption of oxygen and metabolic substrate delivery at the microcirculatory level is essential, however, evidences also suggests that too much oxygen during the stages of reperfusion can exacerbate neuronal injury. This process may last as long as 24 to 48 hours. Despite cerebral microcirculatory failure, macroscopic reperfusion is often hyperaemic in the first few minutes after cardiac arrest because of elevated cerebral perfusion pressure (CPP), decreased cerebral blood flow (CBF), and impaired cerebrovascular autoregulation. This high initial perfusion pressure can theoretically minimize impaired reflow. Yet hyperaemic reperfusion can potentially exacerbate brain oedema and reperfusion injury.

At 6–12 hours after ROSC when early interventions might be most effective, injury pathways are still active and aggressive treatment is typically instituted. The recovery phase is a period beyond 3 days when prognostication can be commented upon and ultimate outcomes are more predictable (Figure 72.3).

A clear and consistent update in the progress and deterioration of the patient should be effectively communicated to the relatives. It is always prudent to wait for at least 72 hours before any conclusions are made.

Specific Therapy

Therapeutic Hypothermia

Therapeutic hypothermia (TH) is a widely used method for neuroprotection. Hypothermia reduces the cerebral metabolic rate for oxygen ($CMRO_2$)/oxygen consumption by 6%–7% for every 1°C reduction in brain temperature >28°C. Also it decreases neutrophil and macrophage functions and free radical production which hence reduces the inflammatory response evoked by ischaemia.[32] Current literature supports the institution of hypothermia to a patient who is unable to follow verbal commands after ROSC immediately within a few hours after resuscitation. It promotes cerebral perfusion with improved neurological and mortality outcomes. International resuscitation guidelines support the use of targeted temperature management for the comatose patient. Neurological injury is the most common cause of death in a patient suffering from anoxic injury. Hypothermia causes profound reduction of active and basal cellular energy requirements, improved blood–brain barrier (BBB) stability with reduced excitotoxic neurotransmitter release, neutrophil infiltration, oxygen-free radical production, and decreased cytokine and leukotriene production protection against cytoskeletal proteolysis.[33] A large database review suggests improved survival benefits for the patient in whom intervention of hypothermia is followed.[34] A recent large randomized controlled trial (RCT) did not find any difference in mortality between the two hypothermic groups targeting 33 and 36 degrees. Core temperature and invasive BP should be monitored with the intervention.

Methods of cooling

Methods of cooling[35] may vary in terms of ease, speed, and availability of measures:

- External or surface cooling can be achieved by circulating cold water blankets, ice packs to the axillae and groins, cooling garments, helmets, etc. This method is faster but costly and relatively takes more time and titration of temperature can be difficult. Furthermore, immersion in ice bath is an effective method in children but it is contraindicated in pulmonary oedema.
- Internal cooling can be achieved by large volume ice cold intravenous (IV) fluid: 30 ml/kg crystalloid cooled to 4°C and infused over 30 mins. Body cavity lavage: gastric 500 ml/10 min, bladder 300 ml/10 min, peritoneal. These methods are time-consuming and invasive. Extracorporeal circuits may be part of continuous renal replacement therapy (CRRT) and invasive.

The patient undergoing TH should be monitored for shivering, bradycardia, and cardiovascular instability, infection, hyperglycaemia (caused by decreased insulin release from the pancreas and insulin resistance), electrolyte abnormalities, and reduced clearance of drugs. Sedation and relaxants will be required for the patient undergoing TH and mechanical ventilation. Blood pressure should be maintained during the cooling phase by optimizing preload as this will be helpful during the warming phase to prevent hypotension from vasodilation. Coagulation abnormalities without significant risk of bleeding may occur during hypothermia. Therefore, it is necessary to monitor prothrombin time (PT), activated partial thromboplastin time (APTT)/international normalized ratio (INR), and platelets.

Actively bleeding patients should be supplemented with platelet concentrates and fresh frozen plasma. Peripheral vasoconstriction puts the patient at risk of skin breakdown, so turning the patient every 4 hours and frequent skin assessment should be followed.

Shivering increases the metabolic rate and oxygen consumption and makes it difficult to achieve target temperature. Signs and symptoms of shivering include a drop in mixed venous oxygen saturation, hyperventilation, EKG artefacts, and muscle fasciculation. Shivering can be managed by analgesia and sedation like benzodiazepines, opioids, propofol, and magnesium sulphate. If relaxants were used for the TH, then it should be stopped as soon as hypothermia is completed or warming is initiated.

Re-warming is done passively like removing ice packs and holding cold IV fluids when surface cooling method is followed. Target a temperature rise of 0.3–0.5 degrees per hour when an endovascular cooling device is used by measuring flux of heat transfer. Avoid rapid re-warming and hyperthermia during the process.

Watch for hypotension and electrolyte imbalances (hypokalaemia, hypomagnesaemia, hypophosphataemia, hypocalcaemia) during the warming phase.

Haemodynamics

Haemodynamic monitoring addressing the needs of vasopressors requirements, clinical end-points of resuscitation, and tissue perfusion goals is indispensable. Inadequate tissue oxygen delivery can even persist after ROSC because of microcirculatory failure.

Aim for optimizing right heart pressures corresponding to central venous pressure (CVP) of 8–13 by optimizing preload and maintaining CPP, keeping in mind that the placement of urinary catheter is helpful in guiding fluid balance.

Hyperglycaemia

Hyperglycaemia[36] is common in post-cardiac-arrest patients and is associated with poor neurological outcome. Elevated post-ischaemic blood glucose concentrations exacerbate ischaemic brain injury. Hyperglycaemia should be controlled using insulin treatment with regular monitoring. Glucose should be controlled at levels less than 150 mg/dL. Tight glycaemic control is usually not encouraged as it carries risk of hypoglycaemia which may further reduce CBF.

Hormone Replacement

Hypoxic ischaemic encephalopathy is a pan-hypopituitary state,[37] and currently there are no recommendations on when to initiate hormone replacement therapy. Replacement of hormone not only helps with improving cardiovascular instability but also improves organ protection. Levothyroxine, methylprednisolone, insulin, and vasopressin are the hormones described in the literature.

Seizures

Seizures in the post-cardiac-arrest period are associated with worse prognosis as they increase cerebral and systemic metabolic demand. Almost a third of the patients sustaining hypoxic-ischaemic insult develop seizures within 24 hours. Good vigilance for seizure activity and EEG should be used to monitor non-convulsive status epilepticus. Post-hypoxic status epilepticus almost invariably results in fatal outcomes.[38]

Prophylactic anticonvulsants are not used routinely. Antiepileptics such as valproate or clonazepam may respond well to myoclonic seizures. Agents like propofol or other benzodiazapenes ensuring adequate sedation should be instituted alongside to reduce the dose of antiepileptics.

Cerebral Oedema

Although transient brain oedema is observed early after ROSC, it is rarely translated with clinically relevant increases in intracranial pressure (ICP).[39]

Rehabilitation

The placement of implantable cardioverter-defibrillators (ICD) in survivors with good neurological recovery[40] and insertion of an ICD is indicated if subsequent cardiac arrests cannot be reliably prevented by other treatments (such as pacemaker for atrio-ventricular (AV) block, transcatheter ablation of a single ectopic pathway, or valve replacement for critical aortic stenosis).

Organ Transplantation

Most of the organ transplantation occurs from the brain dead donors. The successful recovery of viable organs depends on the appropriate identification and medical care of brain dead patients.[41] These donors should ideally be managed in specialized units such as ICUs with continued haemodynamic support and monitoring, and optimized ventilator support to prevent hypoxia or hypercapnia.

CONCLUSIONS

Hypoxic ischaemic encephalopathy can be a consequence of medical illness or accidental and non-accidental injuries. A multidisciplinary approach should be followed including active participation of family members in the treatment plan. Nonetheless, presentation at the time of admission, clinical response to supportive therapy, and prognostic markers may be helpful in decision making.

REFERENCES

1. Busl KM, Greer DM. Hypoxic-ischemic brain injury: Pathophysiology, neuropathology and mechanisms. *NeuroRehabilitation* 2010;26(1):5–13. doi:10.3233/NRE-2010-0531.
2. Gutierrez LG, Rovira À, Portela LAP, Leite C da C, Lucato LT. CT and MR in non-neonatal hypoxic–ischemic encephalopathy: radiological findings with pathophysiological correlations. *Neuroradiology* 2010;52(11):949–76. doi:10.1007/s00234-010-0728-z.
3. Herlitz J, Eek M, Holmberg M, Engdahl J, Holmberg S. Characteristics and outcome among patients having out of hospital cardiac arrest at home compared with elsewhere. *Heart* 2002;88(6):579–82. Available from: http://www.ncbi.nlm.nih.gov/pubmed/12433883. Accessed November 11, 2016.
4. Rea TD, Paredes VL. Quality of life and prognosis among survivors of out-of-hospital cardiac arrest. *Curr Opin Crit*

Care 2004;10(3):218–23. Available from: http://www.ncbi. nlm.nih.gov/pubmed/15166840. Accessed November 11, 2016.

5. de Vreede-Swagemakers JJ, Gorgels AP, Dubois-Arbouw WI, et al. Circumstances and causes of out-of-hospital cardiac arrest in sudden death survivors. *Heart* 1998; 79(4):356–61. Available from: http://www.ncbi.nlm.nih. gov/pubmed/9616342. Accessed November 11, 2016.

6. Dragancea I, Rundgren M, Englund E, et al. The influence of induced hypothermia and delayed prognostication on the mode of death after cardiac arrest. *Resuscitation* 2013; 84(3):337–42. doi:10.1016/j.resuscitation.2012.09.015.

7. Herlitz J, Engdahl J, Svensson L, Young M, Angquist K-A, Holmberg S. Can we define patients with no chance of survival after out-of-hospital cardiac arrest? *Heart* 2004;90(10):1114–18. doi:10.1136/hrt.2003.029348.

8. Weaver WD, Cobb LA, Hallstrom AP, Fahrenbruch C, Copass MK, Ray R. Factors influencing survival after out-of-hospital cardiac arrest. *J Am Coll Cardiol* 1986;7(4):752–7. Available from: http://www.ncbi.nlm. nih.gov/pubmed/3958332. Accessed November 11, 2016.

9. Bunch TJ, Hammill SC, White RD. Outcomes after ventricular fibrillation out-of-hospital cardiac arrest: expanding the chain of survival. *Mayo Clin Proc* 2005;80(6):774–82. doi:10.1016/S0025-6196(11)61532-2.

10. Goldstein S, Landis JR, Leighton R, et al. Characteristics of the resuscitated out-of-hospital cardiac arrest victim with coronary heart disease. *Circulation* 1981;64(5):977–84. Available from: http://www.ncbi.nlm.nih.gov/pubmed/ 7285312. Accessed November 11, 2016.

11. Stub D, Bernard S, Duffy SJ, Kaye DM. Post cardiac arrest syndrome: a review of therapeutic strategies. *Circulation* 2011;123(13):1428–35. doi:10.1161/ CIRCULATIONAHA.110.988725.

12. Vaagenes P, Ginsberg M, Ebmeyer U, et al. Cerebral resuscitation from cardiac arrest: pathophysiologic mechanisms. *Crit Care Med* 1996;24(Suppl 2):S57–68. Available from: http://www.ncbi.nlm.nih.gov/pubmed/ 8608707. Accessed November 11, 2016.

13. Lipton SA, Rosenberg PA. Excitatory amino acids as a final common pathway for neurologic disorders. *N Engl J Med* 1994;330(9):613–22. doi:10.1056/ NEJM199403033300907.

14. Zündorf G, Reiser G. Calcium dysregulation and homeostasis of neural calcium in the molecular mechanisms of neurodegenerative diseases provide multiple targets for neuroprotection. *Antioxid Redox Signal* 2011;14(7): 1275–88. doi:10.1089/ars.2010.3359.

15. Machado C. Diagnosis of brain death. *Neurol Int* 2010; 2(1):e2. doi:10.4081/ni.2010.e2.

16. Estraneo A, Moretta P, Loreto V, et al. Predictors of recovery of responsiveness in prolonged anoxic vegetative state. *Neurology* 2013;80(5):464–70. doi:10.1212/ WNL.0b013e31827f0f31.

17. Wijdicks EFM, Bamlet WR, Maramattom BV, Manno EM, McClelland RL. Validation of a new coma scale:

The FOUR score. *Ann Neurol* 2005;58(4):585–93. doi:10.1002/ana.20611.

18. Rollnik JD, Bertram M, Bucka C, et al. Criterion validity and sensitivity to change of the Early Rehabilitation Index (ERI): results from a German multi-center study. *BMC Res Notes* 2016;9(1):356. doi:10.1186/s13104-016-2154-8.

19. Rollnik JD. The Early Rehabilitation Barthel Index (ERBI). *Rehabilitation (Stuttg)* 2011;50(6):408–11. doi:10.1055/s-0031-1273728.

20. Mahoney FI, Barthel DW. Functional evaluation: the Barthel index. A simple index of independence useful in scoring improvement in the rehabilitation of the chronically ill. *Md State Med J* 1965;14:56–61.

21. Heinz UE, Rollnik JD. Outcome and prognosis of hypoxic brain damage patients undergoing neurological early rehabilitation. *BMC Res Notes* 2015;8:243. doi:10.1186/ s13104-015-1175-z.

22. Westhall E, Rossetti AO, van Rootselaar A-F, et al. Standardized EEG interpretation accurately predicts prognosis after cardiac arrest. *Neurology* 2016;86(16): 1482–90. doi:10.1212/WNL.0000000000002462.

23. Søholm H, Kjær TW, Kjaergaard J, et al. Prognostic value of electroencephalography (EEG) after out-of-hospital cardiac arrest in successfully resuscitated patients used in daily clinical practice. *Resuscitation* 2014;85(11):1580–5. doi:10.1016/j.resuscitation.2014.08.031.

24. Howard RS, Holmes PA. REVIEW 4 Practical neurology hypoxic-ischaemic brain injury. *Pr Neurol* 2011;11:4–18. doi:10.1136/jnnp.2010.235218.

25. Fogel W, Krieger D, Veith M, et al. Serum neuron-specific enolase as early predictor of outcome after cardiac arrest. *Crit Care Med* 1997;25(7):1133–8. Available from: http://www.ncbi.nlm.nih.gov/pubmed/9233737. Accessed November 11, 2016.

26. Rosén H, Rosengren L, Herlitz J, Blomstrand C. Increased serum levels of the S-100 protein are associated with hypoxic brain damage after cardiac arrest. *Stroke* 1998;29(2):473–7. Available from: http://www.ncbi.nlm. nih.gov/pubmed/9472892. Accessed November 11, 2016.

27. Ekmektzoglou KA, Xanthos T, Papadimitriou L. Biochemical markers (NSE, S-100, IL-8) as predictors of neurological outcome in patients after cardiac arrest and return of spontaneous circulation. *Resuscitation* 2007;75(2):219–28. doi:10.1016/j.resuscitation.2007.03.016.

28. Wijdicks EFM, Hijdra A, Young GB, Bassetti CL, Wiebe S. Practice Parameter: Prediction of outcome in comatose survivors after cardiopulmonary resuscitation (an evidence-based review): Report of the Quality Standards Subcommittee of the American Academy of Neurology. *Neurology* 2006;67(2):203–10. doi:10.1212/01. wnl.0000227183.21314.cd.

29. Daubin C, Guillotin D, Etard O, et al. A clinical and EEG scoring system that predicts early cortical response (N20) to somatosensory evoked potentials and outcome after cardiac arrest. *BMC Cardiovasc Disord* 2008;8:35. doi:10.1186/1471-2261-8-35.

30. Kilgannon JH. Association between arterial hyperoxia following resuscitation from cardiac arrest and in-hospital mortality. *JAMA* 2010;303(21):2165. doi:10.1001/jama.2010.707.

31. Vincent WR, Hatton KW. Critically ill patients need 'FAST HUGS BID' (an updated mnemonic). *Crit Care Med* 2009;37(7):2326–7. doi:10.1097/CCM.0b013e3181aabc29.

32. Peberdy MA, Callaway CW, Neumar RW, et al. Part 9: Post–Cardiac Arrest Care. *Circulation* 2010;122(18)(suppl 3): S768–86.

33. Arrich J, Holzer M, Havel C, Müllner M, Herkner H. Hypothermia for neuroprotection in adults after cardiopulmonary resuscitation. In: Arrich J, ed. *Cochrane Database of Systematic Reviews.* Chichester, UK: John Wiley & Sons, Ltd; 2016. doi:10.1002/14651858.CD004128.pub4.

34. Nielsen N, Wetterslev J, Cronberg T, et al. Targeted temperature management at 33°C versus 36°C after cardiac arrest. *N Engl J Med* 2013;23369(5):2197–206. doi:10.1056/NEJMoa1310519.

35. Vaity C, Al-Subaie N, Cecconi M. Cooling techniques for targeted temperature management post-cardiac arrest. *Crit Care* 2015;19(1):103. doi:10.1186/s13054-015-0804-1.

36. Krinsley JS, Grover A. Severe hypoglycemia in critically ill patients: Risk factors and outcomes. *Crit Care Med* 2007;35(10):2262–7. doi:10.1097/01.CCM.0000282073.98414.4B.

37. Dusick JR, Wang C, Cohan P, Swerdloff R, Kelly DF. Pathophysiology of hypopituitarism in the setting of brain injury. *Pituitary* 2012;15(1):2–9. doi:10.1007/s11102-008-0130-6.

38. Novy J, Logroscino G, Rossetti AO. Refractory status epilepticus: A prospective observational study. *Epilepsia* 2010;51(2):251–6. doi:10.1111/j.1528-1167.2009.02323.x.

39. Sakabe T, Tateishi A, Miyauchi Y, et al. Intracranial pressure following cardiopulmonary resuscitation. *Intensive Care Med* 1987;13(4):256–9. doi:10.1007/BF00265114.

40. Birnie DH, Sambell C, Johansen H, et al. Use of implantable cardioverter defibrillators in Canadian and US survivors of out-of-hospital cardiac arrest. *CMAJ* 2007;177(1):41–6. doi:10.1503/cmaj.060730.

41. Todd PM, Jerome RN, Jarquin-Valdivia AA. Organ preservation in a brain dead patient: information support for neurocritical care protocol development. *J Med Libr Assoc* 2007;95(3):238–45. doi:10.3163/1536-5050.95.3.238.

73

Status Epilepticus

L. Koffman, W. Ziai, N. Goettel, and P. W. Kaplan

ABSTRACT

Status epilepticus (SE) is a neurological emergency that should be quickly identified followed by rapid initiation of anti-seizure therapy. Diagnosis and initial treatment of seizures typically begins in the emergency department. Those patients who continue to have seizures or have been determined to be in status epilepticus require admission to the intensive care unit (ICU). This chapter discusses the different phases of treatment for status epilepticus in adults including emergent, urgent, and refractory treatment. In addition to anti-seizure therapies, these patients often require close haemodynamic monitoring and support, mechanical ventilation, and further investigations to identify the aetiology of seizures. Most patients admitted to the ICU should also be on continuous electroencephalographic monitoring while being treated for status epilepticus.

KEYWORDS

Status epilepticus (SE); seizures; anti-epileptic medications; refractory status epilepticus.

CASE STUDY

A 58-year-old woman with a past medical history of chronic pulmonary obstructive disease was found unresponsive at home. She was intubated by paramedics and brought to the emergency room for further evaluation. On initial examination, she was comatose with a dilated left fixed pupil, no corneal reflexes, intact cough, and gag reflexes. The right upper extremity was flexing and all other extremities had extensor posturing (Glasgow Coma Scale [GCS] 5T). Head computed tomography (CT) was done (Figure 73.1) and revealed a subarachnoid haemorrhage, a left-sided subdural haematoma, and a left temporal intra-parenchymal haemorrhage (modified Fisher scale 3). The patient was immediately taken for coiling of a left posterior communicating artery aneurysm and left-sided hemicraniectomy with haematoma evacuation.

On hospital day six, she was noted to be less responsive in her neurological examination with a new gaze preference. She was placed on continuous electroencephalography (EEG) monitoring and was found to be in status epilepticus (Figure 73.2A). Levetiracetam and valproate were administered in addition to intravenous (IV) midazolam. Midazolam was titrated to an EEG burst-suppression pattern (Figure 73.2B) using a maximum infusion rate of 15 mg/hour. After midazolam was weaned, left-sided periodic lateralized epileptiform discharges were noted (Figure 73.2C), but no seizures. As anti-seizure drugs (ASDs) were weaned and the patient became more alert, her EEG pattern improved, showing more EEG background activity (Figure 73.2D).

INTRODUCTION

Status epilepticus (SE) has been historically defined as seizures that persist for at least 30 minutes or multiple seizures without a return to baseline neurological examination.[1] This definition has been modified and while somewhat controversial, the Neurocritical Care

Society guidelines define SE as clinical or electrographic seizures that continue for more than five minutes or multiple seizures without a return to baseline.[2] There are many ways of classifying seizure types based on semiology and aetiology (see Table 73.1).

This chapter covers the treatment of the following types of SE:

• Convulsive Status Epilepticus (CSE): Generalized CSE (GCSE) typically consists of tonic-clonic movement of the extremities with an impairment in mental status which may include confusion, lethargy or coma.

Table 73.1 Various aetiologies to consider for status epilepticus

Acute processes

• Metabolic disturbances
  – Electrolyte abnormalities
  – Hypoglycaemia
  – Renal failure
• Sepsis
• Infection of the central nervous system
  – Meningitis
  – Encephalitis
  – Cerebral abscess
• Stroke
• Intracerebral haemorrhage
• Subarachnoid haemorrhage
• Cerebral sinus thrombosis
• Head Trauma
  – Traumatic brain injury
  – Subdural haematoma
  – Epidural haematoma
• Drugs
  – Toxicity
  – Withdrawal
  – Anti-seizure medication noncompliance
• Hypoxia, cardiorespiratory arrest
• Posterior reversible encephalopathy syndrome (PRES)
• Autoimmune encephalitis
• Paraneoplastic syndrome

Chronic processes
• Known history of epilepsy • Brain tumour • Remote injury of the central nervous system

Sources: (1) Brophy GM, Bell R, Claassen J, et al. Guidelines for the evaluation and management of status epilepticus. *Neurocrit Care* 2012;17:3–23. (2) Chen JWY, Wasterlain CG. Status epilepticus: pathophysiology and management in adults. *Lancet Neurol* 2006;5: 246–56. (3) Alldredge BK. A comparison of lorazepam, diazepam and placebo for the treatment of out-of-hospital status epilepticus. *N Engl J Med* 2001;345:631–7.

• Non-Convulsive Status Epilepticus (NCSE): There may be no clinical convulsive activity witnessed, but there may be subtle signs such a twitches, nystagmus, or gaze deviation.[3] There is evidence of EEG seizures— two subtypes have been described:
  – The awake patient who is confused but otherwise neurologically intact, who carries a good prognosis.[3]
  – The critically ill patient with severe impairment of mental status, or who is comatose, often with subtle motor movements secondary to an underlying neurologic insult.[4,5]
• Refractory Status Epilepticus (RSE): While there is debate over the duration of seizure activity to qualify as RSE, most authors agree to define RSE as clinical or EEG seizures despite adequate doses of standard therapies (including a benzodiazepine and second-line ASDs.[1,2]

Aside from these seizure types, there are other kinds of seizures and patient populations that should also be mentioned:

• *Focal seizures* are seizures that typically cause rhythmic movements of part of the body with preservation of mental status. Focal seizures that persist (epilepsia partialis continua) do not require the aggressive therapies given to patients in GCSE.
• *Paroxysmal Non-epileptic Events* (PNE), formerly known as psychogenic seizures, are seizures that may mimic those of GCSE and are often difficult to differentiate without EEG monitoring. These patients should be treated as GCSE until the diagnosis of PNE can be given with the aid of EEG monitoring. Once established, ASDs may be weaned. There are some clinical features that may raise suspicion for PNE: prolonged convulsions without autonomic disturbance, bilateral convulsions without decreased level of consciousness, absence of post-ictal confusion, and presence of asynchronous or side-to-side movements.[6]
• Patients who suffer cardio-respiratory arrest may have anoxic brain injury and subsequent epileptic activity. Generalized CSE after cardiac arrest may be treated as outlined below, but one must remember that SE in this context usually carries an abysmal prognosis, and more research is needed to help with accurate prognostication in the age of hypothermia protocols.
• There are known risks to using ASDs in pregnancy, but there are few data regarding treatment of SE and pregnancy. Recommendations for urgent and emergent ASDs include lorazepam and fosphenytoin,[7] though there are known risks of birth defects with exposure to

older ASDs (phenytoin, valproate, phenobarbital) in the first trimester when used in the long-term for epilepsy treatment. Some data suggests a lower risk to the foetus with exposure to newer agents prompting consideration for the use of levetiracetam.[8] Consideration should be taken when choosing maintenance doses of ASDs because pregnancy affects the volume of distribution and clearance of medications.

EPIDEMIOLOGY

Status epilepticus is a common neurologic emergency that has a reported incidence of 18–41 patients per year per 100,000 population.[9–11] Of these cases of SE about 31%–43% will become refractory.[12–14] Delay in diagnosis or treatment, focal seizures at onset and NCSE have been identified as predictors of refractoriness.[12,13] Furthermore, NCSE may be under-recognized, with one study reporting that NCSE affected 16% of confused elderly patients in the hospital.[15] A prospective observational study examined patients admitted to a neurointensive care unit (NICU) for altered mental status and diagnosed 21% of patients with either non-convulsive seizures or NCSE.[16]

PATHOPHYSIOLOGY

Status epilepticus should be quickly treated as seizures become more difficult to treat the longer they continue. Status epilepticus occurs due to an imbalance in excitatory and inhibitory mechanisms. Glutamine, its analogues, or other excitatory amino acids are responsible for an increase in excitatory synapses.[6] Gamma-aminobutyric acid (GABA) is the inhibitory neurotransmitter that has been implicated in the modulation of seizure activity.[6] When seizure activity is prolonged, there is a reduction in post-synaptic $GABA_A$ receptors and an increase in inactive $GABA_A$ receptors. As these post-synaptic membrane receptors become inactive, many anti-epileptic agents with GABA-ergic mechanisms lose efficacy.[17,18,20,21]

DIAGNOSTIC EVALUATION

A detailed history should be obtained where possible to assist in identifying a seizure aetiology. A neurological examination should be performed in addition to a complete physical examination. In the early stages, imaging such as CT of the brain may be warranted, if there is no return to baseline level of consciousness, if there is a new focal neurological finding, or if no identifiable cause can be found for the seizures.[19] Appropriate laboratory investigations are listed in Table 73.2. If the clinical

Table 73.2 Laboratory tests to include during initial evaluation

Serologic investigations
• Glucose and basic metabolic panel
• Arterial blood gas and acid-base abnormalities
• Calcium and magnesium
• Liver function panel
• Lactic acid
• Ammonia
• Alcohol level
• Toxicology screen
• Anti-seizure drug levels

history is suggestive of infection, the patient is febrile, or there is concern for subarachnoid haemorrhage, a lumbar puncture should be performed.[19] Cerebrospinal fluid (CSF) should be examined for cell count, glucose, protein, gram stain and culture, as well as other studies as indicated by the clinical history and presentation (i.e., xanthochromia, herpes simplex virus detection, or further studies if there is evidence or a history of immunodeficiency).[6]

Monitoring through EEG is crucial to managing a patient in SE. Guidelines for the management of SE strongly recommend that EEG monitoring should be initiated within an hour of suspected SE and continued until 24 hours after cessation of electrographic seizures or during ASD-weaning trials.[2] Comatose patients should be monitored for at least 48 hours.[2] There is class 1, level B evidence from the guidelines for the evaluation and management of status epilepticus for continuous EEG monitoring of the following indications:[2]

- Recent clinical seizure or SE without a return to baseline after 10 minutes
- Patient in a comatose state (including cardiac arrest)
- Epileptiform activity or periodic discharges on initial emergent EEG
- Suspected non-convulsive seizures in patients with altered mental status

Further imaging studies may be considered if none of the above yields a diagnosis. Magnetic resonance imaging of the brain may be performed. Imaging of other regions of the body may be indicated if there is a possibility of a paraneoplastic syndrome, including CT of the chest, abdomen, and pelvis, as well as ovarian or testicular ultrasound.[6] More thorough screenings for infection, autoimmune, inflammatory, and malignant aetiologies can be performed on serum and CSF. If there is still diagnostic uncertainty, other imaging studies may be considered including a whole-body positron emission tomography (PET) scan, single-photon emission computed tomography (SPECT) or fludeoxyglucose-PET of the brain. If the testing remains inconclusive and there is a lesion of the central nervous system identified on imaging, a brain biopsy may also be considered.[6]

TREATMENT

As previously mentioned, therapy should be implemented as quickly as possible with the aim of terminating clinical and electrographic seizures as soon as possible, preferably within 30–60 minutes.[2] While treating SE using the algorithm (Figure 73.3), airway and haemodynamic support should be provided in parallel, and adequate intravenous access should be established. Many of the medications used to treat SE can cause sedation, respiratory depression, arterial hypotension, and cardiac arrhythmias, warranting close monitoring. Pharmacological interventions have been divided into first-line or emergent therapy, second-line therapy with non-sedating ASDs, and third-line therapy with anaesthetic infusions for the treatment of refractory SE.[2]

There are limited data for efficacy in the treatment of SE, with the exception being the use of benzodiazepines. First-line treatment of SE calls for the use of benzodiazepines. Benzodiazepines may be given via multiple routes (intravenous [IV], intramuscular [IM], rectal, nasal, and oral); however, if IV access is available, this is the preferred route of administration.[2] IV lorazepam and IM midazolam are the expert-recommended therapies (class 1, level A evidence).[2,22–28] Multiple controlled studies have evaluated the use of IV lorazepam against diazepam, phenytoin, phenobarbital, and IM midazolam.[22,23,25,29] Intramuscular midazolam was reported to be non-inferior to IV lorazepam in prehospitalized patients.[29]

Table 73.3 denotes dosing and considerations for benzodiazepine therapy. Adverse effects common to this class of medications include arterial hypotension and respiratory depression.

After patients in SE have received emergent therapy, a second-line therapy (using ASDs) should be used, unless there is an identified and correctable cause for the SE (i.e., hypoglycaemia, hyponatraemia, etc).

There are limited data from randomized controlled trials regarding which ASDs are most efficacious, and many new ASDs have become available. The goal is to provide an IV ASD with a loading dose followed by maintenance dose to stop the SE and prevent recurrent seizures. There are ASD options, with IV access, that can reach therapeutic levels within a short amount of time. Table 73.4 summarizes these agents. The ASD should be chosen based on the patient's medical history and comorbidities. Fosphenytoin is generally considered the preferred agent; however, valproate should be used when there is a history of primary (or idiopathic) generalized epilepsy.

Once second-line therapies have been given, one may continue to give bolus doses intermittently with additional ASDs if the patient is haemodynamically stable and protecting his/her airway, or therapy may need to be escalated to continuous infusion therapy. Continuous EEG monitoring should guide therapy, with medications being titrated to the remission of EEG seizure activity, an EEG burst-suppression pattern, or virtual suppression of EEG brain activity.[2] The usual initial options for the treatment of RSE include propofol, midazolam, and barbiturates. There is no evidence for the most successful agent in termination of seizure activity.[30,31] There are some data to suggest that pentobarbital may treat RSE more effectively than midazolam, but it has a long half-life with multiple significant adverse effects.[32]

Table 73.3 Medications and dosing for emergent control of status epilepticus

Drug	Initial dose	Notes
Diazepam	0.15 mg/kg IV <10 mg/dose, may repeat in 5 minutes	• Rapid distribution with short duration • Active metabolite • IV formulation contains propylene glycol
Lorazepam	0.1 mg/kg IV <4 mg/dose, may repeat in 5–10 minutes	• Dilute 1:1 with saline • IV formulation contains propylene glycol
Midazolam	0.2 mg/kg IM (or IV infused at 2 mg/min) <10 mg/dose	• Active metabolite • Renal elimination • Rapid distribution with short duration

Adapted from: Brophy GM, Bell R, Claassen J, et al. Guidelines for the evaluation and management of status epilepticus. *Neurocrit Care* 2012; 17:3–23.

Table 73.4 Summary of second-line ASD options

Drug	Initial dose	Adverse events	Notes
Phenytoin	20 mg/kg IV, can give additional 5–10 mg/kg bolus	• Arterial hypotension • Cardiac arrhythmias • Purple glove syndrome	• Compatible in only saline • Contains propylene glycol
Fosphenytoin	20 mg/kg PE IV, can give additional 5 mg/kg bolus	• Arterial hypotension • Cardiac arrhythmias	• Compatible in saline, dextrose and lactated Ringer's solution
Valproate	20–40 mg/kg IV, can give additional 5–10 mg/kg bolus	• Hyperammonaemia • Pancreatitis • Thrombocytopenia • Hepatotoxicity	• Cautious use in patients with traumatic brain injury
Levetiracetam	1000–3000 mg IV		• Minimal drug interactions • Requires renal dosing
Lacosamide	200–400 mg IV	• Arterial hypotension • Cardiac arrhythmias	• Minimal drug interactions
Phenobarbital	20 mg/kg IV, can give additional 5–10 mg bolus	• Arterial hypotension • Respiratory depression	• IV formulation contains propylene glycol

Adapted from: Brophy GM, Bell R, Claassen J, et al. Guidelines for the evaluation and management of status epilepticus. *Neurocrit Care* 2012; 17:3–23.

Table 73.5 summarizes the dosing for these agents. Each of these infusions has adverse effects which may influence the choice. Patients on IV infusions of anaesthetic agents may commonly require mechanical ventilation and close cardiac and haemodynamic monitoring. It is important to effectively utilize first-line and second-line therapies prior to initiating a third-line agent, as the addition of anaesthetic infusions has serious multi-systemic adverse effects. Studies have shown that the addition of these third-line agents has an increased risk of poor outcome

Table 73.5 Summary of recommendations for continuous infusions with third line therapies

Drug	Initial dose	Continuous infusion dose	Adverse effects	Notes
Midazolam	0.2 mg/kg	0.05–2 mg/kg/hr ***0.1–0.2 mg/kg bolus, rate increase of 0.05–0.1 mg/kg/hr every 3–4 hours	• Arterial hypotension • Respiratory depression	• Prolonged use can cause tachyphylaxis • Active metabolite • Renal excretion
Pentobarbital	5–15 mg/kg, may give additional 5–10 mg/kg	0.5–5 mg/kg/hr ***5 mg/kg bolus, rate increase by 0.5–1 mg/kg/hr every 12 hours	• Arterial hypotension • Respiratory depression • Paralytic ileus	• Requires mechanical ventilation • Contains propylene glycol • Can cause loss of all neurologic reflexes
Propofol	20 mcg/kg/min with 1–2 mg/kg loading dose	30–200 mcg/kg/min ***Increase by 5–10 mcg/kg/min +/–1 mg/kg bolus	• Arterial hypotension • Respiratory depression • Rhabdomyolysis • Metabolic acidosis • Renal failure	• Requires mechanical ventilation • Monitor for propofol infusion syndrome • Cautious use of high doses for >48 hours
Thiopental	2–7 mg/kg	0.5–5 mg/kg/hr ***1–2 mg/kg bolus and increase rate by 0.5–1 mg/kg/hr every 12 hours	• Arterial hypotension • Respiratory depression	• Requires mechanical ventilation • Metabolized to pentobarbital

Note: These medications are titrated based on continuous EEG findings. Asterisks indicate breakthrough SE and appropriate medication adjustments.
Adapted from: Brophy GM, Bell R, Claassen J, et al. Guidelines for the evaluation and management of status epilepticus. *Neurocrit Care* 2012; 17:3–23.

and death independent of known confounders of poor outcome.[33,34]

Once electrographic seizures have ceased for a period of 24 to 48 hours, continuous infusion of the anaesthetic agent should be titrated, using continuous EEG monitoring for guidance. During this period, maintenance doses of non-sedating ASDs should be administered so that they are at therapeutic target zones during and after the weaning of anaesthetic (sedating) ASDs. As the continuous infusion is weaned, there may be recurrent RSE, in which case the infusion should be increased to cessation of epileptiform activity and maintained for a longer duration with addition of other ASDs. There is no strong evidence to guide duration of this therapy, only a weak recommendation to continue anaesthetic agents for at least another period of 24 to 48 hours. EEG monitoring should again be continued for at least 24 hours after cessation of epileptiform activity or while ASDs are being weaned.[2]

In some cases, RSE may be extremely difficult to treat with standard third-line therapies and alternative treatments may be considered. These therapies (Table 73.6) may be appropriate in some patients, such as RSE secondary to autoimmune encephalitis. These treatments have not been studied as well as previously discussed treatment strategies, and their use is based on case series and anecdotal evidence.

SYSTEMIC COMPLICATIONS

Convulsive seizures can adversely affect many organs in addition to the nervous system. If there is suspicion for trauma, an appropriate orthopaedic survey should be performed to address fractures or dislocations. At least one creatine kinase should be checked to exclude

Table 73.6 Summary of alternative therapies for the treatment of RSE when it does not respond to standard treatment

Pharmacological treatments	Non-pharmacological treatments
• Ketamine • Corticosteroids • Volatile anaesthetics • Immunomodulation (Intravenous Immunoglobulins (IVIG), plasmapheresis)	• Vagal nerve stimulation • Ketogenic diet • Hypothermia • Electroconvulsive therapy • Transcranial magnetic stimulation • Surgical management

Adapted from: Brophy GM, Bell R, Claassen J, et al. Guidelines for the evaluation and management of status epilepticus. *Neurocrit Care* 2012;17:3–23.

rhabdomyolysis. Urinary output should be monitored as renal failure can occur. Aspiration may occur during convulsive seizures. Finally, as with other kinds of neurological illness, there is risk for cardiac injury including stress-induced cardiomyopathy, cardiogenic pulmonary oedema and non-ST elevation myocardial infarction.[6]

PROGNOSIS

Large ranges for mortality at hospital discharge have been reported for CSE (9%–21%), NCSE (18%–52%) and RSE (23%–61%).[2] While RSE was previously associated with worse outcomes, it is now postulated that outcome is largely a reflection of seizure aetiology and seizure type, and not duration of seizure activity beyond the first several hours.[35]

As previously mentioned, seizures in the context of CRA should be considered a separate entity. Both CSE and myoclonic SE secondary to hypoxic-ischaemic encephalopathy are associated with poor outcomes such as decreased survival and recovery of consciousness.[36]

CONCLUSIONS

SE is a neurologic emergency that should be rapidly identified and appropriately treated. Caring for a patient in SE requires multiple parallel treatment algorithms (Figure 73.3) to ensure optimal delivery and titration of medications. While medications for the treatment of SE should be administered without delay, priority should be first given to securement of the airway and stabilization of haemodynamics.

REFERENCES

1. Bleck TP. Refractory status epilepticus. *Curr Opin Crit Care* 2005;11:117–20.
2. Brophy GM, Bell R, Claassen J, et al. Guidelines for the evaluation and management of status epilepticus. *Neurocrit Care* 2012;17:3–23.
3. Shorvon S. What is nonconvulsive status epilepticus, and what are its subtypes? *Epilepsia* 2007;48(Suppl 8):35–8.
4. Towne AR, Waterhouse EJ, Boggs JG, et al. Prevalence of nonconvulsive status epilepticus in comatose patients. *Neurology* 2000;54:340–5.
5. Hirsch LJ. Status epilepticus. *Continuum Lifelong Learn Neurol* 2007;13:121–51.
6. Hocker SE. Status epilepticus. *Continuum* 2015;21:1362–83.
7. Karnad DK, Guntupalli KK. Neurologic disorders in pregnancy. *Crit Care Med* 2005;33:S362–71.
8. Molgaard-Nielsen D. Newer-generation antiepileptic drugs and the risk of major birth defects. *J Am Med Assoc* 2011;305:1996–2002.

9. DeLorenzo RJ, Hauser WA, Towne AR, et al. A prospective, population-based epidemiologic study of status epilepticus in Richmond, Virginia. *Neurology* 1996;46:1029–35.

10. Hesdorffer DC, Logroscino G, Gascino G, Aenegers JF, Hauser WA. Incidence of status epilepticus in Rochester, Minnesota, 1965–1984. *Neurology* 1998;50:735–41.

11. Waterhouse EJ, Garnett LK, Towne AR, et al. Prospective population-based study of intermittent and continuous status epilepticus in Richmond, Virginia. *Epilepsia* 1999;40:752–8.

12. Mayer SA, Claaseen J, Lokin J, Mendelsohn F, Dennis LJ, Fitzsimmons BF. Refractory status epilepticus: frequency, risk factors, and impact on outcome. *Arch Neurol* 2002; 59:205–10.

13. Holtkamp M, Othman J, Buchheim K, Meierkord H. Predictors and prognosis of refractory status epilepticus treated in a neurologic intensive care unit. *J Neurol Neurosurg Psychiatry* 2005;76:534–9.

14. Rossetti AO, Logroscino G, Bromfield EB. Refractory status epilepticus: effect of treatment aggressiveness on prognosis. *Arch Neurol* 2005;62:1698–702.

15. Veran O, Kahane P, Thomas P, Hamelin S, Sabourdy C, Vercueil L. De novo epileptic confusion in the elderly: a 1 year prospective study. *Epilepsia* 2010;51:1030–5.

16. Laccheo I, Sonmezturk H, Bhatt AB, et al. Non-convulsive status epilepticus and non-convulsive seizures in neurological ICU patients. *Neurocrit Care* 2015;22:202–11.

17. Feng H, Mathews GC, Kao C, Macdonald RL. Alterations of GABAA receptor function and allosteric modulation during development of status epilepticus. *J Neurophysiol* 2008;99:1285–93.

18. Deeb TZ, Maguire J, Moss SJ. Possible alterations in GABAA receptor signaling that underlie benzodiazepine-resistant seizures. *Epilepsia* 2012;53(Suppl 9): 79–88.

19. Claassen J, Riviello JJ, Silbergleit R. Emergency neurological life support: status epilepticus. *Neurocrit Care* 2015;23:S136–42.

20. Lowenstein DH. Current concepts: status epilepticus. *N Engl J Med* 1998;338:970.

21. Chen JWY, Wasterlain CG. Status epilepticus: pathophysiology and management in adults. *Lancet Neurol* 2006;5:246–56.

22. Alldredge BK. A comparison of lorazepam, diazepam and placebo for the treatment of out-of-hospital status epilepticus. *N Engl J Med* 2001;345:631–7.

23. Treiman DM, Meyers PD, Walton NY, et al. A comparison of four treatments for generalized convulsive status epilepticus. Veterans affairs status epilepticus cooperative study. *N Engl J Med* 1998;339:792–8.

24. Litt B, Wityk RJ, Hertz SH, et al. Nonconvulsive status epilepticus in the critically ill elderly. *Epilepsia* 1998;39: 1194–202.

25. Leppik IE, Derivan AT, Homan RW, Walker J, Ramsay RE, Patrick B. Double-blind study of lorazepam and diazepam in status epilepticus. *JAMA* 1983;249:1452–4.

26. Treiman DM, Walker MC. Treatment of seizure emergencies: convulsive and non-convulsive status epilepticus. *Epilepsy Res* 2006;68(Suppl 1):S77–82.

27. Appleton R, Sweeney A, Choonara I, Robson J, Molyneux E. Lorazepam versus diazepam in the acute treatment of epileptic seizures and status epilepticus. *Dev Med Child Neurol* 1995;37:682–8.

28. Walker JE, Homan RW, Vasko MR, Crawford IL, Bell RD, Tasker WG. Lorazepam in status epilepticus. *Ann Neurol* 1979;6:207–13.

29. Silbergleit R, Durkalski V, Lowenstein D, et al. Intramuscular versus intravenous therapy for prehospital status epilepticus. *N Engl J Med* 2012;366:591–600.

30. Rossetti AO, Lowenstein DH. Management of refractory status epilepticus in adults: still more questions than answers. *Lancet Neurol* 2011;10:9822–930.

31. Rossetti AO, Fersli M. The treatment of super-refractory status epilepticus: a critical review of available therapies and a clinical treatment protocol. *Brain* 2011;134:2802–18.

32. Claassen J, Hirsch JL, Emeron RG, Mayer SA. Treatment of refractory status epilepticus with pentobarbital, propofol or midazolam: a systematic review. *Epilepsia* 2002;43: 146–53.

33. Kowalsi RG, Ziai WC, Rees RN, et al. Third-line antiepileptic therapy and outcome in status epilepticus: The impact of vasopressor use and prolonged mechanical ventilation. *Crit Care Med* 2012; 40:2677–84.

34. Sutter R, De Marchis GM, Semmlack S, et al. Anesthetics and outcome in status epilepticus: A matched two-center cohort study. *CNS Drugs* 2017;31(1):65–74.

35. Drislane FW, Blum AS, Lopez MR, Gautam S, Schomer DL. Duration of refractory status epilepticus and outcome: loss of prognostic utility after several hours. *Epilepsia* 2002;50:1566–71.

36. Nielsen N, Sunde K, Hovdenes J, et al. Hypothermia Network. Adverse events and their relation to mortality in out-of –hospital cardiac arrest patients treated with hypothermia. *Crit Care Med* 2011;39:57–64.

74

Aneurysmal Subarachnoid Haemorrhage

A. Lele

ABSTRACT

Subarachnoid haemorrhage (SAH) due to rupture of an intracerebral aneurysm is a neurological emergency with widespread implications. A thorough knowledge is needed to make rational clinical decisions which are unique for this dynamic clinical condition. Mortality and morbidity are related to re-bleeding, cerebral vasospasm, and delayed cerebral ischaemia. This chapter provides the reader with basic and advanced practical knowledge related to aneurysmal subarachnoid haemorrhage (aSAH).

KEYWORDS

Subarachnoid haemorrhage (SAH); cerebral aneurysm; clipping; coiling; vasospasm; hydrocephalus; hyponatraemia; re-bleeding.

CASE STUDY

A 56-year-old lady was grocery shopping when she collapsed after complaining of severe headache. Bystanders called emergency services and she was taken to the nearest hospital where non-contrast computed tomography (CT) scan of the brain demonstrated subarachnoid haemorrhage (SAH) filling the anterior interhemispheric fissure and quadrigeminal cisterns with concomitant hydrocephalus, without intraventricular hemorrhage. Her post-resuscitation Hunt and Hess score was 2, and modified Fisher score was 3. An external ventricular drain (EVD) was placed for cerebrospinal fluid diversion. Cerebral angiogram confirmed a 4×6 mm anterior-communicating artery aneurysm, which was successfully coil-embolized via endovascular approach. She received enteral nimodipine 60 mg every 4 hours for 21 days. She was followed in the neurointensive care unit (NICU) with daily transcranial Doppler (TCD) ultrasound, which demonstrated maximal mean flow velocities (MFV) of 120 cm/sec in the anterior cerebral artery (ACA) and 146 cm/sec in the middle cerebral artery (MCA) territory, with a maximal Lindegaard ratio (LR) of 3.8. She was taken for cerebral angiogram due to new leg weakness and received 2 mg of intra-arterial nicardipine for treatment of moderate vasospasm in both the ACA and MCA territories with good post-injection cerebral blood flow (CBF). She underwent removal of her EVD and was discharged to an inpatient rehabilitation facility on post-bleed day 16, with some cognitive but no motor deficit.

INTRODUCTION

Aneurysmal subarachnoid haemorrhage (aSAH) is one of the most devastating neurological emergencies. While significant advances have been made in recognition, early aneurysm securement, and multimodal strategies in the management of cerebral vasospasm, aSAH continues to have significant mortality and morbidity. This chapter presents readers with up to date information regarding the following aspects of aSAH: epidemiology, primary prevention of aSAH, historical landmarks in medical management of aSAH, clinical presentation of aSAH, aSAH severity grading scales, neuroimaging in patients with aSAH, critical care management of patients with aSAH, systemic implications in aSAH, repair of ruptured intracerebral aneurysms, prevention of re-bleeding, cerebral vasospasm, outcomes after aSAH, 30-day readmission, and quality improvement initiatives.

EPIDEMIOLOGY OF ANEURYSMAL SUBARACHNOID HAEMORRHAGE

Worldwide Incidence

The prevalence of intracranial aneurysms is 2.3%.[1] Aneurysmal subarachnoid haemorrhage affects approximately 10.5/100,000 patient years.[2] Finland and Japan have the highest incidence of aSAH at 22–23/100,000 patient years.[2] Interestingly, recent evidence indicates that Finland and Japan do not have higher prevalence of unruptured intracranial aneurysms implicating high risk factors for rupture.[3] Aneurysmal subarachnoid haemorrhage affects women more commonly than men (1.24:1)[4] and has a case fatality of 51/100,000 patient years.[2] Patients with first degree relatives affected with aSAH have a higher relative risk of SAH.[2] Hypertension, smoking, and heavy daily alcohol use (>2 units/day) are significant risk factors.[2]

Non-Modifiable Risk Factors

The incidence of aSAH increases with age and peaks in the fifth or sixth decade.[4] Earlier age of menarche and nulliparity are associated with increased risk for aSAH.[4] African-American and minorities in general have increased risk, with the highest incidence being in the Asian/Pacific Islander males.[4]

Studies conducted on American families found susceptibility locus on chromosome 13q, while in Dutch families, high prevalence of intracranial aneurysms found susceptibility loci at 1p36 and Xp22.[4] Other specific loci including single nucleotide polymorphism (SNP) in exon 7 of the endothelial nitric oxide synthase gene, and G894T, signify genetic factors associated with intracranial aneurysm rupture.[4]

It is believed that aneurysm size is the most significant factor in aneurysm rupture. In the International Study of Unruptured Intracranial Aneurysm (ISUIA), patients without a history of SAH, and size under 10 mm had a very small annual rupture risk (0.05%).[5] However, it is equally important to note that aneurysm rupture has been reported in aneurysms smaller than 10 mm in size, the rupture risk for 2 mm to 6 mm aneurysms is 1.1% annually, and for 6 mm to 9 mm aneurysm is 2.3% annually,[4] implying that the risk of rupture increases with size of aneurysm.

Modifiable Risk Factors

Uncontrolled hypertension is associated with increased risk for rupture of intracranial aneurysms.[6] In the younger population, aSAH is associated with many modifiable risk factors such as hypertension, cigarette smoking, cocaine and marijuana use,[7] and presents us the potential challenge for primary prevention.

Cocaine use has been associated with higher risk of aneurysm rupture (odds ratio 24.97).[4] Ruptures tend to occur at an earlier age (18–49 years)[4] with much smaller aneurysms,[8] with an innately high risk for aneurysm re-rupture,[9] and high risk for seizures.[10] The clinical course is complicated by an increased risk for vasospasm[11,12] and poor outcomes, particularly higher mortality and lower home discharge rates.[9,13,14]

Recreational marijuana (cannabis) use has been independently associated with an 18% increased likelihood of aSAH.[15] Cannabis use has been found to be more frequent among younger patients, males, black patients, and Medicaid enrollees,[15] and has been independently associated with delayed cerebral ischaemia and poor outcome.[16]

In a population-based study from Tromso, high daily coffee consumption (>5 cups per day, odds ratio 3.86) has been shown to be a significant risk factor for aSAH.[17]

Former smokers (odds ratio 2.7) and current smokers (odds ratio 6.1) are at higher risk for aneurysm rupture,[4] and the occurrence of aSAH is inversely proportional to the period of abstinence from smoking. Nicotine replacement therapy is safe with similar rates of cerebral vasospasm and delayed cerebral ischaemia.[18] Lower body mass index (BMI) is associated with higher risk of aSAH.[4]

PRIMARY PREVENTION OF ANEURYSMAL SUBARACHNOID HAEMORRHAGE

Although no one strategy exists for primary prevention of aSAH, the 2012 American Heart Association (AHA) guidelines stress the importance of hypertension treatment, avoidance of tobacco and alcohol, along with consumption of a diet rich in vegetables to reduce the risk of aSAH.[19]

In patients with familial aSAH (at least one first-degree relative), and or history of aSAH, it is reasonable to perform non-invasive screening to diagnose de novo aneurysms.[19] In patients with unruptured cerebral aneurysms, size, location, morphological, and haemodynamic characteristics of aneurysms in addition to the patient's age and health status should be incorporated in the discussion of risks of aneurysm rupture.[19]

Historical landmarks in medical advancement for the management of patients with SAH have been covered in Chapter 84, Appendix.

CLINICAL PRESENTATION OF ANEURYSMAL SUBARACHNOID HAEMORRHAGE

Aneurysmal subarachnoid haemorrhage typically presents with a 'thunder clap' ~ 'worst headache of my life'. While this presenting symptom is widely recognized as being synonymic with aSAH, high index of suspicion is required to perform a thorough workup of the patient for suspected ruptured cerebral aneurysm.[19] Apart from headache, frequently associated symptoms include nausea, vomiting, and transient worsening in the level of consciousness.

Patients intermediately present with signs and symptoms of complications associated with aSAH, such as progressive loss of consciousness associated with acute hydrocephalus, and may present with severe cardiovascular collapse during the ictal event.

The location of SAH and the ruptured aneurysm may contribute to specific clinical presentation syndrome complexes, such as headache and loss of consciousness for posterior circulation aneurysm rupture, and headache and diplopia for the rupture of posterior communicating artery aneurysm.

A thorough clinical examination including a comprehensive neurological examination often reveals nuchal rigidity and the presence of third or sixth cranial nerve paresis. Systemic examination reveals an anxious patient with bifrontal and nuchal pain, and a headache that is unremitting to over-the-counter analgesics, who is often hypertensive, tachycardiac (at times bradycardia in the setting of intracranial hypertension).

It important to grade the clinical severity of aSAH, as historically and traditionally Hunt and Hess (H&H) grading has been used to risk stratify patients for surgical intervention. It must be noted that admission H&H grading should only be performed after aggressive resuscitative attempts, which include airway securement, maintenance of cerebral perfusion pressure (CPP), treatment of acute asymptomatic hydrocephalus by external cerebrospinal fluid diversion achieved with the placement of an external ventricular drain (or lumbar drain).[19] Documentation of clinical severity by one of the grading scales (refer to Chapter 84, Appendix) is recommended in the AHA guidelines, and H&H and Fisher score (refer to Chapter 84, Appendix) is a core reportable measure from certified and designated comprehensive stroke centres (CSC).[19]

Funduscopic examination is an important component of clinical assessment after aSAH. The presence of pre-retinal, retinal, and vitreal haemorrhage has been described to be a part of Terson's syndrome, which are associated with high-grade haemorrhages, are frequently associated with elevated intracranial pressures (ICPs),[20] and thus carry poor prognosis.[21,22] Often under-reported, these abnormalities are thought to occur in about 40% of acute aneurysmal bleeds, and suspected vision loss should alert clinicians to perform a funduscopic examination.[23] The presence of Terson's syndrome on CT scan carries a 50% sensitivity and 98.4% specificity.[20]

GRADING SEVERITY OF SUBARACHNOID HAEMORRHAGE

For grading severity scales refer to Chapter 84, Appendix.

NEUROIMAGING IN PATIENTS WITH aSAH

Non-Contrast CT Scan

Subarachnoid haemorrhage is diagnosed by the demonstration of blood products in the cranial subarachnoid space, such as basal, quadrigeminal cisterns, sylvian and anterior interhemispheric fissures on a non-contrast CT scan of the brain (Figure 74.1). Quantitative assessment of subarachnoid blood is of prognostic value and is used in calculation of Fisher[24] or Claassen modification of Fisher score,[25] and the Hijdra sum score.[26] These scales offer the probability of risk of clinical vasospasm. Non-contrast CT scan is extremely sensitive to diagnose SAH (99%) in the first 24 hours and sensitivity gradually wanes to about 30% by about 3–4 weeks after onset of SAH.

Magnetic resonance imaging (MRI), specifically, fluid-attenuated inversion recovery (FLAIR), proton density, diffusion-weighted sequences, and gradient echo (GRE) sequences are reasonable to perform in patients with aSAH with a non-diagnostic CT scan.[19]

CT Angiogram (CTA)

CT angiography with 3-D reconstruction has enabled clinicians to visualize cerebral aneurysms and offer clinical decision-making of a specific best modality for repair, i.e., coiling vs. clipping,[19] however, it is rarely used as the sole angiographic study prior to final aneurysm securement, and in cases where CTA is negative, a digital subtraction angiography is still recommended.[19]

Digital Subtraction Angiography (DSA)

The location and anatomical characteristics of the cause of aSAH, i.e., ruptured cerebral aneurysm on cerebral angiogram still to this date is considered the gold standard.

Detailed digital subtraction with 3-dimensional rotational cerebral angiography (Figure 74.2) is indicated in patients with suspected aSAH.[19] If the first angiogram is negative, as in 'perimesencephalic subarachnoid haemorrhage' the current practice is to obtain a second angiogram 7–10 days after the first angiogram.

APPROACH TO PATIENTS WHO ARE CT NEGATIVE BUT HAVE HIGH CLINICAL SUSPICION FOR aSAH

A certain subset of patients with aSAH (10%–15%) fail to reveal presence of blood on non-contrast CT scan. These patients most likely have SAH but the ictus is greater than 24 hours old. In these patients if the clinical suspicion is high, admission to a neurocritical care unit is warranted. Cerebrospinal fluid (CSF) analysis performed approximately 12 hours after onset of symptoms demonstrating 'xanthochromia' is considered pathognomonic of aSAH. If the CSF is analysed 'too early' xanthochromia is likely not demonstrated, however, haemorrhagic CSF obtained in these patients is not specific for aneurysmal bleed. Thus, caution must be used to interpret results of CSF which contains RBCs but lacks xanthochromia.

Critical Care Management of a Patient with aSAH

Admission to a dedicated neurocritical care unit is paramount in patients with aSAH. Low volume centres (<10 aSAH per year), should consider early transfer to high-volume centres (>35 aSAH per year) with experienced cerebrovascular surgeons, endovascular specialists, and multidisciplinary neurocritical care services.[19] Serial neurological examinations (neurological wake-up tests) are the gold standard to trend level of consciousness, presence of new cranial nerve, and sensory motor deficits, which reflect evolution of intracranial hypertension (IH) and concurrent reduction in CPP.

Standard intensive care unit (ICU) monitoring includes continuous telemetry, pulse oximetry, non-invasive blood pressure (BP), and respiratory rate.

Perhaps the most important critical care intervention is aggressive monitoring and treatment of systolic and mean BPs, and the preservation of CPP. Due to high risk of aneurysm re-bleeding in the first 24 hours of all the stroke subtypes (acute ischaemic, spontaneous intracerebral, and subarachnoid haemorrhages), patients with suspected aSAH receive the most aggressive BP reduction. Patients with systolic blood pressures (SBPs) in excess of 160 mmHg are at statistically significant risk for aneurysm re-bleeding.[27]

Blood pressure management frequently involves the use of non-invasive BP apparatus or invasive arterial BP catheters.

Medications used to treat blood pressures include nicardipine, labetalol or esmolol. Medications such as nitroglycerine or nitroprusside should not be routinely used in anti-hypertensive regimens, as intense cerebral vasodilation associated with these can significantly elevate ICP.

Target systolic pressures are typically 90–120/140 mmHg. According to the 2012 AHA SAH guidelines, SBP should be maintained under 160 mmHg.[19] In elderly patients and in those with chronic severe hypertension, target systolic pressures are 90–140 mmHg. In either scenario, if there is elevation in ICP, a CPP of at least 60 should be maintained and hypotension avoided.

In patients with evidence of myocardial dysfunction, for example, those with hypotension requiring vasopressors, baseline cardiac enzymes, electrocardiography (EKG), echocardiography, and cardiac output monitoring are recommended.[28]

Routine use of central venous pressures to guide fluid management and routine placement of pulmonary-artery catheters is not recommended.[28] While clinicians may use a variety of non-invasive and invasive monitoring techniques, no one technique has been demonstrated to be superior to the other. Monitoring of volume status may be beneficial,[28] and overall goal should be to maintain euvolaemia with isotonic crystalloids, and hypervolaemia should be avoided.[28] Fludrocortisone or hydrocortisone may be used in patients who maintain a persistent negative fluid balance.[28]

Patients who lack ability to protect their airway, must be promptly intubated to prevent hypoxia and inadvertent hypocarbia or hypercarbia. Caution must be exercised as inadvertent hypocarbia despite presence of stable mean arterial pressures (MAP) may cause significant widening of transmural pressure gradient and promote aneurysm re-bleeding. The common steps in management of aSAH are highlighted in Table 74.1.

SYSTEMIC IMPLICATIONS OF SUBARACHNOID HAEMORRHAGE

Aneurysmal subarachnoid haemorrhage is a systemic disease.[29] Nearly all major organ systems are affected. Perhaps the two most of interest include derangements in cardiopulmonary and endocrine systems. Table 74.2 provides highlights of systemic implications of aSAH.

Cardiopulmonary Complications Associated with aSAH

Neurogenic Cardiac Dysfunction

It is now well recognized that cardiac dysfunction, either in the form of neurogenic stunned myocardium or Tako-Tsubo

Table 74.1 Critical care management of patients with aneurysmal subarachnoid haemorrhage

Early management of aSAH
1. Referral to a high-volume aSAH centre
2. Admit to a neurocritical care unit
3. Hourly neurological checks
4. Maintain airway (prompt intubation in those unable to protect airway) and avoid hypoxia
5. Controlled ventilation (avoid hypocarbia and hypercarbia)
6. Isotonic crystalloids
7. Maintain euvolaemia
8. SBP goal 90–120 (or 90–140) mmHg
9. Order labetalol and infusion of nicardipine (5–15 mg/hr) to achieve SBP goals
10. Swallowing evaluation
11. Oral intake only in the form of medications until definite surgical planning
12. Nimodipine 60 mg every 4 hours (or 30 mg every 2 hours, in patients unable to tolerate a 60-mg dose)
13. Analgesia with fentanyl 25–50 mcg every 1–2 hours in addition to acetaminophen 650 mg every 6 hours (avoid long-acting opioids)
14. Ondansetron 4 mg every 6 hours as needed to nausea
15. Bowel regimen to prevent/relieve constipation and straining
16. Surveillance
• Hourly neurological checks
• Admission labs
– Complete metabolic profile
– Serum magnesium, phosphorus, and ionized calcium
– Type and cross match for blood (2–4 units PRBC)
– Cardiac troponin I in high-grade SAH
– 12-lead EKG in all patients
– Beta-natriuretic peptide in high-grade SAH
– ECHO in patients with suspected myocardial dysfunction and in high-grade SAH
• Electrolyte and glucose goals
– Sodium >135 meq/L
– Magnesium >2 mg
– Potassium >4 meq/L
– Phosphorus >2
– Ionized calcium <1.0
– Serum glucose goal 100–180 mg/dL
• Baseline TCD for vasospasm screening
Post-clipping or coiling management of aSAH
1. Readmit to neurocritical care unit
2. Re-establish SBP goals (90–160 mmHg)
3. Maintain euvolaemia, euglycaemia, eunatraemia, eucarbia
4. Maintain normothermia (normothermia protocol, which includes tiered temperature control measures)
• Acetaminophen, surface or intravascular cooling devices, aggressive anti-shivering measures
5. Fludrocortisone for persistent negative fluid balance
6. Daily TCDs for vasospasm screening for 10–14 days or greater
7. Serial CT scan to screen for hydrocephalus during the clamping period of external ventricular drain

like cardiomyopathy exists in a subset of patients with aSAH.[30–33] Factors associated with cardiomyopathy include severity of grade of presentation (H&H ≥3), presence of elevated troponin on admission,[31] and presence of EKG abnormalities.

Peak troponin (cTI) levels have been associated with increased risk of echocardiographic left ventricular dysfunction,[34] pulmonary oedema, hypotension requiring vasopressors, delayed cerebral ischaemia from vasospasm, and death or poor functional outcome at discharge.[31,35,36]

Echocardiography (ECHO), EKG abnormalities, elevated troponins, and pulmonary oedema have been demonstrated with increased frequency in patients with

Table 74.2 Systemic implications of aSAH

Primary organ system affected	Prevalence of abnormalities	Implications
CARDIOVASCULAR		
Neurogenic stunned myocardium Tako-Tsubo cardiomyopathy Reverse Tako-Tsubo cardiomyopathy[*]	Correlation between ST elevation and transient ECHO abnormalities[**]	Reversibility of ECHO abnormalities and association with cerebral vasospasm[***] Augmenting cardiac output can reverse flow deficits from vasospasm[@] Consider use of IABC in patients with medically refractory cerebral vasospasm and low ejection fraction
Heart rate	39% prolonged elevated heart rate (>95 beats/min >12 hours)[@@]	Prolonged elevated heart rate is associated with major cardiopulmonary event and poor outcome[@@]
EKG abnormalities ST elevation, dispersion, T wave inversion, QT prolongation, dispersion, arrhythmias	Prevalence up to 35%, 5% life-threatening.[@@@] 46% ST-T changes, 30% QT prolongation.[#]	Association with elevated troponin I and ECHO dysfunction Baseline EKG must for all patients
Echo dysfunction LV systolic dysfunction	Prevalence 10–31%.[##] Associated with poor-grade SAH	Restores in 5–10 days after ictus May need IABC to augment CPP.[###] Reasonable to ECHO high risk patients
Elevated CK-MB Elevated troponin I	20%–34% Poor clinical grade, IVH, loss of consciousness at ictus, global cerebral oedema, female gender, large BMI, hypotension, tachycardia, use of phenylephrine.[^^,^]	Associated with ECHO abnormalities.[####,^,**] Poor prognostic marker circulation.[^] Reasonable to screen high-grade SAH.
PULMONARY		
Neurogenic pulmonary oedema	Prevalent in high-grade SAH[^^^] Role of circulating norepinephrine[^^^^] Associated with ECG abnormalities[!] May manifest as loss of heart rate variability[!!]	Higher mortality rate[!!!]
ALI and ARDS	True prevalence unknown	Hypoxaemia independent predictor of poor outcome.[-]
NEUROENDOCRINE		
HPA axis derangement	Derangement of diurnal variation in HPA[--]	
Hyponatraemia (<135 meq/L)	20%–43% SIADH vs CSW	Risk factor for DCI and cerebral infarction, surrogate marker for vasospasm
Hypernatraemia	Na >145, 19% Na >155, 2% Diabetes insipidus, 7%	Independent predictor of outcome at 3 months
Stress hyperglycaemia	Exact incidence unknown	Independent predictor of outcome at 3 months.[-,---]
HAEMATOLOGICAL		
Anaemia (Hb <10 g/d)	Prevalence 37%–57%[@@@] 61.2% patients receive PRBC transfusion.[$]	Intraoperative PRBC transfusion independent predictor of poor outcome at 6 months.[$$] Higher Hb is associated with improved outcomes at 14 days/discharge and 3 months[$$$]

Primary organ system affected	Prevalence of abnormalities	Implications
HAEMATOLOGICAL		
Platelet disorders Thrombocytopenia Platelet aggregation disorders	Mild thrombocytopenia 81,000–120,000 (20.7%).[†] Severe thrombocytopenia 51,000–80,000 (6.2%).[@@@]	Complicates, delays placement of EVD Increased incidence of re-bleeding.[††] Association with DCI.[$$] Anti-platelet agents reduced DCI by 35%.[†††]
INFLAMMATORY		
Fever, leukocytosis SIRS	Prevalence 41%–65%[‡] Presence of EVD, symptomatic vasospasm and older age.[‡] Associated with poor-grade SAH and hyperglycaemia.[‡‡] Prevalence 26%–29% Septic shock seen in 10.3%[†] CSF pro-inflammatory cytokines (TNF-alpha, IL-1 beta, IL-6).[‡‡‡]	40% increase in odds of poor outcome for each additional day of fever.[‡] Associated with poor outcome.[»] Surrogate marker of vasospasm.[»»] Aggressive fever control improved outcome at 6 months.[»»»]

*Waller CJ, Vandenberg B, Hasan D, Kumar AB. Stress cardiomyopathy with an 'inverse' takotsubo pattern in a patient with acute aneurysmal subarachnoid hemorrhage. *Echocardiography* 2013;30(8):E224–6.

**Kono T, Morita H, Kuroiwa T, Onaka H, Takatsuka H, Fujiwara A. Left ventricular wall motion abnormalities in patients with subarachnoid hemorrhage: neurogenic stunned myocardium. *J Am Coll Cardiol* 1994;24(3):636–40.

***Jain R, Deveikis J, Thompson BG. Management of patients with stunned myocardium associated with subarachnoid hemorrhage. *AJNR Am J Neuroradiol* 2004;25(1):126–9.

@Joseph M, Ziadi S, Nates J, Dannenbaum M, Malkoff M. Increases in cardiac output can reverse flow deficits from vasospasm independent of blood pressure: a study using xenon computed tomographic measurement of cerebral blood flow. *Neurosurgery* 2003;53(5):1044–51; discussion 1051–1052.

@@Schmidt JM, Crimmins M, Lantigua H, et al. Prolonged elevated heart rate is a risk factor for adverse cardiac events and poor outcome after subarachnoid hemorrhage. *Neurocrit Care* 2014;20(3):390–8.

@@@Solenski NJ, Haley EC, Jr., Kassell NF, et al. Medical complications of aneurysmal subarachnoid hemorrhage: a report of the multicenter, cooperative aneurysm study. Participants of the Multicenter Cooperative Aneurysm Study. *Crit Care Med* 1995;23(6):1007–17.

#Macrea LM, Tramer MR, Walder B. Spontaneous subarachnoid hemorrhage and serious cardiopulmonary dysfunction—a systematic review. *Resuscitation* 2005;65(2):139–48.

##(1) Davies KR, Gelb AW, Manninen PH, Boughner DR, Bisnaire D. Cardiac function in aneurysmal subarachnoid haemorrhage: a study of electrocardiographic and echocardiographic abnormalities. *Br J Anaesth* 1991;67(1):58–63. (2) Galloon S, Rees GA, Briscoe CE, Davies S, Kilpatrick GS. Prospective study of electrocardiographic changes associated with subarachnoid haemorrhage. *Br J Anaesth* 1972;44(5):511–6.

###(1) Lazaridis C, Pradilla G, Nyquist PA, Tamargo RJ. Intra-aortic balloon pump counterpulsation in the setting of subarachnoid hemorrhage, cerebral vasospasm, and neurogenic stress cardiomyopathy. Case report and review of the literature. *Neurocrit Care* 2010;13(1):101–8. (2) Nussbaum ES, Sebring LA, Ganz WF, Madison MT. Intra-aortic balloon counterpulsation augments cerebral blood flow in the patient with cerebral vasospasm: a xenon-enhanced computed tomography study. *Neurosurgery* 1998;42(1):206–13; discussion 213–214.

####Parekh N, Venkatesh B, Cross D, et al. Cardiac troponin I predicts myocardial dysfunction in aneurysmal subarachnoid hemorrhage. *J Am Coll Cardiol* 2000;36(4):1328–35.

^Naidech AM, Kreiter KT, Janjua N, et al. Cardiac troponin elevation, cardiovascular morbidity, and outcome after subarachnoid hemorrhage. *Circulation* 2005;112(18):2851–6.

^^Tung P, Kopelnik A, Banki N, et al. Predictors of neurocardiogenic injury after subarachnoid hemorrhage. *Stroke* 2004;35(2):548–51.

^^^Saracen A, Kotwica Z, Wozniak-Kosek A, Kasprzak P. Neurogenic pulmonary edema in aneurysmal subarachnoid hemorrhage. *Advances in Experimental Medicine and Biology* 2016;952:35–9.

^^^^Inamasu J, Sugimoto K, Yamada Y, et al. The role of catecholamines in the pathogenesis of neurogenic pulmonary edema associated with subarachnoid hemorrhage. *Acta Neurochir (Wien)* 2012;154(12):2179–84; discussion 2184–2185.

!Chen WL, Huang CH, Chen JH, Tai HC, Chang SH, Wang YC. ECG abnormalities predict neurogenic pulmonary edema in patients with subarachnoid hemorrhage. *The American Journal of Emergency Medicine* 2016;34(1):79–82.

!!Chen WL, Chang SH, Chen JH, Tai HC, Chan CM, Wang YC. Heart rate variability predicts neurogenic pulmonary edema in patients with subarachnoid hemorrhage. *Neurocrit Care* 2016;25(1):71–8.

!!!Muroi C, Keller M, Pangalu A, Fortunati M, Yonekawa Y, Keller E. Neurogenic pulmonary edema in patients with subarachnoid hemorrhage. *J Neurosurg Anesthesiol* 2008;20(3):188–92.

‾Claassen J, Vu A, Kreiter KT, et al. Effect of acute physiologic derangements on outcome after subarachnoid hemorrhage. *Crit Care Med* 2004;32(3):832–8.

‾‾Vespa P. Participants in the International Multi-Disciplinary Consensus Conference on the critical care management of subarachnoid hemorrhage. Endocrine function following acute SAH. *Neurocrit Care* 2011;15(2):361–4.

(Cont'd)

Table 74.2 *(Cont'd)*

˜˜˜Lanzino G, Kassell NF, Germanson T, Truskowski L, Alves W. Plasma glucose levels and outcome after aneurysmal subarachnoid hemorrhage. *J Neurosurg* 1993;79(6):885–91.

$Giller CA, Wills MJ, Giller AM, Samson D. Distribution of hematocrit values after aneurysmal subarachnoid hemorrhage. *J Neuroimaging* 1998;8(3):169–70.

$$Smith MJ, Le Roux PD, Elliott JP, Winn HR. Blood transfusion and increased risk for vasospasm and poor outcome after subarachnoid hemorrhage. *J Neurosurg* 2004;101(1):1–7.

$$$Centers for Disease Control and Prevention. Report from the pediatric mild traumatic brain injury guideline workgroup: systematic review and clinical recommendations for healthcare providers on the diagnosis and management of mild traumatic brain injury among children. 2016. [Accessed 2018 Feb 12]. Available from: https://www.cdc.gov/injury/pdfs/bsc/SystemicReviewCompilation_August_2016.pdf.

†Gruber A, Reinprecht A, Illievich UM, et al. Extracerebral organ dysfunction and neurologic outcome after aneurysmal subarachnoid hemorrhage. *Crit Care Med* 1999;27(3):505–14.

††Juvela S, Kaste M. Reduced platelet aggregability and thromboxane release after rebleeding in patients with subarachnoid hemorrhage. *J Neurosurg* 1991;74(1):21–6.

†††Dorhout Mees SM, Rinkel GJ, Hop JW, Algra A, van Gijn J. Antiplatelet therapy in aneurysmal subarachnoid hemorrhage: a systematic review. *Stroke* 2003;34(9):2285–9.

‡Oliveira-Filho J, Ezzeddine MA, Segal AZ, et al. Fever in subarachnoid hemorrhage: relationship to vasospasm and outcome. *Neurology* 2001;56(10):1299–304.

‡‡Commichau C, Scarmeas N, Mayer SA. Risk factors for fever in the neurologic intensive care unit. *Neurology* 2003;60(5):837–41.

‡‡‡Gruber A, Rossler K, Graninger W, Donner A, Illievich MU, Czech T. Ventricular cerebrospinal fluid and serum concentrations of sTNFR-I, IL-1ra, and IL-6 after aneurysmal subarachnoid hemorrhage. *J Neurosurg Anesthesiol* 2000;12(4):297–306.

"McGirt MJ, Mavropoulos JC, McGirt LY, et al. Leukocytosis as an independent risk factor for cerebral vasospasm following aneurysmal subarachnoid hemorrhage. *J Neurosurg* 2003;98(6):1222–6.

""Rousseaux P, Scherpereel B, Bernard MH, Graftieaux JP, Guyot JF. Fever and cerebral vasospasm in ruptured intracranial aneurysms. *Surg Neurol* 1980;14(6):459–65.

"""Badjatia N, Fernandez L, Schmidt JM, et al. Impact of induced normothermia on outcome after subarachnoid hemorrhage: a case-control study. *Neurosurgery* 2010;66(4):696–700; discussion 700–701.

Note: SIDH: syndrome of inappropriate antidiuretic hormone.

severe neurologic deficits (30%–50%) compared to patients with minimal neurologic deficits (10%–30%).[37]

While several mechanisms have been implicated, most evidence seems to correlate this with high circulating catecholamine levels.[30]

Management of cerebral vasospasm in patients with reduced ejection fraction is complicated as patients are at high risk for cardiopulmonary collapse and pulmonary oedema. In order to maintain CPP, intra-aortic balloon counterpulsation (IABC) device has been placed in patients with severe cerebral vasospasm who are refractory to medical and interventional therapies.[38] An IABC device has been shown to augment CPP,[39,40] preserve autoregulation, and when used in patients with severe medically refractory cerebral vasospasm has been found to be safe overall. The IABC has been shown to reduce the need for vasopressors by 50%.[41]

Neurogenic Pulmonary Dysfunction

Pulmonary oedema is noted to occur in approximately 4%–42% of aSAH patients.[29] Neurogenic pulmonary oedema (NPE) is thought to occur without any direct precipitant of acute lung injury. The criteria proposed for NPE includes the presence of acute structural or functional brain disorder, absence of any direct or indirect precipitant

of acute lung injury, presence of bilateral interstitial or alveolar infiltrates on chest X-ray, $PaCO_2/FiO_2$ ratio <300 and lack of evidence to support cardiogenic pulmonary oedema.[29] The risk for NPE increases with increased age and worsening severity of SAH.[29]

While the exact pathophysiology of NPE is controversial, there is a similar correlation with circulating catecholamines as in cardiogenic dysfunction. Treatment is supportive in terms of positive pressure ventilation and diuretics on a case-by-case basis.

Endocrine Dysfunction

Sodium Imbalance

Hyponatraemia is a common metabolic disturbance after aSAH and has been associated with longer length of stay in the hospital.[42] Mild hyponatremia is found in 36% of patients,[42] and is more commonly associated with anterior communicating aneurysm.[43] Hypovolaemic natriuretic state[44] predominates SAH and is thought to be due to cerebral salt wasting syndrome (CSWS), which is indistinguishable from SIADH, except that patients with CSWS are hypovolaemic and respond to prompt isotonic fluid resuscitation. The nadir for hyponatraemia is frequently associated with peak of vasospasm and hyponatraemia is considered one of the surrogate markers of cerebral vasospasm.[45,46] Hypernatraemia on the other hand is independently associated with poor outcomes.[47,48]

Critical care management of patients with aSAH includes avoidance of intravascular volume contraction, avoidance of hypotonic fluid use, use of fludrocortisone acetate and hypertonic saline solution to prevent and correct hyponatraemia.[19,49]

Glucose Management

Care must be taken to prevent hypoglycaemia[19] and judiciously use glucose management protocols in the ICU. Optimal targets for blood glucose are not well established in aSAH, but there is a general agreement in treating glucose levels >180–200 mg/dL. In a case series of 97 patients, persistent hyperglycaemia (>200 mg/dL for more than 2 days) was seven times more likely to be associated with poor outcomes at a mean of 10 months after aSAH.[50]

Hypothalamic-Pituitary Axis (HPA) Derangement

There is disruption of diurnal variation of HPA with initial supranormal cortisol levels that eventually decrease to near normal or normal levels.[51]

REPAIR OF RUPTURED CEREBRAL ANEURYSM

An early repair of ruptured cerebral aneurysm is recommended to prevent re-bleeding.[28] The techniques available for successful repair of ruptured cerebral aneurysm have undergone significant technological advances in the last 30 years. Preceding endovascular repair, the mainstay was surgical repair in the form or clipping, trapping, or bypass of the ruptured cerebral aneurysm.

While surgical clipping is widely considered as the most complete of aneurysm repair, the advances in endovascular technology allow us to use either techniques as necessary adjuncts in patients who require repair of 'residual' ruptured aneurysm(s).

In a randomized control trial (International Subarachnoid Aneurysm Trial [ISAT]) conducted on 2143 patients with ruptured aneurysm, 23.7% patients who underwent endovascular repair were dependent or dead at 1 year compared to 30.6% who underwent surgical repair, while long-term risks of further bleeding are more frequent with endovascular coiling.[52]

Endovascular therapy was introduced by Guglielmi[53] in 1991. The physiological basis for endovascular repair includes insertion of 'coils' into the aneurysmal sac, and performing thrombosis of the aneurysm and its removal from the Circle of Willis.

The decision to offer endovascular coiling versus surgical clipping of the ruptured cerebral aneurysm is a complex one. This is best reached by a multidisciplinary decision based on characteristics of the patient and aneurysm. The 2012 AHA guidelines place the decision for microsurgical repair in patients who present with large intraparenchymal haematomas and MCA aneurysms, while endovascular coiling is considered in patients >70 years of age, poor-grade World Federation of Neurosurgical Societies (WFNS) classification, and basilar apex aneurysms.[19]

PREVENTING RE-BLEEDING OF RUPTURED CEREBRAL ANEURYSM

Re-bleeding is a devastating complication after the initial rupture of intracerebral aneurysm. It is estimated to occur in about 4%–13.6% of patients and has been shown to occur within the first 3 hours (1/3 of re-bleeds) and within 6 hours (1/2 of re-bleeds).[19,54] Predictors of re-bleeding include grade of SAH (odds ratio 1.92 per grade), aneurysm size (odds ratio 1.07 per mm aneurysm size),[54] and systolic blood pressure >160 mmHg.[19]

Re-bleeding reduces the chance of survival.[54] Hijdra et al. in a study of 176 patients found that the absence of anti-fibrinolytic therapy was the only predictor of re-bleeding.[55] Strategies that may reduce the incidence of re-bleeding include early aneurysm repair, short course of anti-fibrinolytic therapy (<72 hours) with either tranexamic acid or aminocaproic acid, and tight BP control.[28]

CEREBRAL VASOSPASM AFTER ANEURYSMAL SUBARACHNOID HAEMORRHAGE

Cerebral vasospasm, especially the occurrence of delayed cerebral ischaemia (DCI) is a cause of high morbidity after aSAH. Most frequently peaking at 7–10 days after ictus, it may resolve spontaneously after 21 days.[19] There currently exists a body of literature on the lack of benefit of hypervolaemia, but rather euvolemia after aSAH and even in the vasospasm phase.[19] Prophylactic angioplasty and antiplatelet prophylaxis are ineffective at reducing morbidity.[19] Intrathecal thrombolytic therapy does have some benefits although clinical trials have been criticized for methodological flaws.[19]

Unfortunately, there is no one therapy that reliably prevents and treats vasospasm. Nimodipine has shown to improve neurological outcome independent on its effect on narrowing of large vessel.[19]

Clazosentan, an endothelin-1 receptor antagonist, perhaps effective in preventing occurrence of angiographic vasospasm, vasospasm-related delayed ischaemic neurological deficits and vasospasm related mortality and morbidity, and rescue therapy.[56] But a recent meta-analysis failed to document its beneficial effect on occurrence of new cerebral infarction and improvement of functional outcome,[56] and is not used in clinical practice.

Prioritization must be made to maintain CPP. Maintenance of euvolaemia and normal circulating blood volume along with induction of hypertension unless the patient is able to spontaneously mount a hypertensive response or cardiac dysfunction exists.[19] In those patients not responding to hypertensive therapy and in clinical vasospasm, cerebral angioplasty and/or selective intra-arterial vasodilator therapy is usually offered.[19]

Contrary to the historical practice for hypertension, hypervolaemia, and haemodilution, the medical management in today's day and age is essentially to augment cerebral perfusion pressure by 'induced hypertension'. Benefits of hypertension are negated by hypervolaemia and haemodilution[57] and early positive fluid balance has been associated with worse clinical presentation and had greater resource use during the hospital course.[58]

Prophylactic hypervolaemia, in one survey based study was found to be highly associated with centres without dedicated NICUs.[59] In the same survey, hypertension was commonly induced by phenylephrine and norepinephrine with equal variability in targeting MAP versus SBP. Cerebral perfusion pressures <70 mmHg are associated with metabolic crisis and brain tissue hypoxia and may increase risk of secondary brain injury.[60]

Although there is no absolute haemoglobin (Hb) trigger for blood transfusion, evidence from microdialysis based on a study by Oddo et al. demonstrates that Hb concentration less than 9 gm/dl was associated with increased incidence of brain hypoxia and cell energy dysfunction in poor-grade aSAH.[61] Packed red blood cell (PRBC) transfusion has been shown to improve brain tissue oxygenation in patients with SAH, although no correlation was found between Hb concentration and lactate–pyruvate ratios (LPRs).[62]

Screening for Cerebral Vasospasm

Clinical screening includes serial neurological examinations, which form the cornerstone of assessment of all aSAH patients, and this is especially important during the clinical phase of cerebral vasospasm. Doppler ultrasound-guided screening for angiographic vasospasm of cerebral vasculature is considered significant if it can demonstrate presence of isolated elevation in intracranial vessel blood flow velocities, and this forms the basis for use of TCD ultrasound in patients with aSAH. Typically,

TCDs are performed daily starting from the day of bleed to about 10–14 days or longer, depending upon the clinical course. Mean flow velocities in the MCA territories >120 cm/sec and LR (MCA/external internal carotid artery [ICA]) of >3 are used as thresholds for cerebral vasospasm.[63] The American Academy of Neurology (AAN) report from the Therapeutics and Technology Assessment Subcommittee provides sensitivity, specificity, and grading for recommendation on the use of TCDs in aSAH.[63] When compared to conventional angiography, TCDs in general have low to moderate sensitivity (13%–100%) but very high specificity in both anterior and posterior circulations with higher sensitivities (77%–100%), especially for the basilar artery.[63] In a retrospective study of 441 patients with aSAH, 40% of patients with delayed cerebral ischaemia never attained the threshold mean flow velocity of 120 cm/sec during the monitoring period.[64]

Medical Management of Cerebral Vasospasm

Many NICUs combine daily TCD data along with clinical trajectory in adjusting BP goals and establishing thresholds for advanced screening such as CTA[65,66] coupled with CT perfusion[67,68] or conventional angiography. This allows diagnostic and therapeutic options (Figure 74.3), which include balloon angioplasty with intra-arterial injection of cerebral vasodilators such as nicardipine or verapamil. There is low threshold for these advanced imaging in patients with a poor or unreliable baseline neurological examination. Prolonged mean transit time (MTT) and time to peak (TTP) are potential indicators for vasospasm on CT perfusion imaging.[67]

New focal neurological deficits after aSAH should carry a high index of suspicion towards cerebral vasospasm, and clinicians must rule out the presence of hydrocephalus, seizures, and metabolic causes of neurological deficits, which act like 'stroke-mimics' in these patients with clinical vasospasm.

Critical care management of patients with aSAH during the vasospasm phase should focus on maintenance of normal carbon dioxide and avoidance of hypocarbia, in addition to maintenance of normal glucose, sodium, magnesium, and body temperature.

OUTCOMES AFTER ANEURYSMAL SUBARACHNOID HAEMORRHAGE

Functional Outcome

Subarachnoid haemorrhage Physiologic Derangement Score (SAH PDS) incorporating critical care elements such as arterio-alveolar gradient, bicarbonate level, serum glucose and MAP was found in one study to be predictive of outcome at 3 months after aSAH.[69]

A substantial minority of poor-grade SAH patients experience delayed recovery.[70] In a study of 88 poor-grade SAH patients by Wilson et al. demonstrated improvement in 18% and 19% patients between 6–12 months and 12–36 months, respectively, after ictus. Hunt and Hess grade 4 as opposed to H&H grade 5 and absence of large or eloquent stroke was associated with improvement up to and beyond 6 months while absence of large stroke was strongly predictive of improvement beyond 1 year.[70] This has also been corroborated in another small sample study of 52 patients by Navi et al. wherein a substantial proportion of patients with discharge disability appear to have significant functional recovery by 6 months.[71] Available data seems to suggest that substantial proportion of high-grade SAH patients may eventually make a good functional recovery albeit at a slower pace, and this information must be made available to families during goals of care discussions, especially in patients with high-grade SAH (H&H grades 4 and 5).

Early worsening after SAH can occur in up to 35% of patients and is related to amount of blood and is associated with mortality and poor functional outcome at 1 year.[72] Metabolic crisis and brain tissue hypoxia are associated with mortality and poor functional outcomes.[60]

Cognitive Impairment After aSAH

Cognitive impairment has been demonstrated in about a third of patients after aSAH. Age, hydrocephalus, and clinical vasospasm has been demonstrated to influence the overall prognosis after aSAH.[24] Springer et al., in a study of 232 patients with aSAH controlled for effects of age, education, and race/ethnicity, demonstrated that the risk for cognitive impairment was higher in anaemia patients who received blood transfusion, those with any temperature greater than 38.6°C, and in those who experienced delayed cerebral ischaemia.[73] Global cerebral oedema and left-sided infarction are also important risk factors for cognitive dysfunction after aSAH.[74] The volume of blood in the subarachnoid space as quantified by Fisher score was also predictive of severe cognitive dysfunction one year after aSAH.[75] Thus, comprehensive, cognitive, behavioural, and psychosocial evaluation is important in all survivors of aSAH.[19]

30-DAY READMISSIONS AFTER ᴀSAH

Greenberg et al. conducted a retrospective review on 778 patients with aSAH and found an overall 30-day readmission rate of 11.4%.[76] The most common reasons for readmission included acute hydrocephalus, infections, thromboembolic events, or hyponatraemia (16.4%).[76]

In a study by Singh et al. readmission was not associated with admission neurologic grade, NIH stroke scale at 14 days, modified Rankin scale at 3 months, history of cardiovascular disease or radiographic cerebral infarction, but rather associated with longer intensive care stay, hospital length of stay, and presence of external ventricular drain.[77] Regardless, a 30-day readmission should be incorporated as a quality improvement indicator for hospitals caring for patients with aSAH.

QUALITY IMPROVEMENT INITIATIVES

Initiatives towards quality of care improvements with relationship to aSAH are important towards reinforcing institutional, national, and international standards. A vigorous, consistent process should examine quality improvement. Proposed here are some initiatives that are mandated by the Joint Commission, Comprehensive Stroke Certification[78] (marked with *) and others that are equally important and should be tracked.

- Competency of providers caring for the aSAH, obtaining certification in Emergency Neurological Life Support (ENLS) for neurocritical care providers.
- Admission processes:
  - Triaging processes for patients with aSAH
  - Prompt and efficient referral to large volume centres
  - Placement of ventriculostomy for patients at high risk for deterioration during inter-hospital transport
- Admission order set
  - Maintaining aSAH specific admission order set
  - Compliance with ordering nimodipine within 24 hours of admission and documentation for reasons not administering nimodipine*
  - Cardiac enzymes, EKG, and ECHO for high-risk patients
- Severity scales
  - Use of clinical and radiographic severity grading scales (H&H, Fisher)*
  - National Institute of Health Stroke Scale (NIHSS)*
- Outcomes
  - 90-day modified Rankin score (mRS)*
  - Coiling vs. clipping outcomes data
- Infection control
  - Catheter-related urinary tract infection, ventilator-associated pneumonia, catheter-related blood stream infections. External ventricular, lumbar drain, and other ICP monitoring device associated infections.
  - Normothermia protocol
  - Anti-shivering protocol

- Vasospasm
  - Competency of personnel performing TCD ultrasound
  - Clinical pathway for screening and clinical decision tree for medical and endovascular therapeutic options
- Systemic implications
  - Use of bedside ultrasound screening for cardiac dysfunction
  - Clinical pathway for clinical decision tree for patients with low ejection fraction
  - Use of enteral and intravenous supplementation of salt, and use of fludrocortisone in hyponatraemic and hypovolaemic patients
  - Target blood glucose levels and percentage above target range
  - Venous thromboembolism prevention
    o Prompt placement of sequential compression devices upon admission
    o Prompt initiation of chemical prophylaxis after securement of ruptured intracerebral aneurysm

CONCLUSIONS

Subarachnoid haemorrhage, due to rupture of intracerebral aneurysm is a devastating neurological disorder with significant systemic implications. Complexities in diagnosis, therapeutic interventions, treatment of cerebral vasospasm, and challenges in improvement mortality and morbidity are now well recognized, and with continued scientific effort, clinicians can implement optimal care pathways for patients with this condition to reduce mortality and improve morbidity.

REFERENCES

1. Rinkel GJ. Natural history, epidemiology and screening of unruptured intracranial aneurysms. *J Neuroradiol* 2008;35(2):99–103.

2. van Gijn J, Rinkel GJ. Subarachnoid haemorrhage: diagnosis, causes and management. *Brain* 2001;124(Pt 2):249–78.

3. Vlak MH, Algra A, Brandenburg R, Rinkel GJ. Prevalence of unruptured intracranial aneurysms, with emphasis on sex, age, comorbidity, country, and time period: a systematic review and meta-analysis. *Lancet Neurol* 2011;10(7):626–36.

4. Zacharia BE, Hickman ZL, Grobelny BT, et al. Epidemiology of aneurysmal subarachnoid hemorrhage. *Neurosurg Clin N Am* 2010;21(2):221–33.

5. Wiebers DO, Whisnant JP, Huston J, 3rd, et al. Unruptured intracranial aneurysms: natural history, clinical outcome, and risks of surgical and endovascular treatment. *Lancet* 2003;362(9378):103–10.

6. Qian Z, Kang H, Tang K, et al. Assessment of risk of aneurysmal rupture in patients with normotensives,

7. controlled hypertension, and uncontrolled hypertension. *J Stroke Cerebrovasc Dis* 2016;25(7):1746–52.

7. Broderick JP, Viscoli CM, Brott T, et al. Major risk factors for aneurysmal subarachnoid hemorrhage in the young are modifiable. *Stroke* 2003;34(6):1375–81.

8. Nanda A, Vannemreddy PS, Polin RS, Willis BK. Intracranial aneurysms and cocaine abuse: analysis of prognostic indicators. *Neurosurgery* 2000;46(5):1063–7; discussion 1067–1069.

9. Chang TR, Kowalski RG, Caserta F, Carhuapoma JR, Tamargo RJ, Naval NS. Impact of acute cocaine use on aneurysmal subarachnoid hemorrhage. *Stroke* 2013;44(7):1825–9.

10. Chang TR, Kowalski RG, Carhuapoma JR, Tamargo RJ, Naval NS. Cocaine use as an independent predictor of seizures after aneurysmal subarachnoid hemorrhage. *J Neurosurg* 2016;124(3):730–5.

11. Garcia-Bermejo P, Rodriguez-Arias C, Crespo E, Perez-Fernandez S, Arenillas JF, Martinez-Galdamez M. Severe cerebral vasospasm in chronic cocaine users during neurointerventional procedures: A report of two cases. *Interv Neuroradiol* 2015;21(1):19–22.

12. Conway JE, Tamargo RJ. Cocaine use is an independent risk factor for cerebral vasospasm after aneurysmal subarachnoid hemorrhage. *Stroke* 2001;32(10):2338–43.

13. Murthy SB, Moradiya Y, Shah S, Naval NS. In-hospital outcomes of aneurysmal subarachnoid hemorrhage associated with cocaine use in the USA. *J Clin Neurosci* 2014;21(12):2088–91.

14. Howington JU, Kutz SC, Wilding GE, Awasthi D. Cocaine use as a predictor of outcome in aneurysmal subarachnoid hemorrhage. *J Neurosurg* 2003;99(2):271–5.

15. Rumalla K, Reddy AY, Mittal MK. Association of recreational marijuana use with aneurysmal subarachnoid hemorrhage. *J Stroke Cerebrovasc Dis* 2016;25(2):452–60.

16. Behrouz R, Birnbaum L, Grandhi R, et al. Cannabis use and outcomes in patients with aneurysmal subarachnoid hemorrhage. *Stroke* 2016;47(5):1371–3.

17. Isaksen J, Egge A, Waterloo K, Romner B, Ingebrigtsen T. Risk factors for aneurysmal subarachnoid haemorrhage: the Tromso study. *J Neurol Neurosurg Psychiatry* 2002;73(2):185–7.

18. Seder DB, Schmidt JM, Badjatia N, et al. Transdermal nicotine replacement therapy in cigarette smokers with acute subarachnoid hemorrhage. *Neurocrit Care* 2011;14(1):77–83.

19. Connolly ES, Jr., Rabinstein AA, Carhuapoma JR, et al. Guidelines for the management of aneurysmal subarachnoid hemorrhage: a guideline for healthcare professionals from the American Heart Association/American Stroke Association. *Stroke* 2012;43(6):1711–37.

20. Joswig H, Epprecht L, Valmaggia C, et al. Terson syndrome in aneurysmal subarachnoid hemorrhage-its relation to intracranial pressure, admission factors, and clinical outcome. *Acta Neurochir (Wien)* 2016;158(6):1027–36.

21. Czorlich P, Skevas C, Knospe V, Vettorazzi E, Westphal M, Regelsberger J. Terson's syndrome—pathophysiologic considerations of an underestimated concomitant disease in aneurysmal subarachnoid hemorrhage. *J Clin Neurosci* 2016;33:182–6.

22. Lee GI, Choi KS, Han MH, Byoun HS, Yi HJ, Lee BR. Practical incidence and risk factors of terson's syndrome: a retrospective analysis in 322 consecutive patients with aneurysmal subarachnoid hemorrhage. *J Cerebrovasc Endovasc Neurosurg* 2015;17(3):203–8.

23. Hassan A, Lanzino G, Wijdicks EF, Rabinstein AA, Flemming KD. Terson's syndrome. *Neurocrit Care* 2011;15(3):554–8.

24. Fisher CM, Kistler JP, Davis JM. Relation of cerebral vasospasm to subarachnoid hemorrhage visualized by computerized tomographic scanning. *Neurosurgery* 1980;6(1):1–9.

25. Claassen J, Bernardini GL, Kreiter K, et al. Effect of cisternal and ventricular blood on risk of delayed cerebral ischemia after subarachnoid hemorrhage: the Fisher scale revisited. *Stroke* 2001;32(9):2012–20.

26. Hijdra A, Brouwers PJ, Vermeulen M, van Gijn J. Grading the amount of blood on computed tomograms after subarachnoid hemorrhage. *Stroke* 1990;21(8):1156–61.

27. Tang C, Zhang TS, Zhou LF. Risk factors for rebleeding of aneurysmal subarachnoid hemorrhage: a meta-analysis. *PLoS One* 2014;9(6):e99536.

28. Diringer MN, Bleck TP, Claude Hemphill J, 3rd, et al. Critical care management of patients following aneurysmal subarachnoid hemorrhage: recommendations from the Neurocritical Care Society's Multidisciplinary Consensus Conference. *Neurocrit Care* 2011;15(2):211–40.

29. Stevens RD, Nyquist PA. The systemic implications of aneurysmal subarachnoid hemorrhage. *J Neurol Sci* 2007;261(1–2):143–56.

30. Lee VH, Oh JK, Mulvagh SL, Wijdicks EF. Mechanisms in neurogenic stress cardiomyopathy after aneurysmal subarachnoid hemorrhage. *Neurocrit Care* 2006;5(3):243–9.

31. Parekh N, Venkatesh B, Cross D, et al. Cardiac troponin I predicts myocardial dysfunction in aneurysmal subarachnoid hemorrhage. *J Am Coll Cardiol* 2000;36(4):1328–35.

32. Tung P, Kopelnik A, Banki N, et al. Predictors of neurocardiogenic injury after subarachnoid hemorrhage. *Stroke* 2004;35(2):548–51.

33. Waller CJ, Vandenberg B, Hasan D, Kumar AB. Stress cardiomyopathy with an 'inverse' takotsubo pattern in a patient with acute aneurysmal subarachnoid hemorrhage. *Echocardiography* 2013;30(8):E224–6.

34. Deibert E, Barzilai B, Braverman AC, et al. Clinical significance of elevated troponin I levels in patients with nontraumatic subarachnoid hemorrhage. *J Neurosurg* 2003;98(4):741–6.

35. Naidech AM, Kreiter KT, Janjua N, et al. Cardiac troponin elevation, cardiovascular morbidity, and outcome after subarachnoid hemorrhage. *Circulation* 2005;112(18):2851–6.

36. Mayer SA, Lin J, Homma S, et al. Myocardial injury and left ventricular performance after subarachnoid hemorrhage. *Stroke* 1999;30(4):780–6.

37. Macrea LM, Tramer MR, Walder B. Spontaneous subarachnoid hemorrhage and serious cardiopulmonary dysfunction—a systematic review. *Resuscitation* 2005;65(2):139–48.

38. Lazaridis C, Pradilla G, Nyquist PA, Tamargo RJ. Intra-aortic balloon pump counterpulsation in the setting of subarachnoid hemorrhage, cerebral vasospasm, and neurogenic stress cardiomyopathy. Case report and review of the literature. *Neurocrit Care* 2010;13(1):101–8.

39. Nussbaum ES, Heros RC, Solien EE, Madison MT, Sebring LA, Latchaw RE. Intra-aortic balloon counterpulsation augments cerebral blood flow in a canine model of subarachnoid hemorrhage-induced cerebral vasospasm. *Neurosurgery* 1995;36(4):879–84; discussion 884–886.

40. Nussbaum ES, Sebring LA, Ganz WF, Madison MT. Intra-aortic balloon counterpulsation augments cerebral blood flow in the patient with cerebral vasospasm: a xenon-enhanced computed tomography study. *Neurosurgery* 1998;42(1):206–13; discussion 213–214.

41. Al-Mufti F, Morris N, Lahiri S, et al. Use of intra-aortic- balloon pump counterpulsation in patients with symptomatic vasospasm following subarachnoid hemorrhage and neurogenic stress cardiomyopathy. *J Vasc Interv Neurol* 2016;9(1):28–34.

42. Mapa B, Taylor BE, Appelboom G, Bruce EM, Claassen J, Connolly ES, Jr. Impact of hyponatremia on morbidity, mortality, and complications after aneurysmal subarachnoid hemorrhage: a systematic review. *World Neurosurg* 2016;85:305–14.

43. Sayama T, Inamura T, Matsushima T, Inoha S, Inoue T, Fukui M. High incidence of hyponatremia in patients with ruptured anterior communicating artery aneurysms. *Neurol Res* 2000;22(2):151–5.

44. Nakagawa I, Kurokawa S, Takayama K, Wada T, Nakase H. [Increased urinary sodium excretion in the early phase of aneurysmal subarachnoid hemorrhage as a predictor of cerebral salt wasting syndrome]. *Brain Nerve* 2009;61(12):1419–23.

45. Maimaitili A, Maimaitili M, Rexidan A, et al. Pituitary hormone level changes and hypxonatremia in aneurysmal subarachnoid hemorrhage. *Exp Ther Med* 2013;5(6):1657–62.

46. Chandy D, Sy R, Aronow WS, Lee WN, Maguire G, Murali R. Hyponatremia and cerebrovascular spasm in aneurysmal subarachnoid hemorrhage. *Neurol India* 2006;54(3):273–5.

47. Qureshi AI, Suri MF, Sung GY, et al. Prognostic significance of hypernatremia and hyponatremia among patients with aneurysmal subarachnoid hemorrhage. *Neurosurgery* 2002;50(4):749–55; discussion 755–6.

48. Beseoglu K, Etminan N, Steiger HJ, Hanggi D. The relation of early hypernatremia with clinical outcome in patients suffering from aneurysmal subarachnoid hemorrhage. *Clin Neurol Neurosurg* 2014;123:164–8.

49. Suarez JI, Qureshi AI, Parekh PD, et al. Administration of hypertonic (3%) sodium chloride/acetate in hyponatremic patients with symptomatic vasospasm following subarachnoid hemorrhage. *J Neurosurg Anesthesiol* 1999;11(3):178–84.

50. McGirt MJ, Woodworth GF, Ali M, Than KD, Tamargo RJ, Clatterbuck RE. Persistent perioperative hyperglycemia as an independent predictor of poor outcome after aneurysmal subarachnoid hemorrhage. *J Neurosurg* 2007; 107(6):1080–5.

51. Vespa P. Participants in the International Multi-Disciplinary Consensus Conference on the critical care management of subarachnoid hemorrhage. Endocrine function following acute SAH. *Neurocrit Care* 2011;15(2):361–4.

52. Molyneux A, Kerr R, Stratton I, et al. International Subarachnoid Aneurysm Trial (ISAT) of neurosurgical clipping versus endovascular coiling in 2143 patients with ruptured intracranial aneurysms: a randomised trial. *Lancet* 2002;360(9342):1267–74.

53. Guglielmi G, Vinuela F, Sepetka I, Macellari V. Electrothrombosis of saccular aneurysms via endovascular approach. Part 1: Electrochemical basis, technique, and experimental results. *J Neurosurg* 1991;75(1):1–7.

54. Naidech AM, Janjua N, Kreiter KT, et al. Predictors and impact of aneurysm rebleeding after subarachnoid hemorrhage. *Arch Neurol* 2005;62(3):410–16.

55. Hijdra A, van Gijn J, Nagelkerke NJ, Vermeulen M, van Crevel H. Prediction of delayed cerebral ischemia, rebleeding, and outcome after aneurysmal subarachnoid hemorrhage. *Stroke* 1988;19(10):1250–6.

56. Wang X, Li YM, Li WQ, Huang CG, Lu YC, Hou LJ. Effect of clazosentan in patients with aneurysmal subarachnoid hemorrhage: a meta-analysis of randomized controlled trials. *PLoS One* 2012;7(10):e47778.

57. Muench E, Horn P, Bauhuf C, et al. Effects of hypervolemia and hypertension on regional cerebral blood flow, intracranial pressure, and brain tissue oxygenation after subarachnoid hemorrhage. *Crit Care Med* 2007;35(8): 1844–51; quiz 1852.

58. Martini RP, Deem S, Brown M, et al. The association between fluid balance and outcomes after subarachnoid hemorrhage. *Neurocrit Care* 2012;17(2):191–8.

59. Meyer R, Deem S, Yanez ND, Souter M, Lam A, Treggiari MM. Current practices of triple-H prophylaxis and therapy in patients with subarachnoid hemorrhage. *Neurocrit Care* 2011;14(1):24–36.

60. Schmidt JM, Ko SB, Helbok R, et al. Cerebral perfusion pressure thresholds for brain tissue hypoxia and metabolic crisis after poor-grade subarachnoid hemorrhage. *Stroke* 2011;42(5):1351–6.

61. Oddo M, Milby A, Chen I, et al. Hemoglobin concentration and cerebral metabolism in patients with aneurysmal subarachnoid hemorrhage. *Stroke* 2009;40(4):1275–81.

62. Kurtz P, Helbok R, Claassen J, et al. The effect of packed red blood cell transfusion on cerebral oxygenation and metabolism after subarachnoid hemorrhage. *Neurocrit Care* 2016;24(1):118–21.

63. Sloan MA, Alexandrov AV, Tegeler CH, et al. Assessment: transcranial Doppler ultrasonography: report of the Therapeutics and Technology Assessment Subcommittee of the American Academy of Neurology. *Neurology* 2004;62(9):1468–81.

64. Carrera E, Schmidt JM, Oddo M, et al. Transcranial Doppler for predicting delayed cerebral ischemia after subarachnoid hemorrhage. *Neurosurgery* 2009;65(2):316–23; discussion 323–324.

65. Shankar JJ, Tan IY, Krings T, Terbrugge K, Agid R. CT angiography for evaluation of cerebral vasospasm following acute subarachnoid haemorrhage. *Neuroradiology* 2012;54(3):197–203.

66. Anderson GB, Ashforth R, Steinke DE, Findlay JM. CT angiography for the detection of cerebral vasospasm in patients with acute subarachnoid hemorrhage. *AJNR Am J Neuroradiol* 2000;21(6):1011–15.

67. Lin CF, Hsu SP, Lin CJ, et al. Prolonged cerebral circulation time is the best parameter for predicting vasospasm during initial CT perfusion in subarachnoid hemorrhagic patients. *PLoS One* 2016;11(3):e0151772.

68. Zhang H, Zhang B, Li S, Liang C, Xu K, Li S. Whole brain CT perfusion combined with CT angiography in patients with subarachnoid hemorrhage and cerebral vasospasm. *Clin Neurol Neurosurg* 2013;115(12):2496–501.

69. Claassen J, Vu A, Kreiter KT, et al. Effect of acute physiologic derangements on outcome after subarachnoid hemorrhage. *Crit Care Med* 2004;32(3):832–8.

70. Wilson DA, Nakaji P, Albuquerque FC, McDougall CG, Zabramski JM, Spetzler RF. Time course of recovery following poor-grade SAH: the incidence of delayed improvement and implications for SAH outcome study design. *J Neurosurg* 2013;119(3):606–12.

71. Navi BB, Kamel H, Hemphill JC, 3rd, Smith WS. Trajectory of functional recovery after hospital discharge for subarachnoid hemorrhage. *Neurocrit Care* 2012;17(3): 343–7.

72. Helbok R, Kurtz P, Vibbert M, et al. Early neurological deterioration after subarachnoid haemorrhage: risk factors and impact on outcome. *J Neurol Neurosurg Psychiatry* 2013;84(3):266–70.

73. Springer MV, Schmidt JM, Wartenberg KE, Frontera JA, Badjatia N, Mayer SA. Predictors of global cognitive impairment 1 year after subarachnoid hemorrhage. *Neurosurgery* 2009;65(6):1043–50; discussion 1050–1051.

74. Kreiter KT, Copeland D, Bernardini GL, et al. Predictors of cognitive dysfunction after subarachnoid hemorrhage. *Stroke* 2002;33(1):200–8.

75. Orbo M, Waterloo K, Egge A, Isaksen J, Ingebrigtsen T, Romner B. Predictors for cognitive impairment one year after surgery for aneurysmal subarachnoid hemorrhage. *J Neurol* 2008;255(11):1770–6.

76. Greenberg JK, Washington CW, Guniganti R, Dacey RG, Jr., Derdeyn CP, Zipfel GJ. Causes of 30-day readmission after aneurysmal subarachnoid hemorrhage. *J Neurosurg* 2016;124(3):743–9.

77. Singh M, Guth JC, Liotta E, et al. Predictors of 30-day readmission after subarachnoid hemorrhage. *Neurocrit Care* 2013;19(3):306–10.

78. The Joint Commission. Specifications manual for Joint Commission National Quality Measures (v2017B2). Comprehensive Stroke Measures 2018. [Accessed 2018 February 24]. Available from: https://manual.jointcommission.org/releases/TJC2017B2/ComprehensiveStroke.html.

75

Intracerebral Haemorrhage

F. A. Rasulo, R. Bertuetti, and N. Latronico

ABSTRACT

This is the case of a 55-year-old male with a past medical history significant for pulmonary embolism and long-standing arterial hypertension, who suffered a spontaneous right lobar intracerebral haemorrhage (ICH). Although stable at first, he later deteriorated neurologically to the point of requiring decompressive craniectomy due to refractory intracranial hypertension (IH). In such a patient, an important challenge is to limit the growth of the haematoma through control of arterial blood pressure (BP) and reversal of risk factors such as anticoagulation therapy. This case deals with some of the most important complications associated with spontaneous ICH, and the associated prevention and treatment strategies. An update of recent literature is also presented.

KEYWORDS

Spontaneous intracerebral haemorrhage; multimodality monitoring; intracranial hypertension (IH); decompressive craniectomy.

CASE STUDY

A 55-year-old male with a past medical history significant for pulmonary embolism (6 months prior) and long-standing arterial hypertension (in pharmacological treatment with warfarin 5 mg q.d. and an angiotensin converting enzyme inhibitor 25 mg t.i.d.) became suddenly disorientated at his workplace after lifting heavy crates. Upon arrival to the emergency department he had a left hemiparesis, a slight right-sided facial droop, and partial gaze palsy. His pupils were 4 mm in diameter, equal in size and bilaterally reactive to light. He was slightly disorientated in time with mild dysarthria, and at times he did not complete phrases. He was evaluated as having a Glasgow Coma Scale score (GCS) of 13 (3[e], 6[m], 4[v]) and a National Institutes of Health Stroke Scale (NIHSS) score of 9.

The initial vital parameters were oxygen saturation of 99% (with 2L of O_2/min), heart rate (HR) 61 beats per minute (bpm), arterial blood pressure (ABP) 200/96 mmHg, respiratory rate (RR) 15, and temperature 37.8°C. Non-contrast brain computed tomography (CT) showed a large right frontal intraparenchymal haemorrhage with 2-mm right to left midline shift and partial effacement of the basilar cisterns (Figure 75.1). Computed tomography angiography (CTA) of the brain was negative for vascular malformations. Chest X-ray was clear.

According to the intracerebral haemorrhage grading scale, the patient had a score of 2 (corresponding to a 30%–44% 30-day mortality risk).[1,2] Urine toxicology, including alcohol, amphetamines, barbiturates, benzodiazepines, cocaine, heroin, phencyclidine (PCP), and tetrahydrocannabinol (THC) were all negative.

Laboratory Findings

The patient's initial laboratory findings were following:
- White blood cell (WBC) count: $10.9 \times 10^3/\mu L$
- Haemoglobin (Hb): 13.5 g/dL
- Haematocrit (Hct): 38.8%

- Platelets: $287 \times 10^3/\mu L$
- Prothrombin Time (PT): 40 sec
- Partial Thromboplastin Time (PTT): 26 sec
- International Normalized Ratio (INR): 3.1
- Blood Urea Nitrogen (BUN): 23 mg/dL
- Na^+: 138 mEq/L
- K^+: 3.6 mEq/L
- CO_2: 32 mmHg
- Creatinine: 1.1 mg/dL
- Glucose: 200 mg/dL

Hospital Course

During the first two hours following hospital presentation, the patient remained neurologically stable and was therefore admitted to the neurosurgical ward where the neurosurgeon decided not to intervene surgically. Since the patient was on warfarin treatment with an INR of 3.1, Vitamin K 10 mg intravenous (IV) infusion (Class I, Level B)[5] and fresh frozen plasma (FFP) (Class I, Level B)[6] were started in order to achieve an INR <1.5. The patient was hypertensive on arrival to the emergency room (200/96 mmHg) increasing the risk and probability of further increase in size of the haematoma. Arterial BP reduction was obtained pharmacologically with urapidil bolus followed by labetalol infusion within 1 hour following admission and maintained between 140–160 mmHg. SaO_2 was maintained >94% and $PaCO_2$ between 35–45 mmHg. Hyperglycaemia (200 mg/dL) was treated with insulin in order to achieve a target value between 120–140 mg/dL. A transcranial Doppler (TCD) examination was performed which showed an intracranial pressure (ICP) estimation of 32 mmHg, a midline shift of 4 mm and an optic nerve sheath (ONS) diameter of 6 mm. Six hours after admission his neurological condition rapidly deteriorated to a GCS of 11 (2[e],6[m],3[v]). Following an IV bolus of 7.5% saline, the patient was sedated, intubated, and had an intraparenchymal ICP fibreoptic bolt placed which confirmed the presence of intracranial hypertension (ICP of 28 mmHg).

A second CT scan of the brain showed a slight increase in the haematoma size and midline shift with the presence of 'spot sign' due most likely to contrast extravasation.

A radial arterial (RA) catheter was placed to maintain a cerebral perfusion pressure (CPP) (which is equal to mean arterial pressure [MAP] less ICP) between 60 and 70 mmHg.

Multimodality monitoring consisted of invasive ICP, continuous TCD, brain tissue oxygenation, and continuous electroencephalogram (EEG) in order to monitor for non-convulsive seizures. Continuous monitoring of cerebrovascular autoregulation was also initiated and resulted in being compromised.

Over the subsequent 5 hours following the intubation, the patient's ICP raised up to 40 mmHg, despite multiple boluses of 3% saline (Na^+ increased to 147 mEq/dL from 136 mEq/dL on admission) and heavy sedation, paralysis, and active superficial cutaneous cooling to maintain normothermia.

Due to refractory ICP elevation, the decision was made to perform a right fronto-temporo-parietal craniectomy with evacuation of the clot.

The ICP after the hemicraniectomy and clot removal was less than 20 mmHg. The following day, after sedation was again suspended for neurological evaluation, the patient awakened and his right hemiparesis improved rapidly. A swallow evaluation test showed near normal swallowing and he was therefore started on a soft diet. He was transferred to the neurosurgical ward on postoperative day 4, and was later discharged to an acute rehabilitation centre with a persisting but mild left-sided weakness, fluent speech with mild dysarthria, and mild right facial droop.

INTRODUCTION

Since many patients with high level of intracranial hypertension (IH) on hospital presentation are deemed as being inoperable, it is paramount that the clinician is provided with sufficient prognostic information as possible in order to make the correct decision whether to continue or limit medical treatment. Literature demonstrates that this may be possible by performing a

Table 75.1 ICH stroke severity score

Variables		Score
GCS	3 to 4	2
	5 to 12	1
	13 to 15	0
ICH VOL	≥ 30 cm^3	1
	<30 cm^3	0
IV extension	Present	1
	Absent	0
Infratentorial origin	Yes	1
	No	0
Age	≥ 80	1
	<80	0

Reprinted with permission from: Hemphill JC 3rd, Bonovich DC, Besmertis L, Manley GT, Johnston SC. The ICH score: A simple, reliable grading scale for intracerebral hemorrhage. *Stroke*. 2001 Apr;32(4):891–7.

thorough neurological examination with grading scores such as the IH scale which combines the GCS with brain imaging information, clot origin, and age[1,2] (Table 75.1). Grading scales and scores may help select patients who will most likely benefit from certain treatments. These later, combined with multimodality monitoring may help improve outcome of patients with spontaneous intracerebral haemorrhage (ICH) through individualization of treatment strategies.

DISCUSSION

The initial treatment strategy of the patient described in the case study was considered to be conservative, being that the patient's neurological condition was stable. However, indication for surgery was given only after the patient deteriorated neurologically and the diagnosis of IH was made (first non-invasively and then invasively). Regarding surgical indication for patients with spontaneous ICH, the benefits of removing the clot were evaluated in two randomized trials:[3,4] (1) The first was a Surgical Trial in Intracerebral Hemorrhage (STICH 3) where 1033 patients with supratentorial haemorrhage (lobar or ganglionic haematoma) were randomized to either early surgery (<96 hours of ictus) versus standard of care (medical management with delayed surgery if necessary). They found no difference in functional outcome at 6 months (p = 0.414). However, the subgroup of patients who had superficial ICHs (lobar haemorrhage within 1 cm of the cortical surface) and who underwent

surgery had better outcomes. (2) This result led to a second trial, STICH II4, which randomized patients with superficial lobar haematomas (10–100 ml) to early surgery versus medical management with delayed surgery if necessary. IVH or coma patients were excluded. There was a difference in mortality or severe disability with early surgery. Interesting to note, patients with predicted poor prognosis at enrolment were more likely to have a favourable outcome with early surgery compared to initial conservative treatment. In patients with predicted good prognosis at enrolment such a benefit with early surgery was not detected.

Due to a history of pulmonary embolism, our patient was on long-term anticoagulant therapy, which is the reason why his INR on arrival to the emergency room (ER) was 3.1. Since patients with spontaneous ICH on anticoagulant therapy are at greater risk of haematoma growth, his INR was reduced to a value <1.5 through infusion of Vitamin K and FFP (Class I, Level B evidence).[5–8] In fact, despite prompt medical treatment, on the second brain CT his haematoma had grown in diameter compared to the first scan. His blood pressure was also quickly reduced to a target range between 140–160 mmHg.[9–11] As for the second Intensive Blood Pressure Reduction in Acute Cerebral Hemorrhage Trial (INTERACT-2), The Antihypertensive Treatment of Acute Cerebral Hemorrhage II (ATACH-2) study failed to show a higher rate of better functional outcomes in patients randomized to intensive systolic BP (SBP) reduction with a target SBP goal of less than 140 mmHg. If a therapeutic benefit of SBP reduction in patients with ICH was present, the current evidence does not show any benefit with a treatment range between 110 and 139 mmHg compared with goals of 140–179 mmHg. Intensive SBP reduction is associated with a higher rate of renal and other serious adverse events and therefore raises concerns regarding this therapeutic target.

Multimodality neuro-monitoring consisted of transcranial colour coded duplex Doppler, invasive ICP, CPP, and EEG, according to suggested guidelines for the Management of Spontaneous Intracerebral Haemorrhage and a Guideline for Healthcare Professionals From the American Heart Association/American Stroke Association.[11]

Although the treatment strategy followed the updated guidelines (including the management of complications such as hypo-hypergycaemia, hyperthermia, etc.) the patient's neurological condition continued to deteriorate due to his refractory intracranial hypertension caused by further growth of the haematoma.[11–13] The decision was made to perform decompressive craniectomy.[14,15] This caused the patient's ICP to reduce drastically with improvement of cerebral haemodynamics. An important randomized controlled trial (RCT) which will evaluate whether decompressive craniectomy in spontaneous ICH patients improves outcome is underway, 'Decompressive Hemicraniectomy in Intracerebral Hemorrhage (SWITCH)' ClinicalTrials.gov Identifier: NCT02258919.

The patient woke up after two days and was transferred to the ward 5 days after decompressive craniectomy.

CONCLUSIONS

A combination of clinical grading scores and multimodality monitoring in patients with spontaneous ICH may help individualize evidence-based treatment strategies, both medical and surgical, eventually leading to improvement of outcome.

REFERENCES

1. Hemphill JC, Bonovich DC, Besmertis L, Manley GT, Johnston SC, Tuhrim S. The ICH score: a simple, reliable grading scale for intracerebral hemorrhage. *Stroke* 2001;32(4):891–7. doi:10.1161/01.STR.32.4.891.

2. Hwang BY, Appelboom G, Kellner CP, et al. Clinical grading scales in intracerebral hemorrhage. *Neurocrit Care* 2010;13(1):141–51. doi:10.1007/s12028-010-9382-x.

3. Mendelow AD, Gregson BA, Fernandes HM, et al. Early surgery versus initial conservative treatment in patients with spontaneous supratentorial intracerebral haematomas in the International Surgical Trial in Intracerebral Haemorrhage (STICH): a randomised trial. *Lancet* 2005; 365:387–97.

4. Mendelow AD, Gregson BA, Rowan EN, et al. Early surgery versus initial conservative treatment in patients with spontaneous supratentorial lobar intracerebral haematomas (STICH II): a randomised trial. *Lancet* 2013;382(9890):397–408. doi:10.1016/S0140-6736(13)60986-1.

5. Pernod G, Godiér A, Gozalo C, Tremey B, Sié P. French clinical practice guidelines on the management of patients on vitamin K antagonists in at-risk situations (overdose, risk of bleeding, and active bleeding). *Thromb Res* 2010;126(3):e167–74. doi:10.1016/j.thromres.2010.06.017.

6. Hickey M, Gatien M, Taljaard M, Aujnarain A, Giulivi A, Perry JJ. Outcomes of urgent warfarin reversal with frozen plasma versus prothrombin complex concentrate in the emergency department. *Circulation* 2013;128(4):360–4. doi:10.1161/CIRCULATIONAHA.113.001875.

7. Sarode R, Milling TJ, Refaai MA, et al. Efficacy and safety of a 4-factor prothrombin complex concentrate in patients on vitamin K antagonists presenting with major bleeding: a randomized, plasma-controlled, phase IIIb study. *Circulation* 2013;128(11):1234–43. doi:10.1161/CIRCULATIONAHA.113.002283.

8. Ray B, Keyrouz SG. Management of anticoagulant-related intracranial hemorrhage: an evidence-based review. *Crit Care* 2014;18(3):223–3. doi:10.1186/cc13889.

9. Qureshi AI, Palesch YY, Barsan WG, et al. Intensive blood-pressure lowering in patients with acute cerebral hemorrhage. *N Engl J Med* 2016; 375:1033–43.

10. Majidi S, Suarez JI, Qureshi AI, et al. Management of acute hypertensive response in intracerebral hemorrhage patients after ATACH-2 trial. *Neurocrit Care* 2017 Oct;27(2): 249–58. doi:10.1007/s12028-016-0341-z.

11. Hemphill JC III, Greenberg SM, Anderson CS, et al. Guidelines for the management of spontaneous intracerebral hemorrhage. A guideline for healthcare professionals from the American Heart Association/American Stroke Association. *Stroke* 2015;46:000.

12. Du F-Z, Jiang R, Gu M, He C, Guan J. The accuracy of spot sign in predicting hematoma expansion after intracerebral hemorrhage: a systematic review and meta-analysis. *PLoS One* 2014;9(12):e115777–7. doi:10.1371/journal.pone.0115777.

13. Becker KJ, Baxter AB, Bybee HM, Tirschwell DL, Abouelsaad T, Cohen WA. Extravasation of radiographic contrast is an independent predictor of death in primary intracerebral hemorrhage. *Stroke* 1999;30(10):2025–32.

14. Fung C, Murek M, Klinger-Gratz PP, et al. Effect of decompressive craniectomy on perihematomal edema in patients with intracerebral hemorrhage. *PloS One* doi: 10.1371. February 12, 2016.

15. Fischer U, Beck J. Decompressive hemicraniectomy in intracerebral hemorrhage trial (SWITCH). ClinicalTrials.gov Identifier: NCT02258919.

76

Acute Ischaemic Stroke—Hemispheric Middle Cerebral Artery Stroke

H. El Beheiry and D. Rosso

ABSTRACT

Proximal middle cerebral artery (MCA) occlusion is associated with severe stroke and may cause severe disability. This chapter discusses the case management of acute ischaemic hemispheric MCA stroke. Patients with MCA territory ischaemic strokes should be cared for by a specialized team. Intravenous thrombolytic therapy can improve outcome and should be done within 3 hours of time of onset. It can be followed by endovascular thrombectomy and intra-arterial thrombolysis. If the MCA stroke develops into malignant MCA infarct syndrome, surgical decompressive craniectomy should be considered and followed by intensive medical therapy. All stroke patients in the acute phase should receive intensive medical therapy with the goal of maintaining cerebral perfusion of compromised brain tissue, prevention of further arterial occlusion, applying neuroprotective measures, and controlling cerebral oedema and intracranial pressure (ICP) in the case of malignant MCA infarction.

KEYWORDS

Middle cerebral artery (MCA); MCA stroke; decompressive craniectomy; emergency neurological life support (ENLS); endovascular thrombectomy; malignant MCA infarction.

CASE STUDY

A 78-year-old right-handed female had a sudden onset of right-sided weakness with slurred speech that progressed to global aphasia. Her cardiovascular risk factors included hypertension, dyslipidaemia, and paroxysmal atrial fibrillation with a slow ventricular response. She was taking telmisartan 80 mg once daily and metoprolol 25 mg twice daily as well as rosuvastatin 20 mg once daily for the past 8 years. She was not receiving any antiplatelet or anticoagulant medication. She was immediately transferred and admitted to the emergency department of a tertiary university affiliated hospital and the stroke team was activated. She had National Institute of Health Stroke Scale (NIHSS) score of 22. A non-contrast computed tomography (CT) scan confirmed the occurrence of a middle cerebral artery (MCA) stroke with hyperdensity of the M1 on the left side (Figure 76.1). Intravenous tissue plasminogen activator (tPA) was started in the emergency department at 90 minutes of the onset of her stroke symptoms. The patient was then admitted to the neurocritical care unit (NICU). However, she remained globally aphasic and was suffering from dense hemiplegia and hemisensory loss (NIH stroke scale = 24). An urgent CT angiogram showed an occlusive thrombus in the M1 segment of the left MCA. The patient was immediately transferred to the neuro-angiography procedural operating room. Recanalization was attempted by endovascular thrombectomy using the Merci Retrieval device after about 3 hours and 20 minutes of the onset of symptoms. The patient was readmitted to the NICU to receive specialized care for stroke patients. Her oxygenation was maintained above 94% with supplemental oxygen (O$_2$). The blood pressure (BP) was controlled around 140–160 systolic BP (SBP) and the blood sugar was kept within 7–9 mmol/L. After 24 hours she was started on aspirin 81 mg and clopidogrel 75 mg. Over the next 48 hours her aphasia and motor deficits improved substantially. The patient was discharged from the NICU to a rehabilitation facility with a NIHSS score of 6 indicating mild neurological deficit and major improvement from the admission presentation.

INTRODUCTION

Hemispheric MCA ischaemic stroke is the abrupt onset of neurological deficits due to thromboembolism leading to focal ischaemic damage of brain structures located within the MCA blood supply territory. The clinical picture of MCA territory stroke depends on the level of occlusion as well as hemispheric dominance (Table 76.1). The more distal the occlusion of the MCA, milder is the stroke. In contrast, the most proximal occlusions, e.g., blockade of the first segment of the MCA (M1) results in widespread deficits. The latter represents a hemispheric syndrome comprising of contralateral hemiplegia, hemisensory loss, homonymous hemianopia and loss of cortical function. MCA hemispheric syndrome may progress into a clinical picture of malignant MCA infarction associated with cerebral oedema, increased intracranial pressure (ICP), worsening of neurological function, and depressed level of consciousness with high mortality and morbidity.[1]

This chapter is a case study of acute ischaemic hemispheric MCA stroke. It will provide an in-depth and multifaceted exploration of this complex condition. The discussion will focus on the essentials of neurocritical care management of these highly demanding and compromised patients suffering from M1 occlusion.

Table 76.1 Clinical picture of middle cerebral artery (MCA) occlusion

Artery occluded	Clinical picture
MCA – M1 segment	Contralateral hemiparesis (brachiocephalic > lower limb)
	Contralateral hemisensory loss
	Contralateral hemianopia
	Global aphasia if the dominant hemisphere is affected
	Contralateral neglect if the non-dominant hemisphere is affected
Left MCA superficial cortical division	Right face and arm upper motor weakness
	Non-fluent (Broca's area) aphasia[a]
	Possible right face and arm cortical type sensory loss
	Possible fluent (Wernicke's area) aphasia[a]
Right MCA superficial cortical division	Left face and arm upper motor weakness
	Left hemineglect (possible)[b]
	Possible left face and arm cortical type sensory loss
Left MCA inferior cortical division	Wernicke's aphasia[a]
	Right mild weakness of face and arm (possible)
	Right hemisensory loss (face, arm, and possible hand)
	Right hemianopsia—mostly upper quadrants
Right MCA inferior cortical division	Left hemineglect and disturbed spatial perception[b]
	Left mild weakness of face and arm (possible)
	Left hemisensory loss (face, arm, and possible hand)
	Left hemianopsia—mostly upper quadrants
Left MCA lenticulostriate branches	Right pure hemiparesis due to damage to the basal ganglia
	Possible aphasia if infarct extends to cortical areas[a]
Right MCA lenticulostriate branches	Left pure hemiparesis due to damage to the basal ganglia
	Possible aphasia if infarct extends to cortical areas

[a]Assuming left hemispheric dominance.
[b]Assuming right hemispheric non-dominance.

DIAGNOSIS AND INITIAL MANAGEMENT OF ISCHAEMIC STROKE

The overall goal of diagnostic workup is to determine the suitability of the patient presenting with MCA territory stroke for reperfusion therapy in order to salvage penumbral tissue. The first step is to diagnose the aetiology of stroke which is the branching point in the emergency neurological life support (ENLS) protocol for managing acute ischaemic stroke.[2] Accordingly, an initial non-contrast computed tomography (CT) scan will determine whether the stroke is due to subdural haematoma, intracerebral haemorrhage or occlusive stroke (Figure 76.1). If the latter is confirmed, the patient will receive intravenous (IV) tissue plasminogen activator (tPA) therapy as soon as possible and before the transfer to the NICU. The indications and contraindications for IV tPA administration are shown in Table 76.2.[2,3]

The second step is to establish the suitability of the patient to undergo endovascular treatment with mechanical thrombectomy in combination with intra-arterial injection of thrombolytic agents. Endovascular treatment should be offered to patients who have: (1) documented occlusion in the distal internal carotid or the proximal MCA, and (2) have a relatively normal non-contrast head CT scan, severe neurological deficit, and can have intra-arterial thrombectomy within 6 hours since they have been seen as normal.[4] In the case history presented, the patient had most of these indications: occlusion of M1, dense hemiplegia, and global aphasia, and near normal CT scan as well as being ready for the procedure within 6 hours of last seen normal. CT angiography will determine the level of occlusion and its suitability for mechanical thrombectomy. In fact, some centres will perform CT angiography at the same time when the non-contrast CT is done to expedite the identification of large vessel intracranial occlusion and the status of extracranial internal carotid artery.

Specialized CT or magnetic resonance imaging (MRI) protocols establish the degree of tissue injury, the presence of vessel occlusion or stenosis in ischaemic stroke patients.[5] A CT angiography determines the level of vessel occlusion. Diffusion weighted imaging (DWI) sequence identifies the brain tissue that is bioenergetically compromised by ischaemia. In humans, ischaemic changes were detected with DWI as early as 2 hours after onset of symptoms. The changes appear as hyperintense areas representing infarcted brain. DWI is based on the assumption that cytotoxic oedema, which is caused by the accumulation of intracellular water due to cell membrane damage minutes after onset of acute cerebral ischaemia causes a restriction of microscopic proton diffusion. This

Table 76.2 Indications and contraindications for recombinant tissue plasminogen activator (tPA) in acute MCA ischaemic stroke with major persistent neurological deficit

Indications for tPA thrombolysis (NINDS inclusion criteria)
Onset less than 3 hours
Patient more than 18 years of age
No imaging evidence of ICH
Absolute contraindications for tPA thrombolysis
Major head trauma or prior stroke in the last 3 months
History of intracranial or intraspinal surgery in the last 3 months
History of intracranial tumours, neurovascular disorders, or ICH
Evidence of active bleeding or acute trauma
Arterial puncture in a non-compressible site or lumbar puncture in the last 7 days
SBP >185 and/or diastolic BP >110 mmHg
Platelet count <100,000 mm^3
Use of anticoagulant medications in the last 48 hours
Blood sugar <2.7 mmol/L (50 mg/dL) or >22 mmol/L (400 mg/dL)
Relative contraindications for tPA thrombolysis
Stroke symptoms rapidly improving or only minor
Seizures at onset of stroke
Pregnancy
Major surgery or trauma in the last 14 days
Gastrointestinal or urogenital bleeding in the last 21 days
Myocardial infarction in the last 3 months
NIHSS more than 25 (major deficits)

Note: NINDS: National Institute of Neurological Disorders and Stroke.

decrease in water diffusion is presumably reflected in a decrease of the apparent diffusion coefficients which is visualized as a hyperintensity on the diffusion-weighted images. Perfusion-weighted MRI (PWI) detects areas of compromised perfusion as a result of vessel occlusion. PWI is based on rapid imaging of the first pass of the contrast agent (gadolinium). In PWI using dynamic contrast-enhanced MRI, T1-weighted sequence detects an increase in intensity proportional to contrast concentration. Thus normal perfusion areas are more intense in appearance compared to areas with haemodynamic compromise. From DWI and PWI data, the volume of salvageable penumbral tissue can be evaluated by visually subtracting the DWI hyperintense area (infarct core) from the PWI hypointense area (haemodynamically compromised area). The region in which there exists perfusion abnormality but no diffusion abnormality points to salvageable penumbral tissue. If there is an appreciable penumbra, endovascular reperfusion method can improve stroke outcome[6] (Figure 76.2).

NEUROINTENSIVE CARE UNIT ADMISSION

Specialized neurological critical care post-thrombolysis therapy was necessary in the case presented. Indeed, the admission criteria to the NICU for patients with acute MCA stroke include neurologic and non-neurologic indications. Neurologic indications are: (1) post-reperfusion therapy by thrombolysis or endovascular treatment, (2) malignant MCA infarction, (3) haemorrhagic conversion, (4) deteriorating level of consciousness, and (5) worsening neurological symptoms. Non-neurological situations that warrant NICU admission during the course of acute ischaemic stroke comprises: (1) failure to protect the airway, respiratory failure, or need for mechanical ventilation, (2) persistent hypotension, (3) severe hypertension requiring IV therapy, (4) acute myocardial infarction or unstable arrhythmias, and (5) severe systemic bleeding.

Since the establishment of neurological intensive care units in the early 1980s, reports showed that there are several benefits in favour of acute ischaemic stroke patients receiving specialized critical care in the NICU.[7,8] Patients had lower in-hospital mortality, shorter in-hospital length of stay, and better discharge disposition to home compared to a rehabilitation or long-term care facility. Moreover, patients had a trend for lower cumulative mortality and better functional outcome at three-month follow-up after discharge.

MANAGEMENT OF POST THROMBOLYTIC AND THROMBECTOMY COMPLICATIONS

The case presented did not suffer any of the complications of thrombolytic or endovascular thrombectomy. The complications of IV thrombolysis with tPA alone or followed by endovascular treatment are uncommon and include symptomatic intracranial haemorrhage (sICH), major systemic haemorrhage, and angio-oedema in approximately 6%, 2%, and 5% of patients, respectively.[9,10] Due to grave consequences of these uncommon complications, admission to the NICU is indicated for post-thrombolysis and post-thrombectomy management.

Hypersensitivity Reactions to tPA

The tPA hypersensitivity reactions range from localized rash and itchiness to life-threatening orolingual angio-oedema. The risk of orolingual angio-oedema is increased with the use of angiotensin-converting enzyme inhibitor medications and frontal and insular strokes.[11] Hypersensitivity usually occurs after a few minutes of injection and begins with perioral tingling and may progress to orolingual angio-oedema in 1–5% of patients. The latter can be life-threatening because of upper airway compromise that may require intubation or urgent tracheostomy in cases of frank and refractory stridor and progressive decrement in O_2 saturation. Hypersensitivity reactions are treated with steroids, and H1 and H2 blockers. Administration of epinephrine in small subcutaneous doses (0.3 ml of 1:1000) is rarely necessary according to previously published case reports.[12]

Symptomatic Intracranial Haemorrhage

According to a recent meta-analysis of eight multicentre randomized controlled studies, the weighted average incidence of sICH in patients receiving IV tPA followed by endovascular treatment is 2.1–9.4%.[13] All studies included patients with intracranial internal carotid artery or proximal MCA occlusion. The most common presenting symptoms of haemorrhagic conversion in the first 24 hours post treatment are worsening of neurological deficits including new cranial nerve palsies and somnolence. Immediate CT scan should be performed. If sICH is confirmed, neurosurgery should be informed and tPA reversal protocol should be considered. The protocols vary but they usually include the transfusion of fresh frozen plasma, cryoprecipitate, and platelets. If these measures are unsuccessful, the antifibrinolytic tranexamic acid or aminocaproic acid may be recommended (Table 76.3).

Systemic Extracranial Haemorrhage

Extracranial haemorrhage is rare but can complicate thrombolysis. Serious systemic haemorrhage occurred in approximately 1.6% of IV tPA treated patients. The major locations of extracranial haemorrhages include the gingiva, gastrointestinal tract, urogenital organs, retroperitoneal areas, and less commonly the pericardial sac.[14] Cardiac tamponade in this situation is associated with hypotension, bradycardia, and ST and T wave changes on the electrocardiogram (ECG) without the elevation of cardiac enzymes. Gastrointestinal bleeding is associated with acute hypotension and decreasing haemoglobin levels and may be epistaxis, haemoptysis, and melena. Severe haemorrhage from the site of arterial puncture in the groin occasionally occurs including the development of retroperitoneal haematoma. Manual compression of the site of bleeding and volume replacement may be required.

In order to prevent extracranial haemorrhage, care should be taken to avoid ICU procedures involving

Table 76.3 Suggested tPA reversal protocol[a]

1. Stop ongoing tPA infusion.
2. Consult appropriate service for the management of intracranial or extracranial bleeding.
3. Control SBP to 140–150 mmHg.
4. Check haemoglobin, platelets, and coagulation profile (fibrinogen, PT, aPTT, and INR).
5. Cross-check if there is evidence of extracranial bleeding or need for possible craniotomy.
6. Give Amicar (ε-aminocaproic acid) 0.05 gm/kg over 30 min.
7. If the fibrinogen is less than 100 mg/dL, give 0.15 units/kg of cryoprecipitate. Repeat fibrinogen levels 30 minutes later and continue to administer cryoprecipitate until fibrinogen level is >100 mg/dL.
8. If the platelets are:
Less than 150K, give 1 platelet pheresis unit.
Less than 100K, give 2 platelet pheresis units.
9. Check platelets after transfusion and repeat platelet transfusion until platelet count is >150K.

aThe primary goal of the protocol is to replace fibrinogen and clotting factors and the poorly understood antiplatelet effect of tPA.

noncompressible sites for example central and arterial line treatment, nasogastric or urinary catheter placement and endotracheal intubation. If extracranial bleeding is life-threatening, tPA reversal protocols should be considered (Table 76.3) and careful monitoring of vital signs and haematocrit and haemoglobin is vital.

Hypertension

Hypertension occurring post thrombolysis and endovascular treatment is a risk factor for haemorrhagic conversion. Blood pressure targets should be individualized to every patient on the basis of degree of revascularization, collateral flow, concern for hyperaemia or intracranial haemorrhage (ICH), and degree of ischaemia on post-thrombolysis or procedural imaging. The ENLS protocol recommends a target SBP <180 mmHg and diastolic BP <105 mmHg.[2] In other institutions the targets are SBP <140 mmHg and mean arterial pressure (MAP) >70 mmHg in patients who had successful revascularization. For patients who did not achieve successful revascularization, haemodynamic targets may be set to allow permissive hypertension per the AHA/ASA stroke guidelines.[3,15] Small sample sized case series have demonstrated safety and mixed results in efficacy for induced hypertension.[16,17]

Hypertension is treated by titratable IV antihypertensive medications. Nicardipine 2.5–5 mg/hr and titrated to a maximum of 15 mg/hr or labetalol 10 mg IV boluses to achieve the target BP and then followed by an infusion of 20–160 mg/hr. A recent study showed less bradycardia and hypotension with nicardipine compared to labetalol. In contrast, hypertension can be induced in selected cases post thrombolysis by using alpha adrenergic agonists, for

example, phenylephrine 0.5–5 µg/kg/min by IV infusion titrated to target SBP >140 mmHg. It is noteworthy mentioning that spontaneous normalization of BP might be seen in patients with hypertensive disease prior to thrombolysis or endovascular treatment. Probably, this is due to successful reperfusion of the brain and consequently loss of compensatory homoeostatic-induced hypertension that may maintain brain perfusion.[18]

MANAGEMENT OF MALIGNANT MCA INFARCT

CASE STUDY

A 65-year-old uncontrolled diabetic male gradually lost all his strength in the right side of his body and the ability to speak; he was rushed to the emergency room via ambulance. A non-contrast head CT determined he was having an ischaemic stroke in the left MCA territory. After tPA therapy, he regained some motor power in his right lower limb. About 8 hours after tPA therapy, he progressively developed right hemiparesis and depressed consciousness. Another non-contrast CT showed that he was developing increased ICP due to massive cerebral oedema, which was causing partial severe midline shift. Urgent neurosurgical consultation suggested urgent decompressive craniectomy. The family agreed after thorough discussion of the risks and benefits pertaining to the patient's previous wishes. After the operation, he was admitted to the NICU, ventilated, and sedated. Intensive medical therapy was implemented and he was weaned from the ventilator after one week. Five weeks later, he was admitted to a rehabilitation facility with a modified Rankin score of 4 indicating severe disability.

Malignant MCA infarction takes place in 8% of acute ischaemic strokes. It is a syndrome of rapid neurological deterioration resulting from the effects of ominous space-occupying cerebral oedema following total or subtotal MCA territory stroke involving the basal ganglia.[18] The aetiology of the syndrome is the occlusion of the distal internal carotid artery or the proximal MCA trunk (M1). Unfortunately, malignant MCA infarction is associated with high mortality approaching 80% and severe disability with poor quality of life. The syndrome is also known as 'massive MCA infarction', 'cerebral infarction with swelling', 'space occupying MCA infarction', 'brain oedema in stroke', and 'large hemispheric infarction' (Figure 76.3).

There is still uncertainty over the optimal management of malignant MCA infarction. However, progress has been made on two separate tracks; first is the development of evidence-based guidelines for medical and surgical management and second is the conclusion of several randomized controlled trials (RCT) showing improved mortality with surgical decompression compared with strictly medical treatment.[19,20]

Medical Management of Malignant MCA Infarction

Medical management should be implemented in all cases of malignant MCA infarction after surgical therapy or in cases where surgery is not indicated. The goal of medical management is to prevent and reduce brain oedema, cerebral tissue shifts, and secondary increases in the ICP. It is important to realize that acute increase in ICP is secondary to the development of brain oedema.[19] Hence, therapeutic strategies aiming at reducing global ICP, i.e., ventriculostomy is not effective.

Intubation, Mechanical Ventilation, and Tracheostomy

There is no specific data regarding intubation and mechanical ventilation in patients with malignant MCA infarction. Therefore, the indications for intubation should follow general critical care principles. A single prospective cohort study investigating malignant MCA infarction reported that the indications for intubation were Glasgow Coma Scale (GCS) score <10, respiratory failure, and infarct size greater than two-thirds of the MCA territory.[21] In contrast, clinical practice suggests that indications for extubating general critical care population cannot be applied to brain injured ICU patients. Failure to extubate is common in patients with GCS ≤8, dysphagia, and impaired level of consciousness. Extubating stroke patients should be individualized.

Tracheostomy may be required if timely extubation is not achievable. Predictors of tracheostomies

include development of hydrocephalus, haemorrhagic transformation, and the existence of obstructive pulmonary disease requiring treatment. In patients with ischaemic stroke including malignant MCA infarction, early tracheostomies within 7–14 days of intubation has been shown to be safe, associated with less mortality, and slightly better functional neurologic outcome, and decreased sedation needs.[22]

Hyperventilation

In general, there is no convincing data supporting the use of hyperventilation as standard therapy for brain oedema. In malignant MCA infarction, hyperventilation can lead to worsening of ischaemia due to cerebrovascular constriction and rebound cerebrovascular dilatation when normocapnia is restored. Additionally, hyperventilation effect on ICP lasts for a short period of time and may not be adequate for managing stroke patients.[23]

Sedation and Neurological Wake-Up Tests

There are no studies for the need of sedation and analgesia in malignant MCA infarction. Clinical practice showed that initial sedation and analgesia are required to manage pain and decrease agitation. Sedation and analgesia can improve measures to lower ICP and allow uninterrupted line insertion and accomplishment of procedures. Sedation can also terminate seizures and increase the thresholds for seizure activity. Short-acting benzodiazepines, low-dose infusion of propofol, and fentanyl infusion are popular choices, but there is no evidence to implement specific protocols.

In the general ICU, regular wake-up tests show reduction in the duration of mechanical ventilation and easier weaning from ventilator therapy.[24] Nonetheless, such wake-up tests may have adverse effects in patients with malignant MCA infarction, for example, increased ICP and increased levels of stress hormones.

Dysphagia and Feeding

Management of dysphagia and feeding in patients with malignant MCA infarction follows the general approach for stroke patients. Dysphagia screening should be done and has been shown to decrease the incidence of aspiration pneumonia. If dysphagia is detected swallowing therapy and nutritional supplementation through nasogastric tube or percutaneous endoscopic gastrostomy should be considered. Nutritional supplementation in the presence of dysphagia in stroke was associated with reduced pressure sores, and increased energy and protein intake. Nasogastric tube feeding compared with percutaneous endoscopic gastrostomy feeding reduced treatment failures and gastrointestinal bleeding, and had higher feed delivery and albumin concentration.[25] Additionally, early tube feeding might reduce case fatality, but at the expense of increasing the proportion of patients surviving with poor outcome.[26] The available data do not support a policy of early initiation of percutaneous endoscopic gastrostomy feeding in dysphagic stroke patients. Hence, the decision to insert percutaneous endoscopic gastrostomy should be performed in patients who need nasogastric feeding for more than 2 weeks or cannot tolerate nasogastric feeding on more than two occasions.

Control of Blood Glucose

Previous RCTs show a consistent U-shaped relationship between serum glucose concentration and neurological outcomes.[27] Both hypoglycaemia and extreme hyperglycaemia are likely to be harmful. Intensive insulin therapy in neurocritical patients achieving blood glucose target of 80–120 mg/dL (4.4–6.7 mmol/L) increased the incidence of hypoglycaemia, length of stay in the ICU, and non-favourable neurological outcome as well as the likelihood of mortality. Initiating insulin therapy at high blood glucose levels >200 gm/L (<11 mmol/L) are associated with worse neurological outcomes. Thus, intermediate blood glucose targets between 140–180 mg/dL (7.8–10 mmol/L) for patients with malignant MCA infarction is appropriate and supported by literature in critically ill neurological patients.[28]

Optimal Haemoglobin Level

In patients with ischaemic or haemorrhagic stroke, WHO-defined anaemia was a significant risk for poor neurologic outcome including all cause mortality or the composite outcome of disability, discharge to a nursing facility or death.[29] Consequently, several reports recommended liberal transfusion trigger of haemoglobin level about 9 g/dL in patients with traumatic brain injury (TBI), subarachnoid haemorrhage (SAH), and acute ischaemic stroke. There are also studies that suggest that a restrictive transfusion trigger of haemoglobin level about 7–8 g/dL does not worsen outcome and may be beneficial.[30] At this time, the effect of anaemia on the recovery from malignant MCA infarction has not been investigated. Hence, blood transfusion decisions should be guided by risk and benefit analysis that should be determined for each patient. Based on physiological knowledge and available data, haemoglobin levels in malignant MCA infarction should not be allowed to drop below 8 g/dL.

Blood Pressure Management

There are no evidence-based specific targets for BP control established for malignant MCA infarction. However, it is reasonable to apply BP management protocols implemented in early management of acute ischaemic stroke. In the absence of IV or endovascular recanalization, MAP should be kept >85 mmHg and systolic and diastolic BP <220 mmHg and <120 mmHg, respectively.[2] It is also prudent to avoid hypotension in malignant MCA infarction to prevent delayed ischaemia or infarction of the anterior and posterior cerebral artery areas. Blood pressure fluctuations are common in the first 24 hours of ischaemic stroke. It can be associated with infarct extension, neurologic deterioration, worse outcomes, and increased mortality.[31] Therefore, it is important to monitor BP frequently to recognize extreme fluctuations that would need treatment. When lowering the BP during acute ischaemic stroke, hazards to the haemodynamic stability of the cerebral circulation will be minimized by lowering the pressure in a well-controlled manner. Controlled lowering of BP during acute stroke is achieved with intravenous antihypertensive therapies as nimodipine, labetalol or nicardipine. A single optimal medication to lower the BP in all patients with acute stroke has not been determined. Antihypertensive therapy should be individualized for every patient.

Hypothermia

Currently, there are no RCTs that show clinical benefit of mild hypothermia (32–35°C) in the management of malignant MCA infarction. Mild hypothermia can help to control critically elevated ICP values in space-occupying cerebral oedema associated with malignant MCA infarction. The evidence supporting its use is based on its relative safety, feasibility, and mostly non-life-threatening side effects.[32] The side effects reported in few and relatively small observational studies investigating malignant MCA infarction include systemic hypotension, thrombocytopenia, hyperfibrinogenaemia, shivering, and pneumonia.[33] Mild hypothermia is recommended in patients who are not eligible for surgical intervention. It is usually induced using surface cooling that is accomplished with circulating cold water blankets and cold air-forced blankets. Hypothermia should start early and be maintained for 24–72 hours.[33] Rewarming can be passive or may be active using surface warming. The rewarming process should be slow enough to prevent cerebral tissue herniation caused by a secondary rise in ICP after rewarming.

Osmotic Therapy

Hyperosmolar therapy reduces ICP by decreasing the volume of healthy cerebral tissue. Meanwhile, there is no evidence to indicate that mannitol, hypertonic saline or glycerol improves functional outcome or mortality in patients with ischaemic brain swelling.[34] During osmotherapy in malignant MCA infarction, normovolaemia is maintained, guided by central venous pressure or pulmonary artery wedge pressure to ensure optimal cerebral perfusion pressure (CPP) and avoid volume overload.

Mannitol 0.25 to 0.5 g/kg IV administered over 20 minutes lowers ICP and can be given every 6 hours. It is indicated in increased ICP and impending cerebral herniation. During mannitol therapy, plasma osmolality should be kept between 310–320 mOsmol/L. Mannitol decreases water content of brain tissue, decreases blood viscosity, and increases cerebrospinal fluid (CSF) absorption. Side effects include initial hypervolaemia, dehydration, and electrolyte imbalance.

Hypertonic saline 3% is usually given when mannitol becomes ineffective. It shifts water from the extravascular to intravascular compartment. In a pilot stroke study, the use of hypertonic saline in patients with clinical transtentorial herniation caused by various supratentorial lesions, including ischaemic and haemorrhagic stroke was associated with a rapid decrease in ICP.[35] Adverse effects of hypertonic saline include volume overload, hypernatraemia (rare), hypokalaemia, hyperchloremic metabolic acidosis, osmotic demyelenation, and seizures. Hypertonic saline solutions of 2%, 3%, or 7.5% contain equal amounts of sodium chloride and sodium acetate (50:50) to avoid hyperchloremic acidosis. Potassium supplementation (20–40 mEq/L) is added to the solution as needed. Continuous intravenous infusions are begun through a central venous catheter at 1–2 ml/kg/hr. The goal is to increase serum sodium concentration to 145 to 155 mEq/L and maintain that level for 48–72 hours until patients demonstrate clinical improvement or there is a lack of response despite achieving the serum sodium target.[35]

Glycerol is a sugar that has been used as an osmotic agent in large MCA infarcts.[36] As it is metabolised as an alternative energy source, it is assumed that it may not cause rebound ICP increase if it crosses the blood–brain barrier (BBB) compared to mannitol and hypertonic saline. Intravenous glycerol 0.25–1.5 g/kg every 6 hours (10% glycerol solution) will effectively decrease ICP.[36] Its side effects include nausea, vomiting, diarrhoea, haemoglobinuria, and bleeding diathesis.[36]

Surgical Management—Decompressive Hemicraniectomy

The rationale for decompressive surgery in patients with malignant MCA infarction is to relieve the high ICP by creating additional space for the oedematous brain to expand, thus preserving cerebral blood flow and preventing cerebral herniation. The procedure involves wide ipsilateral hemicraniectomy followed by duraplasty (Figure 76.3).

The National Institute for Health and Clinical Excellence (NICE) outlined criteria for patients with malignant MCA infarction who may undergo hemicraniectomy.[37] According to these criteria decompressive hemicraniectomy should be performed within a maximum of 48 hours from symptom onset. Such surgical intervention should be considered in patients who meet all of the following criteria: (1) Age <60 years; (2) National Institutes of Heart Stroke Scale (NIHSS) >15; (3) Depressed level of consciousness, i.e., not alert but aroused by minor stimulation or not alert and only responsive to repeated or strong and painful stimuli; and (4) Infarction of at least 50% of the MCA territory as determined by CT with or without infarction in the territory of the anterior and posterior cerebral arteries, or infarct volume of the MCA territory greater than 145 cm^3 according to diffusion-weighted MRI.[37]

The outcome of surgical treatment for malignant MCA infarction has been studied by several multicentre RCTs entitled DESTINY I, DESTINY II, DECIMAL, HAMLET, and HeADDFIRST.[38–42] The latest pooled analysis of data from these studies shows that surgical decompression for malignant MCA infarction results in large decreases in mortality.[20,43–45] A good number of the survivors will suffer from severe and very severe disability, i.e., unable to ambulate and needing help with all bodily needs. The proportion of patients who demonstrate mild to moderate disability is small. Subgroup analyses suggest that patients >60 years of age will show improved mortality, but the majority of survivors will have substantial disability. Therefore, surgical treatment decisions in all patients should be preceded by a thorough discussion with intensivists, neurosurgeons, and family members, considering any wishes the patient may have held relating to survival, dependency, and quality of life.

CONCLUSIONS

Ischaemic stroke of the MCA territory accounts for about 50% of the total number of strokes. The more distal the MCA occlusion the less severe is the stroke effect. Proximal

MCA occlusion is associated with severe stroke and may cause severe disability. Patients with MCA territory ischaemic strokes should be cared for by a specialized team. Intravenous thrombolytic therapy can improve outcome and should be done within 3 hours of time of onset. It can be followed by endovascular thrombectomy and intra-arterial thrombolysis. If the MCA stroke develops into malignant MCA infarct syndrome, surgical decompressive craniectomy should be considered and followed by intensive medical therapy. All stroke patients in the acute phase should receive intensive medical therapy with the goal of maintaining cerebral perfusion of compromised brain tissue, prevention of further arterial occlusion, applying neuroprotective measures, and controlling cerebral oedema and ICP in the case of malignant MCA infarction.

REFERENCES

1. Rordorf G, Koroshetz WJ, Copen WA, et al. Regional ischemia and ischemic injury in patients with acute middle cerebral artery stroke as defined by early diffusion-weighted and perfusion-weighted MRI. *Stroke* 1998;29(5):939–43.

2. Gross H, Guilliams KP, Sung G. Emergency neurological life support: acute ischemic stroke. *Neurocrit Care* 2015;23(Suppl 2):S94–102.

3. Jauch EC, Saver JL, Adams HP Jr, et al. Guidelines for the early management of patients with acute ischemic stroke: a guideline for healthcare professionals from the American Heart Association/American Stroke Association. *Stroke* 2013;44(3):870–947.

4. Chen CJ, Ding D, Starke RM, et al. Endovascular vs medical management of acute ischemic stroke. *Neurology* 2015;85(22):1980–90.

5. Donnan GA, Davis SM. Neuroimaging, the ischaemic penumbra, and selection of patients for acute stroke therapy. *Lancet Neurol* 2002;1(7):417–25.

6. Albers GW, Goyal M, Jahan R, et al. Relationships between imaging assessments and outcomes in solitaire with the intention for thrombectomy as primary endovascular treatment for acute ischemic stroke. *Stroke* 2015;46(10):2786–94.

7. Bershad EM, Feen ES, Hernandez OH, Suri MF, Suarez JI. Impact of a specialized neurointensive care team on outcomes of critically ill acute ischemic stroke patients. *Neurocrit Care* 2008;9(3):287–92.

8. Knopf L, Staff I, Gomes J, McCullough L. Impact of a neurointensivist on outcomes in critically ill stroke patients. *Neurocrit Care* 2012;16(1):63–71.

9. Albers GW, Bates VE, Clark WM, Bell R, Verro P, Hamilton SA. Intravenous tissue-type plasminogen activator for treatment of acute stroke: the Standard Treatment with Alteplase to Reverse Stroke (STARS) study. *JAMA* 2000;283(9):1145–50.

10. Hill MD, Buchan AM. Canadian Alteplase for Stroke Effectiveness Study (CASES) Investigators. Thrombolysis for acute ischemic stroke: results of the Canadian Alteplase for Stroke Effectiveness Study. *CMAJ* 2005;172(10):1307–12.

11. Hill MD, Lye T, Moss H, et al. Hemi-orolingual angioedema and ACE inhibition after alteplase treatment of stroke. *Neurology* 2003;60(9):1525–7.

12. Pahs L, Droege C, Kneale H, Pancioli A. A novel approach to the treatment of orolingual angioedema after tissue plasminogen activator administration. *Ann Emerg Med* 2016;68(3):345–8.

13. Mokin M, Kan P, Kass-Hout T, et al. Intracerebral hemorrhage secondary to intravenous and endovascular intraarterial revascularization therapies in acute ischemic stroke: an update on risk factors, predictors, and management. *Neurosurg Focus* 2012;32(4):E2.

14. Chang H, Wang X, Yang X, Song H, Qiao Y, Liu J. Digestive and urologic hemorrhage after intravenous thrombolysis for acute ischemic stroke: Data from a Chinese stroke center. *J Int Med Res* 2017;45(1):352–60.

15. McManus M, Liebeskind DS. Blood pressure in acute ischemic stroke. *J Clin Neurol* 2016;12(2):137–46.

16. Koenig MA, Geocadin RG, de Grouchy M, et al. Safety of induced hypertension therapy in patients with acute ischemic stroke. *Neurocrit Care* 2006;4:3–7.

17. Hillis AE, Ulatowski JA, Barker PB, et al. A pilot randomized trial of induced blood pressure elevation: effects on function and focal perfusion in acute and subacute stroke. *Cerebrovasc Dis* 2003;16:236–46.

18. Wijdicks EF, Sheth KN, Carter BS, et al. American Heart Association Stroke Council. Recommendations for the management of cerebral and cerebellar infarction with swelling: a statement for healthcare professionals from the American Heart Association/American Stroke Association. *Stroke* 2014;45(4):1222–38.

19. Torbey MT, Bösel J, Rhoney DH, et al. Evidence-based guidelines for the management of large hemispheric infarction: a statement for health care professionals from the Neurocritical Care Society and the German Society for Neuro-intensive Care and Emergency Medicine. *Neurocrit Care* 2015;22(1):146–64.

20. Cruz-Flores S, Berge E, Whittle IR. Surgical decompression for cerebral oedema in acute ischaemic stroke. *Cochrane Database Syst Rev*. 2012 Jan 18;1:CD003435.

21. Berrouschot J, Rössler A, Köster J, Schneider D. Mechanical ventilation in patients with hemispheric ischemic stroke. *Crit Care Med* 2000;28(8):2956–61.

22. Bösel J1, Schiller P, Hook Y, et al. Stroke-related Early Tracheostomy versus Prolonged Orotracheal Intubation in Neurocritical Care Trial (SETPOINT): a randomized pilot trial. *Stroke* 2013;44(1):21–8.

23. Muizelaar JP, Marmarou A, Ward JD, et al. Adverse effects of prolonged hyperventilation in patients with

severe head injury: a randomized clinical trial. *J Neurosurg* 1991;75(5):731–9.

24. Skoglund K, Enblad P, Marklund N. Effects of the neurological wake-up test on intracranial pressure and cerebral perfusion pressure in brain-injured patients. *Neurocrit Care* 2009;11(2):135–42.

25. Gomes CA Jr1, Andriolo RB, Bennett C, et al. Percutaneous endoscopic gastrostomy versus nasogastric tube feeding for adults with swallowing disturbances. *Cochrane Database Syst Rev.* 2015 May 22;5:CD008096.

26. Dennis MS, Lewis SC, Warlow C. FOOD Trial Collaboration. Effect of timing and method of enteral tube feeding for dysphagic stroke patients (FOOD): a multicentre randomised controlled trial. *Lancet* 2005;365(9461):764–72.

27. Osei E, den Hertog HM, Berkhemer OA, et al. MR CLEAN pretrial investigators. Increased admission and fasting glucose are associated with unfavorable short-term outcome after intra-arterial treatment of ischemic stroke in the MR CLEAN pretrial cohort. *J Neurol Sci* 2016;371:1–5.

28. Kramer AH, Roberts DJ, Zygun DA. Optimal glycemic control in neurocritical care patients: a systematic review and meta-analysis. *Crit Care* 2012;16(5):R203.

29. Tanne D, Molshatzki N, Merzeliak O, Tsabari R, Toashi M, Schwammenthal Y. Anemia status, hemoglobin concentration and outcome after acute stroke: a cohort study. *BMC Neurol* 2010;10:22 (p. 1–7).

30. Carson JL1, Stanworth SJ, Roubinian N, et al. Transfusion thresholds and other strategies for guiding allogeneic red blood cell transfusion. *Cochrane Database Syst Rev.* 2016 Oct 12;10:CD002042.

31. Delgado-Mederos R, Ribo M, Rovira A, et al. Prognostic significance of blood pressure variability after thrombolysis in acute stroke. *Neurology* 2008;71(8):552–8.

32. De Georgia MA, Krieger DW, Abou-Chebl A, et al. Cooling for Acute Ischemic Brain Damage (COOL AID): a feasibility trial of endovascular cooling. *Neurology* 2004;63(2):312–7.

33. Jeong HY, Chang JY, Yum KS, et al. Extended use of hypothermia in elderly patients with malignant cerebral edema as an alternative to hemicraniectomy. *J Stroke* 2016;18(3):337–43.

34. Subramaniam S, Hill MD. Massive cerebral infarction. *The Neurologist* 2005;11(3):150–60.

35. Koenig MA, Bryan M, Lewin JL 3rd, Mirski MA, Geocadin RG, Stevens RD. Reversal of transtentorial herniation with hypertonic saline. *Neurology* 2008;70(13):1023–9.

36. Berger C, Sakowitz OW, Kiening KL, Schwab S. Neurochemical monitoring of glycerol therapy in patients with ischemic brain edema. *Stroke* 2005;36(2):e4–6.

37. National Institute for Health Care and Excellence. Guidance 1.9.2. c2015. Available from: https://www.nice.org.uk/guidance/cg68/chapter/1-Guidance#surgery-for-people-with-acute-stroke.

38. Jüttler E, Schwab S, Schmiedek P, et al. DESTINY Study Group. Decompressive Surgery for the Treatment of Malignant Infarction of the Middle Cerebral Artery (DESTINY): a randomized, controlled trial. *Stroke* 2007;38(9):2518–25.

39. Jüttler E, Unterberg A, Woitzik J, et al. DESTINY II Investigators. Hemicraniectomy in older patients with extensive middle-cerebral-artery stroke. *N Engl J Med* 2014;370(12):1091–100.

40. Vahedi K, Vicaut E, Mateo J, et al. DECIMAL Investigators. Sequential-design, multicenter, randomized, controlled trial of early decompressive craniectomy in malignant middle cerebral artery infarction (DECIMAL Trial). *Stroke* 2007;38(9):2506–17.

41. Hofmeijer J, Kappelle LJ, Algra A, Amelink GJ, van Gijn J, van der Worp HB. HAMLET investigators. Surgical decompression for space-occupying cerebral infarction (the Hemicraniectomy After Middle Cerebral Artery infarction with Life-threatening Edema Trial [HAMLET]): a multicentre, open, randomised trial. *Lancet Neurol* 2009;8(4):326–33.

42. Frank JI, Schumm LP, Wroblewski K, et al. HeADDFIRST Trialists. Hemicraniectomy and durotomy upon deterioration from infarction-related swelling trial: randomized pilot clinical trial. *Stroke* 2014;45(3):781–7.

43. Vahedi K, Hofmeijer J, Juettler E, et al. DECIMAL, DESTINY, and HAMLET investigators. Early decompressive surgery in malignant infarction of the middle cerebral artery: a pooled analysis of three randomised controlled trials. *Lancet Neurol* 2007;6(3):215–22.

44. Back L, Nagaraja V, Kapur A, Eslick GD. Role of decompressive hemicraniectomy in extensive middle cerebral artery strokes: a meta-analysis of randomised trials. *Intern Med J* 2015;45(7):711–7.

45. Alexander P, Heels-Ansdell D, Siemieniuk R, et al. Hemicraniectomy versus medical treatment with large MCA infarct: a review and meta-analysis. *BMJ Open* 2016;6(11):e014390 (p. 1–11).

77

Management of Basilar Artery Stroke

S. Wahlster and M. Souter

ABSTRACT

Basilar artery occlusion (BAO) is a rare type of stroke with potentially devastating outcomes. Early diagnosis and treatment are crucial. Symptoms can vary and include a constellation of cranial nerve deficits, long track signs, and impairments in mental status. A high proportion of patients present with preceding transient ischaemic attacks (TIAs) and prodromal symptoms. Advances in acute stroke treatments include improved secondary prevention after TIA, wider implementation of intravenous tissue plasminogen activator (IV tPA) metrics with faster onset-to-treatment times, and more effective endovascular techniques resulting in better outcomes and decreased fatality rates for BAO patients. The optimal treatment approach is mostly a combination of various available treatments based on the individual case. Recanalization, clinical examination on presentation (presence of impaired consciousness and initial National Institutes of Health Stroke Scale [NIHSS] score), age, clot characteristics, and collateral status are the most significant predictors of outcome. Patients with preserved consciousness should be included in decision-making regarding their care and long-term goals.

KEYWORDS

Stroke; basilar artery; transient ischaemic attacks (TIAs); head impulse; nystagmus and test for skew deviation (HINTS); management.

CASE STUDY 1

A 38-year-old man presents to the emergency department with aggressive behaviour and altered mental status. On initial evaluation his vital signs and laboratory results appear stable. He is acting erratically and violent towards the medical staff. His toxicology screen is positive for marijuana, which he is reported to consume at times, and benzodiazepines, which he takes for anxiety. His medical history is otherwise unremarkable. His friends report that he saw his chiropractor earlier this morning. They met him for lunch and noticed that his behaviour was 'off' and that his speech was slightly slurred. Neurological examination was notable for dysconjugate gaze, but otherwise limited by lack of cooperation and agitation. A non-contrast head computed tomography (CT) scan was unremarkable.

He was admitted to the medicine hospitalist service for observation, assuming a possible toxidrome, with plan for a follow-up brain magnetic resonance imaging (MRI) and electroencephalogram (EEG) if his symptoms do not improve. He is subsequently given several doses of IV haloperidol given his combative behaviour. Overnight, his nurse notices a mild facial asymmetry but is unsure whether this is a new finding. On morning rounds, he appears very sleepy which is attributed to the antipsychotics he received. Later during the day, his mental status further deteriorates and he is noted to be weak in both arms and the left leg. He is intubated for airway protection, a computed tomography angiography (CTA) of the head and neck reveals an occlusive thrombus in his distal BA as well as a left vertebral artery (VA) dissection. Intervention is deferred since the time last seen well is more than 36 hours ago. An MRI scan demonstrates restricted diffusion affecting his thalami and large parts of his midbrain and pons (Figures 77.1 and 77.2).

CASE STUDY 2

A 55-year-old lady with a past medical history notable for hypertension and atrial fibrillation is noted to have a mild facial droop and 'garbled' speech while opening presents at her birthday party. As friends attempt to help her lay down, she suddenly collapses and loses consciousness. Emergency medical services is called for on an urgent basis. On initial evaluation, she is not responding to commands, her pupils are found to be dilated and not reactive. She has a right upper motor neuron facial palsy, withdraws her left leg to painful stimuli but otherwise does not move or localize. She is intubated for a Glasgow Coma Scale (GCS) score of 4 and is taken to a nearby hospital, which is a stroke centre. On arrival, she is evaluated by the acute stroke team in the emergency room. An emergent CT/CTA of her head and neck reveals a fully occlusive thrombus at the 'top of the basilar artery' (Figure 77.3). Her laboratory parameters are notable for an international normalized ratio (INR) of 1.8 (she is taking warfarin) and treatment with intravenous thrombolytics is deferred. The endovascular team decides to perform an emergent thrombectomy. Successful recanalization is achieved within 4 hours from symptom onset (Figures 77.4 and 77.5). She is admitted to the intensive care unit (ICU) for close observation and noted to be moving her lower extremities after the procedure. Overnight she starts following commands. An MRI of the brain shows multiple small embolic cerebellar strokes, but no evidence of residual stroke affecting the brainstem. She is extubated the next day, complaining of dizziness and severe nausea, but otherwise appears neurologically intact. She is discharged from the hospital after a few days. She is also started on a novel anticoagulant instead of warfarin. Five years later, she again celebrates her birthday with her friends. She is also excited to welcome her first grandchild and continues to run half marathons for charitable purposes.

CASE STUDY 3

The patient referenced in Case Study 1 is admitted to the ICU. On examination, he appears alert when sedation is held, has limited eye movements (at times able to sustain upgaze briefly) and can open his eyes to command. He is quadriplegic and his physicians recommend tracheostomy and feeding tube placement. They predict that he will be bedbound and nursing home dependent for the rest of his life. His brothers voice strongly that he had previously said he would never want to live in such a disabled state. His wife and mother agree, but wonder whether he feels different now as he appears emotional and tearful when he sees them. He also has two small children, 1 and 3 years old, and his family thinks he might 'want to be around to see them grow up'.

He is unfortunately not able to consistently communicate his wishes by blinking or with eye movements. His physicians recommend proceeding with tracheotomy and feeding tube placement to give him more time to refine his communication skills. After weeks of working with speech therapists in a rehabilitation unit, he can answer simple questions reliably and indicates that he would like to stay alive, despite significant impairments and care needs. He agrees with permanent placement in a nursing facility.

INTRODUCTION

Accounting for only ~27% of posterior circulation strokes and ~1%–4% of all ischaemic strokes,[1,2] basilar artery occlusion (BAO) is a relatively rare condition, but the potentially devastating outcome requires prompt recognition and management. As the presenting symptoms can be highly variable and non-specific (yet commonly presented), the diagnosis can pose a significant challenge for clinicians.

AETIOLOGY

The most common mechanism of BAO is thought to be due to intrinsic atherosclerotic stenosis resulting in local thrombosis.[2,3] Other frequent causes include embolic occlusions from a cardiac source (up to 35%) and large artery atherosclerosis (up to 36%) affecting the vertebral arteries (VAs).[4,5] Particularly in younger patients, propagation or embolization of a thrombus from a dissected VA can be seen frequently, at times in combination with a recent history of neck trauma, lifting of heavy objects, and other activities causing rapid neck movements or pressure on the neck. A large number of basilar infarcts (up to 35%) remain cryptogenic despite a comprehensive stroke workup.[5]

Rare causes of BAO include arteritis (infectious, giant-cell and other autoimmune forms) and vasculitis, cervical spine or skull base fractures, upper cervical instability in the context of rheumatoid arthritis, meningitis, aneurysms, migraines, neurosyphilis, and iatrogenic complications after an endovascular or neurosurgical procedure.[6–12]

VASCULAR ANATOMY

The VAs originate from the subclavian arteries and join at the ponto-medullary junction to form the basilar artery (BA). The BA ascends the brainstem in the basilar sulcus ventral to the pons and divides into the posterior cerebellar arteries (PCAs) at the ponto-mesencephalic junction. Branches include the anterior inferior cerebellar artery (AICA), pontine paramedian perforating arteries (arising either directly from the dorsal surface or from short circumferential arteries running around and into the pons), superior cerebellar artery (SCA), and in ~15% of cases the labyrinthine artery. The posterior inferior cerebellar artery (PICA) is a direct branch of the VA.

The BA can be divided into a proximal (origin to AICA), middle (AICA to SCA) and distal (SCA to tip) segments, supplying the pons (proximal and middle segment) as well as the midbrain and thalamus (distal segment). The medulla usually receives its supply from branches of the distal VA.

Clinical Presentation

The degree of impairment in patients with BAO varies significantly from mild transient symptoms to the highly disabling 'locked-in syndrome'. The constellation of signs depends on the anatomical structures affected based

Table 77.1 Anatomical structures within the brainstem and their clinical correlates

	Anatomical structures
Reduced consciousness or coma	Ascending reticular activating system
Hemiparesis or quadriparesis, hemiplegia or quadriplegia, extensor plantar sign	Corticospinal tracts in pons or cerebral peduncles
Unilateral or bilateral hypaesthesia or anaesthesia	Medial lemnisci and spinothalamic tracts, thalamic nuclei
Ataxia, loss of coordination of limbs and posture, loss of balance	Cerebellum, cerebellar peduncles, proprioceptive tracts
Vertigo, loss of balance, directional nystagmus	Vestibular nuclei, labyrinth, vestibulocerebellum
Headache, neck pain	Trigeminal fibres of vessels and meninges
Horner's syndrome	Sympathetic fibres in dorsal longitudinal fascicle
Disturbance of respiration, heart rate, and blood pressure	Medullary autonomic nuclei and efferent and afferent fibres
Incontinence	Parasympathetic hypothalamic nuclei, sympathetic and parasympathetic connecting fibres from frontal micturition centre to spinal cord
Oculomotor nerve palsy	Fascicle of oculomotor nerve
Nuclear oculomotor nerve palsy, vertical gaze paresis, bilateral ptosis, anisocoria, non-reactive pupils, vertical oculocephalic reflex loss	Oculomotor nerve nucleus, rostral interstitial nucleus of the medial longitudinal fascicle, dorsal commissure
Internuclear ophthalmoplegia	Medial longitudinal fascicle
Horizontal gaze paresis, horizontal oculocephalic reflex loss	Abducens nerve nucleus, paramedian pontine reticular formation
Gaze-evoked nystagmus	Cerebellum and its connections to brainstem
Double vision, strabismus, skew deviation	Brainstem oculomotor system, eye nerves
Facial palsy	Corticobulbar tract, facial nerve nuclei
Tinnitus, hearing loss	Inner ear, cochlear nuclei, lateral lemnisci
Dysarthria, dysphagia, anarthria, aphagia	Corticobulbar tracts, cerebellum, caudal cranial nerve nuclei
Hemianopia, blindness	Occipital lobes
Disorientation, confusion, memory disturbance	Thalamic nuclei, medial temporal lobes
Extension rigidity, jerking, shaking episodes, convulsive-like seizures	Pyramidal tracts

Reprinted with permission from: Mattle HP, Arnold M, Lindsberg PJ, Schonewille WJ, Schroth G. Basilar artery occlusion. *Lancet Neurol* 2011;10: 1002–14.

on the location of the thrombus, degree of occlusion, and the collateral circulation. Table 77.1 provides a comprehensive overview of various symptoms and their neuroanatomical correlates.

The onset of symptoms in BAO can be abrupt or stuttering, with gradual progression, depending on the extent of occlusion and vascular supply to the brain. When compared to patients with anterior circulation strokes, patients with BAO frequently experience prodromal symptoms. These prodromes can occur as early as several weeks prior to presentation and typically present as vertigo and nausea followed by headaches and neck pain.[2,13,14] They are more frequently encountered in patients with atherosclerotic and then embolic occlusions. A 'herald hemiparesis' is a unilateral transient weakness and can occur in the period prior to stroke. The Basilar Artery International Cooperation Study (BASICS) registry reported prodromal transient ischemic attacks in 19% of patients; another 19% of patients experienced minor strokes in the recent past.[4] In the New England Medical Center Posterior Circulation Registry (NEMC-PCR) 59% of patients with a basilar transient ischaemic attacks (TIA) experienced a subsequent stroke.[2] The ABCD2 score may help stratify patients at high risk. Points are assigned based on age >60; blood pressure (BP) >140/90 mmHg; the presence of weakness, speech disturbance or any other neurological symptom; duration of symptoms; and diabetes. A score of less than 3 has a 1% risk of stroke as opposed to 27% in those scoring over 6.[15]

In general, the presentation of BAO can be very non-specific with symptoms of headaches, vertigo, nausea or vomiting, blurry vision, alterations of consciousness, and, at times, abnormal or bizarre behaviour. However, these symptoms are mostly accompanied by focal neurological signs, even if they appear subtle. In the NEMC-PCR, less than <1% of patients with vertebrobasilar ischaemia had only one presenting symptom or sign.[2] The neurological examination in such patients should therefore include a careful evaluation of the cranial nerves (assess for diplopia, gaze palsies, visual deficits, a skew deviation, pathological nystagmus, facial weakness in an upper motor neuron pattern, dysarthria and dysphagia, or an asymmetric palate) and also screen for concomitant cerebellar dysfunction as well as focal sensory or motor deficits. Some patients present with episodes of twitching, shaking, or posturing that can closely mimic epileptic events.[16]

The clinical decision tool HINTS (Head Impulse, Nystagmus and Test for Skew deviation) is efficient in distinguishing between central and peripheral vertigo and has proven to be more sensitive than MRI in the diagnosis of strokes presenting with 'dizziness'.[17]

TREATMENT
Acute Management

The first crucial steps to prompt management of BAO are quick recognition of the clinical picture and then confirmation of the diagnosis with neuroimaging. In addition to making a rapid diagnosis, it is also essential to establish the time window from last seen well (LSW) or the exact symptom onset early on in order to determine whether the patient is potentially eligible for treatments such as intravenous thrombolysis (IV tPA) and/or endovascular therapy. Contraindications for IV tPA need to be elicited while learning about the patient. If available, the Acute Stroke and Endovascular team on call should be alerted immediately when there is a strong suspicion for BAO.

When initially evaluating the patient, airway, breathing, and circulation should be assessed and stabilized as needed. Particularly in patients with decreased mental status or lower cranial nerve dysfunction, early endotracheal intubation may be necessary. Securing the airway can also be helpful in safely and rapidly obtaining further imaging. In order to maintain cerebral perfusion, BP should be closely monitored avoiding significant reductions (i.e., more than 10% from baseline) on induction or administration of sedation.

In an attempt to enhance cerebral perfusion through collaterals or past a partially occlusive stenosis, the head of bed should be as flat as safely tolerated by the patient. The patient's systolic BP (SBP) target should be at least above 120 mmHg and ideally above 140 mmHg. Fluids or vasopressors can be used to achieve this goal, as appropriate. Generally, fluid deficits should be corrected prior to initiating pressors, but severe hypotension may require early pressor initiation to promote adequacy of cerebral perfusion with subsequent dynamic adjustment as fluids are loaded.

The imaging study to order in the acute setting is usually a CT scan of head and neck with CTA. It is often more rapidly available than an MRI. In patients with renal failure, a magnetic resonance angiography (MRA) can be pursued if immediately available, but ultimately the risk of potentially devastating brain injury and index of suspicion for BAO needs to be weighed against the risk of worsening kidney function. Fluid loading can prelude and accompany contrast studies to reduce chances of contrast nephropathy.[18]

The non-contrast head CT scan, if obtained early on, is frequently unremarkable. Infarcts on CT typically evolve gradually within 6 hours of symptom onset. Ischaemic strokes in the brainstem are also usually difficult to see on CT, especially when small. Additional infarcts from an embolic source might be visualized elsewhere in the brain, and if seen, this finding needs to be taken into account when further therapeutic decisions are made. A hyperdense BA can be visualized in some cases, although at times this finding can be due to artifact or calcifications in the setting of chronic atherosclerosis.[19] Ultimately, a proper vessel imaging study needs to be performed. A CTA confirms the presence of thrombus and one can visualize the extent (fully versus partially occlusive) and exact location of the clot within the BA. Once the diagnosis is confirmed with a CTA, the clinician can make a therapeutic decision based on characteristics of the clot, the collateral vasculature, the severity of neurological deficit on presentation and the timeframe in which the patient presents.

An MRI of the brain can be very helpful in determining the extent of stroke. Interventionalists may occasionally request an MRI prior to proceeding with endovascular clot removal in order to assess the full extent of injury that has already occurred on diffusion-weighted imaging (DWI)/apparent diffusion coefficient (ADC). This approach might help to select patients possibly benefiting from the procedure, especially if the exam on presentation already suggests a stroke affecting large parts of the vascular territory. However, MRI may delay treatment significantly, and false negatives for DWI can occur,[20] with a greater prevalence in the posterior circulation.[21] Cases of DWI reversibility in the brainstem have also been reported.[22] In general, an MRI is obtained after the stages of acute management for prognostic purposes and to evaluate for additional strokes. When dissection is suspected, MRA with a T1 fat saturated sequence can be useful in assessing the vasculature. Transcranial Doppler (TCD) can be helpful in demonstrating absent or reversed flow in the posterior circulation, although the sensitivity is low and BAO cannot be ruled out with this technique. However, TCD might be helpful as a quick bedside screening and for follow-up examinations.

Antiplatelets and Anticoagulation

There are no studies specifically assessing the effect of antiplatelets or anticoagulation versus placebo. They are routinely used, given some evidence of absolute benefit[23–26] and their role in secondary prevention for stroke patients. In a case series assessing patients with BAO treated with antiplatelets or anticoagulation, good outcomes (defined as modified Rankin score [mRS] 0–3) were reported in 20%–59% of patients,[2,27] however, the BASICS registry reported a case fatality of 54% for patients on antiplatelets at 1 month.[4]

There are also no trials comparing antiplatelets and anticoagulation directly for BAO. Studies in other stroke populations, excluding infarcts with a clear cardioembolic aetiology suggest that antiplatelets are not inferior to anticoagulation and carry a lower bleeding risk.[28] The choice of therapy therefore depends on the clinical context—in particular the underlying stroke aetiology, stroke size, a potential source of embolism, the presence of low ejection fraction, atrial fibrillation, a mechanical valve, the extent and location of a dissection (intradural vs extradural), other comorbidities, and bleeding risk. In some instances, if a partially occlusive thrombus is seen on vessel imaging or if continuing embolization is noted with TCDs, clinicians can empirically choose to use anticoagulants with an aim of diminishing the risk of further ischaemic strokes to the brainstem.

Usually, antiplatelets or anticoagulation are considered in the acute phase when a patient is not thought to be a candidate for IV thrombolytics, or alternatively can be initiated as early as 24 hours after IV tPA administration depending on the overall infarct burden, risk for haemorrhagic conversion, and other risk factors.

Intravenous tPA

In the absence of any significant contraindications, IV tPA is considered the standard of care for patients with BAO presenting with acute ischaemic stroke within 4.5 hours from LSW or witnessed symptom onset. The landmark trials demonstrating improved outcomes after 3 months in acute ischaemic stroke[29,30] included patients with posterior circulation strokes, however, there is no detailed information about results of initial vessel imaging nor about effects on recanalization. Within the registries and case series assessing patients with BAO, moderate to good outcomes (mRS 0–3) were reported in up to 63% of cases[4,31,32] with mortalities as high as 50% and haemorrhage rates up to 16%. Within the BASICS registry, patients with mild-moderate deficits have similar outcomes when treated with aspirin versus IV tPA.[4] Patients with severe deficits had much better outcomes after receiving IV tPA. However, the level of efficacy of IV tPA has been noted to vary depending on the site of occlusion and extent of thrombus. A study based on TCD monitoring suggests recanalization rates of only 30% in patients with BAO treated with IV tPA.[33]

Intra-Arterial Thrombolysis (IAT)

The first evidence hinting at a benefit of IAT in vertebrobasilar insufficiency (VBI) and BAO was published in the 1980s.[34,35] These studies suggested improved quality of life and survival. They were also amongst the first reports to demonstrate a significant correlation between recanalization and better outcomes. There is only one small (n = 16) randomized controlled trial (RCT) (the Australian Urokinase Trial) assessing the benefits of urokinase plus full-dose heparin versus just the full-dose heparin.[36] The trial was terminated early as a consequence of slow recruitment and withdrawal of the sale of urokinase in Australia (due to manufacturing quality concerns, it was also withdrawn in other countries and replaced by different fibrinolytic agents). No significant difference was noted in outcome; 4 patients died in each arm and mRS was noted to be better (1 in the urokinase plus heparin group versus 3 in the heparin only group amongst survivors). The number of patients in the trial is certainly too small to draw meaningful conclusions for the general use of IAT. Subsequent case series vary significantly in terms of patient selection and the method of documented outcome. Mortality rates range between 6%–50% with moderate to good outcomes (mRS 0–3) ranging between 17%–50%. Overall, the majority of studies have supported the notion that patients with partial or complete recanalization have significantly better outcomes. A meta-analysis of 10 studies, including 316 patients reported an overall recanalization rate of 65%, mortality of 56% (87% in non-recanalized vs 47% in canalized patients).[37] The largest series to date, a German trial including 180 patients across five centres demonstrated an mRS of 5–6 (severe disability or death) in 86% of patients with no recenalization compared to 43% of patients with partial and 33% of patients with full recanalization.[38]

Two major studies have attempted to compare IV tPA and IAT.[4,32] The rates of death and dependency and survival rates were overall very similar despite significantly higher recanalization rates (65% vs 53%) in the IAT group. Patients with mild or moderate deficits overall had a worse outcome after IAT compared with IV tPA. Outcomes for patients with severe deficits were similar, although a third of patients in the IV tPA group ultimately received both treatments.

Endovascular Mechanical Thrombectomy (EMT)

Recent significant advances in the field of endovascular therapy include the introduction of improved technology for clot retrieval (stent retrievers such as the SOLITAIRE device, Figure 77.6), enabling faster and more effective achievement of recanalization. A series of recent major trials have demonstrated significant improvement of neurologic outcomes in patients with acute ischaemic

stroke and large vessel occlusions, in addition to the benefit provided by IV tPA.[39–43] This marks a paradigm shift towards endovascular therapy as the standard of care for patients with acute ischaemic stroke presenting within 6 hours (in combination with IV tPA). The REVASCAT42 and ESCAPE41 trial even included patients beyond this time window—up to 8 and 12 hours from LSW. Recent studies in BAO, albeit not always using the latest technology have demonstrated extremely high recanalization rates of 78%–100% for EMT.[44–47] The use of a stent retriever for patients with BAO has been associated with better angiographic and clinical outcomes in recent studies.[48,49]

Large crossover rates within trials make it difficult to compare the effects between IV tPA, IAT, and EMT directly—most patients in these studies receive a combination of these therapies. A small retrospective study, comparing outcomes of IAT versus EMT found significantly shorter groin puncture to recanalization times (48.5 vs 92 minutes), higher rates of recanalization (88% vs 42%) and higher rates of good clinical outcome (39% vs 17%, although not statistically significant) in the EMT group.[50]

Many experts hypothesize that the overall better outcomes of BAO reported over the past decades can at least partially be attributed to advances in the field of mechanical recanalization. The exact window of opportunity for EMT in patients with BAO remains controversial and clinical practice varies between experts in the field. The more conservative approach is to remain within 6–8 hours from the LSW point, but many providers consider treating patients as late as 24–48 hours from symptom onset, especially if there is concern for a 'top of the basilar' syndrome given the potentially devastating prognosis. There are reports of patients who had EMT up to 48 hours from LSW with a good prognosis in the absence of extensive baseline ischaemia on imaging.[51] However, literature is probably biased towards reporting positive outcomes. When selecting patients who may benefit from EMT, each case needs to be evaluated individually. Factors that should be weighed include age, NIHSS score, time from LSW, comorbidities and pre-stroke baseline, presence of infarct on CT or MRI, potential risks of the procedure, stenoses or occlusions in the neck vasculature, as well as presence and degree of collaterals. The ENDOSTROKE study reported that young age, lower initial NIHSS score, the absence of hypertension, better collateralization status, treatment with a stent retriever, and the use of MRI prior to EMT were predictors of better outcome. Surprisingly, no significant relationship between onset to treatment time (OTT) and clinical outcome was found; however,

OTT was not always reliably recorded. Patients who received IV tPA and/or IAT in combination with EMT did not have better outcomes, but those patients who improved after treatment with IV tPA were subsequently excluded from the study and not considered as candidates for EMT.[48] While the use of MRI has been associated with better outcomes, most likely by helping to exclude patients who 'already completed their infarct', reversibility of DWI changes in the brainstem after EMT have been reported.[22] Given its limited availability in some institutions and potential to significantly delay treatment, MRI should not be routinely acquired but rather be used as an additional tool in uncertain cases if readily available.

Combination Therapies

There has been some controversy over the past decades regarding the 'best' treatment approach in the acute setting. As stated above, trials are limited by crossover and an RCT comparing IV tPA, IAT, and EMT is realistically not feasible due to ethical concerns of withholding therapies that have proven benefit. Table 77.2, given at the end of the chapter, provides an overview of major studies outlining outcomes for various treatment strategies.

An IV tPA can certainly be administered more quickly compared to IAT or EMT and it is more widely available. The procedural risks of IAT and EMT also need to be considered. However, higher rates of recanalization and lower rates of symptomatic haemorrhage suggest advantages of endovascular therapies. In an attempt to maximize clinical benefit to the patient, many institutions have adopted a 'bridging' approach combining both intravenous and endovascular treatments. The IV tPA or glycoprotein IIb/IIIa inhibitors are being administered before proceeding to IAT and/or EMT. There are a few smaller, non-randomized studies suggesting that IV abciximab in combination with IAT has resulted in improved clinical outcomes compared to IAT alone.[52,53] Some centres have also used tirofiban (which is thought to be safer due to a shorter half-life), but reports are limited to very few patients.[54] A 'drip, ship, and retrieve' approach with patients initially receiving IV tPA in a community hospital followed by IAT in a specialized stroke centre has shown significant benefits when compared to IAT alone or IAT plus tirofiban.[47] This strategy (IV tPA → EMT +/− IAT) has become increasingly common for patients with acute ischaemic stroke after positive trials supporting EMT and will probably become the standard approach for patients with BAO. We suggest the algorithm given in Figure 77.7, based on current data and widely practiced principles, recognizing that clinical practice can vary based on provider opinions and experience, specific considerations for the individual patient, as well as availability of treatments and resources within each institution.

Monitoring and Workup

Patients presenting with basilar TIAs or strokes should be admitted to the hospital for close monitoring and workup. Given the high number of patients with basilar TIAs progressing to subsequent strokes (up to 59%),[2] a careful workup and secondary prevention are warranted. Patients with BA infarcts and persistent stenosis or occlusion of the BA should be admitted to an intensive care setting for vigilant monitoring of BP and neurological examination.

Although some patients may initially present with very mild symptoms, sudden deterioration can occur after admission, and may warrant consideration of EMT. In patients with strokes affecting the thalamus (in some patients partially supplied by branches from the distal BA) or the reticular activating system in the brainstem, dramatic mental status fluctuations are frequently encountered and airway protection may be a concern.

In some cases, most commonly when BAO is due to embolic thrombi from the VA, concomitant cerebellar strokes can be seen. The presence of a large cerebellar stroke warrants close monitoring given the risks for swelling, herniation, and hydrocephalus due to obstruction of the fourth ventricle. Ventriculostomy placement and decompressive suboccipital craniectomy may become necessary in some cases, particularly in patients with infarcts affecting the PICA territory. Therapeutic anticoagulation, even if indicated, may be temporarily unsafe. The risk of further embolic events and necessity of anticoagulation have to be weighed against the risk of haemorrhagic conversion.

Patients who received IV tPA have to be observed closely in an ICU or stroke unit for up to 24 hours given the concern for haemorrhagic complications. After EMT, specific BP goals may be indicated depending on the degree of recanalization after the procedure, presence of coexisting vascular stenoses, and concern for hyperperfusion in revascularized patients. The puncture site and peripheral pulses distal to the puncture site have to be monitored carefully.

A comprehensive stroke workup is indicated with a goal of identifying the underlying aetiology and preventing future infarcts. In addition to imaging of the neck and cranial vasculature (typically acquired in the acute phase), evaluation for cardiac and other embolic sources is warranted. Cerebrovascular risk factors such as hypertension, hyperlipidaemia, and hyperglycaemia should be optimized. Further investigations for less common causes of ischaemic stroke have to be considered in the absence of an established stroke mechanism based on the patient's age, comorbidities, other systemic findings, and history of prior thromboembolic events.

When considered safe, the process of rehabilitation should be initiated. Some patients may benefit from tracheotomy placement. The need for airway protection over longer periods (weeks to years) is usually due to lesions within the reticular activating system or thalamus causing decreased or fluctuating mental status. The caudal cranial nerves are mostly spared, as the medulla typically receives its blood supply from the VAs; and many patients even with large midbrain and pontine infarct have intact respiratory mechanics. Patients with impaired respiratory function due to lower cranial nerve deficits are thought to have a worse outcome.

Infarcts affecting the corticobulbar tracts, cerebellum, and caudal cranial nuclei tend to cause dysarthria and dysphagia, and warrant careful assessment of swallowing function. Placement of a nasogastric tube is frequently necessary, at least in the short-term, to ensure adequate caloric input while further assessments are underway. Continuing evaluation by a speech therapist with expertise in stroke is recommended to help identify the risk of aspiration, providing input about the consistency of food that a patient can tolerate, adequate positioning, frequency of meals, and the predicted need for a percutaneous endoscopic gastrostomy (PEG) tube.

PROGNOSIS

When first described, the outcomes of BAO were thought to be extremely poor with mortality rates as high as 85%–100%.[55–58] Most of these data were obtained by post-mortem analysis, and are therefore biased towards fatal cases. Mortality rates in more recent studies obtained in the era of antithrombotic treatment, thrombolytics, recanalization, and advancement of non-invasive vascular imaging techniques range between 29%–45% with 32% of patients having a good clinical outcome (mRS 3 or less) at 30 days.[2,4] Successful recanalization appears to be the single most important predictor of a good outcome.[31,32,59] Stroke severity (determined by initial NIHSS), age, location, and length of the occlusion, posterior-circulation ASPECT score, the state of collaterals, and presence of symptomatic intraparenchymal

haemorrhage are also significant factors that are thought to influence outcomes.[31,38,51,60–63] Decreased level of consciousness has been reported to be one of the most powerful clinical predictors of poor outcome followed by pupillary dysfunction, tetraparesis, bulbar signs, and dysarthria.[2,64] Early treatment is thought to result in better outcomes, but some studies suggest that late presentation does not preclude treatment and does not universally result in a poor outcome if patients are selected appropriately.[51]

There are few studies focusing on long-term outcomes, with good outcomes (defined as mRS 0–2) reported in about 30% of patients after a median follow-up timeframe of 2.8 years.[5,65] Reports of significant improvement in locked-in patients are rare.[66] Essential components of care for these patients include extensive nursing care and rehabilitation as well as effort to decrease the risk of nosocomial infections and appropriate thromboembolic prophylaxis. Patients with persistent severe disabilities from BAO, including locked-in syndrome, often report being content with their decision to live years later. For the most part, they would not consider the option of euthanasia and perceive their quality of life to be similar to that of age-matched controls.[67,68] These findings stress the importance of allowing patients themselves to participate in decisions regarding their care. Even though families frequently voice that the patient would not have wanted to live with such impairments, it is crucial to remember that locked-in patients usually have preserved cortical function, and should be able to voice their own preference in this situation. Frequently, it does take time, in some cases weeks to months, for patients to learn how to consistently communicate with eye movements and blinks.

There is often a striking contrast between abstract consideration of a possibility versus a real immediacy of disability or death, and patients should be allowed to reconsider prior positions, wherever possible. The substituted judgement standard (i.e., asking family or surrogates to represent the patient's wishes) is a fallback position for circumstances of indefinitely compromised communication and should never be exercised for expediency or convenience.

CONCLUSIONS

Basilar artery occlusion is a rare entity, but with potentially devastating outcomes. It requires prompt recognition and management. As the presenting symptoms can be variable and non-specific, the diagnosis can pose a significant challenge for clinicians.

Table 77.2 Summary of clinical trials

	Patients (n)	Time to treatment (h)†	Good outcome (mRS 0–2 or independence) [%]	Moderate-to-good outcome (mRS 0–3) [%]	Mortality (%)	Symptomatic haemorrhages (%)	Recanalisation rate (%)	Remarks
Antithrombotics								
Schoneville et al.[27]	82	...	...	20	40	...	N/A	Patients from 3 centres
BASICS[4]	104 (mild-to-moderate deficit)	...	37	58	13	0	...	Multicentre registry; outcome assessed at 1 month
BASICS[4]	79 (severe deficit)	...	3	8	54	1	...	Multicentre registry; outcome assessed at 1 month
Intravenous thrombolysis								
Lindsberg and Mattle[32]	76	N/A	22	...	50	11	53‡	Systematic analysis of publications up to 2005
BASICS[4]	49 (mild-to-moderate deficit)	N/A	53	63	16	6	71‡	Multicentre registry; 40 of 121 intravenous thrombolysis patients received rescue intra-arterial thrombolysis; outcome assessed at 1 month
BASICS[4]	72 (severe deficit)	N/A	21	26	46	6	66‡	Multicentre registry; 40 of 121 intravenous thrombolysis patients received rescue intra-arterial thrombolysis; outcome assessed at 1 month
Sairanen et al.[31]	116	8·7	26	36	41	16	65	Large single-centre consecutive intravenous thrombolysis series
Intra-arterial thrombolysis								
Lindsberg and Mattle[32]	344	N/A	24	...	55	8	65	Systematic analysis of publications up to 2005
BASICS[4]	92 (mild-to-moderate deficit)	N/A	30	43	23	14§	83‡	Multicentre registry; outcome assessed at 1 month
BASICS[4]	196 (severe deficit)	N/A	11	17	49	14§	69‡	Multicentre registry; outcome assessed at 1 month

Study	N							Technique
Renard et al.[69]	16	9·2 (3–22)	31	...	50	0	69	Intra-arterial thrombolysis without endovascular mechanical recanalisation
Kashiwagi et al.[70]	18	4·5 (1·3–24·5)	39	...	6	6	94	Intra-arterial thrombolysis with on-demand percutaneous transluminal angioplasty
Yu et al.[71]	52	3–48	42	...	38	12	77	Intra-arterial thrombolysis with on-demand stenting
Chandra et al.[72]	40	7·2	35	50	33	13	83	Intra-arterial thrombolysis with on-demand percutaneous transluminal angioplasty and Merci Retriever (Concentric Medical, Hertogenbosch, Netherlands) endovascular mechanical recanalisation
Jung et al.[5]	106	5·5 (1·3–24·5)	33	44	41	1	70	Intra-arterial thrombolysis with on-demand endovascular mechanical recanalisation
Endovascular mechanical recanalisation								
Lutsep et al.[45]	27	5·4 (1·2–17·3)	33	41	44	19	78	56% received undescribed adjunctive treatments
Pfefferkorn et al.[47]	26	6·0 (1·5)	38	50	31	8	85	Full-dose intravenous alteplase as bridging agent; Penumbra (Penumbra, Alameda, CA, USA), Angiojet (MedRad, Warrendale, PA, USA), or Merci (Concentric Medical) used in 16/26 patients
Miteff et al.[46]	10	4 (0–48)	20	20	30	10	100	Intra-arterial thrombolysis with on-demand microwire disruption or Merci (Concentric Medical) endovascular mechanical recanalisation

(Cont'd)

Table 77.2 (*Cont'd*)

	Patients (n)	Time to treatment (h)†	Good outcome (mRS 0–2 or independence) [%]	Moderate-to-good outcome (mRS 0–3) [%]	Mortality (%)	Symptomatic haemorrhages (%)	Recanalisation rate (%)	Remarks
Costalat et al.[44]	16	<24	44	...	25	2	81	10/16 patients treated with full-dose intravenous alteplase before endovascular treatment; Solitaire (Microtherapeutics, Irvine, CA, USA) stent used in all
Abciximab as bridging agent to intra-arterial thrombolysis								
Eckert et al.[52]§	47	6·0 (3·4–14·2)	...	34	38	13	72	Percutaneous transluminal angioplasty or stenting also used in 15 patients
Nagel et al.[53]	43	5 (2–12)	19	35	58	14	84	...
Barlinn et al.[73]	20	7 (3·5–13)	15	15	45	15	85	...

Studies with a large portion of occlusions at the level of vertebral artery were not included because outcome data were not reported separately for basilar artery.

*Number of participants greater than ten.

†Data for time to treatment are either median (range) or mean.

‡Recanalisation was assessed at end of angiography with intra-arterial thrombolysis, but at a later timepoint with intravenous thrombolysis.

§Number for patients with mild-to-moderate and severe deficits.

¶Good outcome defined as mRS 0–3.

mRS=modified Rankin scale.

N/A=not applicable.

Reprinted with permission from: Mattle HP, Arnold M, Lindsberg PJ, Schonewille WJ, Schroth G. Basilar artery occlusion. *Lancet Neurol* 2011;10:1002–14.

REFERENCES

1. Israeli-korn SD, Schwammenthal Y, Yonash-Kimchi T, et al. Ischemic stroke due to acute basilar artery occlusion: proportion and outcomes. *Isr Med Assoc J* 2010;12(11): 671–5.

2. Voetsch B, DeWitt LD, Pessin MS, Caplan LR. Basilar artery occlusive disease in the New England Medical Center Posterior Circulation Registry. *Arch Neurol* 2004;61(4):496–504.

3. Castaigne P, Lhermitte F, Gautier JC, et al. Arterial occlusions in the vertebro-basilar system. A study of 44 patients with post-mortem data. *Brain* 1973;96(1):133–54.

4. Schonewille WJ, Wijman CA, Michel P, et al. Treatment and outcomes of acute basilar artery occlusion in the Basilar Artery International Cooperation Study (BASICS): a prospective registry study. *Lancet Neurol* 2009;8(8): 724–30.

5. Jung S, Mono ML, Fischer U, et al. Three-month and long-term outcomes and their predictors in acute basilar artery occlusion treated with intra-arterial thrombolysis. *Stroke* 2011;42(7):1946–51.

6. Oshima K, Sakaura H, Iwasaki M, Nakura A, Fujii R, Yoshikawa H. Repeated vertebrobasilar thromboembolism in a patient with severe upper cervical instability because of rheumatoid arthritis. *Spine J* 2011;11(2):e1–5.

7. Sugrue PA, Hage ZA, Surdell DL, Foroohar M, Liu J, Bendok BR. Basilar artery occlusion following C1 lateral mass fracture managed by mechanical and pharmacological thrombolysis. *Neurocrit Care* 2009; 11(2):255–60.

8. Meyding-Lamade U, Rieke K, Krieger D, et al. Rare diseases mimicking acute vertebrobasilar artery thrombosis. *J Neurol* 1995;242(5):335–43.

9. Ruecker M, Furtner M, Knoflach M, et al. Basilar artery dissection: series of 12 consecutive cases and review of the literature. *Cerebrovasc Dis* 2010;30(3):267–76.

10. Feng W, Caplan M, Matheus MG, Papamitsakis NI. Meningovascular syphilis with fatal vertebrobasilar occlusion. *Am J Med Sci* 2009;338(2):169–71.

11. Bauerle J, Zitzmann A, Egger K, Meckel S, Weiller C, Harloff A. The great imitator–still today! A case of meningovascular syphilis affecting the posterior circulation. *J Stroke Cerebrovasc Dis* 2015;24(1):e1–3.

12. Akman-Demir G, Serdaroglu P, Tasci B. Clinical patterns of neurological involvement in Behcet's disease: evaluation of 200 patients. The Neuro-Behcet Study Group. *Brain* 1999;122 (Pt 11):2171–82.

13. Ferbert A, Bruckmann H, Drummen R. Clinical features of proven basilar artery occlusion. *Stroke* 1990;21(8):1135–42.

14. Grad A, Baloh RW. Vertigo of vascular origin. Clinical and electronystagmographic features in 84 cases. *Arch Neurol* 1989;46(3):281–4.

15. Navi BB, Kamel H, Shah MP, et al. Application of the ABCD2 score to identify cerebrovascular causes of dizziness in the emergency department. *Stroke* 2012;43(6): 1484–9.

16. Ropper AH. 'Convulsions' in basilar artery occlusion. *Neurology* 1988;38(9):1500–1.

17. Newman-Toker DE, Kattah JC, Alvernia JE, Wang DZ. Normal head impulse test differentiates acute cerebellar strokes from vestibular neuritis. *Neurology* 2008;70(24 Pt 2):2378–85.

18. Nicola R, Shaqdan KW, Aran K, Mansouri M, Singh A, Abujudeh HH. Contrast-induced nephropathy: identifying the risks, choosing the right agent, and reviewing effective prevention and management methods. *Curr Probl Diagn Radiol* 2015;44(6):501–4.

19. Connell L, Koerte IK, Laubender RP, et al. Hyperdense basilar artery sign-a reliable sign of basilar artery occlusion. *Neuroradiology* 2012;54(4):321–7.

20. Bulut HT, Yildirim A, Ekmekci B, Eskut N, Gunbey HP. False-negative diffusion-weighted imaging in acute stroke and its frequency in anterior and posterior circulation ischemia. *J Comput Assist Tomogr* 2014;38(5):627–33.

21. Simonsen CZ, Madsen MH, Schmitz ML, Mikkelsen IK, Fisher M, Andersen G. Sensitivity of diffusion- and perfusion-weighted imaging for diagnosing acute ischemic stroke is 97.5%. *Stroke* 2015;46(1):98–101.

22. Yoo AJ, Hakimelahi R, Rost NS, et al. Diffusion weighted imaging reversibility in the brainstem following successful recanalization of acute basilar artery occlusion. *J Neurointerv Surg* 2010;2(3):195–7.

23. CAST: randomised placebo-controlled trial of early aspirin use in 20,000 patients with acute ischaemic stroke. CAST (Chinese Acute Stroke Trial) Collaborative Group. *Lancet* 1997;349(9066):1641–9.

24. The International Stroke Trial (IST): a randomised trial of aspirin, subcutaneous heparin, both, or neither among 19435 patients with acute ischaemic stroke. International Stroke Trial Collaborative Group. *Lancet* 1997;349(9065):1569–81.

25. Bousser MG. Aspirin or heparin immediately after a stroke? *Lancet* 1997;349(9065):1564–5.

26. Kay R, Wong KS, Yu YL, et al. Low-molecular-weight heparin for the treatment of acute ischemic stroke. *N Engl J Med* 1995;333(24):1588–93.

27. Schonewille WJ, Algra A, Serena J, Molina CA, Kappelle LJ. Outcome in patients with basilar artery occlusion treated conventionally. *J Neurol Neurosurg Psychiatry* 2005;76(9):1238–41.

28. Adams RJ, Albers G, Alberts MJ, et al. Update to the AHA/ASA recommendations for the prevention of stroke in patients with stroke and transient ischemic attack. *Stroke* 2008;39(5):1647–52.

29. Tissue plasminogen activator for acute ischemic stroke. The National Institute of Neurological Disorders and Stroke rt-PA Stroke Study Group. *N Engl J Med* 1995;333(24):1581–7.

30. Hacke W, Kaste M, Bluhmki E, et al. Thrombolysis with alteplase 3 to 4.5 hours after acute ischemic stroke. *N Engl J Med* 2008;359(13):1317–29.

31. Sairanen T, Strbian D, Soinne L, et al. Intravenous thrombolysis of basilar artery occlusion: predictors of recanalization and outcome. *Stroke* 2011;42(8):2175–9.

32. Lindsberg PJ, Mattle HP. Therapy of basilar artery occlusion: a systematic analysis comparing intra-arterial and intravenous thrombolysis. *Stroke* 2006;37(3): 922–8.

33. Saqqur M, Uchino K, Demchuk AM, et al. Site of arterial occlusion identified by transcranial Doppler predicts the response to intravenous thrombolysis for stroke. *Stroke* 2007;38(3):948–54.

34. Zeumer H, Hacke W, Ringelstein EB. Local intraarterial thrombolysis in vertebrobasilar thromboembolic disease. *AJNR Am J Neuroradiol* 1983;4(3):401–4.

35. Hacke W, Zeumer H, Ferbert A, Bruckmann H, del Zoppo GJ. Intra-arterial thrombolytic therapy improves outcome in patients with acute vertebrobasilar occlusive disease. *Stroke* 1988;19(10):1216–22.

36. Macleod MR, Davis SM, Mitchell PJ, et al. Results of a multicentre, randomised controlled trial of intra-arterial urokinase in the treatment of acute posterior circulation ischaemic stroke. *Cerebrovasc Dis* 2005;20(1):12–17.

37. Smith WS. Intra-arterial thrombolytic therapy for acute basilar occlusion: pro. *Stroke* 2007;38(Suppl 2):701–3.

38. Schulte-Altedorneburg G, Hamann GF, Mull M, et al. Outcome of acute vertebrobasilar occlusions treated with intra-arterial fibrinolysis in 180 patients. *AJNR Am J Neuroradiol* 2006;27(10):2042–7.

39. Berkhemer OA, Fransen PS, Beumer D, et al. A randomized trial of intraarterial treatment for acute ischemic stroke. *N Engl J Med* 2015;372(1):11–20.

40. Goyal M, Demchuk AM, Menon BK, et al. Randomized assessment of rapid endovascular treatment of ischemic stroke. *N Engl J Med* 2015;372(11):1019–30.

41. Saver JL, Goyal M, Bonafe A, et al. Stent-retriever thrombectomy after intravenous tPA vs. tPA alone in stroke. *N Engl J Med* 2015;372(24):2285–95.

42. Jovin TG, Chamorro A, Cobo E, et al. Thrombectomy within 8 hours after symptom onset in ischemic stroke. *N Engl J Med* 2015;372(24):2296–306.

43. Campbell BC, Mitchell PJ, Kleinig TJ, et al. Endovascular therapy for ischemic stroke with perfusion-imaging selection. *N Engl J Med* 2015;372(11):1009–18.

44. Costalat V, Machi P, Lobotesis K, et al. Rescue, combined, and stand-alone thrombectomy in the management of large vessel occlusion stroke using the solitaire device: a prospective 50-patient single-center study: timing, safety, and efficacy. *Stroke* 2011;42(7):1929–35.

45. Lutsep HL, Rymer MM, Nesbit GM. Vertebrobasilar revascularization rates and outcomes in the MERCI and multi-MERCI trials. *J Stroke Cerebrovasc Dis* 2008;17(2):55–7.

46. Miteff F, Faulder KC, Goh AC, Steinfort BS, Sue C, Harrington TJ. Mechanical thrombectomy with a self-expanding retrievable intracranial stent (Solitaire AB): experience in 26 patients with acute cerebral artery occlusion. *AJNR Am J Neuroradiol* 2011;32(6):1078–81.

47. Pfefferkorn T, Holtmannspotter M, Schmidt C, et al. Drip, ship, and retrieve: cooperative recanalization therapy in acute basilar artery occlusion. *Stroke* 2010;41(4):722–6.

48. Singer OC, Berkefeld J, Nolte CH, et al. Mechanical recanalization in basilar artery occlusion: the ENDOSTROKE study. *Ann Neurol* 2015;77(3):415–24.

49. Fahed R, Di Maria F, Rosso C, et al. A leap forward in the endovascular management of acute basilar artery occlusion since the appearance of stent retrievers: a single-center comparative study. *J Neurosurg* 2016:1–7.

50. Jung S, Jung C, Bae YJ, et al. A comparison between mechanical thrombectomy and intra-arterial fibrinolysis in acute basilar artery occlusion: single center experiences. *J Stroke* 2016;18(2):211–9.

51. Strbian D, Sairanen T, Silvennoinen H, Salonen O, Kaste M, Lindsberg PJ. Thrombolysis of basilar artery occlusion: impact of baseline ischemia and time. *Ann Neurol* 2013;73(6):688–94.

52. Eckert B, Koch C, Thomalla G, et al. Aggressive therapy with intravenous abciximab and intra-arterial rtPA and additional PTA/stenting improves clinical outcome in acute vertebrobasilar occlusion: combined local fibrinolysis and intravenous abciximab in acute vertebrobasilar stroke treatment (FAST): results of a multicenter study. *Stroke* 2005;36(6):1160–5.

53. Nagel S, Schellinger PD, Hartmann M, et al. Therapy of acute basilar artery occlusion: intraarterial thrombolysis alone vs bridging therapy. *Stroke* 2009;40(1):140–6.

54. Junghans U, Seitz RJ, Wittsack HJ, Aulich A, Siebler M. Treatment of acute basilar artery thrombosis with a combination of systemic alteplase and tirofiban, a nonpeptide platelet glycoprotein IIb/IIIa inhibitor: report of four cases. *Radiology* 2001;221(3):795–801.

55. Kubik CS, Adams RD. Occlusion of the basilar artery; a clinical and pathological study. *Brain* 1946;69(2):73–121.

56. Labauge R, Pages M, Marty-Double C, Blard JM, Boukobza M, Salvaing P. [Occlusion of the basilar artery. A review with 17 personal cases (author's transl)]. *Rev Neurol (Paris)* 1981;137(10):545–71.

57. Biemond A. Thrombosis of the basilar artery and the vascularization of the brain stem. *Brain* 1951;74(3): 300–17.

58. Cravioto H, Rey B, Prose PH, Feigin I. Occlusion of the basilar artery; a clinical and pathologic study of 14 autopsied cases. *Neurology* 1958;8(2):145–52.

59. Kumar G, Shahripour RB, Alexandrov AV. Recanalization of acute basilar artery occlusion improves outcomes: a meta-analysis. *J Neurointerv Surg* 2015;7(12):868–74.

60. Strbian D, Sairanen T, Silvennoinen H, Salonen O, Lindsberg PJ. Intravenous thrombolysis of basilar artery

occlusion: thrombus length versus recanalization success. *Stroke* 2014;45(6):1733–8.

61. Brandt T, von Kummer R, Muller-Kuppers M, Hacke W. Thrombolytic therapy of acute basilar artery occlusion. Variables affecting recanalization and outcome. *Stroke* 1996;27(5):875–81.

62. Puetz V, Sylaja PN, Coutts SB, et al. Extent of hypoattenuation on CT angiography source images predicts functional outcome in patients with basilar artery occlusion. *Stroke* 2008;39(9):2485–90.

63. Puetz V, Khomenko A, Hill MD, et al. Extent of hypoattenuation on CT angiography source images in basilar artery occlusion: prognostic value in the basilar artery international cooperation study. *Stroke* 2011;42(12):3454–9.

64. Devuyst G, Bogousslavsky J, Meuli R, Moncayo J, de Freitas G, van Melle G. Stroke or transient ischemic attacks with basilar artery stenosis or occlusion: clinical patterns and outcome. *Arch Neurol* 2002;59(4):567–73.

65. Lindsberg PJ, Soinne L, Tatlisumak T, et al. Long-term outcome after intravenous thrombolysis of basilar artery occlusion. *JAMA* 2004;292(15):1862–6.

66. Leemann B, Schnider A. [Unusually favorable recovery from locked-in syndrome after basilar artery occlusion]. *Rev Med Suisse* 2010;6(241):633–5.

67. Lule D, Zickler C, Hacker S, et al. Life can be worth living in locked-in syndrome. *Prog Brain Res* 2009;177: 339–51.

68. Laureys S, Pellas F, van Eeckhout P, et al. The locked-in syndrome : what is it like to be conscious but paralyzed and voiceless? *Prog Brain Res* 2005;150:495–511.

69. Renard D, Landragin N, Robinson A, et al. MRI-based score for acute basilar artery thrombosis. *Cerebrovasc Dis* 2008;25:511–16.

70. Kashiwagi J, Kiyosue H, Hori Y, et al. Endovascular recanalization of acute intracranial vertebrobasilar artery occlusion using local fibrinolysis and additional balloon angioplasty. *Neuroradiology* 2010;52:361–70.

71. Yu YY, Niu L, Gao L, et al. Intraarterial thrombolysis and stent placement for acute basilar artery occlusion. *J Vasc Interv Radiol* 2010;21:1359–63.

72. Chandra RV, Law CP, Yan B, Dowling RJ, Mitchell PJ. Glasgow coma scale does not predict outcome post-intra-arterial treatment for basilar artery thrombosis. *Am J Neuroradiol* 2011;32:576–80.

73. Barlinn K, Becker U, Puetz V, et al. Combined treatment with intravenous abciximab and intraarterial tPA yields high recanalization rate in patients with acute basilar artery occlusion. *J Neuroimaging* 2012;22:167–71.

78

Management of Myasthenia Gravis in ICU

T. Yuyen and O. Chaiwat

ABSTRACT

Myasthenia gravis (MG) is an autoimmune disorder resulting from antibodies attacking on components of the postsynaptic membrane of the neuromuscular junction causing neuromuscular weakness. Myasthenic crisis (MC) is a life-threatening neurological emergency. The crisis is due to the weakening of bulbar or respiratory muscles leading to respiratory failure which requires an admission to the intensive care unit (ICU). The management of MC patients in the ICUs is composed of several modalities including eradication of precipitating factors, evaluation of bulbar and respiratory functions, mechanical ventilatory support, specific immunotherapy (human intravenous immunoglobulin, immunoadsorption, and plasma exchange), prevention and prompt treatment of systemic complications, and establishing a plan for long-term treatment after recovery from the crisis. Due to prompt diagnosis and effective treatment of the disease, nowadays, the mortality rate of MG is less than 5%. Most MG patients have a near-normal life expectancy.

KEYWORDS

Myasthenia crisis; autoimmune disorder; bulbar and respiratory function; respiratory failure; mechanical ventilatory support; immunotherapy.

CASE STUDY

A 35-year-old woman has been diagnosed with myasthenia gravis (MG) for 6 months. The serologic testing indicated her as muscle-specific tyrosine kinase type MG (MuSK-MG). Pyridostigmine 30 mg every 6 hours was prescribed for symptomatic treatment and prednisolone 30 mg/day was given for immunotherapy. She was clinically stable after the treatment. Three days earlier, she had non-productive cough and was diagnosed with acute bronchitis. Clarithromycin 500 mg every 8 hours was taken. After that she developed flaccid dysarthria with hypernasal speech, dysphagia, and fatigued easily when chewing. This morning she felt difficulty to breathe and hurried to the hospital.

In the emergency room (ER), she was found to have shortness of breath, tachypnoea, orthopnoea, tachycardia, restlessness, sweating, and the use of accessory muscles of respiration. The vital signs showed blood pressure (BP) 160/90 mmHg, heart rate 120 beats per minute (bpm), respiratory rate 40 per minute, and oxygen saturation 94% at room air. Arterial blood gas (ABG) demonstrated pH 7.2, PaO_2 80 mmHg, $PaCO_2$ 50 mmHg, HCO_3 24 mmol/L.

She was diagnosed with myasthenic crisis (MC) and was intubated immediately at the ER since she was developing respiratory failure. After that, she was admitted to the ICU. The initial ventilator setting was volume-controlled mandatory ventilation (V-CMV) for full support. The precipitating factor was then evaluated. Clarithromycin was considered to be a trigger and was discontinued. Prednisolone was prescribed continually, meanwhile, pyridostigmine was temporarily discontinued in order to prevent further MC. The plasmapheresis was performed to wash out the antibodies from the plasma.

Five days later, the severity of muscle weakness gradually declined. The ventilatory support was deescalated to pressure support mode. The plasmapheresis was discontinued. Pyridostigmine was resumed to the usual dose. She did not suffer from any systemic complications of MC such as fever, pneumonia, atelectasis, volume overload, and congestive heart failure.

Two days later, she was extubated successfully. The immunosuppressive drugs were adjusted for appropriate long-term treatment. Finally, she was discharged from the ICU.

INTRODUCTION

Myasthenia gravis is one of the diseases causing neuromuscular weakness which may lead to respiratory failure requiring an ICU admission. It is an autoimmune disorder resulting from antibodies attacking on components of the postsynaptic membrane of the neuromuscular junction. The antibodies that bind to the acetylcholine receptor contribute to the abnormal neuromuscular transmission resulting in clinical weakness.[1] The main clinical features of MG are weakness and fluctuated fatiguability of skeletal muscles where repeated or sustained activity worsens the symptoms, however resting can improve the weakness. The weakness can either localize to specific muscle groups or generalize to others. In addition, the involvement of bulbar and respiratory muscles may lead to life-threatening conditions. The most common affected muscles include the *levator palpebrae superioris*, extraocular muscles, proximal muscles of the extremities, muscles of facial expression, and neck extensors.[2]

Myasthenic crisis is the most severe condition of MG. It is a life-threatening neurological emergency. The crisis is composed of the weakening of bulbar or respiratory muscles resulting in ventilation failure which requires an admission to the ICU for non-invasive or invasive respiratory support. It may occur in patients with previous diagnosis of MG, however, the MC may be the first manifestation of MG.[1,3,4]

EPIDEMIOLOGICAL DATA

Myasthenia gravis is the most common disorder affecting the neuromuscular junction (NMJ). Its prevalence has been reported at about 72 per 1,000,000. The incidence of MG is around 0.25 to 2.0 per 1,000,000.[5] The occurrence of MG demonstrates a bimodal distribution with the first peak in the age of 30 to 40 affecting mostly women and the second peak in the age of 60 to 70 affecting mostly men.[2] For patients who are younger than 40 years, the male to female ratio is 3:7. The ratio is equal in the ages of 40 to 49 years and the male to female ratio becomes 3:2 for those who are older than 50 years.[1,6,7]

Approximately 15%–20% of MG patients will develop MC, mostly during the first few years after the diagnosis when the disease is in the active phase.[3,4,8–10] Twenty per cent of MG patients develop MC as the first manifestation of the disease and one-third of the survivors may experience another crisis.[1,3,4]

Untreated MG demonstrated a mortality rate of 30%–70%. Complications such as aspiration, pneumonia, and falls caused by an intermittent impairment of muscle strength can occur. Nowadays, with the advancement in treatment of MG, most MG patients have a near-normal life expectancy. Currently, the mortality rate of MG has decreased to less than 5% because of prompt diagnosis and effective treatment of the disease.[8–12]

PATHOPHYSIOLOGY

Myasthenia gravis is an autoimmune disorder. Autoantibodies develop against components of the postsynaptic membrane (Table 78.1), mainly acetylcholine nicotinic postsynaptic receptors at the skeletal muscles. The cholinergic receptors of smooth and cardiac muscles have different antigenicity and are not affected by the disease. Acetylcholine receptors (AChR) autoantibodies are mainly the IgG1 and IgG3 subtypes which are divalent and complement activating.[13] They bind to the alpha subunit of AChR in the area of the main immunogenic region causing an impairment of the cholinergic nerve conductivity. Consequently, a reduction in both number and density of functional AChR may occur. In addition, the antibodies that cross-link AChR will accelerate the process of endocytosis and degradation of the receptors lead to a destruction of AChR.[2] The other mechanism is an increase in the diffusion distance of acetylcholine molecules at the synaptic junction as a result of destruction of the synaptic membrane by autoantibodies.[8] These changes occur due to the activation of the complement system by the antibody and the process of T-cell-dependent antigen at the postsynaptic membrane of the neuromuscular junction.[1]

There are other target sites for autoantibodies at the neuromuscular junction reported that relate to the

Table 78.1 Clinical subtypes and the presence of the various autoantibodies in the different subgroups of myasthenia gravis

MG subgroup	Age of onset	Thymic histology	Autoantibodies (percentage of patients)			
			AChR	MuSK	Titin	RyR
Early onset non-MuSK non-thymoma	<40	Hyperplasia	+ (100%)	− (100%)	+ (10%)	− (100%)
Late onset non-MuSK non-thymoma	>40	Normal/Thymic atrophy	+ (100%)	− (100%)	+ (58%)	+ (14%)
MuSK positive	<40 (most patients)	Normal	− (100%)	+ (100%)	NA	NA
Seronegative			− (100%)	− (100%)	− (100%)	− (100%)
Thymoma	40–50	Thymoma	+ (100%)	NA	+ (95%)	+ (70%)

Notes: HLA: histocompatibility antigen; AChR: acetylcholine receptor; MuSK: muscle-specific tyrosine kinase; RyR: ryanodin receptor; TAMG: Thymoma-associated myasthenia gravis.
Reprinted with permission from: Godoy DA, Mello LJ, Masotti L, Di Napoli M. The myasthenic patient in crisis: an update of the management in Neurointensive Care Unit. *Arq Neuropsiquiatr.* 2013 Sep;71(9A):627–39. doi:10.1590/0004-282X20130108.

development of MG. Muscle-specific tyrosine kinase is one of the most well-known targeted proteins located at the postsynaptic membrane. The protein tyrosine kinase function of MuSK is activated when agrin, a proteoglycan from the nerve terminal binds to MuSK via its co-receptor low-density lipoprotein receptor-related protein 4 (LRP4) resulting in agrin-MuSK-LRP4 complex, which is responsible for the activation and clustering of AChR at the neuromuscular junction. MuSK also anchors acetylcholinesterase at the synaptic basal lamina. Antibodies against MuSK (Anti-MuSK) are mostly of the non-complement-fixing IgG4 subclass and disrupt neuromuscular transmission by interfering with MuSK-LRP4 interaction, reducing AChR clustering at the muscle endplate.[13,14] The majority of patients with anti-MuSK are female and have a characteristic pattern of weakness involving mainly the bulbar, neck, shoulder, and respiratory muscles, lingual atrophy and relatively mild limb weakness.[1] Antibodies against LRP4 are predominantly of the complement-binding IgG1 and IgG2 subclasses which inhibit the LRP4-agrin interaction and interfere with the clustering of AChR in muscle cells. Antibodies against agrin inhibit agrin-induced MuSK phosphorylation and the clustering of AChR in muscle cells.[15]

Thymomas are the neoplasm of thymic epithelial cells (TECs) with mixed cortical and medullary properties.[15] About 10%–15% of MG patients have a thymoma and about 30% of thymoma patients are thymoma-associated MG (TAMG).[8] Thymoma-associated MG is common in both men and women and can occur at any ages, with peak onset at the age of 50 years.[1] Patients with TAMG show high titers of anti-AChR antibodies, and mostly have anti-Titin antibodies. Titin is a protein which offers a direct link between muscle gene activation and mechanical muscle strain. Over a half of late-onset generalized MG without thymoma patients carry anti-Titin antibodies. Moreover, autoantibodies against Ryanodin receptor (RyR) can be found in 50% of TAMG.[1] The RyR is the calcium channel of the sarcoplasmic reticulum which plays a role in excitation-contraction coupling of skeletal muscle. Patients with RyR antibodies commonly demonstrate weakness of the bulbar, respiratory, and neck muscles. Neck weakness at onset is a typical feature of patients with RyR antibodies. Patients who have symptoms of neck weakness and non-limb bulbar weakness should be suspected for thymoma.[1]

About 10%–20% of MG patients are seronegative which do not have antibodies against AChR and MuSK. The clinical features of these patients are heterogeneous. They can demonstrate purely ocular muscle involvement, mild generalized, or severe generalized disease. Some cases of seronegative patients show similar clinical features, treatment response, and thymus gland pathologies to seropositive patients.[1]

CLASSIFICATION

Myasthenia gravis can be classified by several different criteria including by the onset of the disease, severity of the disease, aetiology of the disease, the thymic pathology, and

Table 78.2 Clinical classifications (with modifications) of the severity of myasthenia gravis

Osserman and Genkins[16]	**Grade I:** Ocular MG **Grade IIa:** Mild generalized MG responding well to therapy **Grade IIb:** Moderate generalized MG responding less well **Grade III:** Severe generalized MG **Grade IV:** Myasthenic crisis with respiratory failure
Myasthenia Gravis Foundation*[17]	**Class I: Ocular myasthenia** (may have weakness of eye closure, all other muscles have normal strength) **Class II: Mild weakness** (affecting muscles beside ocular muscles; may also have ocular muscle weakness of any degree) **Class IIa:** Mostly affecting extremities, axial muscles, or both; may also have involvement of oropharyngeal muscles to a lesser degree **Class IIb:** Mostly involving oropharyngeal, respiratory muscles, or both; may also have involvement of extremities, axial muscles, or both to a lesser or equal degree **Class III: Moderate weakness** (in muscles besides ocular muscles; may also have weakness of any degree of ocular muscles) **Class IIIa:** Involvement is mostly of extremities, axial muscles, or both; may also have involvement of oropharyngeal muscles to a lesser degree **Class IIIb:** Mostly involving oropharyngeal, respiratory muscles, or both; may also have involvement of extremities, axial muscles, or both to a lesser or equal degree **Class IV: Severe weakness** (in muscles besides ocular muscles; may also have weakness of any degree of ocular muscles) **Class IVa:** Involvement is mostly of extremities, axial muscles, or both; may also have involvement of oropharyngeal muscles to a lesser degree **Class IVb:** Mostly involving oropharyngeal, respiratory muscles, or both; may also have involvement of extremities, axial muscles, or both to a lesser or equal degree **Class V: Myasthenic crisis** intubation, with or without mechanical ventilation (except when intubated for routine postoperative management)

*Myasthenia Gravis Foundation of America (MGFA) clinical classification based on neurologic examination. The limitations of clinical classification is fluctuating muscle weakness, so that examiner's subjective classification of mild, moderate, severe classification should be based on most severely affected muscles.
Reprinted with permission from: Godoy DA, Mello LJ, Masotti L, Di Napoli M. The myasthenic patient in crisis: an update of the management in Neurointensive Care Unit. *Arq Neuropsiquiatr* 2013 Sep;71(9A):627–39. doi:10.1590/0004-282X20130108.

serologic status (Table 78.1).[2] The various classification types are detailed as follows:

Onset of the disease:

- Neonatal MG
- Juvenile MG
- Early-onset MG (EOMG)
- Late-onset MG (LOMG)

Severity of the disease (Table 78.2):

- Osserman and Genkins classification[16]
- Myasthenia Gravis Foundation[17]

Aetiology of the disease:

- Acquired autoimmune MG
- Transient neonatal MG
- Drug-induced MG
- Congenital myasthenic syndromes

Thymic pathology:

- Thymic hyperplasia associated MG
- Thymoma associated MG

Serologic status:

- Seropositive
  - Anti-AChR
  - Anti-MuSK
- Seronegative

MYASTHENIC CRISIS

The clinical features of MC are intense weakness of the bulbar muscles which are innervated by cranial nerves and/or respiratory muscles. The weakness of respiratory muscles can contribute to ventilatory failure that require ventilator support. Myasthenic patients who undergo any operations and are unable to extubate within 24 hours because of respiratory weakness are also considered to be in crisis.[8] These cases fall in grade IV in the Osserman classification of MG, and class V of the disease severity staging proposed by the Myasthenia Gravis Foundation of America.[16,17]

The respiratory failure in MC results from severe bulbar weakness and ventilatory muscles weakness. The dysfunction of bulbar muscles affects coughing, swallowing reflexes, and sigh mechanisms. Dysphagia, nasal regurgitation, nasal and staccato speech, jaw and tongue weakness, and bifacial paresis are the common manifestations.[18] The ineffective clearance of secretions in the oropharynx and poor patency of the upper airway increase the possibility of microaspiration and atelectasis.[8–11,18–20] Meanwhile, ventilatory muscle weakness can produce inadequate tidal volume and a decrease in functional residual capacity resulting in basal lung atelectasis and worsening work of breathing. All of these changes have an impact on the ventilation and perfusion relationship causing hypoxaemia and hypercapnia.[1]

The respiratory mechanism parameter changes of respiratory failure in MC are characterized by the decrease of forced vital capacity (FVC) to less than 1 litre and the inability to create negative inspiratory force (NIF) of 20 cm H_2O.[8–11,18–20] The MC patients should be in close monitoring of respiratory status and perform bedside pulmonary function test 4–6 times/day.[9] Arterial blood gas analysis commonly shows hypercapnia before hypoxaemia. Early endotracheal intubation should be considered due to the rapid deterioration of involved bulbar and respiratory muscles.[9]

In MuSK-MG, bulbar weakness always manifests before respiratory failure.[8] In AChR-MG, muscle weakness initially involves the intercostal and accessory muscles and progresses to the diaphragm.[18,20] During a crisis, central ventilatory drive usually remains intact, therefore, all MG patients should be examined for signs of MC although they do not complain of weakness. The signs of respiratory distress can be under-detected because of the generalized weakness. Respiratory muscles may suddenly become fatigued leading to acute respiratory collapse. The signs of limb or bulbar weakness are not proportionally associated with respiratory muscle weakness in some patients. Nevertheless, MC can present with only ventilatory failure in rare cases.[21,22]

INVESTIGATION

Electrophysiological Testing

Repetitive nerve stimulation (RNS) applies repetitive supramaximal electrical stimulations at a frequency 3 Hz to a nerve and measures the response in the distal muscles.[2] In MG patients, RNS demonstrates a decreasing response more than 10% between the first and the fourth compound muscle action potential.[1] RNS decreases ACh storage at the neuromuscular junction reducing successful neuromuscular transmission. Phrenic and long thoracic nerves should be tested in patients with respiratory involvement.[23] The test is almost always positive in generalised MG, but only half of ocular MG cases yield a positive result.[2] Single-fibre electromyography (SFEMG) measures the firing time of two muscle fibres within the same motor unit. The time difference is recorded as 'jitter' (<55 millisecond [ms]).[2] The jitter is usually greater than 100 ms in MG cases. The SFEMG is the most sensitive test for detecting abnormal neuromuscular transmission. However, this test has limitations concerned with time consumption and requirement of special expertise.[24]

Pharmacological Testing

Edrophonium (tensilon test) is a short-acting intravenous acetylcholinesterase inhibitor. Its onset time is within 30 seconds and the duration of action is 5 minutes. This test has a sensitivity of 86% for ocular MG and 95% for generalized MG.[1] Edrophonium temporarily improves muscle strength and is interpreted as a positive result. It is usually performed by two investigators with blinded protocol and also compared to the placebo (normal saline) injection. Firstly, edrophonium 2 mg is given as a test dose, then if there is no response after 30 seconds, another 8 mg is given. If there is improvement in muscle strength within 1 minute of any dose increment, the test is considered as positive and a further dose of edrophonium is unnecessary.[1,2] Common side effects of edrophonium include sweating, tearing, fasciculation, and abdominal cramping. Bradycardia and hypotension are the most important side effects of edrophonium. A pre-test 12-lead EKG should be available and if there is evidence of conduction block or acute cardiac disease, then the test should be avoided. During the test, patients should be monitored with real-time EKG monitoring and atropine should always be available to correct bradycardia. Worsening of bulbar and respiratory symptoms in MuSK-MG after edrophonium test has been reported and could confuse the clinical diagnosis.[7] In addition, positive results can be found in other conditions including motor neuron disease poliomyelitis, peripheral neuropathies, brainstem lesions, and mitochondrial myopathies.[25]

Serological Testing

• Anti-AChR antibody test: 80–85% of these antibodies are found in generalized MG but only 50–60% are demonstrated in ocular MG.[2] The test is strongly specific for MG.

- Anti-MuSK antibody test: If anti-AChR antibodies are not found, MuSK antibodies should be tested. Both antibodies would not be detected in the same patient. MuSK antibodies should also be tested in highly suspicious cases, for example, muscle weakness with bulbar involvement.[2]

Radiological Testing

MG patients with age greater than 40 years may have a thymic tumour.[2] Chest computed tomography (CT) scan should be performed to exclude thymoma in patients with new onset of MG. Chest CT is more sensitive than plain chest radiographs for detecting anterior mediastinal masses. Magnetic resonance imaging (MRI) does not increase diagnostic sensitivity. All radiological testing should be made when the patient is in stable condition.

General Evaluation of Myasthenic Crisis

The management of MC should follow the steps shown in Figure 78.1 according to the European Federation of Neurological Societies guidelines.[26] Early detection of impending respiratory failure is an important step for successful management. The pattern of respiratory muscle weakness in AChR-MG frequently starts at the intercostal and accessory muscles, and is followed by the diaphragm.[18,20] In MuSK-MG, bulbar weakness always presents before respiratory failure.[8]

TRIGGER DETECTION

Most of the patients who develop MC have a precipitating factor, although one-third of the cases are not able to detect associated factors.[1,27] The common precipitating factors for MC include respiratory infections, aspiration, sepsis, surgery, rapid tapering of immunotherapy, starting corticosteroid treatment, exposure to drugs aggravating myasthenic weakness, and pregnancy.[28] Corticosteroid-induced exacerbations of MG may occur after beginning treatment with corticosteroids and result in temporary worsened muscle weakness. The worsened weakness may have an onset within 7–10 days after initiating corticosteroids and remain for about 1 week before strength improves.[28] About 9%–18% of the patients who received corticosteroids develop MC.[29] Therefore, hospital admission is required for close observation of clinical weakness when the patients are initiated on corticosteroid treatment. The patients should receive close monitoring for the first 2 weeks of corticosteroid treatment.

Risk factors of exacerbation from steroids are old age, lower score on Myasthenia Severity Scale, and more severe bulbar and generalized symptoms.[29] Some medications can exacerbate MG (Table 78.3). An antibiotic in the macrolide group, such as telithromycin is contraindicated in MG.[1] Live vaccines should be administered cautiously in MG patients who were receiving immunosuppressive agents.[8,11] MG can be exacerbated by over-replacement with levothyroxine in patients with coexisting thyroid disease. Pregnancy aggravates MG in approximately one-third of all women, and MC in pregnancy carries high perinatal mortality.[8,11,30] Electrolyte imbalance, especially hypokalaemia and hypophosphataemia can worsen muscle weakness.

RESPIRATORY AND BULBAR FUNCTION ASSESSMENT

Respiratory and bulbar dysfunction occur at the same time with generalized muscle weakness of the MG patient. Clinical manifestations include dyspnoea, tachypnoea, orthopnoea, tachycardia, sweating, and paradoxical ventilation.[1]

As a result of respiratory muscle weakness, tidal volume declines progressively. The reduced tidal volume is initially compensated by increased respiratory rate showing the pattern of rapid and shallow breathing. In this setting, the clinical signs of diaphragmatic weakness can be observed by using accessory muscles and paradoxical abdominal movement. An ineffective cough or an inability to count numbers from 1 to 20 within a single breath suggests significant expiratory muscle weakness.[28]

Although upper airway muscle weakness is hard to assess and less important than respiratory muscle weakness, it is necessary to be recognized since it is a common mechanism leading to MC in many cases.[20] Oropharyngeal muscle weakness may cause upper airway collapse with obstruction accompanied with the inability to swallow secretions causing airway obstruction and aspiration.

The signs of bulbar weakness consists of flaccid dysarthria with hypernasality, staccato (horse speech), dysphagia associated with nasal regurgitation, and chewing fatigue. Mouth closure is frequently weak and cannot be upheld against applied pressure by an examiner. In order to assess tongue weakness, ask the patients to protrude their tongue into each cheek. The tongue cannot protrude beyond the lips when there is severe tongue weakness.[28] A dropped head syndrome due to neck extensor weakness may occur, although neck flexors are often weaker. The paralysis of vocal cord abductor muscles may result in upper airway obstruction presented with stridor.

Table 78.3 Medications and drugs that may provoke myasthenia crisis

Drug class	Medication
Antipsychotics	Phenothiazines, sulpiride, atypicals (clozapine)
Neuromuscular-blocking agents	Succinylcholine, Vecuronium
Anticholinergic drugs	Ocular proparacaine
Cardiovascular medications	Cibenzoline Lidocaine (systemic dosing) Procainamide Propranolol (and other beta-blockers) Quinidine Verapamil Bretylium Statins
Neurologic and psychoactive medications	Chlorpromazine Lithium Phenytoin Carbamazepine Trihexyphenidyl Trimethadione
Antibiotics	All aminoglycosides Ciprofloxacin Colistin Lincomycins (e.g., clindamycin) Macrolides Erythromycin Clarithromycin Telithromycin (has risk of exacerbation of MG, including rapid onset of life-threatening acute respiratory failure) Penicillins (include ampicillin and imipenem-cilastatin) Polymyxins Tetracyclines
Other antimicrobial drugs	Emetine Imiquimod Ritonavir
Antirheumatologic and immunosuppressive medications	Chloroquine, penicillamine, prednisone, interferons
Other medication	Aprotinin Iodinated-contrast agents levonorgestrel Magnesium (including magnesium sulphate) Methoxyflurane Pyrantel pamoate Propafenone Dextro carnitine-levocarnitine but not levocarnitine alone Interferon alfa Methocarbamol Transdermal nicotine acetazolamide

Reprinted with permission from: Godoy DA, Mello LJ, Masotti L, Di Napoli M. The myasthenic patient in crisis: an update of the management in Neurointensive Care Unit. *Arq Neuropsiquiatr* 2013;71(9A):627–39. doi:10.1590/0004-282X20130108.

When performing the flow-volume loop test, the inspiratory portion of flow–volume loop is abnormally 'flattened' due to extrathoracic airway obstruction.[28]

The decrease in negative inspiratory pressure and flow measurements may be together presented with the abnormality in flow–volume loop.

MANAGEMENT OF MYASTHENIC CRISIS

Intubation and Mechanical Ventilation

Indications for intubation include evidence of fatigue with increasing tachypnea and declining tidal volumes, hypoxaemia despite supplemental oxygen, hypercapnia, and difficulty with clearing secretions.[28] Some pulmonary function tests can be performed to determine the need for mechanical ventilation such as FVC, negative inspiratory pressure (NIP), and positive expiratory pressure (PEP). The 20/30/40 rule (FVC <20 ml/kg; NIP <30 cmH$_2$O; and PEP <40 cmH$_2$O) is a helpful guide to make a decision for intubation.[1] An FVC of <30 ml/kg may be interpreted as an ineffective cough and followed by poor clearing of secretions and atelectasis. An NIP of <20 cmH$_2$O may be associated with a sign of inspiratory muscles and diaphragm weakness. A PEP of <40 cmH$_2$O indicates weakness of expiratory muscles associated with ineffective cough and poor secretion clearance.[1] However, these examinations are difficult to perform in bulbar weakness patients because of difficulty in covering the lips around the spirometer mouthpiece or by an inability to seal the nasopharynx. Moreover, these threshold values have not been established through well-designed prospective studies which demonstrate them to be reliable predictors of the need for mechanical ventilation.[1] There are some absolute conditions that intubations are necessary such as cardiac arrest, respiratory failure, alteration of consciousness, severe shock, life-threatening arrhythmias, severe blood gas disturbance, and bulbar dysfunction with confirmed aspiration.[12,31] In neuromuscular respiratory failure, hypoxaemia usually occurs late and generally improves with oxygen supplementation. In this setting, the use of bi-level positive airway pressure (BiPAP) is helpful because it overcomes the increased upper airway resistance and prevents alveolar collapse and atelectasis. Myasthenic patients with mild hypercapnia (PaCO$_2$ <50 mmHg) may avoid the need for intubation by using BiPAP. However, severe hypercapnia (PaCO$_2$ >50 mmHg) indicates that muscle fatigue is impending and using BiPAP may not be helpful. Thus, monitoring O$_2$ saturation alone is inadequate. Arterial blood gas assessment with measurement of PaCO$_2$ is necessary. Sometimes, when the clinical criteria for intubation is not clear, elective intubation is recommended to prevent abrupt respiratory failure.

After intubation, the patients should be arranged in a semi-recumbent position with the head of bed up to 30 degrees to decrease the work of breathing. The initial ventilatory support goals are to improve respiratory muscle weakness and to preserve lung expansion. Several modes of mechanical ventilation are appropriate for MC patients including controlled mandatory ventilation (CMV), intermittent mandatory ventilation (IMV), synchronized intermittent mandatory ventilation (SIMV), and pressure support mode with additional positive end-expiratory pressure (PEEP). The preferable presets are low tidal volumes (6–8 mL/kg), respiratory rate 12–16/min, PEEP of 5 cmH$_2$O. Fraction of inspired oxygen (FiO$_2$) should be as least as possible to achieve an oxygen saturation (SpO$_2$) >92% or partial pressure of oxygen in arterial blood (PaO$_2$) >70 mmHg. In case of atelectasis, the strategies to improve hypoxaemia include performing recruitment manoeuvres, the utilization of sighs (1.5 × tidal volume) 3 to 4 times per hour and the application of PEEP.[10] In patients with chronic hypercapnia with compensated metabolic alkalosis, partial pressure of carbon dioxide in arterial blood (PaCO$_2$) should be kept above 45 mmHg to avoid alkalosis and bicarbonate wasting, which lead to difficult weaning.[12] The degree of support is considered individually dependent on clinical conditions and should be adjusted according to arterial blood analysis to achieve normocarbia and prevent hypoxaemia. The ventilator requirement is usually prolonged in MC. Most MC patients often require mechanical ventilation up to 14 days. Predictors of prolonged intubation (more than 14 days) include baseline serum bicarbonate greater than or equal to 30 mmol/L, vital capacity less than 25 ml/kg within the first week after intubation, and age greater than 50 years.[19] A tracheostomy should be considered for patients with prolonged intubation as tracheostomy reduces the risk for ventilator-associated pneumonia (VAP), tracheolaryngeal injury, facilitates suctioning of tracheal secretions, reduces dead space, and the tracheostomy is more comfortable for long-term ventilated patients.[28]

Respiratory Care During Mechanical Ventilation

In MC, bronchodilators such as β2 agonist and terbutaline is beneficial for improving bronchospasm. For myasthenic patients with concomitant chronic obstructive pulmonary disease (COPD), inhaled ipratropium bromide is the bronchodilator of choice due to its ability to reduce bronchial secretions which limit the use of cholinesterase inhibitors.[1]

As the patients have ineffective cough, chest therapy including percussion, vibration, and postural drainage followed by regular suctioning should be implemented.[32] Regular suctioning facilitates the removal of excess oropharyngeal and tracheal secretions and stimulates coughing. Inspired gas humidity is kept around 80% at 37°C to lubricate sticky secretions.

Adequate nutrition should be accomplished to avoid a negative energy balance which worsens the muscle weakness.[1] Enteral feeding is preferable in all patients if there are no contraindications. The goal of nutritional support is 25–35 calories/kg/day. Low carbohydrate feed is preferable in patients with hypercarbia and difficult weaning.[32] Checking blood for electrolyte imbalance, especially hypokalaemia, hypomagnesaemia, and hypophosphataemia is important because these electrolyte derangements can exacerbate MC. Anaemia can also increase weakness, and transfusion trigger at haemoglobin levels less than 9 g/dL is recommended.[33] Deep vein thrombosis (DVT) prophylaxis, maintenance of haemodynamic stability, and optimal glycaemic control are also essential.

Weaning Criteria

The weaning process should be considered when patients demonstrate an improvement of respiratory muscle strength and reasons for mechanical ventilation have been resolved. The daily assessment of general parameters for weaning such as a normal oxygenation and ventilation, stable vital signs with minimal vasopressors, good consciousness, ability to cough effectively, clear of infection, no electrolytes disturbance, no systemic complications, PaO_2–FIO_2 ratio more than 200 and PEEP $\leq$5 cmH$_2$O are recommended.

The respiratory mechanic criteria for weaning include negative expiratory force greater than 20 cmH$_2$O, positive expiratory force greater than 40 cmH$_2$O, and vital capacity greater than 10 ml/kg.[28] The clinical improvement of bulbar and respiratory muscle strength can be assessed by testing for improved strength of neck flexors and other adjunct muscles.[1]

The initial goal of weaning is to de-escalate from controlled ventilation to pressure support mode, then to reduce the amount of pressure support by 2 cmH$_2$O every 3 hours, and finally to try on a T-piece.[28] If the patient develops signs of respiratory fatigue such as rapid and shallow breathing, diaphoresis, tachycardia, or agitation, the weaning trial should be discontinued and assisted ventilation should be reinstituted. An ineffective cough and inadequate airway clearance are the most common causes of extubation failure.

Anticholinesterase Drugs

Anticholinesterase drugs should be temporarily discontinued when the patients are using mechanical ventilator because the overdose of these medications may promote cholinergic crisis.[8,11,19] Cholinergic crisis may produce excessive pulmonary secretions due to muscarinic effects and fasciculations from nicotinic effects, both of which result in exacerbation of muscle weakness and respiratory failure. Furthermore, acetylcholinesterase inhibitors may cause cardiac arrhythmias and myocardial infarction. When the patient demonstrates clinical improvement, it is recommended to resume anticholinesterase drugs before considering weaning of mechanical ventilation.

Immunotherapy

Immunotherapy is considered as a specific treatment for MC patients. Specific immunotherapy includes plasma exchange (PE), immunoadsorption (IA), and human intravenous immunoglobulin (IVIG). All of them have reported similar efficacy, so the decision to use any of them is interchangeable depending on the availability, side effects, costs, experience, and patients' profile.[1,26,34]

Plasma exchange is an effective short-term treatment for MC and to optimize symptomatic myasthenic patients for surgery.[28] The therapeutic effect is derived from the rapid clearance of circulating autoantibodies in plasma. Plasma exchanges are usually performed on five occasions involving 1.5–2 litres each time. The first two exchanges can be performed on consecutive days, but the later exchanges usually require a day off between treatments to avoid coagulopathy or persistent hypocalcaemia.[11] Onset of improvement normally happens within 2 to 3 days. However, the muscle strength is temporarily improved which lasts up to several weeks at maximum. The insertion of a central venous catheter is required which also carries some complications such as vascular injury, venous thrombosis, infection, and pneumothorax. During the procedure, large volume shifts may lead to complications such as hypotension, bradycardia, congestive heart failure, coagulopathy, and hypocalcaemia.[28]

Immunoadsorption can be used instead of plasma exchange for the treatment of MC. The main advantage of immunoadsorption is no requirement for the substitution of plasma proteins and coagulation factors, providing rapid treatment of 2–2.5 times of the plasma volume per day which is a much higher volume than plasma exchange.[34,35]

Both PE and IA demonstrate a rapid clinical response, especially in patients who have no improvement, are worsening, or are suffering from severe complications. Both anti-AChR and anti-MuSK positive patients have a good response to PE and IA.

Intravenous immunoglobulins are composed of pooled polyclonal immunoglobulins derived from a large number of healthy donors.[15] The mechanism of action is unknown. The usual dosage is 0.4 g/kg/day for five consecutive days.[36] The other regimen is 1 g/kg/day for two consecutive days.[37] Intravenous immunoglobulins have provided similar efficacy to PE and IA in terms of shortening the period of mechanical ventilation during MC. Common side effects are fever, nausea, and headache. Due to high oncotic pressure of IVIG, pulmonary oedema from fluid overload can occur. More serious but less frequent complications include aseptic meningitis, dermatitis, renal dysfunction, cardiac arrhythmia, thrombocytopenia, stroke, myocardial infarction, pulmonary embolism, and anaphylaxis, particularly in immunoglobulin A (IgA) deficient patients.[1]

Corticosteroids

Steroids should be continued in patients who have been treated with steroids before the development of crisis. The drug should be given via the oral or nasogastric route because of the risk of developing critical illness myopathy in patients who are given intravenous corticosteroids. Prednisolone is preferred to start after PE or IVIG at a dosage of 1 mg/kg/day.[1] The indication for prednisolone is for patients who cannot be extubated after 2 weeks of specific treatment. Due to delayed action after 2 weeks, prednisone can be given concurrently with PE or IVIG. In contrast, if the patients improve with PE or IVIG, the initiation of prednisolone can be deferred until after extubation and when able to tolerate oral ingestion. The improvement of clinical weakness as a result of prednisolone treatment should occur within 2 weeks.[29] If the patients begin to show improvement, the dose can be tapered down to alternate-day dosing. In septic patients, steroids should be delayed until the infection is effectively controlled. Relative contraindications include poorly controlled diabetes and severe osteoporosis. There are three dose regimens that are recommended for clinical use:[15]

- Start prednisolone 10–20 mg/day and increase 5 mg/day per week until stable clinical improvement is achieved (at about 1 mg/kg/day).
- Start prednisolone 1–1.5 mg/kg/day in combination with immunosuppressive drugs until stable clinical improvement and then dose reduction of 5 mg/day every month with the goal of total cessation of steroid therapy.
- Intravenous pulse methylprednisolone dosage of 500–2000 mg/day for 3–5 consecutive days followed by oral prednisolone tapering off.

Cyclosporine, azathioprine, and mycophenolate are immunosuppressive agents which are necessary in long-term management of MG. These agents are not useful during crisis mainly because of the delayed onset of action.[1]

Surgical Thymectomy

Thymectomy is the only specific treatment for MG providing the chance of complete remission.[6,7] Indications for thymectomy include new onset of generalized MG, failure of long-term conservative therapy, and thymoma.[6,7,26] Patients with age <60 years, seropositivity, and thymic hyperplasia also have great benefit from thymectomy. The role of thymectomy in MuSK patients is unclear.

Postoperative crisis after thymectomy is associated with onset of disease at age >50 years, grade IIA, IIB, and III according to clinical grading of Osserman classification, a history of previous MC, preoperative sign of bulbar weakness, AChR antibody levels >100 nmol/L, and intraoperative blood loss of >1 litre. Other predisposing factors include obesity with BMI >25.6 kg/m^2, higher doses of pyridostigmine >270 mg/day, FVC <2 litre, and history of infection one month before surgery.[38] Less invasive surgery such as video-assisted thoracoscopic thymectomy, cervicotomy, and partial sternotomy shows a reduced risk for postoperative crisis.[39–41]

COMPLICATIONS FROM MYASTHENIC CRISIS

The most common adverse effects of MC are fever (69%), pneumonia (51%), and atelectasis (40%).[28] Additionally, atelectasis, *Clostridium difficile* enterocolitis, anaemia, and congestive heart failure have been found to be associated with prolonged duration of MC.[19] The antibiotic should be prescribed when there is a proved indication to avoid *Clostridium difficile* enterocolitis, which results from a complication of broad-spectrum antibiotic therapy. A fever in MC patients should be investigated for bronchopulmonary infections by chest imaging and sputum cultures. Aggressive respiratory treatment may reduce prolonged respiratory complications of atelectasis and pneumonia and shorten mechanical ventilation duration and length of ICU stay. When compared to non-crisis patients, those who are admitted with MC have an increased incidence of sepsis, DVT, and cardiac complications including congestive heart failure, acute myocardial infarction, arrhythmias, and cardiac arrest.[1]

CONCLUSIONS

Myasthenic crisis is a life-threatening neurological condition. Respiratory and bulbar muscle weakness lead to respiratory failure requiring an ICU admission for mechanical ventilatory support. The cornerstones of treatment include proper ventilatory support, detection and eradication of precipitating factors, specific immunotherapy such as plasma exchange, immunoadsorption, preventing systemic complications, and planning for long-term treatment with immunosuppressive agents. The crisis is a reversible condition which results in no long-term disability if treated promptly and appropriately. With advancement in the treatment of MC patients in an ICU, the outcomes have improved significantly with mortality rate less than 5%.

REFERENCES

1. Godoy DA, Mello LJ, Masotti L, et al. The myasthenic patient in crisis: an update of the management in Neurointensive Care Unit. *Arq Neuropsiquiatr* 2013;71(9A):627–39.

2. Turner C. A review of myasthenia gravis: Pathogenesis, clinical features and treatment. *Current Anaesthesia & Critical Care* 2007;18(1):15–23.

3. Cohen MS, Younger D. Aspects of the natural history of myasthenia gravis: crisis and death. *Ann N Y Acad Sci* 1981;377:670–7.

4. Bedlack RS, Sanders DB. On the concept of myasthenic crisis. *J Clin Neuromuscul Dis* 2002;4(1):40–2.

5. Carr AS, Cardwell CR, McCarron PO, et al. A systematic review of population based epidemiological studies in Myasthenia Gravis. *BMC Neurol* 2010;10:46.

6. Nicolle MW. Myasthenia gravis. *Neurologist* 2002;8(1):2–21.

7. Juel VC, Massey JM. Myasthenia gravis. *Orphanet J Rare Dis* 2007;2:44.

8. Chaudhuri A, Behan PO. Myasthenic crisis. *QJM* 2009; 102(2):97–107.

9. Jani-Acsadi A, Lisak RP. Myasthenic crisis: guidelines for prevention and treatment. *J Neurol Sci* 2007;261(1–2): 127–33.

10. Bershad EM, Feen ES, Suarez JI. Myasthenia gravis crisis. *South Med J* 2008;101(1):63–9.

11. Lacomis D. Myasthenic crisis. *Neurocrit Care* 2005;3(3): 189–94.

12. Wendell LC, Levine JM. Myasthenic crisis. *The Neurohospitalist* 2011;1(1):16–22.

13. Phillips WD, Vincent A. Pathogenesis of myasthenia gravis: update on disease types, models, and mechanisms. F1000 Faculty Rev-1513. *F1000Res* 2016;5:pii.

14. Nicolle MW. Myasthenia gravis and Lambert-Eaton myasthenic syndrome. *Continuum (Minneap Minn)* 2016; 22(6, Muscle and Neuromuscular Junction Disorders): 1978–2005.

15. Melzer N, Ruck T, Fuhr P, et al. Clinical features, pathogenesis, and treatment of myasthenia gravis: a supplement to the Guidelines of the German Neurological Society. *J Neurol* 2016;263(8):1473–94.

16. Osserman KE, Kornfeld P, Cohen E, et al. Studies in myasthenia gravis; review of two hundred eighty-two cases at the Mount Sinai Hospital, New York City. *AMA Arch Intern Med* 1958;102(1):72–81.

17. Jaretzki A, 3rd, Barohn RJ, Ernstoff RM, Kaminski HJ, Keesey JC, Penn AS, Sanders DB. Myasthenia gravis: recommendations for clinical research standards. Task Force of the Medical Scientific Advisory Board of the Myasthenia Gravis Foundation of America. *Neurology* 2000;55(1):16–23.

18. Rabinstein AA, Wijdicks EF. Warning signs of imminent respiratory failure in neurological patients. *Semin Neurol* 2003;23(1):97–104.

19. Thomas CE, Mayer SA, Gungor Y, et al. Myasthenic crisis: clinical features, mortality, complications, and risk factors for prolonged intubation. *Neurology* 1997; 48(5):1253–60.

20. Putman MT, Wise RA. Myasthenia gravis and upper airway obstruction. *Chest* 1996;109(2):400–4.

21. Dushay KM, Zibrak JD, Jensen WA. Myasthenia gravis presenting as isolated respiratory failure. *Chest* 1990;97(1):232–4.

22. Mier A, Laroche C, Green M. Unsuspected myasthenia gravis presenting as respiratory failure. *Thorax* 1990;45(5): 422–3.

23. Lo YL, Leoh TH, Dan YF, et al. Repetitive stimulation of the long thoracic nerve in myasthenia gravis: clinical and electrophysiological correlations. *J Neurol Neurosurg Psychiatry* 2003;74(3):379–81.

24. Medicine AQACAAoE. Practice parameter for repetitive nerve stimulation and single fiber EMG evaluation of adults with suspected myasthenia gravis or Lambert-Eaton myasthenic syndrome: summary statement. *Muscle Nerve* 2001;24(9):1236–8.

25. Dirr LY, Donofrio PD, Patton JF, et al. A false-positive edrophonium test in a patient with a brainstem glioma. *Neurology* 1989;39(6):865–7.

26. Skeie GO, Apostolski S, Evoli A, et al. Guidelines for treatment of autoimmune neuromuscular transmission disorders. *Eur J Neurol* 2010;17(7):893–902.

27. Marquardt J, Reuther P. [Myasthenia gravis. Information for the anesthetist and critical care physician]. *Anaesthesist* 1984;33(5):207–11.

28. Juel VC. Myasthenia gravis: management of myasthenic crisis and perioperative care. *Semin Neurol* 2004;24(1): 75–81.

29. Bae JS, Go SM, Kim BJ. Clinical predictors of steroid-induced exacerbation in myasthenia gravis. *J Clin Neurosci* 2006;13(10):1006–10.

30. Plauche WC. Myasthenia gravis in mothers and their newborns. *Clin Obstet Gynecol* 1991;34(1):82–99.

31. Vianello A, Arcaro G, Braccioni F, et al. Prevention of extubation failure in high-risk patients with neuromuscular disease. *J Crit Care* 2011;26(5):517–24.

32. Varelas PN, Chua HC, Natterman J, et al. Ventilatory care in myasthenia gravis crisis: assessing the baseline adverse event rate. *Crit Care Med* 2002;30(12):2663–8.

33. Kirmani JF, Yahia AM, Qureshi AI. Myasthenic crisis. *Curr Treat Options Neurol* 2004;6(1):3–15.

34. Ahmed S, et al. An update on myasthenic crisis. *Curr Treat Options Neurol* 2005;7(2):129–41.

35. Kohler W, Bucka C, Klingel R. A randomized and controlled study comparing immunoadsorption and plasma exchange in myasthenic crisis. *J Clin Apher* 2011;26(6): 347–55.

36. Imbach P, Barandun S, d'Apuzzo V, et al. High-dose intravenous gammaglobulin for idiopathic thrombocytopenic purpura in childhood. *Lancet* 1981;1(8232):1228–31.

37. Gajdos P, Tranchant C, Clair B, et al. Treatment of myasthenia gravis exacerbation with intravenous immunoglobulin: a randomized double-blind clinical trial. *Arch Neurol* 2005;62(11):1689–93.

38. Chu XY, Xue ZQ, Wang RW, et al. Predictors of postoperative myasthenic crisis in patients with myasthenia gravis after thymectomy. *Chin Med J (Engl)* 2011;124(8):1246–50.

39. Huang CS, Hsu HS, Huang BS, et al. Factors influencing the outcome of transsternal thymectomy for myasthenia gravis. *Acta Neurol Scand* 2005;112(2):108–14.

40. Shrager JB, Deeb ME, Mick R, et al. Transcervical thymectomy for myasthenia gravis achieves results comparable to thymectomy by sternotomy. *Ann Thorac Surg* 2002;74(2):320–6; discussion 326–7.

41. Tomulescu V, Ion V, Kosa A, et al. Thoracoscopic thymectomy mid-term results. *Ann Thorac Surg* 2006; 82(3):1003–7.

79

Guillain-Barré Syndrome

Rossetti Emanuele and Valzani Yvonne

ABSTRACT

Acute polyradiculoneuritis in children may lead to acute respiratory failure and paediatric intensive care unit (PICU) admission. Non-invasive as well as invasive ventilation have been exploited to support respiratory function and weaning-off mechanical ventilation (MV) results in a challenge among these critically ill paediatric patients.

KEYWORDS

Polyradiculoneuritis; Guillain-Barré syndrome (GBS); critical care; invasive ventilation; respiratory care; immunoglobulin; plasmapheresis; paediatric; neurally adjusted ventilatory assist (NAVA).

CASE STUDY

A 6-year-old child reported with Miller–Fisher Syndrome (MFS), a variant of Guillain-Barré syndrome (GBS), due to an Epstein–Barr virus (EBV) infection. After 3 days of fever with cervical lympho-adenomegaly, he complained of diplopia, inappetence, aphonia, and urine incontinence. On day 4, he suddenly fainted due to worsening dysfunction of the autonomic nervous system, and thus required invasive mechanical respiratory support and paediatric intensive care unit (PICU) admission.

In the meanwhile, diagnostic blood and cerebrospinal fluid (CSF) samples were examined, and afterwards cerebral magnetic resonance imaging (MRI) and electromyography (EMG) were performed, and prompt immunoglobulin bolus treatment was assessed, according to international guidelines for acute polyradiculoneuritis management.[1] Hence, in order to provide fast-track weaning-off the mechanical ventilation (MV) and on having a previous experience in paediatric polyradiculoneuritis,[2] the patient was started early on neurally adjusted ventilatory assist (NAVA) on day 3 after PICU admission.

After NAVA catheter was placed, the diaphragmatic electrical activity was less than 0.5 microVolt (μV), and therefore the NAVA level was set at 1.5 cm $H_2O/\mu V$ that corresponded to pressure support (PS) 18 cmH_2O; and the positive end-expiratory pressure (PEEP) was set at 5 cmH_2O. With NAVA, the patient seemed well-synchronized with MV, being calm and collaborative despite midazolam infusion tapering. He maintained stable arterial blood gases (ABGs) progressively and no atelectasis developed. The NAVA led to weaning off invasive MV in 4 days with a NAVA level of 0.5 due to diaphragm electrical activity (Eadi) of 1.8 μV, hence starting non-invasive ventilation (NIV) with helmet interface for the following 5 days.

Finally, the child was discharged to the neuro-rehabilitative ward on day 10 after admission. To date, after intensive rehabilitation efforts, the child is again attending gym time at school.

INTRODUCTION

The Guillain-Barré syndrome (GBS) is the most common cause of flaccid paralysis in children since poliomyelitis has been eradicated, with incidence ranging from 0.5–1.5 cases per 100,000 children. Male children are affected more than female children. The peak age of incidence is from 4 to 8 years, and it affects children younger than 1 year rarely.

HISTORY

In 1859, Jean Landry first described a form of acute ascending polyneuropathy.[3] In 1916, Georges Guillain Jean Alexandre Barrè and Andrè Strohl recognized the main diagnostic aberration of the disease in the albumin–cytological dissociation in CSF.[4] In 1978, plasma exchange was applied for the first time and its benefits demonstrated in 1985; thus in 1988 intravenous (IV) immunoglobulins (IVIG) were introduced.[5]

DEFINITION

Guillain-Barrè syndrome is an acute autoimmune demyelinating polyneuropathy that involves the peripheral nervous system (autonomic, motor, and sensory). Usually the demyelinating process is symmetrical and ascending, clinically resulting in weakness and areflexia of the inferior limbs before the upper limbs and in some cases of the cranial nerves and develops over a few hours to days and weeks. These features are not pathognomonic of the disease and they can underlie different polyneuropathies.

AETIOLOGY AND PATHOGENESIS

The GBS is mostly preceded by a respiratory or gastrointestinal illness. Virus and bacteria generally involved are:

- Epstein–Barr virus
- Cytomegalovirus
- Hepatitis E virus (HEV)
- Varicella–Zoster virus
- *Campylobacter jejuni*
- Human immunodeficiency virus
- *Mycoplasma pneumoniae*
- Japanese Encephalitis virus (JEV)
- *Plasmodium falciparum*
- *Haemophilus influenzae*

In some cases GBS can develop following vaccines (influenza vaccination, hepatitis B, typhoid, and tetanus) or minor surgery. Cross-reaction between endogenous myelin and ganglioside antigens and the constituents of bacteria or virus determines an abnormal T cell and macrophage response directly against peripheral nerve fibres with production of antibodies against myelin by B cell.[6]

DIAGNOSTIC CRITERIA

The early diagnosis of GBS is the cornerstone of successful care of patients. Strict monitoring is essential in patients with suspicion of GBS. After the diagnosis is made, it is mandatory to begin proper treatment as soon as possible, namely plasma-exchange and, if necessary, intravenous immunoglobulin. In fact, it has been reported that prompt treatment can improve the outcome of patients affected by GBS and, in some cases, it may prevent life-threatening events such as respiratory arrest and life-threatening arrhythmias.

Several diagnostic criteria have been proposed that detect GBS early. The Brighton Collaboration—a scientific international board sponsored by the World Health Organization—has revised the most recent criteria[7] (Table 79.1).

Bilateral and flaccid weakness of limbs, decreased or absent deep tendon reflex (DTR) in weak limbs, monophasic course with time between onset—nadir 12 hours to 28 days and absence of alternative diagnosis for weakness are the diagnostic criteria associated with the highest level of diagnostic certainty.[8]

Nevertheless in 2011, Yuki N, et al.[9] found that in patients affected by GBS, DTRs could be normal or hyperexcitable during the entire clinical course. The DTR

Table 79.1 Brighton criteria for Guillain-Barré syndrome

Diagnostic criteria	Level of diagnostic certainty			
	1	2	3	4
Bilateral and flaccid weakness of limbs	+	+	+	+/−
Decreased or absent deep tendon reflexes in weak limbs	+	+	+	+/−
Monophasic course and time between onset-nadir 12 h to 28 days	+	+	+	+/−
CSF cell count <50/µl	+	+*	−	+/−
CSF protein concentration > normal value	+	+/−*	−	+/−
NCS findings consistent with one of the subtypes of GBS	+	+/−	−	+/−
Absence of alternative diagnosis for weakness	+	+	+	+

+, present; −, absent; +/−, present or absent; NCS, nerve conduction studies.

*If CSF is not collected or results not available, nerve electrophysiology results must be consistent with the diagnosis of Guillain-Barré syndrome. Level 1 is the highest level of diagnostic certainty, level 4 is the lowest level of diagnostic certainty. Reproduced with permission from Oxford University Press © Fokke, C. *et al. Brain* 137, 33–43 (2014).
Reproduced with permission from: Fokke C, van den Berg B, Drenthen J, Walgaard C, van Doorn PA, Jacobs BC. Diagnosis of Guillain-Barré syndrome and validation of Brighton criteria. *Brain* 2014 Jan;137 (Pt 1):33–43. doi:10.1093/brain/awt285. Epub 2013 Oct 26.

response should be considered in the diagnostic criteria for GBS to avoid deferment in the management.[10]

VARIANTS

The GBS may be sub-classified into several forms as per clinical features, aetiology, and pathological and electrophysiological studies.

Among the different variants of GBS, MFS is the commonest. It is marked by the clinical triad of ophthalmoplegia, ataxia, and areflexia. Respiratory involvement and relapses are unusual. Patients with MFS variant exhibit good clinical recovery and have no residual deficits.

These are acute inflammatory demyelinating polyradiculoneuropathy (AIDP); axonal forms of GBS, which include acute motor-sensory axonal neuropathy (AMSAN) and acute motor axonal neuropathy (AMAN). The AMAN is associated with rapidly progressive weakness, often with respiratory failure. Nevertheless, patients affected by AMAN usually show a good outcome. On the other hand, the AMSAN is characterized by poorer prognosis and exhibits slow and incomplete recovery.

DIFFERENTIAL DIAGNOSIS

The exclusion of alternative causes of flaccid paralysis is essential to confirm the diagnosis of GBS. Thus, the principal diseases to exclude are:

* Botulism
* *Cauda equina* and *Conus medullaris* syndromes
* Chronic inflammatory demyelinating polyradiculoneuropathy
* Myasthenia gravis
* Lyme disease
* Multiple sclerosis

Botulism

Clostridium botulinum is a gram-positive, spore-forming anaerobe that is able to produce a neurotoxin. The bacillum naturally inhabits soil, dust, newborn gut, and raw or processed food products. All botulinum toxins are zinc-metalloproteases that bind to different membrane proteins involved in fusion of the synaptic vesicle to the presynaptic membrane. This fusion allows the release of acetylcholine into the synaptic junction. Botulinum toxin inhibits this fusion and thereby the cholinergic transmission causing a functional muscle denervation. The toxin is not able to cross the blood–brain barrier (BBB). Clinically, botulism presents with acute areflexic descending paralysis, with the occasional involvement of cranial nerves. It is associated with gastrointestinal signs and symptoms, more frequently constipation. No biochemical alterations are found in the CSF examination. Diagnosis is made after an accurate medical history and the detection of botulinum toxin in gastric secretion, vomitus, or faeces.

Cauda Equina and Conus Medullaris Syndromes

Both these syndromes manifest with neuromuscular and urogenital symptoms resulting from the simultaneous compression of multiple lumbosacral nerve roots, including low back pain, sciatica (unilateral or, usually bilateral), saddle sensory disturbances, bladder and bowel dysfunction, and a variable lower extremity motor and sensory loss. In children *cauda equina* and *conus medullaris* syndromes are rare and associated to traumatic events, congenital malformation, and neoplasm. Surgical decompression needs to be performed in an emergency, so as to avoid permanent neurological sequelae.

Chronic Inflammatory Demyelinating Polyradiculoneuropathy

This is an autoimmune disease with uncertain aetiology. It presents signs, symptoms, electrophysiological findings, and cytological-albumin dissociation like GBS. In contrast to GBS, steroids are most commonly used for treatment because of proven benefits.

Myasthenia Gravis

It is an autoimmune disorder due to the anti-acetylcholine or, more rarely, the muscle-specific kinase (MuSK) receptor antibodies. Ptosis and ophthalmoplegia represent the onset of generalized myasthenia gravis with a proximal to distal progression.[11,12] Nevertheless, Talebian, et al. reported in 2016 favourable outcomes with the use of IVIG in a 10-year-old girl with bilateral ptosis without ophthalmoplegia and subsequent weakness in the extremities. Due to the patient's initial eyelid elevators, myasthenia gravis was ruled out by a Tensilon test and electrophysiological studies. The results of this case divulge the likelihood of isolated ptosis without ophthalmoplegia in GBS.

Lyme Disease

It is caused by a spirochete, *Borrelia burgdorferi*, carried by tick. Neurological symptoms (weakness, flaccid paralysis, and headache) are associated with a distinctive circular rash at the site of the tick bite, usually around 3 to 30 days after the bite. This is known as *erythema migrans*.

The rash appears like a bull's eye on a dartboard, with redness of the affected region of the skin and raised edges (Figure 79.1).[13]

Multiple Sclerosis

A family history of multiple sclerosis, weakness, and optic neuritis should address towards this diagnosis. Confirmation tests are elevated IgG index and oligoclonal bands in CSF and findings in MRI.[14]

SPECIFIC THERAPIES

Corticosteroids

Corticosteroids administration is not proven effective in the treatment of GBS. In January 2016 Hughes, et al. revisited all randomized controlled trials (RCTs) on corticosteroid or adrenocorticotrophic hormone versus placebo in GBS. Variation in disability grade on a 7-point scale at four weeks constituted the primary end-point. Whereas, time from recruitment to recovery of unaided walking and weaning from MV, death, and disability after 1 year and relapse or side effects were the secondary outcomes.

Hughes, et al. found that monotherapy of corticosteroids had insignificant effect on recovery from GBS or long-term outcomes. There was a very low quality evidence to suggest that oral corticosteroids delayed recovery. Furthermore, a high incidence of metasteroid diabetes requiring insulin was found with high quality evidence.[15]

Conversely, steroids can be used for pain relief in children with GBS. Kajimoto M, et al. reported a case of a 10-year-old child affected by GBS. Despite improvement in muscle weakness, he complained of severe needle-like pain in the thighs and buttocks and also painful numbness over the gastrocnemius regions. Acetaminophen and hydroxyzine was not useful, whereas oral administration of prednisolone 0.7 mg/kg/day resulted in significant pain decrease and recovery from muscle weakness.[16]

Plasma Exchange

Plasma exchange (PE) removes and dilutes the humoral antibodies implicated in the pathogenesis of GBS. PE is a well-established modality of treatment in a variety of neurological, haematological, renal, and autoimmune diseases. Plasma exchange has been proven to be safe and effective in adults. However, it is not used in children owing to lack of acceptability and technical issues including difficulty in establishing vascular access, low blood volume, numerous procedural side effects, and poor patient cooperation. Furthermore, dysautonomic alteration in GBS can compromise the application of PE.

Maitrey Gajjar, et al.[17] conducted a study in the Department of Transfusion Medicine of a tertiary care teaching hospital, the Medical College and Civil Hospital of Gujarat, India between January 2013 and July 2014. This study involved both male and female patients from 3 to 15 years of age. A total of 122 therapeutic PE procedures (with an average of the three procedures per patient) were performed on 40 paediatric patients. Among 40 patients, 18 patients showed significant clinical improvement and 3 patients did not show any improvement and were shifted to IVIG therapy when they failed to respond to PE. Complication was seen in 26 patients and minor complications were observed in 14 patients (hypotension, symptomatic hypocalcaemia, allergic reactions, and catheter-related adverse effects).

It was found that therapeutic PE can be performed safely in paediatric patients with GBS and has been shown to be effective: it shortens the course of hospitalization and reduces the mortality and incidence of permanent paralysis.

Sanem Eren Akarcan published a case report in 2016. A 7-month-old boy was brought to the PICU with chief complaints of progressive muscle weakness, feeding difficulty, and constipation since 10 days. He was administered IVIG and PE therapy, which resulted in complete recovery. It was thus suggested that PE may be a safe alternative in infants with GBS.[18]

It is not clear how many sessions of PE are necessary in GBS. Raphael JC, et al. in 2002 found that in mild GBS, two sessions of PE are significantly superior to none. In moderate GBS, four sessions showed better results than two sessions. In severe GBS, six sessions of PE were non-superior to four sessions. Continuous flow PE machines may be superior to intermittent flow machines and albumin to fresh frozen plasma (FFP) as the exchange fluid. Early onset of PE therapy (within 7 days of disease onset) was more beneficial, however, therapy remained effective if initiated within 30 days of disease.[19]

Intravenous Immunoglobulin

Administration of IVIGs represents the replacement therapy in inflammatory and autoimmune diseases. The IVIG treatment is safer and less traumatic for children in comparison to PE. In addition, PE is not available in all centres. Nevertheless, there is no evidence that IVIG or the combination of IVIG and PE is equivalent or superior to PE.

Saad K, et al. led a retrospective study of children diagnosed with GBS who were admitted to the Assiut University Children's Hospital from January 2010 to October 2014. Before 2011, PE was not available at the hospital, so treatment for GBS consisted mainly of IVIG in a dose of 0.4 g/kg/day for 5 consecutive days. From 2011, PE was available and it was applied to the protocol of the North American trial [Guillain–Barré Syndrome Study Group, 1985] in which a total of 200–250 ml/kg is exchanged over 7–10 days. The authors found that the mean duration of hospital stay and the need for MV in patients treated with PE were significantly lower than in cases treated with IVIG.[20]

El-Bayoumi, et al. compared the outcome of intravenous immunoglobulin and PE treatment in children with GBS requiring MV. They found that PE is superior to IVIG regarding the duration of MV, but not PICU stay or the short-term neurological outcome.[21]

Conversely, Shanbag P, et al. in 2003 collected data from 25 children admitted to the PICU with a diagnosis of GBS, treated with IVIG at a dose of 2 g/kg body weight over 2–5 days and it was shown that early initiation of IVIG could decrease mortality and the requirement for intubation and MV.[22]

The IVIG treatment should not be used in patients with congenital IgA deficiency, hyperviscosity syndrome, and congestive heart failure. In this setting of patients, PE represents the treatment of choice.[23]

INTENSIVE CARE ADMISSION

In order to evaluate the severity of illness, five grades for GBS were defined:[24]

- Grade 1:
  - Force of distal lower extremities 3/5
  - Force of proximal lower extremities 4/5
  - DTR of lower extremities decreased
  - DTR of upper extremities normal
  - Gag reflex, crying, phonation, and swallowing normal
- Grade 2:
  - Force of distal lower extremities 3/5
  - Force of proximal lower extremities 3/5
  - Force of distal upper extremities 4/5
  - Force of proximal upper extremities 4/5
  - DTR of upper and lower extremities decreased (especially in lower extremities)
  - Gag reflex, crying, phonation, and swallowing normal
- Grade 3:

- Force of proximal lower extremities 3/5
- Force of distal lower extremities 2/5
- Force of proximal upper extremities 4/5
- Force of distal upper extremities 3/5
- DTR of upper extremities decreased
- DTR of lower extremities decreased or absent
- Gag reflex decreased, crying, and phonation weak, and swallowing normal
- Grade 4:
  - Complete flaccid paralysis in lower extremities
  - Force of distal upper extremities below 2/5
  - Force of proximal upper extremities below 3/5
  - DTR of lower extremities absent
  - Gag reflex decreased, crying weak
  - Mechanical ventilation needed during hospital stay
- Grade 5:
  - Complete flaccid paralysis in upper and lower extremities (flaccid quadriplegic)
  - DTR of upper and lower extremities absent
  - Gag reflex absent
  - Aphonic, needs immediate mechanical ventilation

Children affected by GBS with a grade of severity major than 3 are at high risk for life-threatening respiratory complications and autonomic disturbances. They should be immediately admitted to the intensive care unit (ICU).

Respiratory Care

Respiratory failure is rarely associated with GBS but is the most common life-threatening complication in this setting of patients. It is derived from bulbar and phrenic demyelinating process. About 15% of children with GBS develop respiratory failure and require supportive mechanical ventilation. For this reason, it is important to develop a score system to determine the risk factors of respiratory failure in children with GBS.

Mei-Hua Hu, et al. conducted a retrospective study to identify the variables that led to respiratory failure in children affected by GBS. This study revealed that the predictors of respiratory failure in childhood GBS were the disability score at nadir (Hughes score superior to 3), respiratory distress, and hypotension. At the point of nadir during admission to the hospital, patients were graded using a disability scale modified from Hughes et al: Grade 0 indicates a normal functional state without neurological deficits; Grade 1 is characterized by minor symptoms or signs, but being able to do manual work; Grades 2 and 3 indicate the presence of ambulation without or with assistance, respectively; Grade 4 indicates that the patient is chair- or bed-bound; Grade 5 is applied when the patient requires a mechanical ventilator; and Grade 6 indicates death.[25]

Need for intubation derived from the inability to cough, a vital capacity (measured volume with forceful exhalation after maximal inhalation) below 20 mL/kg, a PImax (maximum inspiratory pressure generated after maximal sucking in through a mouthpiece while occluding the nose) of less than 30 cmH$_2$O or a PEmax (maximum expiratory pressure generated on maximal blowing out) of less than 40 cmH$_2$O warns of imminent respiratory arrest.

The patient's respiratory drive can be modulated with the recent introduction of NAVA (Servo-i, Maquet, Wayne, New Jersey). The functioning involves simple and minimally invasive measure of the electrical activity of the diaphragm (Edi). It delivers pressure to the airways in linear proportionality to Edi through a constant NAVA level (airway pressure delivered per unit of Edi) adjusted by the clinician. NAVA aids in enhancing patient-ventilator synchrony. There is little evidence substantiating preservation of the phrenic nerve-diaphragm unit in patients with GBS or critical illness-associated polyneuromyopathy. Weaning outcomes may be successfully predicted with EDI-derived indices.[26]

In addition, the NAVA mode could also help to adapt the level of pressure support in patients with GBS who have a significant Edi. In the recent paediatric case of a 2-year-old child with GBS, investigators started NAVA on day 17 post intubation. Prior to NAVA, weaning attempts caused patient-ventilator asynchrony with hypercapnia, tachypnea, and hypoxia. Titration of the pressure support level (NAVA level) was based on monitoring the Edi signal. After the NAVA level had been reduced from 1.4 to 1.0 cmH$_2$O/V, weaning and extubation were successful on day 23. The NAVA allowed reduction of patient-ventilator asynchrony, dissynchrony, and associated waste efforts of the child leading to effective weaning from mechanical ventilation. This was associated with a daily reduction in the NAVA level, lower pressure assist but similar tidal volume. This resulted in a well-tolerated increase in the patient's breath effort and Edi. Therefore, under these circumstances, decrease in neuroventilatory efficiency is not suggestive of decreased efficacy, but rather patient recovery. The measure of Edi could help in estimating the progression of inspiratory efforts during the recovery phase of GBS.

In literature, there is no evidence for NIV in respiratory support of children affected by GBS. Wijdicks, et al. discouraged it because of the need of emergency intubation.[27] Tracheostomy is not routinely used in paediatric patients with GBS, however, it may be used in periods of prolonged mechanical ventilation. A notable study in this context was conducted by Freezer, et al. The group collated data of 59 infants and children with GBS in 10 years. Among the patients, 15 were subjected to tracheostomies.

The median duration of assisted ventilation including endotracheal intubation was 21 days and the median duration of tracheostomy was 39 days. All patients were successfully decannulated at the first attempt. As far as complications were concerned only two patients developed croup. The lung parameters such as lung volumes, and inspiratory and expiratory flows were normal. There were no reports of tracheal stenosis or significant tracheomalacia noted.[28]

Cardiovascular Care

Serious and potentially fatal disturbances of autonomic function, including arrhythmias (tachyarrhythmia to asystole) and extreme hypertension or hypotension occur in approximately 20% of patients with GBS.[29]

Pfeiffer, et al. found that bradycardia was preceded by increased daily systolic blood pressure (SBP) variation (>85 mmHg), which thus proved to be a sensitive and prognostically valuable indicator of dysautonomia in GBS.

It is possible that many other individuals suffering from severe forms of GBS, especially those with significant autonomic dysfunction may actually have undiagnosed and therefore untreated pulmonary hypertension. Therefore, it is recommended that clinicians caring for critically ill children with GBS have a high index of suspicion for pulmonary hypertension and should consider echocardiography if there are clinical signs of this potentially fatal process.[30]

Accurate monitoring of cardiovascular assessment of children and correct use of inotropes, vasopressors, and antihypertensive drugs are fundamental in the management of children affected by GBS.

'FAST HUG'

In 2005, Jean-Louis Vincent proposed a useful protocol (Table 79.2) to be used in the ICU as a checklist to verify the quality of patient care at least once a day. It is a mnemonic (little and symbolic acronym) able to complete the visit to the bedside of the patient.[31]

A distinctive issue of children with GBS is visceral dysautonomia. Gastrointestinal autonomic neuropathy that was accompanied by vomiting and constipation caused by adynamic ileus is common in paediatric patients with GBS. As known, enteral nutrition is always to be

Table 79.2 FAST HUG approach

Feeding	Can the patient be fed orally, if not enterally? If not, should we start parenteral feeding?
Analgesia	The patient should not suffer pain, but excessive analgesia should be avoided
Sedation	The patient should not experience discomfort, but excessive sedation should be avoided; 'calm, comfortable, collaborative' is typically the best level
Thromboembolic prevention	Should we give low-molecular-weight heparin or use mechanical adjuncts?
Head of the bed elevated	Optimally, 30° to 45°, unless contraindications
Stress ulcer prophylaxis	Usually H2 antagonists; sometimes proton pump inhibitors
Glucose control	Within limits defined in each ICU

Source: Vincent J-L. Give your patient a fast hug (at least) once a day. *Crit Care Med* 2005 Jun;33(6):1225–9.

preferred to inhabit the bowel thereby reducing bacterial translocation to the bloodstream. If enteral nutrition is not feasible, parenteral nutrition should be started. Impaired feeding is the cause of weaning failure, long mechanical ventilation time, and pneumonia.

PROGNOSIS

Guillain-Barré Syndrome presents a good prognosis, especially in children. However ~25% of patients require artificial ventilation and 20% are still unable to walk unaided after 6 months.[32] In a study by Lee, et al., advancing age, diarrhoea, higher disability rate at the time of presentation, and mechanical ventilation compromised prognostic outcomes. The relevance of F-wave abnormalities as a prognostic factor was also tested in children with GBS.

The name 'F-wave' is derived from initial recordings performed in the small muscles of the foot. The F-wave represents compound action potential evoked by supramaximal antidromic stimulation of a motor nerve. The F-wave pathway involves antidromic excitation of all stimulated motor axons travelling to the spinal cord with reactivation of a small proportion of the anterior horn cell axon hillocks and orthodromic action potentials of one or more motor axons travelling to the muscle. The F-wave is the most sensitive and reliable nerve conduction study for evaluating polyneuropathy and radiculopathy.

Roodbol, et al. examined the long-term outcome in a group of children treated for GBS at the Sophia Children's

Hospital in Rotterdam from 1987 to 2009. They found that most children show good recovery of neurological deficits after GBS, but many have persisting long-term residual complaints and symptoms that may lead to psychosocial problems interfering with participation in daily life.[33]

CONCLUSIONS

In order to improve paediatric critically ill patients outcome and reduce their PICU length of stay, a multidisciplinary approach is essential to provide prompt treatment and vital function support. A recent novel ventilation technique and neurologic monitoring may lead forward the fall of long- and short-term neurologic complications among these polyradiculoneuritis affected children.

REFERENCES

1. Cortese I, Chaudhry V, So YT, et al. Evidence-based guideline update: plasmapheresis neurologic disorders: report of the Therapeutics and Technology Assessment Subcommittee of the American Academy of Neurology. *Neurology* 2011;76:294–300.
2. Rossetti E, Bianchi R, Picardo S, et al. Neurally adjusted ventilatory assist and Guillain-Barré syndrome in a child. *Minerva Anestesiologica* 2014;80(8):972–3.
3. Landry JB. 'Note sur la paralysie ascendante aiguë'. *Gazette Hebdomadaire de Médecine et de Chirurgie* 1859;6:472–4, 486–8.
4. Guillain G, Barré J, Strohl A. 'Sur un syndrome de radiculonévrite avec hyperalbuminose du liquide céphalo-rachidien sans réaction cellulaire. Remarques sur les caractères cliniques et graphiques des réflexes tendineux'. *Bulletins et mémoires de la Société des Médecins des Hôpitaux de Paris* 1916;40:1462–70.
5. Walgaard C, Jacobs BC, van Doorn PA. Emerging drugs for Guillain-Barré syndrome. *Expert Opinion on Emerging Drugs* 2011 March;16(1):105–20.
6. Desai J, Ramos-Platt L, Mitchell WG. Treatment of paediatric chronic inflammatory demyelinating polyneuropathy: Challenges, controversies and questions. *Ann Indian Acad Neurol* 2015;18(3):327–30.
7. Fokke C, van den Berg B, Drenthen J, Walgaard C, van Doorn PA, Jacobs BC. Diagnosis of Guillain-Barré syndrome and validation of Brighton criteria. *Brain* 2014 Jan;137(Pt 1):33–43.
8. Avila-Funes JA, Mariona-Montero VA, Melano-Carranza E. Guillain-Barre syndrome: etiology and pathogenesis. *Rev Invest Clin* 2002 Jul–Aug;54(4):357–63.
9. Yuki N, Kokubun N, Kuwabara S. Guillain-Barré syndrome associated with normal or exaggerated tendon reflexes. *J Neurol* 2012 Jun;259(6):1181–90. 2011 Dec 6.

10. Eung-Bin Lee, Yun Young Lee, Jae Min Lee, et al. Clinical importance of F-waves as a prognostic factor in Guillain-Barré syndrome in children. *Korean J Pediatr* 2016;59(6): 271–5.

11. van der Pluym J, Vajsar J, Jacob FD, et al. Clinical characteristics of pediatric myasthenia: a surveillance study. *Pediatrics* 2013 Oct;132(4):e939–44.

12. Chaudhuri Z, Pandey PK, Bhomaj S, Chauhan D, Rani LU. Childhood myasthenia gravis in an infant. *Br J Ophthalmol* 2002 Jun;86(6):704–5.

13. Sood SK. Lyme disease in children. *Infect Dis Clin North Am* 2015 Jun;29(2):281–94.

14. Patel Y, Bhise V, Krupp L. Pediatric multiple sclerosis. *Ann Indian Acad Neurol* 2009 Oct;12(4):238–45.

15. Hughes RAC, Brassington R, Gunn AA, et al. Corticosteroids for Guillain-Barré syndrome. *Cochrane Database Syst Rev*. 2016 Oct 24;10:CD001446.

16. Kajimto M, Koga M, Narumi H, et al. Successful control of radicular pain in a pediatric patient with Guillain–Barré syndrome. *Brain* 2015;37(9):897–900.

17. Gajjar M, Patel T, Bhatnagar N, Solanki M, Patel V, Soni S. Therapeutic plasma exchange in paediatric patients of Guillain–Barre syndrome: Experience from a tertiary care centre. *Asian Journal of Transfusion* 2016;10(1):98–100.

18. Akarcan SE, İşgüder a R, Yilmaz U, et al. Guillain–Barre syndrome in a 7-month-old boy successfully applied plasma exchange transfusion and apheresis. *Science* 2016;54:139–43.

19. Raphaël JC, Chevret S, Hughes RA, Annane D. Plasma exchange for Guillain-Barré syndrome. *Cochrane Database Syst Rev*. 2002;(2):CD001798.

20. Saad K, Mohamad IL, Abd El-Hamed MA, et al. A comparison between plasmapheresis and intravenous immunoglobulin in children with Guillain-Barré syndrome in Upper Egypt. *Ther Adv Neurol Disord* 2016;9(1):3–8.

21. El-Bayoumi, El-Refaey AM, Abdelkader AM, et al. Comparison of intravenous immunoglobulin and plasma exchange in treatment of mechanically ventilated children with Guillain Barré syndrome: a randomized study. *Critical Care* 2011;15:R164.

22. Shanbag P, Amirtharaj C, Pathak A. Intravenous immunoglobulins in severe Guillian-Barre syndrome in childhood. *Indian J Pediatr* 2003 Jul;70(7):541–3.

23. Karimzadeh P. High and low dose intravenous immunoglobulin therapy in Guillain-Barre syndrome children: a comparison. *Iran J Child Neurology* June 2006;1(1):23–31.

24. Sladky JT. Guillain-Barre syndrome in children. *J Child Neurol* 2004;19:191–200.

25. Mei-Hua Hu, Chiung-Mei Chen, Kuang-Lin Lin, et al. Risk factors of respiratory failure in children with Guillain-Barré syndrome. *Pediatrics and Neonatology* 2012;53:295e–299.

26. Dugernier J, Bialais E, Reychler G, Vinetti M, Hantson P. Neurally adjusted ventilatory assist during weaning from respiratory support in a case of Guillain-Barré syndrome. *Respir Care* 2015 Apr;60(4):e68–72.

27. Wijdiks, Roy TK. BiPAP in early Guillain-Barre syndrome may fail. *Can J Neurol Sci* 2006;33(1):105–6.

28. Freezer NJ, Robertson CF. Tracheostomy in children with Guillain-Barre syndrome. *Crit Care Med* 1990 Nov;18(11):1236–8.

29. Pfeiffer G, Schiller B, Kruse J, et al. Indicators of dysautonomia in severe Guillain-Barré syndrome. *J Neurol* 1999 Nov;246(11):1015–22.

30. Rooney KA, Thomas NJ. Severe pulmonary hypertension associated with the acute motor sensory axonal neuropathy subtype of Guillain-Barré syndrome. *Pediatr Crit Care Med* 2010 Jan;11(1):e16–9.

31. Vincent J-L. Give your patient a fast hug (at least) once a day. *Crit Care Med* 2005;33(6):1225–9.

32. van Doorn PA, Kuitwaard K, Walgaard C, et al. IVIG treatment and prognosis in Guillain-Barré syndrome. *J Clin Immunol* 2010;30(Suppl 1):S74–8.

33. Roodbol J, de Wit MC, Aarsen FK. Long-term outcome of Guillain-Barré syndrome in children. *J Peripher Nerv Syst* 2014 Jun;19(2):121–6.

80

Cerebral Hyperperfusion Syndrome

M. S. Tandon and M. U. Sharma

ABSTRACT

Cerebral hyperperfusion syndrome (CHS) is an infrequent, but potentially catastrophic complication of cerebral revascularization procedures, such as carotid artery endarterectomy or stenting. It is also known to occur after resection/embolization of cerebral vascular malformations, e.g., arteriovenous and Galen vein malformation. In this condition, rapid restoration or a sudden increase in cerebral perfusion to an area of the brain which was previously chronically hypoperfused and has a 'pressure passive circulation', leads to sudden hyperaemia, and consequently, an increased risk of cerebral oedema, swelling, and/or intracerebral haemorrhage (ICH). Clinical symptoms range from headache, seizures, neurological deficits (e.g., aphasia, hemiparesis), to acute neurological deterioration. Hypertension is common and plays an important role in the occurrence of ICH as well as in aggravating the neurologic injury. Brain imaging, perfusion imaging, and vascular imaging techniques help to confirm the diagnosis. Early recognition of this condition along with aggressive management of hypertension and elevated cerebral perfusion pressures (CPPs) are critical to the clinical outcome; while cerebral swelling and oedema are potentially reversible with aggressive management, occurrence of ICH often heralds a grim prognosis.

KEYWORDS

Cerebral hyperperfusion syndrome (CHS); reperfusion syndrome; hyperperfusion; reperfusion; carotid artery stenting; carotid endarterectomy; cerebral blood flow (CBF); normal perfusion pressure breakthrough (NPPB); venous occlusion hyperaemia; transcranial Doppler (TCD); arteriovenous malformation; intracerebral haemorrhage (ICH); cerebral oedema.

CASE STUDY

A 76-year-old man was transferred to the neurointensive care unit (NICU) after undergoing an uneventful left internal carotid artery (ICA) angioplasty and stenting for severe left proximal ICA stenosis. He had a history of multiple transient ischaemic attacks (TIAs) in the preceding six months, and hypertension and dyslipidaemia for the past 10 years. His medications included metoprolol (100 mg OD), amlodipine (5 mg OD), atorvastatin (20 mg OD) for the past 10 years; and aspirin (75 mg OD) with clopidogrel (75 mg OD) for the past 6 months. Preoperative magnetic resonance imaging (MRI) showed multiple old infarctions in the bilateral parieto-occipital junctions and left internal border zone area. Magnetic resonance angiography (MRA) showed severe bilateral ICA stenosis (95% in right ICA, 85% in left ICA).

On arrival in the NICU, he was awake, alert, had stable vital parameters (heart rate 84/min, invasive blood pressure (BP) 144/96 mmHg, respiratory rate 14 breaths/min, oxygen saturation (SpO_2) 99%), and a normal neurological examination. However, 12 hours later, he became restless and complained of severe throbbing headache on the left side of his head. His BP was 200/110 mmHg; labetolol boluses (20 mg IV) were administered. Shortly thereafter, he had focal seizures in the left arm, became aphasic and developed right-sided paresis. He subsequently required an emergent endotracheal intubation because of deterioration in his mental status and an inability to maintain his airway.

An urgent computed tomography (CT) scan revealed a 9-mm midline shift; left frontal, parietal, and occipital hypodensities, predominantly in the white matter; and sulcal effacement of the overlying cortex along with some cortical hyperdensities which were suggestive of petechial haemorrhages. Transcranial Doppler (TCD) sonography revealed a marked increase in the mean flow velocity (MFV) of the left middle cerebral artery (MCA) (post-intervention 178 cm/sec; pre-intervention 42 cm/sec). A colour Doppler ultrasound of the left common carotid artery and left ICA revealed visibly patent vessels. Subsequent axial T2-weighted MRI showed diffuse oedema of the left hemisphere; perfusion-weighted MRI imaging (PWI) showed hyperperfusion of the left hemisphere. Absence of hyperintensities in the left cerebral hemisphere on diffusion weighted MRI imaging (DWI) ruled out an acute cerebral infarction and was suggestive of vasogenic oedema.

A diagnosis of cerebral hyperperfusion syndrome (CHS) was made. Aggressive antihypertensive (labetolol, nicardipine), antiepileptic (phenytoin), and cerebral decongestant (mannitol, furosemide, and hyperventilation) measures were initiated. Four days later, MCA-MFV was 92 cms/sec and a repeat CT scan showed a decrease in the oedema. The patient showed neurological improvement and was discharged three weeks later with a mild hemiparesis.

INTRODUCTION

Cerebral hyperperfusion syndrome is an uncommon, but potentially catastrophic complication of cerebral revascularization procedures; it can also occur after resection/embolization of cerebral vascular malformations, such as arteriovenous malformation (AVM), and Vein of Galen malformation.[1–4] It is characterized by acute cerebral hyperaemia (due to either rapid restoration or a sudden increase in cerebral perfusion) in an area of the brain, which has been chronically hypoperfused, has severely impaired vasoreactivity and a 'pressure passive' circulation.[3] The consequent reperfusion injury results in cerebral oedema, swelling, and/or intracerebral haemorrhage (ICH). While the cerebral oedema is potentially reversible with aggressive management, occurrence of ICH heralds a grim prognosis; hence, early recognition of this condition is critical. Strict control of BP can limit the rise in cerebral perfusion pressure (CPP) and prevent ICH, and hence forms the cornerstone of both prevention and management of CHS.[3,4]

CEREBRAL HYPERPERFUSION SYNDROME AFTER CEREBRAL REVASCULARIZATION PROCEDURES

This syndrome was initially reported in patients undergoing carotid endarterectomy (CAE); it is now a well-recognized complication of several surgical and endovascular cerebral revascularization procedures, such as carotid and vertebral angioplasty alone or with stenting; clipping or endovascular flow diversion for intracranial aneurysms; aorto-carotid bypass surgery; external carotid artery (ECA)-ICA bypass procedures (e.g., for Moyamoya disease or for giant aneurysms);

and after thrombolytic therapy for acute ischaemic stroke.[1–5] While the guiding principles are relevant for all these mentioned procedures, the following discussion focuses largely on the occurrence of CHS after carotid revascularization.

CEREBRAL HYPERPERFUSION, CEREBRAL HYPERPERFUSION SYNDROME, AND CEREBRAL REPERFUSION SYNDROME

After the cerebral vascularization procedure, there is an almost inevitable increase in perfusion to the revascularized area of the brain. Quantitatively, when the increase in ipsilateral cerebral blood flow (CBF) (on the treated side) is $\geq 100\%$ of preoperative/baseline values, it is termed as 'cerebral hyperperfusion'.[2] The CHS is the clinical manifestation of 'cerebral hyperperfusion' (hence, presence of clinical manifestations is an essential diagnostic criterion for CHS).[3,6] Further, since some patients can become symptomatic at moderate CBF elevations (<100% increase in CBF as compared to baseline/preoperative values), CHS is also referred to as 'reperfusion syndrome'.[7]

Pathophysiology

The exact pathophysiology of CHS is not completely understood, but a combination of factors seem to play a role in its occurrence. The key event is a sudden and significant increase in CBF to a chronically ischaemic cerebral hemisphere, in the setting of an impaired cerebrovascular reserve (due to critical vessel stenosis and poor collateral circulation), a damaged blood–brain barrier (BBB), and an iatrogenic baroreceptor dysfunction; both pre- and post-procedural hypertension play a critical role in the occurrence of ICH and exacerbation of the neurological injury.[6,8]

Chronic hypoperfusion due to high-grade stenosis in a carotid artery induces compensatory vasodilatation of the distal vessels. However, over time, the distal arterioles become maximally dilated and their vasoreactivity becomes impaired. Ultimately, vasomotor paralysis (inability to vasoconstrict/vasodilate in response to alterations in mean arterial pressure [MAP]/CPP) occurs, and the CBF becomes directly dependent on the systemic BP. The dysautoregulation is reportedly mediated by vasodilatory substances, such as nitric oxide, which are produced in response to cerebral ischaemia; nitric oxide (NO) also causes endothelial dysfunction, increases microvascular permeability, and damages the BBB.[9]

Post-revascularization, the sudden restoration/increase in blood flow to the chronically ischaemic region results in a 'flash flood' like situation. Inability of the dilated arterioles to vasoconstrict and protect the capillary bed, with consequent overwhelming of venous return and pooling of blood in the capillary bed, predisposes to vascular engorgement and rupture.[10] In addition, reperfusion-induced oxygen-derived free radical production, complement activation, and cytokine release further aggravate the endothelial damage and microvascular permeability, resulting in vasogenic oedema and breakdown of the BBB.[8,11,12] In fulminant cases, ICH (intracerebral or subarachnoid haemorrhage [SAH]) occurs due to vascular disruption.[3,8,13] Pre-existing hypertensive microangiopathy contributes to dysfunctional BBB, and is associated with a higher likelihood of postoperative hypertension.[8] Refractory post-procedure hypertension is common after carotid revascularization procedures and is mostly attributed to iatrogenic baroreceptor dysfunction/denervation.[8] Postoperatively, an acute rise in BP, in the presence of an impaired cerebrovascular reserve can result in a profound increase in CPP, which increases the risk of ICH, especially in an infarcted or ischaemic area of the brain.[8]

Incidence

While 9%–13% patients develop cerebral hyperperfusion after carotid revascularization procedures, the incidence of CHS and ICH, however, is not very high.[6] Moulakkis, et al. in a review analysis of published series on post-carotid revascularization CHS (between 2003 and 2008), reported a post CAE incidence of CHS and ICH as 1.9% (range 0.4%–14%) and 0.37% (range, 0%–1%), respectively; the incidence of CHS and ICH after carotid artery stenting (CAS) was 1.16% (range, 0.44%–11.7%) and 0.74% (range, 0.36%–4.5%), respectively.[6]

Diagnosis

Cerebral hyperperfusion syndrome should be suspected if a patient develops clinical symptoms suggestive of unilateral focal neurological injury (ipsilateral to the treated side) in the post-procedure period; it is confirmed by diagnostic neuro-imaging that demonstrates the presence of cerebral hyperperfusion and absence of cerebral ischaemia.[6]

Clinical Presentation

Cerebral hyperperfusion syndrome can occur at any time from the immediate revascularization period until up to about a month later, though most patients become symptomatic within the first 5–7 post-intervention days.[3,14] The onset of symptoms tends to be earlier with CAS than after CAE. Ogaswara, et al. reported a peak incidence at 12 hours and 6 days after CAS and CAE, respectively; ICH shows the same pattern with a peak incidence of 1.7 ± 2.1 days after CAS and 10.7 ± 9.9 days after CEA.[15]

The clinical presentation is a manifestation of the underlying pathologies, cerebral oedema and, in severe cases, ICH. It includes a spectrum of clinical symptoms ranging from the classical triad of ipsilateral headache, ipsilateral seizures and focal neurological deficits, to confusion, nausea and vomiting, and in fulminant cases, loss of consciousness, and even death.[3,16,17]

Ipsilateral headaches in temporal, frontal, or retro-orbital regions are usually the heralding sign, and sometimes, the only clinical manifestation of CHS. They are generally severe, with a throbbing migraine-like character, though they can be mild or intermittent, in addition; the headaches tend to improve when the patient is made to sit upright.[3] Seizures are usually focal, but can become generalized. Neurological deficits can vary; cortical deficits, e.g., visual, motor deficits, aphasia, hemiplegia, and hemianopia are most common, though psychotic alterations and/or long-term cognitive deficits have also been reported. Post-procedural hypertension is another significant (though not essential) feature, which is observed in most of the symptomatic patients, especially those who develop ICH.[3,6,14,18]

Intracerebral haemorrhage is the most feared complication with a mortality and morbidity of 50% and 30%, respectively.[8] A special condition called 'Hyperacute ICH' has been reported after CAS. It typically manifests as a basal ganglia bleed, within a few hours of the procedure (usually 8 minutes to 8 hours), and often without any prodromal symptoms. Its mortality is very high and affected patients usually have high-grade vessel stenosis along with microangiopathy.[6]

Differential Diagnosis

An important diagnostic dilemma in patients who develop a new onset, post-procedure neurological deficit or neurological deterioration after a carotid revascularization procedure is whether it is due to CHS, an intracranial haematoma, or an ischaemic stroke/TIA (due to vascular occlusion, restenosis, or thromboembolism). A combination of transient neurological deficits, seizures, and altered consciousness usually favours the diagnosis of CHS. Brain imaging, perfusion imaging, and vascular imaging techniques help to confirm the diagnosis.[6,7,14,18]

Investigations

Confirmatory investigations for CHS include brain imaging (CT/MRI scan), perfusion imaging [DWI, PWI, TCD, single-photon emission computed tomography (SPECT), perfusion CT imaging (Xenon-enhanced CT and CT perfusion scans)], and vascular imaging [carotid Doppler ultrasound, duplex scan, digital subtraction angiography (DSA)].[6,7,14,18]

Conventional CT scan findings are highly suggestive of, but not pathognomonic for CHS. Nevertheless, a CT scan is still useful, considering that it is the initial investigation for most of the neurological events that occur in the post-intervention period; it detects haemorrhage and also provides clues that help to exclude an ischaemic aetiology. In CHS, it may reveal ipsilateral, sulcal effacement, diffuse or patchy white matter oedema, mass effect, and petechial haemorrhages. Findings from CT are usually normal after a TIA and are often normal within hours after a stroke, while MRI findings show white matter oedema, focal infarction, and local or massive haemorrhage. However, normal findings on CT or MRI scan do not conclusively exclude the presence of CHS. Hyperacute ischaemic lesions may be ruled out using DWI.[7]

Hyperperfusion can be assessed with perfusion imaging techniques. A TCD measures CBF velocities (peak systolic velocity, end-diastolic velocity, MFV, pulsatility index [PI]) and provides real-time information about CBF. A >100% increase in post-revascularization MCA flow velocities as compared to preoperative/baseline values is indicative of cerebral hyperperfusion.[6] Being a non-invasive, bedside, and easily reproducible technique, it is very widely used to predict, diagnose, and monitor the course of CHS in the ICU.[18] Methods such as SPECT, PWI, and perfusion CT imaging reveal markedly increased perfusion in the ipsilateral hemisphere, as compared with the baseline or the contralateral hemisphere; measurement of 'relative inter-hemispheric differences' in CBF enables a quantitative assessment of perfusion differences between cerebral hemispheres.[14]

In addition, a duplex scan/carotid Doppler/DSA is required for ruling out vascular restenosis, thrombotic occlusion or thromboembolism; in CHS, the vessels are patent.

Risk Factors

Several factors predispose to the development of CHS after a cerebral revascularization procedure (Table 80.1), the most critical of these, probably, is an impaired cerebrovascular reserve.[3,6,16–18] Severity of dysautoregulation is usually proportional to the duration and degree of regional cerebral hypoperfusion; this in turn is largely determined by a combination of two factors—severity of ipsilateral vascular stenosis (>90%) and the extent of collateral flow (Table 80.1). An elevated post-procedure BP is also a very significant risk factor for development of both CHS and ICH.[14–16,18] Bourri, et al. reported an 81% incidence of ICH in patients who

Table 80.1 Risk factors for cerebral hyperperfusion syndrome

Preoperative factors	Impaired cerebral vasoreactivity: Critical ipsilateral ICA stenosis (>90%) or occlusion in conjunction with a poor collateral flow (e.g., severe contralateral carotid stenosis/occlusion, advanced occlusive disease in other extracranial cerebral vessels, incomplete circle of Willis) Microangiopathy (e.g., due to chronic hypertension, diabetes mellitus) with insufficient intracranial collateralization Age >75 yrs Female sex Recent contralateral CEA or carotid puncture (within the past 3 months) Recent stroke or ischaemia
Intraoperative factors	Distal carotid artery stump pressure of <40 mmHg Intraoperative ischaemia (e.g., prolonged ICA clamp) Peri-procedural cerebral infarction High doses of volatile halogenated hydrocarbon anaesthetics Markedly increased cerebral perfusion (MCA flow velocity or pulsatility) after flow restoration
Postoperative factors	Postoperative hypertension Administration of anticoagulants or antiplatelet agents

had a post-operative systolic blood pressure (SBP) >180 mmHg.[14] Other important risk factors include advanced age, recent stroke, and/or ischaemia, brief interval between ischaemic symptoms, and revascularization, recent procedure on the contralateral vessel, and microangiopathy due to chronic hypertension, and/or diabetes mellitus. While some studies report an increased incidence of CHS with the use of antiplatelet agents or other anticoagulants, the available evidence, however, is rather inconclusive.[13] Analysis through TCD, SPECT, and MRI (PWI, T2 flair images) can help in identifying patients who have a high risk of developing postoperative CHS.[6,8,17]

On TCD evaluation, a >150% increase in the MCA-MFV compared with preoperative levels, and/or a significant increase in mean ICA volume flow (MICAVF) have a high predictive accuracy for the occurrence of CHS.[6,8] Preoperatively, a significant reduction in the mean flow MCA velocity compared with baseline values indicates hypoperfusion, and is associated with high risk of postoperative hyperperfusion.[19] Preoperative SPECT reveals a characteristic diffuse asymmetric pattern of ipsilateral reduced CBF; postoperatively, ipsilateral hyperperfusion lasting for at least three days predisposes to development of CHS.[20] The presence of cerebral microbleeds (latent vascular damage) on a preoperative MRI is also predictive of CHS.

Evaluating the cerebral vasoreactivity through TCD, SPECT, Xenon CT, and MR perfusion imaging can be done by assessing the CBF variation in response to hypercarbia. In a normal person, induction of hypercarbia by breath-holding, carbon dioxide (CO_2) inhalation or administration of acetazolamide causes cerebral vasodilatation, and consequently, a rapid increase in CBF. Reduced (<20%), absent, or even reversed preoperative vasoreactivity is predictive of postoperative hyperperfusion and CHS.[3,8,12]

Management

Cerebral hyperperfusion syndrome is potentially reversible in its early stages; however, occurrence of ICH can be fatal. Hence, early recognition is important so that prompt measures can be taken before cerebral oedema or ICH occurs. Vigilant monitoring of invasive BP and strict regulation of BP should be ensured, especially in high-risk patients. If CHS occurs, the goal is to aggressively control the BP to prevent a further increase in the CBF, and effectively manage cerebral oedema and seizures. A management strategy is shown in Figure 80.1.

Meticulous BP control forms the cornerstone of prevention and management of CHS, however, there are no definitive guidelines regarding the target BP, what drugs to use, and for how long the BP needs to be controlled.[14] Bouri, et al. performed a systematic review to evaluate the efficacy of BP control in preventing CHS after CEA; they reported that while a postoperative SBP >150 mmHg was associated with an increase in the cumulative incidence of CHS and ICH, there were no documented cases of CHS at SBP <135 mmHg.[14] Abou-Chebl, et al. reported a decrease in incidence of CHS and ICH following CAS, when BP was maintained below 140/90 mmHg and 120/80 mmHg in lower risk and high risk patients, respectively.[18] Several other studies also report markedly decreased odds for ICH when target SBP is maintained at <140–160 mmHg or at <20% of preoperative values.[15]

Several antihypertensive drugs have been used for CHS, however, there are no randomized controlled trials recommending use of a specific drug for optimal BP control. Labetalol, α1, β1, and β2-adrenergic antagonist decreases MAP and CPP without directly altering the CBF. Beta blockers such as esmolol and metoprolol reduce BP and have little effect on intracranial pressure (ICP) within the autoregulatory range, though they may exacerbate bradycardia that can occur after CAS. Clonidine, an alpha-2 adrenergic agonist with central sympatholytic effects has the distinct advantage of decreasing CBF, and is commonly used after CEA (associated with raised cranial and plasma catecholamine concentrations).[8] These drugs are probably preferable to vasodilatory antihypertensive agents such as calcium channel blockers, sodium nitroprusside, glycerol trinitrate, and angiotensin II inhibitors, which can increase CBF and can potentially worsen CHS. However, most importantly, close monitoring and prompt titration of BP is probably the key consideration, rather than a specific choice of an antihypertensive agent.

Strict BP control must be maintained until cerebral autoregulation is restored; TCD can assess recovery of vasoreactivity and guide antihypertensive therapy. Since CHS can occur until up to a month after the intervention, BP monitoring is strongly recommended for at least two weeks after the procedure.

Cerebral oedema should be aggressively treated (Table 80.2); seizures are controlled with anticonvulsant drugs; however, prophylactic antiepileptic medication is not indicated (Figure 80.1).[6] Evacuation of ICH is generally not required unless it causes a significant mass effect. Corticosteroids and barbiturates have been used, though their effect on clinical outcome is uncertain.[6]

Table 80.2 Management of cerebral oedema and intracranial hypertension

Medical management	
General measures	Maintain normoxia (PaO$_2$ >95 mmHg; SaO$_2$ >93%), normocapnia (PaCO$_2$ 35–40 mmHg)
	Normovolaemia (with isotonic, glucose-free crystalloids), normothermia, haematocrit 30%–35%
	Normoglycaemia (serum glucose: 80–180 mg/dL)
Specific measures	Controlled hyperventilation: (PaCO$_2$ 30 mmHg)
	Diuretics: Osmotic diuretics—Mannitol (0.25–1.0 mg/kg bolus over 10–15 mins; repeat dosing every 6 hours); 23% hypertonic saline (250 ml bolus for refractory ICH); Serum osmolality goal: 300–320 mOsm/L; Serum sodium goal: 145–155 mEq/L
	Loop diuretics—Furosemide (0.1 to 0.2 mg/kg IV bolus; usually in combination with osmotherapy)
	Analgesia, sedation, neuromuscular blockade: Fentanyl (25–100 μgm bolus/titratable infusion @25–100 mcg/hr); propofol infusion (1–3 mg/kg/hr); non-depolarizing muscle relaxants (vecronium, atracrurium, rocuronium)
	Pharmacological coma: Barbiturates (pentobarbital: 3–10 mg/kg IV bolus, followed by a continuous infusion 0.5–3.0 mg/kg/hr); Thiopentone (3–10 mg/kg bolus over 10–15 minutes followed by infusion of 1–2 mg/kg/hr)
	or Propofol (2 mg/kg bolus followed by 100–200 μg/kg/min) doses titrated to sustain ICP reduction/burst suppression on EEG.
	Controlled CSF drainage: (if intraventricular ICP catheter in situ)
Surgical management	
Evacuation of haematoma	
Decompressive craniectomy	

Notes: PaO$_2$: Partial pressure of arterial oxygen; PaCO$_2$: Partial pressure of arterial carbon dioxide; SaO$_2$: Arterial oxygen saturation; ICP: Intracranial pressure; EEG: Electroencephalogram.

Temporary withdrawal of antithrombotic therapy may be considered, if patients are symptomatic or if the MCA velocities are more than twice their baseline value, till the symptoms have resolved and optimal BP control has been achieved.[13]

CHS AFTER SURGICAL RESECTION OR ENDOVASCULAR EMBOLIZATION OF CEREBRAL VASCULAR MALFORMATIONS

Pathophysiology

Several processes including 'normal perfusion pressure breakthrough' (NPPB) and passive 'venous occlusion hyperaemia', collectively also referred to as 'arterial–capillary–venous hypertensive syndrome, contribute to occurrence of CHS after obliteration of cerebral vascular malformations, e.g., AVM and vein of Galen malformations.

Normal perfusion pressure breakthrough (NPPB) or circulatory breakthrough

In an AVM, blood is directly shunted from arterioles to medium-sized veins without an intervening capillary network. This luxurious high flow, low resistance system 'steals' blood from adjacent circulatory beds (which derive their blood supply from the same parent artery, which feeds the AVM) and consequently results in ischaemia of the surrounding brain parenchyma. Compensatory vasodilatation of the peri-nidal resistance arterioles initially helps to maintain the perfusion in these chronically ischaemic regions, but gradually, maximal vasodilatation occurs, their autoregulatory capacity becomes exhausted and the flow becomes pressure-dependant (vasomotor paralysis).[21] In addition, neovascularization also takes place, but the newly formed vessels are both structurally and functionally abnormal (increased fragility, deficient vascular tone, impaired autoregulatory mechanisms).

Following removal of the AVM and redistribution of blood to the surrounding cerebral vessels, the perfusion pressure in the ischaemic peri-nidal region is suddenly restored to 'normal'; but the pressure–naive circulatory bed is unable to constrict and regulate the CBF, which leads to hyperperfusion. Consequently, cerebral swelling, vasogenic oedema and sometimes, massive ICH occur due to the intravascular engorgement, BBB breakthrough and vascular disruption, respectively.[21] An impaired autonomic perivascular innervation of vessels proximal and distant to the AVM, and a leftward shift of the cerebral autoregulatory curve, also contribute to symptomatic hyperaemia.[22]

Venous Occlusion Hyperaemia

Postoperatively, a passive 'occlusive hyperaemia' can also occur, either because of stagnation and obstruction of arterial flow in former AVM feeders and their parenchymal branches and/or due to flow restriction and spontaneous thrombosis in the draining veins adjacent to the AVM.[23] The consequent capillary disruption and BBB breakthrough can cause or aggravate the cerebral swelling, oedema, and haemorrhage.[23] Occlusion of a main draining vein by a propagating thrombus or a nidus remnant can result in rapid neurological deterioration due to development of malignant cerebral oedema.[24]

Diagnosis

Clinical Presentation

The clinical presentation can vary from nonspecific symptoms such as nausea, headache, and vomiting to serious manifestations including seizures, neurological deficits (e.g., aphasia, hemiparesis) and even life-threatening, acute deterioration in the neurological status.[23–26] Symptoms of CHS; brain swelling due to retraction oedema or a venous infarct; vasospasm and haemorrhage from a residual AVM can be quite similar; differentiation between these conditions can be made by confirmatory neuroimaging.[27–29]

Investigations

The CT scan and MRI scan usually reveal localized or generalized cerebral oedema, hyperaemia, and focal or multifocal intracranial haemorrhage.[25–28] TCD may demonstrate vasomotor paralysis (less than 10% change in MCA-MFV with CO_2 or acetazolamide challenge; or if the flow velocity changes with BP over physiological ranges).[25–28] Cerebral angiography may show stagnation and/or thrombosis in the feeders and draining veins of the resected AVM and delayed circulation.[25–29]

Risk Factors

Preoperatively, patients who demonstrate ischaemic rather than haemorrhagic symptoms; a reduced cerebrovascular reserve on TCD and/or SPECT evaluation; CT/MRI features of hypoperfusion-induced cerebral atrophy; angiographic evidence of large (>3.5 cms), high-flow AVMs (>20 cm³), border zone AVMs (rolandic, inferior limbic, and insular region), large-calibre or deep feeding arteries, and/or vascular steal from other vessels; Spetzler Martin Grade III–V AVMs (>3 cm, located in eloquent cortex and/or have a deep venous drainage) are at risk of developing CHS in the post-intervention period.[30,31]

Management

A management strategy for these patients is suggested in Figure 80.2. Patients should be observed for at least 24 hours in the NICU; high-risk patients merit continuous care and monitoring for a longer duration (7 days or more because delayed haemorrhage can occur within this period).[25–29,32] Management includes careful assessment for any change in the neurological status; intensive monitoring (invasive arterial BP, TCD, oxygen saturation, electrocardiogram (EKG), heart rate); aggressive BP control; maintenance of euvolaemia, and prophylactic antiepileptic therapy. ICP monitoring is desirable in high-risk patients and in those in whom a clinical examination is not feasible; an angiogram should also be also performed postoperatively to confirm complete resection of the AVM.[25–29]

Control of BP is vital for prevention as well as management of CHS. Systolic BP is maintained slightly lower than the patient's baseline values, preferably between 90–110 mmHg; escalating doses of parenteral antihypertensives (e.g., labetolol, esmolol, metoprolol, nicardipine) may be required for adequate BP control. The management of hypertension is described in Figure 80.1.[25–29] Due to the increased incidence of postoperative seizures, prophylactic antiepileptic therapy (e.g., phenytoin, levetiracetam) is usually initiated, especially if seizures were occurring preoperatively also. Dehydration predisposes to further venous thrombosis, hence normovolaemia should be maintained; and a serum haematocrit of <35 is desirable.[25–29]

If the patient develops pertinent clinical symptoms, an emergent CT scan should be done to rule out haemorrhage or hydrocephalus; an MRI brain with DWI should be obtained if the CT scan is negative for haemorrhage, and there is suspicion of cerebral infarction. Treatment focuses on management of hypertension (Figure 80.1), cerebral oedema (Table 80.2), and ICH. Mild cerebral oedema can be managed with diuretics, but malignant brain oedema and intracranial hypertension require aggressive measures including endotracheal intubation, sedation, hyperventilation, controlled CSF drainage, and pharmacological coma with thiopental/propofol (titrated to a burst suppression pattern on the electroencephalogram). A combination of propofol and labetalol is commonly used for the management of these patients.[25] A large intracranial bleed requires emergent surgical evacuation. Decompressive craniectomy may be considered as a last resort for ICP control in patients with refractory malignant brain swelling. Since impaired vasoreactivity can take a few days to recover, withdrawal of these intensive measures should be guided by clinical signs of neurological recovery, ICP, and TCD monitoring.

CONCLUSIONS

CHS can cause serious postoperative morbidity and mortality in patients undergoing cerebrovascular revascularization procedures (e.g., CAE, CAS) or obliteration of cerebral vascular malformations (e.g., arteriovenous and Galen vein malformation). The key pathophysiological process in this condition is a sudden and significant increase in the CBF to an area of the brain which is chronically hypoperfused, has a 'pressure passive circulation' (impaired cerebrovascular autoregulation), and a damaged BBB; in addition, 'venous occlusion hyperaemia' may also contribute to the occurrence of CHS after an AVM obliteration procedure. This acute cerebral hyperaemia predisposes to the development of severe cerebral oedema, brain swelling, and/or ICH. Hypertension plays an important role in occurrence of ICH as well as in aggravating the neurologic injury. Patients can present with headache, seizures, neurological deficits, and/or an acute deterioration in the neurological status. Early recognition of CHS is important to prevent and/or effectively manage the ensuing cerebral oedema, seizures, and ICH. TCD, a non-invasive, bedside, and easily reproducible technique is very widely used to diagnose, monitor the course, and guide the therapy for CHS. Aggressive BP management forms the cornerstone of prevention and management of CHS. Mild cerebral oedema can be treated with diuretics, but malignant brain oedema and intracranial hypertension often require aggressive measures including endotracheal intubation, sedation, hyperventilation, controlled CSF drainage, pharmacological coma, and rarely, a decompressive craniectomy. Evacuation of ICH is generally not required, unless it causes a significant mass effect. Prophylactic antiepileptic therapy is indicated in patients who have undergone an obliteration procedure for a cerebrovascular malformation.

REFERENCES

1. Sundt TM Jr, Sandok BA, Whisnant JP. Carotid endarterectomy: Complications and preoperative assessment of risk. *Mayo Clin Proc* 1975;50(6):301–6.

2. Sundt TM Jr, Sharbrough FW, Piepgras DG, Kearns TP, Messick JM Jr, O'Fallon WM. Correlation of cerebral blood flow and electroencephalographic changes during carotid endarterectomy: with results of surgery and hemodynamics of cerebral ischemia. *Mayo Clin Proc* 1981; 56(9):533–43.

3. Adhiyaman V, Alexander S. Cerebral hyperperfusion syndrome following carotid endarterectomy. *QJM* 2007; 100(4):239–44.

4. Gupta AK, Purkayastha S, Unnikrishnan M, Vattoth S, Krishnamoorthy T, Kesavadas C. Hyperperfusion syndrome after supraaortic vessel interventions and bypass surgery. *J Neuroradiol* 2005;32(5):352–8.

5. Zhao WG, Luo Q, Jia JB, Yu JL. Cerebral hyperperfusion syndrome after revascularization surgery in patients with moyamoya disease. *Br J Neurosurg* 2013;27(3):321–5.

6. Moulakakis KG, Mylonas SN, Sfyroeras GS, Andrikopoulos V. Hyperperfusion syndrome after carotid revascularization. *J Vasc Surg* 2009;49(4):1060–8.

7. Karapanayiotides T, Meuli R, Devuyst G, et al. Postcarotid endarterectomy hyperperfusion or reperfusion syndrome. *Stroke* 2005;36(1):21–6.

8. Farooq MU, Goshgarian C, Min J, Gorelick PB. Pathophysiology and management of reperfusion injury and hyperperfusion syndrome after carotid endarterectomy and carotid artery stenting. *Exp Transl Stroke Med* 2016;8(1):7. DOI 10.1186/s13231-016-0021-2.

9. Janigro D, West GA, Nguyen TS, Winn HR. Regulation of blood-brain barrier endothelial cells by nitric oxide. *Circ Res* 1994;75(3):528–38.

10. Ascher E, Markevich N, Schutzer RW, Kallakuri S, Jacob T, Hingorani AP. Cerebral hyperperfusion syndrome after carotid endarterectomy: Predictive factors and hemodynamic changes. *J Vasc Surg* 2003;37(4):769–77.

11. Ogasawara K, Inoue T, Kobayashi M, Endo H, Fukuda T, Ogawa A. Pretreatment with the free radical scavenger edaravone prevents cerebral hyperperfusion after carotid endarterectomy. *Neurosurg* 2004;55(5):1060–7.

12. Suga Y, Ogasawara K, Saito H, et al. Preoperative cerebral hemodynamic impairment and reactive oxygen species produced during carotid endarterectomy correlate with development of postoperative cerebral hyperperfusion. *Stroke* 2007;38(10): 2712–17.

13. Abou-Chebl A, Yadav JS, Reginelli JP, Bajzer C, Bhatt D. Intracranial hemorrhage and hyperperfusion syndrome following carotid artery stenting: risk factors, prevention, and treatment. *J Am Coll Cardiol* 2004; 43(9):1596–601.

14. Bouri S, Thapar A, Shalhoub J, et al. Hypertension and the post-carotid endarterectomy cerebral hyperperfusion syndrome. *Eur J Vasc Endovasc Surg* 2011;41(2): 229–37.

15. Ogasawara K, Sakai N, Kuroiwa T, et al. Intracranial hemorrhage associated with cerebral hyperperfusion syndrome following carotid endarterectomy and carotid

artery stenting: retrospective review of 4494 patients. *J Neurosurg* 2007;107(6):1130–6.

16. Lieb M, Shah U, Hines GL. Cerebral hyperperfusion syndrome after carotid intervention: a review. *Cardiol Rev* 2012;20(2):84–9.

17. van Mook WN, Rennenberg RJ, Schurink GW, et al. Cerebral hyperperfusion syndrome. *Lancet Neurol* 2005; 4(12):877–88.

18. Abou-Chebl A, Reginelli J, Bajzer CT, Yadav JS. Intensive treatment of hypertension decreases the risk of hyperperfusion and intracerebral hemorrhage following carotid artery stenting. *Catheter Cardiovasc Interv* 2007; 69(5):690–6.

19. Keunen R, Nijmeijer HW, Tavy D, et al. An observational study of pre-operative transcranial Doppler examinations to predict cerebral hyperperfusion following carotid endarterectomies. *Neurol Res* 2001;23(6):593–8.

20. Ogasawara K, Yukawa H, Kobayashi M, et al. Prediction and monitoring of cerebral hyperperfusion after carotid endarterectomy by using single-photon emission computerized tomography scanning. *J Neurosurg* 2003; 99(3):504–10.

21. Spetzler RF, Wilson CB, Weinstein P, Mehdorn M, Townsend J, Telles D. Normal perfusion pressure breakthrough theory. *Clin Neurosurg* 1978;25:651–72.

22. Young WL, Kader A, Ornstein E, et al. Cerebral hyperemia after arteriovenous malformation resection is related to 'breakthrough' complications but not to feeding artery pressure. The Columbia University Arteriovenous Malformation Study Project. *Neurosurgery* 1996;38(6):1085–95.

23. Al-Rodhan NR, Sundt TM Jr, Piepgras DG, Nichols DA, Rufenacht D, Stevens LN. Occlusive hyperemia: a theory of the hemodynamic complications following resection of intracerebral arteriovenous malformations. *J Neurosurg* 1993;78(2):167–75.

24. Wilson CB, Hieshimia G. A new way to think about an old problem. *J Neurosurg* 1993;78:165–6.

25. Chyatte D. Normal pressure perfusion breakthrough after resection of arteriovenous malformation. *J Stroke Cerebrovasc Dis* 1997;6(3):130–6.

26. Cata JP, Kurz A. Postoperative normal perfusion pressure breakthrough. In: Mashour GA, Farag E eds. *Case Studies in Neuroanesthesia and Neurocritical Care*. 1st ed. Cambridge: Cambridge University Press, 2011; pp. 83–4.

27. Morgan M. Therapeutic decision making. In: Win HR ed. *Youmans Neurological Surgery*. 6th ed. Philadelphia PA: Elsevier Saunders, 2011; pp. 4034–48.

28. Kretschmer T, Heros RC. Microsurgical management of arteriovenous malformations. In: Win HR ed. *Youmans Neurological Surgery*. 6th ed. Philadelphia PA: Elsevier Saunders, 2011; pp. 4072–87.

29. Malik G, Bhangoo S. Vascular malformations (arteriovenous malformations and dural arteriovenous fistulas). In: Ellenbogen RG, Abdulrauf SI, Sekhar LN eds. *Principles of Neurosurgery*. 3rd ed. Philadelphia, PA: Elsevier Saunders, 2012; pp. 229–47.

30. Pasqualin A, Barone G, Cioffi F, Rosta L, Scienza R, Da Pian R. The relevance of anatomic and hemodynamic factors to a classification of cerebral arteriovenous malformations. *Neurosurgery* 1991;28(3):370–9.

31. Hamilton MG, Spetzler RF. The prospective application of a grading system for arteriovenous malformations. *Neurosurgery* 1994;34:2–7.

32. Morgan MK, Sekhon LH, Finfer S, et al. Delayed neurological deterioration following resection of arteriovenous malformations of the brain. *J Neurosurg* 1999; 90:695–701.

81

Cerebral Venous Thrombosis

M. A. Kirkman

ABSTRACT

Cerebral venous thrombosis (CVT) is an uncommon form of stroke that preferentially affects young females. The diagnosis is often delayed, in part due to the associated wide clinical spectrum that ranges from isolated headaches to coma and death. The CVT can be associated with intracerebral haemorrhage (ICH), infarction, and oedema. The mainstay of treatment of CVT relies on anticoagulant therapy, although in selected cases there may be a role for systemic thrombolysis, endovascular therapy, and surgery. Although mortality and functional outcomes following CVT have improved over time, more patients are being admitted to intensive care in part due to an increasing role for endovascular treatment approaches. This chapter describes the investigation and management of a patient with CVT, followed by a review of literature on this important and under-recognized condition. Further high-quality research is required to better define optimal treatment of CVT and its associated complications.

KEYWORDS

Anticoagulation; cortical vein thrombosis; dural sinus thrombosis; endovascular therapy; intracranial hypertension (IH); stroke; thrombolysis; thrombophilia.

CASE

A 31-year-old female project manager presented to the emergency department with a 2-month history of headaches. Over the preceding 48 hours, the headaches had progressively increased in severity, associated with the development of blurred vision and nine episodes of vomiting. She described the headaches as being like 'a tight band across the forehead'. In addition, she was photophobic with neck stiffness. Her past medical history comprised exclusively of depression. She had regularly taken an anti-depressant (sertraline 100 mg daily) and a combined oral contraceptive pill (ethinylestradiol 0.03 mg/drospirenone 3 mg) for several years. The patient rarely drank alcohol, was a non-smoker, and denied illicit drug use. Her family history was not significant.

On examination, the patient was clearly in discomfort and photophobic. Heart rate, blood pressure, temperature, oxygen saturation, and respiratory rate were within normal limits. Her Glasgow Coma Scale (GCS) score was 15. Fundoscopic examination revealed bilateral papilloedema, and she had diplopia on lateral gaze bilaterally, but the remainder of the cranial nerve examination was normal. She had increased tone and reflexes in all four limbs, but normal power, sensation, and coordination. Plantar response was upgoing consistent with Babinski's sign, and clonus was present. Kernig's sign was negative. Examination of the cardiovascular, respiratory, and abdominal system was unremarkable. Her calves were soft and non-tender.

A computed tomography (CT) scan of the head was performed, which demonstrated a hyperdensity extending along the torcular, right transverse and sigmoid sinuses (Figure 81.1). The patient then proceeded to a CT venogram (CTV), which confirmed an occlusive thrombus in the torcular extending throughout the right transverse sinus into the sigmoid sinus and proximal right internal jugular vein (Figure 81.1). In addition, there was non-occlusive thrombus in the posterior portion of the superior sagittal sinus (SSS). The cortical veins and remainder of the sinus system were patent.

Blood tests, including full blood count, coagulation, and urea and electrolytes were normal. As per advice from the local neurology physicians, the patient was admitted to the Stroke Unit, underwent a lumbar puncture, and then commenced treatment-dose of the low molecular weight heparin (LMWH) tinzaparin, dosed according to weight at 175 units/kg of body weight. At lumbar puncture, the opening pressure was 41 cmH$_2$O and, through cautious cerebrospinal fluid (CSF) drainage, this was reduced to a closing pressure of 17 cmH$_2$O. The patient was commenced on the carbonic anhydrase inhibitor acetazolamide (500 mg twice daily) for raised intracranial pressure (ICP), and the vitamin K antagonist warfarin (dosage to target Internationalised Normal Ratio [INR]: 2.0–3.0). A thrombophilia screen performed during the admission was positive for lupus anticoagulant.

Shortly after admission, magnetic resonance imaging (MRI) of the head was performed which did not identify any underlying cause for CVT, or any associated abnormalities such as haemorrhage or infarction (Figures 81.2 and 81.3). Her conscious level deteriorated on the ward and she proceeded to endovascular therapy (intrasinus thrombolysis) after which she was transferred to the intensive care unit (ICU) for ongoing monitoring and management. She improved clinically and was stepped down to the stroke unit several days later, prior to discharge home. In order to fulfil the consensus diagnostic criteria for antiphospholipid antibody syndrome, lupus anticoagulant testing was repeated three months after the initial test and found to be negative.

The patient continued to experience severe headaches secondary to intracranial hypertension (Figure 81.3) requiring regular therapeutic lumbar punctures and, subsequently, a lumboperitoneal shunt. She had follow-up imaging within six months of the initial diagnosis and by 18 months the SSS had largely recanalized and the venous sinus thrombotic burden had reduced (Figures 81.3 and 81.4). Formal catheter angiography performed at this time identified a tentorial dural arteriovenous fistula (DAVF; Figure 81.5). The DAVF was treated with endovascular occlusion and the patient made a complication-free recovery. Her headaches have improved significantly and she remains under regular clinic follow-up.

INTRODUCTION

Cerebral venous thrombosis (CVT) is a relatively uncommon but serious form of stroke that can affect the dural sinuses and/or cerebral veins. It preferentially affects young female adults and the diagnosis is often delayed, owing in part to the myriad non-specific symptoms it is associated with. Although the majority of treated patients have a good outcome, a proportion do not respond or deteriorate following treatment. Although mortality and functional outcomes following CVT have improved over time,[1] more patients are being admitted to intensive care in part due to an increasing role for endovascular treatment approaches, as has been observed in acute ischaemic stroke (AIS).[2]

This chapter describes the investigation and management of a patient with CVT followed by a review of the literature on this important and under-recognized condition.

EPIDEMIOLOGY

Cerebral venous thrombosis is more common than previously thought, in part due to improved imaging techniques identifying less severe cases, with a recent estimated annual incidence of 15.7 cases per million people.[3]

Nevertheless, CVT is a rare cerebrovascular disorder, accounting for only 0.5%–1% of all strokes. The female–male ratio of CVT in adults has increased over time and is currently approximately 3:1, with an increasing female–male ratio over the years likely due to increased oral contraceptive use.[4] Cerebral venous thrombosis also has a predilection for younger patients; in the large International Study on Cerebral Vein and Dural Sinus Thrombosis (ISCVT), over three-quarters of patients were under the age of 50.[5]

PATHOPHYSIOLOGY

A detailed review of the pathophysiology of CVT is beyond the scope of this chapter. However, briefly, one can consider the pathophysiology of CVT as two distinct mechanisms: (1) thrombosis of the cerebral sinuses, and (2) thrombosis of the cortical veins; both of these pathophysiological processes may result in intracranial hypertension, infarction, and/or haemorrhage from increased venous pressure.[6]

A thrombus in the cerebral sinuses impairs venous outflow from the brain and diminishes effective blood flow to the area, with resulting venous engorgement leading to white matter oedema.[7] Since the cerebral sinuses also have a role in the transport of CSF, occlusion of the cerebral sinuses can result in impaired CSF transport.[7] A thrombus in the cortical veins obstructs the drainage of blood from adjacent brain tissue, which can lead to increased venous and capillary pressure as well as blood-brain barrier disruption.[8]

RISK FACTORS AND UNDERLYING CAUSES OF CVT

The risk factors and underlying aetiology of CVT can be largely considered in light of Virchow's triad—that is, those which result in changes in the vessel wall, composition of the blood, or stasis of the blood (Table 81.1).[9] In the absence of specific risk factors, it is highly likely that the patient has an undiagnosed myeloproliferative disorder.[10]

CLINICAL PRESENTATION

Clinical findings in CVT can result from increased ICP secondary to impaired venous drainage and/or focal brain injury related to venous ischaemia/infarction or haemorrhage.[7] The CVT is associated with a wide clinical spectrum[9] ranging from isolated headaches, visual or auditory disturbances, to motor deficits, impaired consciousness, and death (Table 81.2). Headaches are the prominent feature, present in approximately 90% of cases[9] and, although most are diffuse and slowly progressive in severity over days to weeks, some patients present with an acute severe headache akin to that typically associated with subarachnoid haemorrhage (SAH), and up to a quarter of patients with CVT present with isolated

Table 81.1 Risk factors associated with the development of CVT

Risk factor or predisposing cause	Proportion of CVT cases (%)
Thrombophilia • Genetic, e.g., antithrombin III deficiency, protein C deficiency, protein S deficiency, mutation G20210A of factor II, resistance to activated protein C and factor V Leiden • Acquired, e.g., antiphospholipid and anticardiolipin antibodies, nephrotic syndrome, hyperhomocysteinaemia	34.1
Pregnancy and puerperium*	20.1
Medications • Oral contraceptives* • Others, e.g., hormone replacement therapy, steroids, cytotoxic agents	54.3 7.5
Malignancy • Including central nervous system, solid tumour outside the CNS, and haematological	7.4
Vascular abnormalities • Including dural fistula, venous anomaly, and arteriovenous malformation	1.9
Haematological abnormalities • Including polycythaemia, thrombocythaemia, and anaemia	12
Inflammatory systemic disorders • Vasculitis, e.g., associated with systemic lupus erythematosus, Behçet disease, and rheumatoid arthritis • Inflammatory bowel disease • Sarcoidosis	3 1.6 0.2
Other systemic disorders • Including thyroid disease	2.4
Infection • Including of the central nervous system, ear, sinus, mouth, face, and neck	12.3
Dehydration	1.9
Mechanical precipitants • Including lumbar puncture, cranial trauma, jugular catheter occlusion, and neurosurgery	4.5
Surgery	2.7
None identified	12.5

*Percentages derived from the total number of female patients aged under 50.

Note: Figures do not sum to 100% as some patients in ISCVT had more than one risk factor.

Derived from: Ferro JM. Prognosis of cerebral vein and dural sinus thrombosis: results of the international study on cerebral vein and dural sinus thrombosis (ISCVT). *Stroke* 2004;35:664–70.

Table 81.2 Symptoms and signs of cerebral venous thrombosis

Symptom or sign	Proportion of CVT cases (%)
Headaches	89
Seizure (focal or generalized)	39
Motor deficit*	37
Papilloedema	28
Mental status disorders	22
Aphasia	19
Diplopia	14
Stupor or coma	14
Visual loss	13
Sensory disturbance	5
Other focal cortical sign	3

*including bilateral motor deficit in 4%.

Note: Figures do not sum to 100% as some patients in ISCVT had more than one symptom or sign.

Derived from: Ferro JM. Prognosis of cerebral vein and dural sinus thrombosis: results of the international study on cerebral vein and dural sinus thrombosis (ISCVT). *Stroke* 2004;35:664–70.

headaches.[11] Seizures occur in approximately 40% of patients with CVT,[9] a rate higher than most other forms of cerebrovascular disease. Other unique features of CVT relative to other cerebrovascular pathologies include the relatively slow onset of symptoms, and the frequency of bilateral cerebral involvement (bilateral motor signs are present in ~4%).[9]

The clinical presentation may indicate the location of the occlusion. The most commonly affected vessels are the SSS and transverse sinuses (Figure 81.6).[9] Superior sagittal sinus occlusion tends to present clinically with headaches, intracranial hypertension, papilloedema, motor deficit, and/or seizures.[12] Transverse sinus occlusion may present with symptoms related to an underlying associated condition such as otitis media (e.g., fever, ear discharge), as well as otalgia, pain in the mastoid region, and headaches.[13] Occlusion involving the deep cerebral venous system can lead to thalamic or basal ganglia infarction and often leads to rapid neurological decline.[14,15]

INVESTIGATIONS

Blood Testing

Routine blood studies including biochemistry, full blood count, and coagulation studies should be performed in all patients with suspected CVT. This may identify evidence of a hypercoagulable state or indicate an infective aetiology. An underlying haematological cause for the

CVT requires a hypercoagulability assessment for: factor V Leiden, prothrombin gene mutation, antithrombin III levels, protein C and protein S activity and levels, and antiphospholipid antibodies (lupus anticoagulant and anticardiolipin). However, these tests rarely change acute management. Acute phase reactants can be elevated in the presence of acute thromboembolism and thus repeat testing at least 12 weeks apart is recommended as per the international consensus guidelines for the confirmation of antiphospholipid syndrome.[16] Furthermore, testing for antithrombin III and protein C and S should be delayed to 2–4 weeks after anticoagulant therapy, since the results are unreliable in the context of warfarin use.

A recent meta-analysis of 636 patients evaluated the role of D-dimer in excluding CVT in 'low-risk' patients with isolated headache.[17] In the absence of focal neurological deficits and risk factors for CVT, as well as a normal cranial CT scan, D-dimer values were found to have high negative predictive value (99.8%, 95% confidence interval [CI]: 98.9%–100%). Sensitivity was lower (97.8%, 95% CI: 88.2%–99.6%), but comparable to the values accepted in deep vein thrombosis (DVT) and pulmonary embolism (PE). This suggests that normal D-dimers in low-risk patients may reduce unnecessary imaging, although a normal D-dimer should not preclude further evaluation if the clinical suspicion of CVT remains high.

Imaging

Imaging is required to diagnose CVT, but can also help look for an underlying aetiology such as an intracranial tumour. The main imaging modalities used to diagnose CVT are plain CT, CTV, MRI, magnetic resonance venography (MRV), and cerebral digital subtraction angiography (DSA; Table 81.3). Ultrasound has a role in paediatric patients, and may be used for routine monitoring of thrombus and parenchymal changes in association with transcranial Doppler (TCD).[18]

In a non-contrast CT, acute CVT can appear as hyperdensity of a cortical vein or dural sinus.[19] Thrombosis of the posterior SSS can result in the so-called 'empty delta sign' on contrast imaging, which results from a central hypointensity due to very slow or absent flow within the sinus, surrounded by contrast enhancement in a triangular shape in the posterior aspect of the SSS.[20] This may appear only several days after symptom onset, but can persist for several weeks.[19]

The commonest associated radiological findings in CVT include intracerebral haemorrhage (ICH), cerebral oedema, and infarction (Figure 81.7). Rarely, subdural haemorrhage and SAH may be present. Intracerebral haemorrhage can manifest in multiple ways, typically as an area of oedema

Table 81.3 The commonest imaging modalities used to investigate for cerebral venous thrombosis

Imaging modality	Comment
CT	• Useful in the initial evaluation of CVT, but a normal result does not exclude CVT
CTV	• As good as MRV in the detection of CVT,[*] but has the advantage of being more accessible in many centres, and less expensive

MRI	• Useful in the initial evaluation of CVT, but a normal result does not exclude CVT
	• Superior to CT for the detection of parenchymal lesions
	• Susceptibility-weighted images can improve the diagnostic yield, and are particularly helpful in cortical vein thrombosis[@]
	• Thrombus signal intensity on MRI varies over time:[#]
	  – Acute thrombus: hypointense on T2* imaging (T1 and T2 sequences may be falsely reassuring)
	  – Subacute thrombus: hyperintense on all sequences (T1, T2, T2*, FLAIR, diffusion)
	  – Chronic thrombus: typically isointense on T1 imaging and iso/hyperintense on T2 imaging, but significant variability exists

MRV	• As good as CTV in the detection of CVT,[*] but has the advantage of no radiation dosage • Time-of-flight sequences are most often employed, although contrast-enhanced MRV can better delineate the venous system[$]
DSA	• Invasive and becoming less commonly used • Useful when CTV or MRV are inconclusive but clinical suspicion remains high[^] • Can also be used when endovascular intervention is planned

*Ozsvath RR, Casey SO, Lustrin ES, et al. Cerebral venography: comparison of CT and MR projection venography. *American Journal of Roentgenology* 1997;169:1699–707.
@Boukobza M, Crassard I, Bousser MG, et al. MR imaging features of isolated cortical vein thrombosis: diagnosis and follow-up. *AJNR Am J Neuroradiol* 2009;30:344–8.
#Leach JL, Fortuna RB, Jones BV, et al. Imaging of cerebral venous thrombosis: current techniques, spectrum of findings, and diagnostic pitfalls. *Radiographics* 2006;26(Suppl 1):S19–41–discussion S42–3.
$Farb RI, Scott JN, Willinsky RA, et al. Intracranial venous system: gadolinium-enhanced three-dimensional MR venography with auto-triggered elliptic centric-ordered sequence—initial experience. *Radiology* 2003;226:203–9.
^Saposnik G, Barinagarrementeria F, Brown RD, et al. Diagnosis and management of cerebral venous thrombosis: a statement for healthcare professionals from the American Heart Association/American Stroke Association. *Stroke* 2011;42:1158–92.

with patchy areas of haemorrhage within it. The oedema is often reversible.[21] Focal oedema without haemorrhage is seen in approximately 8% of CT and 25% of MRI scans of CVT, and focal parenchymal changes with oedema and haemorrhage in up to 40% of patients.[19] Juxtacortical haemorrhage is very specific for CVT, occurring almost exclusively in association with SSS occlusion.[22] It manifests as small haemorrhages, with little/no oedema, at the junction of the superficial and deep venous drainage systems.

Repeated venographic imaging should be performed in patients with persistent or evolving symptoms despite treatment, and in those with symptoms suggestive of clot propagation.[19] Follow-up CTV or MRV 3–6 months after diagnosis to evaluate for recanalization of occluded cortical veins and/or sinuses is recommended in the American Stroke Association (ASA) guidelines.[19]

MANAGEMENT OF CVT

In addition to treatment of the underlying cause of CVT (e.g., tumour, infection) where possible, the following principles should be followed to optimize outcomes.

Location of Care

There is class I evidence, as shown in a Cochrane systematic review and meta-analysis,[23] that care of stroke patients in dedicated stroke units managed by multidisciplinary teams results in improved patient outcomes. Although these data relate primarily to AIS, given the relative rarity of CVT, it is reasonable to assume that patients with CVT would also benefit from specialized care in high-volume centres. In particular, high risk patients with risk factors for poor outcome (Table 81.4) should be in a setting with easy access to critical care, interventional radiological or neurosurgical services, and thrombolysis.

Anticoagulation

The purpose of anticoagulant therapy in CVT is to prevent thrombus growth, facilitate recanalization, and prevent DVT or PE. Anticoagulation is widely considered as the first-line treatment for CVT and recommended in the US[19] and European[24] guidelines. This is based on the results of two randomized controlled trials (RCTs) including 79 patients, one with unfractionated heparin (UFH) as the treatment arm,[25] and the other LMWH.[26] A Cochrane systematic review incorporating the two RCTs found anticoagulation to be safe and associated with a reduction in the risk of death or dependency compared to controls (pooled relative risk: 0.46, 95% confidence interval [CI]: 0.16–1.31)—this was not significant, possibly a result of the small number of patients

Table 81.4 Predictors of death or dependence after CVT

Demographic factors:
• Age >37 years
• Male gender
Clinical factors:
• Coma and decreased level of consciousness
• Encephalopathy
• Neurological deficit and severity (NIHSS), including weakness
• Seizures
Neuroimaging factors:
• Haemorrhage on admission CT
• Thrombosis of the deep cerebral venous system
• Straight sinus involvement
• Venous infarction
• Posterior fossa lesion
Risk factors:
• Central nervous system infection
• Cancer
• Underlying coagulopathy

Note: NIHSS: National Institutes for Health Stroke Scale.
Sources: (1) Canhão P, Ferro JM, Lindgren AG, et al. Causes and predictors of death in cerebral venous thrombosis. *Stroke* 2005;36:1720–5. (2) Ferro JM. Prognosis of cerebral vein and dural sinus thrombosis: results of the international study on cerebral vein and dural sinus thrombosis (ISCVT). *Stroke* 2004;35:664–70. (3) Saposnik G, Barinagarrementeria F, Brown RD, et al. Diagnosis and management of cerebral venous thrombosis: a statement for healthcare professionals from the American Heart Association/American Stroke Association. *Stroke* 2011;42:1158–92. (4) Ferro JM, Lopes MG, Rosas MJ, et al. Long-term prognosis of cerebral vein and dural sinus thrombosis. Results of the VENOPORT study. *Cerebrovasc Dis* 2002;13:272–8. (5) Breteau G, Mounier-Vehier F, Godefroy O, et al. Cerebral venous thrombosis 3-year clinical outcome in 55 consecutive patients. *J Neurol* 2003;250:29–35. (6) de Bruijn SF, De Haan RJ, Stam J. Clinical features and prognostic factors of cerebral venous sinus thrombosis in a prospective series of 59 patients. For The Cerebral Venous Sinus Thrombosis Study Group. *J Neurol Neurosurg Psychiatry* 2001;70:105–8. (7) Appenzeller S, Zeller CB, Annichino-Bizzachi JM, et al. Cerebral venous thrombosis: influence of risk factors and imaging findings on prognosis. *Clinical Neurology and Neurosurgery* 2005;107:371–8.

recruited.[27] No new symptomatic ICH were observed in the studies, although one major gastrointestinal haemorrhage did occur following heparin treatment. PE, an important cause of death in patients with CVT prior to anticoagulation use, did not occur in any patient treated with heparin in the two trials, but caused one fatality in a patient in the placebo arm of one of the trials.

After commencing heparin treatment, a patient with CVT is typically commenced on an oral anticoagulant for a pre-specified period of time. The duration of anticoagulant therapy is usually dictated by the underlying aetiology of CVT and consideration of the risks of bleeding due to long-term anticoagulant therapy (Table 81.5). ASA

guidelines recommend the use of vitamin K antagonists (e.g., warfarin) with a target INR of 2.0–3.0, irrespective of the duration of therapy.[19] There is no class I evidence for or against the use of newer, direct oral anticoagulants, including direct factor Xa inhibitors (e.g., rivaroxaban, apixaban) and direct thrombin inhibitors (e.g., dabigatran) in CVT. Unlike warfarin, these agents have no requirement for serum level monitoring, but they also have no specific reversal agent. Two recent small retrospective studies found rivaroxaban[28] and dabigatran[29] to provide similar outcomes to warfarin. Class I evidence from the use of direct oral anticoagulants for stroke prevention in atrial fibrillation[30] and for acute venous thromboembolism[31] indicate a significantly reduced risk of ICH compared to warfarin. Prospective evaluation of their use in CVT should therefore be a priority.

Escalation of Therapy

A subset of patients with CVT do not respond to anticoagulation; in the ISCVT study, approximately 13% of patients experienced a bad outcome despite anticoagulant therapy.[9] In high-risk patients who deteriorate further or do not respond to anticoagulant therapy, more aggressive therapy may be warranted, including systemic thrombolysis, endovascular therapy or surgery. In such cases it would be important to exclude other causes of deterioration or apparent failure to respond, including developing or worsening ICH, oedema, and/or infarction.

Systemic Thrombolysis

A recent systematic review of 16 non-randomized studies including 26 patients found insufficient evidence to assess the efficacy of thrombolysis in CVT, and highlighted the not insignificant risk of mortality from serious bleeding.[32] Although 88% of patients regained independence, there were three cases of serious bleeding (11.5%), two of whom died. Furthermore, the optimal intervention, dosage, and route or method of thrombolysis administration remain unknown.

Endovascular Therapy

Examples of endovascular therapy used in CVT include intrasinus thrombolysis, mechanical thrombectomy, and balloon angioplasty. A recent systematic review of 42 studies including 185 cases of CVT treated with mechanical thrombectomy with or without intrasinus thrombolysis found good outcomes in 156 (84%) patients (modified Rankin score [mRS] 0–2), whilst 22 (12%) died. Only nine (5%) patients showed no evidence of recanalization, whereas 137 (74%) had near to complete recanalization. New or increased ICH occurred in 18 (10%) cases.[33]

Table 81.5 Aetiology of CVT and recommended duration of anticoagulant therapy

Underlying aetiology	Minimum recommended duration of therapy
Transient (reversible) risk factor e.g., pregnancy, puerperium	3 months[*]/3–6 months[#]
'Mild' thrombophilia e.g., heterozygous factor V Leiden or prothrombin G20210A mutation, high plasma levels of factor VIII	6–12 months
'Severe' thrombophilia e.g., anti-thrombin, protein C or S deficiency, homozygous factor V Leiden or G20210A mutation, antiphospholipid antibodies, or combined abnormalities, two or more episodes of idiopathic objectively documented extracerebral venous thrombosis	Long-term/indefinite treatment

Sources and notes: #Saposnik G, Barinagarrementeria F, Brown RD, et al. Diagnosis and management of cerebral venous thrombosis: a statement for healthcare professionals from the American Heart Association/American Stroke Association. *Stroke* 2011;42:1158–92. *Einhaupl K, Stam J, Bousser MG, et al. EFNS guideline on the treatment of cerebral venous and sinus thrombosis in adult patients. *Eur J Neurol* 2010;17:1229–35.

Despite these promising findings, there remains no class I evidence supporting the use of endovascular therapy in CVT. An ongoing RCT comparing thrombolysis with or without mechanical clot removal and standard therapy (therapeutic heparin) to standard therapy alone (Thrombolysis Or Anticoagulation for Cerebral venous Thrombosis study [TO-ACT]) will hopefully clarify if, and in which patients, endovascular therapy is beneficial.[34]

Surgery

The major cause of death in CVT is herniation associated with unilateral mass effect, and there may be a role for early decompressive craniectomy in those with impending herniation.[35] Data from a systematic review and retrospective registry of 69 acute-severe CVT patients treated with decompressive craniectomy, haematoma removal, or both found surgery to often be life-saving and result in good overall functional outcomes; 39 (57%) were independent after a median follow-up of 12 months, whilst 11 (16%) patients died.[36] Three of the nine patients with bilateral fixed pupils recovered completely. This supports the notion that selected patients with severe CVT should be treated aggressively. The ongoing DECOMPRESS-2 study, a prospective registry of CVT patients that undergo decompressive craniectomy will hopefully provide better delineated optimal indications and outcomes of surgical intervention in CVT.

SPECIFIC CHALLENGES IN CVT MANAGEMENT

Intracranial Haemorrhage

Approximately 30%–50% of patients with CVT have ICH of varying sizes. Evidence to guide decision-making about anticoagulation in this setting is limited, but ICH is not a contraindication to anticoagulant use.[19,24]

In one RCT, of the 15 patients with CVT and ICH given LMWH, there was no clinical worsening or new symptomatic ICH.[26] In another retrospective analysis of 43 patients with CVT and ICH,[25] four of 27 (15%) patients treated with UFH died and 14 (52%) completely recovered, whereas in the 13 not receiving heparin, nine (69%) died and only three (23%) completely recovered.

Long-term anticoagulants can be commenced once the patient is confirmed to be clinically stable and sequential neuroimaging of ICH is satisfactory.

Pregnancy and Puerperium

Pregnancy and puerperium accounts for approximately 20% of CVT cases,[9] with the highest risk in the first two weeks postpartum. Pregnancy is associated with a hypercoagulable state, although specific pathophysiological mechanisms are not completely understood. The ASA guidelines recommend full anticoagulation with treatment-dose LMWH throughout pregnancy and continuation of treatment, either LMWH or a vitamin K antagonist (target INR: 2.0–3.0) for at least six weeks postpartum to a total minimum duration of therapy of six months.[19] Unfractionated heparin can be considered before delivery, especially if caesarean section is planned and can be started at 36 weeks. Anticoagulation can be resumed six hours after vaginal delivery and 12 hours after caesarean section. As for non-pregnancy related CVT, the presence of ICH is not a contraindication to anticoagulation. If the patient has a history of CVT, LMWH prophylaxis can be administered during pregnancy through to the postpartum period.[37]

INTENSIVE CARE MANAGEMENT

There are several reasons why a patient with CVT may require admission to ICU (Table 81.6). There are no

Table 81.6 Possible indications for intensive care admission in patients with CVT

- Need for airway/ventilatory support, e.g., due to:
  - Deterioration in conscious level
  - Prevention of aspiration pneumonia
  - Adjuvant therapy for intracranial hypertension or significant cerebral oedema
  - Uncontrolled seizures
- Following endovascular therapy or surgery
- Management of complications arising from treatment, e.g., haemorrhagic transformation
- Need for invasive haemodynamic monitoring or support, e.g., if unstable blood pressure
- Need for invasive neurological monitoring
- Postoperatively for intensive monitoring
- High risk features indicating severe CVT (see Table 81.4)
- Facilitate the early detection and treatment of mass effect in patients deemed high-risk

existing guidelines or significant evidence base to guide the ICU management of patients with CVT, but it is reasonable to adopt some of the general principles used for AIS (Table 81.7).

COMPLICATIONS OF CVT

In addition to venous infarction and haemorrhage, CVT can result in several sequelae that can be divided into early and late complications (Table 81.8). Seizures are a common presenting feature of CVT and can also begin weeks and months after the diagnosis of CVT (see Table 81.9 for prevalence and risk factors at different time points). Chronic headaches affect around 50% of patients with CVT during follow-up,[38,39] and in over 10% the headaches may be severe enough to require bed rest or hospital admission.[9,38] Follow-up MRV may show stenosis in a previously

Table 81.7 Intensive care management of cerebral venous thrombosis: general principles

Domain	Management principles	Comment
Oxygenation and ventilation	Maintain oxygen saturations >94% If intubated: target $PaCO_2$ 35–45 mmHg (higher if chronic pulmonary disease and CO_2 retention)	No specific high-quality evidence available for CVT; based on AIS recommendations[*,#]
Blood pressure	Maintain normal BP, avoiding extremes and rapid BP lowering where possible Continuous arterial line BP measurements if cardiovascular instability or mechanically ventilated Consider lowering BP to <185/110 mmHg prior to thrombolysis and for at least 24 hours after	No specific high-quality evidence for BP targets in CVT Reducing BP for thrombolysis based on recommendations for AIS[*]
Cardiac function	Continuous ECG	
Blood glucose monitoring	Hourly blood glucose measurements Use of continuous insulin infusion to maintain serum glucose 140–180 mg/dL (8–10 mmol/L)	Serum glucose target based on AIS[#] Admission hyperglycaemia has been shown to strongly predict poor outcomes in CVT[@]
Temperature control	Avoid pyrexia (>37.5°C) Investigate and treat suspected infections	No specific evidence to guide temperature management in CVT
Fluid management	Individualised—maintain euvolaemia with isotonic saline	
Blood transfusion	Avoid anaemia Avoid aggressive transfusion practices	No robust data to support specific haemoglobin thresholds or targets
Neuromonitoring	Frequent monitoring of clinical status (GCS, pupils, neurological examination where possible) Routine ICP monitoring not recommended ICP monitoring may be used if significant oedema, haemorrhage or infarct volumes	CPP-guided therapy not evidence-based in CVT No evidence for use of other neuromonitoring tools

*European Stroke Organisation (ESO) Executive Committee, ESO Writing Committee. Guidelines for management of ischaemic stroke and transient ischaemic attack 2008. *Cerebrovasc Dis* 2008;25:457–507.

#Jauch EC, Saver JL, Adams HPJ, et al. Guidelines for the early management of patients with acute ischemic stroke: a guideline for healthcare professionals from the American Heart Association/American Stroke Association. *Stroke* 2013;44:870–947.

@Zuurbier SM, Hiltunen S, Tatlisumak T, et al. Admission hyperglycemia and clinical outcome in cerebral venous thrombosis. *Stroke* 2016;47:390–6.

Adapted due to a lack of specific evidence for CVT from: Kirkman MA, Citerio G, Smith M. The intensive care management of acute ischemic stroke: an overview. *Intensive Care Med* 2014;40:640–53.

Notes: CPP: cerebral perfusion pressure; ECG: electrocardiography.

Table 81.8 Complications associated with CVT and management

	Complication	Management	Comment
Early complications	Seizures	Early initiation of antiepileptic medications following first seizure in patients with CVT Routine use of anticonvulsants in patients with CVT but no history of seizures is not recommended	No high-quality evidence has studied the optimal timing, choice, and duration of anticonvulsants in CVT Risks of anticonvulsant use in those without a history of seizures probably outweigh the benefits
	Intracranial hypertension	Administration of acetazolamide if raised intracranial pressure is suspected Monitor for progressive visual loss with urgent treatment if present	Treatments for progressive visual loss include lumbar puncture, optic nerve decompression, and shunt Decompressive craniectomy can be used if neurological deterioration occurs due to severe mass effect or intracranial haemorrhage Surgery will preclude anticoagulation for the immediate postoperative period
	Hydrocephalus	CSF diversion through a ventriculostomy and, where required long-term, through shunt insertion	Communicating hydrocephalus can occur due to failure of CSF absorption from defective arachnoid granulations Obstructive hydrocephalus can occur (less commonly) as a result of intraventricular haemorrhage
Late complications	Seizures	As above	As above
	Headaches	Evaluate for recurrence of CVT or intracranial hypertension	Headaches in the follow-up period are commoner in patients with CVT who presented acutely with isolated intracranial hypertension If MRI is normal, lumbar puncture may be required to exclude raised intracranial pressure
	Visual loss	Complete neuro-ophthalmological assessment, including visual acuity and formal visual fields testing	Visual defects more common in patients with papilloedema and those with intracranial pressure at presentation Delayed diagnosis is associated with increased risk of subsequent visual deficit Treatments for progressive visual loss include lumbar puncture, optic nerve decompression, and shunt
	Dural arteriovenous fistula	Cerebral angiography—may be amenable to endovascular occlusion	Exact incidence unknown Can close with successful recanalization

Source: Saposnik G, Barinagarrementeria F, Brown RD, et al. Diagnosis and management of cerebral venous thrombosis: a statement for healthcare professionals from the American Heart Association/American Stroke Association. *Stroke* 2011;42:1158–92.

Table 81.9 Prevalence and risk factors for seizures in CVT

	Pre-diagnosis seizure	Early seizure (≤2 weeks after diagnosis)	Remote seizure (>2 weeks after diagnosis)	Post-CVT epilepsy (>1 seizure)
Patients affected, %	39	7	11	5
Risk factors	Supratentorial lesion Cortical vein thrombosis Sagittal sinus thrombosis Puerperal CVT	Supratentorial lesion Presenting seizures	Haemorrhagic lesion on admission CT/MRI Early seizure Paresis	Haemorrhagic lesion on admission CT/MRI Early seizure Paresis

Abbreviations: CVT: cerebral venous thrombosis; CT: computed tomography; MRI: magnetic resonance imaging.
Sources: (1) Ferro JM. Prognosis of cerebral vein and dural sinus thrombosis: results of the international study on cerebral vein and dural sinus thrombosis (ISCVT). *Stroke* 2004;35:664–70. (2) Ferro JM, Canhão P, Bousser M-G, et al. Early seizures in cerebral vein and dural sinus thrombosis. *Stroke* 2008;39:1152–8. (3) Ferro JM, Vasconcelos J, Canhão P, et al. Remote seizures in acute cerebral vein and dural sinus thrombosis (CVT): incidence and associated conditions. *Cerebrovasc Dis* 2007;23:48.

occluded sinus, although whether this is related to the development of headaches remains unclear.[19] Severe visual loss due to CVT is unusual (2%–4% of cases) but papilloedema can cause transient visual impairment which, if prolonged, can lead to optic atrophy and blindness;[19] visual deficit is more likely with diagnostic delay.[40] Dural arteriovenous fistulae can result from CVT (Figure 81.5),[41] but cause and effect can be difficult to establish as DAVF can also contribute to the development of CVT.

RECURRENCE AND OTHER VENOUS THROMBOEMBOLISM

New thrombotic events, including stroke, transient ischaemic attack, acute limb ischaemia, PE, and limb or pelvic venous thrombosis occur in approximately 4% of patients. Additional thromboses can occur even whilst the patient is on anticoagulant therapy.[9] The risk of CVT recurrence is low overall. In a systematic review of 13 studies with a follow-up duration ranging from 12 to 145 months, two-thirds of patients recanalized in the first few months following presentation, and a recurrence rate of 2.8% was found.[42]

OUTCOMES AND PROGNOSIS

Although CVT has historically been considered a condition with a grave prognosis, there has been a clear decline in mortality over time[1] and most patients have a good outcome. This decline in mortality is likely to be due to a number of factors, including improved recognition of less severe cases as well as improved treatment options. The current overall mortality rate for CVT is between 5% and 10%.[1,6,42] Approximately 80% of patients recover without functional disability, although many survivors are left with chronic symptoms such as headaches and concentration difficulties which negatively affect their quality of life.[9,43] Even in patients requiring ICU admission, although mortality is higher than general CVT cohorts (25%–34%)[44,45] the vast majority (80%–92%)[44,45] of survivors have an acceptable functional outcome (mRS 0–3).

Favourable prognostic factors include CVT associated with pregnancy, puerperium, oral contraceptive pill use, and hormone replacement therapy, a Glasgow Coma Scale score of 14 or 15 on admission, complete or partial intracranial hypertension syndrome (including isolated headache) as the only manifestation of CVT, and absence of aphasia.[38,39] Poor prognostic factors for CVT are shown in Table 81.4.

CONCLUSIONS

CVT is a relatively uncommon but serious form of stroke. Although the majority of treated patients have a good outcome, a proportion do not respond or deteriorate following treatment. The increasing use of endovascular treatments, among other reasons, has resulted in increasing numbers of patients with CVT being admitted to the ICU. High-quality studies are required to better define the indications for, and relative effectiveness of, the different therapeutic modalities for CVT, including endovascular therapy. In addition, a strong evidence base to guide the management of CVT in the ICU, and the complications associated with CVT, is currently lacking and urgently required.

REFERENCES

1. Coutinho JM, Zuurbier SM, Stam J. Declining mortality in cerebral venous thrombosis: a systematic review. *Stroke* 2014;45:1338–41.
2. Kirkman MA, Citerio G, Smith M. The intensive care management of acute ischemic stroke: an overview. *Intensive Care Med* 2014;40:640–53.
3. Devasagayam S, Wyatt B, Leyden J, et al. Cerebral venous sinus thrombosis incidence is higher than previously thought. *Stroke* 2016;47:2180–2.
4. Zuurbier SM, Middeldorp S, Stam J, et al. Sex differences in cerebral venous thrombosis: A systematic analysis of a shift over time. *Int J Stroke* 2016;11:164–70.
5. Canhão P, Ferro JM, Lindgren AG, et al. Causes and predictors of death in cerebral venous thrombosis. *Stroke* 2005;36:1720–5.
6. Coutinho JM. Cerebral venous thrombosis. *J Thromb Haemost* 2015;13(Suppl 1):S238–44.
7. Agrawal K, Burger K, Rothrock JF. Cerebral sinus thrombosis. *Headache: The Journal of Head and Face Pain* 2016;56:1380–9.
8. Ungersböck K, Heimann A, Kempski O. Cerebral blood flow alterations in a rat model of cerebral sinus thrombosis. *Stroke* 1993;24:563–9–discussion 569–70.
9. Ferro JM. Prognosis of cerebral vein and dural sinus thrombosis: results of the international study on cerebral vein and dural sinus thrombosis (ISCVT). *Stroke* 2004;35:664–70.
10. Artoni A, Bucciarelli P, Martinelli I. Cerebral thrombosis and myeloproliferative neoplasms. *Curr Neurol Neurosci Rep* 2014;14:496.
11. Crassard I, Bousser MG. Headache in patients with cerebral venous thrombosis. *Rev Neurol (Paris)* 2005;161:706–8.

12. Biousse V, Ameri A, Bousser MG. Isolated intracranial hypertension as the only sign of cerebral venous thrombosis. *Neurology* 1999;53:1537–42.

13. Teichgraeber JF, Per-Lee JH, Turner JS. Lateral sinus thrombosis: a modern perspective. *Laryngoscope* 1982;92: 744–51.

14. Crombé D, Haven F, Gille M. Isolated deep cerebral venous thrombosis diagnosed on CT and MR imaging. A case study and literature review. *JBR-BTR* 2003;86: 257–61.

15. van den Bergh WM, van der Schaaf I, van Gijn J. The spectrum of presentations of venous infarction caused by deep cerebral vein thrombosis. *Neurology* 2005;65: 192–6.

16. Miyakis S, Lockshin MD, Atsumi T, et al. International consensus statement on an update of the classification criteria for definite antiphospholipid syndrome (APS). Blackwell Science Inc, 2006(4):295–306.

17. Alons IME, Jellema K, Wermer MJH, et al. D-dimer for the exclusion of cerebral venous thrombosis: a meta-analysis of low risk patients with isolated headache. *BMC Neurol* 2015;15:118.

18. Schwartz N, Monteagudo A, Bornstein E, et al. Thrombosis of an ectatic torcular herophili: anatomic localization using fetal neurosonography. *Journal of Ultrasound in Medicine* 2008;27:989–91.

19. Saposnik G, Barinagarrementeria F, Brown RD, et al. Diagnosis and management of cerebral venous thrombosis: a statement for healthcare professionals from the American Heart Association/American Stroke Association. *Stroke* 2011;42:1158–92.

20. Ford K, Sarwar M. Computed tomography of dural sinus thrombosis. *American Journal of Neuroradiology* 1981;2:539–43.

21. Leach JL, Fortuna RB, Jones BV, et al. Imaging of cerebral venous thrombosis: current techniques, spectrum of findings, and diagnostic pitfalls. *Radiographics* 2006;26(Suppl 1):S19–41–discussionS42–3.

22. Coutinho JM, van den Berg R, Zuurbier SM, et al. Small juxtacortical hemorrhages in cerebral venous thrombosis. *Ann Neurol* 2014;75:908–16.

23. Stroke Unit Trialists' Collaboration. Organised inpatient (stroke unit) care for stroke. *Cochrane Database Syst Rev.* 2013;9:CD000197.

24. Einhaupl K, Stam J, Bousser MG, et al. EFNS guideline on the treatment of cerebral venous and sinus thrombosis in adult patients. *Eur J Neurol* 2010;17:1229–35.

25. Einhaupl KM, Villringer A, Meister W, et al. Heparin treatment in sinus venous thrombosis. *Lancet* 1991;338:597–600.

26. de Bruijn SF, Stam J. Randomized, placebo-controlled trial of anticoagulant treatment with low-molecular-weight heparin for cerebral sinus thrombosis. *Stroke* 1999; 30:484–8.

27. Coutinho J, de Bruijn SF, Deveber G, et al. Anticoagulation for cerebral venous sinus thrombosis. Stam J (ed.). *Cochrane Database Syst Rev.* 2011:CD002005.

28. Geisbüsch C, Richter D, Herweh C, et al. Novel factor Xa inhibitor for the treatment of cerebral venous and sinus thrombosis: first experience in 7 patients. *Stroke* 2014;45:2469–71.

29. Mendonça MD, Barbosa R, Cruz-e-Silva V, et al. Oral direct thrombin inhibitor as an alternative in the management of cerebral venous thrombosis: a series of 15 patients. *Int J Stroke* 2015;10:1115–8.

30. Chatterjee S, Sardar P, Biondi-Zoccai G, et al. New oral anticoagulants and the risk of intracranial hemorrhage. *JAMA Neurol* 2013;70:1486–90.

31. van Es N, Coppens M, Schulman S, et al. Direct oral anticoagulants compared with vitamin K antagonists for acute venous thromboembolism: evidence from phase 3 trials. *Blood* 2014;124:1968–75.

32. Viegas LD, Stolz E, Canhão P, et al. Systemic thrombolysis for cerebral venous and dural sinus thrombosis: a systematic review. *Cerebrovasc Dis* 2014;37:43–50.

33. Siddiqui FM, Dandapat S, Banerjee C, et al. Mechanical thrombectomy in cerebral venous thrombosis: systematic review of 185 cases. *Stroke* 2015;46:1263–8.

34. Coutinho JM, Ferro JM, Zuurbier SM, et al. Thrombolysis or anticoagulation for cerebral venous thrombosis: rationale and design of the TO-ACT trial. *Int J Stroke* 2013;8:135–40.

35. Coutinho JM, Majoie CBLM, Coert BA, et al. Decompressive hemicraniectomy in cerebral sinus thrombosis: consecutive case series and review of the literature. *Stroke* 2009;40:2233–5.

36. Ferro JM, Crassard I, Coutinho JM, et al. Decompressive surgery in cerebrovenous thrombosis: a multicenter registry and a systematic review of individual patient data. *Stroke* 2011;42:2825–31.

37. Bushnell C, McCullough LD, Awad IA, et al. Guidelines for the prevention of stroke in women: a statement for healthcare professionals from the American Heart Association/American Stroke Association. *Stroke* 2014; 45:1545–88.

38. Ferro JM, Lopes MG, Rosas MJ, et al. Long-term prognosis of cerebral vein and dural sinus thrombosis. Results of the VENOPORT study. *Cerebrovasc Dis* 2002;13: 272–8.

39. Breteau G, Mounier-Vehier F, Godefroy O, et al. Cerebral venous thrombosis 3-year clinical outcome in 55 consecutive patients. *J Neurol* 2003;250:29–35.

40. Ferro JM, Canhão P, Stam J, et al. Delay in the diagnosis of cerebral vein and dural sinus thrombosis: influence on outcome. *Stroke* 2009;40:3133–8.

41. Phatouros CC, Halbach VV, Dowd CF, et al. Acquired pial arteriovenous fistula following cerebral vein thrombosis. *Stroke* 1999;30:2487–90.

42. Dentali F, Gianni M, Crowther MA, et al. Natural history of cerebral vein thrombosis: a systematic review. *Blood* 2006;108:1129–34.

43. Dentali F, Poli D, Scoditti U, et al. Long-term outcomes of patients with cerebral vein thrombosis: a multicenter study. *J Thromb Haemost* 2012;10:1297–302.

44. Soyer B, Rusca M, Lukaszewicz A-C, et al. Outcome of a cohort of severe cerebral venous thrombosis in intensive care. *Ann Intensive Care* 2016;6:1–8.

45. Kowoll CM, Kaminski J, Wei V, et al. Severe cerebral venous and sinus thrombosis: clinical course, imaging correlates, and prognosis. *Neurocrit Care* 2016:1–8.

82

Management of Spinal Cord Injury

A. M. Benson, C. Gray, E. Farag, and A. Khanna

ABSTRACT

Spinal cord injury (SCI) is usually the result of trauma. However, non-traumatic causes are often a complex combination of a medical syndrome or a surgical misadventure. Whatever the underlying cause, these patients need specialized care in the intensive care unit (ICU). The first year after injury has the highest probability of mortality and complications. This chapter describes the acute and chronic complications, as well as management of SCI in the ICU in the context of a descriptive clinical vignette.

KEYWORDS

Spinal cord injury (SCI); neurosurgery; complications; postoperative care; intensive care; perioperative period.

CASE STUDY

A 20-year-old man is brought to the emergency department after falling from more than 25 feet in a climbing accident. He is awake, alert, and oriented, has appropriate speech, but is unable to move any of his extremities. His head and neck are immobilized. Cranial nerve examination appears intact, but muscle stretch reflexes and sensory reflexes in upper and lower extremities are absent. There are no other injuries except superficial scrapes on primary and secondary examination. Vital signs on initial exam: blood pressure (BP) 88/55 mmHg, heart rate 57 beats per minute (bpm), respirations 25 breaths per minute, and temperature 36.4°C. Laboratory results are normal except for mild respiratory acidosis. Imaging reveals a C4/5 burst fracture with evidence of cord compression. An arterial line is placed and he is brought to the operating room for surgical stabilization. His airway is secured with an awake, fibreoptic intubation, maintaining in-line stabilization of his cervical spine.

After surgery, the patient is brought to a neurointensive ICU (NICU) where support is provided for his hypothermia and hypotension with fluid and vasopressors as his spinal shock worsens over the subsequent hours. Despite appropriate DVT prophylaxis, he develops a common femoral DVT and pulmonary embolism on hospital day 10. He is unable to wean from the ventilator and requires a tracheostomy, as well as a gastrostomy tube for long-term feeding, and a suprapubic catheter for urinary drainage. He has minimal neurologic recovery despite aggressive medical treatment and is ultimately discharged to a spinal rehabilitation facility on hospital day 23.

INTRODUCTION

Despite advances in the understanding and management of spinal cord injury (SCI), it remains a devastating event, often resulting in severe and permanent disability, in addition to enormous healthcare costs. In the United States, the National Spinal Cord Injury Statistical Center has been collecting data about SCI since 1973. As of 2016, the annual incidence of SCI was approximately 17,000 cases, with males accounting for 80% of new SCIs and an average age of 42 years at injury, increased from 29 years in the 1970s.[1] Motor vehicle accidents are the leading cause of injury (38%) with alcohol playing a role in at least 25% cases, followed by falls (30.5%), violence (primarily gunshot wounds, 13.5%), and recreation activities (9%).[1,2] Non-traumatic causes of SCI include transverse myelitis, infection (examples: staphylococcus, tuberculosis), intraoperative spinal cord ischaemia during aortic surgery, and primary or secondary tumours.[3] Cervical SCI accounts for more than 50% of cases, with subsequent complete or incomplete tetraplegia.[1,3,4] Survival depends on age at injury, aetiology of injury, severity of neurological deficit, and requirement for long-term mechanical ventilation.[2,5] In general, mortality is highest in the first year after SCI (6.4%) and decreases thereafter (1%–2% per year). Leading causes of death include respiratory complications, septicaemia, pulmonary embolism, and suicide.[1,2,4]

PATHOPHYSIOLOGY

Primary versus Secondary Injury

The majority of traumatic SCIs involve both fracture and dislocation of the bony elements from one or more vertebral levels. Primary injury involves the initial neuronal disruption from mechanical forces and haemorrhage into and around the spinal cord.[2,3,6] This sets off an inflammatory cascade, with cytokine, free radical, and prostaglandin production, lipid peroxidation, ionic shifts, impaired mitochondrial function, hypoxia, ischaemia, and apoptosis, which result in spinal cord oedema and secondary injury.[2,6,7] Secondary injury leads to worsening of the initial neurological status.[2,3] It starts minutes after primary injury and usually peaks at 48 to 72 hours.[2,3,6,8] As the inflammatory process subsides, glial scar tissue remains, leaving persistent neurologic injury and making regeneration difficult.[3,7] To date, there is no evidence that any pharmacologic agents significantly protect against this process of secondary neuronal injury in humans.[2,9]

Patterns of Spinal Cord Injury

The American Spinal Injury Association (ASIA) classification (A, B, C, D, and E) of SCI has been widely adopted.[2,4,9,10] Complete SCI is classified as ASIA A and is defined as the absence of sensory or motor function in the perianal sacral segments S4–5 for more than 48 hours, and accounts for approximately 45% of SCI.[4] Incomplete injuries (ASIA B through E) account for the majority of SCI and are associated with significantly more favourable prognosis than complete injuries. Classification category ASIA B includes patients with preserved sensory function in S4–5.[4] ASIA C and D are incomplete SCIs with preserved motor function below the level of injury in more than half of key muscles.[4] Finally, ASIA E refers to patients with SCI but without any neurological deficits

detectable on examination.[4] In all cases, the level of injury is described as the highest with normal neurological function.

In addition to the five classes of SCI, ASIA also describes several specific clinical syndromes of incomplete injury:[2–4]

- *Central cord syndrome* is the most common incomplete SCI (10% of all cases). Elderly with pre-existing cervical spondylosis and hyperextension injuries represent the majority of cases. As the injury typically affects the mid and lower cervical spine, the upper extremities have more neurologic impairment than the lower extremities. Respiratory dysfunction is common due to phrenic nerve involvement.
- *Brown-Sequard syndrome* is uncommon. It results from traumatic hemisection of the cord or very rarely, lesions within the lateral vertebral canal. Patients present with ipsilateral loss of motor, touch, and vibration sense, as well as contralateral pain and temperature loss below the level of injury.
- *Anterior cord syndrome* causes loss of motor as well as pain and temperature sensation below the level of injury but with preservation of vibration and joint-position sensation from the posterior columns.
- *Cauda equina syndrome* results from damage or inflammation of the lumbar spinal nerves below L2. Potential causes include haematoma, trauma, tumour or compressive lesions in the lumbar spinal canal, prolapsed intervertebral disc, and lumbar spinal stenosis. Clinical presentation includes bowel and bladder dysfunction, low back pain, saddle or perineal anaesthesia, and motor and sensory deficits in the lower extremities. Surgical decompression within 6 to 8 hours of symptom onset gives the best chance of clinical recovery.
- *Conus medullaris syndrome* results from injury to conus medullaris (T12–L1) and presents similarly to cauda equina syndrome with bowel and bladder dysfunction but without significant motor weakness or sensory loss in the lower extremities.

Regardless of the type of SCI, early management is aimed at immobilization, treatment of accompanying life-threatening injuries, airway protection, maintenance of oxygenation, and blood pressure control.[3,4,9,10] All SCI patients should receive the standard 'three-view radiographic series' (lateral, anteroposterior, and odontoid/open-mouth) of the cervical spine, which detects approximately 95% of cervical spine injuries.[2,4,9–11] Computed tomography (CT) scans better assess lower cervical injuries and spinal cord compression.[2,4,9,11]

Magnetic resonance imaging (MRI) provides the best assessment of ligamentous and soft tissue injury.[2,4,9,10] However, it is time-consuming and thus reserved for after initial stabilization. Emergency neurosurgical intervention is indicated if there is spinal cord compression or unstable injuries with evolving neurologic deficits.[2,10,12,13] Meta-analyses and the Surgical Timing in Acute Spinal Cord Injury Study (STASCIS) have shown that early decompression within 24 hours, reduces secondary injury and improves neurological outcomes, particularly in incomplete SCI.[9,12]

ACUTE CONSIDERATIONS

There are several specific acute cardiopulmonary and other physiological disturbances common to patients with acute SCI that require close monitoring and management in an intensive care unit (ICU). The most significant of these are described in the following paragraphs.

Spinal Shock and Cardiovascular Effects

Haemodynamic alterations occur after SCI due to disruption of the autonomic nervous system.[4,14] Immediately after injury, there is a massive sympathetic discharge that leads to hypertension, tachycardia, and pulmonary hypertension.[2,3] Subsequently, within 30–60 minutes, spinal shock develops to varying degrees depending on the level of injury.[2,9] The sympathetic nervous system extends from T1 to L2 with cardio-accelerator fibres originating from T1 to T4.[3,15] Hypotension, with vasodilation and decreased myocardial contractility, develops due to lack of sympathetic outflow below the level of injury.[6,9,14] Bradycardia and heart block, sometimes requiring treatment with anticholinergic medications or temporary pacemakers are common with injuries above T4.[4,5,9,14] The unopposed vagal influence can be exacerbated by parasympathetic stimulation such as tracheal suctioning, positional changes, and intra-abdominal distension.[2,3] Nearly all patients with cervical SCI have a resting heart rate less than 60 bpm and almost 70% have a heart rate below 45 bpm.[6,15] Despite the predominance of bradyarrhythmias, tachyarrhythmias can also be seen.[2]

As nearly all SCI patients experience haemodynamic instability acutely, invasive BP monitoring is often required, with or without central venous pressure monitoring.[3,14] Maintenance of tight BP control with mean arterial pressure (MAP) of at least 85–90 mmHg is essential to optimize spinal cord perfusion due to loss of blood flow autoregulation after SCI.[3,6,14,15] Induced hypertension is recommended for 7 days after injury and is associated

with reduced morbidity and improved neurological outcomes after SCI.[2,5,14,15] Although careful volume resuscitation is helpful, typically vasopressors, with or without inotropes, are required to restore vascular tone and cardiac function.[2,3,15] No vasopressor has been shown to be superior in these patients.[3] Spinal shock and bradycardia usually resolves by 5 to 7 days after injury, however, it can persist for several weeks.[2,15]

Respiratory Concerns

Pulmonary complications, both early and late, account for the majority of deaths after SCI.[4,16,17] The degree of respiratory compromise depends greatly on the level of injury and the patient's pre-existing respiratory status.[4,17,18] Initial respiratory dysfunction and failure can result from direct chest trauma, pneumothorax, haemothorax, flail chest from rib fractures, diaphragm rupture, or pulmonary contusions.[4] Additionally, the initial sympathetic surge after injury can cause neurogenic pulmonary oedema.[2,3]

In the absence of direct pulmonary trauma, ventilation can be significantly impaired by disruption of the nerves innervating the diaphragm (phrenic nerve: C3–5, with accessory contribution from C6), and accessory muscles of respiration such as the scalene muscles (C3–8), sternocleidomastoid (C1–4), and intercostal muscles (T1–11).[17–19] In addition, impairment of the cough reflex (involving abdominal and respiratory muscles) results in significant morbidity as patients are unable to clear their secretions.[3,17,19] This makes them prone to mucus plugs, hypoxia, aspiration, pneumonia, and increased work of breathing.[3,9] Autonomic dysfunction with increased parasympathetic tone makes patients prone to bronchospasm and increased secretions.[3,6] For patients with SCI above C5, vital capacity can be reduced to 10%–20% predicted and respiratory failure requiring mechanical ventilation is required in 80%–90%.[3,9,18] Patients with injury at C2 or higher have instant respiratory paralysis and will die if not immediately intubated and ventilated at the scene.[6,18]

Close monitoring of respiratory function in the acute period is critical, as it is common for respiratory function to deteriorate over the first 3 to 4 days after injury.[2,3,9,11,16,18] This occurs due to atelectasis, weak cough reflex with increased secretions, increased work of breathing, and respiratory muscle fatigue.[2,3,17] In addition, cranial extension of neurological dysfunction occurs due to spinal cord oedema and secondary injury.[17,18] For patients with mid-cervical SCI, this can mean loss of diaphragm function and 65% of vital capacity (VC) several days after initial injury.[17,18]

Monitoring of VC is the most useful to evaluate evolving respiratory dysfunction.[9] Patients with a predicted VC of 20%–30% require very close monitoring, as those with a VC less than 20% require mechanical ventilation.[3,5] Peak cough flow, maximal inspiratory pressure, and trends in arterial carbon dioxide (CO_2) and oxygen (O_2) tensions are also useful assessments of respiratory function.[3]

It is essential to ensure adequate oxygenation and normocapnia after SCI to avoid worsening of spinal cord ischaemia and other organ dysfunction. Due to a significantly increased risk of pneumonia, patients should have strict adherence to standard ventilator care bundles and aspiration precautions.[3] If mechanical ventilation is not required, intensive respiratory therapy should be pursued with deep breathing exercises and incentive spirometry.[2,9] Nebulized bronchodilators such as ipratropium and albuterol as well as mucolytics are often useful.[2] Intermittent non-invasive positive pressure ventilation may be required to temporarily reduce the work of breathing.[16] Chest physiotherapy along with cough assist devices may be helpful in the acute post-injury period as well.[2,3,5,9] However, these should not be relied upon for respiratory failure or ongoing issues with poor clearance of secretions.

Endotracheal intubation should be pursued in patients with worsening VC, hypercarbia or hypoxia, as well as those too weak to clear their secretions effectively.[2,5,6,9] Approximately one-third of patients with cervical SCI will require intubation within the first 24 hours after injury.[6] As these patients have an inherent risk factor for a difficult airway, intubation is best done under a controlled setting, prior to the development of critical respiratory distress.[3,18] Succinylcholine muscle relaxation should be avoided more than 24 to 48 hours after injury due to the risk of hyperkalaemic cardiac arrest.[3,9] With unstable cervical spine patients, there is no demonstrated difference between fibreoptic oral or nasotracheal intubation and direct laryngoscopy with manual in-line immobilization, provided that there are no other indicators of a difficult airway.[11]

Gastrointestinal and Urinary Concerns

There are several gastrointestinal (GI) and urinary complications frequently seen in patients with SCI. In the immediate post-injury period, paralytic ileus is common due to autonomic dysfunction, as well as opioid analgesia and if present, intra-abdominal pathology.[2,3,5] Ileus in these patients is resistant to the usual prokinetic and stool softening agents.[3] Unfortunately, bowel function often remains compromised in the long term.[2] As the majority of patients with cervical SCI will require enteral feeding, it is important to carefully select the type of feed with

fibre supplements and closely monitor GI function and metabolic needs.[3,9,10]

In addition to ileus, SCI patients, especially those who are mechanically ventilated, are at high risk for stress ulcers and should receive prophylaxis with either a proton pump inhibitor or H2-receptor blocker for at least four weeks after injury.[5,9] Aspiration is also a concern due to impaired swallow reflexes and delayed gastric emptying. Nasogastric tube placement for decompression can help reduce the risk of aspiration and improve pulmonary mechanics. Patients should have a formal swallow evaluation prior to oral intake.[9]

Bladder dysfunction causing urinary retention and requiring catheterization is expected after acute SCI.[9] Urinary drainage is important, as bladder distension is a common cause for autonomic dysreflexia in the subacute and chronic phases of SCI.[3,5] Long-term bladder spasms with detrusor and sphincter hyperactivity and dyssynergy lead to issues with incontinence, urgency, and incomplete emptying. The majority of SCI patients require some assistance with bladder function.[5] This includes intermittent catheterization, occasionally a chronic indwelling catheter, and medications such as anticholinergics (oxybutynin) and alpha-blockers (prazosin) to reduce bladder spasms and aid in sphincter relaxation.[9] Urinary tract infections (UTIs) and urosepsis represent a major cause of morbidity for SCI patients, so appropriate genitourinary management is essential.[3]

Temperature

After SCI, hypothermia is expected. Vasodilation due to sympathectomy, combined with muscle atony (inability to generate heat by shivering), and loss of afferent temperature input below the injury result in rapid heat loss.[2,3] Core body temperature should be monitored, as peripherally patients may be warm due to vasodilation.[9] Although hypothermia is a much more common finding, patients can also have recurrent fevers without infection due to dysautonomia.[5] Conversely, infection may be present without a fever as well.[3] Hyperthermia, if it occurs, should be aggressively treated, as it is associated with worsening of neurologic outcomes.[2]

Thromboprophylaxis and Pressure Ulcers

Deep venous thrombosis (DVT) prophylactic therapy is essential in SCI patients due to high incidence of DVT and pulmonary embolism relative to other patient populations.[4,9,10,20] This occurs due to abnormal venous blood flow patterns combined with immobility.[14] Prophylaxis should include bilateral lower extremity sequential compression devices and chemoprophylaxis with low-molecular weight heparin recommended over subcutaneous unfractionated heparin.[4,14,20] The incidence of DVT is highest between 72 hours and 2 weeks after the injury. For this reason, it is recommended to start prophylactic heparin within 72 hours and continue it for a minimum of 8 weeks after injury.[5,9,14] Patients with high cervical injury may not present with typical tachypnoea, dyspnoea, chest pain, or tachycardia in the event of a pulmonary embolism due to impaired afferent pathways.[3] For this reason, a high level of suspicion must be present in these patients.[5] With appropriate prophylaxis, the incidence of DVT in SCI patients can be reduced from approximately 80% to 5%.[2] However, pulmonary embolism still represents the third leading cause of death in these patients.[20]

Pressure sores are another major cause of morbidity in SCI patients.[2,3,5,9] There are several factors that predispose these patients to pressure ulcers:

- Loss of afferent sensory input
- Immobility and reliance on others for repositioning
- Muscle atony and atrophy
- Impaired autoregulation and cutaneous blood flow

As in other patient populations, the areas most prone to pressure sores are the heels, sacrum, and ischium.[3,5] The occiput is also of concern in quadriplegic patients. Patient care should include pressure-relief mattresses, rotational beds, padding of bony prominences, and repositioning every two hours.[2,3,5,9] If early signs of pressure sores are detected, aggressive care is needed to avoid infection and further ulceration. This includes wound care, debridement, and antibiotics if needed, pressure relief measures, and optimized nutrition.[9] Even with these therapies, pressure sores are slow to heal and not uncommonly a cause of sepsis in the long-term care of patients with SCI.[3]

Acute Neuroprotection

As mentioned previously, there are currently no pharmacologic or non-pharmacologic measures that have proven benefit for improving neurologic outcomes after SCI.[2,3,7,9] Steroids have been widely used for acute SCI in the past due to the belief that it would decrease secondary injury by reducing inflammatory mediators, stabilizing membranes, decreasing lipid peroxidation, and improving blood flow.[3,8,21–23] Studies including the National Acute Spinal Cord Injury Studies (NASCIS II, 1990 and III, 1997) of methylprednisolone 30 mg/kg followed by 5.4 mg/kg/hr for 24 to 48 hours after injury, started within 3 to 8 hours of injury, showed improvement in motor scores

at 6 weeks and 6 months but no significant difference at 1 year.[8,21] Importantly, subsequent analyses of these and other studies showed patients who received high-dose steroids had increased rates of wound infection, pulmonary embolism, pneumonia, sepsis, and death.[4,8,22,23] Current guidelines now list high-dose steroids as a 'treatment option' in acute SCI rather than a standard of care due to concerns of harmful effects without solid evidence for long-term improvement in neurological outcomes.[3,5–7,23] Importantly, guidelines recommend against glucocorticoids in patients with SCI and moderate to severe traumatic brain injury or multisystem trauma, as it is associated with increased mortality in these patient subsets.[8,9]

Other agents have been studied to decrease secondary injury after SCI including GM1-ganglioside, thyrotropin releasing hormone, naloxone, minocycline, hyperbaric oxygen, and erythropoietin.[2,3,6–8] However, none of these has shown significant clinical benefit.[2,9] Animal studies indicate moderate hypothermia may be beneficial, but there have been no studies demonstrating this effect in humans.[6,24] Given the potential negative circulatory, metabolic, and immunologic side effects of hypothermia, this therapy is not currently recommended after SCI.[2,24] However, hyperthermia is clearly detrimental.[24] There are ongoing studies to evaluate whether stem cell transplantation could be a future therapy to induce spinal cord regeneration.[2,3] Currently, the most important intervention for these patients in terms of neuronal recovery remains strict management of haemodynamics, oxygenation and ventilation, with early and aggressive rehabilitation at a certified facility.[2,15]

LONG-TERM CONSIDERATIONS

Many of the long-term considerations in patients after SCI are similar to the acute issues including ileus, urinary retention, and propensity to develop thrombosis and pressure ulcers due to immobilization. Other sequelae of SCI include ongoing autonomic disturbances, respiratory issues, and development of spasticity due to loss of descending inhibitory neuronal pathways and increased sensitivity of spinal cord reflex arcs. Several of these chronic issues are explored in more detail below.

Autonomic Hyperreflexia

The sympathetic nervous system derives its pre-ganglionic innervation from the levels of T1 through approximately L2. When there is a SCI above the level of T6, there is significant disruption of sympathetic outflow.[3,6,25] As described previously, in the acute period, this leads to spinal shock with decreased vascular tone, hypotension, and bradycardia.[14,25] However, after the acute period, autonomic dysreflexia or hyperreflexia can occur. Although variable, it typically starts 6 weeks after injury and is more common in patients with complete cord injury.[6,14]

With autonomic hyperreflexia, sympathetic stimuli below the level of injury cause rapid and exaggerated sympathetic outflow due to denervation hypersensitivity of sympathetic pathways, as well as the loss of supraspinal inhibitory input.[3,14,25] Typical stimuli include bladder or colonic distension, faecal impaction, abdominal or pelvic surgery, uterine contractions during labour, or any cause of somatic pain.[2,3,14,25] Physiologically, this presents with profound hypertension (increase in systolic blood pressure at least 20% above baseline) due to peripheral vascular constriction below the level of injury and reflex bradycardia or arrhythmias due to intact baroreceptors from cranial nerves IX and X.[6,14,25] Above the level of injury, reflex autonomic responses attempt to counteract the sympathetic surges from below with vasodilation resulting in cutaneous flushing, sweating, headache, blurred vision, nausea, and nasal congestion.[3,14]

Major adverse effects of autonomic dysreflexia beyond patient discomfort include myocardial ischaemia, seizures, and intracerebral haemorrhage (ICH) related to the sudden, profound hypertension.[3,6,25] Treatment involves removal of the stimulus and administration of rapid-onset vasodilator medications to lower BP.[3,14,25] Some useful medications include sublingual nifedipine or captopril, nitrates (sublingual, transdermal, or intravenous), labetalol, hydralazine, and magnesium.[2,14,25] In the setting of labour or abdominal/pelvic surgery, epidural and spinal anaesthesia have been well documented as effective in preventing autonomic dysreflexia due to blockade of afferent input and sympathetic outflow.[2,3,25] If patients are able, change in position from lying down to sitting or standing can help also to acutely lower BP.[14] Prophylactic antihypertensives are not recommended due to typically low baseline BP from sympathoparesis.[3]

Chronic Respiratory Issues

Most patients with cervical SCI require mechanical ventilation in the acute period and are often slow to wean from the ventilator due to residual respiratory muscle weakness.[5,18,19] This improves somewhat as spinal cord oedema resolves and there is transition from acute flaccid paralysis to chronic increased muscle tone and spasticity, with improved chest wall stability several weeks after injury.[3,5,6] Interestingly, in contrast to healthy patients, VC actually improves in the supine position for those with cervical SCI.[3] Initial ventilator weaning in the

supine position or with an abdominal binder can improve success in these patients.[3] Additionally, kinetic therapy or rotational beds are helpful in improving pulmonary function.[2,3,5]

Of those who are initially ventilator-dependent, the majority can eventually be weaned to tolerate periods off the ventilator.[3] However, as this can take some time, tracheostomy should be considered early.[2,3,9,18] Approximately 1%–2% of all patients with SCI remain ventilator-dependent, with the highest rates in those with high cervical levels of initial injury.[3] This has a substantial effect on morbidity and mortality. Patients who remain ventilator dependent have only 30%–40% survival at one year.[3,5]

It can be difficult to predict which patients will be ventilator-dependent in the long-term. Surprisingly, a significant proportion of patients with injuries above C4 can still be weaned from the ventilator by one year post-injury.[3,18] Phrenic nerve pacing is helpful in some of these patients.[3,19] Although expensive, these implantable devices can aid in ventilator liberation and decrease the incidence of respiratory tract infections and subsequently, decrease hospitalizations.

Pain Control and Spasticity

Although SCI patients have acute pain from the initial injury, the more challenging issue in these patients is a disabling, chronic neuropathic pain that often develops and is difficult to treat.[2] Opioids are a less effective long-term option compared to other medications. Several agents with some efficacy for neuropathic pain control include:[2,3]

- Antiepileptics such as gabapentin, pregabalin, topiramate, valproate, or lamotrigine
- Tricyclic antidepressants such as amitriptyline, nortriptyline, desipramine, and doxepin
- Serotonin norepinephrine reuptake inhibitors such as venlafaxine or duloxetine
- Topical lidocaine or capsaicin

In addition to neuropathic pain, persistent spasticity develops in the chronic phase of SCI due to loss of inhibitory descending spinal pathways.[10,26] This makes sensorimotor reflex arcs below the level of injury very sensitive to minor stimuli, similar to the exaggerated responses seen with autonomic hyperreflexia. Some degree of spasticity and muscle tone is helpful to maintain muscle activity, bulk, and protection from pressure sores.[3] However, often the spasms and spasticity are excessive and require treatment. Physical therapy is generally the first line of treatment, however, several pharmacologic agents have been used for SCI-related spasticity.[26] The most commonly used is baclofen, a gamma-aminobutyric acid (GABA)-B agonist, which activates inhibitory interneurons at the level of the spinal cord.[3,26] Baclofen is slowly up-titrated until spasms are manageable. The most common side effects are drowsiness and weakness. Other side effects include nausea, headache, constipation, frequent urination, confusion, and less frequently transaminitis, rash, or chest pain.[26] When a patient has significant systemic side effects or poor control of spasms on high doses of baclofen, they can undergo a trial of intrathecal baclofen and if successful, an intrathecal baclofen pump can be placed.[27]

There are two potential emergencies associated with indwelling intrathecal baclofen pumps.[3,26,27] The first is baclofen overdose due to malfunction or misprogramming of the pump. Depending on the degree of overdose, presentation would include ascending weakness, flaccid paralysis, nausea, vomiting, confusion, respiratory muscle weakness, as well as potential for coma, and cardiorespiratory arrest if baclofen reaches the brainstem.[3] Patient may require invasive support for up to 48 hours until the baclofen recedes. The second emergency occurs if there is complete pump failure or if the catheter breaks and leaks baclofen outside of the intrathecal space.[3,27] In both instances, there is a sudden withdrawal of baclofen. This can cause extreme hyperspasticity, hyperthermia, autonomic dysreflexia, disorientation, agitation, and respiratory failure due to spasm of respiratory muscles.[27] If not detected and treated appropriately, patients can develop respiratory arrest, rhabdomyolysis, and subsequent renal and multiorgan system failure.[3] Treatment includes benzodiazepines to reduce spasms, while restarting baclofen via systemic or intrathecal routes.[27] If benzodiazepines are initially ineffective, propofol or other sedatives with or without neuromuscular blockade may be required in the short term to break the spasms and allow reintroduction of baclofen. Although the symptoms closely resemble the presentation of neuroleptic malignant syndrome (NMS), dantrolene and other treatments for NMS are ineffective for baclofen withdrawal syndrome.[27]

Another systemic option for spasticity is dantrolene.[3,26] Developed initially as a muscle relaxant and used for the treatment of malignant hyperthermia and NMS, dantrolene causes diffuse impairment of excitation-contraction coupling at the level of the sarcoplasmic reticulum in myoctyes. Benzodiazepines, such as diazepam or clonazepam, can also be used for spasms.[3,26] These are typically dosed at night due to their sedative effects. Tizandine and clonidine are centrally-acting alpha-2 agonists that are sometimes used alone or in combination with baclofen.[3,26] Finally, in recent years, there has been some interest in cannabinoids, which may provide some relief of spasticity and pain for these patients.[3,26]

CONCLUSIONS

SCI represents a devastating event, often in young, otherwise healthy individuals. There is still much research needed to fully elucidate the mechanisms of secondary injury and potential therapeutic approaches to minimize long-term neurological damage. Cornerstones of acute SCI management involve cervical immobilization, aggressive treatment of expected cardiopulmonary derangements, airway protection, ventilatory support if needed, surgical intervention for unstable fractures or cord compression, early rehabilitation, and prophylaxis for stress ulcers and DVT. Long-term SCI patients face a variety of challenges. Knowledge and anticipation of these issues and their management is essential to provide optimal care for SCI patients, who inevitably present for procedures and require re-hospitalization throughout their lives.

REFERENCES

1. National Spinal Cord Injury Statistical Center. Spinal cord injury facts and figures at a glance. Nov 2016. Available from: https://www.nscisc.uab.edu/.

2. Cottrell J, Young W. Neurosurgical disease and trauma of the spine and spinal cord: anesthetic considerations. *Cottrell and Young's Neuroanesthesia*. 5th Ed. Mosby Elsevier. 2010:343–89.

3. Matta BF, Menon DK, Smith M. Neurointensive care. *Core Topics in Neuroanaesthesia and Neurointensive Care* Cambridge University Press. 2011:271–84.

4. Taghva A, Hoh DJ, Lauryssen CL. Advances in the management of spinal cord and spinal column injuries. *Handbook of Clinical Neurology* 2012;109(3):105–30.

5. Wuermser L-A, Chester HH, Chiodo AE, et al. Spinal cord injury medicine: 2: Acute care management of traumatic and nontraumatic injury. *Arch Phys Med Rehabil* 2007;88(Suppl 1): S55–61.

6. Evans LT, Lollis SS, Ball PA. Management of acute spinal cord injury in the neurocritical care unit. *Neurosurg Clin N Am* 2013;24:339–47.

7. Onose G, Anghelescu A, Muresanu DR, et al. A review of published reports on neuroprotection in spinal cord injury. *Spinal Cord* 2009;47:716–26.

8. Sayer FT, Kronvall E, Nilsson OG. Methylprednisolone treatment in acute spinal cord injury: The myth challenged through a structured analysis of published literatures. *Spine J* 2006;6:335–43.

9. Consortium for Spinal Cord Medicine. Early acute management in adults with spinal cord injury: a clinical practice guideline for healthcare providers. *J Spinal Cord Med* 2008;31(4):403–79.

10. AANS/CNS Joint Guidelines Committee. Guidelines for the management of acute cervical spine and spinal cord injuries: 2013 update. *Neurosurgery* 2013;60(Supp 1): 82–91.

11. Crosby ET. Airway management in adults after cervical spine trauma. *Anesthesiology* 2006;104:1293–318.

12. Fehlings MG, Vaccaro A, Wilson JR, et al. Early versus delayed decompression for traumatic cervical spinal cord injury: results of the surgical timing in acute spinal cord injury study (STASCIS). *PLoS One* 2012;7(2):e32037.

13. La Rosa G, Conti A, Cardali S, et al. Does early decompression improve neurological outcome of spinal cord injured patients? Appraisal of the literature using a meta-analytical approach. *Spinal Cord* 2004;42:503–12.

14. Furlan JC, Fehlings MG. Cardiovascular complications after acute spinal cord injury: pathophysiology, diagnosis, and management. *Neurosurg Focus* 2008;25(5):E13.

15. Ploumis A, Yadlapalli N, Fehlings MG, et al. A systematic review of the evidence supporting a role for vasopressor support in acute SCI. *Spinal Cord* 2010;48:356–62.

16. Berney S, Bragge P, Granger C, et al. The acute respiratory management of cervical spine cord injury in the first 6 weeks after injury: a systematic review. *Spinal Cord* 2010;49:17–29.

17. Winslow C, Rozovsky J. Effect of spinal cord injury on the respiratory system. *Am J Phys Med Rehabil* 2003;82: 803–14.

18. Como JJ, Sutton ER, McCunn M, et al. Characterizing the need for mechanical ventilation following cervical spinal cord injury with neurological deficit. *J Trauma* 2005;59:912–16.

19. Zimmer MB, Nantwi K, Goshgarian HG. Effect of spinal cord injury on the respiratory system: basic research and current clinical treatment options. *J Spinal Cord Med* 2007; 30(4):319–30.

20. Geerts WH, Berggvist D, Pineo GF, et al. Prevention of venous thromboembolism: ACCP evidence-based clinical practice guidelines, 8th ed. *Chest* 2008;133(Suppl 6): 381S–453S.

21. Bracken MB, Shepard MJ, Collins WF, et al. A randomized, controlled trial of methylprednisolone and naloxone in the treatment of acute spinal cord injury. *NEJM* 1990; 322(20):1405–11.

22. Bracken MB, Shepard MJ, Holdford TR, et al. Administration of methylprednisolone for 24 or 48 hours or tirilazadmesylate for 48 hours in the treatment of acute spinal cord injury: Results of the Third National Acute Spinal Cord Injury Randomized Controlled Trial. *JAMA* 1997;277:1597–604.

23. Short DJ, El Masry WS, Jones PW. High dose methylprednisolone in the management of acute spinal cord injury—a systematic review from a clinical perspective. *Spinal Cord* 2000;38(5):273–86.

24. Inamasu J, Nakamura Y, Ichikizaki K. Induced hypothermia in experimental traumatic spinal cord injury: An update. *J Neurol Sci* 2003;209:55–60.

25. Krassioukov A, Warburton DE, Teasell R, et al. A systematic review of the management of autonomic dysreflexia after spinal cord injury. *Arch Phys Med Rehab* 2009;90: 682–95.

26. Adams MM, Hicks AL. Spasticity after spinal cord injury. *Spinal Cord* 2005;43:577–86.

27. Coffey RJ, Edgar TS, Francisco GE, et al. Abrupt withdrawal from intrathecal baclofen: recognition and management of a potentially life-threatening syndrome. *Arch Phys Med Rehabil* 2002;83:735–41.

83

Intensive Care Unit–Acquired Muscle Weakness

N. Latronico, N. Fagoni, F. A. Rasulo

ABSTRACT

Intensive care unit (ICU)-acquired weakness (ICUAW) defines a clinical syndrome characterized by generalized and symmetrical weakness. This condition affects both limb and respiratory muscles and is associated with prolonged mechanical ventilation and ICU stay, and increased ICU, hospital and 1-year mortality. Long-term physical dysfunction can persist for months or years after ICU discharge. One quarter to 50% of patients who require prolonged mechanical ventilation develop ICUAW, but incidence is even higher, up to 64%, in patients with sepsis. We present the case of a patient who had ICUAW with tetraparesis and prolonged ventilator dependency as well as delirium following severe, community-acquired *Legionella pneumophila* pneumonia complicated by sepsis and multiple organ failures. Clinical history and electrophysiological investigations helped clarify the diagnosis, excluding Guillain-Barré syndrome (GBS) as the cause of paralysis. At a 1-year follow-up, the patient still had physical and cognitive impairments indicating that the consequences of critical illness can be long-lasting.

KEYWORDS

Muscle weakness; sepsis; Guillain-Barré syndrome (GBS); community-acquired pneumonia; *Legionella pneumophila* pneumonia; delirium.

CASE STUDY

A 67-year-old previously healthy man presented to the emergency department due to a febrile illness of 6-day duration, nausea, vomiting, and watery diarrhoea. Over the past two days, the patient had experienced progressive dyspnoea and severe fatigue, and had developed a productive cough with yellow-brown sputum.

Past medical history was unremarkable, but the patient was a heavy smoker of approximately one pack of cigarette a day in the last 40 years. Pulse was 108 beats per minute (bpm), respiratory rate 35 to 40 breaths per minute, blood pressure (BP) 155/85 mmHg, and arterial oxygen saturation of 82% on room air which increased to 92% when breathing 50% oxygen via face mask. At physical examination, the patient was febrile (body temperature of 38.8°C) and in respiratory distress. He appeared mildly confused and with reduced attention but awake and oriented. Pulmonary examination showed bilateral crackles throughout lung fields. His cardiovascular examination was normal apart from mild tachycardia, as was his abdomen examination. Musculoskeletal examination, including muscle strength, was normal despite the patient complaining of fatigue. Skin was warm and moist with good capillary refill (<2 sec).

Laboratory studies showed hyponatraemia with serum sodium of 125 mmol/L, chloride of 96 mmol/L, blood urea nitrogen of 7.1 mmol/L (20 mg/dL), and creatinine of 115 μmol/L (1.3 mg/dL). His complete blood count showed leukocytosis with white cell count of 13.4×10^9/L and platelet count of 372×10^9/L. Chest X-ray revealed alveolar opacities in both lungs, mainly basal.

Blood gas demonstrated a pH of 7.30, pressure of arterial carbon dioxide ($PaCO_2$) of 29 mmHg, and pressure of arterial oxygen (PaO_2) of 69 mmHg with a fraction of inspired oxygen (FiO_2) of 0.5. The patient was admitted to the intensive care unit (ICU) and was rapidly intubated and mechanically ventilated. Initial empiric antibiotic treatment with ceftriaxone and azithromycin was changed to levofloxacin when the patient's urine *Legionella pneumophila* antibody assay returned positive.

In the ICU, the patient was managed according to the ABCDEF bundle with optimized analgesia (fentanyl 0.7–10 µg/kg/hr as needed) and sedation (first propofol 5–50 µg/kg/min, then dexmedetomidine 0.2–0.7 µg/kg/hr), daily spontaneous awakening and breathing trials, twice-a-day delirium assessment, and early goal-directed mobilization.[1,2] With minimal dexmedetomidine sedation, hypoactive delirium was documented on days 3, 4, and 5. Starting on day 7, severe weakness was also documented, with the patient unable to move his arms against gravity and resistance and his limbs against gravity (Medical Research Council [MRC] sum score was 30/60),[3] and unable to breathe spontaneously. Neurological consultation suggested electroneurography (ENG), electromyography (EMG), and lumbar puncture to exclude a Guillain-Barré syndrome (GBS). Differentiating weakness as the cause of ICU admission from weakness complicating the ICU stay ENG-EMG indicated a severe axonal sensory-motor neuropathy with signs of myopathy, so that the lumbar puncture was cancelled. Final diagnosis was ICUAW caused by critical illness polyneuropathy (CIP) and critical illness myopathy (CIM). On day 9, since the patient could not be weaned from the ventilator, a tracheostomy was performed and the patient was transferred to a rehabilitation unit. It took 3 more weeks for the patient to be weaned from artificial ventilation and tracheostomy. During this period, the patient's muscle strength progressively improved and after 3 months he had regained full MRC sum score of 60. When lastly seen at 12-month follow-up, the patient complained of severe fatigue that was limiting his daily activities despite normal MRC. Fatigue severity score confirmed severe fatigue,[4] but ENG-EMG was normal. The physical and mental component scores of Medical Outcomes Study 36-item Short-Form General Health Survey (SF-36)[5] were lower than the mean scores for an age-matched and sex-matched control population, and the patient performed suboptimally at the 6-minute walk distance[6] and at The Montreal Cognitive Assessment (MoCA),[7] indicating persisting physical and cognitive impairments.

INTRODUCTION

Intensive care unit (ICU)-acquired weakness (ICUAW) is a complication of critical illness and may represent 'the extreme end of a spectrum of weakness that begins with any serious illness regardless of care location' (2017). This condition is common, affecting 25%–50% of patients with prolonged mechanical ventilation and up to 64% of patients with sepsis, and is a serious complication, being associated with prolonged mechanical ventilation and ICU stay, and increased ICU, hospital, and 1-year mortality.

In the case study, we presented a patient who had ICUAW with flaccid paralysis of all four limbs and prolonged ventilator-dependency following community-acquired *Legionella pneumophila* pneumonia. Clinical history and electrophysiological investigations of peripheral nerves and muscles helped clarify the diagnosis, excluding GBS. Despite successful weaning of the patient from the ventilator and progressive improvement of muscle strength, the patient had physical and cognitive impairments still persisting at one year, indicating that the consequences of critical illness can be long-lasting.

DISCUSSION

The term ICUAW defines a 'clinically detected weakness in critically ill patients in whom there is no plausible etiology other than critical illness'.[8] Muscle weakness is generalized and symmetrical, and affects both limbs and respiratory muscles. As such, failure to wean patients from the ventilator and tetraparesis or tetraplegia with reduced deep tendon reflexes can be the prevailing clinical signs. Criteria where ICUAW should be excluded includes:[9] distribution of muscle weakness is asymmetrical (for example, in patients with hemiplegia); clinical signs suggest a central nervous system (CNS) disorder (for example, Babinski signs or spasticity); facial muscles are involved; progression of muscle weakness has a specific pattern, such as ascending or descending, or is fluctuating and worsens after brief exercise; concurrent signs, such as skin rash, abdominal pain or dysautonomia suggest systemic disorders; and neuromuscular blocking agents or other drugs affecting the peripheral nerve, the neuromuscular transmission, and the muscle have been used for prolonged periods.

Diagnosis and Epidemiology of ICUAW

The MRC sum score is usually used to achieve the diagnosis.[10] The MRC muscle strength is assessed in 12 muscle groups: a summed score below 48/60 designates ICUAW or significant weakness,[10] and an MRC score below 36/48 indicates severe weakness.[11] Handgrip dynamometry measures isometric muscle strength and can be used as an alternative to MRC as a quick diagnostic test. Cut-off scores of less than 11 kg (interquartile range [IQR] 10–40) in males and less than 7 kg (IQR 0–7.3) in females indicates ICUAW (Figure 83.1).[12] The ICUAW is a serious complication being associated with prolonged mechanical ventilation and ICU stay, as well as increased ICU, hospital, and 1-year mortality.[3] Moreover, long-term impairment of physical function can persist for months or even years after ICU discharge.[13] It is estimated that one-quarter to a half of patients who require prolonged mechanical ventilation develop ICUAW.[14] Based on this, more than 75,000 patients in the United States and up to 1 million worldwide may develop ICUAW.[15]

Sepsis and Failure of the Brain, the Peripheral Nerves, and Muscles

The incidence is significantly higher, up to 64%, in patients with severe sepsis.[15] The Third International Consensus Definitions for Sepsis and Septic Shock (Sepsis-3) recently defined sepsis as a life-threatening organ dysfunction due to a dysregulated host response to an infection, thus emphasizing that sepsis is invariably associated with some degree of organ dysfunction.[16] In clinical practice, sepsis is more often recognized from the associated organ dysfunction than from the more difficult to identify infection. The patient described here had respiratory failure in response to an infection, and hence sepsis. He also had neurologic dysfunction, as indicated by confusional state and inattention. Inattention is a cardinal feature of delirium, a 'brain dysfunction' that commonly complicates the early stage of sepsis,[17] clearly indicating that the patient had multiple organ dysfunctions involving the respiratory system, as well as the central and peripheral nervous system and muscles. Neurologic dysfunction is important to detect and monitor in patients with sepsis as it strongly increases the risk of death after living hospital discharge.[18]

The Differential Diagnosis

Interestingly, the patient from our case study complained of fatigue, a subjective symptom, without demonstrable muscle weakness on physical examination. Fatigue is a common symptom in many medical conditions, including infection and cancer.[13] Together with infectious signs and diarrhoea preceding respiratory failure, fatigue also suggested the diagnosis of GBS, an acute, auto-immune, post-infectious polyradiculoneuropathy, which can be a cause of acute neuromuscular respiratory failure requiring ICU admission.[19] However, muscle weakness clearly followed the development of sepsis, which is a critical step to define ICUAW (Figure 83.1).[12] Electrophysiological investigations helped clarify the diagnosis by showing an axonal sensory-motor polyneuropathy and myopathy, thus excluding typical GBS which is characterized by motor nerve demyelination without acute myopathy. Differential diagnosis between GBS and CIP/CIM is usually easy; however, if GBS is rapidly progressive, diagnosis can be difficult.[20] To further complicate this issue, *Legionella pneumophila*[21] and *Pneumococcus pneumonia*[22] can rarely be complicated by GBS, and GBS can be axonal rather than demyelinating.[23] In such cases, accurate clinical history and neurological evaluation are of paramount importance together with electrophysiological investigations and lumbar puncture to achieve a correct and timely diagnosis.

Since ICUAW represents the dysfunction or failure of peripheral neuromuscular system during critical illness,[3] this patient had multiple organ dysfunctions including respiratory as well as central and peripheral nervous system dysfunction. Onset of ICUAW can be early during the ICU stay, and is often associated with acute muscle wasting.[24] In the Italian multicentre critical illness myopathy or neuropathy (CRIMYNE) study, median time of onset of CIP diagnosed with ENG was 6 days.[25] In this patient, ICUAW detected clinically with use of the MRC sum score was diagnosed on day 6, however, delirium precluded an earlier assessment. In fact, diagnosis of ICUAW requires that the patient is awake and cooperative, and hence, diagnosis is often delayed because of sedation or delirium.[13] There is no evidence that delirium has a direct impact on ICUAW; however, delirium and ICUAW possibly interact with each other because early rehabilitation in the ICU improves physical function and may reduce the duration of delirium (Figure 83.2).[13]

ICUAW and the Post-Intensive-Care Syndrome

Many ICU survivors experience long-term physical, cognitive, and mental health complications directly associated with critical illness and pre-ICU condition. This has been termed post-intensive-care syndrome.[26] Onset of ICUAW during the acute stage of critical illness is associated with increased 1-year mortality in survivors of critical illness.[27] ICU-acquired delirium is a recognized risk factor for late cognitive impairment, as experienced by our patient; longer duration of delirium is associated with worse global cognition and executive function up to 1 year after ICU discharge.[28] Fatigue, which was an important symptom at the onset of acute disease, was still vexing the patient at 1-year follow-up. Fatigue is described in 70% of acute respiratory distress syndrome (ARDS) survivors and is often associated with psychiatric disorders, pain, and cognitive impairments but specific pathophysiological mechanisms remain elusive.[13] Axonal loss detected using specialized neurophysiological techniques such as motor unit number estimation is associated with fatigue in patients with GBS,[29] but mechanisms in survivors of critical illness are unknown and likely to be multifactorial.[13]

CONCLUSIONS

The ICUAW is a common and clinically relevant complication of critical illness which is associated not only with important short-term outcomes such as increased duration of mechanical ventilation and ICU stay, and increased ICU and hospital mortality, but also with long-term physical impairment and reduced quality of life in survivors of critical illness. As such, it is important that clinicians are aware of it and predispose to diagnose it at an early stage of ICU stay. Early diagnosis is the essential precondition to prevent or reduce the occurrence of ICUAW and its serious consequences.

REFERENCES

1. Balas MC, Vasilevskis EE, Olsen KM, et al. Effectiveness and safety of the awakening and breathing coordination, delirium monitoring/management, and early exercise/mobility bundle. *Crit Care Med* 2014 May;42(5):1024–36.

2. Schaller SJ, Anstey M, Blobner M, et al. Early, goal-directed mobilisation in the surgical intensive care unit: a randomised controlled trial. *Lancet* 2016;388(10052):1377–88.

3. Latronico N, Bolton CF. Critical illness polyneuropathy and myopathy: a major cause of muscle weakness and paralysis. *Lancet Neurol* 2011;10(10):931–41.

4. Wessely S, Powell R. Fatigue syndromes: a comparison of chronic 'postviral' fatigue with neuromuscular and affective disorders. *J Neurol Neurosurg Psychiatry* 1989;52(8):940–8.

5. Ware JJ, Kosinski M, Gandek B. SF-36 health survey manual & interpretation guide. Lincoln, RI: Quality Metric;2005.

6. Dolmage TE, Hill K, Evans RA, Goldstein RS. Has my patient responded? Interpreting clinical measurements such as the 6-minute-walk test. *Am J Respir Crit Care Med* 2011;184(6):642–6.

7. Nasreddine ZS, Phillips NA, Bedirian V, et al. The Montreal Cognitive Assessment, MoCA: a brief screening tool for mild cognitive impairment. *Journal of the American Geriatrics Society* 2005;53(4):695–9.

8. Stevens RD, Marshall SA, Cornblath DR, et al. A framework for diagnosing and classifying intensive care unit-acquired weakness. *Crit Care Med* 2009;37(Suppl. 10):299–308.

9. Sharshar T, Citerio G, Andrews PJD, et al. Neurological examination of critically ill patients: a pragmatic approach. Report of an ESICM expert panel. *Intensive Care Med* 2014;40(4):484–95.

10. De Jonghe B, Sharshar T, Lefaucheur JP, et al. Paresis acquired in the intensive care unit: a prospective multicenter study. *JAMA* 2002;288(22):2859–67.

11. Hermans G, Clerckx B, Vanhullebusch T, et al. Interobserver agreement of Medical Research Council sum-score and handgrip strength in the intensive care unit. *Muscle Nerve* 2012;45(1):18–25.

12. Latronico N, Gosselink R. A guided approach to diagnose severe muscle weakness in the intensive care unit. *Rev Bras Ter Intensiva* 2015;27(3):199–201.

13. Latronico N HM, Hopkins RO, et al. The ICM research agenda on intensive care unit acquired weakness. *Intensive Care Med* 2017;43:1270–81.

14. Latronico N. Critical illness polyneuropathy and myopathy 20 years later. No man's land? No, it is our land! *Intensive Care Med* 2016;42(11):1790–3.

15. Fan E, Cheek F, Chlan L, et al. An official American Thoracic Society Clinical Practice guideline: the diagnosis of intensive care unit-acquired weakness in adults. *Am J Respir Crit Care Med* 2014;190(12):1437–46.

16. Seymour CW, Liu VX, Iwashyna TJ, et al. Assessment of clinical criteria for sepsis: for the third international consensus definitions for sepsis and septic shock (Sepsis-3). *JAMA* 2016;315(8):762–74.

17. Barr J, Fraser GL, Puntillo K, et al. Clinical practice guidelines for the management of pain, agitation, and delirium in adult patients in the intensive care unit: Executive summary. *Am J Health Syst Pharm* 2013;70(1):53–8.

18. Schuler A, Wulf DA, Lu Y, et al. The impact of acute organ dysfunction on long-term survival in sepsis. *Crit Care Med* 2018;46(6):843–9.

19. Latronico N, Fagoni N. Neuromuscular disorders and acquired neuromuscular weakness. In: Smith Martin M. CG, Kofke Andrew W, eds. *Oxford Textbook of Neurocritical Care*. Oxford, England: Oxford University Press; 2016.

20. Cabrera Serrano M, Rabinstein AA. Causes and outcomes of acute neuromuscular respiratory failure. *Arch Neurol* 2010;67(9):1089–94.

21. Landau D, Kiarashi J, Robbins M, Farmakidis C. Guillain-Barre syndrome after legionella pneumonia: case report and literature review. 2016;86(16 Supplement P1.308).

22. Bianchi G, Domenighetti G. Pneumococcus pneumoniae infection and Guillain-Barre syndrome: fortuitous or specific association? *Intensive Care Med* 2006;32(2):338–9.

23. Willison HJ, Jacobs BC, van Doorn PA. Guillain-Barre syndrome. *Lancet* 2016;388(10045):717–27.

24. Puthucheary ZA, Rawal J, McPhail M, et al. Acute skeletal muscle wasting in critical illness. *JAMA* 2013; 310(15):1591–600.

25. Latronico N, Bertolini G, Guarneri B, et al. Simplified electrophysiological evaluation of peripheral nerves in critically ill patients: the Italian multi-centre CRIMYNE study. *Crit Care* 2007;11(1):R11.

26. Needham DM, Davidson J, Cohen H, et al. Improving long-term outcomes after discharge from intensive care unit: Report from a stakeholders' conference. *Critical Care Med* 2012;40(2):502–9.

27. Hermans G, van Mechelen H, Bruyninckx F, et al. Predictive value for weakness and 1-year mortality of screening electrophysiology tests in the ICU. *Intensive Care Med* 2015;41(12):2138–48.

28. Pandharipande PP, Girard TD, Jackson JC, et al. Long-term cognitive impairment after critical illness. *N Engl J Med* 2013;369(14):1306–16.

29. Drenthen J, Jacobs BC, Maathuis EM, van Doorn PA, Visser GH, Blok JH. Residual fatigue in Guillain-Barre syndrome is related to axonal loss. *Neurology* 2013;81(21): 1827–31.

Part XX

Appendix

84

Scales and Scores

A. Khandelwal, V. Singhal, and I. Kapoor

ABSTRACT

This chapter provides a structured summary of commonly used scales and scores in neuroanaesthesia and neurointensive care. The list of classifications is divided into sections: (1) neuroanaesthesia and neurointensive care; (2) neurological and neurosurgical; (3) neuroradiological; and (4) outcome.

KEYWORDS

Scales; scores; neurointensive care; neurosurgery; neuroradiology; health assessment; discharge criteria; pain assessment; sedation assessment.

Scores/Scales	References
I. Neuroanaesthesia and neurointensive care	
Mallampati Score for Airway Assessment	Mallampati SR, Gatt SP, Gugino LD, et al. A clinical sign to predict difficult tracheal intubation: A prospective study. *Can Anaesth Soc J* 1985;32:429–34.
Cormack-Lehane Classification for Airway Assessment	Cormack RS, Lehane J. Difficult tracheal intubation in obstetrics. *Anaesthesia* 1984;39:1105–11.
ASA (American Society of Anesthesiologists) Physical Status Classification System	Hurwitz EE, Simon M, Vinta SR, et al. Adding examples to the ASA-physical status classification improves correct assignment to patients. *Anesthesiology* 2017;126:614–22.
Modified Aldrete Recovery Score	Aldrete JA. The post-anesthesia recovery score revisited. *J Clin Anesth* 1995;7:89–91.
Modified Post-anaesthesia Discharge Scoring (PADS) System	Chung F, Chan VW, Ong D. A post-anesthetic discharge scoring system for home readiness after ambulatory surgery. *J Clin Anesth* 1995;7:500–6.
Ramsay Sedation Scale (RSS)	Ramsay MA, Savege TM, Simpson BR, Goodwin R. Controlled sedation with alphaxalone-alphadolone. *Br Med J* 1974;2:656–9.
Richmond Agitation-Sedation Scale (RASS)	Sessler CN, Gosnell MS, Grap MJ, et al. The Richmond Agitation-Sedation Scale: validity and reliability in adult intensive care unit patients. *Am J Respir Crit Care Med* 2002;166:1338–44. Ely EW, Truman B, Shintani A, et al. Monitoring sedation status over time in ICU patients: reliability and validity of the Richmond Agitation-Sedation Scale (RASS). *JAMA* 2003;289:2983–91.
Numeric Rating Scale for Pain Assessment	McCaffery M, Beebe A. *Pain: Clinical Manual For Nursing Practice*. Mosby-Year Book; 1989.
Behavioural Pain Scale	Payen JF, Bru O, Bosson JL, et al. Assessing pain in critically ill sedated patients by using a behavioral pain scale. *Crit Care Med* 2001;29:2258–63.

(Cont'd)

(Cont'd)

Scores/Scales	References
The Nociception Coma Scale	Schnakers C, Chatelle C, Vanhaudenhuyse A, et al. The Nociception Coma Scale: a new tool to assess nociception in disorders of consciousness. *Pain* 2010;148:215–9.
Intensive Care Delirium Screening Checklist	Bergeron N, Dubois MJ, Dumont M, Dial S, Skrobik Y. Intensive Care Delirium Screening Checklist: evaluation of a new screening tool. *Intensive Care Med* 2001;27:859–64.
II. Neurological and Neurosurgical	
Glasgow Coma Scale (GCS) for Consciousness Assessment	Teasdale G, Jennett B. Assessment of coma and impaired consciousness. A practical scale. *Lancet* 1974;2:81–4.
FOUR SCORE (Full Outline of UnResponsiveness) for Consciousness Assessment	Wijdicks EF, Bamlet WR, Maramattom BV, Manno EM, McClelland RL. Validation of a new coma scale: The FOUR score. *Ann Neurol* 2005;58: 585–93.
American Spinal Injury Association (ASIA) Impairment Scale	Kirshblum SC, Burns SP, Biering-Sorensen F, et al. International standards for neurological classification of spinal cord injury (revised 2011). *J Spinal Cord Med.* 2011;34:535–46.
Cognard Classification for Dural Arteriovenous Fistula	Cognard C, Gobin YP, Pierot L, et al. Cerebral dural arteriovenous fistulas: clinical and angiographic correlation with a revised classification of venous drainage. *Radiology* 1995;194:671–80.
Borden Classification for Dural Arteriovenous Fistula	Borden JA, Wu JK, Shucart WA. A proposed classification for spinal and cranial dural arteriovenous fistulous malformations and implications for treatment. *J Neurosurg* 1995;82:166–79.
Barrow Classification for Caroticocavernous Fistula	Barrow DL, Spector RH, Braun IF, Landman JA, Tindall SC, Tindall GT. Classification and treatment of spontaneous carotid-cavernous sinus fistulas. *J Neurosurg* 1985;62:248–56.
Botterell's Clinical Grades for Aneurysmal Subarachnoid Haemorrhage	Botterell EH, Lougheed WM, Scott JW, Vandewater SL. Hypothermia, and interruption of carotid, or carotid and vertebral circulation, in the surgical management of intracranial aneurysms. *J Neurosurg* 1956;13:1–42.
Modified Hunt & Hess Grading System for Aneurysmal Subarachnoid Haemorrhage	Hunt WE, Hess RM. Surgical risk as related to time of intervention in the repair of intracranial aneurysms. *J Neurosurg* 1968;28:14–20.
Modified Hunt and Kosnik Grading System for Aneurysmal Subarachnoid Haemorrhage	Hunt WE, Kosnik EJ. Timing and perioperative care in intracranial aneurysm surgery. *Clin Neurosurg* 1974;21:79–89.
World Federation of Neurological Surgeons' (WFNS) Grades for Aneurysmal Subarachnoid Haemorrhage	*Teasdale GM, Drake CG, Hunt W*, et al. A universal subarachnoid hemorrhage scale: report of a committee of the World Federation of Neurosurgical Societies. *J Neurol Neurosurg Psychiatry* 1988;51:1457.
Spetzler-Martin Grading for Arteriovenous Malformation	Spetzler RF, Martin NA. A proposed grading system for arteriovenous malformations. 1986. *J Neurosurg* 2008;108:186–93.
Modified National Institutes of Health Stroke Scale (mNIHSS) for Stroke Assessment	Lyden PD, Lu M, Levine SR, Brott TG, Broderick J. NINDS rtPA Stroke Study Group. A modified National Institutes of Health Stroke Scale for use in stroke clinical trials: preliminary reliability and validity. *Stroke* 2001;32:1310–17.
ABCD Score for Prediction of Stroke	Rothwell PM, Giles MF, Flossmann E, et al. A simple score (ABCD) to identify individuals at high early risk of stroke after transient ischaemic attack. *Lancet* 2005;366:29–36.
ABCD2 Score for Prediction of Stroke	*Johnston SC, Rothwell PM, Nguyen-Huynh MN*, et al. Validation and refinement of scores to predict very early stroke risk after transient ischaemic attack. *Lancet* 2007;369:283–92.
III. Neuroradiological scores/scales	
Grading of Diffuse Axonal Injury	*Adams JH, Doyle D, Ford I, Gennarelli TA, Graham DI, McLellan DR.* Diffuse axonal injury in head injury: definition, diagnosis and grading. *Histopathology* 1989;15:49–59.

Fisher Scale for Aneurysmal Subarachnoid Haemorrhage	*Fisher CM, Kistler JP, Davis JM*. Relation of cerebral vasospasm to subarachnoid hemorrhage visualized by computerized tomographic scanning. *Neurosurgery* 1980;6:1–9.
Modified Fisher Scale for Aneurysmal Subarachnoid Haemorrhage	Frontera JA, Claassen J, Schmidt JM, et al. Prediction of symptomatic vasospasm after subarachnoid hemorrhage: the modified Fisher scale. *Neurosurgery.* 2006;59:21–7; discussion 21–7.
Anderson-D'Alonzo Classification for Odontoid Fracture	Hsu WK, Anderson PA. Odontoid fractures: update on management. *J Am Acad Orthop Surg* 2010;18:383–94.
MRI Classification of Cavernous Malformation	*Zabramski JM, Wascher TM, Spetzler RF*, et al. The natural history of familial cavernous malformations: results of an ongoing study. *J Neurosurg* 1994;80:422–32.
Marshall CT Classification of Traumatic Brain Injury (TBI)	Marshall LF, Marshall SB, Klauber MR, et al. The diagnosis of head injury requires a classification based on computed axial tomography. *J Neurotrauma* 1992;9(Suppl 1):S287–92.
IV. Outcome scores/scales	
Glasgow Outcome Scale	Jennett B, Bond M. Assessment of outcome after severe brain damage. *Lancet* 1975;1:480–4.
Extended Glasgow Coma Scale	Wilson JT, Pettigrew LE, Teasdale GM. Structured interviews for the Glasgow Outcome Scale and the extended Glasgow Outcome Scale: guidelines for their use. *J Neurotrauma* 1998;15:573–85.
Modified Rankin Scale	Rankin J. Cerebral vascular accidents in patients over the age of 60. II. Prognosis. *Scott Med J.* 1957;2:200–15. *Farrell B, Godwin J, Richards S, Warlow C*, et al. The United Kingdom transient ischaemic attack (UK-TIA) aspirin trial: final results. *J Neurol Neurosurg Psychiatry* 1991;54:1044–54.
Barthel Index	Mahoney FI, Barthel DW. Functional Evaluation: The Barthel Index. *Md State Med J.* 1965;14:61–65.

Index

Page numbers followed by *t* indicate tables.